INDEX OPHTHALMOLOGICUS

DIRECTORY

OF THE INTERNATIONAL FEDERATION
OF OPHTHALMOLOGICAL SOCIETIES
INCLUDING
OPHTHALMOLOGICAL ASSOCIATIONS, OPHTHALMOLOGISTS,
OPHTHALMOLOGICAL CLINICS, INSTITUTES, JOURNALS

EDITED BY THE

INTERNATIONAL COUNCIL OF OPHTHALMOLOGY

SEVENTH EDITION

1974
H. E. STENFERT KROESE BV, PUBLISHERS
PIETERSKERKHOF 38, LEIDEN, THE NETHERLANDS

INDEX OPHTHALMOLOGICUS

IN QUO RECENSENTUR
FOEDERIS SOCIETATUM ARTIS OPHTHALMOLOGICAE
MEDICI INSTITUTA EDITA

EDITIO SEPTA
EDIDIT CONCILIUM OPHTHALMOLOGICUM UNIVERSALE
ANNO MCMLXXIV

STENFERT KROESE – LEIDEN

ISBN 978-90-207-0401-3   ISBN 978-94-010-1964-4 (eBook)
DOI 10.1007/978-94-010-1964-4

PRAEFATIO

This seventh Index continues the series after an eight years intermission. It comprises the data of those countries, the National Societies of which constitute the International Federation of Ophthalmological Societies. We are greatly indebted to their secretaries for furnishing the material required.

May this Index again be an instrument for facilitating the mutual relations within our profession throughout the world.

Ce septième Index continue la série après une trève de huit ans. Il contient les données des pays dont les Sociétés Nationales constituent la Fédération Internationale des Sociétés Ophtalmologiques. Nous sommes profondément obligés aux Secrétaires des dites Sociétés Nationales pour nous avoir procuré le matériel nécessaire.

Puisse cet Index devenir à nouveau un instrument pour faciliter les relations mutuelles en notre profession parmi le monde entier.

Dieser siebente Index setzt die Serie nach achtjähriger Pause fort. Er enthält Angaben diejenigen Länder, deren nationale Gesellschaften den Internationalen Verband der Ophthalmologischen Gesellschaften bilden. Den Schriftführern dieser Gesellschaften sind wir für die Beschaffung des benötigten Materials zu grossem Dank verpflichtet.

Möge dieser Index abermals ein Instrument zur Erleichterung der wechselseitigen Beziehungen innerhalb unserer Berufsgemeinschaft auf der ganzen Welt werden.

Este el septo Index está continuando la serie después de un intervalo de ocho años. Contiene los datos de aquellos países, cuyos sociedades nacionales constituyen la Federación Internacional de Sociedades Oftalmológicas. Debemos mucho a sus secretarios por habernos procurado los datos necesarios.

Que este Index sirva otra vez para facilitar las relaciones mutuales dentro de nuestra profesión por todo el mundo.

Zutphen (Holland)   A. C. Copper

May 1974   *Adj.-Secr.*

CONSPECTUS

CONCILIUM OPHTHALMOLOGICUM UNIVERSALE

Président honoraire à vie: Sir Stewart Duke Elder, London
Président: Prof. J. François, Gand (Belgique)
Vice-président: Dr. M. J. Hogan, San Francisco (U.S.A.)
Secrétaire: Prof. A. Dubois-Poulsen, 8 Av. Daniel Lesueur, Paris VII (France)
Trésorier: Prof. B. Streiff, Lausanne (Suisse)
Ancien Président de Conseil: Prof. J. Charamis, Athenes (Grèce)

Membres ex officio:

Président de la Ligue Internationale contre le Trachome: Prof. G. B. Bietti, Roma
Président de l'Association Internationale de Prophylaxie de la Cécite: Prof. G. Von Bahr, Uppsala (Sweden)
Président de l'Association Panaméricaine d'Ophtalmologie: Prof. E. Maumenee, Baltimore (U.S.A.)
Ancien Président du Congrès International 1970: Dr. M. Puig Solanes, Mexico 7, D.F.
Représentant de la Société Européenne d'Ophtalmologie: Prof. J. François, Gand (Belgique)
Président du Congrès International 1974: Prof. P. Bregeat, Paris XVII (France)

Membres ordinaires:

Mrs. Prof. S. Vannas, Helsinki (Finland)
Prof. H. Sautter, Hamburg (DBR)
Dr. H. Moutinho, Lisboa (Portugal)
Dr. S. N. Cooper, Bombay (India)
Prof. G. W. Crock, East Melbourne (Australia)
Prof. Mme. M. Radnot, Budapest (Hongrie)
Prof. H. Rocha, Belo Horizonte (Brasil)
Prof. S. Miller, London W.1. (England)

Secrétaire-adjoint pour l'Index:

Dr. A. C. Copper, Coehoornsingel 42, Zutphen (Nederland)

FOEDERATIO SOCIETATUM UNIVERSALIS

STATUTA

1. Statutes of the International Federation of Ophthalmological Societies

Article I

The International Federation of Ophthalmological Societies is an association constituted in conformity with Article 60 and onwards of the Swiss Civil Code.

Article II

The aim of the International Federation of Ophthalmological Societies (hereinafter called 'The Federation') is to promote the science of Ophthalmology among all peoples and nations, and in furtherance of this to ensure permanent co-operation between representative Ophthalmological Societies of different countries and with their Governments and the various international bodies concerned with the organization of educational, scientific and cultural matters. For these purposes it shall elect, through its members, the International Council of Ophthalmology which shall act as its executive body.

Article III

The registered office of the Federation is at the domicile of the Treasurer. The duration of the Federation is unlimited.

Article IV

An Ophthalmological Society recognized as of good standing shall be entitled to join the Federation as an Affiliated Society subject to the approval of the International Council provided it has paid its due subscription.

Article V

Each Society joining the Federation shall appoint one of its members as delegate who shall hold office during the interim between two International Congresses, unless a reappointment is made by his Society. Any change in the delegate should be notified to the Secretary of the Council immediately. The name of the delegate to attend the meeting of the Federation shall be confirmed to the Secretary of the Council at least six months before each International Congress.

In the event of one country, (together with its colonies, dependencies and trusteeship territories), having more than one Society affiliated to the Federation and thus being represented thereon by more than one delegate, only one of these, to be chosen among themselves, shall have voting powers.

Article VI

At each International Congress these delegates shall sit with the members of the International Council to form a Joint Meeting to transact the business of the Federation and elect new members to the Council. The President of the Council shall be the Chairman of this Joint Meeting. All members of both bodies shall have equal voting powers and the Chairman shall have a casting vote.

Article VII

The further duties of a delegate shall be:

(a) To act as a liaison officer between the International Council and his Society in the interval between two International Congresses.

(b) To supply the Secretary of the International Council, periodically or on request, with the names and addresses of the oculists of his country and such other matters as are required for the Index Ophthalmologicus.

(c) To be responsible for collecting and forwarding the annual subscription of his Society to the Treasurer of the International Council.

Article VIII

The subscription of each Affiliated Society shall be proportional to the number of its national members, the amount being determined at the Joint Meeting of the Federation and Council to be held during each International Congress. The subscription shall remain unchanged in the years between two Congresses unless the International Council finds that unforeseen circumstances make other financial arrangements necessary. The annual subscription is due in advance on the Ist of January of each year. Any Society not up to date with its subscription shall, ipso facto, but without prejudice to its liability to the Federation, cease to be an affiliated Society and to participate, through its delegate, in the activities of the Federation, unless the Council is satisfied that reason for its default is unavoidable.

Article IX

Joint Meetings of the Federation and Council shall be conducted in the administrative languages agreed for the particular Congress at which the meetings are held, but speakers, whether making propositions or participating in discussions, may use the language they prefer.

Article X

Amendments and additions to these Statutes shall be valid only if they are recommended at least six months in advance by the International Council (a majority of 2/3 in that body being necessary) or by four delegates of the Federation whose appointments have been confirmed to the Secretary of the Council as in Article V, and if they are accepted by a majority of 2/3 at the joint meeting of the Council and Federation. Such amendments shall be distributed five months in advance to the delegates.

Article XI

The dissolution of the Federation can be effected by a vote of 2/3 of its members. In the event of dissolution the assets of the Federation shall be vested in a project of public interest the aims of which conform with those of the Federation.

2. Statutes of the International Council of Ophthalmology

Article I

The International Council of Ophthalmology (hereinafter known as 'The Council') is the executive body of the Federation. It shall consider and, if deemed advisable, implement recommendations of the International Federation, promote international co-operation in all matters pertaining to ophthalmology, initiate and supervise arrangements for periodical International Congresses and maintain an Index Ophthalmologicus of ophthalmologists and opthalmological institutions throughout the world.

Article II

A New Council shall assume office one year after the conclusion of each International Congress and shall consist of:
1. Ex-officio members:
   (I)   The President of the Council.
   (II)   The Vice-President of the Council.
   (III)   The Secretary of the Council.
   (IV)   The Treasurer of the Council.
   (V)   The President of the Association for the Prevention of Blindness.
   (VI)   The President of the Organization against Trachoma.
   (VII)   A representative of each of such supra-national Ophthalmological Societies as are approved by the joint meeting of the Federation and Council.
   (VIII) The immediate Past President of the Council.
   (IX)   The immediate Past Secretary of the Council.
   (X)   The retiring President of the previous Congress.
   (XI)   The President-elect of the forthcoming Congress.
2. Ten ordinary members.
3. Any honorary life member(s) proposed by the Council which the joint meeting of the Federation and Council may from time to time determine to elect.

Article III

Of the ex-officio members, the President, Vice-President, Secretary and Treasurer shall be elected (or re-elected) by the Joint Meeting of the Federation and Council at each International Congress; they need not be chosen from the delegates of the Federation or the members of the Council. The number of the ex-officio members may be less than the number indicated in Art. II if one or more Councillors serve in more than one capacity. The immediate Past-President and Past Secretary of the Council remain members of the Council until the next Congress.

Article IV

In the appointment of new officers and new councillors it will be the duty of the Council to present nominations to the joint meeting of the Council and Federation; these will be voted upon together with any other nomination proposed by the delegates of the Federation.

Article V

Of the ten ordinary members, the five who have been longest in office shall retire after each International Congress and shall be replaced by new members elected by the Joint Meeting of the Federation and Council. In cases of equality of tenure the retiring member or members shall be determined by casting lots.
If any Councillor is absent from any two consecutive ordinary meetings, unless in extraordinary circumstances, he shall be considered as having resigned.
Any vacancy in the Council occurring in the intervening years between Congresses shall be filled by the Council, the appointment being held temporarily until the next session of the Federation, whereat these appointments shall be confirmed or new members elected in their place. In such cases the Councillor thus appointed shall be deemed to carry the seniority of the member he replaced in deciding length of tenure of office.

Article VI

No one shall be eligible for election to the Council unless he belongs to a Society affiliated to the Federation and honoring its annual subscription, unless the reasons for the Society's default are acceptable to the Council. Nominations by Affiliated Societies for such appointments should be sent to the Secretary of the Council six months before the appropriate meeting of the Federation. No country, together with its colonies, dependencies and trusteeship territories, shall be represented by more than one ordinary member of Council.

Article VII

Sessions of the Council shall be directed in such language as appear necessary to the President for the convenience of members of the Council, but Councillors may use any language they choose in making propositions and taking part in discussions.

Article VIII

The President in consultation with the Secretary shall have the power to decide what business may be transacted by correspondence between meetings of the Council.

Article IX

The aim of the Council shall be to arrange periodically for the issue of a new edition of the Index Ophthalmologicus at a price or prices to be determined from time to time by the Council.

Article X

The secretary of the Council shall supply the delegates with copies of the minutes of the meetings of the Council and the Federation.

Article XI

Amendments and additions to these Statutes shall be valid only if they are recommended at least six months in advance by the International Council (a majority of 2/3 in that body being necessary) or by four delegates of the Federation whose appointments have been confirmed to the Secretary of the Council as in Article V of the Statutes of the Federation and if they are accepted by a majority of 2/3 at the joint meeting of the Council and Federation. Such amendment shall be distributed five months in advance to the delegates.

3. Statuts du Congrès International d'Ophtalmologie

Article I

Le but du Congrès est de contribuer au progrès de l'Ophtalmologie et de fournir l'occasion de rencontres et de discussions aux personnes s'intéressant à cette science.

Article II

La date et le siège du Congrès sont fixés par le Conseil International, en accord avec la Fédération ou, éventuellement, par le Conseil seul. L'invitation de tenir un Congrès dans un pays ne pourra être prise en considération que si elle émane d'une Société Nationale d'Ophtalmologie membre de la Fédération et pouvant prouver qu'elle a l'appui de son gouvernement pour le Congrès éventuel.

Article III

Avant chaque Congrès le Conseil International décide du nombre de langues administratives qui seront utilisées et les choisit.

Article IV

L'organisation du Congrès est confiée à un Comité National constitué dans le pays siège du Congrès. Ce Comité National travaille de concert avec le Conseil International.

Article V

Le Président du Congrès est désigné par le Conseil International, sur proposition du pays organisateur.

Article VI

Peuvent seuls être inscrits comme membres titulaires du Congrès:
(1) Les docteurs en médecine;
(2) Les personnalités ayant rendu des services à la cause de l'Ophtalmologie et dont le Comité National souhaiterait la participation. Le Comité National se réserve le droit de veto pour chaque demande individuelle d'inscription et sans être tenu de justifier sa décision, mais toute personne refusée peut en appeler au Conseil International.

Article VII

Peuvent être inscrits comme membres associés, les parents et amis des membres titulaires. Ils ne peuvent participer aux séances scientifiques et aux séances d'affaires, mais ils peuvent prendre part aux réceptions et activités de caractère amical ou mondain.

Article VIII

Peuvent être inscrites comme membres associés-scientifiques les personnes que le Comité National considérera comme pouvant ne verser qu'une cotisation réduite, soit en raison de leur âge, soit du fait qu'elles se consacrent uniquement à la recherche scientifique, soit pour toute autre raison. Ces membres associés-scientifiques peuvent participer aux réunions scientifiques et assister aux séances solennelles d'ouverture et de clôture, mais non nécessairement aux réceptions et activités de caractère amical ou mondain.

Article IX

Le montant des cotisations est fixé par le Conseil International, d'accord avec le Comité National. Il y a trois catégories de cotisations:
(1) Une cotisation ordinaire pour les membres titulaires appartement à l'une des Sociétés affiliées à la Fédération à l'époque du Congrès.
(2) Une cotisation extraordinaire (supérieure d'environ 10% à la cotisation ordinaire) pour les membres titulaires n'appartenant pas à l'une des Sociétés affiliées à la Fédération, à l'époque du Congrès.
(3) Une cotisation réduite (environ 1/3 de la cotisation ordinaire) pour les membres associés et associés-scientifiques.
Le Trésorier du Congrès est tenu de reverser au Trésorier du Conseil, les sommes versées à titre d'excédents par les membres payant une cotisation extraordinaire.

Article X

Les séances sont dirigées dans l'une des langues administratives du Congrès et les Rapports rédigés dans l'une de ces même langues. Pour les communications et les discussions, le choix de la langue est libre.

Article XI

Un Comité de rédaction decide de la publication intégrale, ou seulement résumée, des communications et des discussions.

Article XII

Un compte-rendu imprimé des travaux du Congrès sera adressé à chacun des membres titulaires et des membres associés-scientifiques. Le Comité National est chargé de faire établir et d'envoyer ces Comptes-rendus.

Article XIII

Le Comité National a la responsabilité de la gestion financière du Congrès.
Après la clôture du Congrès et la publication des Comptes-Rendus, le Comité National fait parvenir un relevé des comptes, certifié conforme, au Conseil International qui le conserve dans se archives. Après paiement de tous les frais et clôture des comptes, s'il reste à la disposition du Comité National un solde créditeur, celui-ci est reversé au Conseil International.
Après cette clôture des comptes du Comité National, le produit de la vente éventuelle des volumes de Comptes-Rendus sera versé directement au Trésorier du Conseil International.

Article XIV

Des modifications ou des additions aux Status ne pourront entrer en vigeur qu'après avoir été acceptées par le Conseil à une majorité des 2/3 et votées à la même majorité des 2/3, les membres du Conseil et les Délégués de la Fédération siégeant ensemble.

4. Règlement Interieur du Congrès

I. – Communications originales

1. Les membres désirant faire une communication doivent en notifier le sujet au Secrétaire du Comité National et lui en faire parvenir un résumé au moins 6 mois avant la date du Congrès afin d'en permettre l'impression et la distribution préalables.
Le Comité National institue une Commission du Programme qui a le droit de refuser des communications; elle doit, en effet, s'assurer que leur intérêt est suffisant et veiller à ce que leur nombre soit en rapport avec le temps disponible.
2. Ces résumés doivent être rédigés dans chacune des langues administratives du Congrès.
3. Les communications doivent être originales. Jusqu'à la parution du volume des Comptes-Rendus, le texte des communications demeure la propriété du Comité National. Les communications dont le texte intégral doit être publié dans le volume des Comptes-Rendus, ne doivent pas être publiées ailleurs.
4. Le Comité de Rédaction décide de la publication intégrale ou abrégée des communications. Si le Comité décide de n'inprimer qu'un résumé, l'auteur est autorisé à publier ailleurs, et sans délai, le texte intégral de sa communication.
5. Les séances sont dirigées dans l'une des langues administratives du Congrès, mais pour les communications et les discussion, le choix de la langue est libre.
6. Le texte des communications, avec ses figures, doit être remis au Secrétaire avant la fin de chaque séance.
Tour membre ayant pris part à la discussion doit en faire parvenir un résumé au Secrétaire au plus tard le lendemain.
7. Il est accordé 10 minutes pour chaque communication. Tout membre désirant participer à la discussion doit faire connaître son nom par écrit au Président de Seance et se limiter à 5 minutes.
8. Les auteurs peuvent obtenir des tirages à part, à leurs frais, et jusqu'à concurrence de 200. Ils doivent les commander à l'imprimeur en renvoyant leurs épreuves corrigées.

II. – Rapports

9. Les sujets de rapport et les Rapporteurs sont choisis par le Conseil International.
10. Les rapports doivent être rédigés dans l'une des langues administratives du Congrès et les Rapporteurs doivent en fournir un résumé dans le autres. Pour les discussions le choix de la langue est libre.
11. Chaque Rapporteur a 15 minutes pour son exposé. Tout membre participant à la discussion doit faire connaître son nom par écrit au Président de séance et se limiter à 5 minutes. L'article 6 est également applicable aux Rapports et à la discussion des rapports.
12. Le Conseil, en accord avec le Comité National, pourra organiser des Symposia.

III. – Séances Annexes

13. En annexe aux séances scientifiques, le Comité National peut organiser des séances de films, des expositions d'instruments, ou toute autre démonstration pouvant intéresser les membres du Congrès.

Ces Statuts ont été adoptés par la Fédération internationale des Sociétés d'Ophtalmologie, à New-Delhi, le 3 décembre 1962.

INSTITUTA UNIVERSALIA

International Organization against Trachoma

Address: c/o Clinica Oculistica Univ. di Roma, Via Cesare Beccaria 18, Roma
President: Prof. G. B. Bietti (Roma)
Ist. Vice-President: Dr. Phillips Thygesou (U.S.A.)
IInd. Vice-President: Dr. Roger Nataf (France)
Secretary-General: G. Coscas
Treasurer: R. Pages
Vice-Presidents for geographical areas: Y. Mitsui (Japan), A. M. Soliman (Egypt), Aouchiche (Algeria), Graham-Scott
Bibliography: Transactions of the International Congresses.
Revue Internationale du Trachome, published jointly with *La Ligue contre le Trachome* (Président: Dr. Roger Nataf)

Association Internationale de Prophylaxie de la Cécité

President: Gunnar von Bahr (Uppsala, Sweden)
Vice-President: A. E. Maumenee (Baltimore, Md., U.S.A.)
Secretary General: William John Holmes, Suite 280, 1013 Bishop St., Honolulu Hawaii 96813, U.S.A.
Treasurer: William S. Hunter (Toronto, Canada)

Regional Secretaries: Sabri Kamel (Cairo, Egypt)
Osvaldo Velasquez (Panama)
David O. Tonkin (Adelaide, Australia)
Henning Skydsgaard (Copenhagen, Denmark)
Members at large: G. de Ocampo (Manila, Philippines), Isak Salin (Salemba, Indonesia), T. Mascati (Bombay, India), Calvin Ring (Auckland, New Zealand), Simone Delthil (Paris, France), J. Schappert-Kimmijser (Den Haag, Netherlands), A. M. Soliman (Cairo, Egypt), Isaac C. Michaelson (Jerusalem, Israel), F. C. Rodger (Great Britain), Archangelsky (Moskau, USSR)
Members ex officio: Jules François (Gand, Belgium), Pres. Int. Council Ophth.; André Dubois-Poulsen (Paris, France) Secr. Int. Council Ophth.; Giam-Battista Bietti (Roma, Italy) Pres. League Prev. Trach.; G. Coscas, Secr. Gen. League Prev. Trach.; John Wilson (Haywards Heath, England) Chairman, Com. f. Prev. of Blindness, W.C.W.B.
Honorary Vice-Presidents: B. Courtis, (Buenos-Aires, Argentine), Frank W. Law (London, England), Alexander E. MacDonald (Toronto, Canada), J. K. Muller (Bonn, West-Germany), A. M. Soliman (Cairo, Egypt)

International Association of Secretaries of Ophthalmological and Otolaryngological Societies

President: Joseph West
Secretary: Milton W. Erdel, 2 E. White St., Frankfort, Ind. 46041 (U.S.A.)

SOCIETATES SUPRANATIONALES

Pan American Association of Ophthalmology

President: Dr. A. Edward Maumenee, Johns Hopkins Hospital, Baltimore, Md. 21205
Vice-President: Dr. Louis J. Girard, 1700 E. Holcombe Blvd., Houston, Texas 77025
Executive Director: Dr. Benjamin F. Boyd, Apartado 1189, Panama 1, R.P.
Secretary-Treasurers:
  for North of Panama: Dr. Robert C. Drews, 211 N Meramee Avenue, Clayton, Missouri 63105, U.S.A.
  for South of Panama: Dr. Juan Arentsen S., Augustinas 1141, Santiago, Chili
President Congress 1975: Dr. Guillermo Pico, San Juan, Puerto Rico

Societas Ophthalmologica Europæa

President: Mme. Prof. M. Radnot, Budapest VIII (Hongrie)
Secretary-General and Treasurer: Prof. J. François, de Smet de Naeyerplein, 15, B-9000 Gent (Belgique)
Honorary Members: Prof. I. Abramowicz, ul. Debinki 7a, Gdansk-Wrzeszcz (Pologne). Dr. N. Ayberk, Taksim Cumhuriyet, Cad. 27–2, Istanbul (Turquie). Prof. L. Coppez, 17 avenue de l'Horizon, B–1150 Bruxelles (Belgique). Prof. H. Ehlers, Dag Hammarskjöldalle I, København Ø (Denmark). Prof. A. Hagedoorn, Apollolaan 129, Amsterdam–Z. (Netherlands). Dr. F. W. Law, Flat 14, 59, Weymouth Street, London W1N 3LH (England). Prof. Petre Vancea Sr., Bd. Schitu Magureanu 3, Bucuresti (Roumanie). Prof. V. Vejdovsky, Cs. Lekarské Spolecnosti J. Ev. Purkyne, I. P. Pavlova 6, Olomouc (Tchécoslovaquie). Dr. L. E. Werner, 32 Fitzwilliam Square, Dublin 2 (Ireland). Prof. V. N. Archangelski, 435 Bolshaya Pirgavskaya, 2/6 Glaznaya Klinika, I. Medizinski Institut, Im. Setchenova, Moskva (URSS)
Members: Prof. J. Böck, II. Universitäts-Augenklinik, Alserstrasse 4, Wien IX (Austria). Prof. A. Dubois-Poulsen, 8 avenue Daniel Lesueur, Paris VII (France). Prof. G. Meyer-Schwickerath, Universitäts-Augenklinik, Hufelandstrasse 55, 43 Essen-Holsterhausen (DBR). Prof. T. Thomassen, Øyeavdelingen – Rikshospitalet, Oslo (Norway). Prof. Petre Vancea Jr., rue Decebal 22, Iassy (Roumanie). Prof. Mme. S. Vannas, P. Rante 10A, Helsinki (Finland). Prof. J. Vanysek, Divadelni, 3, Brno (Tchécoslovaquie). Prof. G. Von Bahr, Swartbäcksgatan 1B, 75320 Uppsala (Sweden). Prof. N. Konstantinoff, Rue Dante 1, Sofia (Bulgarie). Prof. J. Charamis, 1 rue Lycabette, Athenes (Grèce). Prof. N. Ayberk Jr., Taksim Cumhuriyet, Cad. 27/2, Istanbul (Turquie). Prof. P. Danis, 15 avenue de la Folle Chanson, B-1050 Bruxelles (Belgique). Prof. M. Blagojevic, Clinique Ophtalmologique Universitaire, Dz. Vasingtona 19, Beograd (Yougoslavie). Prof. A. Grignolo, Direttore Clinica Oculistica Universitari, Via Flora 9, Genova (Italie). Dr. F. Alves, Av. da Liberdade 224 r/c esq., Lisboa (Portugal). Dr. D. P. Greaves, 56 Wimpole Street, London W.1. (Great Britain). Prof. J. Casanovas, 77 Lauria A° 1, Barcelona 9 (Espagne). Prof. T. Krwawicz, ul. Krak. Przedmiéscie 49, Dublin (Pologne). Prof. H. Henkes, Oog-

ziekenhuis, Schiedamsevest 180, Rotterdam (Netherlands). Prof. B. Streiff, 2 Mont-
bénon, Lausanne (Suisse). Prof. B. Braendstrup, Sortedam Dossering 95B, København Ø (Denmark). Prof. P. Dwyer-Joyce, 11 Merrion Square, Dublin 2 (Ireland).
Prof. K. E. Kruger, Universitäts-Augenklinik, Leninallee 8, 802 Halle a.d. Saale
(DDR). Prof. E. Avetisov, Helholtz Institute of Ophthalmology, Sadovaya Cher-
nogrisskaya Street 14–19, Moscow B-64 (URSS)

European Ophthalmic Pathology Society

Honorary Life President: Prof. Norman Ashton, Institute of Ophthalmology, Judd
    Street, London, W.C. 1H, 9QS, England
President: Prof. Dr. H. Fanta, Ferstelgasse 4, A 1090 Wien IX, Austria
Corresponding Secretary: Dr. G. Naumann, Univ. Augenklinik, Martinistrasse 52,
    2 Hamburg 20, Germany
Organizing Secretary 1973/1974: Prof. Dr. P. Bec, 34, Rue Remusat, 31000 Toulouse,
    France

The Asia-Pacific Academy of Ophthalmology

President: Dr. Akira Nakajima, Tokyo, Japan
Vice-President: Dr. P. Sivasubramaniam, Columbo, Ceylon; Dr. Isak Salim, Djakarta,
    Indonesia; Dr. Gerard Crock, Victoria, Australia
Secretary-General: William John Holmes, Suite 280, 1013 Bishop Street, Honolulu,
    Hawaii 96813, U.S.A.
Regional Secretaries: Dr. John C. N. Chang, 148 Prince Edward Rd., 3rd Floor,
    Kowloon, Hong Kong; Dr. Kuang Hui Lim, 16 Pasir Panjang Hill, Singapore 5; Dr.
    B. D. Telang, 395 Lamington Road, Bombay, India; Dr. Ian F. Robertson, 2 Collins
    Street, Melbourne, Australia

Afro-Asian Congress of Ophthalmology

Permanent Council:

President: Professor I. Abboud, 26 Sherif Pasha Street, Cairo.
Vice-Presidents: Professor Y. Mitaui, Department of Ophthalmology, Tokushima
    University School of Medicine, Kuramoto-Machi, Tokushima, Japan. Professor
    L. P. Agarawal, All India Institute of Medical Sciences, New-Delhi, India
Secretary: Dr. Sabri Kamel, 44 Opera Square, Cairo, Egypt
Treasurer: Prof. A. Mortada, 18(A), 26 July Street, Cairo
Members:
    Prof. M. A. M. Labib, 56 Abdel-Khalek Sarwat Street, Cairo
    Prof. Y. El-Gammal, 21, 26 July Street, Cairo
    Prof. A. El-Massri, 32 El-Falaki Street, Cairo
    Prof. Moussabecova Umnissa, Kirova 21, KV 33, Baku, USSR
    Prof. M. Aouchiche, 5 Rue de Tanger, Alger, Algeria
    Prof. I. Salim, Djalan Djeruk 4, Djakarta, Indonesia
    Dr. Hadi Rais, Institut d'Ophtalmologie, Tunis

Dr. El-Bagir Ibrahim, Khartoum, Sudan
Dr. Leon Asmar, P.O. Box 795, Aleppo, Syria
Dr. Mulhim Hassan, Asseili Building, Riad El-Solh Square, Beirut, Lebanon
Prof. A. Nakejima, Department of Ophthalmology, Juntendo University, Hongo, Tokyo, Japan
Dr. A. Zalzala, El-Karkh, Bagdad, Iraq
Prof. C. Orgen, Hal Karisi, Yeni Kersi, Kat 2D, 99, Ankara, Turkey
Prof. Kobchai Prommindaroj, Department of Ophthalmology, Chulalongkorn hospital faculty of medicine, Chulalongkorn University, Bangkok, Thailand
Dr. E.O. Akinsete, Ophthalmological Society of Nigeria, P.O. Box 4092, Lagos, Nigeria

Sociedad Interamericana de Oftalmologia (S.I.D.O.)

Address: Eucken # 16–201, México 5.D.F.
President: Dr. Roberto Wallentin (Mexico)
Vice-President: Dr. Wellington Amaya (Guatemala)
Treasurer: Dr. Fco. Lopez B. (El Salvador)
Secretary: Dr. Carlos Elvir (Honduras)

International Society for Clinical Electroretinography (ISCERG)

Address: Schiedamse Vest 180, Rotterdam, Netherlands
President: Prof. H. E. Henkes, Rotterdam
Vice-President: J. François, Ghent, Belgium
Secretary-General: G. H. M. van Lith, Rotterdam
Secretary, Western Hemisphere: J. Pearlman, Los-Angeles, U.S.A.
Secretary, Far East: A. Nakajima, Tokyo
Treasurer-General: W. Straub, Bonn
Treasurer, Socialist Countries: E. Schmöger, Erfurt, D.D.R.
Editor Newsletter: J. H. Jacobson, Ogdensburg, U.S.A.
Member-at-Large: I. Rendahl, Stockholm
Number of members: 240

The Society of Eye Surgeons

Director: John Harry King Jr.
Executive Secretary: James J. Lawlor, 5255 Longborough Rd., N.W., Washington D.C. 20016, U.S.A.

International College of Surgeons, Section on Ophthalmology and Otolaryngology

President: Hans von Leden
Secretary-Treasurer: Richard A. Perritt, 30 N Michigan Ave, Chicago 60602, U.S.A.

International Strabismological Association

President: Hermann M. Burian
Secretary-Treasurer: Gunter K. von Noorden, Texas Children's Hospital, Texas Medical Center, Houston 77025, Texas

European Contact-Lens Society of Ophthalmologists

Honorary President: Jules François, Gent
President: Montague Ruben, London
Vice-President: Paul Cochet, Paris
Vice-President: Hermann Kemmetmüller, Wien
Secretary-General: Hanfried Laue, D-8 München 2
Treasurer: Jürgen Rix, Rosenheim

SOCIETATES OPHTHALMOLOGICAE, NOMINA ET DOMICILIA MEDICORUM, NOSOCOMIA, INSTITUTA SCHOLAEQUE RECENSAE

AEGYPTUS

SOCIETATES OPHTHALMOLOGICAE

Ophthalmological Society of Egypt

President: Prof. Dr. El Said Khalil Abu Shousha
Vice-President: Dr. Ahmed Ezzeldin Naim
Honorary Secretary: Dr. Ahmed Amin El-Gamal
Honorary Treasurer: Prof. Dr. Abd El-Rahim Ali Fouad
Honorary Assistant Secretary: Dr. Khalid Ahmed Eyada
Members: Prof. Dr. Anwar El Masri, Prof. Dr. Wafic Mohamed Hifni, Dr. Mohamed Sobhy, Dr. Ahmed Safwat
Bureau: Dar El-Hekma, 42, Kasr El-Ainy Street, Cairo

NOMINA ET DOMICILIA MEDICORUM AB OCULIS

Abbas, Salwa Riad	23, El Hassan Dokki	Cairo
Abbas, Samira Abd El-Hamid	76, Mohi Abou El Ez St.	Douki
Abbassi, Ahmad Fahmi	33, Abd El Khalik Tharwat Pasha Street	Cairo
Abboles, Samira		Lybia
Abboud, Ibrahim Ahmad	26, Sherif Pasha St.	Cairo
Abdalla, Ahmed Shafik	21, Abdel Megid El-Labban St.	Sayeda Zeinab
Abdallah, Mohammad Ibrahim	30, Rashid St.	Heliopolis
Abd El-Ahad, Dib	12, Sayed Darwish Street	Cairo
Abd El-Ati, Ahmad Abd El-Salam	22, Abd El-Hamid El-Dib St.	Sarwat, Alexandria
Abd El-Ghani, Maamoun Hassan	6, Gomhoria Street	Khartoum
Abd El-Halim, Mohammad Mihriz		Kina
Abd El-Kerim, Mohammad Alam El-Din		Koussia
Abd El-Khalik Mohammad Abd El-Momein	15, El-Mekias El-Roda	Cairo
Abd El-Malek, Edwar Shehata	Oph. Hosp.	Samalout
Abd El-Malek, Samir Labib	2, Mahad El-Tewlid Street	Alexandria
Abd El-Malek, Wadih Ishak		Shebin El Kom
Abd El-Massih, Kamel		Sohag
Abd El-Megid, Mohamed Zaki	Oph. Hosp.	Assiut
Abd El-Rahman, Ibrahim Zohid		Manfalout
Abd El-Rahman, Mostafa Said	12, 28 Street	Agouza
Abd El-Razik, Iglal	12, Noubar Street	Cairo
Abd El-Rehim, Mohamed Hassan	28, Abasa Street	Heliopolis
Abd El-Salam, Mohammad Nagib	2, Sherif El-Kébir Street	Cairo

Abd El-Salam, Abd El-Aziz .	13, Youssef El Guindi Street ...	Cairo
Abdel-Salam, Wageeh	12, El-Dewan Str	Garden City
Abdel-Sayed, Michael I.....	31, Mist and Sudan Str.	Cairo
Abd El Shafi, Laila	....	Mahalla
Abd El-Wahab, Hassan Saad		
El-Din	....	El-Sudan
Abdin, Gamal El-Din Farid .	28, July 26 Street	Cairo
Abdou Ibrahim Essa	7, Ali Ben Radwan	Heliopolis
Abdu Mohammad Moham-		
mad	Kalawon O. H.	Cairo
Abid, Abd El-Fattah Ahmad	El-Mahallah O. H.	
Abou El-Einin, Gamal I.....	Univ. Hosp.	Kasr El-Aini
Abu El-Fadl, Mahmoud ...	....	Cairo
Abu Shousha, El-Said Khalil	1, Morally Street	Alexandria
Adib Gamal Habib	7, Khalil Agha St.	Garden City, Cairo
Adly Alfons Gorgi	7, Kobet El Hawa St.	Shoubra, Cairo
Ahmad, Mostafa Gomah ...	....	Mit Ghamr
Ahmad, Refat Mansour	11, Abd El-Salam El-Kharbotly	Zitoon
Amara, Mohamed Hassanein		
Moahmed	16, Sh. Mahmoud Azmi	Zamalek
Anton, Khalil Gamal	12 Sh. Rashid	Heliopolis
Armanious, Fawzia, Misid ..	29, Abd El-Hamid Basha El-Dib .	Alexandria
Assaad, M. S. Mohammad ..	....	Minia El-Kamh
Ata, Amin Gad El-Rab	16, Madinet Nasr	Cairo
Atalla Nabil Shoukry	Balyana Ophth. Hospital	
Ata, Riad Georgi	....	Tanta
Atia, Hazem Ezzat	13, Yafi Ben Zeid Street	Douki
Attiah, Kasdy Youssef	20 A, El-Gisr Street	Shoubra
Awad, Awad Milik	....	Tima
Ayoub, Ahmad Mohammad	4, Aboul Sourour El-Bakry Street	Manshiet El-Bakry
Ayoub, Hanna	71, Kasr El-Aini Street	Cairo
Ayoub, Mohamed Ibrahim .	2, Mamal El-Soukar	Garden City
Aziz Samia Nashid	15, Shehata Tawadros St.	Shoubra, Cairo
Badir, Gamal	26, El-Kanisah El-Morquosiah Street	Cairo
Badr, Ahmad El-Dessouky .	16, Hassan Mazhar Street	Heliopolis
Badr, Mohamed Mahmoud .	....	Menouf
Bakeed, Mahmoud Helmi		
Ibrahim	475, Haram Street	Cairo
Bakhoum, Mamdouh Fakhri	19, Ebn Sina	Heliopolis
Bakhoum, Mumtaz Fakrhy .	El-Nozha Square	Heliopolis
Bakri, El-Sayed Mohamed ..	23, Said Zul Fakar Street	Manial, Cairo
Balamon, Armia Barsoom ..	....	Tamia
Barada, Mohammad Aziz ..	117, Gamei El-Attarin Street ...	Alexandria
Barhoum, A. Gamal	29, El-Guindy Street	Helwan
Barradah, Mohammad Ala-		
El-Din	9, Emad El-Din Street	Cairo
Barsoum, Emad	202, Mehatat El-Souk	Baqos, Alexandria
Barsoum, Fahim	66, Abou Bakr El-Sedic Str.	Heliopolis
Basali, Megali	....	El-Shohada
Bashat, Khaled Mohamed ..	13, El-Mahad El-Eshtraki	Heliopolis
Basili, Fouad	....	Dissouk
Basili, Toma	3, Mohamed Ali El-Bakli	Heliopolis
Bastawros, Kamel Girgis ...	26, Shoubra Street	Cairo
Benzahin, Selim	41, El-Nabil Danial Street	Alexandria

Beshay, Youssef Welson ...	El-Horria St.	Abou Tig
Bishai, Abdel Sayed	13, Mossadak St.	Dokki
Bishay, Abdel Sayed	4, Iskandar Marcel St.	Heliopolis
Bishay, Samir Iskandar	....	El Minia
Bondok, Busayna Hassan ..	7, El-Der Street	Cleopatra, Alexandria
Daoud, Kamal Habib	56, Abd El-Khalek Sarwat St. ...	Cairo
Deeb, Nabil Anton	27, El-Zaher Street	Cairo
Deryas, Lewis	87 A, Shoubra Street	Cairo
Disouki, Abd Rabbo	....	Benha
Disouki, Ismail	12, Aischa El-Taymouria Street .	Garden City
Dos, Shafik	725, Port Said Street	Ghamra, Cairo
Ebeid Rafik Nashid	70, Misr Wal Soudan St.	Koubba, Cairo
Effat Soraya Josef	25, Koubba St.	Heliopolis
El-Aarabi, Mohyi El-Din Ab- dallah	11, El-Falaky Square	Cairo
El-Agizy, Hamed Moham- mad Kamal	33, Sh. Ahmad Massoud	El-Dokki, Cairo
El-Antabli, Said Abd El- Ghani	4, Moustafa Fadel St.	Cairo
El-Aswad, Mohamed Ali Has- san	214, Sh. Ramsis	Cairo
El-Ayadi, Badr El-Din	Kalawon O. H.	Cairo
El-Bahnasawi, Samiha Abd El-Badie	El-Giza Ophth. Hospital	Cairo
El-Banna, M. Mohamed	34, Port Said Street	El-Shatbi, Alexandria
El-Dabagh, Mostafa Sadek .	....	Kafr El-Dawar
El-Dabh, Noshi Ghorbal ...	....	Maghagha
El-Dairy, Fakhri Hanna	8, Osman Ibn Affan Str.	Heliopolis
El-Damouhy, Mohammad El- Gemeiy	....	El-Delengat
El-Dars, Mohammad Hassan	....	Mehalla El-Kobra
El-Difrawi, Hamid	....	Kuwait
El Deiry Maged Moh.	11, El Mahallawi St.	Dokki, Cairo
El-Fahham, Zaki El-Hamawi	Gadet El-Darwishia Hos.	Damascus
El-Gamal, Ahmad Amin ...	6, Mahad El-Sahara	Heliopolis
El-Gamal, Hamid Ali El-Said	9, Abd El-Al St.	Ard El-Naam, Mataria, Cairo
El-Gammal, Magdolin Yehia	93, Oad 103	Maadi, Cairo
El-Gammal, Yehia Abd El- Rahman	....	Cairo
El-Ghandour, Mohammad Husni Hafez	21, July 26 Street	Tanta
El-Ghonemi, Mohyi El-Din Riad	66, 104 St.	Maadi, Cairo
El-Guindi, Nabil Mahmoud .	131, Misr-Melwan Street	Maadi
El-Goul, Hussein Mohammad	....	Sherbin
El-Gwini, Hohamed Haher Abd El-Hamid	24, El-Goumhoria Square	Cairo
El Hag Eid Taha Abdel Ha- mid	57, Khoufo St.	Giza
El-Hakim, Hassan Husni Aly	56, Al Gesr Es Sewess Street	Heliopolis
El-Hawari, Golzamin Moha- med Ragheb	6, Madinet Nasr	Cairo
El-Hofi, Osama Ahmed	7, Mansoora Street	Manial El-Roda, Cairo
El-Hoseiny, Mohammad Khalil	7, El-Sheikh Hassan Street	Heliopolis
El-Hoshy, Mohamed Hassan	10, Al-Imam Ali Street	Heliopolis

El-Kalawi, Hassan Mohamed Selim	58, El-Montazah Street	Heliopolis
El-Kateb, Mohamed Abd-Alla	....	Damahour
El-Kholy, Aziz	Research Centre	Qualiub
El-Korashi, Mohamed Medhat	2, Sh. Yong.	Alexandria
El-Koussi Nagia Hossein ...	449, Ramses St.	Cairo
El-Labban, Ibrahim Mohammad Ibrahim	Deherness	Dakahlia
El-Maghrabi, Mohamed Atef Amin	9, Hod El-Labban Street	Garden City
El-Marzouki, Momtaz, Mohamed	....	Shebin El-Kom
El-Masri, Anwar Mohammad Amin	32, El-Falaki Street	Bab El-Louk, Cairo
El-Mofti, Ali Abd El-Monem	30, Shagaret El-Dor St.	Zamalek, Cairo
El-Naggar, Abd El-Baset Ahmed	5, Abou El-Nehar Mahmoud Hamza Street	Alexandria
El-Nashar, Hassan Kamel Abdel-Halim	3, Hassouna El-wawawy Street ..	Heliopolis
El-Obary Nabil Abdel Ghani	9, Souria St.	Roushdi, Alexandria
El-Refai, Mohamed El-Sayed	18, Maher Pasha Street	Abbassia
El-Rifai, Ahmad Amin	Ophthalmic Department, Univ. Hospital	Alexandria
El-Roubi, Ahmad Mohammad	77, Shoubra Street	Cairo
El-Sayed, Ateyat Mostafa ..	5, El-Doctor Abd El-Halim Helmi, Gesr El-Suis	Zaytoun, Cairo
El-Seiddy, El-Sayed Mostafa	....	Samaloot
El-Sessy, Salah El-Din Hamid Mustafa	....	Belbeis
El-Shama, Nabil Awad	....	Kafr El-Sheikh
El-Shenawi, M. Mohamed ..	Oph. Hosp.	Beni Suef
El-Sheyati, Mohamed Fawzi	11, Midan El-Falaki	Cairo
El-Shiwy, Taha Mohamed ..	4, Maris Street	Manial, Cairo
El-Tyty, Sady Hassan Abd El-Halim	....	Nablus, Jordan
El-Zind, Hassan Ali	....	El-Manzalah
Estefanos, Layla Youssef ..	3 A, Mohamed Mazhar St.	Zamalek, Cairo
Eyada, Khalid Ahmad	26, Adly Street	Cairo
Ezz El-Arab, Sami Mahmoud	....	El-Mahalla
Fahmi, Fayek	56, Abdel-khalek Sarwat Street .	Cairo
Fahmi, Nabila Mohamed ...	261, Port Said St.	Cleopatra, Alexandria
Farag, Samir Labib	....	Beni Suef
Farahat, Hassan	Giza Ophth. Hospital	Cairo
Fares, Nabil Bouless	Oph. Hosp.	Somosta
Farghali, Ibrahim Ahmed Sabri	329, Tareek El-Horria	Alexandria
Farouk, Ahmad	157, El-Tatweeg Street	Alexandria
Fattouh, Fattouh Mohammad	32, El-Falaki Street	Bab El-Louk, Cairo
Firgani, Gamil Mabrouk ...	....	Fayoum
Flatas, Rifaat Nazmi	....	Faraskour
Fouad, Abd El-Rehim Ali ..	28, 26 July Street	Cairo

Fouad, Azmi		Beba
Gaafar, Hassan Hosni	11, Yashbak Street	El-Abbassia, Cairo
Gaber, Aly	47, Ramsis Street, Pfizer Scientific Office	Cairo
Gadallah, A. M. A.	11, Midan El-Tahrir	Cairo
Gamal El-Din, Mahmoud		Damanhour
Gawdat, Ismail	8, Mohamed Sidky Shafie	Roda, Cairo
Gayed Eskandar Ishak	215, Ramses Street	Cairo
Ghabaros, Edwar Abd El-Malek	4, Italian Hosp. Str.	Fayoum
Gharbawi, Fahim Tadros		
Gharbawi, Kamal Fahim Tadros		Shebin El-Kanater
Ghattas, Salah El-Din Ayoub	32 A, Shoubra Street	Cairo
Ghobrial, Hanna Salib		El-Monira
Ghobrial, Fouad Gorgi	Karmooz	Alexandria
Ghobrial, Sadik Hanna		Kottor
Girgis, Emil Hanna	9, Sh. Beniswef	Kamp Shizar, Alexandria
Girgis, Ishak Bisada	Luxor O.H.	
Girgis, Girgis Tadros		El-Wasta
Girgis, Samir Nashid		El-Simbelawen
Gubran, Mufid	249, El-Geish Street	Cairo
Graiss, Amin Yassa	Memorial Institute for Ophthalmic Research	Giza
Guirgis, Aziz Fahim	5, Baghdad Str.	Heliopolis
Guirgis, Aziz Habib	Oph. Hosp.	Mahmoudeya
Guirgis, Botros Youssef		Edfina
Guwaida, Bahgat Badawi	3, El-Senbellawen Street	Camp Shezar, Alexandria
Habashi, Nagat S.	3 A, Halab Street	Heliopolis
Habashi, Stani	41, Kasr El-Nil Street	Cairo
Habashi, Waguih Zikry		Mashtal El-Souk
Habib, Ezzat Shalabi		Tanta
Habib, Moheb Kamal	21, Ezzat Street	Zaytoon
Hakim, Emil Soryal	Oph. Hosp. Markaz Badr. Moderiet	El-Tahrir
Hakim, Salah El-Din	Azhar O. H.	Cairo
Hamada, Youssef Mohammad Eid	Oph. Hosp.	Embaba
Hamdan, Yehia Mohammad	Garet El-Mandoura Street	Roda, Cairo
Hamid, Hassan Hilmy	O.H.	Giza
Hammouda, Ibrahim Mostafa	58, Kasr El-Aini Str.	Cairo
Hammouda, Ismail Kamel	115, Manial Street	Cairo
Hanafi, Fathi Ahmad Helmi Khalaf	14, Manfiss Str.	Camp Shezar, Alexandria
Hanna, Adel Wagdi	9, Obersh Street	Alexandria
Hanna, Lucy Shafik	18, Shambilion Str.	Cairo
Hanna, Onsi Farag	7, Hassan Shaker Street	Giza
Hanna, Sami Mina	Oph. Hosp.	Edko
Hanna, Tadros Youssef		Etsa Fayoum
Hassaballa, Nadra Shaaban	11, El-Emari Str.	Bab El-khalk, Cairo
Hassan, Ibrahim Mohammed	18, Mohamed Salah Str.	Dokki
Hassan, Ibrahim Mohammed	2, El-Kadi El-Fadel Str.	Cairo
Hassan, Adel Mohammad	El-Sawra Street	El-Mansoura
Hefzi, M. Y.	16, El-Makreezy Street	Saray El-Kobbah, Cairo
Hegab, Ibrahim Ali Yousef		Zakazik
Hegab, Samiha M. A.	37, Farid Street	Heliopolis

Hegazy, Momtaz A.	5, Kasr El-Nil Street	Cairo
Helal, Yehya Moustafa	12, Ahmed Shafik St.	Koubba
Helmi, Esmat Riad	O.H.	Rod El-Farag
Hifny, Wafik Mohammad ..	12, Latif Mansour Street	Heliopolis
Higazy, Nadia Abdel Hamid	5, Mahmoud Sidki Street	Zamalek
Hilmy, Fayek	16, Abd El-Aziz Street	Cairo
Hilmy, Saad Aziz	....	Ashmoun
Hosni, Farouk	3, Beirut Street	Heliopolis
Hosni, Farouk Hosni	....	Saoudi Arabia
Hussein, Hussein Ahmad ...	....	Khartoum, Sudan
Ibrahim, Adli Abadeer	5, Diomides Street	Ramleh Station, Alexandria
Ibrahim, El-Bakir	....	Khartoum, Sudan
Ibrahim, Ibrahim Selim	2, Istanboul Street	Alexandria
Ibrahim, Kamil Girgis	23, Midan El-Tahrir	Alexandria
Ibrahim, Mahmoud Hamdi .	Ain Shams University	
Ibrahim, M. Salah El-Din ..	39, El-Foza Str.	Heliopolis
Ibrahim, Mostafa Ismail ...	....	El-Santa
Ibrahim, Talaat Zaki	5, El-Edfay St.	Heliopolis, Cairo
Idris, Abd El-Rehim Ali ...	....	Kom Ombo
Iskandar, Gamal Abdel Magid	....	Abou Hommoss
Ismail, Abd El-Magid Abd El-Rahman	23, 9th Street	Maadi, Cairo
Ismail, Barakat Hassan	Medical Commission	Cairo
Ismail, Mohammad El-Fatih Sayed	29, Yacoub Street	Dawawin, Cairo
Ismail, Mohammad Tawfik .	41, Abdel-Khalek Sarwat Street .	Cairo
Istifanous, Maher Labib ...	....	Marsa Matrouh
Kabil, Hassan Kamal Abd El-Magid	....	Aswan
Kaddis, Maher Riad	....	Damanhour
Kamali, Khalifa Abd El-Latif	....	Ramses Square, Cairo
Kamel, Ahmad Hussein	....	Mallawi
Kamel, Ibrahim Dia El-Din .	42, Ragi Street	Bolkly, Alexandria
Kamel, Sabri	44, El-Gumhuria Str.	Opera Square, Cairo
Kamel, Sabri Kamel	11, Ghinia Str.	Heliopolis, Cairo
Kamel, Abd El-Fattah Mustafa	13, Dr. Mohammad Bey Raafat Street	Zaghloul Square, Alexandria
Karas, Monir Latif	45, Sh. Hossin El-Swifi	Saray El-Kobba, Cairo
Karas, Latif Tadros	....	Assiout
Kassem, Mahmoud Ahmad .	5, El-Doctor Abd El-Halim Helmi	Gisr El-Suis Zaytoon, Cairo
Kassem, Rashad Mohamed Mohamed	10, Sh. Kasr El-Mukhtar	Cairo
Kelani, Abd El- Moneim Abd El-Aziz	....	Shebin El-Kom
Keriakos, Nazmi Zaki	....	Beirot, Lebranon
Khaki, Farouk Mohammad Tawfik	34, Rod El-Rarag Street	Shubra, Cairo
Khalifa, Sherif Ahmed Ali .	4, Ibrahim Osman, Madinet El-Mohandes in Dokki	Cairo
Khalil, Mahmoud Fahmi ...	42, El-Samma St.	Abbassia, Cairo
Kirollos, Fawzi	....	Assiout
Korra, A.	17, Rami Station Square	Alexandria
Kosman, Hanna Louis	....	Gerga
Labib, Magdi Helmi	....	Khanka

Labib, Mohammad Abd El-Moneim	56, Abd El-Khalek Tharwat Pasha Street	Cairo
Labib, Thabet		Isna
Latif, Talaat Nagi	16, Salah El-Din Street	Heliopolis
Longiuotto, M. B.		Jedda, Soudi Arabia
Louis, Pamela Elen	56, Abdel Khalek Sarwat Street	Cairo
Mahmoud, Mohamed Tawfik	2, Okba Street	Dokki
Makarem, Fatma	7, Mostafa Reda Street	Manial
Mankarious, Adly		Beni Suef
Masoud, Farid	29, Emad El-Din Street	Cairo
Masoud, Wagiehah Hassan	10, Dr. Handousah Street	Garden City
Megali, Raouf Amin	16, Ismail Street	Zamalek, Cairo
Mehasseb, Hosam El-Din Hussein	47, Giza Street	Cairo
Mekkawi, Mohammad Fathy	Ain Shams University	Cairo.
Messiha, Nabil Wadieh	Sawra Str.	Assiout
Mikhail, Farid Halim		Zauriet El Naoura
Mikhail, Henry Fahmy		Dayrout
Mikhail, Nodaki Ibrahim	Ophth. Hospital	Tanta
Mina, Emad Hamdi	24, Massara St.	Shoubra, Cairo
Mishriki, Ramses	20, Lazoghly Str.	Helwan
Mohammad, Abd. El-Aziz	Azhar University D.S.	Cairo
Monir, Amira Mohamed	24, Mohamed Youssef El-Kadi Str.	Heliopolis, Cairo
Morad, Adel El-Sayed	Oph. Hosp.	Fayoom
Mortada, Ali	18 A, 26 July Street	Cairo
Mostafa, Ahmed Safwat	Port Said Hospital	Port Said
Mostafa, Hassan Negm	12, Sayed Darwish Str.	Cairo
Mostafa, Mahmoud Salah El-Din	93, Roda 103	Maadi, Cairo
Mostafa, Mohamad Ismail	1, El-Nahda Str.	Sohag
Mostafa, Mohamed Samir		Koos
Mourgan, Attiah Hamed	El-Husseinia	Sharkia
Moussa, Ahmad Fikri	5, Sherif Street	Cairo
Moris, El-Sayed Ekram Abd El-Samad	55, Abd El-Aziz Al Seoud	Manial El-Roda, Cairo
Moza, Faris Saman	Kalawon O.H.	Cairo
Nabih, Fayek Nast		El-Fashn
Nagib, Ihab Fathi	Oph. Hosp.	Ebashaway
Naim, Ahmad Izz El-Din	Kalawon O.H.	Cairo
Nakhla, Marie Garas		Kafr El-Zayat
Nashid, Alfonse	127, Ramses Street	Cairo
Noman, Hossni Talaat	Borg El-Maadi	Maadi
Omar, Gamalat	5, Zakaria El-Ansari Street	Pyramids, Cairo
Osman, Zenab Mahmoud	4, El-Soudi Str.	Manshiet Al Bakri, Cairo
Rabie, Hamid Abd El-Hamid	4, Momen St.	Abbasia, Cairo
Radwan, Mohammad Salah El-Din	15, 47 Street	Maadi
Ragab, M. Hafez	216, Port Said Street	Cleopatra, Alexandria
Rashed, Mohamed Omar Mohamed	Oph. Section, Ein Shams University	Cairo
Rifaat, Aida	18, Dar El- Shefa Str.	Cairo
Rifaie, M. El-Sayed	18, Maher Pasha Str.	Abbassia
Riskallah, Fathy		Shabrakheit
Rofail, Naguib Farag		Minia

Rofail, Tomas Botros	5, Kamel Sedki Street	Fagalla, Cairo
Rushdy, Maher Salib	15, Liwa Fatin Street	Shoubra
Saad, Mohammad Ahmad ..	....	Banha
Saad El-Din, Abd El-Aziz Mohammad	27, El-Badrawy Ashour Street ..	Douki, Cairo
Saad, Nawal Samuel	40, El-Mahata St.	Giza
Saad, Abdalla Fawzi	35, Kawkeb St.	Moharam Bey, Alexandria
Sabri, Ismat	Ahmad Maher Hospital	Cairo
Sabri, Nabil Ibrahim	14, El-Eskandar El-Akbar Str. ...	Azarita, Alexandria
Sabri, Wadi Said	44, Sherif Street	Cairo
Sachs, Rudolf	....	
Sachs, Willy	....	
Sadek, Ahmad	Spinning & Weaving Misr Comp. .	El-Mahalla
Sadek, Tvon	Aswan O.H.	Aswan
Sadek Wafik Zaki	Ophth. Hospital	Kasr El-Dawar
Said, Ahmed Hassan	183, Tahrir Street	Cairo
Said, Mohammad Mohyi El-Din	40, Safiya Zaghloul Street	Alexandria
Said, Widad	28, 26 July Str.	Cairo
Said El-Din, Sayed	8, Abbassia Street	El-Daher
Sawiris, Fouad Amin	....	Mit-Ghamr
Salama, Maher Michail	1, Moustafa Kamel Square	Samouha, Alexandria
Saleh, Mohamed Fathi Mo-hamed	449, Ramsis Street	Cairo
Salem, Taghrid Ahmad	....	Zagazig
Samuel, Habib	....	Sohag
Sayed, Mohamed Abd El-Moneim El-Montasah, Sidi Beshr	593, Kebli Al Sekak Al Hadid ...	Alexandria
Sayed, Mohammad Ezz El Din	7, El-Rifai Street	Citadel, Cairo
Sakla, Fouad Ragheb	....	Abu El-Matamir
Siam, Abd El-Latif Hussein .	62, Abbassia Street	Cairo
Shaaban, Sami Mohamed Ahmed	....	El-Ismailia
Shalabi, Tadros	Fouad Hospital	Alexandria
Shalash, Bahai El-Din	3, Diwan Street	Garden City, Cairo
Shawki, Mohammad	Oph. Hospital	Tanta
Shawki, Mohamed Rashed Ahmed	Oph. Hospital	Abou Kebir
Sherif, Zeinab Hafez	Memorial Institute for Ophth. Research	Giza
Sheta, Ahmed Sabri	13, El-Kalsa Street	Alexandria
Shinouda, Adli Abdou	....	Beni Suef
Shinouda, Samuel Nagib ...	19, Waboor El-Talg Street	El-Mahalla
Shoman, Eglal Mohamed ..	5, Nobar Street	Cairo
Sidhom, Mansour Salib	13, El-Malek El-Mozzafar Str. ...	Rodah
Sidhom, Kamal Girgis	6, El-Moukhtar Street	Roda
Sidky, Samir Ghobrial	....	Nabaroh
Sidky, Shaker Fouad	Memorial Institute for Ophthal-mic Research	Giza
Siganos, E.	16, Boustan Street	Cairo
Sobhy, Mohamed M. I.	54, Abd El-Khalek Sarwat Str. ..	Cairo
Soliman, Abd El-Mohsen ..	174, El-Tahrir Street	Cairo
Soliman, Farag	....	Maghagha
Soliman, Fatma M.	24, Masnaa El-Tarabeesh St.	Cairo

Soliman, Mohamed M. A. H.	7, Abdel-Aziz Str.	Aguzah
Soliman, Iskandar Hanna ..	Giza Oph. Hospital	Cairo
Tadros, George Sami	41, Soliman Street	Cairo
Tadros, Samir Anis	Monira Hospital	Cairo
Taha, Mohamed Salah El-Din	....	El-Minsha Sohag
Taher, Mohamed Abou El-Maali Mohamed	90, Riad Street	Assiout
Taher, Zakaria	1, Mohamad Mazloum Pasha Street	Cairo
Tantawi, Ezz El-Din Hassan El-Soufy	Oph. Hospital	Sohag
Tashkandi, Abd El-Aziz ...	Nasria Hosp.	El-Riad
Tawadros, Shihata Habib ..	Mansheyet El-Bakri Hosp.	
Tharwat, Ahmed Osman ...	....	Tanta
Tiba, Ahmed Mohamed	....	Mansoura
Tiba, Mohammad Kamal El-Din Mustafa	....	Mansoura
Tolba, Osman Ghaleb	Giza Oph. Hospital	Cairo
Toubia, Samir	11, Adly Yakan St.	Mazloum, Alexandria
Wahba, Edward Azer	....	Minia
Wasfi, Ismail Ahmad	3, 10 Street	Maadi
Wassef, Nessim Labib	16, Street, Vella 22	Sidi Beshr, Alexandria
Wazir, Ahmed Mohamed ...	Manial Oph. University Hosp. ...	Cairo
Weshahi Mohamed Abdel Ghani	11, Haroun St.	Dokki, Cairo
Yassa, Nagi Soliman	10, 26 July Street	Cairo
Youssef Layla Osman	5, Ben Radwan St.	Giza
Youssef, Mohammad Osman	33, Abd El-Khalek Sarwat Pasha Street	Cairo
Youssef, Nabil Fahmy Said .	....	Fakoos
Youssef. Nagat Akhnoukh .	141, Masr and Soudan St.	Hadayek El-Kobba, Cairo
Zaki, Hoda Abd El-Aziz ...	Afrah El-Angal Street	Monira, Cairo
Zaki. Fvza Abdalla	Gamhoria Street ....,...	Maghagha
Zanati, Mahmoud Osman ..	....	Tanta
Zayed, Amin Ismail	84, Abou Bakr El-Sedik	Heliopolis
Zayed, Mohamed Ali	Damietta Oph. Hospital.	
Zein-Eddin, Esam Said	18, Ismail Sabri Str.	Heliopolis
Zidan, Abd El-Kader El-Said	17, Badawi St.	Maharam Bey, Alexandria
Zohdi, Mohamed Mohamed	....	Kom Hamada

NOSOCOMIA QUIBUS OCULIS AEGRI CURANTUR

Eye departments in all General Hospitals

INSTITUTA SCHOLAEQUE CAECIS DESTINATAE

Centre for the rehabilitation of the blind:
302, Tereet El-Gabal, Zaytoon, Cairo.
Covering 28 schools and institutes with a total of 5476 pupils.

AFRICA MERIDIONALIS (Union of S. Africa)

SOCIETATES OPHTHALMOLOGICAE

Ophthalmological Society of South Africa

President: Dr. J. L. van Selm
Vice-President: Dr. S. Sacks
Immediate Past President: Prof. H. Meyer
Members: Dr. S. Etzine, Dr. J. G. Louw, Dr. N. H. Welsh
Secretary: Dr. E. T. Meyer, 1207 Lister Building, 195 Jeppe Street, Johannesburg
Number of members: 128

NOMINA ET DOMICILIA MEDICORUM AB OCULIS

Abel, S.	308 Medical Centre, Heerengracht	Cape Town
Adler, S.	204 Osler Chambers, Jeppe Street	Johannesburg
Amoils S. P.	1202 Medical Arts Building, Jeppe Street	Johannesburg
Ancker, E.	Ophthalmology Department, Tygerberg Hospital	Tiervlei, Cape
Appleton, S. C.	411 Medical Centre, Heerengracht	Cape Town
Barlow, G. B.	P.O. Box 636	Vereeniging, Tvl.
Been, L. M.	25 van Riebeeck Building, Schoeman Street	Pretoria, Tvl.
Blumenthal, C. J.	28 St. James Road	East London
Bosch, A. H.	1105 Oasim North, Havelock Street	Port Elizabeth
Boshoff, P.	21a, Main Road	Port Alfred, C.P.
Botha, P. J. L.	1021 Medipark, Hertzog Boulevard, Foreshore	Cape Town
Bradfield, I. L.	401 Union Castle Building, Adderley Street	Cape Town
Bristow, J. H.	801 Lancet Hall, Jeppe Street ...	Johannesburg
Brody, H. v. D.	1025 Medipark, Hertzog Boulevard, Foreshore	Cape Town
Brown, M. E.	401 Union Castle Building, Adderley STreet	Cape Town
Chait, H.	509 Salisbury House, West Street	Durban
Chouler, N. J. G.	318 Medical City, 160 Eloff Street	Johannesburg
Clarke, P. A.	101 Medical Centre, 331 Burger Street	Pietermaritzburg, Natal
Coetzee, D. C.	3rd Floor, Medical Centre, 5th Avenue	Springs, Tvl.
De Kock, J.	719 Medipark, Hertzog Boulevard, Foreshore	Cape Town
De Kock, J. K.	719 Medipark, Hertzog Boulevard, Foreshore	Cape Town
De Moor, S.	P.O. Box 259	Pretoria, Tvl.

De Villiers, G. F.	Octron Building	Potchefstroom, Tvl
Du Plessis, G. G.	1003 Lancet Hall, Jeppe Street ..	Johannesburg
Du Toit, P. B.	730 Medipark, Hertzog Boulevard, Foreshore	Cape Town
Dold, N. E.	331 Sanlam Building, Jones Street	Kimberley, C.P.
Douglas, W. H. G.	Brenthurst Clinic, Park Lane, Parktown	Johannesburg
Epstein, E.	P.O. Box 2565	Johannesburg
Etzine, S.	802 Lister Building, Jeppe Street	Johannesburg
Ferreira, A. B. W.	724 Medipark, Hertzog Boulevard, Foreshore	Cape Town
Frampton, G.	Brenthurst Clinic, Park Lane, Parktown	Johannesburg
Framks, M.	208 Medical Centre, Jeppe Street	Johannesburg
Garber, I.	1 Medical Centre, Jeppe Street ..	Johannesburg
Gelman, H. Z.	802 Medical Towers, Jeppe Street	Johannesburg
Golden, B.	Dept. of Ophthalmology, Medical School, Hospital Hill	Johannesburg
Goldin, C.	506 Medipark, Hertzog Boulevard, Foreshore	Cape Town
Gordon, T. D.	1214 United Buildings, Cnr. Smith & Gardiner Streets ...	Durban
Haarburger, O. M.	P.O. Box 27	Bergvliet, C.P.
Hamelberg, H. J.	422 Medical Centre, Jeppe Street	Johannesburg
Howes, G. R.	18 St. James Road	East London
Hutten, J. B.	307 van Riebeeck Building, Schoeman Street	Pretoria, Tvl
Israel, E. B.	202 Cranwell Hall, 2nd Street, Killarney	Johannesburg
Jacobs, D. J.	41 van Riebeeck Building, Schoeman Street	Pretoria, Tvl
Johnson, P. A.	14th Floor, Denor House, Cnr. Smith & Field Street	Durban
Joubert, A.	P.O. Box 840	Klerksdorp, Tvl
Judes, D.	301 Medical Centre, Jeppe Street	Johannesburg
Kay, B.	National Mutual Building, Church Square	Cape Town
Kaye, H.	1 Medical Centre, Jeppe Street ..	Johannesburg
Kooy, C.	82 Church Street	Worcester, Cape
Kopelowitz, N.	1309 Lister Building, Jeppe Street	Johannesburg
Kriel, P. J.	P.O. Box 845	Pietersburg, Tvl
Kruger, L. P.	1112 Medical City, 160 Eloff Street	Johannesburg
Küpper, F. J.	712 Medipark, Hertzog Boulevard, Foreshore	Cape Town
Kuming, B. S.	716 Tower Hill, Cnr. Kotze & Klein Streets, Hillbrow	Johannesburg
Leiman, G.	705 Harley Chambers, Jeppe Street	Johannesburg
Lecuona, M. A.	Suite E, Medical Centre, 331 Burger Street	Pietermaritzburg, Natal
Le Roux, L.	730 Medipark, Hertzog Boulevard, Foreshore	Cape Town
Levy, R.	305 Lancet Hall, Jeppe Street ...	Johannesburg
Levy, W. M.	714 Medical Centre, Jeppe Street	Johannesburg

Loubser, M. v. R.	431 Robert Koch Medical Building, Pretorius Street	Pretoria, Tvl.
Louw, C.	P.O. Box 234	Welkom, O.F.S.
Louw, J. G.	808 Medical Centre, Heerengracht	Cape Town
Luntz, M. H.	Medical School, Hospital Hill ...	Johannesburg
MacEwan, I. C.	114 Park Drive	Port Elizabeth
Marais, C. F.	620 U.B.S. Building, Maitland Street	Bloemfontein, O.F.S.
Marais, I	422 Medical Centre, Jeppe Street	Johannesburg
McCartney, D. R.	1 Medical Centre, Jeppe Street ..	Johannesburg
Meyer, E. T.	1207 Lister Building, Jeppe Street	Johannesburg
Meyer, H.	316 van Riebeeck Building, Schoeman Street	Pretoria, Tvl.
Meyer, J. M. Durr.	P.O. Box 123	Klerksdorp, Tvl.
Meyer, P. L.	Frere Hospital	East London
Meyerson, L.	723 Medical Centre, Jeppe Street	Johannesburg
Miller, E.	318 Barclays Bank Building, 68 Main Street	Port Elizabeth
Molteno, A. C. B.	Plumtree Cottage, Palmboom Road	Newlands, Cape
Morrish, D. H.	1004 S. A. Mutual Building, Gardiner Street	Durban
Murray, N. L.	504 Medical Centre, Pretorius Street	Pretoria, Tvl.
Neethling, A. C.	506 Medipark, Hertzog Boulevard, Foreshore	Cape Town
Phillips, G. I.	1408 Eagle Building, West Street	Durban
Pienaar, B. T.	216 Sanlam Building, Bok Street	Welkom, O.F.S.
Potgieter, G. J.	P.O. Box 587	Kroonstad, O.F.S.
Pretorius, G. H. M.	Saambou Building, Merriman Avenue	Vereeniging, Tvl.
Pullar, A. J. G.	P.O. Box 330	Salisbury, Rhodesia
Quirke, P. D. G.	1306 Durdoc Centre, 460 Smith Street	Durban
Rakusin, W.	303 Medical Towers, Jeppe Street	Johannesburg
Ross, M. Park.	12th Floor, United Building, Cnr. Gardiner & Smith Streets ...	Durban
Rubidge, L. A.	P.O. Box H 139, Hatfield	Salisbury, Rhodesia
Sacks, S.	National Mutual Building, 17 Church Square	Cape Town
Schaffer, M.	509 Colonial Mutual Building, West Street	Durban
Scott, J. G.	105 Benmore Gardens, West Street	Sandton, Tvl.
Schrire, L.	517 Medical Centre, Heerengracht	Cape Town
Scribante, S. E.	208 Sentrakor Building, 173 Pretorius Street	Pretoria, Tvl.
Sevel, D.	Dept. of Ophthalmology, Groote Schuur Hospital	Observatory, Cape
Shochet, S.	205 Lancet Hall, Jeppe Street ...	Johannesburg
Stange, H.	15th Floor, Eagle Building, Murchies Passage, off West Street	Durban
Staples, W. E.	44 Veld Street, P.O. Box 176 ...	Ficksburg, O.F.S.
Staz, L.	714 Medical Centre, Jeppe Street	Johannesburg
Steinitz, E.	704 Church Square House, Cnr. Church Square & Spin Street .	Cape Town

Steven, P. S. C.	Groote Schuur Hospital	Observatory, Cape
Steyn, A. L	Themba Hospital, Private Bag 816	White River, Tvl.
Swartz, J.	605 Medical Arts Building, Jeppe Street	Johannesburg
Talerman, H. J.	307 Oasim South	Port Elizabeth
Townsend, R. L. H.	National Mutual Building, 17 Church Square	Cape Town
Trichard, G. L	3rd Floor, Medfontein Building, 155 St. Andrew Street	Bloemfontein, O.F.S.
Trichard, L.	1ste Floor, Sanlam Building	Queenstown, C.P.
Trope, R. A.	1 Medical Centre, Jeppe Street	Johannesburg
Truter, S. R.	Durban Road Medical Centre	Bellville, Cape
Van Biljon, E. H.	507 U.B.S. Building, Maitland Street	Bloemfontein, O.F.S.
Van Dam, A.	P.O. Box 2451	Windhoek, S.W.A.
Van der Merwe, J. R.	422 Medical Centre, Jeppe Street	Johannesburg
Van der Merwe, S. P.	15th Floor, Eagle Building, Murchies Passage, off West Street	Durban
Van Duyn, J.	402 Nedpark Medical Centre, Trevenna Street, Sunnyside	Pretoria, Tvl.
Van Heerde, J.	P.O. Box 840	Klerksdorp, Tvl.
Van Huyssteen, M. P.	411 Medical Centre, Pretorius Street	Pretoria, Tvl.
Van Niekerk, P. S.	P.O. Box 263, 39 Marais Street	Strand, Cape
Van Rensburg, S. F. J.	622 van Riebeeck Building, Schoeman Street	Pretoria, Tvl.
Van Rooyen, M. M. B.	5 Danie Theron Street	Parow North, C.P.
Van Rooyen, R. A.	406 Nedpark, Trevenna Street, Sunnyside	Pretoria, Tvl.
Van Selm, J. L	401 Union Castle Building, Adderley Street	Cape Town
Van Soelen, P. N.	122 York Street	George, Cape
Von Geyso, M. F. W.	1140 Louis Pasteur, 374 Schoeman Street	Pretoria, Tvl.
Victor, A.	308 S.A.P.M. Building, Jones Street	Kimberley, C.P.
Warren, R. St. H.	Tudor Court, 14 St. Matthews Road	East London
Welsh, N. H.	509 Salisbury House, West Street	Durban
Wentzel, P. R.	Oasim, Pearson Street	Port Elizabeth
Wessels, J. H. W.	620 U.B.S. Building, Maitland Street	Bloemfontein, O.F.S.
Wolff, J. E.	1302 Lister Building, Jeppe Street	Johannesburg

NOSOCOMIA QUIBUS OCULIS AEGRI CURANTUR

St. John Eye Hospital: Baragwanath, Transvaal, South Africa.   no. of beds: 100
Provincial Hospitals and Mission Hospitals have eye-departments.

INSTITUTA SCHOLAEQUE CAECIS DESTINATAE

The South African National Council for the Blind. Societies Affiliated to the Council:
Athlone School for the Blind, Kasselsvlei Road, Bellville, C.P. 131 Pupils.

Beacon Club for the Blind, P.O. Box 8, Grassy Park, Cape Town.
Bosele School for Bantu Blind, P.O. Mpudule, via Middelburg, Tvl. 79 Pupils.
Cape Town Civilian Blind Society, 45 Salt River Road, Salt River, C.P. Employ 103 Blind.
Civilian Blind Society of the O.F.S., 331 C.N.A. Buildings, Maitland Street, Bloemfontein.
Coloured and Indian Blind Welfare Association, P.O. Box 42181, Fordsburg, Johannesburg. Employ 21 Blind.
East London Society for the Civilian Blind, 75 Princess Alice Drive, East London.
Efata School for Blind and Deaf Bantu Children, P.O. Box 177, Umtata. 69 Pupils.
Goldfields (O.F.S.) Civilian Blind Society, P.O. Box 560, Welkom.
Grahamstown Civilian Blind Society, P.O. Box 91, Grahamstown.
Johannesburg Society to Help Civilian Blind, P.O. Box 20, Linmeyer, Johannesburg. Employ 56 Blind.
Kimberley and Northern Cape Civilian Blind Society, P.O. Box 784, Kimberley. Employ 30 Blind.
King William's Town Society for the Civilian Blind, P.O. Box 273, King William's Town. Employ 30 Blind.
League of Friends of the Blind, P.O. Box 3, Athlone, C.P. 10 Accommodated.
Lighthouse Club for the Blind, 1005 Medical Centre, Heerengracht, Cape Town.
Natal Bantu Blind Society, Private Bag, Ntokozweni, Natal. Employ 98 Blind.
Natal European and Coloured Civilian Blind Association, 194 Umbilo Road, Durban. Employ 45 Blind.
Natal Indian Blind and Deaf Society, P.O. Box 1109, Durban. Employ 42 Blind.
New Horizon School for the Blind, 87 Royston Road, Mountain Rise, Pietermaritzburg.
Port Elizabeth Society for the Blind (Civilian), Lower Mount Road, Port Elizabeth. Employ 53 Blind.
Pretoria Society to Help Civilian Blind, 331 Boom Street, Pretoria. Employ 28 Blind.
Prinshof School for the Partially Sighted and Preparatory School for the Blind, P.O. Box 2817, Pretoria. 57 Pupils.
S.A. Blind Workers' Organisation, P.O. Box 2360, Johannesburg.
S.A. Guidedogs Association for the Blind, P.O. Box 65120, Benmore, Tvl.
The S.A. Library for the Blind, P.O. Box 115, Grahamstown.
Siloe School for Bantu Blind Children, Private Bag 7354, Pietersburg. 91 Pupils.
Stellenbosch Society for the Blind, 2 Swawel Avenue, Stellenbosch.
Tape-Aids for the Blind, P.O. Box 3858, Durban.
Transvaal Bantu Blind Society, P.O. Box 76, Ga-Rankuwa, Tvl. Employ 198 Blind.
Vela Langa Association for the Blind, P.O. Lovedale, Alice, C.P.
Vuleka School for Blind and Deaf Zulu Children, P.O. Nkandla, Zululand. 26 Pupils.
Workshop and Homes for the Blind, Worcester, P.O. Box 231, Worcester. Employ 94 Blind.
School for the Blind Worcester, 20 Adderley Street, Worcester. 232 Pupils.

AMERICA SEPT. (U.S.A.)

SOCIETATES OPHTHALMOLOGICAE

Nationales

American Ophthalmological Society

President: A. Gerald DeVoe
Secretary-Treasurer: Robert W. Hollenhorst, 200 First St. S.W., Rochester, Minn. 55901

American Academy of Ophthalmology and Otolaryngology

President: Kenneth L. Roper
Executive Secretary-Treasurer: C. M. Kos, 15 Second St. S.W., Rochester, Minn. 55901

American Medical Association, Section on Ophthalmology

Chairman: Bernard Becker
Secretary: Thomas Duane, 1025 Walnut St., Philadelphia 19107

American Association of Ophthalmology

President: Henry F. Allen
Secretary: Albert C. Esposito, Medical Center Bldg., 420-22 11th St., Huntington, WVa 25701

Association for Research in Vision and Ophthalmology

Chairman: Jay M. Enoch
Secretary: Robert D. Reinecke, Department of Opthalmology, Albany Medical College, Albany, N.Y. 12208

American Society of Ophthalmologic and Otolaryngologic Allergy

President: Jack D. Clemis
Secretary: Hamish M. Mann, Medical Arts Bldg., 1600 University Ave., Grand Forks, N.D. 58201

American Society of Ophthalmic plastic and reconstructive Surgery

President: Charles K. Beyer
Secretary: George F. Buerger, Apartm. Tower Center 1F, Pittsburg 15219

Contact-Lens Association of Ophthalmologists, inc.

President: Whitney G. Sampson
Corresponding-Secretary: G. Peter Halberg, 40 W. 77th. St., New York 10024

National Society for the Prevention of Blindness, inc.

President: Bradford A. Warner
Secretary: Thomas R. Moore
Executive Director: Virginia S. Boyce, 79 Madison Ave., New York 10016

Society of Military Ophthalmologists

President: Col. Budd Appleton
Secretary: Lester Stein, P.O. Box 1137, Steubenville, Ohio 43952

Association of University Professors of Ophthalmology

Membershiplist obtainable through the American Association of Ophthalmology

Regionales

Ark-la-tex Oto-ophthalmic Society

President: Steve G. Kirkikis
Secretary: John K. Graham, 2751 Virginia Ave, Shreveport, La. 71103

Louisiana-Mississippi Ophthalmological and Otolaryngological Society

President: Ralph A. Sneed
Secretary: Arthur V. Hays, PO Box 1018, Gulfport, Miss. 39501

New England Ophthalmological Society

President: Harry E. Braconier
Secretary: Albert R. Frederick, Jr., 10 Hawthorne Pl, Boston 02114

Pacific Coast Oto-Ophthalmological Society

President: Orson W. White
Secretary: Daniel G. Vaughan, Room 495U, University of California Medical Center, San Francisco 94122

Southern Medical Association, Section on Ophthalmology

Chairman: William R. Hudson
Secretary: R. Dean Williams, 305 W 43rd St, Kansas City, Mo. 64111

Wisconsin-upper Michigan Society of Ophthalmology and Otolaryngology

President: John A. Ottum
Secretary: James C. Allen, Eye Clinic, University Hospitals, Madison, Wis. 53706

In all states and major cities ophthalmological societies do exist. For reference: The Directory of Societies, issued by the American Academy of Ophthalmology and Otolaryngology.

NOMINA ET DOMICILIA MEDICORUM AB OCULIS

See also supplementum on page 129

Aaberg, Thomas M.	Marquette Medical School, 8700 W. Wisconsin Ave.	Milwaukee, Wisc. 53226
Abbott, Albert J.	203 E. Green St.	Nanticoke, Pa. 18634
Abbott, Orville L.	219 N. Main St.	Bloomington, Ill. 61701
Abell, Harry D.	Box 1243	Paducah, Ky. 42001
Abernethy, Lynn D.	653 N. State St.	Jackson, Miss. 39201
Abernethy, Paul M.	Vaughn Rd., Medical Village	Burlington, N. C. 27215
Abernethy, Rodney E.	215 N. San Mateo Dr.	San Mateo, Cal. 94401
Abraham, Raymond A.	5220 Clark Ave.	Lakewood, Cal. 90712
Abraham, Robert K.	16542 Ventura Blvd.	Encino, Cal. 91316
Abraham, Samuel V.	9201 Sunset Blvd.	Los Angeles, Cal. 90069
Abrahams, I. Willard	95 E. Main St.	Meriden, Conn. 06450
Abrahamson, Ira A., Sr. . . .	36 E. 4th St.	Cincinnati, O. 45202
Abrahamson, Ira A., Jr. . . .	36 E. 4th St.	Cincinnati, O. 45202
Abrams, Henry	253 Witherspoon St.	Princeton, N. J. 08540
Abramson, Victor	111 N. Wabash	Chicago, Ill. 60602
Acers, Thomas E.	Pasteur Bldg.	Oklahoma City, Okla. 73103
Ackerman, Albert L.	1016 Fifth Ave.	New York, N. Y. 10028
Ackerman, Calvin	523 Forest Ave.	Paramus, N. J. 07652
Ackerman, Frederick F. . . .	Cobb Medical Ctr.	Seattle, Wash. 98101
Ackerman, Martin	30 E. 40th St.	New York, N. Y. 10016
Ackerman, Walter G.	6841 W. Cermak Rd.	Berwyn, Ill.
Ackermann, Kurt	Medical Towers South	Louisville, Ky. 40202
Adair, Bonnie L.	105, Westbank Expressway	Gretna, La. 70053
Adair, Frank	Central Medical Bldg.	St. Paul, Minn. 55104
Adalman, Philip	74-01 34th Ave.	Jackson Heights, N. Y. 11372
Adams, Curtis L.	211 W. Main St.	Dothan, Ala. 36301
Adams, Raymond E.	108 W. Collings Ave.	Collingswood, N. J. 08108
Adams, Scharrold O.	1820 Prof. Dr.	Sacramento, Cal. 95825
Adamski, M. S.	408 North St.	Logansport, Ind. 46947
Addington, Charles H.	85 High St.	Buffalo, N. Y. 14203
Adelman, Benjamin B.	320 S. Harrison St.	East Orange, N. J. 07018
Adelstein, Nelson J.	13861 Cedar Rd.	Cleveland, O. 44118
Adkins, Howard E.	1129 Bellevue	Boise, Ida. 83706
Adler, Francis H.	8870 Towanda St.	Philadelphia, Pa. 19118
Adler, William M.	2415 High School Ave.	Concord, Cal. 94520
Adrain, John H.	1834 W. Lincoln Ave.	Anaheim, Cal. 92801
Aebi, Ernest P.	5th General Hospital, APO	N. Y. 09154
Aebli, Rudolf	E. 40th St.	New York, N. Y. 10016
Afeman, Chas. E.	1260 Main St.	Baton Rouge, La. 70802
Agatston, Howard J.	444 Community Dr.	Manhasset, N. Y. 11030
Agin, Lambert J.	36 Chestnut St.	Battle Creek, Mich. 49017
Aherne, William E.	1409 Forest Dr.	Annapolis, Md. 21403
Ahlers, Hartwig W.	2300 California St.	San Francisco, Cal. 94109
Ahmed, Quzi M.	3700 Fifth Ave.	Pittsburgh, Pa. 15213
Aicher, D. Craig	337 Wyoming Ave.	Kingston, Pa. 18704
Aiello, John S.	926 E. McDowell Rd.	Phoenix, Ariz. 85006
Aiello, Lloyd M.	108 Bay State Rd.	Boston, Mass. 02215
Aijian, Karl M.	307 West Mistletoe Pl.	San Antonio, Tex. 78212
Aiken, Samuel D.	1154 Montgomery Dr.	Santa Rosa, Cal. 95405

Ainsworth, Wm. N.	1550 Riverside Ave.	Jacksonville, Fla. 32204
Ajello, Dominick A.	1 Nevins St.	Brooklyn, N. Y. 11217
Alba, Anthony	132 Pleasant St.	Woburn, Mass. 01801
Albaugh, Clarence H.	321 N. Larchmont Blvd.	Los Angeles, Cal. 90004
Albaugh, Kathryn L.	321 N. Larchmont Blvd.	Los Angeles, Cal. 90004
Alberstadt, Norbert F.	Baldwin Bldg.	Erie, Pa. 16501
Albert, Dan G.	1515 Chain Bridge Rd.	McLean, Va. 22101
Albert, Daniel M.	789 Howard Ave.	New Haven, Conn. 06510
Albrecht, John G.	212 Oak Meadow Dr.	Los Gatos, Cal. 95030
Albright, Arnold A.	131 E. Columbia	Battle Creek, Mich. 49015
Alcorn, Harry W.	Medical Arts Ctr.	Mason City, Ia. 50401.
Alden, John C.	2915 Telegraph Ave.	Berkeley, Cal. 94705
Aldous, Richard A.	857 E. Second South St.	Salt Lake City, Utah 84108
Aldrich, Harry D.	5506 E. 16th St.	Indianapolis, Ind. 46218
Aldrich, Robert C.	Oak Hills Med. Bldg.	San Antonio, Tex. 78229
Alecce, Paul M.	550 Brickell Ave.	Miami, Fla. 33131
Alexander, Chas. M.	930 W. Sproul Rd.	Springfield. Pa. 19064
Alexander, Chas. S.	Hermann Prof. Bldg.	Houston, Tex. 77025
Alexander, Harold B.	14 W. Valerio St.	Santa Barbara, Cal. 93101
Alexander, Robt. L.	1810 Prof. Dr.	Sacramento, Cal. 95825
Alexander, Stephen J.	408 W. Market	Crawfordsville, Ind. 47933
Alfano, Jos. E.	111 N. Wabash Ave.	Chicago, Ill. 60602
Alford, T. Dale	5700 W. Markham St.	Little Rock, Ark. 72205
Alger, Leon J.	1st Pasadena St. Bk. Bldg.	Pasadena, Tex. 77502
Alkoff, Louis	713 E. Genesee St.	Syracuse, N. Y. 13210
Allain, Donald	139 Lincoln St.	Framingham, Mass. 01701
Allain, Jas. J.	2022 Swift, N.	Kansas City, Mo. 64116
Allan, Wm. B.	139 E. 66th St.	New York, N. Y. 10021
Allen, Benjamin I.	13 Park St.	Norwalk, Conn. 06851
Allen, Donald G.	1021 Prospect	Cleveland, O. 44115
Allen, Griffin M.	1949 E. 105	Cleveland, O. 44106
Allen, Henry F.	243 Charles St.	Boston, Mass. 02114
Allen, Homer B.	1202 Coggin	Brownwood, Tex. 76801
Allen, Jas. C.	Univ. Hospitals	Madison, Wisc. 53706
Allen, Jas. H.	1430 Tulane Ave.	New Orleans, La. 70112
Allen, Robt. L.	1036 N. Dearborn St.	Chicago, Ill. 60610
Allen, Robt. T.	34 S. 7th St.	Richmond, Ind. 47374
Alliband, Geo. T.	Doctors Bldg.	Omaha, Nebr. 68131
Allington, John H.	411 30th St.	Oakland, Cal. 94609
Alpar, John J.	2300 W. Seventh Ave.	Amarillo, Tex. 79106
Alper, Melvin G.	2141 K. St. N.W.	Washington, D. C. 20037
Alperin, Benjamin J.	154 Hempstead Ave.	Rockville Center, N. Y. 11570
Alpert, D. Robert	1101 Beacon St.	Brookline, Mass. 02146
Alport, Benjamin	120 Maple St.	Springfield, Mass. 01103
Alter, Albert J., Sr.	3626 Monroe St.	Toledo, O. 43606
Alterman, Morton A.	104 Fulton Ave.	Poughkeepsie, N. Y. 12603
Alvelais, G. R.	414 Navarro St.	San Antonio, Tex. 78205
Alvis, Bennett Y.	211 N. Meramec Ave.	St. Louis, Mo. 63105
Alvis, David L.	822 Hume-Mansur Bldg.	Indianapolis, Ind. 46204
Alvis, Edmond O.	Hume Mansur Bldg.	Indianapolis, Ind. 46204
Alvis, Edmund B.	211 N. Meramec Ave.	St. Louis, Mo. 63105
Ambrose, Anthony	64 Maple Ave.	Morristown, N. J. 07960
Ambrose, Melton Crosby ..	416 N. Seminary	Florence, Ala. 35630
Amdur, Jos	3392 Coral Way	Miami, Fla. 33145
Amdur, Louis	270 Henderson St.	Jersey City, N. J. 07302

Amelkin, Robert S.	34 Plaza St.	Brooklyn, N. Y. 11238
Amicucci, Vincent A.	324 Fuller Ave.	Helena, Mont. 59601
Anaclerio, Angelo M.	917 N. Walnut St.	Danville, Ill. 61832
Anderman, David A.	414 Miller Ave.	Brooklyn, N. Y. 11207
Anderson, Douglas R.	1638 N.W. 10th Ave.	Miami, Fla. 33136
Anderson, Edward E.	303 Professional Arts Bldg.	Davenport, Ia. 52803
Anderson, Edwin R.	514 W. Third Ave.	West Warren, Pa. 16365
Anderson, Elbert C.	Murchison Bldg.	Wilmington, N. C. 28401
Anderson, Frank G., Jr. ...	2026 Texas Ave.	Bryan, Tex. 77801
Anderson, H. Gordon	2312 15th St.	Troy, N. Y. 12180
Anderson, John Rutherford .	2909 St. Anthony Blvd.	Minneapolis, Minn. 55418
Anderson, Oscar D.	103 N. Broad St.	Mankato, Minn. 56001
Anderson, Paul D.	815 S. 10th St.	LaCrosse, Wisc. 54601
Anderson, Ralph D., Jr. ...	550 Washington St.	San Diego, Cal. 92103
Anderson, Robt. G.	1132 Waukegan Rd.	Glenview, Ill. 60025
Anderson, Russell H.	East Range Clinic	Virginia, Minn. 55792
Anderson, Thomas W.	1125 E. 17th St., N-254	Santa Ana, Cal. 92701
Anderson, W. Banks, Jr. ...	Duke Univ. Medical Ctr.	Durham, N. C. 27706
Anderson, W. Banks, Sr. ...	1241 University Dr.	Durham, N. C. 27707
Anderson, W. Clayton	212 W. Boscawen	Winchester, Va. 22601
Anderson, W. Dale	2322 Marlborough Rd.	Colorado Springs, Colo. 80909
Anderson, Wm. F.	1312 Main St.	Lubblock, Tex. 79401
Anderson, William H., Jr. ..	116 S. W. 15th St.	Ocala, Fla. 32670
Andrew, James M.	303 E. Town St.	Columbus, O. 43215
Andrew, Reed C.	417 S. Monroe	Green Bay, Wisc. 54301
Andrew, Robt. B.	20 S. Park	Madison, Wisc. 53715
Andrews, Edson J.	205 E. College Ave.	Tallahassee, Fla. 32301
Andrews, John H.	807 W. Sterling	Baytown, Tex. 77520
Angiuoli, Domenic N.	472 Berkeley Ave.	Orange, N. J. 07050
Annesley, Wm. H., Jr.	39 Glendale Rd.	Upper Darby, Pa. 19082
Anthony, Daniel H.	220 S. Claybrook	Memphis, Tenn. 38117
Anthony, Eugene W.	451 S. 4th St.	Fulton, N. Y. 13069
Anthony, Marc	Old Nat'l Bank Bldg.	Spokane, Wash. 99201
Anthony, Robt. A.	22 N. Pauline St.	Memphis, Tenn. 38105
Antine, Bartley E.	3370 Rivers Ave.	Charleston Heights, S. C. 29405
Antle, Robt. C.	101 W. John	Bay City, Mich. 48707
Antony, Moss L.	3600 Prytania Street	New Orleans, La. 70115
Antuna, Juan	137 Broad St.	Claremont, N.H. 03743
Apisson, John G.	635 Belle Terre Rd.	Port Jefferson, N.Y. 11777
Appelbaum, Alfred	P. O. Box 2003	Laguna Hills, Cal. 92653
Apple, Carl	55 E. Washington St.	Chicago, Ill. 60602
Applebaum, David I.	6228 W. Manchester Ave.	Los Angeles, Cal. 90045
Appleton, Budd	Walter Reed Gen. Hosp.	Washington, D.C. 20012
Apt, Leonard	UCLA School of Medicine	Los Angeles, Cal. 90024
Apter, Julia T.	1753 W. Congress Pkwy.	Chicago, Ill. 60612
Aquavella, Jas. V.	1160 Chili Ave.	Rochester, N. Y. 14624
Aragones, Jaime V.	134 W. University Dr.	Rochester, Mich. 48063
Archambeau, Paul L.	50 Santa Rosa Ave.	Santa Rosa, Cal. 95404
Archer, D. Dale	1415 18th St.	Lake Charles, La. 70601
Arendshorst, Wm.	144 W. 26th St.	Holland, Mich. 49423
Arenson, Kenneth J.	6325 Topanga Canyon	Woodland Hills, Cal. 91364
Armaly, Mansour F.	George Washington Univ. Med. Ctr., 2150 Pennsylvania ave. N.W. .	Washington, D.C. 20037
Armenia, John V.	7906 Buffalo Ave.	Niagara Falls, N. Y. 14304

Armstrong, Jas. R.	14701 Detroit Ave.	Lakewood, O. 44107
Armstrong, John R.	911 Sixth Ave.	Ft. Worth, Tex. 76104
Armstrong, Richard C.	595 E. Colorado Blvd.	Pasadena, Cal. 91101
Armstrong, William R.	955 North State St.	Jackson, Miss. 39201
Arnold, Chas. O.	1808 High	Denver, Colo. 80218
Arnold, Harry D., Jr.	1293 Peachtree St., N.E.	Atlanta, Ga. 30309
Arnold, I. Lee	Medical Arts Bldg.	Chattanooga, Tenn. 37402
Arnold, Morton	29 North St.	Willimantic, Conn. 06226
Aronberg, Chas	465 N. Roxbury Dr.	Beverly Hills, Cal. 90210
Aronson, Samuel B.	San Francisco Gen. Hosp.	San Francisco, Cal. 94110
Aronstam, Robert H.	Guthrie Clinic	Sayre, Pa. 18840
Arribas, Neva P.	640 S. Kingshighway	St. Louis, Mo. 63108
Arrington, James Millard	15the Ave. & Lake	San Francisco, Cal. 94118
Arteaga, Oliver	384 Peachtree St. N. E.	Atlanta, Ga. 30308
Asbill, David S., Jr.	1417 Barnwell St.	Columbia, S. C. 29201
Asbill, David S., Sr.	1417 Barnwell St.	Columbia, S. C. 29201
Asbury, Mary K.	2401 Ingleside	Cincinnati, O. 45206
Asbury, Taylor	250 Wm. H. Taft Rd.	Cincinnati, O. 45219
Ascher, Karl W.	1404 E. McMillan	Cincinnati, O. 45206
Ashley, Byron J.	1616 W. 8th St.	Topeka, Kans. 66606
Ashley, B. John, Jr.	1616 W. 8th St.	Topeka, Kans. 66606
Ashley, Richard W.	5711 8th Ave.	Kenosha, Wisc. 53141
Ashline, John	81 W. 84th Ave.	Denver, Colo. 80221
Ashodian, Mila J.	Lankenau Med. Bldg.	Philadelphia, Pa. 19151
Askren, Edward L., Jr.	Peachtree Med. Bldg.	Atlanta, Ga. 30308
Asregadoo, Edward R.	1515 Newell Ave.	Walnut Creek, Cal. 94596
Atchoo, Peter D.	220 Seaview Ave.	Jersey City, N. J. 07305
Atkinson, Marshall, B.	450 Sutter St.	San Francisco, Cal. 94108
Atkinson, Thomas E.	Professional Bldg.	Springfield, Mo. 65806
Atkinson, Walter S.	146 Mullin St.	Watertown, N. Y. 13601
Audette, J. Paul	1851 Tahiti	Costa Mesa, Cal. 92626
Austin, Frederick L., Jr.	U. S. Naval Hospital	Oakland, Cal. 94627
Auten, Hanford L.	251 Elm St.	Claremont, N. H. 03743
Aventuro, Louis J.	50 Samsondale Plaza	West Haverstraw, N. Y. 10993
Avizonis, V.	51 Maple Ave.	Bayshore, N. Y. 11706
Axe, Paul W.	1762 N. Waterman Ave.	San Bernardino, Cal. 92404
Ayash, John J.	123 2nd Ave., S.E.	Minot, N. D. 58701
Azar, Robt. F.	Maison Blanche Bldg.	New Orleans, La. 70112
Babacz, Teofil	450 Gay St.	Phoenixville, Pa. 19460
Back, Marcel E.	300 N. Main St.	Spring Valley, N. Y. 10977
Backer, Gordon L.	614 First St.	Wausau, Wisc. 54401
Backer, William D.	614 First St.	Wausau, Wisc. 54401
Bacon, Lewis H.	300 Mahantongo St.	Pottsville, Pa. 17901
Bade, Craig P.	2806 N. Navarro	Victoria, Tex. 77901
Baer, Alvin J.	751 E. 63rd St.	Kansas City, Mo. 64114
Baer, D. Theodore	Allenmore Med. Ctr.	Tacoma, Wash. 98405
Bailey, Arby L.	98 Clinton St.	Greenville, Pa. 16125
Bailey, John H.	270 Jay St.	Brooklyn, N. Y. 11238
Bailey, Jos. C.	511 Memorial Blvd.	Murfreesboro, Tenn. 37130
Bailey, Paul F., Jr.	511 S. W. 10th	Portland, Ore. 97205
Bailey, William R., Jr.	501 20th St.	Knoxville, Tenn. 37916
Bain, James B.	465 Cherry Ave.	Waynesboro, Va. 22980
Bair, Hugo L.	200 First St., S.W.	Rochester, Minn. 55901
Baker, Charles Robert	1411 N. Flagler Dr.	W. Palm Beach, Fla. 33401
Baker, Larry E.	325 E. Main St.	Lafayette, La. 70501

Baker, Philip H.	11633 S. Hawthorne Blvd.	Hawthorne, Cal. 90250
Baker, Robert E.	10405 E. Northwest Hwy.	Dallas, Tex. 75238
Baldeck, Eugene M.	627 6th Ave.	Lewiston, Ida. 83501
Balding, Grant	101 S. Madison	Pasadena, Cal. 91101
Balding, Thomas L.	U. S. Naval Hospital	Long Beach, Cal. 90801
Balding, Willard V.	101 S. Madison	Pasadena, Cal. 91101
Baldone, Jos. A.	Claiborne Towers	New Orleans, La. 70112
Baldridge, Max	Box 431	Heber Springs, Ark. 72543
Baldwin, Gertrude W.	116 N. Main St.	Greensburg, Pa. 15601
Baldzikowski, Ralph A.	2066 Clarmar Way	San Jose, Cal. 95128
Balen, Robert F.	27 S. State St.	Lake Oswego, Ore. 97034
Balent, Alvan	E. Oakland Park Blvd.	Fort Lauderdale, Fla. 33306
Balfour, Robert V.	2522 Dana St.	Berkeley, Cal. 94704
Balian, John V.	134 W. University Dr.	Rochester, Mich. 48063
Balistocky, Marvin H.	1320 Dekalb St.	Norristown, Pa. 19401
Ball, Charles J.	551 Millburn Ave.	Short Hills, N. 1. 07078
Ball, Danald N.	Professional Bldg.	Princeton, W. Va. 24740
Ball, William L.	514 W. Third Ave.	Warren, Pa. 16365
Ballen, Peter H.	1300 Union Tpke.	New Hyde Park, N. Y. 11040
Baller, Robert S.	1008 N. Main	Bloomington, Ill. 61701
Ballin, Norman	300 Homer Ave.	Palo Alto, Cal. 94301
Ballintine, Elmer J.	10515 Carnegie Ave.	Cleveland, O. 44106
Ballou, Robert A.	3810 River Rd.	Point Pleasant, N. J. 08742
Balsis, Bernard A.	226 W. State St.	Trenton, N. J. 08608
Balstad, Paul D.	1646 Elmira St.	Aurora, Colo. 80010
Bankes, Claude W.	742 Centre Ave.	Reading, Pa. 19601
Banks, Thomas L.	18597 W. Ten Mile Rd.	Southfield, Mich. 48075
Banks, William S. III	1616 Memorial Professional Bldg.	Houston, Tex. 77002
Banoff, Harry	431 Monterey Ave.	Los Gatos, Cal. 95030
Baraff, Albert A.	1680 N. Vine St.	Los Angeles, Cal. 90028
Baragry, Richard A.	1801 State St.	Santa Barbara, Cal.
Baras, Irving	783 Park Ave.	New York, N. Y. 10021
Barasch, Kenneth R.	783 Park Ave.	New York, N. Y. 10021
Barbour, Fleming A.	Mott Foundation Bldg.	Flint, Mich. 48502
Bard, Eli	Republic Bldg.	Denver, Colo. 8020
Bard, Leslie A.	251 E. Baltimore St.	Hagerstown, Md. 21740
Barest, Herman D.	332 Main St.	Mt. Kisco, N. Y. 10549
Bargmeyer, Ernest M.	1903 Bancroft	Missoula, Mont. 59801
Barkan, Thomas A.	4141 Geary Blvd.	San Francisco, Cal. 94118
Barker, John S.	8850 Ralston Rd.	Arvada, Colo. 80002
Barkwill, Bernard G.	390 San Antonio St.	San Diego, Cal. 92106
Barlis, Arthur A.	741 Broadway	Somerville, Mass. 02144
Barmatz, Hirsh E.	2121 E. Eighteenth Ave.	Denver, Colo. 80206
Barnert, Alan H.	1047 Park Ave.	New York, N. Y. 10028
Barnes, C. Keith	800 5th Ave.	Fort Worth, Tex. 76104
Barnes, Charles R.	200 S. 'A' St.	Oxnard, Cal. 93030
Barnes, William J.	Medical Arts Bldg.	Pittsburgh, Pa. 15213
Barnet, Ronald W.	550 West Thomas Rd.	Phoenix, Ariz. 85013
Barnshaw, Harold D.	526 Cooper St.	Camden, N. J. 08102
Barr, Richard N.	6100 Mart Way	Mission, Kans. 66202
Barranco, Anthony J.	116 Lincoln Rd.	Brooklyn, N. Y. 11225
Barrett, Charles V.	636 Church St.	Evanston, Ill. 60201
Barrett, Earl L.	1107 N. E. 45th St.	Seattle, Wash. 98105
Barron, Gerald J.	14935 Rinaldi St.	Mission Hills, Cal. 91344
Barron, Stewart S.	217 Mound St.	Nacogdoches, Tex. 75961

Barros, Paul R.	701 W. 55th Ave.	Gary, Ind. 46410
Barsam, Paul C.	279 Massachusetts Ave.	Arlington, Mass. 02174
Barsky, David	100 Oak St.	Wyandotte, Mich. 48192
Bartholomew, Henry H.	333 S. 9th E.	Salt Lake City, Utah 84102
Bartlett, Robert E.	1001 Gayley Ave.	Los Angeles, Cal. 90024
Bartley, Max D.	Hume Mansur Bldg.	Indianapolis, Ind. 46204
Barton, Arnold	21700 W. Soledad Canyon Rd.	Saugus, Cal. 91350
Barton, Stanley L.	50 West Gay St.	Columbus, O. 43215
Baruch, Richard	28055 Grosse Point Dr.	Sun City, Cal. 92381
Bassen, Edw. J.	70 E. 66th St.	New York, N. Y. 10021
Bastien, Henry L.	3801 N. Fairfax Dr.	Arlington, Va. 22203
Bates, Thomas R.	Naval Hospital	Orlando, Fla. 32813
Battles, Morris L.	363 E. Town St.	Columbus, O. 43215
Bauer, Thomas W.	550 W. Thomas Rd.	Phoenix, Ariz. 85013
Baum, Gilbert	333 King St.	Port Chester, N.Y. 10527
Baum, Jules L.	171 Harrison Ave.	Boston, Mass. 02111
Baum, Robert D.	940 Park Ave.	Lake Park, Fla. 33403
Baum, William W.	645 Medical Center Dr.	Salem, Ore. 97301
Bauman, Lucian	3553 16th St., N.W.	Washington, D. C. 20010
Baumgarten, O. Charles	4527 College Ave.	San Diego, Cal. 92115
Baumgartner, Wilbur W.	120 N. Chestnut St.	Kewanee, Ill. 61443
Bausch, Carl P.	85 Jefferson St.	Hartford, Conn. 06106
Bayadi, George El	Geisinger Medical Center	Danville, Pa. 17821
Bayard, Walter L.	230 C Pacolet	Tryon, N. C. 28782
Baylis, Henry I.	5353 Balboa	Encino, Cal. 91316
Beale, John P., Jr.	1801 Bush St.	San Francisco, Cal. 94109
Beall, John G.	1105 E. Front St.	Traverse City, Mich. 49684
Beallo, Allen	706 D St.	San Rafael, Cal. 94901
Beam, A. Duane	20160 Mack Ave.	Grosse Point, Mich. 48236
Beaman, Thomas C.	Coronado Bldg.	Santa Fe, N. M. 87501
Beams, Ralph H.	Medical Center Bldg.	Ft. Wayne, Ind. 46802
Beard, Crowell	240 Meridian Ave.	San Jose, Cal. 95126
Beard, Hallard	166 Crest Rd.	Glen Ellyn, Ill.
Beasley, C. Harold	1212 West Presidio	Ft. Worth, Tex. 76102
Beasley, Frank J.	915 Middle River Dr.	Ft. Lauderdale, Fla. 33304
Beasley, Jos. O., Jr.	131 Marlin Dr.	Spartanburg, S. C. 29302
Beattie, Canfield	1020 S. W. Taylor	Portland, Ore. 97205
Beauchaump, Joseph O.	835 4th Ave.	Naples, Fla. 33940
Beaudette, Robert P.	116½ S. 2nd St.	Raton, N. M. 87740
Bechert, Charles H.	2540 N. E. 9th St.	Ft. Lauderdale, Fla. 33304
Bechtel, Edward J.	351 Hospital Rd.	Newport Beach, Cal. 92660
Beck, Paul M.	620 Francis St.	St. Joseph, Mo. 64501
Beck, Peter	43 Austin St.	Portsmouth, N. H. 03801
Beck, William	125-10 Queens Blvd.	Kew Gardens, N. Y. 11415
Becker, Bernard	660 S. Euclid Ave.	St. Louis, Mo. 63110
Becker, Edward F.	Professional Bldg.	Wilmington, Dela. 19803
Becker, Jerome H.	Kaiser Richmond	Richmond, Cal.
Becker, Rolfe A.	601 E. 63rd St.	Kansas City, Mo. 64110
Becker, Sidney F.	174 Nemaha	Pomona, Cal. 91767
Becker, Stanley C.	3720 Washington Blvd.	St. Louis, Mo. 63108
Beckman, Hugh	20001 Greenfield	Detroit, Mich. 48235
Beckner, William M., Jr.	251 E. Baltimore St.	Hagerstown, Md. 21740
Bedell, Arthur J.	344 State St.	Albany, N. Y. 12210
Bedell, Rowland H. S.	5415 Cedar Ln.	Bethesda, Md. 20014
Bedrick, Morton	302 State St.	New London, Conn. 06320
Bedrossian, E. Howard	4501 State Rd.	Drexel Hill, Pa. 19026

Bedrossian, Paul B.	131 S. Ocean Ave.	Freeport, N. Y. 11520
Bedrossian, Robert H.	3200 Main St.	Vancouver, Wash. 98663
Bee, Rudolf W.	88 Goodwin St.	Bristol, Conn. 06010
Beehler, Cecil C.	1542 Carson St.	Fort Myers, Fla. 33901
Beeler, Robert V.	1950 Arlington St.	Sarasota, Fla. 33579
Beem, John W.	208 S. 6th Ave.	W. Reading, Pa. 19602
Beery, Edwin N.	96 Remsen St.	Brooklyn, N. Y. 11201
Beetham, William P.	108 Bay State Rd.	Boston, Mass. 02215
Behle, Charles F.	1060 E. 1st South	Salt Lake City, Utah 84102
Behrens, Herbert C.	6712 S. Friends Ave.	Whittier, Cal. 90601
Beideman, Joseph E.	17 E. Airy St.	Norristown, Pa. 19401
Beigelman, Maurice N.	327 S. Lorraine	Los Angeles, Cal. 90033
Beitel, Robert J., Jr.	1026 Hamilton St.	Allentown, Pa. 18101
Belau, Paul G.	Mayo Clinic	Rochester, Minn. 55901
Belcher, William T., Jr.	2754 N. Decatur Rd.	Decatur, Ga. 30030
Belevetz, David R.	7015 Keene Mill Rd.	Springfield, Va. 22150
Belknap, Wilford H.	1101 S. W. Main	Portland, Ore. 97205
Bell, Alan E.	1720 N. 'E' St.	Pensacola, Fla. 32501
Bell, Bernard T.	234 Beach Dr., N.E.	St. Petersburg, Fla. 33701
Bell, Dudley P.	411 30th St.	Oakland, Cal. 94609
Bell, Nelson C.	1708 N. Garey Ave.	Pomona, Cal. 91767
Bellamy, Earl D.	725 De Shong Dr.	Paris, Tex. 75460
Bellet, Jerome	505 Wanaque Ave.	Pompton Lakes, N. J. 07442
Bellows, John G.	30 N. Michigan Ave.	Chicago, Ill. 60602
Belmont, Owen	5723 Park Ave.	Philadelphia, Pa. 19141
Belmont, William S.	1880 Arlington	Sarasota, Fla. 33579
Belson, Michael J.	923 Eliza St.	Green Bay, Wisc. 54301
Belyeu, J. H.	1931 Boulevard	Jacksonville, Fla 32206
Bending, G. C.	2020 N. Waterman Ave.	San Bernardino, Cal. 92404
Benedict, Walter H.	Blount Prof. Bldg.	Knoxville, Tenn. 37920
Benjamin, Kenneth W.	1419 Spruce St.	Philadelphia, Pa. 19102
Benkwith, Karl B.	234 S. Hull St.	Montgomery, Ala. 36104
Bennett, Arthur L.	147 Linwood Ave.	Buffalo, N. Y. 14209
Bennett, B. Kent	Univ. Med. Center	Ann Arbor, Mich. 48104
Bennett, Edwin H.	130 Lincoln St.	Worcester, Mass. 01605
Bennett, James E.	5500 Ridge Rd.	Cleveland, O. 44129
Bennett, Nicholas G.	1544 'B' St.	Hayward, Cal. 94541
Bennett, Wayne E.	2001 4th Ave.	San Diego, Cal. 92101
Bennett, William H.	524 Main St.	Racine, Wisc. 53403
Benson, Clifton E.	Sheridan Village	Bremerton, Wash. 98310
Benson, Paul J.	2355 Fort St.	Lincoln Park, Mich. 48146
Bentley, Maxwell D.	828 Oak St.	Cadillac, Mich. 49601
Benton, Curtis D., Jr.	1800 E. Las Olas Blvd.	Ft. Lauderdale, Fla. 33301
Benz, Carl A.	308 N. Broad St.	Adrian, Mich. 49221
Berbos, James N.	1321 North Harbor Blvd.	Fullerton, Cal. 92632
Beresky, Tibor A.	100 Casa St.	San Luis Obispo, Cal. 93401
Berg, Edward F.	8064 Watkins Dr.	Clayton, Mo. 63105
Berg, Herman B.	107-21 Queens Blvd.	Forest Hills, N. Y. 11375
Berg, John A.	1810 Professional Dr.	Sacramento, Cal. 95825
Berg, Joseph L.	121 Oglethorpe Ave.	Albany, Ga. 31702
Berg, Leonard	711 Delaware Ave.	Ft. Pierce, Fla. 33450
Bergam, Miroslav	7002 7th Ave.	Brooklyn, New York, N. Y.
Berge, Richard E.	4717 Engle Rd.	Carmichael, Cal. 95608
Berger, Allan M.	2375 E. Main St.	Columbus, O. 43209
Berger, Harold J.	1680 Meridian Ave.	Miami Beach, Fla. 33139
Berger, John V., Jr.	1025 Regent St.	Madison, Wisc. 53715

Berger, Leonard H.	1101 N. Calvert St.	Baltimore, Md. 21202
Berger, Louis	950 W. Peachtree St., N.W.	Atlanta, Ga. 30309
Bergman, Gary D.	26615 Greenfield	Southfield, Mich. 48075
Bergmann, Milton B.	33 Melbury Rd.	Babylon, N. Y. 11702
Bergmann, Robert B.	595 Hicksville Rd.	Massapequa, N. Y. 11758
Berk, Myles M.	9102 Babcock Blvd.	Pittsburgh, Pa. 15237
Berke, Raynold N.	Stanford University Medical Center	Palo Alto, Cal. 94305
Berkeley, Ralph G.	Hermann Prof. Bldg.	Houston, Tex. 77025
Berkley, William L.	411-414 Allied Arts Bldg.	Lynchburg, Va.
Berkman, Ronald	3520 Fifth Ave.	Pittsburg. Pa. 15213
Berkow, Joseph W.	4419 Falls Rd.	Baltimore, Md. 21211
Berler, David K.	2141 K St., N. W.	Washington, D. C. 20037
Berlin, Allison J., Jr.	5500 Ridge Road	Cleveland, O. 44129
Berliner, Milton L.	57 W. 57th St.	New York, N. Y. 10019
Berman, Gerald	Medical Towers Bldg.	Louisville, Ky. 40202
Berman, Martin B.	29925 W. Six Mile Rd.	Livonia, Mich. 48152
Bernard, Henri S.	414 David Whitney Bldg.	Detroit, Mich. 48221
Bernasconi, Ezio J.	726 Broad St.	Providence, R. I. 02907
Berner, Richard A.	1515 State St.	Santa Barbara, Cal. 93104
Berney, Irving V.	31 Lincoln Park	Newark, N. J. 07102
Bernfield, Michael	1601 N. Tucson Blvd.	Tucson, Ariz. 85716
Bernie, David L.	655 Salem Ave.	Dayton, O. 45406
Bernstein, Ellen H.	525 Irvington Ave.	Elizabeth, N. J. 07208
Bernstein, Howard N.	10401 Old Georgetown Rd.	Bethesda, Md. 20014
Bernstein, Louis	11600 Wilshire Blvd.	Los Angeles, Cal. 90025
Bernstein, Martin	344 Main St.	Mount Kisco, N. Y. 10549
Berrocal, Jose A.	303 De Diego Ave.	Santurce, P. R. 00909
Berry, Erwin A.	223 E. Charles	Oelwein, Ia. 50662
Berry, F. Dean	1045 'S' St.	Fresno, Cal. 93721
Berry, Frank D.	762 Altos Oaks Dr.	Los Altos, Cal. 94022
Berry, Jack J.	2010 E. 102nd St.	Cleveland, O. 44106
Berry, Juanedd	1901 Oak Park Blvd.	Lake Charles, La. 70601
Berson, Eliot L.	243 Charles St.	Boston, Mass. 02114
Berson, Paul	16 Murray Ave.	Annapolis, Md. 21401
Bertolucci, Frank A.	3691 E. Shields Ave.	Fresno, Cal. 93726
Bertrand, George J.	73 Main St.	Montpelier, Vt. 05601
Bertuglia, Sebastian	1668 Putnam Ave.	Brooklyn, N. Y. 11227
Best, Milton	1249 Fifth Ave.	New York, N. Y. 10029
Bethel, Robert D.	2767 Olive Hwy.	Oroville, Cal. 95965
Bettman, Jerome W.	3910 Sand Hill Rd.	Woodside, Cal. 94062
Bettman, Jerome W. Jr. ...	1112 Burke Dr.	Gallup, N. M. 87301
Betz, Richard N.	37 N. Brevard Ave.	Cocoa Beach, Fla. 32931
Beucler, Wade F.	600 Coffee Rd.	Modesto, Cal. 95350
Beuerman, Virgil A.	2600 Greenbush	Lafayette, Ind. 47905
Beyer, Charles K.	1493 Cambridge St.	Cambridge, Mass. 02139
Beyrer, Charles R.	375 E. Main St.	Bay Shore, N. Y. 11706
Bialik, Michael H.	14853 Michigan	Dearborn, Mich. 48127
Bick, Malcolm W.	33 Mulberry St.	Springfield, Mass. 01105
Bickerton, John H.	1030 Pearl St.	La Jolla, Cal. 92037
Biegel, Albert C.	3909 12th St.	Riverside, Cal. 92501
Bierman, Edward O.	1212 7th St.	Santa Monica, Cal. 90401
Biggs, Robert D.	670 W. Market	Lima, O. 45801
Biklé, Charles E.	9 Elizabeth St.	Auburn, N. Y. 13021
Bilello, James A.	21 Jefferson St.	Brooklyn, N. Y. 11206
Billet, Edwin	3200 Grand Concourse	Bronx, N. Y. 10458

Billig, Stuart L.	213 Madison Ave.	New York, N. Y. 10016
Billings, Robert J.	Jenkins Arcade	Pittsburgh, Pa. 15222
Billingsley, C. B.	400 Fairview	Ponca City, Okla. 74601
Billingsley, John A.	1225 N. 78th St.	Kansas City, Kans. 66112
Binder, Donald K.	1706 Eastern Pkwy.	Schenectady, N. Y. 12309
Binder, Hertha F.	12793 Taylor-Wells Rd.	Chardon, O. 44024
Binder, Rudolf F.	4568 Mayfield Rd.	S. Euclid, O. 44121
Binion, Warren W.	1401 Ballinger St.	Fort Worth, Tex.
Binkhorst, Richard D.	125 E. 74th St.	New York, N. Y. 10021
Birge, Henry L.	664 Farmington Ave.	Hartford, Conn. 06105
Bishop, David W.	1715 Forest Ave.	Durango, Colo. 81301
Bishop, John W.	630 12th Ave. E.	Eugene, Ore. 97401
Bishop, Stanley E.	284 N. Riverside Ave.	Rialto, Cal. 92376
Bisno, Daniel	8000 Bonhomme	St. Louis, Mo. 63105
Biswell, Roderick	220 Meridian Ave.	San Jose, Cal. 95126
Bitner, Daniel G.	625 Broadway	San Diego, Cal. 92101
Bivins, Thomas E.	600 Central Ave.	Great Falls, Mont. 59401
Bixler, Donald P.	1931 Brown St.	Anderson, Ind. 46014
Bizzell, James W.	Borden Bldg.	Goldsboro, N. C. 27530
Black, Chester J.	172 Schiller	Elmhurst, Ill. 60126
Black, Robert C.	1900 Mowry Ave.	Fremont, Cal. 94538
Black, Vernon A.	2100 N. Fulton	Wharton, Tex. 77488
Blackhurst, Robert T.	233 E. Larkin St.	Midland, Mich. 48640
Blackmon, L. W.	1516 Gregg St.	Columbia, S. C. 29201
Blaine, Richard M.	5330 W. Devon Ave.	Chicago, Ill. 60646
Blair, Charles J.	Medical Arts Bldg.	Richmond, Va. 23218
Blair, Edwin	1050 W. Pacific Coast Hwy.	Harbor City, Cal. 90710
Blair, Frank W.	369 Green Lane	Philadelphia, Pa. 19128
Blais, Bernard R.	Box 76, Naval Hospital	San Diego, Cal. 92134
Blak, Paul S.	909 Hyde St.	San Francisco, Cal. 94109
Blalock, Raymond B.	1400 13th St.	Huntsville, Tex. 77340
Bland, Robert P., Jr.	21 E. Calhoun St.	Sumter, S. C. 29150
Blankstein, Samuel S.	2040 W. Wisconsin Ave.	Milwaukee, Wisc. 53233
Blanton, Frederick M.	4701 N. Federal Hwy.	Ft. Lauderdale, Fla. 33308
Blau, Robert I.	17822 Beach Blvd.	Huntington Beach, Cal. 92646
Blaydes, James E.	107 Federal St.	Bluefield, W. Va. 24701
Blaydes, J. Elliott, Jr.	107 Federal St.	Bluefield, W. Va. 24701
Blazar, Howard A.	1101 Beacon St.	Brookline, Mass. 02146
Blender, William	300 E. War Mem'l Dr.	Peoria, Ill. 61614
Bloch, Charles L.	Medical Towers	Louisville, Ky. 40202
Bloch, Fritz J.	155 Crary Ave.	Mount Vernon, N. Y. 10550
Bloch, Malcolm H.	8 Shunpike Rd.	Madison, N. J. 07940
Blocker, Donald R.	1415 18th St.	Lake Charles, La. 70601
Blodget, Rush M., Jr.	1950 Court St.	Redding, Cal. 96001
Blodi, Frederick C.	University Hosp.	Iowa City, Ia. 52240
Blondis, Robert R.	11811 Shaker Blvd.	Cleveland, O. 44120
Bloom, Henry R.	546 Shirley St.	Winthrop, Mass. 02152
Bloomberg, Louis	Home Savings & Loan Bldg.	Youngstown, O. 44503
Bloomenthal, John	233 A St.	San Diego, Cal. 92101
Bloomenthal, S. R.	100 N. State College Blvd.	Fullerton, Cal. 92631
Bloomfield, Sylvan	1010 Fifth Ave.	New York, N. Y. 10028
Bloomgarden, Charles I.	181 Main St.	Huntington, N. Y. 11743
Blouin, Alfred R.	144 Central St.	Gardner, Mass. 01440
Blount, Richard L.	440 E. Woodrow Wilson Ave.	Jackson, Miss. 39216
Blum, Fred G., Jr.	20 S. Park St.	Madison, Wisc. 53715

Blum, Jerome V.	885 Scott Blvd.	Santa Clara, Cal. 95050
Blum, M. Barry	The Quadrangle	Baltimore, Md. 21210
Blumberg, Elliott J.	1116 W. Randol Mill Rd.	Arlington, Tex. 76010
Blumenthal, Gerald	181 Main St.	Huntington, N. Y. 11743
Bocci, Jerrold C.	2325 Ocean Ave.	San Francisco, Cal. 94010
Bocian, Franklin L.	650 Main St.	New Rochelle, N. Y. 10801
Bock, Rudolf H.	850 Middlefield Rd.	Palo Alto, Cal. 94301
Bockoven, John B.	Third National Bldg.	Dayton, O. 45402
Bockoven, Sterling	1525 18th St. N. W.	Washington, D. C. 20036
Bodian, Martin	135 Eastern Pkwy.	Brooklyn, N. Y. 11238
Boehlke, Russell R.	1017 Robertson St.	Fort Collins, Colo. 80521
Boland, Stanley W.	303 Medical Arts Building	Scranton, Pa. 18503
Boldizar, Albert G.	3720 Washington Blvd.	St. Louis, Mo. 63108
Boldt, Henry A.	31526 N. California	Peoria, Ill. 61603
Boles, Donald J.	55 E. Washington St.	Chicago, Ill. 60602
Boles, James H.	Center & Cherokee	Kingsport, Tenn. 37662
Boles, Wm. McD.	1206 Pere Marquette Bldg.	New Orleans, La. 70112
Bolger, James V., Jr.	102 E. Main St.	Waukesha, Wisc. 53186
Boling, Richard C.	1332 W. Indiana Ave.	Elkhart, Ind. 46514
Bolheimer, Donald A.	623 Medical Center Bldg.	Ft. Wayne, Ind. 46802
Bolman, Harold R.	6½ S. Main St.	Monroeville, O. 44847
Bonaccolto, Girolamo	123 E. 61st St.	New York, N. Y. 10021
Bonadia, Calogero	1822 70th St.	Brooklyn, N. Y. 11204
Bonatti, William D.	800 Pine Dr.	New Kensington, Pa. 15068
Bond, Floyd M.	625 Broadway	San Diego, Cal. 92101
Bond, John B.	214 Medical Arts Bldg.	Nashville, Tenn. 37212
Bond, John W. L.	120 E. Birch	Walla Walla, Wash. 99362
Bond, Sidney D., Jr.	USN, Bur. of Med. & Surg.	Pensacola, Fla. 32508
Boniuk, Isaac	4989 Barnes Hospital Plaza	St. Louis, Mo. 63110
Boniuk, Milton	1200 Moursund Ave.	Houston, Tex. 77025
Bonner, John L.	524 3rd Ave. N.W.	Grand Rapids, Mich. 55744
Bonner, William R.	3 W. White St.	Summit Hill, Pa. 18250
Bonser, William H.	219 15th St.	Toledo, O. 43624
Bontley, Jack R.	21 E. State St.	Columbus, O. 43215
Boomer, Robert B.	850 Middlefield Rd.	Palo Alto, Cal. 94301
Booth, Edgar W.	1513 Line Ave.	Shreveport, La. 71101
Booth, Geo R.	Highland Ave. & Gateway Blvd.	Westville, N. J. 08093
Booth, Lee N.	1138 Elm St.	Manchester, N. H. 03101
Boozan, Charles W.	33 De Witt Rd.	Elizabeth, N. J. 07208
Bores, Leo D.	974 Fisher Bldg.	Detroit, Mich. 48202
Borger, Jules H.	Hermann Prof. Bldg.	Houston, Tex. 77025
Born, John H.	115 E. 61st St.	New York, N. Y. 10021
Boruchoff, S. Arthur	192 Bay State Rd.	Boston, Mass. 02215
Bosilevac, Fred N.	155 S. 18th St.	Kansas City, Kans. 66102
Boss, Eugene G.	336 Long Hill St.	Springfield, Mass. 01108
Bostwick, James E.	1479 Ygnacio Valley Rd.	Walnut Creek, Cal. 94598
Bosworth, Wesley F.	11858 Rosecrans	Norwalk, Cal. 90650
Botsford, Daniel R.	3240 Main St.	Buffalo, N. Y. 14214
Bounds, George W., Jr.	1211 21st Ave. S.	Nashville, Tenn. 37212
Bourne, Malcolm G.	Hotel Jamestown Bldg.	Jamestown, N. Y. 14701
Bousquet, Franklyn P., Jr.	701 Abercorn St.	Savannah, Ga. 31402
Bouvier, Marianne	1501 Locust St.	Pittsburgh, Pa. 15219
Bovenmyer, Samuel D.	638 Black Bldg.	Waterloo, Ia. 50703
Bowen, Jesse W., Jr.	Medical Arts Bldg.	Tacoma, Wash. 98402
Bowen, Stephen F., Jr.	16 Hampton Village	St. Louis, Mo. 63109
Bowers, Bruce T.	12614 La Noche	San Antonio, Tex. 78233

Bowers, Jack F.	359 Main St.	Haverhill, Mass. 01830
Bowlds, Joseph H.	Naval Hospital Boston	Chelsea, Mass. 02150
Bowman, John H.	601 N. Duke St.	Lancaster, Pa. 17602
Boyce, David C.	515 Lakeside Dr., S.E.	Grand Rapids, Mich. 49506
Boyd, Charles G.	1410 E. Broward Blvd.	Ft. Lauderdale, Fla. 33301
Boyd, Charles W.	111 W. Adams St.	Jacksonville, Fla. 32202
Boyd, Herschell H.	1051 116th N.E.	Bellevue, Wash. 98004
Boyd, James L.	8 Medical Plaza	Glen Cove, N. Y. 11542
Boyden, Blaine S.	4141 Geary Blvd.	San Francisco, Cal. 94118
Boyden, Douglas G.	Naval Hospital	San Diego, Cal. 92134
Boylan, Charles E.	1601 16th Ave.	Seattle, Wash. 98122
Boyle, Samuel F.	33 Winship Ave.	San Anselmo, Cal. 94960
Brachman, Edwin F.	100 N. State College Blvd.	Fullerton, Cal. 92631
Bracken, Franklin	140 Arlington Ave.	Brooklyn, N. Y. 11207
Brackup, Alvin H.	30-74 36th St.	Long Island City, N. Y. 11133
Braconier, Harry E.	1180 Beacon St.	Brookline, Mass. 02146
Bradbrook, Charles	2615 Eye St.	Sacramento, Cal. 95816
Bradford, John F.	4320 Wornall	Kansas City, Mo. 64111
Bradford, Ray T.	2328 Auburn Ave.	Cincinnati, O. 45219
Bradish, Robert F.	1712 Raeford Rd.	Fayetteville, N. C. 28305
Bradley, Arvid J.	Setauket Med. Ctr.	E. Setauket, L. I., N. Y. 11733
Bradley, Francis J.	1503 St. Georges Ave.	Colonia, N. J. 07067
Brady, Harry R.	Northland Medical Bldg.	St. Louis, Mo. 63136
Braley, Alson E.	227 N. Dubuque St.	Iowa City, Ia. 52240
Brandon, Sylvan	Medical Arts Bldg.	Houston, Tex. 77002
Brandt, John P.	316 N. Grove St.	Lock Haven, Pa. 17745
Brandwan, Samuel R.	Rose Bldg.	Cleveland, O. 44115
Branigan, C. Hugh	17 Kraft Ave.	Bronxville, N. Y. 10708
Brannin, Dan	Medical Arts Bldg.	Dallas, Tex. 75201
Brannon, Daniel R.	108 Thisted Center	Great Falls, Mont. 59401
Branower, Gerald M.	36 Barstow Rd.	Great Neck, N. Y. 11021
Brant, Carl E.	121 N. Main St.	Greensburg, Pa. 15601
Brasseur, Eugene V. H.	Paulsen Med. & Dental Bldg.	Spokane, Wash. 99201
Brasuk, Virginia M.	633 Washington Rd.	Pittsburgh, Pa. 15228
Braufman, Harvey S.	111 Church St.	St. Louis, Mo. 63135
Braum, F. Gene	Westcliff Professional Bldg.	Dallas, Tex. 75224
Braun, William	406 Cooper St.	Camden, N. J. 08102
Braunstein, Edgar G.	1009 79th St.	N. Bergen, N. J. 07047
Braunstein, Richard B.	1785 San Carlos Ave.	San Carlos, Cal. 94070
Brauston, Bruce B.	10 Beech St.	Berea, O. 44017
Brav, Solomon S.	5575 N. Park Ave.	Philadelphia, Pa. 19141
Braveman, Bernard L.	515 Sinclair St.	McKeesport, Pa. 15132
Braver, David A.	7 Church Ln.	Baltimore, Md. 21208
Braverman, Sheldon P.	224 W. Evergreen	San Antonio, Tex. 78212
Breakey, Arnold S.	718 Park Ave.	New York, N. Y. 10021
Breakstone, Gerald J.	12840 Riverside Dr.	N. Hollywood, Cal. 91607
Breed, Frederic B.	15 Florence St.	Danvers, Mass. 01923
Breffeilh, Louis A.	2515 Line	Shreveport, La. 71104
Breger, Barbara C.	86-15 Queens Blvd.	Elmhurst, N. Y. 11373
Breinin, Goodwin M.	550 First Ave.	New York, N. Y. 10016
Brennan, James W.	549 Linwood Ave.	Buffalo, N. Y. 14209
Breslin, Harvey J.	36 Barstow Rd.	Great Neck, N. Y. 11021
Bresnick, George H.	812 Pine St.	Philadelphia, Pa. 19107
Brewer, A. L.	400 N. 17th St.	Birmingham, Ala. 35203

Brewer, Malcolm I	11711 N. E. Glisan	Portland, Ore. 97220
Brewer, Ray L.	8830 Long Point Rd.	Houston, Tex. 77055
Brewer, Schiele Alcuin	452 Main St.	Oneida, N. Y. 13421
Brewster, William B., Jr.	85 Jefferson St.	Hartford, Conn. 06106
Bribach, Eugene J.	121½ N. 5th.	Atchison, Kans. 66002
Bricca, Constantine R., Jr.	909 Hyde St.	San Francisco, Cal. 94109
Bridges, William Z.	451 Park Ave. N.	Winter Park, Fla. 32789
Briggs, Henry H.	309 Doctor's Bldg.	Asheville, N. C. 28801
Brikates, Peter	140 E. 54th St.	New York, N. Y. 10022
Brinckerhoff, Albert J.	1615 Hill Rd.	Novato, Cal. 94947
Brindley, B. I.	304 W. Washington Ave.	Madison, Wisc. 53703
Brinker, William R.	250 S. Chestnut	Ravenna, O. 44266
Brinton, Sherman S.	508, E. South Temple St.	Salt Lake City, Utah 84102
Bristow, Jack H.	3838 Jackson	Riverside, Cal. 92503
Bristow, Walter J.	203 S. Waccaman Ave.	Columbia, S. C. 29205
Brobeck, Von H.	106 E. St. Vrain	Colorado Springs, Colo. 80902
Broccoli, Anthony C.	1524 Atwood Ave.	Johnston, R. I. 02919
Brock, Charles L.	625 N. Grandview Ave.	Daytona Beach, Fla. 32018
Brockhurst, Robert J.	100 Charles River Plaza	Boston, Mass. 02114
Brodersen, James D.	7905 Calumet Ave.	Munster, Ind. 46321
Brodstein, Robert S.	3955 Harrison Blvd.	Ogden, Utah 84403
Brody, Michael	228 Livingston Ave.	New Brunswick, N. J. 08902
Brody, Yale	127 E. Acacia St.	Stockton, Cal.
Broggi, Richard J.	33 Lancaster St.	Worcester, Mass. 01608
Broman, Charles R.	702 Ninth St. N.	Texas City, Tex. 77590
Bronk, Henry N.	Jenkins Arcade Bldg.	Pittsburgh, Pa. 15222
Bronson, Nathaniel R. II	186 Old Town Rd.	Southampton, N. Y. 11968
Bronstein, Melvin	27 Ludlow St.	Yonkers, N. Y. 10705
Brooks, Earl B.	2323 S. 22nd St.	Lincoln, Nebr. 68502
Brooks, Norman F.	Bank of America Bldg.	San Diego, Cal. 92101
Brooks, Roosevelt	200 E. 75 th St.	Chicago, Ill. 60619
Brosnan, D. Wm., III	417 Biltmore Ave.	Asheville, N C. 28801
Broussard, Wm. J.	1341 S. Hickory St.	Melbourne, Fla. 32901
Brown, Andrew G.	DuPont Bldg.	Miami, Fla. 33131
Brown, Christopher J.	393 N. Dunlap St.	St. Paul. Minn. 55104
Brown, Delatus E.	Fidelity Medical Bldg.	Dayton, O. 45402
Brown, D. V. L.	122 S. Michigan Ave.	Chicago, Ill. 60603
Brown, Dwight H.	17000 W. North Ave.	Brookfield, Wisc. 53005
Brown, Frank J.	116½ N. Bridge St.	Chippewa Falls, Wisc. 54729
Brown, George	125 S. College Ave.	Ft. Collins, Colo. 80521
Brown, H. Zane	520 N. Duke St.	Lancaster, Pa. 17602
Brown, Harold E.	333 E. State St.	Columbus, O. 43215
Brown, Harold W.	15 Park Ave.	New York, N. Y. 10016
Brown, Harry F.	612 W. Duarte Rd.	Arcadia, Cal. 92660
Brown, Howard D. H.	525 E. 68th St.	New York, N. Y. 10019
Brown, James P.	Lowry Medical Arts Bldg.	St. Paul, Minn. 55113
Brown, James W.	110 E. Diamond St.	Butler, Pa. 16001
Brown, Oscar A.	David Whitney Bldg.	Detroit, Mich. 48226
Brown, Paul R.	2243 McGregor Blvd.	Ft. Myers, Fla. 33901
Brown, Richard E.	347 S. Ripley St.	Montgomery, Ala. 36104
Brown, Robert A., Jr.	10 Summer St.	Greenville, S. C. 29601
Brown, Russell N.	1126 S. Main St.	Dayton, Ohio 45409
Brown, Stuart I.	525 E. 68th St.	New York, N. Y. 10021
Brown, William C.	3260 Beard Rd.	Napa, Cal. 94558
Brown, William C.	651 W. State St.	Trenton, N. J. 08608

Brown, Wootten	210 Medical Park Tower	Austin, Tex. 78705
Brownell, Robert D.	1750 El Camino Real	Burlingame, Cal. 94010
Browning, Carroll W.	836 N. Zang Blvd. at Sixth St. ..	Dallas, Tex. 75208
Browning, Charles W.	1010 Duane St.	Astoria, Ore. 97103
Brownsberger, Sidney B. ...	1530 E. Chevy Chase Dr.	Glendale, Cal. 91206
Brubaker, Richard F.	The Mayo Clinic	Rochester, Minn. 55901
Bruce, Charles O., Jr.	121 S. Sherrin Ave.	Louisville, Ky. 40207
Bruce, Robert A.	1126 S. Main St.	Dayton, O. 45409
Bruce, Robert G.	9777 Ferguson Rd.	Dallas, Tex. 75228
Bruechert, Robert W.	Oregon City Eye Clinic, 421 High St.	Oregon City, Oregon 97045
Brugge, E. Homer	426 17th St.	Oakland, Cal. 94612
Brugman, R. Barry	1019 Madison Medical Bldg.	Seattle, Wash. 98104
Bruhl, Martin G.	300 Central Medical Bldg.	St. Paul, Minn. 55104
Brumback, George F.	348 N. Elm St.	Greensboro, N. C. 27401
Brumback, Joseph E., Jr. ..	Medical Arts Bldg.	Baltimore, Md. 21201
Brumbaugh, John D.	75 N. Wheaton Rd.	Akron, O. 44313
Brumm, Lewis P.	2328 Auburn Ave.	Cincinnati, O. 45219
Brunemeier, Faylon M.	1950 Court St.	Redding, Cal. 96001
Bruner, Blackwell S.	9509 Milstead Dr.	Bethesda, Md. 20034
Bruner, Claude R.	Professional Bldg.	Columbia, Mo. 65201
Brunner, G. Harmon	Medical Professional Bldg.	San Antonio, Tex. 78205
Bruno, Mary G.	737 Front St.	Hempstead, N. Y. 11550
Brunton, Robert I.	410 W. 5th Ave.	Olympia, Wash. 98501
Brusegard, James F.	1121 East Ave.	Red Wing, Minn. 55066
Bryan, Bert C.	8210 Walnut Hill Ln.	Dallas, Tex. 75201
Bryan, James H.	950 Francis Pl.	Clayton, Mo. 63105
Bryant, Frederick W.	3535 W. 13 Mile	Royal Oak, Mich. 48072
Bryant, Winston M., Jr.	5900 Spruce St.	Philadelphia, Pa. 19139
Bryant, W. R.	7275 E. Southgate Dr.	Sacramento, Cal. 95823
Bryce, William F.	116 E. Franklin St.	Richmond, Va. 23219
Bryson, J. Gordon	3166 Reid Dr.	Corpus Christi, Tex. 78404
Bryson, Jerry M.	Daniel Boone Clinic	Harlan, Ky. 40831
Buchanan, William S.	216 N. Third St.	Sterling, Colo. 80751
Buck, Robert H.	602 Babcock Rd.	San Antonio, Tex. 78201
Buckhaults, Wendell W. ...	905 Abercorn St.	Savannah, Ga. 31401
Buckley, Eugene T.	520 Franklin Ave.	Garden City, L. I., N. Y. 11530
Buckman, Lewis T.	26 W. River St.	Wilkes-Barre, Pa. 18702
Buckman, Samuel T.	70 S. Franklin St.	Wilkes-Barre, Pa. 18701
Buesseler, John A.	Texas Tech U. School of Med. ..	Lubbock, Tex. 79409
Buhrman, Charles M.	1126 S. Main St.	Dayton, O. 45409
Buka, Theodore E.	3024 Burnet Ave.	Cincinnati, O. 45219
Bullington, S. J.	56 Baribeau Dr.	Brunswick, Me. 04011
Bullington, Walter G.	Doctor's Bldg.	Charlotte, N. C. 28207
Bullis, John A. E.	400 Newport Center Dr. E.	Newport Beach, Cal. 92660
Bullwinkel, George A. Jr. ..	70 Mill River St.	Stamford, Conn. 06902
Bullwinkel, H. G.	86 State Circle	Annapolis, Md. 21401
Bunting, Richard F.	3500 Kensington Ave.	Richmond, Va. 23221
Bunyor, Agnes K.	Physicians Bldg., Warm Springs Ave.	Huntington, Pa. 16652
Burch, G. William	908 Hospital Dr.	Tyler, Tex. 75701
Burch, Peter G.	477 S. Broad St.	Meriden, Conn. 06450
Burde, Ronald M.	517 S. Euclid	St. Louis, Mo. 63110
Burden, Alfred L., Jr.	Nix Professional Bldg.	San Antonio, Tex. 78205
Burell, Vincent A.	256 Roseberry St.	Phillipsburg, N. J. 08865

Burgess, Roy E.	555 W. Catalina Dr.	Phoenix, Ariz. 85013
Burhans, John B.	515 Lakeside Dr., S.E.	Grand Rapids, Mich. 49506
Burian, Hermann M.	University Hospitals	Iowa City, Ia. 52240
Burke, Daniel W.	Brown Bldg.	Louisville, Ky. 40202
Burke, Jordan D.	120 Summit Ave.	Summit, N. J. 07901
Burman, Daniel	1938 Grand Concourse	New York, N. Y. 10457
Burnes, James E.	928 Gallatin Rd.	Madison, Tenn. 37115
Burnett, Arthur B.	312 Burr Bldg.	New Castle, Ind. 47362
Burnett, Edmund L.	3838 Hillcroft	Houston, Tex. 77027
Burnham, Charles J.	1529 N. 25th St.	Birmingham, Ala. 35234
Burns, C. L., Jr.	133 W. Boscawen St.	Winchester, Va. 22601
Burns, Charlotte Ann	University Hospital	Iowa City, Ia. 52240
Burns, Donald T.	1500 Penn Ave.	Wyomissing, Pa. 19610
Burns, John A.	303 E. Town St.	Columbus, O. 43215
Burns, Lucille R.	210 E. 63rd St.	New York, N. Y. 10021
Burns, Robert P.	3181 S. W. Sam Jackson Park Rd.	Portland, Ore. 97201
Burns, Thomas A.	4212 N. E. Broadway	Portland, Ore, 97213
Burns, William P.	3400 Spruce St.	Philadelphia, Pa. 19104
Burnside, R. M.	4105 Live Oak	Dallas, Texas 75221
Burr, Sherwood P.	490 N. Alvernon Way	Tucson, Ariz. 85711
Burris, James E.	170 Maple Ave.	White Plains, N. Y. 10601
Burroughs, Ralph B.	406 Fulton St.	Troy, N. Y. 12180
Burroughs, Roswell G.	David Whitney Bldg.	Detroit, Mich. 48226
Burrows, Herbert L.	8215 Van Nuys Blvd.	Panorama City, Cal. 91402
Burstein, Frank	355 Meisel Ave.	Springfield, N. J. 07081
Burton, Edwin W.	1400 Jefferson Park Ave.	Charlottesville, Va. 22903
Burton. Jack S.	172 Schiller St.	Elmhurst, Ill. 60126
Burton, Thomas C.	Dept. of Ophthalmology, University Hospitals	Iowa City, Iowa 52240
Bushard, Wilfred J.	4550 51st Ave. N.	Phoenix, Ariz. 85015
Bushnell, Theodore L.	3700 East-West Hwy.	Hyattsville, Md. 20782
Bussey, Frank R.	375 E. Main	Bay Shore, N. Y. 11706
Bussey, Joe L.	1201 W. Presidio	Ft. Worth, Tex. 76102
Buten, Robert E.	1001 York St.	Newport, Ky. 41071
Butler, Frederick C., Jr.	Murchison Bldg.	Wilmington, N. C. 28401
Butler, James E.	2177 W. Grand Blvd.	Detroit, Mich. 48208
Butler, Jay B. V.	919 S. W. Taylor St.	Portland, Ore. 97205
Butler, Richard G.	1922 Monroe	Dearborn, Mich. 48124
Butler, William E.	1221 N. 26th St.	Billings, Mont. 59102
Button, Richard R.	1901 Westcliff	Newport Beach, Cal. 92660
Butz, Robert C.	V. A. Hosp.	Northport, N. Y. 11768
Buxeda, Fernando L.	1302 Ponce de Leon Ave.	Santurce, P. R. 00908
Buxeda, Roberto	Ashford Medical Center	San Juan, P. R. 00907
Buxton, Jorge N.	648 Park Ave.	New York, N. Y. 10021
Buys, Norman S.	877 W. Fremont Ave.	Sunnyvale, Cal. 94087
Buzzard, Josiah F.	1110 13th Ave.	Altoona, Pa. 16601
Byer, Norman E.	3400 W. Lomita Blvd.	Torrance, Cal. 90505
Byerly, Baxter H.	108 Holbrook St.	Danville, Va. 24541
Byers, Barton	246 Saratoga Ave.	Los Gatos, Cal. 95030
Byers, Jerome L.	1114 N. Bishop	Dallas, Tex. 75208
Byland, Samuel S.	1808 San Miguel Dr.	Walnut Creek, Cal. 94596
Byrne, Harry V.	301 Essex St.	Lawrence, Mass. 01840
Byrnes, Victor A.	234 Beach Dr. N. E.	St. Petersburg, Fla. 33701
Byron, Herve M.	220 Engle St.	Englewood, N. J. 07631
Caballero, Mariano C.	25 S. E. 2nd Ave.	Miami, Fla. 33131
Cabitt, Henry L.	60 Charlesgate W.	Boston, Mass. 02215

Caccamise, William C.	233 Alexander St.	Rochester, N. Y. 14607
Cacioppo, Leonard R.	7704 Fourth Ave.	Brooklyn, N. Y. 11209
Cadan, Henry	308 N. Osceola	Okeechobee, Fla. 33472
Cady, Frederick J., Jr.	402 S. Jefferson	Saginaw, Mich. 48607
Cahill, James F.	600 E. Genesee St.	Syracuse, N. Y. 13202
Cahill, John E.	196 Main St.	Brockton, Mass. 02401
Cahill, William F.	135 S. Kenilworth	Elmhurst, Ill. 60126
Cahn, Peter H.	Hume Mansur Bldg.	Indianapolis, Ind. 46204
Caldemeyer, Everett S.	1515 Chain Bridge Rd.	McLean, Va. 22101
Caldwell, Pearson C.	3155 Stagg Dr.	Beaumont, Tex. 7701
Caldwell, William T.	31 Leroy Pl.	Red Bank, N. I. 07701
Calenda, Alexander M.	171 Broadway	Providence, R. I. 02903
Calhoun, F. Phinizy, Jr.	1365 Clifton Rd., N.E.	Atlanta, Ga. 30322
Calkins, James P.	490 N. Alvernon	Tucson, Ariz. 85711
Calkins, Larry L.	7301 Mission Rd.	Prairie Village, Kans. 66208
Callahan, Alston	903 S. 21st St.	Birmingham, Ala. 35205
Callis, Charles M.	550 N. Bumby Ave.	Orlando, Fla. 32803
Calnan, Arthur F.	605 Commonwealth Ave.	Boston, Mass. 02215
Calvert, Raymond R.	314 N. 6th St.	Lafayette, Ind. 47901
Calvy, William J.	801 N. Harbor Blvd.	Anaheim, Cal. 92805
Cameron, Ronald B.	21350 Hawthorne Blvd.	Torrance, Cal. 90503
Cammisa, James J. V.	53 Bay State Rd.	Boston, Mass. 02115
Campbell, Allen D., Jr.	1202 N. Beckley	Dallas, Tex. 75203
Campbell, Bernard E.	1861 Wadsworth Blvd.	Lakewood, Colo. 80215
Campbell, Charles J.	635 W. 165th St.	New York, N. Y. 10032
Campbell, E. Malcolm	207 E. Watauga Ave.	Johnson City, Tenn. 37601
Campbell, Francis P.	140 E. 54th St.	New York, N. Y. 10022
Campbell, J. E., Jr.	600 W. Main Ave.	Knoxville, Tenn. 37902
Campbell, John R.	Medical Dental Bldg.	Seattle, Wash. 98101
Campbell, Lamar M.	Baptist Med. Center, Montclair	Birmingham, Ala. 35213
Campbell, Malcolm D.	435 Ridgewood Rd.	Key Biscayne, Fla. 33149
Campbell, Maury		Inez, Tex. 77968
Campbell, Milton F.	Dearheld Medical Bldg.	Greenwich, Conn. 06830
Campbell, Peter C.	Medical Towers South	Louisville, Ky. 40202
Campbell, Robert E.	900 N. W. 10th St.	Oklahoma City, Okla. 73106
Campbell, Sherburne	1192 E. Main St.	Meriden, Conn. 06450
Campbell, Thomas E.	Medical Towers	Louisville, Ky. 40202
Campbell, W. Leigh	421 High St.	Oregon City, Ore. 97045
Campell, Henry S.	749 E. Church St.	Martinsville, Va. 24112
Campion, George S.	490 Post St.	San Francisco, Cal. 94102
Canaan, Samuel A., Jr.	4901-A Easton Ave.	St. Louis, Mo. 63113
Cancilla, Michael L.	195 South St.	Pittsfield, Mass. 01201
Cangelosi, Robert J.	3024 Gentilly Blvd.	New Orleans, La. 70122
Canniff, James C.	51 Main St.	Torrington, Con. 06790
Cannon, Edward J.	1321 Spruce St.	Philadelphia, Pa. 19107
Cannon, Robert L.	311 E. Main St.	Galesburg, Ill. 61401
Caplan, Harold E.	3320 Plainview	Pasadena, Tex. 77504
Capocchi, Leo H.	1548 Stockton St.	San Francisco, Cal. 94133
Capone, Salvatore J.	415 Bay Ridge Pkwy.	Brooklyn, N. Y. 11209
Capper, Stanley A.	16550 Ventura Blvd.	Encino, Cal. 91316
Cappetta, Domenico	103 E. 84th St.	New York, N. Y. 10028
Capriotti, Octavius A.	404 E. Broad St.	Souderton, Pa. 18964
Capus, Bertram	4131 MacDonald Ave.	Richmond, Cal. 94805
Carabelle, R. William	3570 25th St.	Port Arthur, Tex. 77640
Carboy, David T.	22 E. Mall Plaza	Carnegie, Pa. 15106
Cárdenas, Alfonso	18161 Morris Ave.	Homewood, Ill. 60430

Carelli, Paul V.	5248 W. North Ave.	Chicago, Ill. 60639
Carey, J. David	2799 W. Grand Blvd.	Detroit, Mich. 48128
Carey, Thomas F.	1300 Spring St.	Seattle, Wash. 98104
Carl, E. Franklin	2500 N. Mayfair Rd.	Wauwatosa, Wisc. 53226
Carlisle, Joseph R.	400 29th St.	Oakland, Cal. 94609
Carlisle, O. B.	3158 Maple Dr. N. E.	Atlanta, Ga. 30305
Carlson, A. Eugene	925 W. 9th Ave.	Albany, Ore. 97321
Carlson, Frederick B.	Box 110, 14th Naval Dist., FPO .	San Francisco, Cal. 96610
Carlson, Roland D.	3070 Mayfield Rd.	Cleveland, O. 44118
Carman, Henry F.	93 Morningside Dr.	San Francisco, Cal. 94122
Carmichael, Paul L.	601 E. Main St.	Lansdale, Pa. 19446
Carmody, Raymond F.	5284 Broadway	Gary, Ind. 46408
Carr, Ronald E.	566 First Ave.	New York, N. Y. 10016
Carriker, Frederick R.	1313 N. 2nd St.	Phoenix, Ariz. 85004
Carroll, Frank D.	66 Milton Rd.	Rye, N. Y. 10580
Carroll, G. T.	1014 San Juan Ave.	Exeter, Cal. 93221
Carroll, James R.	6465 S. Yale Ave.	Tulsa, Okla. 74135
Carroll, John M.	1493 Cambridge St.	Cambridge, Mass. 02139
Carroll, Michael E.	2800 W. 87th	Chicago, Ill. 60652
Carson, Willis T.	506 N. Alleghaney	Odessa, Tex. 79760
Carter, Charles B.	3200 Main St.	Vancouver, Wash. 98663
Carter, George Z.	30 E. 60th St.	New York, N. Y. 10022
Carter, Leland F.	David Whitney Bldg.	Detroit, Mich. 48226
Cater, Robert C.	4010 Sepulveda Blvd.	Torrance, Cal. 90505
Cater, Vincent, Jr.	179 Cedar Lane	Teaneck, N. J. 07666
Cartwright, William H.	1105 E. Front St.	Traverse City, Mich. 49684
Caruthers, Samuel B.	127 S. Main St.	Grenada, Miss. 38901
Case, Paul H	555 W. Catalina	Phoenix, Ariz. 85013
Case, William F.	11201 Colorado	Kansas City, Mo. 64137
Casebeer, Harvey L.	320 S. Clark	Butte, Mont. 59701
Casey, Edwin J.	4424 Hampton	St. Louis, Mo. 63109
Casey, Ernest R.	1005 S.W. 2nd Ave.	Gainesville, Fla. 32601
Casey, William J.	490 Post St.	San Francisco, Cal. 94102
Cassady, J. Vernal	Sherland Bldg.	South Bend, Ind. 46601
Cassady, John R.	Sherland Bldg.	South Bend, Ind. 46601
Casserly, George B.	571 7th St.	San Pedro, Cal. 90731
Castagno, Marion M.	215 Washington St.	Hartford, Conn. 06106
Castaneda, David J.	1338 S. W. 8th St.	Miami, Fla. 33130
Gasteen, William F.	2007 17th	Bakersfield Cal. 93301
Casten, Virgil G.	412 Beacon St.	Boston, Mass. 02115
Castroviejo, Ramon	9 E. 91st St.	New York, N. Y. 10028
Caterini, Joseph M.	779 Bergen Ave.	Jersey City, N. J. 07306
Cation, Vivian A.	4640 Marine Dr.	Chicago, Ill. 60640
Caulfield, John D.	201 S. Linn	New Hampton, Ia. 50659
Cavaliere, Joseph T.	1929 New Hyde Park Rd.	New Hyde Park, N. Y. 11040
Cavero, Rafael	1249 Fifth Ave.	New York, N. Y. 10029
Caygill, Wayne M.	357 30th St.	Oakland, Cal. 94609
Cefaratti, Michael D.	232 N. 5th St.	Reading, Pa. 19601
Cerny, F. J.	80 Sheboygan St.	Fond du Lac, Wisc. 54935
Cetner, John A.	668 Madison Ave.	Albany, N. Y. 12208
Chaimov, Alan L.	530 N. W. 27th St.	Corvallis, Ore. 97330
Chalfin, J. Eugene	41 E. Parkway	Brooklyn, N. Y. 11238
Chalkley, Thomas F. H. . . .	700 N. Michigan Ave.	Chicago, Ill, 60611
Chamberlain, Calvin B.	174 Nemaha St.	Pomona, Cal. 91767
Chamberlain, Webb P.	1422 Euclid Ave.	Cleveland, O. 44115

Chambers, Arthur L., II ...	27 Ludlow St.	Yonkers, N. Y. 10705
Chambers, Benjamin M. ...	44 Broad St., N.W.	Atlanta, Ga. 30303
Chambers, John D.	2601 M Ave.	Anacortes, Wash. 98221
Chamblee, H. Royster, Jr. ..	704 Professional Bldg.	Raleigh, N. C. 27601
Chambless, Wm. S.	2811 Lemmon Ave. E.	Dallas, Tex. 75204
Chamichian, Souren L.	117 S. University Ave.	Mt. Pleasant, Mich. 48858
Chamikles, Saebert L.	1490 Ocean Ave.	Brooklyn, N. Y. 11230
Chamlin, Max	8 E. 77th St.	New York, N. Y. 10021
Chan, Guy H., Jr.	Wills Eye Hospital, 1601 Spring Garden	Philadelphia, Pa. 19130
Chandler, Arthur C.	1215 Quarrier St.	Charleston, W. Va. 25301
Chandler, Arthur C., Jr. ...	Duke University Medical Center .	Durham, N. C. 27704
Chandler, Clinton B.	3010 Hampton Ave.	Brunswick, Ga. 31520
Chandler, Paul A.	5 Bay State Rd.	Boston, Mass. 02215
Chapman, Jules B.	867 Cypress Lake Circle	Ft. Myers, Fla. 33901
Chapman, Lawrence I.	760 Arlington Heights Rd.	Elk Grove Village, Ill. 60007
Chapman, Richard B.	92 Highland St.	Milton, Mass. 02186
Charap, Bertram W.	114 Continental Ave.	Forest Hills, N. Y. 11375
Charlap, Myron	138 Dubois St.	Newburgh, N. Y. 12550
Chase, David S.	355 Pearl St.	Burlington, Vt. 05401
Chase, Robert C.	1212 W. 2nd	Grand Island, Nebr. 68801
Chastanet, Denis V. P.	2044 Bridgeport Ave.	Milford, Conn. 06460
Chatow, Jerome A.	22330 S. Hawthorne Blvd.	Torrance, Cal. 90505
Chatterley, J. Garth	72 W. Harding Ave.	Cedar City, Utah 84720
Chatzinoff, Albert B.	2035 Lakeville Rd.	New Hyde Park, N. Y. 11040
Cheij, Abraham P.	Bennie Dillon Bldg.	Nashville, Tenn. 37203
Chen, George D.	School of Aerospace Medicine, Brooks AFB	San Antonio, Tex. 78235
Chen, John E.	120 E. Pine	Caldwell, Ida. 83605
Chenault, Oran W.	2846 Polk St.	San Francisco, Cal. 94109
Cheng, George P.	3116 W. Beverly Blvd.	Montebello, Cal. 90640
Chenoweth, Richard G. ...	Box 175, Valley Forge Gen. Hospital	Phoenixville, Pa. 19460
Cherr, Donald	1501 East Ave.	Rochester, N. Y. 14610
Chessen, Gerald J.	601 N. Wilmot Rd.	Tucson, Ariz. 85711
Chiapella, Karl J.	260 Cohasset Ln.	Chico, Cal. 95926
Chickering, Donald H.	2414 Youngstown Rd. S. E.	Warren, O. 44484
Childers, Melvin D., Jr.	1928 Randolph Rd.	Charlotte, N. C. 28207
Childers, Stanley G.	830 W. Abriendo Ave.	Pueblo, Colo. 81005
Childrey, Edgar, Jr.	501 E. Franklin St.	Richmond, Va. 23219
Chin, Newton B.	333 E. 34th St.	New York, N. Y. 10016
Chinn, Chester W.	209 W. 125th St.	New York, N. Y. 10027
Chiques, Carlos M.	First Federal Bldg.	Santurce, P. R. 00909
Chirls, I. Allen	109 S. Munn Ave.	East Orange, N. J. 07018
Chisholm, Donald E.	10425 W. North Ave.	Wauwatosa, Wisc. 53226
Chisholm, Julian F., Jr., ...	59 Sandy Valley Rd.	Dedham, Mass. 02026
Chisholm, Leslie L., Jr.	5206 N. Armenia Ave.	Tampa, Fla. 33603
Chizek, David J.	U. S. Army Hospital, Okinawa, Box 123 APO	San Francisco, Cal. 96331
Cholst, Mortimer R.	40 Park Ave.	New York, N. Y. 10016
Chopin, Richard M.	120 Millburn Ave.	Millburn, N. J. 07041
Choy, Martin F.	2500 Hospital Dr.	Mountain View, Cal. 94040
Christenberry, Kenneth W. .	501 W. Church Ave.	Knoxville, Tenn. 37902
Christensen, Clarence A. ...	2209 Lloyd Ctr.	Portland, Ore. 97232
Christensen, Gerald R.	Univ. of Texas Medical Branch ..	Galveston, Tex. 77550

Christensen, Leonard	3181 S. W. San Jackson Park Rd.	Portland, Ore. 97201
Christensen, Llewellyn E. ..	Doctor's Bldg.	Minneapolis, Minn. 55402
Christensen, Robert E	800 Westwood Plaza	Los Angeles, Cal. 90024
Christerson, John W.	621 E. Campbell Ave.	Campbell, Cal. 95030
Christiansen, Gunnar E. ...;	1834 W. Lincoln Ave.	Anaheim, Cal. 92801
Christman, Ernest H.	223 E. Palace Ave.	Santa Fe, N. M. 87501
Christoferson, Kent W.	132 E. Broadway	Eugene, Ore. 97401
Ciccarelli, Eugene C.	Cape Cod Medical Center	Hyannis, Mass. 02601
Cimino, Eugene A.	20 N. Goodman St.	Rochester, N. Y. 14607
Cimmino, Gerald N.	121 Wakelee Ave.	Ansonia, Conn. 06401
Cinelli, Albert B.	420 Oak Hill Ave.	Youngstown, O. 44502
Cinotti, Alfonse A.	3285 Kennedy Blvd.	Jersey City, N.J. 07307
Clahassey, Erwin G.	50 College Ave.	Grand Rapids, Mich. 49503
Clahr, George D.	799 Park Ave.	New York, N. Y. 10021
Clark, Charles E.	211 S. Saratoga St.	New Orleans, La. 70112
Clark, George A.	23 E. Ohio St.	Indianapolis, Ind. 46204
Clark, Graham	420 W. 116th St.	New York, N. Y. 10027
Clark, Howard E.	1088 Cass	Monterey, Cal. 93940
Clark, Ivor G.	1989 W. Fifth Ave.	Columbus, O. 43212
Clark, Lee A., Jr.	Wilson Clinic	Wilson, N. C. 27893
Clark, Randall L.	851 McClelland Dr., MacDill AFB	Tampa, Fla. 33608
Clark, Robert M.	2809 W. Godman Ave.	Muncie, Ind. 47304
Clark, S. William, Jr.	502 Isabella St.	Waycross, Ga. 31501
Clark, W. Bruce	545 W. 7th St.	St. Paul. Minn. 55102
Clark, Williard C.	249 Chatham Dr.	Dayton, Ohio 45429
Clark, William B.	211 S. Saratoga St.	New Orleans, La. 70112
Clarke, Clement C.	240 Bradley St.	New Haven, Conn. 06510
Clarke, David L.	559 Glen St.	Glens Falls, N. Y. 12801
Clarke, Samuel T.	130 N. Virginia	Reno, Nev. 89501
Clay, Richard A.	415 N. W. 11	Oklahoma City, Okla. 73103
Cleasby, Gilbert W.	2400 Clay St.	San Francisco, Cal. 94115
Clegg, William R.	301 N. Prairie Ave.	Inglewood, Cal. 90056
Clement, Charles C.	Mease Manor	Dunedin, Fla. 33518
Clements, Richard K.	568 Park Ave.	New York, N. Y. 10021
Cleveland, Albert F.	615 Morgan Ave.	Drexel Hill, Pa. 19026
Cleveland, Willard H.	1004 Beverly Dr.	Rockledge, Fla. 32955
Clevenger, Charles E.	The Medical Center Clinic	Pensacola, Fla. 32502
Cline, J. William	1110 W. Main St.	Durham, N. C. 27701
Close, James S.	1492 N. Main St.	Wheaton, Ill. 60187
Clothier, William L.	732 Washington Ave.	Pocatello, Ida. 83201
Cloud, Thomas M.	Hermann Prof. Bldg.	Houston, Tex. 77025
Clough, Dexter, J., II	224 State St.	Bangor, Me. 04401
Clough, Howard K.	Lankenau Med. Bldg.	Philadelphia, Pa. 19151
Clough, Joseph M.	266 Beacon St.	Boston, Mass. 02116
Clower, James W.	1012 Volusia Ave.	Daytona Beach, Fla. 32014
Cloyd, David H.	128 S. Hickory St.	Escondido, Cal. 92025
Clune, John P.	632 Eastland Professional Bldg. .	Harper Woods, Mich. 48236
Cluskey, Donald J.	5121 Garfield Dr.	La Mesa, Cal. 92041
Cobots, Joseph C.	423 E. Ninth St.	Chester, Pa. 19013
Coburn, Sheldon A.	16542 Ventura Blvd.	Encino, Cal. 91316
Cockerham, Walter D.	1408 Penna	Fairfield. Cal. 94533
Coe, Richard O., Jr.	7301 Mission Rd.	Prairie Village, Kans. 66208
Cofer, Hershel	Box 'O' Balboa Heights	Canal Zone, Panama
Cogan, David G.	243 Charles St.	Boston, Mass. 02114
Cogan, James R.	2080 Century Park E.	Los Angeles, Cal. 90069
Cogswell, Thomas G.	46 Pleasant St.	Concord, N. H. 03301

Cohan, Bruce E.	2355 E. Stadium Blvd.	Ann Arbor, Mich 48104
Cohen, Harold H.	308 Glessner Ave.	Mansfield, O. 44903
Cohen, Irving	54 Grand Ave.	Poughkeepsie, N. Y. 12603
Cohen, Irwin J.	50 E. 72nd St.	New York, N. Y. 10021
Cohen, J. H.	708 Johnstown Bank & Trust Bldg.	Johnstown, Pa. 15901
Cohen, Louis B.	1320 Arrott St.	Philadelphia, Pa. 19124
Cohen, Samuel W.	522 Ocean Ave.	Brooklyn, N. Y. 11226
Coiro, Vittorio	115 E. 89th St.	New York, N. Y. 10028
Colbert, John J.	1127 11th St.	Sacramento, Cal. 95814
Cole, Helen G.	780 Park Ave.	New York, N. Y. 10021
Cole, J. Gordon	780 Park Ave.	New York, N. Y. 10021
Cole, Nathaniel B.	104 Market St.	Perth Amboy, N. J. 08861
Cole, Roger W.	490 N. Alvernon Way	Tucson, Ariz. 85711
Cole, Ronald J.	David Grant Medical Center	Travis AFB, Cal. 04535
Coleman, D. Jackson	635 W. 165th St.	New York, N. Y. 10032
Coleman, Denzil R.	166 Park Ave.	Port Richmond, N. Y. 10302
Coleman, H. Reese	22 W. Washington St.	Lexington, Va. 24450
Coleman, Robert R.	89-18 146th St.	Jamaica, N. Y. 11435
Coleman, Stan L.	807 Cathedral St.	Baltimore, Md. 21201
Coles, Robert S.	125 E. 72nd St.	New York, N. Y. 10021
Collier, Robert H.	12892 Palm St.	Garden Grove, Cal. 92640
Collier, Robert W., Jr.	250 Baltic St.	Brooklyn, N. Y. 11201
Collins, Braswell E.	800 First St.	Macon, Ga. 31201
Collins, Elmer C.	3600 Olentagy River Rd.	Columbus, O. 43214
Collins, Raymond C.	144 S. Harrison St.	East Orange, N. J. 07018
Collinson, Arthur W.	8 Porter St.	Melrose, Mass. 02176
Collis, William J.	1800 Nicholasville Rd., Suite 302	Lexington, Ky. 40503
Colliton, Patrick A.	920 Holiday Dr.	Moorhead, Minn. 56560
Colquhoun, Graham F.	188 College St.	Battle Creek, Mich. 49017
Colson, Z. William	301 Essex	Lawrence, Mass. 01840
Colyear, Bayard H., Jr.	3627 California St.	San Francisco, Cal. 94119
Combs, Luke	2007 Earhart St.	Charlottesville, Va. 22901
Conboy, John E.	200 Cabrini Blvd.	New York, N. Y. 10033
Connell, Evan S.	922 Walnut	Kansas City, Mo. 64106
Connole, John F.	319 N. Logan Blvd.	Altoona, Pa. 16602
Connolly, Edward B.	605 Commonwealth Ave.	Boston, Mass. 02215
Connor, Robert W.	601 E. Main St.	Lansdale, Pa. 19446
Conoan, Eduardo A.	316 Medical Arts Bldg.	Omaha, Nebr. 68102
Conrad, William C.	2401 Broadway	Boulder, Colo. 80302
Constans, George M.	2961 Arriba Way	Santa Barbara, Cal. 93105
Constantine, Elizabeth F.	215 E. 64th St.	New York, N. Y. 10021
Constantine, Frank H.	215 E. 64th St.	New York, N. Y. 10021
Conway, John E.	59 Racine St.	Menasha, Wisc. 54952
Conway, William S.	Burns Clinic	Petoskey, Mich. 49770
Cook, Martin J.	1054 E. High St.	Springfield, O. 45505
Cook, Raymond C.	601 Scott St.	Little Rock, Ark. 72201
Cook, Robert D.	220 Meridian Ave.	San Jose, Cal. 95126
Cook, T. William Jr.	2300 N. Rockton Ave.	Rockford, Ill. 61101
Cooley, Beamon S., Jr.	1016 S. 18th St.	Birmingham, Ala. 35205
Cooley, Carl C.	Medical Tower	Norfolk, Va. 23507
Cooley, William C.	16 Center St.	Northampton, Mass. 01060
Coombs, James W.	42 Main St.	Park Ridge, Ill. 60068
Cooper, Charles F., Jr.	478 Peachtree St. N. E.	Atlanta, Ga. 30308
Cooper, Edmond L.	4200 N. Woodward Ave.	Royal Oak, Mich. 48072
Cooper, Frank B.	102 Mocksville Ave.	Salibury, N. C. 28144

Cooper, Fred B.	Medical Professional Bldg.	San Antonio, Tex. 78212
Cooper, George M.	420 10th St.	Tuscaloosa, Ala. 35401
Cooper, Jack C.	Medical Arts Bldg.	Dallas, Tex. 75201
Cooper, James H.	351 E. Boundary St.	Perrysburg, O. 43551
Cooper, Robert R.	825 S. Eighth St.	Minneapolis, Minn. 55404
Cooper, William C.	73 E. 71st St.	New York, N. Y. 10021
Cooperman, Harold O.	9615 Brighton Way	Beverly Hills, Cal. 90210
Cope, Paul T.	415 7th St., S.	St. Petersburg, Fla. 33701
Copeland, Gary B.	1629 Owen Dr.	Fayetteville, N. C. 28304
Copeland, Robert L.	230 Hilton Ave.	Hempstead, N. Y. 11550
Copenhaver, Richard M. ...	560 Avenue K, S. E.	Winter Haven, Fla. 33880
Copps, James M.	4105 Live Oak St.	Dallas, Tex. 75204
Corbett, Thomas D.	625 W. Santa Fe Dr.	Merced, Cal. 95340
Corcoran, George B., Jr. ...	91 School St.	Springfield, Mass. 01105
Corin, Norman	10350 W. Bay Harbor Dr.	Miami Beach, Fla. 33154
Corn, Marvin	10 Benton Ave.	Middletown, N. Y. 10940
Cornelius, George R.	900 N.W. 10th	Oklahoma City, Okla. 73106
Corwin, Martin E.	65 E. Northfield Rd.	Livingston, N. J. 07039
Cosentino, Robert T.	300 Kensington Ave.	New Britain, Conn. 06052
Cosgrove, James F.	390 Main St.	Worcester, Mass. 01608
Cosgrove, K. W., Jr.	516 Scott	Little Rock, Ark. 72201
Costenbader, Frank D.	1605 22nd·St., N.W.	Washington, D. C. 20008
Costner, Alfred N.	207 E. Watauga Ave.	Johnson City, Tenn. 37601
Coston, Tullos O.	Pasteur Medical Bldg.	Oklahoma City, Okla. 73103
Cotlier, Edward	2801 N. Sheridan Rd.	Chicago, Ill.
Cotner, Jerry B.	304 S. Cottonwood	Richardson, Tex. 75080
Coughlan, Charles H.	1003 Central Ave.	Ft. Dodge, Ia. 50501
Coulter, William H.	14 W. Valerio St.	Santa Barbara, Cal. 93101
Cousar, George R., Jr.	606 Pendleton St.	Greenville, S. C. 29601
Couvillion, Glynne C.	1532 Anacapa St.	Santa Barbara, Cal. 93101
Covell, Lester L.	27 Chestnut St.	Wakefield, Mass. 01880
Covey, John K.	115 S. Spring St	Bellefonte, Pa. 16823
Covitz, Edward E.	475 Commonwealth Ave.	Boston, Mass. 02215
Cowan, Claude L.	1802 11th St. N. W.	Washington, D. C. 20009
Cowan, Robert F.	2230 Lynn Rd.	Thousand Oaks, Cal. 91360
Cowan, Thomas H.	1930 Chestnut St.	Philadelphia, Pa. 19103
Cowan, Thomas W.	1667 Chuckanut Dr.	Bellingham, Wash. 98225
Cowen, Homer C.	1570 Humboldt St.	Denver, Colo. 80218
Cowen, Jack P.	111 N. Wabash Ave.	Chicago, Ill. 60602
Cowger, Robert	4280 S. W. Celar Hills Blvd.	Beaverton, Ore. 97005
Cowley, I. Jack	5301 F. St.	Sacramento, Cal. 95819
Cowper, Alexander R.	543 Franklin St.	Buffalo, N. Y. 14202
Cox, James H.	203 Angell St.	Providence, R. I. 02906
Cox, J. Robert	261 Salem-Woodstown Rd.	Salem, N. J. 08079
Cox, Kelly	Medical Arts Bldg.	Dallas, Tex. 75201
Cox, Morton S., Jr.	University Med. Ctr.	Ann Arbor, Mich. 48104
Cox, Ronald A.	1779 Massachusetts N.W.	Washington, D. C. 20036
Coyle, John J.	2 E. Broad St.	Hazelton, Pa. 18201
Coyle, J. Terrence	1300 116th N. E.	Bellevue, Wash. 98004
Cozean, Charles H., Jr.	937 Broadway	Cape Girardeau, Mo. 63701
Crage, Francis M.	724 Indian Beach Ln.	Sarasota, Fla. 33580
Craig, Paul C.	232 N. Fifth St.	Reading, Pa. 19601
Crain, A. Penn, Jr.	East Physicians and Surgeons Bldg.	Shreveport, La. 71101
Crampton, H. Jerome	130 Parker St.	Lawrence, Mass. 01843
Cramton, Edward A.	28 Underclyffe Rd.	St. Johnsbury, Vt. 05819

Crane, Cyril V.	442 James St.	Dunedin, Fla. 33528
Crane, Donald V.	2651 E. 21st St.	Tulsa, Okla. 74114
Crapotta, Joseph A.	88-25 148 St.	Jamaica, N. Y. 11435
Crawford, Clifford N.	123 Congress St.	Pasadena, Cal. 91105
Crawford, Elisabeth S.	10 Oakdale	Houston, Tex. 77006
Crawford, J. Brooks	490 Post St.	San Francisco, Cal. 94102
Crawford, James H.	930 N. 1350 West	Provo, Utah 84601
Crawford, Joseph W.	490 Post St.	San Francisco, Cal. 94102
Crawford, Mark E.	Stuart Bldg.	Lincoln, Nebr. 68508
Crawford, Walter J.	4296 Orange St.	Riverside, Cal. 92501
Crawford, William J.	Savings & Loan Bldg.	Middletown, O. 45042
Cregar, John S.	44 S. Munn Ave.	E. Orange, N. J. 07018
Creighton, J. Burns, Jr.	3000 W. Buffalo Ave.	Tampa, Fla. 33607
Creswell, Wiltie A., Jr.	800 Fifth Ave.	Ft. Worth, Tex. 76104
Crigler, Fielding J.	1400 Jefferson Park Ave.	Charlottesville, Va. 22903
Crilley, Francis J., Jr.	4400 E. West Hwy.	Bethesda, Md. 20014
Crisman, Homer R.	515 Kensington	Missoula, Mont. 59801
Croasdale, Raymond E.	Bronson Medical Center	Kalamazoo, Mich. 49006
Crockett, Charles A.	155 S. 18th St.	Kansas City, Kans. 66102
Crockett, Douglas H.	207 E. Watauga Ave.	Johnson City, Tenn. 37601
Croffead, George S.	31 Smith St.	Charleston, S. C. 29401
Croll, Leo J.	12703 W. Seven Mile Rd.	Detroit, Mich. 48235
Croll, Maurice	12703 W. Seven Mile Rd.	Detroit, Mich. 48235
Cronin, Thomas P.	94 Pleasant St.	Arlington, Mass. 02174
Cross, Albion B., Jr.	1260 Main St.	Baton Rouge, La. 70802
Cross, Junius B.	500 S. University Ave.	Little Rock, Ark. 72205
Crossen, Robert J.	20867 Mack Ave.	Grosse Pointe Woods, Mich. 48236
Crosswell, Hal H., Jr.	1520 Laurel St.	Columbia, S. C. 29202
Crowder, John I.	Sansum Medical Clinic	Santa Barbara, Cal. 96102
Crowder, Miles S.	603 Main Ave.	Knoxville, Tenn. 37902
Crowgey, Junius E.	711 S. Jefferson St.	Roanoke, Va. 24008
Crowley, Frederick A.	1008 N. Main St.	Bloomington, Ill. 61701
Cruciani, Dominick A., Jr.	303 Medical Arts Bldg.	Scranton, Pa. 18503
Cuadra, Gilbert	5015 Whittier Blvd.	Los Angeles, Cal. 90022
Cuadra, Marie E.	9209 S. Colima Rd.	Whittier, Cal. 90605
Cube, Ernesto M.	P. O. Box 928	Radford, Va. 24141
Culton, Julian C.	1600 E. Third St.	Charlotte, N. C. 28204
Cultron, Frank T.	800 E. Crawford St.	Salina, Kans. 67401
Culver, James F.	134 Heritage Hills Dr.	Prattville, Ala. 36067
Culver, Warren T.	1203 Iowa	Lawrence, Kans. 66044
Cummings, Edward J.	915 19th St., N.W.	Washington, D. C. 20006
Cundy, Donald T.	825 S. 8th St.	Minneapolis, Minn. 55404
Cunningham, John C.	49 S. Winooski Ave.	Burlington, Vt. 05401
Cunningham, Richard D.	2401 S. 31st St.	Temple, Tex. 76501
Curcio, Michael	320 N. 63rd St.	Philadelphia, Pa. 19139
Curnyn, Arnold D.	601 W. Central Rd.	Mt. Prospect, Ill. 60056
Curran, Desmond	925 Grand Ave.	Kansas City, Mo. 64106
Currey, Thomas A.	210 Jackson	Memphis, Tenn. 38105
Curry, Henry F., Jr.	2951 Sycamore Dr.	Semi Valley, Cal. 93065
Curtin, Brian J.	115 E. 61st St.	New York, N. Y. 10021
Curtin, Thomas L.	3230 Waring Ct.	Oceanside, Cal. 92054
Curtin, Victor T.	1638 N. W. 10th Ave.	Miami, Fla. 33136
Curtis, James L.	Geisinger Medical Ctr.	Danville, Pa. 17821
Curts, Calvin J.	4320 Wornall Rd	Kansas City, Mo. 64111
Curts, James H.	1205 N. Michigan Ave.	Saginaw, Mich 48602

Cury, Dahar	3621 E. Century Blvd.	Lynwood, Cal. 90262
Cusick, Paul L.	15901 9 Mile Rd.	Southfield, Mich. 48075
Cuthbert, Marvin	3266 N. Meridian St.	Indianapolis, Ind. 46208
Cutino, Rodolph M.	Box 307, R. D. 1	Lake Hopatcong, N. J. 07849
Cutino, Rudolph L.	1880 Arlington St.	Sarasota, Fla. 33579
Cutler, Morton	206 Martin St.	Twin Falls, Ida. 83301
Cutler, Norman L.	1300 Harrison St.	Wilmington, Dela. 19806
Cutler, William M.	800 S. Adams	Birmingham, Mich. 48011
Czarnecki, Casimir	9412 Academy Rd.	Philadelphia, Pa. 19114
Dabezies, Oliver H., Jr.	4440 Magnolia St.	New Orleans, La. 70115
Dahl, Mary M.	1062 E. 21st St.	Salt Lake City, Utah 84106
Dahlene, Oscar, Jr.	924 S. 18th St.	Birmingham, Ala. 35205
Dailey, Edward G.	618 N. 3rd St.	Harrisburg, Pa. 17101
Daily, Charles D.	599 Sir Francis Drake Blvd.	Kentfield, Cal. 94904
Daily, Louis	Medical Towers Bldg.	Houston, Tex. 77025
Daily, Ray K.	Medical Towers Bldg.	Houston, Tex. 77025
Dalburg, Lewis A., Jr.	300 Kensington Ave.	New Britain, Conn. 06050
D'Alena, Peter	45 S. 17th St.	San Jose, Cal. 95112
Dalton, H. M.	Kinston Clinic	Kinston, N. C. 28501
Dalton, John T.	67 Coddington St.	Quincy, Mass. 02169
D'Amato, Fredric R.	Central Tower Bldg.	Youngstown, O. 44503
D'Ambrosio, Francis A.	John Cuming Bldg.	Concord, Mass. 01742
Dame, Lawrence R.	78 Federal St.	Greenfield, Mass. 01301
D'Amico, Robert A.	737 Park Ave.	New York, N. Y. 10021
D'Amico, Thomas V.	208 Passaic Ave.	Passaic, N. J. 07055
Damitz, John C.	656 W. Market St.	Akron, O. 44303
Dan, Julius M.	1362 President St.	Brooklyn, N. Y. 11213
Dan, Lewis R.	835 N. E. 79th St.	Miami, Fla. 33138
Danforth, Edward P.	19 Old Mamaroneck Rd.	White Plains, N. Y. 10605
D'Angelo, Thomas M.	92-11 35th Ave.	Jackson Heights, N. Y. 11372
Daniel, Ruby K.	Medical Arts Bldg.	Dallas, Tex. 75201
Danielski, John J.	30900 Ford Rd.	Garden City, Mich. 48135
Danielson, Ralph W.	5770 E. Third Ave.	Denver, Colo. 80220
Dardis, Walter T.	830 W. Abriendo Ave.	Pueblo, Colo. 81005
Dark, Anthony J.	750 E. Adams St.	Syracuse, N. Y. 13210
Darnell, Clarence A.	1777 Vine St.	Hollywood, Cal. 90028
Darr, Joseph L.	Walter Reed Gen. Hospital	Washington, D. C. 20012
Darrell, Richard W.	635 W. 165th St.	New York, N. Y. 10032
da Silva, Lionel B.	440 Fair Dr.	Costa Mesa, Cal. 92626
Daukas, Charles	809 Main St.	E. Hartford, Conn. 06108
Daukas, Nicholas J.	124 Washington St.	Middletown, Conn. 06457
Davey, Gerald P.	2030 Schiller Ave.	Cuyahoga Falls, O. 44223
Davidorf, Bernard	22030 Sherman Way	Canoga Park, Cal. 91393
Davidson, Alan	P. O. Box 250	New Bern, N. C. 28560
Davidson, Bernard	7232 Van Nuys Blvd.	Van Nuys, Cal. 91405
Davidson, Gene L.	1225 Miccosukee Rd.	Tallahassee, Fla. 32302
Davidson, John A.	660 S. Euclid	St. Louis, Mo. 63110
Davidson, L. Stacy, Jr.	304 Delta Ave.	Cleveland, O. 38732
Davidson, Richard	21297 Foothill Blvd.	Hayward, Cal. 94541
Davidson, Richard A.	The Everett Clinic, Colby at 39th.	Everett, Wash. 98201
Davidson, Sheldon	777 E. Brill St.	Phoenix, Ariz. 85006
Davies, Gerald T.	5224 St. Antoine	Detroit, Mich. 48202
Davies, Robert H.	633 Washington Rd.	Pittsburgh. Pa. 15228
Davies, Windsor S.	28 W. Adams Ave.	Detroit, Mich. 48226

Davies, Bradford L.	USAF Regional Hospital	Carswell AFB, Tex. 76127
Davis, C. Truman	1150 N. Country Club Dr.	Mesa, Ariz. 85201
Davis, Dale George	1638 N.W. 10th Ave.	Miami, Fla. 33136
Davis, David B., II	420 Estudillo Ave.	San Leandro, Cal. 94577
Davis, Frederick J.	1025 Regent St.	Madison, Wisc. 53715
Davis, Frederick S., Jr.	3500 Kensington Ave.	Richmond, Va. 23221
Davis, Jerome D.	19075 Middlebelt Rd.	Livonia, Mich. 48152
Davis, Matthew D.	1025 Regent St.	Madison, Wisc. 53715
Davis, Michael J.	2601 W. Lincoln Hwy.	Olympia Fields, Ill. 60461
Davis, Robert Howard	93 Arch St.	Redwood City, Cal. 94062
Davis Robert J. ...٢......	South 427 Bernard	Spokane, Wash. 99204
Davis, Robert V., Jr.	31 Leroy Pl.	Red Bank, N. J. 07701
Davis, W. L.	P.O. Box 1226	Orangeburg, S. C. 29115
Dawson, Chandler R.	F. I. Proctor Foundation, University of California	San Francisco, Cal. 94122
Dawson, Robert E.	512 Simmons St.	Durham, N. C. 27701
Day, Robert	2000 Massachusetts Ave. N. W. ...	Washington, D. C. 20036
Day, Robert M.	108 E. 68th St.	New York, N. Y. 10021
Day, Roy W.	First National Bank Bldg.	Glenwood Springs, Colo. 81601
Dayton, Glenn O.	10921 Wilshire Blvd.	Los Angeles, Cal. 90024
Dean, Abbott M.	536 First Ave.	Council Bluffs, Ia. 51501
Dean, Alfred	....	Sagola, Mich 4988
Dean, Wynant	250 E. Liberty St.	Louisville, Ky. 40202
Deas, Ralph H.	3312 Piedmont Rd. N.E.	Atlanta, Ga. 30305
DeCarlo, Joseph D.	1815 Grand Concourse	New York, N. Y. 10453
Decker, Joseph H.	45 S. 17th St.	San Jose. Cal. 95112
Deer, Philip J., Jr.	601 Scott St.	Little Rock, Ark. 72201
Deering, Donald W.	2335 Monroe St.	Milwaukie, Ore. 97222
De Francois, Walter	122 S. Michigan Ave.	Chicago, Ill. 60603
De Golia, Pershing	1515 Montgomery Dr.	Santa Rosa, Cal. 95405
De Haven, Charles R.	826 S. Fleishel	Tyler, Tex. 75701
Deichler, John W.	1930 Chestnut St.	Philadelphia, Pa. 19103
Deitch, Robert D.	23 E. Ohio St.	Indianapolis, Ind. 46204
Deitch, Ronald S.	1234 19th St., N. W.	Washington, D. C. 20036
Deiter, Paul D.	16542 Ventura Blvd.	Encino, Cal. 91316
Deitz, Michael R.	155 S. 18th St.	Kansas City, Kans. 66102
de Juan, Eugene	1563 Springhill Ave.	Mobile, Ala. 36604
de la Motte, Walter	1275 Olentangy River Rd.	Columbus, O. 43212
Delaney, James H.	225 W. 25th St.	Erie, Pa. 16502
Delaney, William V., Jr. ...	109 S. Warren St.	Syracuse, N. Y. 13202
de la Vega, Felix	168 S. E. 1st St.	Miami, Fla. 33133
Delevie, Jaap B.	Riker Bldg.	Pontiac, Mich. 48058
Delgado, Robert E.	2100 N. Orange Ave.	Orlando, Fla. 32804
Dellaporta, Angelos	Stanford Medical Center	Stanford, Cal. 94305
Dello Russo, Joseph Y.	170 Washington Ave.	Dumont, N. J. 07628
Delman, Martin	8301 Bay Pkwy.	Brooklyn, N. Y. 11214
DeLong, Samuel L.	234 E. College Ave.	State College, Pa. 16801
Delp, James R.	P. O. Box 681	Williamson, W. Va. 25661
Demby, Allen M.	42 N. Franklin Tnpk	Ramsey, N. J., 07446
Demming, James H.	135 Broadway	Daytona Beach, Fla. 32018
Demorest, Byron H.	5301 F St.	Sacramento, Cal. 95819
Dempsey, Edmund V.	450 Sutter	San Francisco, Cal. 94108
Denicke, Ernest W.	1530 5th St.	San Rafael, Cal. 94901
Dennis, Patrick H.	Ashley House, 1C	Charleston, S. C. 29401
Dennis, Richard H.	33 College Ave.	Waterville, Me. 04901

Dennis, Robert P.	1002 Gore Blvd.	Lawton, Okla. 73501
Denny, Lorin W.	215 N. San Mateo Dr.	San Mateo, Cal. 94401
DeNote, Anthony P.	1175 N. E. 125th St.	North Miami, Fla. 33161
Depp, Donald S.	2600 Capitol Ave.	Sacramento, Cal. 95816
Derivaux, Joseph H.	401 Lowell Dr. S. E.	Huntsville, Ala. 35801
de Roetth, Andrew, Jr.	635 W. 165th St.	New York, N. Y. 10032
Derose, Louis F.	780 Chestnut St.	Springfield, Mass. 01107
Derrick, Geo. L.	1520 Laurel St.	Columbia, S. C. 29201
Dersh, Jerome	232 N. 5th St.	Reading, Pa. 19601
Despain, Robert V.	211 S. 7th E.	Salt Lake City, Utah 84102
Dessoff, Joseph	1302 18th St., N.W.	Washington, D. C. 20036
de Suto-Nagy, Ilona Krasso	139 Alston Ave.	New Haven, Conn. 06515
Deters, Curtis F.	700 N. Michigan	Chicago, Ill. 60611
Deutch, Marcella G.	321 N. Main St.	Fall River, Mass. 02720
Deutch, Sydney S.	321 N. Main St.	Fall River, Mass. 02720
Deutsch, Alice R.	1308 Commerce Title Bldg.	Memphis, Tenn. 38103
Deutsch, Frederic H.	155 E. 76th St.	New York, N. Y. 10021
Deutsch, William E.	30 N. Michigan Ave.	Chicago, Ill. 60602
de Venecia, Guilermo B.	1300 University Ave.	Madison, Wisc. 53706
De Voe, Arthur G.	635 W. 165th St.	New York, N. Y. 10032
De Vol, Russell A.	302 S. Bailey Ave.	North Platte, Nebr. 69101
Deweese, Melvin W.	1320 Linden Ave.	Memphis, Tenn. 38104
Diamond, Marshall A.	50 W. Edmonston Dr.	Rockville, Md. 20852
Diamond, Stanley	490 Post St.	San Francisco, Cal. 94102
Diana, Louis N.	1541 E. Clark	Pocatello, Ida. 83201
Dias, John F.	52 Brigham St.	New Bedford, Mass. 02740
Diaz-Bonnet, Victor M.	400 Domenech Ave.	Hato Rey, P. R. 00918
Di Cello, Anthony J.	150 Mentor Ave.	Painesville, O. 44077
Dickerman, Frederick A.	1138 Elm St.	Manchester, N. H. 03101
Dickerson, Donald E.	2021 Santa Monica Blvd.	Santa Monica, Cal. 90404
Dickerson, John W.	Medical Tower	Norfolk, Va. 23507
Dickey, C. Allen	450 Sutter St.	San Francisco, Cal. 94108
Dickey, Robert L.	Medical Ctr.	Salisbury, Md. 21801
Dickinson, Ralph H.	131 Fulton Ave.	Hempstead, N. Y. 11550
Dickinson, Richard K.	753 James St.	Syracuse, N. Y. 13203
Dickinson, Thomas G.	1880 Arlington St.	Sarasota, Fla. 33579
Dickinson, Thomas J.	15366 Eleventh St.	Victorville, Cal. 92392
Dickson, Owen C.	2320 Channing Way	Berkeley, Cal. 94704
DiFrancesco, John G.	7902 4th Ave.	Brooklyn, N. Y. 11209
Dillahunt, Jack A.	2201 San Pedro Dr. N. E.	Albuquerque, N. M. 87110
Dillon, Ronald W.	127 McClanahan St.	Roanoke, Va. 24014
DiMaio, Alphonse	42-27 Union St.	Flushing, N. Y. 11355
Dimmitt, Frank W.	154 Waterman St.	Providence, R. I. 02906
Dimun, Michael F.	337 E. Main	Carnegie, Pa. 15106
Dinsdale, Howard A.	630 N. Cotner Blvd.	Lincoln, Nebr. 68505
Diorio, Philip C.	3400 Lomita Blvd.	Torrance, Cal. 90505
Dippé, Donald W.	Alska Native Med. Center	Anchorage, Alaska 99501
Diskan, Samuel M.	1616 Pacific Ave.	Atlantic City, N. J. 08401
Dismukes, Henry M.	1359 Spring Hill Ave.	Mobile, Ala. 36604
Dix, Harold C.	405 N. Charles St.	Baltimore, Md. 21201
Dixon, Gerald R.	3141 N. W. Expressway	Oklahoma City, Okla. 73112
Dixon, John B.	Brick & Tile Bldg.	Mason City, Ia. 50401
Dixon, Joseph M.	Medical Arts Bldg.	Birmingham, Ala. 35205
Dobbie, J. Graham	707 N. Fairbanks Ct.	Chicago, Ill. 60611
Dobbs, Charles E.	Memorial Prof. Bldg.	Houston, Tex. 77002
Dobies, Richard J.	1126 S. Main St.	Dayton, O. 45409

Docter, Luebert L.	Medical Arts Bldg.	Grand Rapids, Mich. 49502
Doctor, Daniel W.	129 Kings Hwy.	Westport, Conn. 06880
Doctrow, William M.	128 E. Main St.	Riverhead, N. Y. 11901
Dodd, Elbert W., Jr.	1835 Eye St. N. W.	Washington, D. C. 2006
Dodds, H. Thomas	Wills Eye Hospital, 1601 Spring Garden St.	Philadelphia, Pa. 19130
Dodick, Jack M.	6 E. 76th St.	New York, N. Y. 10021
Dodson, John W.	Meyer Bldg.	Hot Springs, Ark. 71901
Does, Charles W.	110 Lockwood St.	Providence, R. I. 02903
Dohlman, Claes H.	243 Charles St.	Boston, Mass. 02114
Dole, John A.	513 Neal Ave.	Ironton, O. 45638
Dolmage, G. H.	168 Aurora Ave.	St. Paul, Minn. 55103
Dolphin, Murray	83 S. Franklin St.	Wilkes-Barre, Pa. 18701
Domanskis, Alina A.	9948 S. Western Ave.	Chicago, Ill. 60643
Dominique, Gerard L.	1110 N. Green St.	McHenry, Ill. 60050
Donahue, Hugh C.	280 Washington St.	Boston, Mass. 02135
Donald, Russell A.	1245 R. St.	Fresno, Cal. 93721
Donaldson, David D.	243 Charles St.	Boston, Mass. 02114
Dong, Emma O.	535 E. Romie Lane	Salinas, Cal. 93901
Donin, Jerry F.	1774 Alameda St.	Pomona, Cal. 91767
Donn, Anthony	635 W. 165th St.	New York, N. Y. 10032
Donnelly, Wm. L.	661 N. Long Beach Rd.	Rockville Ctr., N. Y. 11570
Donoghue, William F.	67 Chestnut St.	Springfield, Mass. 01103
Donohue, Robert J.	188 Chestnut St.	Holyoke, Mass. 01040
Donovan, Bernard F.	1360 Mt. Hope Ave.	Rochester, N. Y. 14620
Donovan, Richard J.	465 Walnut St.	Fall River, Mass. 02720
Doolittle, John W.	110 E. Main St.	Madison, Wisc. 53703
Doolittle, Uri, Jr.	120 E. Washington St.	Syracuse, N. Y. 13202
Dorenbush, Martin	1180 Route 46	Parsippany, N. J. 07054
Dorge, Richard	1111 Nicollet Ave.	Minneapolis, Minn. 55402
Dorsch, William E.	2844 Summit St.	Oakland, Cal. 94609
Dorton, David H., Jr.	Medical Arts Bldg.	Louisville, Ky. 40217
Dortzbach, Richard K.	1025 Regent St.	Madison, Wisc. 53715
Dougan, Archie F.	330 S. 5th St.	Enid, Okla. 73701
Dougherty, Malvin J.	34 Copley Rd.	Upper Darby, Pa. 19082
Dougherty, Raymond A. ..	213 S. 17th St.	Mattoon, Ill. 61938
Doughman, Donald J.	77 Warren St.	Boston, Mass. 02135
Douglas, Edward M.	87-85 153rd St.	Jamaica, L. I., N. Y. 11432
Douvas, Nicholas G.	4200 Gratiot Ave.	Port Huron, Mich. 48060
Dow, David S.	2223 Austin Ave.	Waco, Tex. 76701
Dow, Julian N.	435 N. Bedford Dr.	Beverly Hills, Cal. 90210
Dowling, Joseph L., Jr.	159 Waterman St.	Providence, R. I. 02906
Downey, Harold, R.	2000 Mass. Ave., N. W.	Washington, D. C. 20036
Downing, Arthur H.	604 Locust St.	Des Moines, Ia. 50309
Downing, John E.	Naval Hospital	Jacksonville, Fla. 32114
Dozier, Horace B.	2701 Napoleon Ave	New Orleans, La. 70115
Draheim, Jerry W.	3939 Monroe St.	Toledo, O. 43606
Drake, Henry P.	2525 W. Bancroft	Toledo, O. 43607
Drews, Robert C.	211 N. Meramec Ave	Clayton, Mo. 63105
Driver, L. Rowe	Mid State Medical Ctr.	Nashville, Tenn. 37203
Droegemueller, William H. .	2000 16th St.	Greeley, Colo. 80631
Drucker, Arnold P.	333 N. San Mateo Dr.	San Mateo, Cal. 94401
Druckrey, Gerald R.	1146 Grant St.	Beloit, Wisc. 53511
Dryden, James S.	1835 Eye St., N. W.	Washington, D. C. 20006
Dryden, Robert M.	10220 Glen Rd.	Potomac, Md. 20854
Duane, Thomas D.	1025 Walnut St.	Philadelphia, Pa. 19107

Dubins, Henry B.	23 Hackett Blvd.	Albany, N. Y. 12208
DuBose, L. Moultrie	615 Roswell St., N. E.	Marietta, Ga. 30060
Dubroff, Seymour	1111 Spring St.	Silver Spring, Md. 20910
Duehr, Peter A.	1025 Regent St.	Madison, Wisc. 53715
Duel, Arthur B., Jr.	200 N. Village Ave.	Rockville Centre, N. Y. 11570
Duffner, Lee R.	3816 Hollywood Blvd.	Hollywood, Fla. 33021
Duffy, Frank K.	16 King St.	Palmer, Mass. 01069
Dugan, Robert B.	225 W. 25th St.	Erie, Pa. 16502
Duggan, J. Winston	220 Meridian Ave.	San Jose, Cal. 95126
Duggan, Paul M.	6319 Castle Pl.	Falls Church, Va. 22044
Duggan, Walter F.	258 Genesee St.	Utica, N. Y. 13502
Duke, James R.	14 W. Mount Vernon Pl.	Baltimore, Md. 21201
Dukes, T. Earl, Jr.	Watson Clinic	Lakeland, Fla. 33802
Dumler, Larry J.	2750 Broadway	Boulder, Colo. 80302
Dunbar, John C.	Empire Bldg.	Pittsburgh, Pa. 15222
Duncan, Charles R., Jr.	24 Vardry St.	Greenville, S. C. 29601
Duncan, Frank B.	305 Polk St.	Amarillo, Tex. 79101
Duncan, James A.	280 Mamaroneck Ave.	White Plains, N. Y. 10605
Duncan, J. Harry	701 Abercorn St.	Savannah, Ga. 31402
Duncan, Perry E.	218 E. Stetson Dr.	Scottsdale, Ariz. 85251
Dunker, George O.	7008 W. Greenfield Ave.	Milwaukee, Wisc. 53214
Dunlap, Edward A.	525 E. 68th St.	New York, N. Y. 10021
Dunlap, Henry A.	7815 E. Jefferson Ave.	Detroit, Mich. 48214
Dunlap, Lawrence G.	3013 Louise Ln.	Springfield, Ill. 62702
Dunn, Paul P.	1030 President Ave.	Fall River, Mass. 02720
Dunn, Ralph O.	6200 Hillcroft	Houston, Tex. 77036
Dunn, Shepard N.	1520 Laurel St.	Columbia, S. C. 29201
Dunnavan, Floyd L.	P. O. Box 790	Vancouver, Wash. 98663
Dunnigan, William J.	2572 Atlantic	Long Beach, Cal. 90806
Dunnington, John H.	1 E. 71st St.	New York, N. Y. 10021
Dunphy, Edwin B.	75 Mt. Auburn St.	Cambridge, Mass. 02138
Dunphy, Robert N.	1125 E. 17th	Santa Ana, Cal. 92701
Dunworth, R. Lawrence	1116 Fifth Ave.	Huntington, W. Va. 25719
duPrey, Robert E.	10090 Main St.	Fairfax, Va. 22030
Durham, Davis G.	Professional Bldg.	Wilmington, Dela. 19803
Durk, Irving	135 Ocean Ave.	Brooklyn, N. Y. 11225
Durocher, Normand E.	35 S. Johnson St.	Pontiac, Mich. 48053
Durrani, Jehangir	2 Holcomb St.	Hartford, Conn. 06112
Dushay, Frederick	720 East Ave.	Rochester, N. Y. 14607
Duszynski, Leonard R.	2908 Elmwood Ave.	Kenmore, N. Y. 14217
Du Vall, Clyde H., Jr.	1115 S. W. Taylor	Portland, Ore. 97221
Dvorak, Joseph E.	Ins. Exch. Bldg.	Sioux City, Ia. 51101
Dyar, E. W.	1010 E. 86th St.	Indianapolis, Ind. 46240
Dyar, Robert W.	1010 E. 86th St.	Indianapolis, Ind. 46240
Dye, Robert A.	124 Fulton St., E.	Grand Rapids, Mich. 49502
Dyer, John A.	Mayo Clinic	Rochester, Minn. 55901
Dykstra, Frederick	USPHS Hosp.	Staten Island, N. Y. 10304
Eaddy, Norman O.	201 N. Washington St.	Sumter, S. C. 29150
Eagle, Frank L.	8300 Dodge St.	Omaha, Nebr. 68114
Eareckson, Vincent O., Jr.	129 N. Washington St.	Easton, Md. 21601
Easom, Harry, A.	2266 N. Prospect Ave.	Milwaukee Wisc. 53202
Easton, Mahlon T.	70 Carlton St.	Brookline, Mass. 02146
Eaves, R. Spencer	224 New Hope Rd.	Gastonia, N. C. 28052
Ebel, Ronald G.	560 Winter St. S. E.	Salem, Ore. 97301
Eber, Carl T.	610 Locust St.	St. Louis, Mo. 63101

Ebert, Reinhold O.	....	Pine River, Wisc. 54965
Ebert, Stanley	76 S. Central Ave.	Valley Stream, N. Y. 11580
Eby, T. M.	100 E. Valencia Mesa Dr.	Fullerton, Cal. 92632
Eckdahl, Robert W.	2942 Fresno St.	Fresno, Cal. 93721
Eckley, Robert	Scott-White Clinic	Temple, Tex. 76501
Economon, Joanne W.	915 19th St. N. W.	Washington, D. C. 20006
Edelstein, Isidore S.	135 Willow St.	Brooklyn, N. Y. 11201
Eden, John	132 E. 76th St.	New York, N. Y. 10021
Edgar, Erwood G.	12462 Brookhurst St.	Garden Grove, Cal. 92640
Edward, William O.	303 Mulberry, N. E.	Albuquerque, N. M. 87106
Edwards, David L.	Utica Square Medical Ctr.	Tulsa, Okla. 74114
Edwards, David L., Jr.	312 Utica Square Medical Center	Tulsa, Okla. 74114
Edwards, John E.	701 E. Colfax Ave.	Denver, Colo. 80203
Edwards, Thomas J.	Lowry Med. Arts Bldg.	St. Paul, Minn. 55102
Edwards, Thomas L.	670 W. Market St.	Lima, O. 45801
Edwards, Thomas S.	Marshall Taylor Doctors Bldg. ..	Jacksonville, Fla. 32207
Edwards, William C.	323 E. Chestnut St.	Louisville, Ky 40202
Edwards, William T.	34 Tenth St., N. E.	Atlanta, Ga. 30309
Edwin, Russell L.	602 First National Bank Bldg. ..	Great Falls, Mont 59401
Egan, John A.	2045 E. 18th Ave.	Denver, Colo. 80206
Egenhofer, Albert W.	141 E. Palace Ave.	Santa Fe, N. M. 87501
Eggert, James F.	400 29th St.	Oakland, Cal. 94609
Eggleston, Robert B.	170 S. Main	Harrisonburg, Va. 22801
Eggleston, Thomas F.	11745 Olive Blvd.	Creve Coeur, Mo. 63141
Egleston, DuBose	560 Oak Ave.	Waynesboro, Va. 22980
Ehlers, Charles W.	13847 E. 14th St.	San Leandro, Cal. 94578
Ehrenfeld, Edward	2840 S. County Rd.	Palm Beach, Fla. 33480
Ehrhardt, John A.	2811 Lemmon Ave. E.	Dallas, Tex. 75204
Ehrlich, Bernard	321 Prince George St.	Laurel, Md. 20810
Ehrlich, Leon H.	444 E. Boston Post Rd.	Mamaroneck, N. Y. 10543
Ehrlich, Max	721 N. Broad St.	Elizabeth, N. J. 07208
Ehrmann, Evelina W.	72 S. La Grange Rd.	La Grange, Ill. 60525
Eifrig, David E.	Mayo Memorial Hospital	Minneapolis, Minn. 55455
Eigner, Edwin H.	5 Severance Cir.	Cleveland Heights, O. 44118
Eilert, John H.	8706 Preston Pl.	Chevy Chase, Md. 20015
Einaugler, Richard B.	46 Maple Ave.	Morristown, N. J. 07960
Eisenberg, I. J.	2806 Green St.	Harrisburg, Pa. 17110
Eisenhower, Charles E.	426 W. Market St.	York, Pa. 17404
Eisenlohr, John E.	2811 Lemmon Ave. E.	Dallas, Tex. 75204
Eisenschmid, John A.	1360 Mt. Hope Ave.	Rochester, N. Y. 14620
Eissler, Rolf	2340 Sutter St.	San Francisco, Cal. 94115
Elander, Richard	2080 Century Park E.	Los Angeles, Cal. 90067
Elder, Orr J.	550 W. Main St.	Boonton, N. J. 07005
Elgin, Lee W., Jr.	1330 Miccosukee Rd.	Tallahassee, Fla. 32303
Elgin, Stephen S.	8710 Old Georgetown Rd.	Bethesda, Md. 20014
Elias, Mark H.	2206 Genesee St.	Utica, N. Y. 13502
Elias, Stanton B.	660 Lincoln Ave.	Pittsburgh, Pa. 15202
Eliasoph, Ira	35 E. 85th St.	New York, N. Y. 10028
Ellenberger, Carl	14701 Detroit Ave	Lakewood, O. 44107
Ellermann, Norman C.	2905 E. Tahquitz McCallum Way .	Palm Springs, Cal. 92262
Elliff, John E.	216 N. 3rd St.	Sterling, Colo. 80751
Ellingsen, Donald A.	S. 427 Bernard	Spokane, Wash. 99204
Ellingson, Frederick Thomas	405 E. Broadway	Bismarck, N. D. 58501

Ellingson, Richard B.	Doctors Bldg.	Minneapolis, Minn. 55402
Elliott, James H.	Vanderbilt Univ. Hosp.	Nashville, Tenn. 37203
Elliott, Richard L.	1125 E. 17th St.	Santa Ana, Cal. 92701
Ellis, George S.	812 Maison Blanche Bldg.	New Orleans, La. 70112
Ellis, Orwyn H.	635 S. Westlake Ave.	Los Angeles, Cal. 90057
Ellis, Philip P.	4200 E. Ninth Ave.	Denver, Colo. 80220
Ellis, Richard A.	255 S. 17th St.	Philadelphia, Pa. 19103
Ellis, Robert C.	3805 N. High St.	Columbus, O. 43214
Ellis, Van M.	1528 Spruce St.	Philadelphia, Pa. 19102
Ellison, Paul D.	Prudential Plaza	Salina, Kans. 67401
Ellman, Donald	1554 Northern Blvd.	Manhasset, N. Y. 11030
Ellsasser, Michael G.	1312 Main St.	Lubbock, Tex. 79401
Ellsworth, Robert M.	635 W. 165th St.	New York, N. Y. 10032
Ellsworth, Roy J.	2402 W. Jefferson	Boise, Ida. 83702
Elser, Otto H.	10901 Winner Rd.	Independence, Mo. 64052
Elvin, Norris C.	81 Willow St.	Garden City, N. Y. 11535
Emerson, Eugene	235 Alexander St.	Rochester, N. Y. 14607
Emerson, George O.	255 N. Lakemont Ave.	Winter Park, Fla. 32789
Emerson, John A.	25 S. E. 2nd Ave.	Miami, Fla. 33131
Emerson, Samuel M.	1415 18th St.	Lake Charles, La. 70601
Emrich, Paul S.	456 Mt. Vernon	Oshkosh, Wisc. 54901
Enders, Walter R.	421 High St.	Oregon City, Ore. 97045
Endres, Bernard J.	150 Mentor Ave.	Painesville, O. 44027
Engler, Carl H.	3737 Moraga	San Diego, Cal. 92117
Enns, James H.	317 S. E. 2nd	Newton, Kans. 67114
Eppler, William R.	20160 Mack Ave.	Grosse Pointe Woods, Mich. 48236
Epstein, Eugene B.	340 Main St.	Worcester, Mass. 01608
Epstein, Howard N.	383 W. State St.	Trenton, N. J. 08618
Epstein, Jerome L.	27 S. Prospect St.	Ypsilanti, Mich. 48197
Epstein, Sidney S.	2021 Grand Concourse	New York, N. Y. 10453
Erami, Mohammad	75 High St.	Bristol, Conn. 06010
Erbaugh, John K.	V. A. Hospital	Fresno, Cal. 93907
Erdbrink, Wayne L.	2018 Webster St.	San Francisco, Cal. 94115
Erickson, Raymond L.	939 Oak St., S.	Salem, Ore. 97301
Ernest, J. Terry	Walter Reed Army Institute of Research	Washington, D. C. 20010
Ernsting, Harry C.	VA Hosp.	Big Spring, Tex. 79720
Errgong, William H.	88 Huntington St.	New Brunswick, N. J. 08903
Esbin, Leo	1228 Wantagh Ave.	Wantagh, N. Y. 11793
Eschenbrenner, John W. ...	510 E. Stoner	Shreveport, La. 71101
Esposito, Albert C.	420-422 11th St.	Huntington, W. Va. 25701
Espy, John W.	945 Lexington Ave.	New York, N. Y. 10021
Esterly, Daniel B.	104 N. Madison Ave.	Pasadena, Cal. 91101
Esterly, Harold D., Jr.	3939 Iowa St.	San Diego, Cal. 92104
Esterman, Benjamin	1300 Cornaga Ave.	Far Rockaway, N. Y. 11691
Estes, Robert T.	1601 N. Tucson Blvd.	Tucson, Ariz. 85716
Estlow, Bert R.	1616 Pacific Ave.	Atlantic City, N. J. 08401
Etherington, John L.	915 E. Mulberry St.	Goldsboro, N. C. 27530
Eubank, Miriam D.	636 Church St.	Evanston, Ill. 60201
Eubank, Will R.	6700 Troost Ave.	Kansas City, Mo. 64131
Eubanks, William L.	490 Peachtree St.	Atlanta, Ga. 30308
Evans, Daniel R.	1101 E. Glendale Blvd.	Valparaiso, Ind. 46383
Evans, David, J.	2828 H St.	Bakersfield, Cal. 93301
Evans, Fred S.	Naval Aeromedical Institute	Pensacola, Fla. 32512
Evans, Gerald	100 Central Ave.	Staten Island, N. Y. 10301

Evans, Gomer P.	David Whitney Bldg.	Detroit, Mich. 48226
Evans, Peter Y.	3800 Reservoir Rd., N. W.	Washington, D. C. 20007
Evans, Thomas M.	550 Grant St.	Pittsburgh, Pa. 15219
Evatt, Clay W., Jr.	91 Rutledge Ave.	Charleston, S. C. 29401
Everett, William G.	Jenkins Arcade	Pittsburgh, Pa. 15222
Everton, Marta V.	185 S. Euclid Ave.	Pasadena, Cal. 91101
Ewald, Roger A.	Carle Clinic and Carle Foundation Hospital	Urbana, Ill. 61801
Ey, Richard C.	1753 W. Congress Pkwy.	Chicago, Ill. 60612
Ezell, Roy C.	2531 Park Dr.	Nashville, Tenn. 37214
Fackler, Charles L.	600 Country Club Rd.	York, Pa. 17403
Fagan, William J.	1801 House, Argyle Sq.	Babylon, N. Y. 11702
Fager, Charles B.	126 Walnut St.	Harrisburg, Pa. 17108
Faier, Herman I.	9730 Wilshire Blvd.	Beverly Hills, Cal. 90212
Faier, Robert G.	8300 Dodge St.	Omaha, Nebr. 68114
Faier, Samuel Z.	1500 Dodson Ave.	Ft. Smith, Ark. 72901
Failing, Willard N.	258 Genesee St.	Utica, N. Y. 13502
Fair, John R.	1502 Anthony Rd.	Augusta, Ga. 30904
Fairbanks, Bryce J.	34 S. 5th E.	Salt Lake City, Utah 84102
Fairbanks, E. B.	34 S. 5th E.	Salt Lake City, Utah 84102
Fairbanks, Stephen	P. O. Box 46	Wellston, Mich. 49689
Fairfax, Kenneth T.	423 Main St.	Geneva, N. Y. 14456
Fairfax, Walter A., Jr.	645 Medical Center Dr. N. E.	Salem, Ore. 97301
Falls, Harold F.	Univ. Med. Ctr.	Ann Arbor, Mich. 48104
Falls, Richard A.	200 Little Falls St.	Falls Church, Va. 22046
Fantl, Eric W.	111 N. Wabash Ave.	Chicago, Ill. 60602
Farber, David N.	134 N. Fifth St.	Reading, Pa. 19601
Farber, Sanders M.	303 E. Town St.	Columbus, O. 43215
Farish, Henry G.	12027 Riverside Dr.	North Hollywood, Cal. 91607
Farkas, Tibor G.	950 E. 59th St.	Chicago, Ill. 60637
Farmer, Howard	2866 N. E. 30th St.	Ft. Lauderdale, Fla. 33306
Farr, William F.	11737 S. W. 88th Ave.	Tigard, Ore. 97223
Farrant, Floyd H.	28 S. Mountain Ave.	Montclair, N. J. 07042
Farrell, James I.	250 Genesee St.	Utica, N. Y. 13502
Farrington, Nolley C.	1407 S. Carrollton Ave.	New Orleans, La. 70118
Farris, R. Linsy	635 W. 165th St.	New York, N. Y. 10032
Farson, Clyde	3901 Las Posas Rd.	Camarillo, Cal. 93010
Fasanella, Rocko M.	842 Howard Ave.	New Haven, Conn. 06519
Fasano, Carl V.	Fifth Ave. at 105th St.	New York, N. Y. 10029
Fastenberg, William	115 E. 86th St.	New York, N. Y. 10028
Fattel, Henry C.	8300 Kennedy Blvd.	North Bergen, N. J. 07047
Faulk, Wallace H.	1211 21st Ave. S.	Nashville, Tenn. 37212
Faulkner, Robert F.	23 Baldwin Ave.	San Mateo, Cal. 94401
Faust, Arland K.	414 S. Broadway	McAllen, Tex. 78501
Faust, Joseph M.	9735 Wilshire Blvd.	Beverly Hills, Cal. 90212
Faust, Kenneth J.	Naval Hospital	Pensacola, Fla. 32512
Fawcett, Keith R.	205 W. 2nd St.	Duluth, Minn. 55802
Fawcett, R. Alan	75 12th St.	Wheeling, W. Va. 26003
Fay, Stuart S.	80 Grove St.	Fitchburg, Mass. 01420
Fay, Thomas M.	U. S. Naval Hospital	Oakland, Cal. 94627
Faye, Eleanor E.	121 E. 60th St.	New York, N. Y. 10022
Feamster, Robert C.	6306 Woodbrook Lane	Houston, Tex. 77008
Fecko, Paul	189 Townsend Ave.	Birmingham, Mich. 48011
Feidler, Herbert D.	509 Norfolk Ave.	Norfolk, Nebr. 68701
Feiman, Lawrence H.	425 E. Wisconsin Ave.	Milwaukee, Wisc. 53202

Fein, William	465 N. Roxbury Dr.	Beverly Hills, Cal. 90210
Feinberg, Louis	1440 N. Lakeshore Dr.	Chicago, Ill. 60602
Feinhandler, Harold S.	111 N. Wabash	Chicago, Ill. 60602
Feldberg, Irving	28 Elm St.	Hornell, N. Y. 14843
Felding, Howard A.	Pecksland Rd.	Greenwich, Conn. 06830
Feldman, A. William	10734 Paramount Blvd.	Downey, Cal. 90241
Feldman, Jerald	8120 Walnut Hill Ln.	Dallas, Tex. 75231
Feldman, Mark S.	3521 W. Broward Blvd.	Ft. Lauderdale, Fla. 33312
Feldman, Noah	1060 Sanford Ave.	Irvington, N. J. 07111
Feldman, Ross	5222 Balboa	San Diego, Cal. 92117
Feldman, Victor F.	104 W. Clark St.	Champaign, Ill. 61820
Feldstein, Morris	55 E. 86th St.	New York, N. Y. 10028
Fellows, M. Fording	324 W. Superior St.	Duluth, Minn. 55802
Fellows, Victor G., Jr.	595 Buckingham Way	San Francisco, Cal. 94132
Felt, Robert S.	Medical Arts Bldg.	Salt Lake City, Utah 84111
Fenneman, Robert J.	402 S. E. Seventh St.	Evansville, Ind. 47713
Fenske, H. David	412 Phoenix St.	South Haven, Mich. 49090
Fenton, Robert H.	690 Howard Ave.	New Haven, Conn. 06519
Fercho, Calvin K.	Medical Arts Bldg. ..,.......	Fargo, N. D. 58102
Ferguson, Edward C.	Univ. of Tex. Med. Br.	Galveston, Tex. 77550
Ferguson, William H.	121 W. Underwood St.	Orlando, Fla. 32806
Ferguson, William J., Jr. ...	490 Post St.	San Francisco, Calif. 94102
Fernandez, Guillermo J. ...	160 Ponce De Leon Ave.	San Juan, P. R. 00901
Fernandez, Luis J.	Box 2206	San Juan, P. R. 00903
Fernández, Rafael O.	160 Ponce de Leon Ave.	San Juan, P. R. 00903
Fernandez, Ricardo F.	160 Ponce de León Ave.	San Juan, P. R. 00903
Ferrero, Jose V.	572 Munoz Rivera Ave.	Hato Rey, P. R. 00918
Ferry, Andrew P.	Fifth Ave. & 100th St.	New York, N. Y. 10029
Ferry, John F.	308 S. Tyler St.	Covington, La. 70433
Ferwerda, James R.	8020 Sheridan Rd.	Kenosha, Wisc. 53140
Fethke, Norbert	54 Church St.	Amsterdam, N. Y. 12010
Feuerman, Martin N.	605 N. Federal Hwy.	Hollywood, Fla. 33020
Fezza, Michael L.	2447 Whitney Ave.	Hamden, Conn. 06518
Fial, Edward A.	330 Buffalo Rd.	E. Aurora, N. Y. 14052
Fiedler, Howard W.	2040 W. Wisconsin Ave.	Milwaukee, Wisc. 53233
Field, Homer B.	13000 S. Maple Ave.	Blue Island, Ill. 60406
Fields, H. Maxwell	405 N. Bedford Dr.	Beverly Hills, Cal. 90210
Fields, Jack	4418 Vineland Ave.	North Hollywood, Cal. 91602
Filante, William J.	1300 S. Eliseo Dr.	Greenbrae, Cal. 94904
Filar, Alfred A., Jr.	611 Park Ave.	Baltimore, Md. 21201
File, Thomas M.	11 W. Monument Ave.	Dayton, O. 45402
Filkins, John C.	The Doctors Bldg.	Omaha, Nebr. 68131
Filmer, George A.	1955 Pennsylvania St.	Denver, Colo. 80203
Finder, Anthony G.	3034 W. Peterson Ave.	Chicago, Ill. 60645
Fine, Abraham	23 Soundview Dr.	Port Jefferson, N. Y. 11777
Fine, Ben S.	915 19th St. N.W.	Washington, D. C. 20006
Fine, Lawrence M.	2107 Third Ave.	San Diego, Cal. 92101
Fine, Max	2233 Post St.	San Francisco, Cal. 94115
Finegan, James F.	558 N. Avenida Sevilla	Laguna Hills, Cal. 92653
Fingerman, Louis H.	1056 Fourth St.	Des Moines, Ia. 50314
Fink, Austin I.	110 Remsen St.	Brooklyn, N. Y. 11201
Fink, Robert J.	4450 W. 76th St.	Edina, Minn. 55435
Finkel, Stanley	20392 Town Center Lane	Cupertino, Cal. 95014
Finkelstein, Elliot	636 Beacon St.	Boston, Mass. 02215
Finlay, James W.	218 S. Trenton Ave.	Pittsburgh, Pa. 15221

Finlay, John R.	49 Lake Ave.	Greenwich, Conn. 06830
Finley, John K.	51 Kings Hwy. W.	Haddonfield, N. J. 08033
Finley, Ralph M., Jr.	602 Julia St.	New Iberia, La. 70560
Finney, Nancy E.	998 S. Monroe	Xenia, O. 45385
Finnin, John J.	47 Forest St.	Medford, Mass. 02155
Finton, Max A.	211 S. High St.	Northport, Mich. 49670
Fiol-Bigas, José	67 Concordia St.	Ponce, P. R. 00731
Fischer, Frank J.	560 Avenue K, S. E.	Winter Haven, Fla. 33880
Fischer, Robert E.	511 S. W. Tenth Ave.	Portland, Ore. 97205
Fish, John H.	207 E. 7th St.	Big Spring, Tex. 79720
Fisher, Albert	1121 Somerville Rd., S. E.	Decatur, Ala. 35601
Fisher, Alvin	3816 Hollywood Blvd.	Hollywood, Fla. 33021
Fisher, Daniel F.	220 S. Claybrook	Memphis, Tenn. 38104
Fisher, George W., Jr.	1629 Owen Dr.	Fayetteville, N. C. 28304
Fisher, H. Noland	505 Clark Ave.	Billings, Mont. 59101
Fisher, John T.	234 E. College Ave.	State College, Pa. 16801
Fisher, Julian J.	2600 Capitol Ave.	Sacramento, Cal. 95816
Fisher, Lawrence C.	469 W. Market St.	York, Pa. 17404
Fisher, Norman F.	25 N. 14th St.	San Jose, Cal. 95112
Fisher, Robert D. A.	116 N. Tucson Blvd.	Tucson, Ariz. 85716
Fisher, Roscoe L.	813 Madison Ave.	York, Pa. 17404
Fishkoff, Daniel	132 Market St.	Perth Amboy, N.J. 08861
Fishman, Gordon R. A. ...	25721 Coolidge	Oak Park, Mich. 48237
Fishman, Ronald S.	106 Irving St. N. W.	Washington, D. C. 20010
Fissell, George McG.	188 Roseville Ave.	Newark, N. J. 07107
Fite, J. Donald	542 Church St.	Decatur, Ga. 30030
Fitzgerald, George T.	3900 W. 95th St.	Evergreen Park, Ill. 60642
Fitzgerald, Gerald P.	124 S. Third St.	Delavan, Wisc. 53115
Fitzgerald, John R.	1360 Mt. Hope Ave.	Rochester, N. Y. 14620
Fitzgerald, J. Robert	6429 W. North Ave.	Oak Park, Ill. 60302
Fitzpatrick, John J.	4951 Center St.	Omaha, Nebr. 68106
Fixott, Richard S.	2131 N. Tejon St.	Colorado Springs, Colo. 80907
Fjordbotten, Alf L.	3801 N. Fairfax Dr.	Arlington, Va. 22203
Flack, Clarence E.	Box 486	Saugatuck, Mich. 49453
Flack, J. Vincent	650 Main St.	New Rochelle, N. Y. 10801
Fladen, Jerome D.	1320 N. Market	Canton, O. 44714
Flagg, Geddes B.	Gulf National Bank Bldg.	Gulfport, Miss. 39501
Flaherty, Norman W.	3677 Fort St.	Lincoln Park, Mich. 48146
Flaherty, Walter T.	17502 Irvine Blvd.	Tustin, Cal. 92680
Flanagan, Joseph C.	39 Glendale Rd.	Upper Darby, Pa. 19082
Flanagan, Roger M.	Shamrock Bldg.	Coos Bay, Ore. 97420
Flanary, Lemuel M.	530 W. 20th St.	Houston, Tex. 77008
Flatley, Robert E.	829 15th St.	Moline, Ill. 61265
Fleckner, Richard A.	1300 Union Tpke.	New Hyde Park, N. Y.
Fleischner, Alois L.	2488 Grand Concourse	Bronx, N. Y. 10458
Fleming, Robert J.	120 1st Capitol Dr.	St. Charles, Mo. 63301
Fletcher, Mary C.	2215 Dorrington St.	Houston, Tex. 77025
Fletcher, Thomas A.	2320½ Dowling St.	Houston, Tex. 77004
Flick, Edward	18532 Firland Way N.	Seattle, Wash. 98133
Flick, John J.	668 E. 38th St.	Indianapolis, Ind. 46205
Flitman, D. Blake	6601 S. W. 80th St.	Miami, Fla. 33143
Flocks, Milton	1101 Welch Rd.	Palo Alto. Cal. 94304
Flom, Leonard	1700 Post Rd.	Fairfield, Conn. 06430
Florentz, Theodore R.	1011 Idaho St.	Boise, Ida. 83702
Flowers, Jeremiah T.	Medical Towers	Louisville, Ky. 40202

Floyd, Glen	508 E. Fifth	Bartlesville, Okla. 74003
Floyd, Paul E.	2 Middle St.	Farmington, Me. 04938
Flynn, Gregory E.	401 Peachtree St., N. E.	Atlanta, Ga. 30308
Flynn, John B.	506 Stanford Rd.	Burbank, Cal. 91504
Flynn, John E.	340 E. Main St.	Bay Shore, N. Y. 11706
Flynn, John T.	1638 N. W. 10th Ave.	Miami, Fla. 33152
Flynn, Martin A.	104 N. Madison Ave.	Pasadena, Cal. 91101
Fogarty, Terence P.	30 E. 40th St.	New York, N. Y. 10016
Fogg, Gary R.	1053 R St.	Fresno, Cal. 93721
Fokes, Robert E. Jr.	1303 4th St., S. W.	Moultrie, Ga. 31768
Folk, Eugene R.	64 Old Orchard	Skokie, Ill. 60076
Fonda, Donald A.	20 Wilsey Sq.	Ridgewood, N. J. 07450
Fonda, Gerald E.	551 Millburn Ave.	Short Hills, N. J. 07078
Fonken, H. A.	1032 Luke St.	Fort Collins, Colo. 80521 ..
Foohey, Fleur C.	146 Jefferson St.	Hartford, Conn. 06103
Foote, C. M.	422 N. Hastings Ave.	Hastings, Nebr. 68901
Foote, William D.	5225 Connecticut Ave. N. W.	Washington, D. C. 20015
Forbes, Max	635 W. 165th St.	New York, N. Y. 10032
Forbush, John J.	1010 Cass St.	Monterey, Cal. 93940
Ford, Donald P.	Hermann Prof. Bldg.	Houston, Tex. 77025
Ford, H. L.	18 Numi Dr.	Fort Lauderdale, Fla 33301
Ford, James C.	3875 Wilshire Blvd.	Los Angeles, Cal. 90005
Fordon, Leona R.	1944 S. Euclid	Berwyn, Ill. 60402
Foree, Kenneth, III	Medical Arts Bldg.	Dallas, Tex. 75201
Forney, Claudius L.	1226 Hyde Park Blvd.	Chicago, Ill. 60615
Forrest, Arnold W.	61 Maple Ave.	White Plains, N. Y. 10601
Forrest, Robert L.	1125 E. 17th St.	Santa Ana, Cal. 92701
Forster, H. Walter, Jr.	37 S. 20th St.	Philadelphia, Pa. 19103
Fortier, Norman L.	85 Jefferson St.	Hartford, Conn. 06106
Foss, Richard H.	21100 Southgate Park Blvd.	Maple Heights, O. 44137
Foss, Robert H.	Equitable Bldg.	Des Moines, Ia. 50309
Fossas, Rafael	First Federal Bldg.	Santurce, P. R. 00909
Foster, Clarence B.	139 E. Pennsylvania Ave.	Southern Pines, N. C. 28387
Foster, George C.	First National Bank Bldg.	Fargo, N. D. 58102
Foster, J. Thomas	24 Second Ave., N. E.	Hickory, N. C. 28601
Foster, Juanita E.	Box 66038	Houston, Tex. 77006
Fountain, Newland W.	400 N. Main St.	Warsaw, N. Y. 14569
Fowler, James G.	412 Linwood Ave.	Buffalo, N. Y. 14209
Fowler, Mary Jane	815 E. Main St.	Medford, Ore. 97501
Fowler, Nathaniel E.	Wyoming Bldg.	Casper, Wyo. 82601
Fox, Francis H.	206 Martin	Twin Falls, Ida. 83301
Fox, J. Robert	637 S. Governors Ave.	Dover, Dela. 19901
Fox, Nathan H.	3172 N. Sheridan Rd.	Chicago, Ill. 60657
Fox, Ralph M.	800 S. Adams Rd.	Birmingham, Mich. 48011
Fox, Samuel L.	1205 St. Paul St.	Baltimore, Md. 21202
Fox, Sherwin A.	3034 W. Peterson	Chicago, Ill. 60645
Fox, Sidney A.	11 E. 90th St.	New York, N. Y. 10028
Foxworthy, Laurel	509 Olive Way	Seattle, Wash. 98101
Fradin, Seymour	20 E. 9th St.	New York, N. Y. 10003
Fralick, F. Bruce	Univ. Medical Ctr.	Ann Arbor, Mich. 48104
Francisco, Manuel	175 N. Jackson Ave.	San Jose, Cal. 95116
Frank, Gordon D.	3707 Gaston Ave.	Dallas, Tex. 75246
Frank, Herman W.	520 Chestnut St.	Gadsden, Ala. 35901
Frank, Joseph J.	State Tower Bldg.	Syracuse, N. Y. 13202
Frank, Paul E.	300 N. York Rd.	Hatboro, Pa. 19040
Frank, Robert L.	York Rd. & Summit Ave.	Hatboro, Pa. 19040

Frank, Walter L.	1515 W. Walnut St.	Jacksonville, Ill. 62650
Frankel, Henry	229 60th St.	West New York, N. J. 07093
Frankel, Jerome	1185 Dundee Ave.	Elgin, Ill. 60120
Frankel, Samuel	20 Washington Pl.	Newark, N. J. 07102
Frankfurt, Majer	104-60 Queens Blvd.	Forest Hills, N. Y. 11375
Franklin, C. Ray	10 E. 90th St.	New York, N. Y. 10028
Franklin, Daniel	4201 E. 22nd Ave.	Denver, Colo. 80207
Franklin, Isadore	238 W. Wisconsin Ave.	Milwaukee, Wisc. 53203
Franklin, John B.	85 Jefferson St.	Hartford, Conn. 06106
Franks, Myron B.	Medical Arts Bldg.	Jamestown, N. Y. 14701
Fratkin, Max	20 Plaza St.	Brooklyn, N. Y. 11238
Fraunfelder, Frederick T. ..	Univ. of Ark. Med. Center	Little Rock, Ark. 72201
Frayer, William C.	829 Spruce St.	Philadelphia, Pa. 19107
Frazin, Lawrence N.	777 E. Brill St.	Phoenix, Ariz. 85006
Fread, Bernard	45 E. 85th St.	New York, N. Y. 10028
Frederick, Albert R., Jr. ...	10 Hawthorne Pl.	Boston, Mass. 02114
Freed, Charles C., Jr.	108 Holbrook Ave.	Danville, Va. 24541
Freedman, Jerome K.	123 York St.	New Haven, Conn. 06511
Freedman, Ruth S.	4910 Forest Park Blvd.	St. Louis, Mo. 63108
Freeman, David	210 Prospect St.	New Haven, Conn. 06511
Freeman, David M.	211 N. Meramec	St. Louis, Mo. 63105
Freeman, H. MacKenzie ...	100 Charles River Plaza	Boston, Mass. 02114
Freeman, Jerre Minor	322 Doctor's Bldg., Methodist Hospital	Memphis, Tenn. 38104
Freemond, Alan S.	19 Garfield Pl.	Cincinnati, O. 45202
Freese, Carl G., Jr.	328 Washington St.	Wellesley Hills, Mass. 02191
Freilich, Dennis B.	20 E. 68 St.	New York, N. Y. 10021
Freimark, Louis	1409 Albemarle Rd.	Brooklyn, N. Y. 11226
Freiwald, Milton J.	222 Rittenhouse Sq. W.	Philadelphia, Pa. 19103
Frell, Albert C.	1008 N. Main	Bloomington, Ill. 61701
French, Alfred R.	52 E. Monterey Way	Phoenix, Ariz. 85012
French, Harry J.	52 E. Monterey Way	Phoenix, Ariz. 85012
Frenkel, Henry H.	827 North Ave.	Bridgeport, Conn. 06606
Frenkel, Marcel	122 S. Michigan Ave.	Chicago, Ill. 60603
Frey, James L.	Northland Medical Bldg.	Southfield, Mich. 48076
Frey, Thomas	6231 Leesburg Pike	Falls Church, Va. 22044
Frey, Walter D.	200 W. 2nd St.	Lexington, Ky. 40507
Frey, Walter W.	641 Medical Arts Bldg.	Nashville, Tenn. 37212
Fricker, Stephen J.	243 Charles St.	Boston, Mass. 02114
Fried, Joseph J.	5 W. 86th St.	New York, N. Y. 10024
Freidland, Walter	289 Essex St.	Hackensack, N. J. 07601
Friedlander, Miles H.	1419 Delachaise St.	New Orleans, La. 70115
Friedman, Alan J.	120 E. 36th St.	New York, N. Y. 10016
Friedman, Benjamin	3 E. 74th St.	New York, N. Y. 10021
Friedman, Bernard B.	Jones Bldg.	Corpus Christi, Tex. 78401
Friedman, Bernard S.	6510 Hillcroft Ave.	Houston, Tex. 77036
Friedman, Ephraim	750 Harrison Ave.	Boston, Mass. 02118
Friedman, Harry S.	Doctors Bldg.	Minneapolis, Minn. 55402
Friedman, Joseph J.	57 Midwood St.	Brooklyn, N. Y. 11225
Friedman, M. Wallace	2233 Post St.	San Francisco, Cal. 94115
Friedman, Michael H.	520 Westfield Ave.	Elizabeth, N. J. 07208
Friedson, Bernard	495 Broadway	Saratoga Springs, N. Y. 12866
Friendly, David S.	Children's Hospital of the District of Columbia	Washington, D. C. 20009
Frisch, Frederick B.	7 S. Dudley Ave.	Ventnor, N. J. 08406

Frisch, Michael R.	2021 Santa Monica Blvd.	Santa Monica, Cal. 90404
Fritch, John M.	710 S. 21st St.	Lafayette, Ind. 47905
Fritsche, Theodore R.	510 First North St.	New Ulm, Minn. 56073
Fritz, Milo H.	2235 Vanderbilt Cir.	Anchorage, Alaska 99504
Frost, John B.	Doctors' Bldg.	Minneapolis, Minn. 55402
Fry, John R.	Doctors' Bldg.	Asheville, N. C. 28801
Fry, Wilfred E.	1930 Chestnut St.	Philadelphia, Pa. 19103
Frydman, Joseph E.	130 E. Randolph Ave.	Chicago, Ill. 60601
Fuelling, James L.	131 N. Washington St.	Marion, Ind. 46952
Fuerste, Frederick, Jr.	1360 Dodge St.	Dubuque, Ia. 52001
Fuhring, S. A.	801 E. Chapel	Santa Maria, Cal. 93454
Fuhs, John C.	Carew Tower	Cincinnati, O. 45202
Fullenwider, Charles G.	Barnes Bldg.	Muskogee, Okla. 74401
Fulmer, John M.	5410 W. Markham St.	Little Rock, Ark. 72205
Fulton, Harry C.	339 N. Duke St.	Lancaster, Pa. 17602
Fung, Wayne E.	2400 Clay St.	San Francisco, Cal. 94115
Funk, Harold A.	1073 Cass St.	Monterey, Cal. 93940
Furgiuele, Francis P.	5430 Greene St.	Philadelphia, Pa. 19144
Fusco, John A.	9209 Colima Rd.	Whittier, Cal. 90605
Gabriel, Carson K.	2421 Kentucky Rd.	Quincy, Ill. 62301
Gabriels, J. A. C.	485 Western Ave.	Albany, N. Y. 12203
Gaddy, George D.	1608 Memorial Dr.	Burlington, N. C. 27217
Gadomski, Casimir F.	331 S. Broad St.	Elizabeth, N. J. 07202
Gage, Tracy D.	4020 21st St.	Lubbock, Texas 79410
Gager, Walter E.	8700 W. Wisconsin Ave.	Milwaukee, Wisc. 53226
Gagliardi, George R.	56 Proctor St.	Framingham, Mass. 01701
Gahagan, Lawrence O.	6120 Sherry Ln.	Dallas, Tex. 75225
Gaida, Joseph B.	Physicians & Surgeons' Bldg.	St. Cloud, Minn. 56301
Gaines, Shelley R.	211 S. Saratoga St.	New Orleans, La. 70112
Gaines, Thos. R.	P. O. Box 1226	Anderson, S. C. 29621
Galantowicz, Thomas H.	23601 Ford Rd.	Dearborn, Mich. 48128
Galas, Stanley M.	Madigan Gen. Hosp.	Ft. Lewis, Wash. 98433
Galin, Miles A.	1249 Fifth Ave.	New York, N. Y. 10029
Gallaher, David M.	Irving Zuelke Bldg.	Appleton, Wisc. 54911
Gallaher, John A.	1808 San Miguel Dr.	Walnut Creek, Cal. 94596
Gallizzi, D. Vincent	643 Charles Ave.	Kingston, Pa. 18704
Galman, Barry D.	406 Cooper St.	Camden, N. J. 08102
Galt, John	222 South St.	Pittsfield, Mass. 01201
Galyon, Frank B., Jr.	715 Walnut St.	Knoxville, Tenn. 37902
Gambacorta, Humbert M.	605 Broad St.	Newark, N. J. 07102
Gambill, Harold D.	240 Meridian Ave.	San Jose, Cal. 95126
Gamble, Lyne S.	344 Arnold Ave.	Greenville, Miss. 38701
Gammill, Ralph R.	4809 College Ave.	Lubbock, Tex. 79413
Gan, Walter S.	8101 Bradford St.	Philadelphia, Pa. 19152
Gans, Jack S.	505 Wanaque Ave.	Pompton Lakes, N. J. 07442
Gans, Jerome A.	1020 Huron Rd.	Cleveland, O. 44115
Gans, Morris E.	1621 Euclid Ave.	Cleveland, O. 44115
Gans, Robert I.	26615 Greenfield	Southfield, Mich. 48075
Garabedian, Vahe	86-88 Walnut St.	Binghamton, N. Y. 13905
Garcia, George E.	636 Beacon St.	Boston, Mass. 02213
Garden, John W.	180 Market St.	Lexington, Ky. 40507
Gardiner, Frederick S.	6475 Alvarado Rd.	San Diego, Cal. 92120
Garfinkle, Carl	1430 N. Arlington Hts. Rd.	Arlington Hts., Ill. 60004
Garland, Leslie C.	3640 Lomita Blvd.	Torrance, Cal. 90505
Garland, Marvin A.	1433 W. Merced	West Covina, CAl. 91790
Garner, Lawrence L.	P. O. Box 1608	Milwaukee, Wisc. 53201

Garnier, William H.	815 S. Pine St.	Stillwater, Okla. 74074
Garnish, John A.	780 Blossom Rd.	Rochester, N. Y. 14534
Garrett, Edwin E.	Memorial Profess. Bldg.	Houston, Tex. 77002
Garrett, Frank E.	877 W. Fremont	Sunnyvale, Cal. 94087
Garrett, Spencer R.	203 Kerneywood	Lakeland, Fla. 33803
Garrison, Leland M.	4817 E. Second St.	Long Beach, Cal. 90803
Garron, Levon K.	426 17th St.	Oakland, Cal. 94612
Gart, Peter	50 E. 72nd St.	New York, N. Y. 10021
Garten, Joseph L.	308 Doctors Bldg.	Minneapolis, Minn. 55402
Gartner, Samuel	1749 Grand Concourse	New York, N.Y. 10453
Garvin, Edward J.	1614 S. Byrne Rd.	Toledo, O. 43614
Garvin, William J.	576 N. Broadway	Yonkers, N.Y. 10701
Gaskin, Ernest R.	101 Doctors Bldg.	Charlotte, N.C. 28207
Gass, John D. M.	1638 N.W. 10th Ave.	Miami, Fla. 33136
Gaston, Ira E.	Medical Dental Bldg.	Portland, Ore. 97205
Gates, Charles L.	427 S. Bernard	Spokane, Wash. 99203
Gates, Lawrence K.	167 E. 2nd N.	Logan, Utah 84321
Gates, Ronald F.	2617 E. 21st St.	Tulsa, Okla. 74114
Gatto, Frank M.	121 S. Highland Ave.	Pittsburgh, Pa. 15206
Gaudreau, Honoré E.	293 Bridge St.	Springfield, Mass. 01103
Gay, Andrew J.	211 N. Meramec Ave.	St. Louis, Mo. 63105
Gaynes, Philip M.	1700 Post Rd.	Fairfield, Conn. 06430
Gaynin, Henry T.	200 W. 58th St.	New York, N. Y. 10019
Gaynon, Irwin E.	231 W. Wisconsin Ave.	Milwaukee, Wisc. 53203
Gazala, Joseph R.	6001 Lakeside Ave.	Richmond, Va. 23228
Gebel, Emile L.	Post Office Box 1469	Shelby, N. C. 28150
Geeseman, George R.	756 Osage Rd.	Pittsburgh, Pa. 15243
Gehring, John R.	328 Washington St.	Wellesley Hills, Mass. 02181
Gelber, Philip J.	2558 Fourth Ave.	San Diego, Cal. 92103
Geltzer, Athur I.	159 Waterman St.	Providence, R. I. 02906
Gentry, James H.	5125 E. Yale	Denver, Colo. 80222
George, Anastasios B.	616 Asylum Ave.	Hartford, Conn. 06105
George, Craig W.	537 E. Market St.	Alliance, O. 44601
George, Lewis C.	23315 Washington	Colton, Cal. 92324
George, Theo. R.	1912 16th St., N.W.	Washington, D. C. 20011
Gerber, Edward P.	6945 Fair Oaks Blvd.	Carmichael, Cal. 95608
Gerber, Margaret	2500 Ridge Ave.	Evanston, Ill. 60201
Gerberg, Israel	1 Nevins St.	Brooklyn, N.Y. 11217
Gerneth, George J.	422 Library St.	Braddock, Pa. 15104
Gernon, William	106 N. 'M' St.	Lake Worth, Fla. 33460
Gerstel, Frederick J.	4 E. 84th St.	New York, N. Y. 10028
Gerstenfeld, J.	4303 Hylan Blvd.	Staten Island, N. Y. 10312
Gess, Lowell A.	221 N. 5th St.	Bismarck, N. D. 58501
Gessler, William F.	402 Boone Ln.	Fairhope, Ala. 36532
Gettelfinger, Ralph A.	Brown Bldg.	Louisville, Ky. 40202
Gettes, Bernard C.	1930 Chestnut St.	Philadelphia, Pa. 19103
Ghent, Thomas D.	1518 Elizabeth Ave.	Charlotte, N. C.
Gianarelli, Emilio	8 North St.	Barre, Vermont 05641
Giannasio, Joseph	2630 Kennedy Blvd.	Jersey City, N. J. 07306
Gibb, W. Blake	1515 State St.	Santa Barbara, Cal. 93104
Gibbins, George W.	1029 Christine Ave.	Anniston, Ala. 36201
Gibson, Glen G.	2031 Locust St.	Philadelphia, Pa. 19103
Gibson, Harry C.	725 Sixth Ave. E.	Kalispell, Mont. 59901
Gibson, William J.	168 Marine St.	St. Augustine, Fla. 32084
Gieser, E. Paul	188 College St.	Battle Creek, Mich. 49017
Gieser, P. Kenneth	1492 N. Main St.	Wheaton, Ill. 60187

Gifford, Byron L.	215 W. Pueblo St.	Santa Barbara, Cal. 93105
Gifford, Edward S., Jr.	1913 Spruce St.	Philadelphia, Pa. 19103
Gifford, Harold	8300 Dodge St.	Omaha, Nebr. 68114
Gilbert, Ralph H.	26 Sheldon Ave. S. E.	Grand Rapids, Mich. 49502
Gilbert, S. Clifford	2701 W. Alameda	Burbank, Cal. 91505
Gilbert, Walter R., Jr.	2535 Riverside Ave.	Jacksonville, Fla. 32204
Gilbert, William S.	106 Irving St. N. W.	Washington, D. C.
Gilcrest, Harry R.	1448 E. Center	Pocatello, Ida. 83201
Giles, Conrad L.	Northland Medical Bldg.	Southfield, Mich. 48075
Giles, Newell W.	1 Atlantic St.	Stamford, Conn. 06901
Gill, Theodore M.	Freeborn Bank Bldg.	Albert Lea, Minn. 56007
Giller, Herbert	2040 W. Wisconsin Ave.	Milwaukee, Wisc. 53233
Gillespie, Frederick D.	1205 Market St.	Parkersburg, W. Va. 26101
Gillette, David R.	7222 Owensmouth Ave.	Canoga Park, Cal. 91303
Gilliam, Robert D.	516 Cassidy St.	Oceanside, Cal. 92054
Gilligan, John H., Jr.	1707 Osage St.	Alexandria, Va. 22302
Gilliland, Donald C.	3434 N. W. 56	Oklahoma City, Okla. 73112
Gillim, Parvin D.	Hume Mansur Bldg.	Indianapolis, Ind. 46204
Gillis, Marion H., Jr.	206 Walnut St.	Salisbury, Md. 21801
Gillman, A. Marvin	54 E. 72nd St.	New York, N. Y. 10021
Gillis, Richard J.	989 James St.	Syracuse, N. Y. 13203
Gillman, Marvin A.	54 E. 72nd St.	New York, N. Y. 10021
Gills, James P.	4312 U. S. Hwy. 19, N.	Tarpon Springs, Fla. 33589
Gilroy, Francis J.	53 Main St.	Binghamton, N. Y. 13905
Gilroy, Regina V.	131 Fulton Ave.	Hempstead, N. Y. 11550
Ginsberg, Joseph	2837 Burnet Ave.	Cincinnati, O. 45219
Giotta, Peter J.	328 Maple St.	San Diego, Cal. 92103
Giovinco, Joseph	706 Franklin St.	Tampa, Fla. 33602
Gipner, John F.	277 Alexander St.	Rochester, N. Y. 14607
Girard, Louis J.	1200 Moursund Ave.	Houston, Tex. 77025
Girard, Paul H.	258 Genesee St.	Utica, N. Y. 13502
Gitter, Kurt A.	1514 Delachaise St.	New Orleans, La. 70115
Givner, Isadore	108 E. 66th St.	New York, N. Y. 10021
Glaser, Joel S.	1638 N. W. 10th Ave.	Miami, Fla. 33136
Glass, William I.	881 Lafayette St.	Bridgeport, Conn. 06603
Glassman, Leonard H.	185 Cedar Lane	Teaneck, N. J. 07666
Gleichauf, John G.	105 E. Marcy St.	Santa Fe, N. M. 87501
Gleitsman, Louis A.	434 High St., N.E.	Warren, O. 44481
Glenn, Leland K.	2301 W. First St.	Ft. Myers, Fla. 33901
Glew, William B.	7700 Connecticut Ave.	Chevy Chase, Md. 20015
Glins, Richard J.	213 Dayton St.	Hamilton, O. 45011
Glotfelty, John W.	1247 Lakeland Hills Blvd.	Lakeland, Fla. 33801
Glover, Clarence K.	2301 Fall Hill Ave.	Fredericksburg, Va. 22401
Glueck, Sidney J.	41 W. McCreight	Springfield, O. 45504
Goad, Robley R.	101 Iowa Ave.	Muscatine, Ia. 52761
Goar, Everett L.	Memorial Professional Bldg.	Houston, Tex. 77002
Goble, Joan H.	101 S. San Mateo Dr.	San Mateo, Cal. 94401
Goble, John L.	101 S. San Mateo Dr.	San Mateo, Cal. 94401
Gocke, Jack T.	Prunty Bldg.	Clarksburg, W. Va. 26301
Goduti, Richard J.	9 Deering St.	Portland, Me. 04101
Godwin, Edmund D.	Professional Bldg.	Long Beach, Cal. 90813
Goetzman, Arthur C.	604 Sunnyside Ct.	Ft. Myers, Fla. 33901
Goff, John L.	11600 Wilshire Blvd.	West Los Angeles, Cal. 90025
Goff, John R.	737 Broadway	Fargo, N. D. 58102
Gold, Allen B.	675 Broadway	Paterson, N. J. 07514

Gold, Arthur A.	893 Central Ave.	Woodmere, N. Y. 11598
Gold, Herbert	99 Pratt St.	Hartford, Conn. 06103
Goldberg, Bernard	213 Madison Ave.	New York, N. Y. 10016
Goldberg, Harry	88-02 150th St.	Jamaica, N. Y. 11435
Goldberg, Harry F.	37 St. Andrews Pl.	Yonkers, N. Y. 10705
Goldberg, Herman K.	807 Cathedral St.	Baltimore, Md. 21201
Goldberg, Jack L.	81 S. Fifth St.	Columbus, O. 43215
Goldberg, Julian R.	6609 Reisterstown Rd.	Baltimore, Md. 21215
Goldberg, Louis	515 W. Main St.	Norristown, Pa. 19401
Goldberg, Morton F.	Illinois Eye and Ear Infirmary	Chicago, Ill.
Goldberg, Richard E.	1333 Buck Rd.	Feasterville, Pa. 19047
Goldberg, Robert T.	142-10 Roosevelt Ave.	Flushing, N. Y. 11354
Goldberg, Sol	Jenkins Bldg.	Pittsburgh, Pa. 15222
Goldblum, Abraham D.	3347 Forbes Ave.	Pittsburgh, Pa. 15213
Goldcamp, John S.	Dollar Bank Bldg.	Youngstown, O. 44503
Golden, John J.	10 W. Martin Ave.	Naperville, Ill. 60540
Golden, Stanley	93 Arch St.	Redwood City, Cal. 94062
Goldfarb, Harold J.	101 S. 17th St.	Allentown, Pa. 18104
Goldman, Henry	627 Salem Ave.	Dayton, O. 45406
Goldman, Irving S.	3347 Forbes Ave.	Pittsburgh, Pa. 15213
Goldman, Jerome	1033 S. W. Yamhill St.	Portland, Ore. 97205
Goldman, Jerome N.	2150 Pennsylvania Ave. N. W.	Washington, D. C. 20037
Goldor, Howard	600 Coffee Rd.	Modesto, Cal. 95350
Goldsby, Henry H., Jr.	1600 Fairfield	Shreveport, La. 71101
Goldsmith, Charles P.	501 N. 17th St.	Allentown, Pa. 18104
Goldsmith, Jacob	30 E. 60th St.	New York, N. Y. 10022
Goldsmith, Maximilian O.	1261 Central Ave.	Far Rockaway, N. Y. 11691
Goldsmith, Robert I.	Michigan Theatre Bldg.	Ann Arbor, Mich. 48108
Goldstein, Arthur M.	2301 S. Broad St.	Philadelphia, Pa. 19148
Goldstein, Edward S.	1880 N. E. 163rd St.	Miami, Fla. 33162
Goldstein, Homer E.	503 E. Park Ave.	Libertyville, Ill. 60048
Goldstein, Jack E.	3791 Katella Ave.	Los Alamitos, Cal. 90720
Goldstein, Jacob W.	193 Ocean Ave.	Brooklyn, N. Y. 11225
Goldstein, Jerome J.	260 Edwards Blvd.	Long Beach, N. Y. 11561
Goldstein, Joseph H.	450 Clarkson Ave.	Brooklyn, N. Y. 11203
Goldstein, Marvin F.	400 E. 91st St.	Kansas City, Mo. 64131
Goldstein, Paul H.	2040 W. Wisconsin Ave.	Milwaukee, Wisc. 53233
Goldstrohm, Robert G.	834 Philadelphia St.	Indiana, Pa. 15701
Gollance, Robert B.	150 Hinchman Ave.	Wayne, N. J. 07470
Gollihar, William P.	598 Westwood Dr.	Abilene, Tex. 79603
Gomon, Louis D.	1203 N. Michigan Ave.	Saginaw, Mich. 48602
González, Caleb	Ashford Med. Ctr.	Santurce, P. R. 00907
Gonzalez-Jimenez, Enrique	Munoz Rivera 30	Caguas, P. R. 00625
Gonzalez, Ubaldo, U. G.	350 S. Broadway	Hicksville, L. I., N. Y. 11801
Good, Palmer W.	715 Lake St.	Oak Park, Ill. 60301
Good, Philip S.	112 Prospect St.	Waterbury, Conn. 06702
Good, Robert C.	112 Prospect St.	Waterbury, Conn. 06702
Goodall, Edwin B.	N. Main St.	Wolfeboro, N. H. 03894
Goodman, Edward	1882 Grand Concourse	Bronx, N. Y. 10457
Goodman, Edward F.	236 Highland Ave.	Somerville, Mass. 02143
Goodman, George	375 E. Main St.	Bayshore, N. Y. 11706
Goodman, Sanders A.	4955 Van Nuys Blvd.	Sherman Oaks, Cal. 91403
Goodner, Ernest K.	95 Kirkham St.	San Francisco, Cal. 94122
Goodside, Victor	1777 Grand Concourse	New York, N. Y. 10453
Goodstein, Seymour	209-11 Union Tnpke.	Bayside, N. Y. 11364
Goodwin, Ralph A., Jr.	33 Court St.	Auburn, Me. 04210

Goodwin, Rufus C.	2000 Van Ness Ave.	San Francisco, Cal. 04109
Goorchenko, V. A.	215 Avenida Del Norte	Redondo Beach, Cal. 90277
Gordon, Betty C.	99 Lafayette Ave.	Brooklyn, N. Y. 11217
Gordon, Carl J.	6333 Wilshire Blvd.	Los Angeles, Cal. 90048
Gordon, Dan M.	441 E. 68th St.	New York, N. Y. 10021
Gordon, Devitt L.	Ohio Bldg.	Akron, O. 44308
Gordon, Orville E.	6450 N. California Ave.	Chicago, Ill. 60645
Gordonson, Lewis C.	1300 Union Tpke.	New Hyde Park, N. Y. 11040
Goren, Seymour B.	Prudential Plaza	Chicago, Ill. 60601
Gorin, Edward F.	841 W. San Bruno Ave.	San Bruno, Cal. 94066
Gorin, George	585 W. End Ave.	New York, N. Y. 10024
Gorin, Malcolm	141 Broad St.	Middletown, Conn. 06467
Gorrilla. L. Vincent	2665 Walnut St.	Huntington Park, Cal. 90255
Goss, Vernon V.	1120 Medical Dr.	Tyler, Tex. 75701
Gostin, Seymour B.	4500 S. Lancaster Rd.	Dallas, Tex. 75205
Gottlieb, Fred	499 Ocean Ave.	Brooklyn, N. Y. 11226
Gottlieb, Louis N.	1210 Reynolds Bldg.	Winston-Salem, N. C. 27101
Gould, Edward L.	470 Tollgate Rd.	Warwick, R. I. 02886
Gould, Herbert L.	90 Greenridge Ave.	White Plains, N. Y. 10605
Goulston, Ralph N.	1720 Marco Polo Way	Burlingame, Cal. 94010
Goumas, Melto	1303 San Carlos Ave.	San Carlos, Cal. 94070
Grabow, Emil F.	7905 Calumet Ave.	Munster, Ind. 46321
Grace, Eugene V.	911 Broad St.	Durham, N. C. 27705
Graether, John M.	309 E. Church St.	Marshalltown, Ia. 50158
Graff, Henry F.	115 N. Potomac St.	Hagerstown, Md. 21740
Grafflin, Allan L.	2 Orchard Lane	Danvers, Mass. 01923
Grafton, Edwin G.	8226 Douglas	Dallas, Tex. 75225
Graham, Donald A.	Medical Arts Bldg.	Tacoma, Wash. 98402
Graham, George A.	842 Carroll St.	Brooklyn, N.Y. 11215
Graham, John H.	5370 Pearl Rd.	Parma, O. 44129
Graham, Robert W.	1000 Pine St.	Klamath Falls, Ore. 97601
Graham, Walter R.	1012 Kings Dr.	Charlotte, N. C. 28207
Grana, Philip C.	422 Library St.	Braddock, Pa. 15104
Grant, Charles P.	924 S. 18th St.	Birmingham, Ala. 35205
Grant, William D.	25100 Euclid Ave.	Euclid, O. 44117
Grant, William F.	309 Roseville Ave.	Newark, N. J. 07107
Grant, William F., Jr.	138 Buckingham Rd.	Upper Montclair, N. J. 07043
Grant, W. Morton	243 Charles St.	Boston, Mass. 02114
Grassi, Anthony J.	20316 Collegewood Dr.	Walnut, Cal. 91789
Grave de Peralta, Jose I. ...	2740 Hollywood Blvd.	Hollywood, Fla. 33020
Graves, Orville M., Jr.	1020 Prospect St.	La Jolla, Cal. 92037
Gray, Claude C.	2701 Eye St.	Sacramento, Cal. 95816
Gray, H. William	4501 Connecticut Ave. N.W. ...	Washington, D. C. 20008
Gray, Joseph W.	993 Cass St.	Monterey, Cal. 93940
Grayman, Harry M.	2912 Fresno St.	Fresno, Cal. 93721
Grayson, Merrill	Indiana University Medical Center	Indianapolis, Ind. 46202
Greco, Gabriel J.	161 St. Nicholas Ave.	New York, N. Y. 10011
Greear, James N., Jr.	975 Ryland St.	Reno, Nev. 89502
Green, Carl A.	VA Hospital	Columbia, S. C. 29201
Green, Earl W.	705 Hall Ave.	Hattiesburg, Miss. 39401
Green, Frank M.	165 N. Village Ave.	Rockville Centre, N. Y. 11570
Green, Hyman S.	6420 N. California Ave	Chicago, Ill. 60645
Green, John E.	Box 1230	Hattiesburg, Miss. 39401

Green, Kenneth O.	301 W. Lincoln St.	Belleville, Ill. 62220
Green, Manuel	831 Plymouth Ave.	Schenectady, N. Y. 12308
Green, Marvin F.	2307 N. W. Overton	Portland, Ore. 97210
Green, Ray L.	220 St. Louis	Plainview, Tex. 79072
Green, Robert D.	214 Engle St.	Engelwood, N. J. 07631
Green, William R.	Armed Forces Inst. of Path.	Washington, D. C. 20305
Greenberg, Maynard M.	1421 Dodge St.	Omaha, Nebr. 68102
Greenberg, Milton	875 Central Ave.	Far Rockaway, N. Y. 11691
Greenberg, Richard S.	Medical Arts Bldg.	Omaha, Nebr. 68102
Greenberger, Merrill H.	64 Old Orchard	Skokie, Ill. 60076
Greene, Maurice L.	821 Quince Ave.	McAllen, Tex. 78501
Greene, Philip B.	422 Riverside	Spokane, Wash. 99201
Greene, Richard W.	633 Nye Ave.	Irvington, N. J. 07111
Greenfield, Philip	7711 Louis Pasteur	San Antonio, Tex. 78229
Greenfield, S. Jerome	2130 Millburn Ave.	Maplewood, N. J. 07040
Greenlee, Max R.	2750 Broadway	Boulder, Colo. 80302
Greenspan, David A.	904½ E. Southmore	Pasadena, Tex. 77502
Greenspan, Martin E.	3051 Long Beach Rd.	Oceanside, N. Y. 11572
Greenwood, M. Allen	707 Jewett Ave.	Staten Island, N. Y. 10314
Greetham, James S.	313 Bradford St.	Marion, O. 43302
Gregg, Frank H.	1015 E. 32nd St.	Austin, Tex. 78705
Gregory, Eugene B.	Hermann Professional Bldg.	Houston, Tex. 77025
Gressette, James H.	920 Holly St.	Orangeburg, S. C. 29115
Gridley, Lawrence J.	214 W. 27th St.	Scottsbluff, Nebr. 69361
Griesemer, Laurence C.	230 W. Jersey St.	Elizabeth, N.J. 07202
Griesemer, Z. Lawrence	515 Locust St.	Rozelle, N. J. 07203
Griffey, Edward W.	Medical Towers	Houston, Tex. 77025
Griffin, Carlton Gonrad	118 Hospital Dr.	Lafayette, La. 70501
Griffin, Richard M.	27 13th Ave., N.E.	Hickory, N. C. 28601
Griffin, Robert M.	90 E. Main St.	Norwich, N. Y. 13815
Griffith, Don G.	2402 W. Jefferson St.	Boise, Ida. 83702
Griffith, Perry P.	520 Franklin Ave.	Garden City, N. Y. 11530
Griffiths, Anthony	1, Atlantic St.	Stamford, Conn. 06901
Griggs, Walter C.	2 Maynard St.	Hanover, N. H. 03755
Grimaldi, Americo J.	1609 Pasadena Ave. S.	St. Petersburg, Fla. 33707
Grimes, M. Osmond	57 Kay St.	Newport, R. I. 02840
Grindle, Lincoln	32331 Coast Hwy.	South Laguna, Cal. 92677
Grisham, Richard S. C.	Price Tower	Bartlesville, Okla. 74003
Grivas, Plato J.	2021 Ygnacio Valley Rd.	Walnut Creek, Cal. 94598
Grizzard, Henry T.	5050 Poplar	Memphis, Tenn. 38117
Groom, Joseph J.	4950 S.W. LeJeune Rd.	Coral Gables, Fla. 33146
Grossmann, Erwin E.	836 N. 12th St.	Milwaukee, Wisc. 53233
Groth, Robert C.	14031 Ambaum Blvd. S. W.	Seattle, Wash. 98166
Grove, Bruce A.	426 W. Market St.	York, Pa. 17404
Grove, Raymond F.	Murchison Bldg.	Wilmington, N. C. 28401
Grove, William K.	426 W. Market St.	York, Pa. 17404
Grow, Kenneth A.	1031 N. Palm Canyon Dr.	Palm Springs, Cal. 92262
Gruber, Ellis	1675 Monroe Ave.	Rochester, N. Y. 14618
Gsell, George F.	3244 E. Douglas	Wichita, Kans. 67208
Gualtieri, S. J.	550 W. Thomas Rd.	Phoenix, Ariz. 85013
Guber, Donald	1021 E. Robinson St.	Orlando, Fla. 32801
Guerry, DuPont, III	2015 Monument Ave.	Richmond, Va. 23220
Guibor, George P.	615 W. Main St.	Ottawa, Ill. 61350
Guida, Anthony J.	420 Estudillo Ave.	San Leandro, Cal. 94577
Guida, Francis P.	1441 Chapel St.	New Haven, Conn. 06511
Guido, Angelina	7719 Rocton Ave.	Chevy Chase, Md. 20015

Guiduli, Robert C.	308 Pearl St.	Burlington, Vt. 05401
Guillette, James L.	390 Main St.	Worcester, Mass. 01608
Guldjord, Knute M.	Box 2125, Sheridan Village	Bremerton, Wash. 98310
Gulyash, Joseph J. F.	756 S. Dora St.	Ukiah, Cal. 95482
Gumm, Melvin L.	1805 Walnut St.	Red Bluff, Cal. 96080
Gump, Millard E.	411 30th St.	Oakland, Cal. 94609
Gundersen, Trygve	720 Harrison Ave.	Boston, Mass. 02118
Gunderson, Ernest O.	2511 Hearst	Berkeley, Cal. 94709
Gundzik, John D.	223 E. Palace Ave.	Santa Fe, N. M. 87501
Gunzburg, Julian	193 N. Robertson Blvd.	Beverly Hills, Cal. 90211
Gurau, Henry H.	Des Moines Bldg.	Des Moines, Ia. 50309
Gurland, Bernard B.	146 W. 37th St.	Bayonne, N. J. 07002
Gurwin, Bernard J.	1800 Eye St., N.W.	Washington, D. C. 20006
Gussler, C. Gordon	Mayo Arcade	Ashland, Ky. 41101
Gustafson, Olga F.	185 N. Wabash Ave.	Chicago, Ill. 60601
Gutman, Froncie A.	Cleveland Clinic, 2020 E. 93rd St.	Cleveland, O. 44106
Gutow, Richard F.	University of Michigan Medical Center	Ann Arbor, Mich. 48104
Gutstein, Naphtali	4801 Church St.	Skokie, Ill. 60076
Guttuso, Thomas J.	225 Bewley Bldg.	Lockport, N. Y. 14094
Guy, Loren P.	1324 Richmond Rd.	Williamsburg, Va. 23185
Guyton, Jack S.	Henry Ford Hosp.	Detroit, Mich. 48202
Guzek, Joseph T.	431 Wyoming Ave.	Scranton, Pa. 18503
Gwathemey, Tayloe	1017 E. Robinson Ave.	Orlando, Fla. 32801
Haas, Joseph S.	1725 W. Harrison St.	Chicago, Ill. 60612
Habeeb, Albert F. W.	Pere Marquette Bldg.	New Orleans, La. 70112
Haddad, Heskel, M.	Beth Israel Medical Center	New York, N. Y. 10003
Hadlund, Ralph L.	2001 Kimball Ave.	Waterloo, Ia. 50702
Haffly, Gilbert N.	509 Olive Way	Seattle, Wash. 98101
Hafner, John N.	1169 Eastern Parkway	Louisville, Ky. 40217
Haft, Abraham S.	1100 Grand Concourse	Bronx, N. Y. 10456
Hagele, James,	152 Catherine Ln.	Grass Valley, Cal. 95945
Hagens, Walter E.	1400 W. 47th St.	La Grange, Ill. 60525
Hagigh, M. Reza	1111 Park Ave.	Baltimore, Md. 21201
Hagler, William S.	Emory Univ. Clinic	Altanta, Ga. 30322
Hagood, Daniel S.	750 Washington Ave.	Montgomery, Ala. 36104
Hagopian, Varant	129 Mt. Auburn St.	Cambridge, Mass. 02138
Hague, Eliott B.	1109 Delaware Ave.	Buffalo, N. Y. 14209
Hahn, Robert E.	8601 W. Dodge Rd.	Omaha, Nebr. 68114
Hahn, William H.	71 Valley St.	South Orange, N. J. 07079
Haik, George M.	812 Maison Blanche Bldg.	New Orleans, La. 70112
Haik, Hilliard M.	Maison Blanche Bldg.	New Orleans, La. 70012
Haines, Robert W.	15 N. Main St.	West Hartford, Conn. 06107
Haire, Paul G.	585 Main St.	Malden, Mass. 02148
Haisten, M. Wyatt	Doctors Bldg.	Beamont, Tex. 77701
Halasa, Adnan H.	University of Iowa	Iowa City, La. 52240
Halberg, G. Peter	40 W. 77th St.	New York, N. Y. 10024
Halden, Harry E. III	600 South Street	New Orleans, La. 70130
Hale, Channing W.	174 Nemaha St.	Pomona, Cal. 91767
Hale, L. Morgan	UNC School of Medicine	Chapel Hill, N. C. 27514
Hale, Philip N.	3955 Harrison Blvd.	Ogden, Utah 84403
Hales, Robert H.	1275 N. University Ave.	Provo, Utah 84601
Haley, Warren D.	78 Church St.	Winchester, Mass. 01890
Hall, Donald S.	First National Bank Bldg.	Vicksburg, Miss. 39180
Hall, George A.	1541 N. W. 54th	Seattle, Wash. 98107
Hall, J. Herod	264 Cohasset Lane	Chico, Cal. 95926

Hall, James M.	914 E. Jefferson Blvd.	South Bend, Ind. 46617
Hall, Lawrence H.	1520 Oak St.	South Pasadena, Cal. 91030
Hall, Robert C.	654 W. Forest Ave.	Jackson, Tenn. 38301
Hall, Thomas G.	3637 Sacramento	San Francisco, Cal. 94108
Halle, Margaret A.	3364 Poplar	Memphis, Tenn. 38111
Hallett, Joseph W.	Medical Arts Bldg.	Philadelphia, Pa. 19102
Hallock, Earle K.	174 S. Grove St.	Freeport, N. Y. 11520
Hallum, Alton V.	490 Peachtree St., N.E.	Atlanta, Ga. 30308
Hallum, Basil A.	1812 N. Oregon	El Paso, Tex. 79902
Halpern, Jesse I.	209 S. Broadway	Nyack, N. Y. 10960
Hamdi, Turgut N.	2004 Delancey Pl.	Philadelphia, Pa. 19103
Hamilton, Quentin P.	20905 Greenfield	Southfield, Mich. 48075
Hamilton, Ralph S.	Exchange Bldg.	Memphis, Tenn. 38103
Hammerman, Murray F.	11125 Rockville Pike	Rockville, Md. 20852
Hammerstad, Lynn M.	EENT Clinic, 607 Tenth Ave.	Fairbanks, Alaska 99701
Hamrick, George V.	Atlas Bldg.	Charleston, W. Va. 25301
Hamtil, Lawrence W.	3700 W. 83rd St.	Prairie Village, Kans. 66208
Haney, David G.	210 S. Grand	Glendora, Cal. 91740
Haney, Lawrence O.	104 E. St. Vrain St.	Colorado Springs, Colo. 80902
Haney, Robert F.	2330 N. W. Flanders	Portland, Ore. 97210
Haney, William P.	3702 Fourth Ave.	San Diego, Cal. 92103
Hanhausen, Edward H.	418 E. Lancaster Ave.	Wayne, Pa. 19087
Hanley, William J.	315 W. Clay Ave.	Muskegon, Mich. 49441
Hanna, William H.	1185 Dundee Ave.	Elgin, Ill. 60120
Hannah, Frank T.	209 Lee St.	Shelby, N. C., 28150
Hannah, Harry W.	23315 Washington	Colton, Cal. 92324
Hannon, John F.	Seven Corners Medical Bldg.	Falls Church, Va. 22044
Hannon, R. Emmet	Hanna Bldg.	Cleveland, O. 44115
Hans, Clarence L.	Provident Bank Bldg.	Cincinnati, O. 45202
Hansen, Alma K.	490 N. Alvernon Way	Tucson, Ariz. 85711
Hansen, Axel C.	Meharry Medical College	Nashville, Tenn. 37208
Hansen, Erling W.	16408 Hidden Valley Rd.	Minnetonka, Minn. 55343
Hansen, Terry L.	246 N. 18th Ave.	Pocatello, Ida. 83201
Hanser, S. Albert	6829 Clayton Ave.	St. Louis, Mo. 63139
Hanson, A. George	P.O. Box 1200	Santa Barbara, Cal. 93105
Hanson, F. Charles	10 Elmgrove Ave.	Providence, R. I. 02906
Harbater, Melvin	444 Community Dr.	Manhasset, N. Y. 11030
Harbert, Fred	Jefferson Med. College	Philadelphia, Pa. 19107
Harbin, Tom S.	1825 Martha Berry Blvd.	Rome, Ga. 30161
Hardenbergh, Firmon E.	2401 Broadway	Boulder, Colo. 80302
Hardesty. Hiram H.	5 Severance Cir.	Cleveland, O. 44118
Hardie, Bradford	El Paso National Bank Bldg.	El Paso, Tex. 79901
Hardie, George C.	724 W. Michigan Ave.	Jackson, Mich. 49201
Harding, Glen F.	460 23rd St.	Ogden, Utah 84401
Harding, M. Richard	3949 Meadows Dr.	Indianapolis, Ind. 46205
Hare, E. Treen, Jr.	21 Cherry St.	Milford, Conn. 06460
Hare, Robert	9735 Wilshire Blvd.	Beverly Hills, Cal. 90212
Harger, Robert W.	23 E. Ohio St.	Indianapolis, Ind. 46204
Hargett, Herbert P.	435 Spring St.	Jeffersonville, Ind. 47130
Hargis, Edward L.	1221 N. 26th	Billings, Mont. 59102
Hargiss, James L.	1601 16th Ave.	Seattle, Wash. 98122
Hargitt, Charles A.	17 Schermerhorn St.	Brooklyn, N. Y. 11201
Hargrove, Carey J.	Memorial Prof. Bldg.	Houston, Tex. 77002
Harkey, Michael E.	210 State St.	New Orleans, La. 70118
Harley, Robinson D.	1601 Spring Garden St.	Philadelphia, Pa. 19130

Harmon, Lewis G.	1775 E. 14 Mile Rd.	Birmingham, Mich. 48008
Harms, Edwin M.	609 N. Broadway	Wichita, Kans. 67214
Harms, Harold H.	Green Clinic	Ruston, La. 71270
Harnack, Klaus E.	2601 Lincoln Hwy.	Olympia Fields, Ill. 60461
Harper, John Y., Jr.	224 W. Evergreen	San Antonio, Tex. 78212
Harper, William H.	Billings Clinic	Billings, Mont. 59103
Harrington, David O.	490 Post St.	San Francisco, Cal. 94108
Harrington, James L.	161 Clinton St.	Watertown, N. Y. 13601
Harrington, M. Ray	2811 Lemmon Ave. E.	Dallas, Tex. 75204
Harris, Carl B.	23 E. Ohio	Indianapolis, Ind. 46204
Harris, John E.	Mayo Memorial Hospital	Minneapolis, Minn. 55455
Harris, Jonathan L.	V. A. Hosp.	East Orange, N. J. 07019
Harris, Louis D.	242 Trumbull St.	Hartford, Conn. 06103
Harris, Morris	102 Broad St.	Bloomfield, N. J. 07003
Harris, Ronald B.	707-711 S. Jefferson St.	Roanoke, Va. 24011
Harris, Stanley L.	195 Hempstead Ave.	Rockville Centre, N. Y. 11570
Harris, William R.	110 E. 'A' St.	Newton, N. C. 28658
Harris, William S.	2811 Lemmon Ave. E.	Dallas, Tex. 75214
Harrison, Glen H.	1616 Grand Ave.	Waukegan, Ill. 60085
Harrison, Raymond	140 E. 54th St.	New York, N. Y. 10022
Harrison, Stratton W.	2740 Carnegie Ave.	Cleveland, O. 44115
Harrison, Thomas J.	825 L St.	Anchorage, Alaska 99501
Hart, Brandon	Parkhurst Medical Bldg.	Beverly, Mass. 01915
Hart, Clinton E.	1601 Foster	Lake Charles, La. 70601
Hart, Edward E.	1301 Trumansburg Rd.	Ithaca, N. Y. 14850
Hart, James C.	5th St. & Walnut	Murray, Ky. 42071
Hart, N. Leon	116 S. Jefferson Davis Pkwy. ...	New Orleans, La. 70119
Hart, Maurice D.	655 Sutter St.	San Francisco, Cal. 94102
Hart, Patrick T.	18 Haines St.	Newark, Dela. 19711
Hart, William M.	Univ. Med. Ctr.	Columbia, Mo. 65201
Hartford, John J.	6931 Stockton Ave.	El Cerrito. Cal. 94530
Hartman, Deane C.	3875 Wilshire Blvd.	Los Angeles, Cal. 90005
Hartman, Eugene C.	418 Avery St.	Parkersburg, W. Va. 26101
Hartman, Ronald H.	5220 Clark Ave.	Lakewood, Cal. 90712
Hartstein, Jack	8631 Delmar Blvd.	St. Louis, Mo. 63124
Harvey, Elmer F.	Westgate Medical Arts Ctr.	Cleveland, O. 44126
Harvey, Lyman B.	13000 S. Maple Ave.	Blue Island, Ill. 60406
Harwin, Murray N.	10501 Wilshire Blvd.	Los Angeles, Cal. 90024
Harwood, David M.	3637 E. Century Blvd.	Lynwood, Cal. 90262
Harwood, Samuel C.	645 E. Aerick St.	Inglewood, Cal. 90301
Haseltine, Charles P.	2 W. Fern Ave.	Redlands, Cal. 92373
Hatch, Joseph L.	465 E. South Temple	Salt Lake City, Utah 84111
Hatcher, William F.	127 McClanahan St., S. W.	Roanoke, Va. 24014
Hathcock, W. C.	401 Peachtree St., N.E.	Atlanta, Ga. 30308
Hauck, Dale L.	1700 Brooklyn Ave.	Los Angeles, Cal. 90033
Haug, James A.	877 W. Fremont Ave.	Sunnyvale, Cal. 94087
Hauk, William L.	218 S. Trenton Ave.	Pittsburgh, Pa. 15221
Hauser, Maurice J.	7411 Third Ave.	Detroit, Mich. 48202
Hauser, Paul J.	2500 Ridge Ave.	Evanston, Ill. 60201
Hausler, Richard C.	206 S. Webster	Saginaw, Mich. 48602
Hausmann, Gertrude S.	Republic Bldg.	Denver, Colo. 80202
Haven, Walter K.	Medical Arts Bldg.	Minneapolis, Minn. 55402
Havener, William H.	320 W. 10th Ave.	Columbus, O. 43210
Havre, Dale C.	36001 Euclid Ave.	Willoughby, O. 44094
Hawkins, W. Rex.	Hermann Professional Bldg.	Houston, Tex. 77025

Hawn, Hugh W.	624 Gate City Bldg.	Fargo, N. D. 58102
Hayashi, D. T.	291 Geary St.	San Francisco, Cal. 94102
Hayden, Gould D.	1025 Pacific St.	San Luis Obispo, Cal. 93401
Hayes, Harrison F.	Franklin Medical Center	Denver, Colo. 80205
Hayes, Jess D., Jr.	4315 Lockwood Dr.	Houston, Tex. 77026
Hayter, Dale W.	234 W. Beauregard	San Angelo, Tex. 76901
Healy, J. P.	425 W. 5th Pl.	Mesa, Ariz. 85201
Healy, Maurice J.	4020 21st	Lubbock, Tex. 79410
Heath, Parker	....	Sullivan Harbor, Me. 04682
Heath, Scott A.	5 Via Joaquin	Monterey, Cal. 93940
Heath, William D.	1211 N. Shartel	Oklahoma City, Okla. 73103
Heatwole, Eugene W.	316 Main St.	Newport News, Va. 23601
Hecht, Sanford D.	42 Weston St.	Waltham, Mass. 02154
Hechter, Raymond H.	111 N. Wabash	Chicago, Ill. 60602
Heckert, Frank B.	Bank of Lansing Bldg.	Lansing, Mich. 48933
Hedemark, Norman G.	3222 Overland Rd.	Boise, Ida. 85705
Hedges, Charles C., Jr.	3411 N. Fifth Ave.	Phoenix, Ariz. 85013
Hedges, Thomas R.	330 S. 9th St.	Philadelphia, Pa. 19107
Hedgpeth, Edward McGowan, Jr.	1110 W. Main St.	Durham, N. C. 27701
Heidelman, George B.	575 Island Dr.	Palm Beach, Fla. 33480
Heidelman, Joseph M.	2350 Auburn Ave.	Cincinnati, O. 45219
Helberg, David S.	1702 Washington St.	Waukegan, Ill. 60085
Held, Robert A.	11 Carleton Ave.	Islip Terrace, N. Y. 11752
Helfgott, J. L.	915 19th St., N.W.	Washington, D. C. 20006
Helfrich, Mart L., Jr.	140 Hill St.	Bucyrus, O. 44820
Helm, John E.	600 E. Main St.	Olney, Ill. 62450
Helmick, Ernest D.	2612 N. 3rd St.	Harrisburg, Pa. 17110
Helsabeck, Belmont A.	Reynolds Bldg.	Winston-Salem, N.C. 27101
Helveston, Eugene M.	110 W. Michigan St.	Indianapolis, Ind. 46202
Henderson, Charles H.	200 Kline Bldg.	Norton, Va. 24273
Henderson, John W.	200 First St., S.W.	Rochester, Minn. 55901
Henderson, John Woodworth	Univ. Med. Ctr.	Ann Arbor, Mich. 48104
Henderson, Lawrence E. ...	194 Thompson Blvd.	Watertown, N. Y. 13601
Hendricks, Clifford A.	1953 First Ave., S.E.	Cedar Rapids, Ia. 52402
Hendricks, Louis J.	4551 Montgomery Ave.	Norwood, O. 45212
Henkind, Paul	111 E. 210th St.	Bronx, N. Y. 10467
Henrich, Mary I.	3240 Main St.	Buffalo, N. Y. 14214
Henry, Daniel W.	617 Diagonal	Clarkston, Wash. 99403
Henry, Forrest, Jr.	516 Scott	Little Rock, Ark. 72201
Henry, L. Murphey	602 Garrison Ave.	Ft. Smith, Ark. 72901
Henry, Louise McC.	602 Garrison Ave.	Ft. Smith, Ark. 72901
Henry, Margaret	384 Post	San Francisco, Cal. 94108
Henry, Marvin D.	25 E. Washington St.	Chicago, Ill. 60602
Henry, Morriss M.	203 S. East St.	Fayetteville, Ark. 72701
Henry, Randall W.	Paulsen Medical Dental Bldg. ...	Spokane, Wash. 99201
Henry, Robert T.	East 110 Canyon	Colfax, Wash. 99111
Hensley, Donald T.	1173 E. 42nd St.	Odessa, Tex. 79760
Henton, George H.	511 S. W. 10th Ave.	Portland, Ore. 97205
Hepler, Robert S.	U.C.L.A. Center for Health Sciences	Los Angeles, Cal. 90024
Herbert, Edna E.	303 Josephine St.	Denver, Colo. 80206
Herm, Robert J.	331 Main St.	Keene, N. H. 03431
Hermann, Ernest	7 North St.	Canandaigua, N.Y. 14424
Hermann, John S.	40 Park Ave.	New York, N. Y. 10016

Hermayer, Stephen	220 S. E. Seventh St.	Evansville, Ind. 47713
Hernandez, Eliseo R.	330 W. 58th St.	New York, N. Y. 10019
Herndon, Bruce Wayne	1203 Poplar Ave.	Memphis, Tenn. 38104
Herrick, Donald W.	Lowry Medical Arts Bldg.	St. Paul, Minn. 55102
Herring, Emmett M.	705 Hall Ave.	Hattiesburg, Miss. 39402
Herron, Warren L., Jr.	1720 N. 'E' St.	Pensacola, Fla. 32501
Hersey, James M.	1861 Wadsworth	Lakewood, Colo. 80215
Hersh, Stanley	2309 Austin Ave.	Waco, Tex. 76701
Hertner, John E.	1408 S. Andrews Ave.	Fort Lauderdale, Fla. 33316
Hertzog, Francis C., Jr.	2865 Atlantic Ave.	Long Beach, Cal. 90806
Herzog, Max	Cleaveland Bldg.	Rock Island, Ill. 61201
Heslin, Thomas M.	7 Wirt St.	New Brundwick, N. J. 08901
Hessburg, Philip C.	2799 W. Grand Blvd.	Detroit, Mich. 48202
Hessing, Ernest E.	8 Stonewall Rd.	Berkeley, Cal. 94705
Hester, Marion W.	1255 Lakeland Hills Blvd.	Lakeland, Fla. 33801
Hetherington, John, Jr.	490 Post St.	San Francisco, Cal. 94102
Heuser, Harold H.	Davidson Bldg.	Bay City, Mich. 48706
Heydt, Ernest H., Jr.	216 Summit Ave.	Jenkintown, Pa. 19046
Heyner, Conrad S.	15901 W. Nine Mile Rd.	Southfield, Mich. 48075
Heyner, Frederick J.	15901 W. Nine Mile Rd.	Southfield, Mich. 48075
Hiatt, Roger L.	858 Madison Ave.	Memphis, Tenn. 38103
Hicks, Avery M.	490 Post St.	San Francisco, Cal. 94102
Hicks, John D.	1121 Columbia St.	Seattle, Wash. 98104
Hicks, Robb R.	420 W. Rowland	Covina, Cal. 91722
Hicks, Vonnie M., Sr.	Glenwood Prof. Village	Raleigh, N. C. 27608
Higbee, John W.	150 E. Broad St.	Columbus, O. 43215
Hilding, Anderson C.	St. Luke's Hosp.	Duluth, Minn. 55805
Hildreth, H. Rommel	950 Francis Pl.	St. Louis, Mo. 63105
Hiles, David A.	3520 Fifth Ave.	Pittsburgh, Pa. 15213
Hilgartner, Henry L.	202 W. 13th St.	Austin, Tex. 78701
Hilgermann, George O.	Medical Arts Bldg.	Minneapolis, Minn. 55402
Hill, Charlotte W.	1573 University Ave.	St. Paul, Minn. 55104
Hill, Edwin P.	9730 Wilshire Blvd.	Beverly Hills, Cal. 90212
Hill, Howard F.	325A Kennedy Memorial Dr.	Waterville, Me. 04901
Hill, James E.	A. C. Office Bldg.	Arkansas City, Kans. 67005
Hill, John M.	108 Bay State Rd.	Boston, Mass. 02215
Hill, Kevin	325 A Kennedy Memorial Dr.	Waterville, Me. 04901
Hill, Robert V.	1329 Broadway	Longview, Wash. 98632
Hill, William R.	28 W. Scribner Ave.	DuBois, Pa. 15801
Hilton, George F.	355 30th St.	Oakland, Cal. 94609
Himelfarb, Hillard M.	180 E. Queen St.	Chambersburg, Pa. 17201
Himes, Ralph F., Jr.	501 Howard Ave.	Altoona, Pa. 16601
Himmel, Sanford	97th General Hospital, APO	New York, N. Y. 09757
Hinckley, Ralph H.	2000 Washington St.	Newton, Mass. 02162
Hing, Gloria M.	280 W. MacArthur Blvd.	Oakland, Cal. 94611
Hinken, Michael V.	2300 N. Rockton Ave.	Rockford, Ill. 61103
Hinman, Louis F.	666 E. Penn St.	Philadelphia, Pa. 19144
Hinton, Golden S.	220 N. Milledge Ave.	Athens, Ga. 30601
Hinton, John L.	120 Louiselle St.	Mobile, Ala. 36607
Hipp, Walter	11 Middle Rd.	Port Washington, N. Y. 11050
Hirsch, Lee	130 Maple St.	Springfield, Mass. 01103
Hirschfelder, Max K.	408 W. Second St.	Centralia, Ill. 62801
Hirschman, Henry	5211 Arbor Rd.	Long Beach, Cal. 90808
Hirshman, Marshall	3200 Dempster	Des Plaines, Ill. 60016
Hirst, William R.	2241 Central Ave.	Alameda, Cal. 94501

Hitch, Oliver M.	417 S. Monroe	Green Bay, Wisc. 54301
Hitz, John B.	2040 W. Wisconsin Ave.	Milwaukee, Wisc. 53233
Hix, Ivan E., Jr.	2500 Youngfield St.	Lakewood, Colo. 80215
Hobach, George B.	2100 16th St. N.	St. Petersburg, Fla. 33704
Hobach, John P.	2210 4th St. N.	St. Petersburg, Fla 33704
Hobbs, Frank I.	2255 Langhorne Rd.	Lynchburg, Va. 24501
Hodge, John H.	1130 Forest St.	Bellingham, Wash. 98225
Hodgkinson, B. J.	243 Charles St.	Boston, Mass. 02114
Hodgkinson, Charles P., II .	Med. Arts Bldg.	Grand Rapids, Mich. 49502
Hoefle, Frank B.	430 Bay Ridge Pkwy.	Brooklyn, N. Y. 11209
Hoeltgen, Maurice M.	1836 W. 87th St.	Chicago, Ill. 60620
Hoffman, Eugene F., Jr. ...	301 W. Bastanchury Rd.	Fullerton, Cal. 92632
Hoffman, Franklin D.	550 Grant St.	Pittsburgh, Pa. 15219
Hoffman, Lawrence D.	16000 Harden Cir.	Southfield, Mich. 48075
Hoffman, Parker M.	134 E. First St.	Corning, N. Y. 14830
Hoffman, Richard A.	2328 Auburn Ave.	Cincinnati, O. 45219
Hoffman, Robert M.	15744 E. Imperial Hwy.	La Mirada, Cal. 90638
Hoffman, Theodore E.	1506 Westfield St.	West Springfield, Mass. 01089
Hoffman, Walter F.	6331 Hampton Rd.	Seattle, Wash. 98118
Hoffman, Walter L.	6533 Drew Ave. S.	Minneapolis, Minn. 55435
Hoffmeyer, Iris M.	328 Maple St.	San Diego, Cal. 92103
Hoffner, Herbert H.	18-15 Cornaga Ave.	Far Rockaway, N. Y. 11691
Hofling, Charles A.	506 E. 4th St.	Cincinnati, O. 45202
Hogan, Michael J.	95 Kirkham St.	San Francisco, Cal. 94122
Hogan, Thomas F., Jr.	414 Navarro St.	San Antonio, Tex. 78205
Hogan, Walter L.	750 Main St.	Hartford, Conn. 06103
Hogan, Walter L., Jr.	2324 Bath St.	Santa Barbara, Cal. 93105
Hogenson, Clifford D.	8 S. Second	Walla Walla, Wash. 99362
Hogg, Raymond E.	2909 E. Grand River	Lansing, Mich. 48912
Hogsett, S. Fuller	Medical Ctr. Bldg.	Spokane, Wash. 99204
Hohensee, Edward W.	7531 Seneca St.	E. Aurora, N. Y. 14052
Hohn, Anselm C.	705 Juniper	Atlanta, Ga. 30308
Hok, Roland	5 S. State St.	Concord, N. H. 03301
Holl, Paul F.	Jenkins Bldg.	Pittsburgh, Pa. 15222
Hollabaugh, C. Fowier	1915 Church St.	Nashville, Tenn. 37203
Holladay, George E.	525 Bryan St.	Denton, Tex. 76201
Holland, Charles R.	926 E. McDowell Rd.	Phoenix, Ariz. 85006
Holland, Juergen E.	2018 W. North Ave.	Chicago, Ill. 60647
Holland, John J.	Bondi Bldg.	Galesburg, Ill. 61401
Holland, Malvern C.	125 Mallard St.	Greenville, S. C. 29601
Holland, Monte G.	1430 Tulane Ave.	New Orleans, La. 70112
Holland, William T. Jr.	899 Grove St.	Meadville, Pa. 16335
Hollander, Edward M.	USAF Academy Hospital	USAF Academy, Colo. 80840
Hollenhorst, Robert W.	Mayo Clinic	Rochester, Minn. 55902
Hollister, John F.	2720 Capitol Ave.	Sacramento, Cal. 95816
Holloway, Jonathan A.	Rockwood Clinic, West 312, 8th Ave.	Spokane, Wash. 90204
Holly, John H., Jr.	175 N. E. 96th St.	Miami Shores, Fla. 33138
Holm, Arvid G.	2515 N. Main	Santa Ana, Cal. 92701
Holm, Knut U.	7540 Fourth Ave.	Brooklyn, N. Y. 11209
Holmes, Dorothy B.	1816 R St., N.W.	Washington, D. C. 20009
Holmes, John P.	4515 Poplar Ave.	Memphis, Tenn. 38117
Holmes, Richard L.	910 Via de la Paz	Pacific Palisades, Cal. 90272
Holmes, Wendell B.	210 N. Front	McComb, Miss. 39648

Holowin, Joseph S.	718 S. Brookhurst St.	Anaheim, Cal. 92804
Holstein, Theodore	3401 Folsom Blvd.	Sacramento, Cal. 95816
Holt, Helen	720 N. Michigan Ave.	Chicago, Ill. 60611
Holt, John A. B.	1306 Kanawha Blvd. E.	Charleston, W. Va. 25301
Holt, Lawrence B.	2240 Cloverdale Ave.	Winston-Salem, N. C. 27103
Holt, Robert G.	4th & Chestnut	Halstead, Kans. 67056
Holtz, Marvin J.	6512 S. Painter Ave.	Whittier, Cal. 90601
Holzer, William F.	23 Birchwood Cir.	Bedford, N. H. 03102
Hombach, Frank J.	19 W. Micheltorena St.	Santa Barbara, Cal. 93104
Honan, Paul R.	1720 N. Lebanon St.	Lebanon, Ind. 46052
Honard, Richard J.	5370 Pearl Rd.	Cleveland, O. 44129
Honig, Alan J.	St. James Bldg.	Jacksonville, Fla. 32202
Honstein, Clyde E., Jr.	301 E. Perkins Dr.	Las Cruces, N. M. 88001
Hook, Robert F.	836 Miami Rd.	Jacksonville, Fla. 32207
Hooker, Lyle, ...	2909 Hillcroft	Houston, Tex. 77027
Hoon, William L.	Jenkins Arcade Bldg.	Pittsburgh, Pa. 15222
Hooper, R. James	645 First St.	Macon, Ga. 31201
Hoops, Lillian H.	2201 Paradise Rd.	Las Vegas, Nev. 89105
Hootman, J. Kenneth	633 Washington Rd.	Pittsburgh, Pa. 15228
Hoover, Richard E.	14 W. Mt. Vernon Pl.	Baltimore, Md. 21201
Hopen, Joseph M.	3419 Johnson St.	Hollywood, Fla. 33021
Hopkins, Charles E. R.	88-26 193rd St.	Hollis, N. Y. 11423
Hopkins, Edward D., Jr. ...	1520 Laurel St.	Columbia, S. C. 29201
Hopkins, Robert E.	4255 Pacific Ave.	Stockton, Cal. 95207
Hopkins, William G.	405 W. 15th	Pueblo, Colo. 81003
Hopper, Kenneth C.	155 Bay St.	Glens Falls, N. Y. 12801
Horn, Maurice ....,.....	2200 O'Farrell St.	San Francisco, Cal. 94115
Hornblass, Albert	Kimbrough Army Hosp.	Ft. George G. Meade, Md. 20755
Hornbogen, Daniel P.	Savings Bank Bldg.	Marquette, Mich. 49855
Horns, Richard C.	822 Marquette Ave.	Minneapolis, Minn. 55402
Hornyak, William J.	1303 San Carlos Ave.	San Carlos, Cal. 94070
Horowitz, Alexander S. ...	4512 Kennedy Blvd.	Union City, N. J. 07087
Horowitz, Irving I.	110-45 Queens Blvd.	Forest Hills, N. Y. 11375
Horsfield, Russell T.	700 Broadway	Seattle, Wash. 98122
Horsley, Margaret E.	Stoneham Medical Bldg., 61 Main St.	Stoneham, Mass. 02180
Horwich, Harry	2695 Le Jeune Rd.	Coral Gables, Fla. 33134
Horwitz, Irving D.	9201 Sunset Blvd.	Los Angeles, Cal. 90069
Hoshiwara, Isao	1608 E. Earll Dr.	Phoenix, Ariz, 85016
Hoskins, H. Dunbar, Jr. ...	Medical College of Va.	Richmond, Va. 23219
Hoskins, Leon C.	616 W. Hill Ave.	Knoxville, Tenn. 37902
Hosner, James W.	Surburban Square Bldg.	Ardmore, Pa. 19003
Houck, Richard J.	501 Warren Bldg.	Michigan City, Ind. 46360
Houck, Virgil L.	3007 E. Oakland Ave.	Bloomington, Ill. 61701
Hough, Mac J.	1012 Kings Dr.	Charlotte, N. C. 28207
Houle, Roland E.	3 Hawthorne Pl.	Boston, Mass. 02114
House, Ben F. ;	680 W. Forest	Jackson, Tenn. 38301
House, Rex C.	2455 Morgan Ave.	Corpus Christi, Tex. 78405
Houston, William H.	441 Marshall Taylor Doctors Bldg.	Jacksonville, Fla. 32207
Houston, William R. M. ...	456 W. Park Ave.	Mansfield, O. 44906
Hovland, Kenneth R.	1115 Republic Bldg.	Denver, Colo. 80202
Howard, Donald O.	959 N. Emporia	Wichita, Kans. 67214
Howard, George M.	635 W. 165th St.	New York, N. Y. 10032
Howard, H. Carlton	2700 S. W. Third Ave.	Miami, Fla. 33129

Howard, Jed L.	2622 Nasa Rd. 1	Seabrook, Tex. 77586
Howard, Royal M.	100 Central Ave.	Staten Island, N. Y. 10301
Howard, Rufus O.	Yale Medical School	New Haven, Conn. 06520
Howard, William H.	9138 Commercial Ave.	Chicago, Ill. 60617
Howard, William J.	389 Linwood Ave.	Buffalo, N. Y. 14209
Howard, William M.	389 Linwood Ave.	Buffalo, N. Y. 14209
Howarth, Charles, H.	1129 Bellevue St.	Boise, Ida. 83706
Howe, Archibald W.	2902 N. 27th	Tacoma, Wash. 98407
Howe, Charles A.	2804 Main St.	Buffalo, N. Y. 14214
Howell, Homer P.	3022 E. 14th St.	Oakland, Cal. 94601
Howell, J. Franklin, Jr.	2300 W. 7th Ave.	Amarillo, Tex. 79106
Howitt, David A.	1175 N.E. 125th St.	N. Miami, Fla. 33161
Hoy, James E.	326 Front St.	Marietta, O. 45750
Hoyt, William F.	95 Kirkham St.	San Francisco, Cal. 94122
Hubbard, William B.	Paterson Bldg.	Flint, Mich. 48502
Hubbard, William C.	Paterson Bldg.	Flint, Mich. 48502
Hudnell, Armstead B.	Forsyth Med. Park	Winston-Salem, N. C. 27103
Hudock, John P.	208 Jefferson Ave.	Endicott, N. Y. 13760
Hudson, Kenneth E.	726 McCullough Ave.	San Antonio, Tex. 78215
Hughes, Calvin T., Jr.	85 Jefferson St.	Hartford, Conn. 06106
Hughes, Philip C.	1126 S. Main St.	Dayton, O. 45409
Hughes, Robert P., Jr.	1214 North B St.	Fort Smith, Ark. 72901
Hughes, William F.	1753 W. Congress Pkwy.	Chicago, Ill. 60612
Hughson, Donald T.	10425 W. North Ave.	Milwaukee, Wisc. 53226
Hull, Forrest E.	1741 W. Avenue J.	Lancaster, Cal. 93534
Hull, Frank W.	1408 Pennsylvania Ave.	Fairfield, Cal. 94533
Hull, Frederick H.	2020 N. Waterman Ave.	San Bernardino, Cal. 92404
Hull, Jess S.	2040 W. Bethany Home Rd.	Phoenix, Ariz. 85015
Hull, Stephen Nelson	1741 W. Avenue 'J', Box 1928 ..	Lancaster, Cal. 93534
Hulquist, C. Richard	10921 Wilshire Blvd.	Los Angeles, Cal. 90024
Hultgen, Francis J.	3860 W. 95th St.	Evergreen Park, Ill. 60642
Hultgen, William J.	2450 4th Ave.	Yuma, Ariz. 85364
Hummel, Alvin L.	Santa Barbara Medical Clinic, Calle Real & San Marcos Pass Rd.	Santa Barbara, Cal. 93102
Hummel, Anton J.	5203 Chippewa	St. Louis, Mo. 63109
Hummel, Robert A.	4200 S. Douglas	Oklahoma City, Okla. 73109
Humphreys, John A.	3535 Cherry Creek N. Dr.	Denver, Colo. 80209
Humphreys, John L., Jr. ...	705 Juniper St. N. E.	Atlanta, Ga. 30308
Humphries, Marion K., Jr. .	1400 Jefferson Park Ave.	Charlottesville, Va. 22903
Huneke, John W.	1201G E. 5th	Ada, Okla. 74820
Hungerford, Louis N., Jr. ..	1118 9th Ave.	Seattle, Wash. 98101
Hunsberger, Charles L., Jr. .	406 Main St.	Johnstown, Pa. 15905
Hunt, Carson E.	221 W. E. St.	Encinitas, Cal. 92024
Hunt, Harold E.	150 8th S. E.	Paris, Tex. 75460
Hunt, Wayne A.	1216 Guarantee Savings Bldg. ...	Fresno, Cal. 93721
Hunt, William T., Jr.	1617 John F. Kennedy Blvd. ...	Philadelphia, Pa. 19103
Hunter, Herman J.	2010 Wilshire Blvd.	Los Angeles, Cal. 90057
Hunter, William A.	1146 5th Ave. N.	St. Petersburg, Fla. 33705
Huq, Md. Nasrul	Meharry Medical College Hospital	Nashville, Tenn. 37208
Hurite, Francis G.	550 Grant St.	Pittsburgh, Pa. 15219
Hurley, Paul D.	1101 Beacon St.	Brookline, Mass. 02146
Hursh, M. Douglas	1492 N. Main St.	Wheaton, Ill. 60187
Hurt, Arthur C.	715 Lake St.	Oak Park, Ill. 60302
Hurwitz, Paul	55 E. Washington St.	Chicago, Ill. 60602
Huss, Robert J.	4531 Tactical Hospital	Homestead AFB, Fla. 33030

Hutcherson, J. Kenneth ...	814 Lincoln Federal Bldg.	Louisville, Ky. 40202
Hutchinson, B. Thomas ...	10 Hawthorne Pl.	Boston, Mass. 02114
Hutchinson, Ben B.	3121 20th St.	Lubbock, Tex. 79410
Hutson, Clare F.	1025 Regent St.	Madison, Wisc. 53705
Huwe, Eugene L.	2135 W. Ball Rd.	Anaheim, Cal. 92804
Hyde, Lawrence L.	4620 J. C. Nichols Pkwy.	Kansas City, Mo. 64112
Hyman, Joseph J.	734 Ocean Ave.	Brooklyn, N. Y. 11226
Hyman, Richard D.	2600 Park Ave.	Concord, Cal. 94520
Hymes, Charles	3015 Utah Ave. S.	Minneapolis, Minn. 55426
Hyndiuk, Robert A.	20 Staniford St.	Boston, Mass. 02114
Hynes, Edward A.	62 Columbian St.	South Weymouth, Mass. 02190
Ianacone, Samuel J.	20 N. Goodman St.	Rochester, N. Y. 14607
Ide, Carl H.	Univ. of Mo. Med. Ctr.	Colbumbia, Mo. 65201
Iliff, Charles E.	14 W. Mt. Vernon Pl.	Baltimore, Md. 21201
Inciardi, James A.	149 Midwood St.	Brooklyn, N. Y. 11225
Ingalls, Raymond G.	297 Pleasant St.	Berlin, N. H. 03570
Insabella, John	200 Ivy St.	Newark, N. J. 07106
Insel, H. Herbert	6201 Greenbelt Rd.	College Park, Md. 20740
Ioratti, John B.	157 S. Lincoln Ave.	Aurora, Ill. 60505
Irgens, Edwin R.	519 Ship St.	St. Joseph, Mich. 49085
Irizarry, Jaime E.	P. O. Box 12367 Loiza Sta.	Santurce, P.R. 00914
Irvine, A. Ray, Jr.	3875 Wilshire Blvd.	Los Angeles, Cal. 90005
Irvine, A. Rodman	Letterman Gen. Hosp., The Presidio	San Francisco, Cal. 94129
Irvine, John W.	9503 E. 63rd St.	Kansas City, Mo. 64133
Irvine, Paul S.	1893 Sheridan Rd.	Highland Park, Ill. 60035
Irvine, S. Rodman	9730 Wilshire Blvd.	Beverly Hills, Cal. 90212
Irvine, Wendell C.	3875 Wilshire Blvd.	Los Angeles, Cal. 90005
Irwin, Edward S.	366 Pearl St.	Burlington, Vt. 05401
Irwin, William D.	2333 Sheffield Drive	Kalamazoo, Mich. 49001
Isaacson, Jo D.	Northland Medical Bldg.	Southfield, Mich. 48075
Isaeff, Wayne B.	Loma Linda University Hospital .	Loma Linda, Cal. 92354
Isbell, D.	535 McCallie Ave.	Chattanooga, Tenn. 37402
Isbey, Edward K., Jr.	3C Doctors Park	Asheville, N. C. 28801
Isenstein, Charles	51 Brattle St.	Cambridge, Mass. 02138
Iser, Gilbert	3420 W. Peterson Ave.	Chicago, Ill. 60645
Iverson, Donald G.	P. O. Box 407	Cheyenne, Wyo. 82001
Iverson, Herman A.	2414 Buhne St.	Eureka, Cal. 95501
Ivey, David M.	Malcolm Grow USAF Medical Center, Anfrews AFB	Washington, D. C. 20331
Ivy, H. B.	600 S Glenstone	Springfield, Mo. 65802
Iwantsch, Alfred E.	537 E. Market St.	Alliance, O. 44601
Jack, M. Kim	1121 Columbia St.	Seattle, Wash. 98104
Jacklin, Harold N.	914 N. Elm St.	Greensboro, N. C. 27401
Jackson, Andrew H.	1704 W. Manchester Ave.	Los Angeles, Cal. 90047
Jackson, G. Keefe	1160 Chili Ave.	Rochester, N. Y. 14624
Jackson, J. Truett	1235 Forest Ave.	Montgomery, Ala. 36106
Jackson, William E.	2045 Franklin St.	Denver, Colo. 80203
Jackson, Zach W.	478 Peachtree St., N.E.	Atlanta, Ga. 30308
Jacobius, Henry F.	21st & Fairview Ave.	Easton, Pa. 18042
Jacobs, Clyde H.	370 Market St.	Sunbury, Pa. 17801
Jacobs, Harvey A.	120 Oakbrook Center Mall	Oak Brook, Ill. 60521
Jacobs, Milton	122 S. Michigan Ave.	Chicago, Ill. 60603
Jacobson, Jerry H.	12 E. 68th St.	New York, N. Y. 10021
Jacobson, Leslie W.	6533 Drew Ave. S.	Minneapolis, Minn. 55435

Jacobson, Payson B.	268 Elm St.	Biddeford, Me. 04005
Jaeckle, Charles E.	1133 E. Second St.	Defiance, O. 43512
Jaeger, Edward A.	Media Clinic	Media, Pa. 19063
Jaegers, Kenneth R.	Wilford Hall, U.S.A.F. Hospital .	San Antonio, Tex. 78236
Jaffe, Benjamin	201 St. Pauls Ave.	Jersey City, N. J. 07306
Jaffe, Charles R.	2128 Ocean Ave.	Brooklyn, N. Y. 11229
Jaffe, Morris	11 5th Ave.	New York, N. Y. 10003
Jaffe, Norman S.	1680 Meridian Ave.	Miami Beach, Fla. 33139
Jagerman, Louis S.	101 S. San Mateo Dr.	San Mateo, Cal. 94491
Jahnke, Paul G.	134 W. 6th St.	McMinnville, Ore. 97128
Jakobovits, Rafael	450 Sutter St.	San Francisco, Cal. 94108
Jalbuena, Robert C.	2300 Garrett Rd.	Drexel Hill, Pa. 19026
James, Brien P.	6220 S. Broadway	Littleton, Colo. 80120
James, Burton R.	2914-A Fresno St.	Fresno, Cal. 93721
James, George R.	202 E. 2nd St.	Casper, Wyo. 82601
Jampel, Robert S.	635 W. 165th St.	New York, N. Y. 10032
Jampolsky, Arthur	2340 Clay St.	San Francisco, Cal. 94115
Janes, Charles L.	3875 Wilshire Blvd., Suite 1307 Wilshire Prof. Bldg.	Los Angeles, Cal. 90005
Jansen, Donald H.	7777 Montgomery Rd.	Cincinnati, O. 45236
Jardinico, Robert E.	206 S. Webster St.	Saginaw, Mich. 48602
Jaros, Duval B.	1350 S. Eliseo Dr.	Greenbrae, Cal. 94904
Jarratt, W. Devereaux	626 First St.	Macon, Ga. 31201
Jarrett, William H.	Emory University Clinic	Atlanta, Ga. 30322
Jarvis, Jerome A.	86-01 Homelawn St.	Jamaica, N. Y. 11432
Jeans, Park C., Jr.	1419 Gwinnett St.	Augusta, Ga. 30902
Jenkins, Robert D.	Washington Bldg.	Springfield, Ill. 62701
Jennings, Aubrey L.	5401 Western Ave. N. W., Washington Clinic	Washington, D. C. 20015
Jennings, David T.	21 W. 3rd St.	Williamsport, Pa. 17701
Jensen, Carl D. F.	1601 16th Ave.	Seattle, Wash. 98122
Jensen, Robert L.	167 E. Second N.	Logan, Utah 84321
Jenson, Mark B.	1029 N. 500th W.	Provo, Utah 84601
Jepson, C. Neal	616 S. Tejon	Colorado Springs, Colo. 80901
Jerome, Bourne	1750 Medical Arts Bldg.	Minneapolis, Minn. 55402
Jerrold, S. Harrison	2 Frost Ave. W.	Edison, N. J.
Jervey, E. Darrell	709 Dunbar St.	Greenville, S. C. 29601
Jervey, J. W.	709 Dunbar St.	Greenville, S. C. 29601
Jesberg, Davied O.	350 Parnassus	San Francisco, Cal. 94117
Jessel, Erwin	206-25 Hillside Ave.	Queens Village, N. Y. 11427
Jester, Royal F., Jr.	3011 Ave. A.	Kearney, Nebr. 68847
Jewett, E. Porter	25 Oak Ave.	Worcester, Mass. 01605
Jiroch, John T.	1119 Marshall	Manitowoc, Wisc. 54420
Joe, Shirley	47 Truitt Ln.	Oakland, Cal. 94618
Joffe, William S.	211 N. Meramec Ave.	Clayton, Mo. 63105
Johannsen, Robert A.	933 S. Sunset Ave.	West Covina, Cal. 91790
Johanson, Raymond R. ...	2140 Shattuck Ave.	Berkeley, Cal. 94704
John, Robert H.	Eugene Medical Ctr.	Eugene, Ore. 97401
Johnson, A. Richard	1701 26th St.	Bakersfield, Cal. 93301
Johnson, Albin W.	1300 St. Mary's St.	Raleigh, N. C. 27605
Johnson, Carl C.	3 Hawthorne Pl.	Boston, Mass. 02114
Johnson, Chester D.	1420 7th St.	Moline, Ill. 61265
Johnson, Craig B.	4647 Ingersoll St.	Houston, Tex. 77027
Johnson, David S.	79 Highland Ave.	Salem, Mass. 01970
Johnson, Don R.	3611 Branch Ave. S. E.	Hillcrest Heights, Md. 20031

Johnson, Donald C.	211 N. Market St.	Washington, N. C. 27889
Johnson, Donald R.	321 Greenwood	Bend, Ore. 97701
Johnson, Douglas L.	518 Washington St.	Brainerd, Minn. 56401
Johnson, Elmer E.	4513 Vernon Blvd.	Madison, Wisc. 53705
Johnson, Ernest D.	330 N. Garfield Ave.	Alhambra, Cal. 91801
Johnson, Frank W.	1000 Pine St.	Klamath Falls, Ore. 97601
Johnson, Henrietta May	342 S. Madison	Pasadena, Cal. 91106
Johnson, Jerry	3155 Stagg Dr.	Beaumont, Tex. 77701
Johnson, Lorand V.	10515 Carnegie Ave.	Cleveland, O. 44106
Johnson, Louis L.	509 W. Main St.	Dothan, Ala. 36301
Johnson, Lowell E.	1893 Sheridan Rd.	Highland Park, Ill. 60035
Johnson, Marshall	2107 Hayes St.	Nashville, Tenn. 37203
Johnson, M. Harvey	2330 N. W. Flanders St.	Portland, Ore. 97210
Johnson, Nicholas J.	6681 Ridge Rd.	Parma, O. 44129
Johnson, R. Marion	Hermann Prof. Bldg.	Houston, Tex. 77025
Johnson, Robert C.	2340 Clay St.	San Francisco, Cal. 94115
Johnson, Robert M., Jr.	105 Main St.	Kirkland, Wash. 98033
Johnson, Roger H.	Cobb Bldg.	Seattle, Wash. 98101
Johnson, Samuel B.	1151 N. State	Jackson, Miss. 39201
Johnson, Thomas H.	167 Nelson Rd.	Scarsdale, N. Y. 10583
Johnson, Tom L.	1341 N.W. Expressway	Oklahoma City, Okla. 73112
Johnson, Wendell A.	12th & Douglas	Ames, Ia. 50010
Johnson, W. Rayner	230 W. Boscawen St.	Winchester, Va. 22601
Johnston, Glen P.	4989 Barnes Hospital Plaza	St. Louis, Mo. 63110
Johnston, Neil V.	13346 Ravanna Rd.	Chardon, O. 44024
Johnston, Theodore L.	1805 E. 19th St.	Cheyenne, Wyo. 82001
Johnston, Thomas S.	26 S. Church St.	West Chester, Pa. 19380
Johnston, William H.	715 Market St.	St. Joseph, Mich. 49085
Johnstone, William W.	30 W. El Rose Dr.	Petaluma, Cal. 94952
Joiner, James C., III	755 Columbia Dr.	Decatur, Ga. 30030
Jones, Carlton E.	Mease Clinic	Dunedin, Fla. 33528
Jones, C. Henry	431 Wyoming Ave.	Scranton, Pa. 18503
Jones, David H.	1300 St. Mary's St.	Raleigh, N. C. 27605
Jones, Edley H.	1301 Washington St.	Vicksburg, Miss. 39180
Jones, Edward T.	400 E. Grand	Beloit, Wisc. 53511
Jones, Edward T.	120 Broadway	Richmond, Cal. 94804
Jones, Frank W.	22½ Union Ave.	Schenectady, N. Y. 12308
Jones, George H.	4550 North Blvd.	Baton Rouge, La. 70806
Jones, George R.	U. S. Naval Hosp., Box 536	Portsmouth, Va. 23708
Jones, Ira S.,	E. 71st. St.	New York, N. Y. 10021
Jones, James H.	634 N. Grand Blvd.	St. Louis, Mo. 63103
Jones, John A.	849 Washington Ave.	Montgomery, Ala. 36104
Jones, Kenneth B.	1513 Line Ave.	Shreveport, La. 71101
Jones, Lester T.	Medical Arts Bldg.	Portland, Ore. 97205
Jones, Ottiwell W., III	S. 427 Bernard St.	Spokane, Wash. 99204
Jones, Reed W., Jr.	2301 S. Austin Ave.	Denison, Tex. 75020
Jones, Rheim M.	530 S. Holmes	Idaho Falls, Idaho 83401
Jones, Robert C.	515 Soquel Ave.	Santa Cruz, Cal. 95060
Jones, Samuel T.	4620 J. C. Nichols Pkwy.	Kansas City, Mo. 64112
Jones, Thomas C.	2300 Garrison Blvd.	Baltimore, Md. 21216
Jones, Vincent L.	634 N. Grand	St. Louis, Mo. 63103
Jones, W. Mead	Somerset House	Fort Washington, Pa. 19034
Jones, William M.	5234 S. Michigan Ave.	Chicago, Ill.60615
Jones, W. Yerby	849 Humboldt Pkwy.	Buffalo, N. Y. 14208
Jordan, Arthur C.	Medical Dental Bldg.	Seattle, Wash. 98101
Jordan, James S.	225 N. Washington Ave.	Scranton, Pa. 18503

Jordan, Joseph M.	225 W. Madison Ave.	El Cajon, Cal. 92020
Jordan, Lewis G.	3261 S. Stafford St.	Arlington, Va. 22206
Jordan, Ray C.	106 Circle Way	Lake Jackson, Tex. 77566
Jorgensen, Donald R.	Lowry Medical Arts Bldg.	St. Paul, Minn. 55102
Jorgenson, Ralph E.	79 E. 300 North St.	Provo, Utah 84601
Joselson, Gerald A.	23 Forster Pkwy.	Mt. Vernon, N. Y. 10552
Joseph, Alfred L.	39 N. Ohio Ave	Columbus, O. 43203
Joseph, Robert H.	3660 Arlington Ave.	Riverside, Cal. 92506
Josey, John S.	3010 Hampton Ave.	Brunswick, Ga. 31520
Joy, Harold H.	424 State Tower Bldg.	Syracuse, N. Y. 13202
Judd, J. Hewitt	Doctors' Bldg.	Omaha, Nebr. 68131
Judge, Harry M.	23 Hackett Blvd.	Albany, N. Y. 12208
Judisch, G. Frank	2409 Towncrest Dr.	Iowa City, Ia. 52240
Jukofsky, S. Lawrence	217 Old Hook Rd.	Westwood, N. J. 07675
Jungschaffer, Otto H.	12840 Riverside Dr.	North Hollywood, Cal. 91607
Jurevics, Ingrid E.	2040 W. Wisconsin Ave.	Milwaukee, Wisc. 53233
Juska, Aldona A.	8058 S. Western Ave.	Chicago, Ill. 60620
Kadin, Maurice	10718 White Oak Ave.	Granada Hills, Cal. 91344
Kaebnick, E. Elliott	302 Medical Arts Bldg.	Oak Ridge, Tenn. 37830
Kafka, Adolph J.	1808 High St.	Denver, Colo. 80218
Kahan, Edmund	400 W. End Ave.	New York, N. Y. 10024
Kahn, Cyrus I.	U. S. Naval Hospital	Key West, Fla. 33040
Kahn, Paul, Jr.	1411 W. Olive Ave.	Burbank, Cal. 91506
Kahn, Walter, J.	139 Broad St.	Red Bank, N. J. 07701
Kaiser, Robert F.	1130 Forest St.	Bellingham, Wash. 98225
Kaiser, Rober J.	301 E. Walnut St.	Louisville, Ky. 40202
Kalb, Irvin M.	9735 Wilshire Blvd.	Beverly Hills, Cal. 90212
Kalil, Rodney F.	1514 Jefferson Hwy.	New Orleans, La. 70123
Kalin, Joshua	523 Capitol Trail	Newark, Dela. 19711
Kalina, Robert E.	Univ. of Washington Sch. of Med.	Seattle, Wash. 98105
Kalvin, Nicholas H.	773 4th Ave. N.	Naples, Fla. 33940
Kambara, George K.	321 E. Second St.	Los Angeles, Cal. 90012
Kameen, A. J.	United Penn Bank Bldg.	Wilkes-Barre, Pa. 18701
Kamen, Sheldon D.	21100 Southgate Park Blvd.	Maple Heights, O. 44137
Kamerling, Wm.	423 Clements Bridge Rd.	Barrington, N. J. 08007
Kanarek, Irwin E.	Brookdale Hospital Center	Brooklyn, N. Y. 11212
Kanut, Ray E.	6700 Troost	Kansas City, Mo. 64131
Kane, David S.	111 N. Wabash Ave.	Chicago, Ill. 60602
Kangas, Onni C.	11 Maple St.	Rockland, Me. 04841
Kanner, Albert V.	110 E. Main St.	Madison, Wisc. 53703
Kanofsky, F. J.	1801 State St.	Santa Barbara, Cal. 93102
Kansas, Peter G.	301 S. Allen St.	Albany, N. Y. 12208
Kant, Alfred	104 Paddock St.	Watertown, N. Y. 13601
Kantar, Bruce L.	Physicians & Surgeons Bldg.	Minneapolis, Minn. 55402
Kanter, Philip D.	104-40 Queens Blvd.	Forest Hills, N. Y. 11375
Kanter, Richard S.	1700 Grand Concourse	Bronx, N. Y. 10457
Kanter, Yale C.	451 N. Dunlap	St. Paul. Minn. 55104
Kantor, Samuel	Rockhill Medical Bldg., 6700 Troost	Kansas City, Mo. 64131
Kapetansky, Frederick M. ..	303 E. Town St.	Columbus, O. 43215
Kaplan, Aaron S.	181 Speedwell Ave.	Morristown, N.J. 07960
Kaplan, Arnold M.	1775 Walters Ave.	Northbrook, Ill. 60062
Kaplan, Donald H.	350 Montauk Ave.	New London, Conn. 06320
Kaplan, Joel A.	111 N. Wabash Ave.	Chicago, Ill. 60602
Kaplan, Leon	881 Lafayette St.	Bridgeport, Conn. 06603

Kaplan, Morris	3705 E. Colfax Ave.	Denver, Colo. 80206
Kaplan, Philip	41 Maple Ave.	Bay Shore, N. Y. 11706
Kapustiak, Wendell A.	8058 S. Western Ave.	Chicago, Ill. 60620
Kara, Gerald B.	654 Madison Ave.	New York, N. Y. 10021
Karakashian, Nubar A.	539 E. Allegheny Ave.	Philadelphia, Pa. 19134
Karan, David S.	144-24 37th Ave.	Flushing, N. Y. 11354
Karickhoff, John R.	6060 Arlington Blvd.	Falls Church, Va. 22044
Karlin, David B.	132 E. 76th St.	New York, N. Y. 10021
Karlin, Frank L.	95 N. Main St.	Waterbury, Conn. 06702
Kartch, Matthew C.	330 Ratzer Rd.	Wayne, N. J. 07470
Kasner, David	2695 LeJeune Rd.	Coral Gables, Fla. 33134
Kasper, Richard L.	303 N. Glenoaks Blvd.	Burbank, Cal. 91502
Kasser, Max D.	101 S. 20th St.	Philadelphia, Pa. 19103
Kastelic, Robert	1729 S. 11th St.	Milwaukee, Wisc.
Katlan, Nathaniel R.	56-38 Main St.	Flushing, N. Y. 11355
Katowitz, James A.	1930 Chestnut St.	Philadelphia, Pa. 19103
Katz, Dewey	29 North St.	Willimantic, Conn. 06226
Katz, I. Herbert	713 E. Genesee St.	Syracuse, N. Y. 13210
Katz, Irving M.	9920 S. W. Regal Dr.	Portland, Ore. 97225
Katz, Jacob	Med. Arts Bldg.	Philadelphia, Pa. 19102
Katz, Joseph L.	440 E. Broad St.	Westfield, N. J. 07090
Katz, Sidney L.	22330 Hawthorne Blvd.	Torrance, Cal. 90505
Katzin, Herbert M.	178 E. 71st. St.	New York, N. Y. 10021
Kauffman, M. Luther	Med. Arts Bldg.	Jenkintown, Pa. 19046
Kaufman, Herbert E.	Col. of Med., Univ. of Fla	Gainesville, Fla. 32601
Kaufman, Ira H.	444 Community Dr.	Manhasset, N. Y. 11030
Kaufman, Samuel	57 Maple Ave.	Bay Shore, N. Y. 11706
Kaufmann, Werner C.	34-20 Parsons Blvd.	Flushing, N. Y. 11354
Kaye, Raymond J.	301 S. Illinois St.	Belleville, Ill. 06220
Kayes, Jack	211 N. Meramec	St. Louis, Mo. 63105
Kazdan, Philip	Severance Medical Arts Bldg.	Cleveland Heights, O. 44118
Kearney, William F.	540 Chestnut St.	Manchester, N. H. 03101
Kearns, Thomas P.	Mayo Clinic	Rochester, Minn. 55901
Keates, Edwin U.	2385 Cheltenham Ave.	Philadelphia, Pa. 19150
Keates, Richard H.	410 W. 10th Ave.	Columbus, O. 43210
Keck, C. A.	2902 Fairfield Ave.	Ft. Wayne, Ind. 46807
Keefe, Robert J.	2325 Ocean Ave.	San Francisco, Cal. 94127
Keefe, Wm. J.	205 E. Sidney Ave.	Mount Vernon, N. Y. 10550
Keefe, Wm. P.	240 Ashley St.	Hartford, Conn. 06105
Keeler, Lansing H.	89-04 148 St.	Jamaica, N. Y. 11435
Keeney, Arthur H.	1601 Spring Garden St.	Philadelphia, Pa. 19130
Keil, Francis C.	155 E. 62nd St.	New York, N. Y. 10021
Keipp, James V.	110 Pine Ave.	Long Beach, Cal. 90802
Keislar, Henry D.	6253 Hollywood Blvd.	Los Angeles, Cal. 90028
Keith, Frank R.	3635 Professional Dr.	Port Arthur, Tex. 77640
Keizer, John P.	2330 N.W. Flanders	Portland, Ore. 97210
Kellan, Robert E.	125 Amesbury St.	Lawrence, Mass. 01840
Keller, A. Paul, Jr.	1010 Prince Ave.	Athens, Ga. 30601
Kellerman, Leo	61-34 188th St.	Flushing, N. Y. 11365
Kelley, Robert R.	1 Aspen Ct.	Lafayette, Cal. 94549
Kellie, Thomas E.	110 Remsen St.	Brooklyn, N. Y. 11201
Kelly, Blanche M.	P. O. Box 247	Herrin, Ill. 62948
Kelly, Francis B.	Box 3366 N.	Johnson City, Tenn. 37601
Kelly, John J.	101 Chestnut St.	Rockford, Ill. 61101
Kelly, Stephen J.	1830 14th Ave., S.	Birmingham, Ala. 35205
Kelly, Vincent J.	450 Kennedy Dr.	Kankakee, Ill. 60901

Kelly, Wm. J.	10 Union Ave.	Lynbrook, N. Y. 11563
Kelman, Charles D.	215 E. 64th St.	New York, N. Y. 10021
Kelson, Ralph H.	333 E. Nutwood St.	Inglewood, Cal. 90301
Kemp, Gordon B.	1181 E. State St.	Sharon, Pa. 16146
Kemper, Robert A.	Central Trust Tower	Cincinnati, O. 45202
Kendrick, Dan L.	730 N. Main Ave.	San Antonio, Tex. 78205
Kenneally, Elmer V.	Med-Optic Bldg., Main St. Montague City	Turners Falls, Mass. 01376
Kennedy, John A.	165 Clinton St.	Watertown, N. Y. 13601
Kennedy, John E.	551 Millburn Ave.	Short Hills, N. J. 07078
Kennedy, John J.	1515 Union St.	Schenectady, N. Y. 12309
Kennedy, Keith B.	316 Tyler	W. Memphis, Ark. 72301
Kennedy, Patrick J.	32 Hampden Rd.	Upper Darby, Pa. 19082
Kennedy, Robert E.	235 Alexander St.	Rochester, N. Y. 14607
Kennedy, Roscoe J.	2020 E. 93rd St.	Cleveland, O. 44106
Kennerdell, Edward H.	303 E. 6th Ave.	Tarentum, Pa. 15084
Kennerdell, John S.	230 Lothrop St.	Pittsburgh, Pa. 15213
Kenney, David B.	5506 E. 16th St.	Indianapolis, Ind. 46218
Kennon, Beverley R., III	530 Pembroke Ave.	Norfolk, Va. 23507
Kent, Louis R.	104 W. Clark St.	Champaign, Ill. 61820
Kent, Richard B.	17 S. Church St.	W. Chester, Pa. 19380
Keppen, Ford F.	180 Broadway	Richmond, Cal. 94804
Kera, Henry M.	3333 Eastchester Rd.	Bronx, N. Y. 10469
Kern, Athur S.	50 Union Ave.	Irvington, N. J. 07111
Kern, William A.	40300 Date St.	Hemet, Cal. 92343
Kerns, Thomas C.	1110 W. Main St.	Durham, N. C. 27701
Kerr, Lawrence M.	Valley Forge Gen. Hosp.	Phoenixville, Pa. 19460
Kerrison, Horry H.	31 Smith St.	Charleston, S. C. 29401
Kershner, Calvin M.	510 Main Ave.	Brookings, S. D. 57006
Kerstine, Richard S.	8040 Reading Rd.	Cincinnati, Ohio 45237
Kerwin, Raymond W.	316 Dixie Hwy.	Chicago Heights, Illinois 60411
Kesinger, Herbert F.	740 E. Park St.	Sandusky, O. 44870
Keskey, C. W.	3100 S. 37th St.	Milwaukee, Wisc. 53215
Keskey, G. Richard	2266 N. Prospect	Milwaukee, Wisc. 53202
Ketels, C. F. B.	121 E. 60th St.	New York, N. Y. 10022
Key, Charles B.	8226 Douglas Ave.	Dallas, Tex. 75225
Key, Sam N., Jr.	1301 W. 38th St.	Austin, Tex. 78705
Keyes, John E. L.	22199 McCauley Rd.	Cleveland, O. 44122
Keys, Marshall P.	Eye Clinic, Walson Army Hosp.	Ft. Dix, N. J. 08640
Kfoury, Mitchell E.	353 Lafayette St.	Salem, Mass. 01970
Khodadoust, Ali A.	Johns Hopkins Hosp.	Baltimore, Md. 21205
Kiechler, Richard J.	9200 Colima Rd.	Whittier, Cal. 90605
Kielar, Richard A.	University of Kentucky Med. Center	Lexington, Ky. 40506
Kiesel, Robert	3710 Hamilton St.	Cetronia (Allentown), Pa. 18104
Kiesel, Robert D.	5015 Lee Hwy.	Arlington, Va. 22207
Kiess, Robert D.	3939 Monroe St.	Toledo, O. 43606
Kiffney, G. Thomas, Jr.	906 Broad St.	Durham, N. C. 27705
Kilborn, Kenneth S.	5920 100th St., S. W.	Tacoma, Wash. 98499
Kilmann, Martin H.	30 Central Park S.	New York, N. Y. 10019
Kilpatrick, Wm. R. J.	111-4th St., S. E.	Huron, S. D. 57350
Kim, Joseph C.	585 Main St.	Malden, Mass. 02148
Kimball, Paul	2465 S. Downing St.	Denver, Colo. 80210
Kimmel, Merl F.	3002 Union Ave.	Altoona, Pa. 16602

Kimmelman, David B.	10 Downing St.	New York, N. Y. 10014
Kimura, Samuel J.	University of California, School of Medicine	San Francisco, Cal. 94122
Kinder, Robert S. L.	210 Angell St.	Providence, R. I. 02906
King, Arnold D.	61-34 188th St.	Fresh Meadows, N. Y. 11365
King, Charles M.	20 S. Dudley St.	Memphis, Tenn. 38103
King, Christopher M.	537 E. Market St.	Alliance, O. 44601
King, Clair B.	214 Dartmouth Ave., S. W.	Canton, Ohio 44710
King, James C.	663 E. Grand Ave.	Escondido, Cal. 92025
King, John H.	6000 Wisconsin Ave.	Chevy Chase, Md. 20015
King, John T., Jr.	416 Gordon Ave.	Thomasville, Ga. 31792
King, Lawrence M., Jr.	Mass. Eye and Ear Infirmary	Boston, Mass. 02114
King, Merrill, J., Jr.	Vinal Rd.	W. Rockport, Me. 04865
King, Robert E.	217 Manatee Ave.	Bradenton, Fla. 33505
King, Robert G., Jr.	Medical College of Virginia	Richmond, Va. 23219
King, Robert W.	900 N.W. 10th St.	Oklahoma City, Okla. 73106
King, Walter F.	527 Delaware Ave.	Buffalo, N. Y. 14202
Kingston, Louis C.	6 North St.	Barre, Vt. 05641
Kinn, William F.	607 Tenth Ave.	Fairbanks, Alaska 99701
Kiplin, Lydell C.	Box 35, USAF Hospital	Wiesbaden, APO N. Y. 09220
Kirber, H. P.	9 Waterman Ave.	Philadelphia, Pa. 19118
Kirby, Thomas J.	Mayo Clinic	Rochester, Minn. 55901
Kirchgeorg, Clemens	409 E. Wisconsin Ave.	Neenah, Wisc. 54956
Kirk, Harold Q.	715 Lake St.	Oak Park, Ill. 06301
Kirk, Phillip B.	1341 S. Hickory St.	Melbourne, Fla. 32901
Kirk, Robert C.	15644 Madison Ave.	Lakewood, O. 44116
Kirkconnell, Waite S.	3000 W. Buffalo Ave.	Tampa, Fla. 33607
Kirkeeng, Melvin J.	2034 E. Charleston Blvd.	Las Vegas, Nev. 89104
Kirkegaard, Rodger S.	1710 W. 10th St.	Topeka, Kansas 66604
Kirkegaard, Virgil G.	501 Insurance Exchange Bldg. ..	Sioux City, Ia. 51101
Kirkland, Theo N.	7714 Second Ave. S.	Birmingham, Ala. 35206
Kirkpatrick, Joseph F.	414 E. Main St.	Lancaster, O. 43130
Kirsch, Ralph E.	1335 Biscayne Blvd.	Miami, Fla. 33132
Kirschner, Robert J.	1900 Spruce St.	Philadelphia, Pa. 19103
Kirshner, Harold	40 Park Ave.	New York, N. Y. 10016
Kissling, Arthur C.	2040 W. Wisconsin Ave.	Milwaukee, Wisc. 53233
Kistler, Warren D.	Professional Arts Bldg.	Chambersburg, Pa. 17201
Kitchen, Calvin B.	303 E. Town St.	Columbus, O. 43215
Kitchen, Clyde K.	5000 W. 39th St.	Minneapolis, Minn. 55416
Klages, Ralph F.	540 N. Central Ave.	Glendale, Cal. 91203
Klapper, Raphael M.	241 Central Park, W.	New York, N. Y. 10024
Klayman, Joel	140 Lockwood Ave.	New Rochelle, N. Y. 10801
Kleckner, James F.	2080 Century Pk. E.	Los Angeles, Cal. 90067
Kleefeld, Georges	115 Central Park, W.	New York, N. Y. 10023
Kleh, Thomas R.	404 Pearl St.	Burlington, Vt. 05401
Klein, Harvey Z.	15330 S. Wood St.	Harvey, Ill. 60426
Klein, Irving	7000 Cutler N. E.	Albuquerque, N. M. 87110
Kleinfeld, Jerome	801 Encino Pl. N. E.	Albuquerque, N. M. 87110
Kleinhandler, W. Wolfgang .	2400 21st St.	Troy, N. Y. 12180
Kleis, Walter	Ashford Med. Ctr.	Santurce, P. R. 00907
Klien, Bertha A.	30 N. Michigan Ave.	Chicago, Ill. 60602
Klika, R. Riggs	21100 Southgate Park Blvd.	Maple Heights, O. 44137
Klina, Jacob M.	4955 Van Nuys Blvd.	Sherman Oaks, Cal. 91403
Kline, Oram R., Jr.	406 Cooper St.	Camden, N. J. 08102
Kling, Robert P.	600 Hillwood Ave.	Falls Church, Va. 22042

Klingel, Robert W.	595 Buckingham Way	San Francisco, Cal. 94132
Klodell, Carl B.	1005 Belmont Ave.	Youngstown, O. 44504
Klotz, Hugh A.	1293 Peachtree St. N. E.	Atlanta, Ga. 30328
Klotz, Jeremiah A., Jr.	Wainwright Bldg.	Norfolk, Va. 23510
Klotz, Wm. F.	1661 Madison Ave.	Memphis, Tenn. 38104
Kluger, Joachim A. K.	1431 Highland Dr.	Silver Spring, Md. 20910
Klunzinger, Willard R.	326 W. Ionia St.	Lansing, Mich, 48933
Kluver, Herman C.	Wraywood Manor 331	Fort Dodge, Ia. 50501
Knaggs, James G.	Eye Clinic, USA Hospital	Nurnberg, APO N. Y. 09696
Knapp, Arthur A.	907-5th Ave.	New York, N. Y. 10021
Knapp, Frederick W.	2210 Mesa Dr.	Oceanside, Cal. 92054
Knapp, James W.	2300 Sutter St.	San Francisco, Cal. 94115
Knapp, Philip	635 W. 165th St.	New York, N. Y. 10032
Knauer, Wm. J.	2535 Riverside Ave.	Jacksonville, Fla. 32204
Knauer, Wm. J., Jr.	2535 Riverside Ave.	Jacksonville, Fla. 32204
Knisely, Samuel W.	1410 N. Second St.	Harrisburg, Pa. 17102
Knobloch, Wm. H.	412 S.E. Union St.	Minneapolis, Minn. 55414
Knolle, Guy E., Sr.	1010 Louisiana St.	Houston, Tex. 77002
Knolle, Guy E., Jr.	Memorial Professional Bldg.	Houston, Tex. 77002
Knopf, Merrill M.	117 E. 8th St.	Long Beach, Cal. 90813
Knorr, James E.	Marysville Medical Clinic, 800 Third St.	Marysville, Cal. 95901
Knott, Stuart A.	100 Oak St.	Wyandotte, Mich. 48192
Knowles, Wm. F.	4036 Fifth Ave.	San Diego, Cal. 92103
Knox, David L.	Johns Hopkins Hosp.	Baltimore, Md. 21205
Kobley, Donald E.	245 S. E. First St.	Miami, Fla. 33131
Kobs, Robert J.	720 W. Franklin	Jackson, Mich. 49201
Koch, John C.	1305 Frank Ave.	Lufkin, Tex. 75901
Kochman, Marvin C.	470 Ocean Ave.	Brooklyn, N. Y. 11226
Kochman, Richard S.	501 W. 113th St.	New York, N. Y. 10025
Koenig, Harry	540 E. Division St.	Ishpeming, Mich. 49849
Koenig, Marvin I.	Northland Med. Bldg.	Jennings, Mo. 63136
Koenig, Robert P.	33 N. River Road W.	St. Cloud, Minn. 56301
Kogan, Leonard L.	1106 Spring St.	Silver Spring, Md. 20910
Kogut, Henry V.	50 Ridgefield Ave.	Bridgeport, Conn. 06610
Kogut, Lewis V.	Bowling Green University	Bowling Green, O. 43402
Kohl, Darwin L.	123 2nd Ave., S. E.	Minot, N. D. 58701
Kohl, J. Wm.	2600 Capitol Ave.	Sacramento, Cal. 95816
Kohler, Henry J.	5118 N. Broad St.	Philadelphia, Pa. 19141
Kohlmeyer, Frederick C. ..	1600 S. Western Ave.	Sioux Falls, S. D. 57105
Kohn, Howard D.	3461 Warrensville Center Rd. ...	Shaker Heights, O. 44122
Kohn, Joseph J.	28 W. State St.	Trenton, N. J. 08608
Kohn, Ralph B.	20032 Lake Chabot Rd.	Castro Valley, Cal. 94546
Kohtio, August G.	57 W. 57th St.	New York, N. Y. 10019
Koke, Martin P.	304 Hawthorn St.	San Diego, Cal. 92101
Kolbert, Gerald S.	3455 Steuben Ave.	Bronx, N. Y. 10467
Kolker, Allan E.	4901 Barnes Hospital Plaza	St. Louis, Mo. 63110
Kolker, Ronald H.	1601 N. Tucson Blvd.	Tucson, Ariz. 85716
Koller, Hermann M.	Medical Arts Bldg.	Minneapolis, Minn. 55402
Kolodny, George R.	Hermann Professional Bldg.	Houston, Tex. 77025
Konicoff, Donald S.	49 S. E. Third St.	Boca Raton, Fla. 33432
Koons, Jess W.	Box 1419	Liberal, Kans. 067901
Koop, Richard H.	4352 Sylvania	Toledo, O. 43623
Kopf, George M.	2315 Maple Ave.	Zanesville, O. 43701
Koppel, Zoltan I.	21 Bay St.	Glens Falls, N. Y. 12801
Koransky, David S.	6860 Hohman	Hammond, Ind. 46324

Kornzweig, Abraham L.	1 E. 63rd St.	New York, N. Y. 10021
Korstanje, Marion C.	Post Office Box 366	Huntington, W. Va. 25708
Kortemeier, Elwood F.	1110 S. Park Blvd.	Freeport, Ill. 61032
Kossmann, Richard J.	635 W. 168th St.	New York, N. Y. 10032
Koster, Charles K.	14583 Madison Ave.	Lakewood, O. 44107
Kottler, Saul	3550 Warrensville Center Rd. . . .	Cleveland, O. 44122
Koven, Arthur L.	101 W. Broad St.	Hazelton, Pa. 18201
Kozil, Donald J.	940 Lee St.	Des Plaines, Ill. 60016
Kraff, Manus C.	4958 W. Irving Pk. Rd.	Chicago, Ill. 60641
Kraft, Frederick W.	1119 Pajaro St.	Salinas, Cal. 93901
Kraft, James E.	3102 S. Harvard	Tulsa, Okla. 74135
Krall, J. Thomas	85 N. Lansdowne Ave.	Landsdowne, Pa. 19050
Kramár, Piroska O.	USPHS Hospital	Seattle, Wash. 98114
Kramer, Aaron	81 Ocean Pkwy.	Brooklyn, N. Y. 11218
Kramer, Robert L.	Utica Sq. Med. Ctr.	Tulsa, Okla. 74114
Kratka, Wm. H.	1401 Pennsylvania Ave.	Wilmington, Del. 19806
Kratz, Richard P.	15225 Vanowen St.	Van Nuys, Cal. 91405
Kraus, Albert M.	85 High St.	Buffalo, N. Y. 14202
Krause, Arlington C.	953 Minnehaha St.	Memphis, Tenn. 38117
Kraushar, Marvin F.	565 Park Ave.	New York, N. Y. 10021
Kravitz, Daniel	1 Hanson Pl.	Brooklyn, N. Y. 11217
Kreft, Alfred J.	Portland Med. Ctr.	Portland, Ore. 97205
Kreft, Warrren W.	940 Lee St.	Des Plaines, Ill. 60016
Kreiger, Allan E.	1000 W. Carson St.	Torrance, Cal. 90509
Kremen, Abraham	Sutton Place L-6, 1111 Park Ave.	Baltimore, Md. 21201
Krenz, Marlin P.	803 Hackley Bank Bldg.	Muskegon, Mich. 49440
Kresca, Frank J.	208 W. Green	Champaign, Ill. 61820
Kreshon, Martin J.	1600 E. 3rd St.	Charlotte, N. C. 28204
Krichbaum, Franklin M. . . .	2310 Kipling St.	Lakewood, Colo. 80215
Krieger, A. A.	4627 Fifth Ave.	Pittsburgh, Pa. 15213
Krill, Alex E.	950 E. 59th St.	Chicago, Ill. 60637
Krimmer, Burton M.	5736 W. North Ave.	Chicago, Ill. 60639
Krimsky, Emanuel	103-05 Seaview Ave.	Brooklyn, N. Y. 11236
Krishna, Narendra	584 E. Chestnut St.	Coatesville, Pa. 19320
Krohn, David L.	30 E. 40th St.	New York, N. Y. 10016
Kroll, Arnold J.	7 Whittier Pl.	Boston, Mass. 02114
Kroll, Michael	2016 Forest Ave.	San Jose, Cal. 95128
Kronenberg, Bernard	605 Park Ave.	New York, N. Y. 10021
Kronthal, Alfred	611 Park Ave.	Baltimore, Md. 21201
Krug, Joseph H.	988 Fifth Ave.	New York, N. Y. 10021
Krupski, John G.	125 W. 21st St.	Lorain, O. 44052
Kubitschek, Wm. R.	2310 Kipling St.	Denver, Colo. 80215
Kublin, John G.	1414 W. Fair	Marquette, Mich. 49855
Kuglen, Craig C.	1604 E. Carey Dr.	Harlingen, Tex. 78550
Kuhlman, Wm. K.	209 S. Nevada Ave.	Colorado Springs, Colo. 80902
Kuhn, Hedwig S.	7142 Hohman Ave.	Hammond, Ind. 46324
Kuhns, Thomas R.	120 E. 36th St.	New York, N. Y. 10016
Kulczycki, Edward	Guthrie Clinic	Sayre, Pa. 18840
Kummer, William M.	1247 Lakeland Hills Blvd.	Lakeland, Fla. 33801
Kundert, Karl F.	1106 Pacific St.	San Luis Obispo, Cal. 93401
Kunkel, Cooper D.	701 Professional Dr.	New Bern, N. C. 28560
Kunkel, James A.	Marshfield Clinic	Marshfield, Wisc. 54449
Kunkle, F. Albert	3333 E. Central	Wichita, Kans. 67208
Kupersmith, Harry S.	22030 Sherman Way	Canoga Park, Cal. 91303
Kupfer, Carl	Eye Institute, N.I.H.	Bethesda, Md. 20014

Kuppinger, John C.	1515 Ed Carey Dr.	Harlingen, Tex. 78550
Kurstin, M. Joseph	2695 Le Jeune Rd.	Coral Gables, Fla. 33134
Kurtzman, Joseph L.	48 Rutledge Ave.	Charleston, S. C. 29401
Kurz, George H.	Hunterdon Med. Ctr.	Flemington, N. J. 08822
Kustrup, William J.	1418 S. Broad St.	Trenton, N. J. 08610
Kwedar, Edward W.	615 S. 7th St.	Springfield, Ill. 62703
Laauwe, Roger C.	500 Market St.	Paterson, N. J. 07501
Laborde, Philip M. ....'	4116 Jackson St.	Alexandria, La. 71301
Labriola, Charles	141 Noble St.	Brooklyn, N. Y. 11222
Lachman, Bernard E.	1140 Walnut St.	Allentown, Pa. 18102
Lachman, George S.	450 Sutter St.	San Francisco, Cal. 94108
Lachterman, Alfred	310 Lexington Ave.	New York, N. Y. 10016
Lack, Cyrus	1730 President St.	Brooklyn, N. Y. 11213
Lack, David C.	1983 Crompond Rd.	Peekskill, N. Y. 10566
Ladenheim, Jacob	503 S. Oak Park Ave.	Oak Park, Ill. 60304
LaForte, Peter	70 Mill River St.	Stamford, Conn. 06902
LaGattuta, Frank	2488 Grand Concourse	New York, N. Y. 10458
Lahey, Duane D.	3535 Cherry Creek North Dr. ...	Denver, Colo. 80209
Laibson, Peter R.	1601 Spring Garden St.	Philadelphia, Pa. 19130
Laing, Anna C.	126 Sterling Pl.	Amityville, N. Y. 11701
Laird, Archibald	12 Main St.	Wellsboro, Pa. 16901
Laird, R. G.	435 Cherry S. E.	Grand Rapids, Mich. 49503
Lake, Max S.	United Bldg.	Salina, Kans. 67401
Lakritz, A.	408 S. River St.	Janesville, Wisc. 53545
Lalli, Richard A.	511 S.W. 10th Ave.	Portland, Ore. 97205
Lamberson, Robert E.	57 N. Ottawa St.	Joliet, Ill. 60431
Lambrecht, Paul	3816 Ingersoll Ave.	Des Moines, Ja. 50312
LaMotte, William O., Jr. ...	1303 Delaware Ave.	Wilmington, Dela. 19806
Lancaster, Mary A.	Medical Arts Bldg.	Dallas, Tex. 75201
Landegger, George P.	3875 Wilshire Blvd.	Los Angeles, Cal. 90005
Landers, Gardner H. ......'	318 Thompson	El Dorado, Ark. 71730
Landers, Maurice B. III i	Duke Univ. Medical Center	Durham, N. C. 27706
Landers, Philip H.	53 Main St.	Binghamton, N. Y. 13905
Landesberg, Jacques	625 Ocean Ave.	Brooklyn, N. Y. 11226
Landholm, Wallace M.	440 Fair Dr.	Costa Mesa, Cal. 92626
Landhuis, Leo R.	113 W. Broadway	Columbia, Mo. 65201
Landis, C. B.	2211 South St.	Lafayette, Ind. 47902
Landowski, Jules	123 E. 83rd St.	New York, N. Y. 10028
Landrigan, Frederick L. ...	520 Commonwealth Ave.	Boston, Mass. 02215
Lane, George F.	600 Park Ave.	Plainfield, N. Y. 07060
Lange, Adolph C.	607 N. Grand Blvd.	St. Louis, Mo. 63103
Lanning, Charles D.	975 Ryland St.	Reno, Nev. 89502
Lanou, William W.	73 North St.	Pittsfield, Mass. 01202
Lansche, Richard K.	7946 Ivanhoe Ave.	La Jolla, Cal. 92037
LaPierre, Warren W.	5 Clinic Dr.	Norwich, Bonn. 06360
Large, Henry R.	11 Alderson Ave.	Billings, Mont. 59102
Large, John S.	350 W. 10th St.	Erie, Penna. 16502
Larkin, Ernest W., Jr.	211 N. Market St.	Washington, N. C. 27889
La Rocca, Vito	30 Park Ave.	New York, N. Y. 10016
Larson, Bertil F.	222 Talbott Tower	Dayton, O. 45402
Larson, Darell H.	1022 W. Ivy	Moses Lake, Wash. 98837
Larson, Dean W.	210 S. Grand Ave.	Glendora, Cal. 91740
Larson, Ernest J., Jr.	528 Southdale Medical Bldg. ...	Edina, Minn. 55435
Larson, G. Donald	1500 Eighth St.	Wichita Falls, Tex. 76301
LaRue, Roger P.	New England Bldg.	Winter Park, Fla. 32789
Laschever, E. Frederick ...	193 N. Harrison St.	Princeton, N. J. 08540

Lashmet, Michael H.	Hume Mansur Bldg.	Indianapolis, Ind. 46204
Lasky, Mortimer A.	1 Nevins St.	Brooklyn, N. Y. 11217
Lassiter, Lawrence H.	Provident Bldg.	Chattanooga, Tenn. 37402
Last, Jeremiah	87-01 148th St., Jamaica	New York, N. Y. 11435
Lateiner, Robert	1077 North Ave.	New Rochelle, N. Y. 10804
LaTessa, Anthony J.	218 State Tower Bldg.	Syracuse, N.,Y. 13202
Laties, Alan M.	Hosp. of the Univ. of Pa.	Philadelphia, Pa. 19104
Latta, C. Rex	Doctors Bldg.	Omaha, Nebr. 68131
Latto, Ira S.	8215 Van Nuys Blvd.	Panorama City, Cal. 91402
Laughlin, Robert C.	1117 Minor	Seattle, Wash. 98101
Lauppe, Frederick A.	1801 David Whitney Bldg.	Detroit, Mich. 48226
Lauren, George P.	2850 Sixth Ave.	San Diego, Cal. 92103
Lava, Irving M.	632 S. San Bicente Blvd.	Los Angeles, Cal. 90048
Laval, Joseph	136 E. 64th St.	New York, N. Y. 10021
Lavine, Oscar	4101 Underwood St.	W. Hyattsville, Md. 20782
Lawaczeck, Elmar M. J.	1023 S. 20th St.	Birmingham, Ala. 35205
Lawler, Donald J.	1500 16th Ave. Ct.	Greeley, Colo. 80631
Lawlor, Peter P., Jr.	205 Dorset St.	S. Burlington, Vt. 05401
Lawlor, Robert C.	174 Central St.	Lowell, Mass. 01852
Lawrence, Carteret	1102 Columbia St.	Seattle, Wash. 98104
Lawrence, Granville A.	Med. Arts Bldg.	Nashville, Tenn. 37212
Lawrence, Harry M.	American National Bank Bldg.	Chattanooga, Tenn. 37402
Lawrence, James M.	3500 Lafayette Rd.	Indianapolis, Ind. 46222
Lawson, Edgar C.	1400 Jefferson Park Ave.	Charlottesville, Va. 22903
Lawson, Lawrence J.	723 Elm St.	Winnetka, Ill. 60093
Lawwill, Stewart, Jr.	Med. Arts Bldg.	Chattanooga, Tenn. 37402
Lawwill, Theodore	301 E. Walnut St.	Louisville, Ky. 40202
Layton, George A.	87-17 168th Pl.	Jamaica, N. Y. 11432
Lazerson, Howard E.	645 E. Aerick	Inglewood, Cal. 90301
Lazich, Bronislav M.	10921 Wilshire	Los Angeles, Cal. 90024
Lazor, Edward B.	6360 Wilshire Blvd.	Los Angeles, Cal. 90048
Lea, Martha E.	913 Ave. C.	Marrero, La.
Leahey, Brendan D.	9 Central St.	Lowell, Mass. 01852
Leaman, John C.	3285 Kennedy Blvd.	Jersey City, N. J. 07307
Learn, Richard N.	225 W. Madison Ave.	El Cajon, Cal. 92020
Leavenworth, Richard O., Jr.	5000 W. 39th St.	St. Louis Park, Minn. 55416
Lebensohn, James E.	4010 W. Madison St.	Chicago, Ill. 60624
LeBow, Erwin E.	314 E. Hillcrest Blvd.	Inglewood, Cal. 90301
Leckert, Edmund L., Jr.	4500 Magnolia St.	New Orleans, La. 70115
Ledden, John V.	185 N. 4th St.	Lander, Wyo. 82520
Lederman, Ira R.	7312 Granby St.	Norfolk, Va. 23505
Lee, Charles, J., Jr.	P.O. Box 9207	Santurce, P. R. 00908
Lee, Henry Y.	1401 S. Hope St.	Los Angeles, Cal. 90015
Lee, Jack B.	409 Camden	San Antonio, Tex. 78215
Lee, King Y.	U. S. Army Hospital	Ft. Devens, Mass. 01433
Lee, Myron S.	Professional Village	Missoula, Mont. 59801
Lee, Otis S.	Utica Sq. Med. Ctr.	Tulsa, Okla. 74114
Lee, Parker H., Jr.	1900 Tate Spring Rd.	Lynchburg, Va. 24501
Leech, Vernon M.	9450 Central Prak Ave.	Evanston, Ill. 60203
Leenhouts, Thomas M.	1355 N. Beaver St.	Flagstaff, Ariz. 86001
Lees, Charles R.	600 W. 10th St.	Fort Worth, Tex. 76102
Legett, Carey, Jr.	1707 Colorado	Austin, Tex. 78701
Legge, W. Reynolds	214 W. Boscawen St.	Winchester, Va. 22601
Leggett, Albert E.	Fincastle Bldg.	Louisville, Ky. 40202
Leggett, Albert E., Jr.	Fincastle Bldg.	Louisville, Ky. 40202
Lehman, Mary D.	Box 12021	Pittsburgh, Pa. 15240

Lehman, Robert N.	VA Hospital, University Drive C.	Pittsburgh, Pa. 15240
Lehman, Roger H.	V. A. Ctr.	Wood, Wisc. 53193
Lehner, Robert H.	312 Seventh St.	Racine, Wisc. 53403
Lehwalder, Laurus W.	515 Kensington	Missoula, Mont. 59801
Leib, Dorothy B.	429 Montauk Ave.	New London, Conn. 06320
Leibold, James E.	3705 E. Colfax Ave.	Denver, Colo. 80206
Leibowitz, Howard M.	750 Harrison Ave.	Boston, Mass. 02118
Leigh, Richard E., Jr.	Medical Towers	Houston, Tex. 77025
Leight, Harold C.	1245 E. Colfax Ave.	Denver, Colo. 80218
Leinfelder, Joseph T.	1420 7th St.	Moline, Ill. 61265
Leinfelder, Placidus J.	University Hospitals	Iowa City, Ia. 52240
Leiphart, Clarence D.	336 N. Duke St.	Lancaster, Pa. 17602
Leitch, Gordon B.	919 S. W. Taylor St.	Portland, Ore. 97205
LeMaster, Theodore R.	Hume Mansur Bldg.	Indianapolis, Ind. 46204
Lemcke, Harald H.	490 Post St.	San Francisco, Cal. 94102
Lemoine, Albert N., Jr.	4620 J. C. Nichols Pkwy.	Kansas City, Mo. 64112
Lemp, Michael A.	3800 Reservoir Rd., N.W.	Washington, D. C. 20007
Lempert, Philip	1301 Trumansburg Rd.	Ithaca, N. Y. 14850
Lenartz, Henry F.	305 South Drive	Mountain View, Cal. 94040
Lensink, Everett R.	Medical Arts Ctr.	Bozeman, Mont. 59715
Lenz, Charles R.	405 First St.	Jackson, Mich. 49201
Lenzen, Aloysius F.	555 Second St.	La Salle, Ill. 61301
Leonard, Arthuer L., Jr. ...	52 College Way	Auburn, Cal. 95603
Leonard, Robert E.	1109 Telfair St.	Augusta, Ga. 30901
Leone, Charles R. Jr.	401 M & S. Tower	San Antonio, Tex. 78205
Leopold, Irving H.	Mt. Sinai School of Medicine, City Clinic of N. Y., Fifth Ave. & 100th St.	New York, N. Y. 10029
Lepard, Cecil W.	David Whitney Bldg.	Detroit, Mich. 48226
Le Peter, Alan J.	1138 Second St. S. W.	Roanoke, Va. 24016
Lepley, Frederick J.	19803 Mack Ave.	Grosse Pointe Woods, Mich. 48236
Lerner, Hobart A.	720 E. Ave.	Rochester, N. Y. 14607
Lerner, Leonard H.	26615 Greenfield	Southfield, Mich. 48075
Lerner, Melvin L.	14401 Hamlin St.	Van Nuys, Cal. 91401
Lesko, William S.	1030 Clifton Ave.	Clifton, N. J. 07013
Leslie, Samuel B.	Veterans Administration Hospital	Albuquerque, N. M. 87101
L'Esperance, Francis A., Jr. .	1 E. 71st St.	New York, N. Y. 10021
Lessell, Simmons	750 Harrison Ave.	Boston, Mass. 02118
Lesser, Donald Y.	15955 Samaritan Dr.	San Jose, Cal. 95124
Lester, Harvey A.	2065 Adelbert Rd.	Cleveland, O. 44106
Lester, Jesse C.	478 Peachtree St., N.E.	Atlanta, Ga. 30308
Lester, Robert H.	549 Marshall Taylor Bldg.	Jacksonville, Fla. 32207
Letson, Holton C.	2309 Maple Ave.	Zanesville, O. 43701
Letson, Robert D.	Mayo Memorial Hospital	Minneapolis, Minn. 55455
Letts, Neil F.	1561 Garden	Titusville, Fla. 32780
Leubuscher, Kurt	8301 Bay Pkwy.	Brooklyn, N. Y. 11214
Levatin, Paul	280 W. MacArthur Blvd.	Oakland, Cal. 94610
Levene, Ralph Z.	560 First Ave.	New York, N. Y. 10016
Levenson, David S.	2754 N. Decatur Rd.	Decatur, Ga. 30030
Levi, George A.	1629 Owen Dr.	Fayetteville, N.C. 28304
Levieff, Leo	2875 Main St.	Strafford, Conn. 06497
Levin, Aaron H.	1134 Beacon St.	Brookline, Mass. 02146
Levin, Abram A.	Carew Tower	Cincinnati, O. 45202
Levin, Joseph M.	5889 Colerain Ave.	Cincinnati, O. 45239
Levine, Alan M.	2025 Kings Hwy.	Brooklyn, N. Y. 11229

Levine, Alexander	966 A Park St.	Stoughton, Mass. 02072
Levine, Donald J.	136 E. 64th St.	New York, N. Y. 10021
Levine, George	50 Maple St.	Brooklyn, N. Y. 11225
Levine, Julius	1020 Levine Ct.	Hayward, Cal. 94541
Levine, Meyer R.	280 Broadway	New York, N. Y. 10007
Levine, Oscar	1335 Biscayne Blvd.	Miami, Fla. 33132
Levine, Robert A.	111 N. Wabash Ave.	Chicago, Ill. 60602
Levine, Robert E.	3875 Wilshire Blvd.	Los Angeles, Cal. 90005
Levitt, Jesse M.	515 Ocean Ave.	Brooklyn, N. Y. 11226
Levitzky, Munro J.	566 First Ave.	New York, N. Y. 10016
Levy, Abram	106 E. Union Ave.	Bound Brook, N. J. 08805
Levy, Chauncey F., Jr.	1299 Portland Ave.	Rochester, N. Y. 14621
Levy, Irvin	383 W. State St.	Trenton, N. J. 08618
Levy, Mark R.	2312 15th St.	Troy, N. Y. 12180
Levy, Philip L.	3965 J St.	Sacramento, Cal. 95819
Levy, Phillip M.	316 Main St.	Newport News, Va. 23601
Lewallen, William M., Jr. ..	402 Colorado Ave.	Pueblo, Colo. 81005
LeWin, Thurber	112 Linwood Ave.	Buffalo, N. Y. 14209
Lewin, W. Howard	906 Olive St.	St. Louis, Mo. 63101
Lewis, Donald L.	1275 Olentangy River Rd.	Columbus, O. 43221
Lewis, Earl L.	375 W. Huntington Dr.	San Marino, Cal. 91108
Lewis, Harvey J.	99 Waltham St.	Lexington, Mass. 02173
Lewis, Philip M.	Exchange Bldg.	Memphis, Tenn. 38103
Lewis, Samuel D.	85 Jefferson St.	Hartford, Conn. 06106
Ley, John A.	101 W. John	Bay City, Mich. 48706
Lhotka, Frank M.	6005 Cermak Rd.	Cicero, Ill. 60650
Liao, Cheung-Kuo	15330 S. Wood St.	Harvey, Ill. 60426
Libby, John T.	723 Congress St.	Portland, Me. 04102
Lichter, Paul R.	Bethesda Naval Hospital	Bethesda, Md. 20034
Liddicoat, Douglas A.	135 Monte Vista	Watsonville, Cal. 95076
Lide, Lanneau D.	161 W. Cheves St.	Florence, S. C. 29501
Lidster, Donald K.	1950 Court St.	Redding, Cal. 96001
Liebenberg, Henry S.	123 S. 3rd St.	San Jose, Cal. 95113
Liebergall, Gordon S.	23 Lawrence St.	Spring Valley, N. Y. 10977
Lieberman, Howard L.	1000 Sheridan Rd.	Glencoe, Ill. 60022
Lieberman, Theodore W. ..	11 E. 100th St.	New York, N. Y. 10029
Lieberman, Warren J.	2695 Le Jeune Rd.	Coral Gables, Fla. 33134
Lieberthal, Paul R.	220 S. Suffolk St.	Ironwood, Mich. 49938
Liebesman, Wm. P.	203 Elm St.	Westfield, N. J. 07090
Liebman, Sumner D.	1180 Beacon St.	Brookline, Mass. 02146
Liebowitz, Solomon, ...	41 Park Ave.	New York, N. Y. 10016
Lieurance, Richard E.	411 30th St.	Oakland, Cal. 94609
Light, Arthur	4640 N. Marine Dr.	Chicago, Ill. 60640
Lightfoot, Vernon F.	1120 Montgomery Dr.	Santa Rosa, Cal. 95405
Liioi, Joseph A.	17000 W. Eight Mile Rd.	Southfield, Mich. 48075
Lill, Frank J.	771 Briarwood Dr.	Daytona Beach, Fla. 32014
Lilly, Milton J.	1306 Kanawha Blvd., E.	Charleston, W. Va. 25301
Limaye, Suresh R.	3800 Reservoir Rd. N. W.	Washington, D. C. 20007
Lincoff, Harvey	440 E. 57th St.	New York, N. Y. 10022
Lincoff, Milton H.	685 Third Ave.	Chula Vista, Cal. 92010
Lincoff, Wm.	317 E. 9th St.	Chester, Pa. 19013
Lindberg, Vernon L.	Southdale Med. Bldg.	Minneapolis, Minn. 55435
Lindberg, Winston R.	Doctors Bldg.	Minneapolis, Minn. 55402
Lindblom, Alton E.	839 Belgrade Ave.	Mankato, Minn. 56001
Lindeke, Harold I.	1127 Wilshire Blvd.	Los Angeles, Cal. 90017
Linfesty, John W.	1919 S. University Blvd.	Denver, Colo, 80210

Lingeman, Byron S.	328 Washington St.	Wellesley Hills, Mass. 02181
Linger, Harry T.	224 Court St.	Clarksburg, W. Va. 26301
Linhart, Randolph W.	105 Emerson Ave.	Pittsburgh, Pa. 15215
Linhart, Wm. O.	3515 Fifth Ave.	Pittsburgh, Pa. 15213
Linksz, Arthur	6 E. 76th St.	New York, N. Y. 10021
Linn, Jay G.	Jenkins Bldg.	Pittsburgh, Pa. 15222
Linn, Jay G., Jr.	Jenkins Bldg.	Pittsburgh, Pa. 15222
Linn, Merritt L.	2525 N.W. Lovejoy	Portland, Ore. 97210
Linnell, Paul C.	1200 Michigan Ave.	E. Lansing, Mich. 48823
Lipani, John G.	1 Hanson Pl.	Brooklyn, N. Y. 11217
Lippas, John	1717 Pacific Ave.	Dallas, Tex. 75201
Lippmann, Otto	9 Med. Arts Sq.	Austin, Tex. 78705
Lipsich, Michael P.	4554 N. Broadway	Chicago, Ill. 60640
Lipsius, Edward I.	319 S. 16th St.	Philadelphia, Pa. 19102
Lisman, Jack V.	140 E. 56th St.	New York, N. Y. 10022
Liss, George	8830 Cameron St.	Silver Spring, Md. 20910
Litch, Melvin, Jr.	5050 Poplar Ave.	Memphis, Tenn. 38117
Little, C. R.	1415 Third St.	Corpus Christi, Tex. 78404
Little, Henry O.	455 Warren St.	Hudson, N. Y. 12534
Little, Hunter L.	Palo Alto Med. Clinic.	Palo Alto, Cal. 94301
Little, Milton F.	85 Jefferson St.	Hartford, Conn. 06103
Littwin, C. Stuart	950 Queen Anne Rd.	Teaneck, N. J. 07666
Litwin, Richard L.	11161 Crenshaw Blvd.	Inglewood, Cal. 90303
Liva, Edward L.	385 S. Maple Ave.	Ridgewood, N. J. 07450
Liva, Vinicio G.	391 Summit Ave.	Hackensack, N. J. 07602
Livant, Saul	5823 Liebig Ave.	New York, N. Y. 10471
Livingston, Alan W.	2030 Monroe Ave.	Rochester, N. Y. 14618
Livingston, Wiley K.	1715 9th Ave. S.	Birmingham, Ala. 35213
Llovera, E. Irene N. De. ...	325 Park Ave.	Huntington, N. Y. 11743
Lobell, Stephen M.	1015 Park Ave.	Plainfield, N. J. 07060
Lobsenz, Nathan P.	294 Broadway	Paterson, N. J. 07501
Locken, Gail A.	8255 W. Huron River Dr.	Dexter, Mich. 48130
Lockhart, George, III	800 McKinley Ave.	Canton, O. 44703
Lockwood, Chester C.	721 E. Charleston Blvd.	Las Vegas, Ney, 89104
Loden, James P.	21st & Hayes Med. Bldg.	Nashville, Tenn. 37203
Loder, Leonel L.	406 Hackley Union National Bank Bldg.	Muskegon, Mich. 49440
Lodge, Edmund A.	29 Pleasant	Gloucester, Mass. 01930
Lodge, John	8132 Old Georgetown Rd.	Bethesda, Md. 20014
Loeb, Donald R.	450 Sutter St.	San Francisco, Cal. 94108
Loewe, Walter R.	1 E. 69th St.	New York, N. Y. 10021
Loftis, John R., Jr.	210 Mobberly	Longview, Tex. 75601
Lomas, Richard W.	1126 112th N. E.	Bellevue, Wash. 98004
London, Merritt E.	325 Broad St.	Red Bank, N. J. 07701
London, William	3020 29th St.	Astoria, L. I., N. Y., 11102
Lonergan, Robert C., Jr. ...	144 Pine St.	Kingston, N. Y. 12401
Long, Albert E.	1707 Osage St.	Alexandria, Va. 22302
Long, Ira M.	908 Medical Arts Bldg.	Chattanooga, Tenn. 37402
Long, John C.	1215 Monaco Pkwy.	Denver, Colo. 80220
Long, Robert A.	2731 Napoleon Ave.	New Orleans, La. 70115
Long, Ruth S.	737 Park Ave.	New York, N. Y. 10021
Long, Theo. K.	327 Cumberland St.	Lebanon, Pa. 17042
Longfellow, Don W.	218 E. Stetson Dr.	Scottsdale, Ariz. 85251
Longway, Ralph E.	831 University Blvd., E.	Silver Spring, Md. 20903
Lonn, Lawrence I.	45 Castro St.	San Francisco, Cal. 94114
Lopez, Eduardo A.	10 Prospect St.	Nashua, N. H. 03060

LoPresti, Joseph J.	216 South St.	Oyster Bay, N. Y., 11771
Lordan, John P.	133 S. Lasky Dr.	Beverly Hills, Cal. 90213
Lorenzen, Robert F.	550 W. Thomas Rd.	Phoenix, Ariz. 85013
Losada, Fernando	535 Plandome Rd.	Manhasset, N. Y. 11030
Lossef, Samuel	462 Beach 126th St.	Belle Harbor, N. Y. 11694
Louis, Harold J.	235 Alexander St.	Rohester, N. Y. 14607
Loutfallah, Michel	1826 State St.	Santa Barbara, Cal. 93101
Lovekin, Louise G.	240 Bradley St.	New Haven, Conn. 06510
Loveless, Phil H.	Marcus Lawrence Memorial Hospital	Cottonwood, Ariz. 86322
Lowe, Percy E.	Memorial Prof. Bldg.	Houston, Tex. 77002
Lowe, Reginald S.	107 S. 5th St.	Clarksville, Tenn. 37040
Lowe, Stanley W.	1133 College Ave.	Manhattan, Kans. 66502
Lowry, Austin, Jr.	Rt. 2, Box 503	Lorton, Va. 22079
Lowrey, Daniel B.	1201 S. Highland Ave.	Clearwater, Fla. 33516
Lowrey, James R.	1201 S. Highland Ave.	Clearwater, Fla. 33516
Lowrey, Blackburn W.	706 Franklin St.	Tampa, Fla. 33602
Loy, Arthur W.		Grandview, Tenn. 37337
Lubeck, Marvin J.	3865 Cherry Creek N. Dr.	Denver, Colo. 80209
Lubkin, Virginia	41 Park Ave.	New York, N. Y. 10016
Lubow, Martin	Fitzsimons Gen. Hosp.	Denver, Colo, 80240
Lubowitz, Richard M.	Benson E.	Jenkintown, Pa. 19046
Lucas, Howard C.	560 Avenue K., S.E.	Winter Haven, Fla. 33880
Luce, Cyril M.	102 W. Front St.	Media, Pa. 19063
Lucic, Hugo	P. O. Box 42	La Jolla, Cal. 92037
Lucidi, Edgar A.	601 E. Whittier Blvd.	La Habra, Cal. 90631
Ludes, B. F.	Mayo Clinic	Rochester, Minn. 55901
Ludmerer, Sol	3736 Atlantic Ave.	Long Beach, Cal. 90807
Ludwig, Paul E.	408 W. Market St.	Crawfordsville, Ind. 47933
Lufkin, Murray W.	852 Lowry Medical Arts Bldg.	St. Paul, Minn. 55102
Lugay, Antonio T.	523 N. 4th St.	Steubenville, O. 43952
Luhr, John P.	1914 Colvin Blvd.	Tonawanda, N. Y. 14150
Lundblad, Robert M.	307 S. 12th Ave.	Yakima, Wash. 98902
Lundvick, Cyril V.	7425 Ruby Dr. S. W.	Tacoma, Wash. 98498
Lutman, Frank C.	33 E. Chestnut Hill Ave.	Philadelphia, Pa. 19118
Luton, James P.	430 N. W. 12th St.	Oklahoma City, Okla. 73103
Luxemberg, Malcolm N.	2707 N. Flagler Dr.	W. Palm Beach, Fla. 33407
Lyda, Wood	1601 16th Ave.	Seattle, Wash. 98122
Lyle, Donald J.	411 Oak St.	Cincinnati, O. 45219
Lyle, Philip L.	2000 Church St.	Nashville, Tenn. 37203
Lyman, Howard W.	630 E. 12th Ave.	Eugene, Ore. 97401
Lymberis, Marvin N.	1600 E. Third St.	Charlotte, N. C. 28204
Lynch, Joseph S.	115 E. 15th St.	Chester, Pa. 19013
Lynn, Bernard A.	Price Tower	Bartlesville, Okla. 74003
Lynn, John R.	5323 Harry Hines Blvd.	Dallas, Tex. 75235
Lyon, Ernst F.	133 E. 58th St.	New York, N. Y. 10022
Lyon, James M.	980 Trancas St.	Napa, Cal. 94558
Lyons, Benjamin E.	10 Mott Ave.	Norwalk, Conn. 06850
Lyster, Norman C., Jr.	Medical Arts Bldg.	Norwich, N. Y. 13815
Mabee, Judson O.	305 N. Sanborn	Mitchell, S. D. 57301
Macdonald, Roderick	306 W. Oakland Ave.	Rock Hill, S. C. 29730
Macdonald, Roderick, Jr.	301 E. Walnut St.	Louisville, Ky. 40202
MacDuffee, Frederic D.	3362 Loma Vista Rd.	Ventura, Cal. 93003
MacGlashan, Charles B., Jr.	501 E. Romie Ln.	Salinas, Cal. 93901
Mackay, Alan B.	W. 312 8th Ave.	Spokane, Wash. 99204
MacKenzie, Roland C.	Bedford Rd.	Lincoln Centre, Mass. 01773

MacLaughlin, Charles H. ...	780 Broadway	Everett, Mass. 02149
MacLean, Angus L.	1201 N. Calvert St.	Baltimore, Md. 21202
MacMillan, Karl D.	5901 Lakeshore Dr.	Columbia, S. C. 29206
Macnie, John P.	19536 Bainter Way	Los Gatos, Cal. 95030
MacVicar, Ernest L., Jr. ...	Walton Avenue Bldg.	Racine, Wisc. 53402
MacVicar, James E.	Bronson Med. Ctr.	Kalamazoo, Mich. 49006
Maddalena, Michael A.	1750 El Camino Real	Burlingame, Cal. 94010
Maddox, John D.	Sixth & Pearl	Joplin, Mo. 64801
Maddox, S. Fleetwood	800 First St.	Macon, Ga. 31201
Madeley, H. Randall	1727 Sonoma Blvd.	Vallejo, Cal. 94590
Madsen, George J.	637 E. Sahara	Las Vegas, Nev. 89105
Maestre, Federico J.	1605 Ponce De Leon	Santurce, P. R. 00909
Magaro, Joseph E.	77, Pondfield Rd.	Bronxville, N. Y. 10708
Magee, Alfred J.	Atlas Bldg.	Charleston, W. Va. 25301
Magee, George F.	329 W. 6th St.	Reno, Nev. 89503
Magee, George R.	329 W. 6th St.	Reno, Nev. 89503
Magenheimer, Richard J. ..	317 W. Pueblo St.	Santa Barbara, Cal. 93102
Magnuson, Robert H.	150 E. Broad St.	Columbus, O. 43215
Magoon, Robert C.	1688 Meridian Ave.	Miami Beach, Fla. 33139
Magovern, Malcolm, J., Jr. .	Ft. Jackson Army Hospital	Columbia, S. C. 29206
Magruder, G. Brock	1017 E. Robinson Ave.	Orlando, Fla. 32801
Mahaffy, Steve R.	27400 Hesperian Blvd.	Hayward, Cal. 94545
Maher, Robert C.	S. 427 Bernard St.	Spokane, Wash. 99204
Maher, Walter J.-	440 E. 20th St.	New York, N. Y. 10009
Maier, Paul	723 Congress St.	Portland, Me. 04102
Maislen, Sidney E.	114 Bellevue Ave.	Springfield, Mass. 01108
Major, James C.	427 Biltmore Way	Coral Gables, Fla. 33134
Makley, Torrence A., Jr. ...	410 W. 10th Ave.	Columbus, O. 43210
Malec, Henry W.	50 Pershing St.	Cumberland. Md. 21502
Malkin, Robert D.	1300 Union Turnpike	New Hyde Park, N. Y. 11040
Malloy, David J.	9215 W. Center St.	Milwaukee, Wisc. 53222
Maloney, John J.	1300 N. Ventura Rd.	Oxnard, Cal. 93030
Malouf, George S.	5802 Baltimore Ave.	Hyattsville, Md. 20781
Mamelok, Alfred E.	115 E. 61st St.	New York, N. Y. 10021
Mancall, Irwin T.	21 Woodland St.	Hartford, Conn. 06105
Manchester, Thomas	1938 Peachtree	Atlanta, Ga. 30309
Mandelbaum, Joseph	101 Lafayette Ave.	Brooklyn, N. Y. 11226
Mandeville, Jack W.	2000 Tacoma Mall	Tacoma, Wash. 98409
Manjoney, Vincent A.	2708 Main St.	Bridgeport, Conn. 06606
Mankin, William J.	1655 N. 7th St.	Terre Haute, Ind.
Manley, Donelson R.	1601 Spring Garden St.	Philadelphia, Pa. 19130
Manly, Basil, IV	2A Vardry St. Med. Ct.	Greenville, S. C. 29601
Mann, John L.	6211 Edgemere	El Paso, Tex. 79925
Mann, Mortimer	3426 N. Meridian	Indianapolis, Ind. 46208
Mann, William A.	251 E. Chicago Ave.	Chicago, Ill. 60611
Mannis, Aaron A.	685 Third Ave.	Chula Vista, Cal. 92010
Mansheim, Bernard J.	212 S. 11th	La Crosse, Wisc. 54601
Manson, Richard A.	557B Connor Rd., USMA	West Point, N. Y. 10996
Mansur, Harl D., Jr.	1400 8th St.	Wichita Falls, Tex. 76301
Manzanero, Fortunato M. ..	822 Pecan Ave.	McAllen, Tex. 78501
Maoury, Stanley D.	9611 Champion Ct.	Manassas, Va. 22110
Marchman, Oscar M.	3434 Swiss Ave.	Dallas, Tex. 75204
Marcotte, Dale D.	1130 Alpine	Boulder, Colo. 80302
Marcove, Maurice E.	Republic Bldg.	Denver, Colo. 80202
Marcus, Arthur, A.	46 Deepdale Dr.	Great Neck, N. Y. 11021

Marcus, Hubert C.	1515 Trousdale Dr.	Burlingame, Cal. 94010
Mardesich, Nicholas A.	336 E. Hillcrest	Inglewood, Cal. 90301
Margarida, Carlos J.	Prof. Bldg.	Santurce, P. R. 00909
Margo, Rodolfo E.	Mid Valley Medical Arts Bldg. ..	Weslaco, Tex. 78596
Maris, Charles S. G.	131 Fulton Ave.	Hempstead, N. Y. 11550
Maris, Peter J. G.	131 Fulton Ave.	Hempstead, N. Y. 11550
Mark, Harry H.	2 Church St., S.	New Haven, Conn. 06519
Markey, Frank R.	14853 Michigan	Dearborn, Mich. 48126
Markley, Richard E.	1130 S. W. Morrison	Portland, Ore. 97205
Markman, David A.	4223 W. Redondo Beach Blvd. ..	Lawndale. Cal. 90260
Markowitz, Louis	380 Park Ave.	Paterson, N. J. 07504
Marks, Paul L.	1260 Main St.	Baton Rouge, La. 70802
Marks, Salvo P.	6860 Hohman Ave.	Hammond, Ind. 46324
Markstone, David H.	1100 W. Michigan St.	Indianapolis, Ind. 46202
Marr, Wm. G.	10 E. Chase St.	Baltimore, Md. 21202
Marron, James M.	117 Broadway	Norwood, Mass. 02062
Marron, James W.	Prudential Bldg.	Chicago, Ill. 60601
Marsden, Wilson C.	99 N. Franklin	Wilkes-Barre, Pa. 18701
Marshall, Alexander W.	65 Gadsden, St.	Charleston, S. C. 29401
Marshall, Don	Bronson Med. Ctr.	Kalamazoo, Mich. 49006
Marshall, Ernest T.	9210 E. 14th St.	Oakland, Cal. 94603
Marshall, Hubert A.	1400 Jefferson Park Ave.	Charlottesville, Va. 22903
Marshall, J. R., Jr.	20160 Mack Ave.	Grosse Pointe Woods, Mich. 48236
Marshall, Victor M.	1127 Wilshire Blvd.	Los Angeles, Cal. 90017
Marshburn, Theodore F. ...	9200 Colima Rd.	Whittier, Cal. 90605
Martens, Theodore G.	Mayo Clinic	Rochester, Minn. 55901
Martin, Berkeley H., Jr. ...	1805 Monument Ave.	Richmond, Va. 23220
Martin, John J.	85 Main St.	North Adams, Mass. 02147
Martin, John O.	745 Pine St.	Macon, Ga. 31201
Martin, John T.	845 Eighth St., N.E.	Massillon, O. 44646
Martin, Sidney A.	235 Maple Ave.	Smithtown, N. Y. 11787
Martin, Theodore	577 Lincoln Ave.	Glen Rock, N. J. 07452
Martin, Thomas A.	1300 Brookside Dr.	Raleigh, N. C. 27604
Martin, W. Charles	1510 N. Coast Hwy.	Laguna Beach, Cal. 92651
Martin, William O., Jr.	422 Doctors Bldg.	Atlanta, Ga. 30308
Martin, William O. III	490 Peachtree St.	Atlanta, Ga. 30308
Martinez-Roig, Hugo E. ...	112 Arzuaga	Rio Piedras, P. R. 00928
Martinez-Tapia , Antonio C.	18 N. Union St.	Lambertville, N. J. 08530
Martola, Eeva-Liisa M.	328 Washington St.	Wellesley, Mass. 02181
Marton, Herbert M.	245 Engle St.	Englewood, N. J. 07631
Martyn, Lois J.	2600 N. Lawrence	Philadelphia, Pa. 19144
Martz, George E.	608 N. 3rd St.	Harrisburg, Pa. 17101
Marwill, Lawrence R.	23 Hackett Blvd.	Albany, N. Y. 12208
Masaryk, Joseph A.	524 Park Ave.	Barberton, O. 44203
Masi, Anthony V.	Kenner Army Hospital	Ft. Lee, Va. 23801
Mason, Charlotte E.	1918 Rodman St.	Hollywood, Fla. 33020
Mason, Gordon L.	207 E. Watauga Ave.	Johnson City, Tenn. 37601
Masor, Philip L.	130 E. 18th St.	New York, N. Y. 10003
Mastan, Peter F.	571 W. Seventh St.	San Pedro, Cal. 90731
Masters, J. M.	Hume Mansur Bldg.	Indianapolis, Ind. 46204
Masters, Robert J.	Hume Mansur Bldg.	Indianapolis, Ind. 46204
Masters, Stanley	161 Orchard St.	Plainview, L. I., N. Y. 11803
Mastman, Gary J.	5150 Graves Ave.	San Jose, Cal. 95129
Mastny, Val J.	2475 E. 22nd St.	Cleveland, O. 44115
Mather, Robert L.	805 Purdue National Bank Bldg. .	Lafayette, Ind. 47901

Mather, Robert W.	303 Holton Ave.	Yakima, Wash. 98902
Matheus, Charles G.	2244 Ave. A.	Yuma, Ariz. 85364
Mathias, Daniel W.	First National Tower	Akron, O. 44308
Matthews, John L.	Nix Prof. Bldg.	San Antonio, Tex. 78205
Matthews, Robert B.	762 Altos Oaks Dr.	Los Altos, Cal. 94022
Mattis, Robert D.	1325 S. Grand Ave.	St. Louis, Mo. 63104
Matusak, Lucian R.	7030 W. Belmont Ave.	Chicago, Ill. 60634
Maumenee, A. Edward	Johns Hopkins Hosp.	Baltimore, Md. 21205
Maxey, Ellis F.	Medical Arts Bldg., West Ave. ...	Newport News, Va. 23607
Maxwell, Earl	1212 Presidio	Fort Worth, Tex. 76102
Maxwell, Hal W.	Med. Arts Bldg.	Dallas, Tex. 75201
Maxwell, Harvey C.	1585 S. Coast Hwy.	Laguna Beach, Cal. 92651
Maxwell, James C.	3191 S. Broadway	Englewood, Colo. 80110
Maxwell, Joseph S.	95 Fairmont Ave.	Fairmont, W. Va. 26554
May, James W.	425 E. 63rd St.	Kansas City, Mo. 64110
Mayer, James T.	Hanna Bldg.	Cleveland, O. 44115
Mayer, Leo L.	113 Elcrest St.	Jackson, Miss. 39209
Mayer, Walter	501 E. Franklin St.	Richmond, Va. 23219
Maylath, Florian R.	65 E. Elizabeth Ave.	Bethelem, Pa. 18018
Maynard, Robert E.	4300 Talbot Rd.	Renton, Wash. 98055
Mays, J. Lamar	401 Peachtree St., N.E.	Atlanta, Ga. 30308
Mazow, Malcolm L.	Hermann Professional Bldg.	Houston, Tex. 77025
Mazzocco, Thomas R.	450 Sutter St.	San Francisco, Cal. 94108
McAffee, Don B.	508 E. S. Temple	Salt Lake City, Utah 82102
McAllister, Harry M.	2400 H St., N.W.	Washington, D. C. 20037
McAlpine, Paul T.	120 Summit Ave.	Summit, N. J. 07901
McArtor, James R.	2301 Fall Hill Ave.	Fredericksburg, Va. 22401
McBain, Earle H.	1530 5th Ave.	San Rafael, Cal. 94901
McBee, Alexander V. W. ...	500 N. Dalmont	Hobbs, N. M. 88240
McBride, J. P.	1052 W. 6th St.	Los Angeles, Cal. 90017
McBride, Noel S.	407 Merchants Bank Bldg.	Terre Haute, Ind. 47801
McCaffery, James N.	607 N. Central Ave.	Glendale, Cal. 91203
McCall, James D.	Medical-Dental Center	Mineral Wells, Tex. 76067
McCall, Marion G.	8401 Woodward	Detroit, Mich. 48202
McCallum, George C.	630 E. 12th Ave.	Eugene, Ore. 97401
McCally, Ward	33 W. 1st St.	Dayton, O. 45402
McCann, Donald S.	174 Pleasant St.	Attleboro, Mass. 02703
McCann, James W., Jr.	1800 E. Las Olas Blvd.	Ft. Lauderdale, Fla. 33301
McCann, Thomas P.	1650 Wantagh Ave.	Wantagh, N.Y. 11793
McCannel, Malcolm A.	Doctors Bldg.	Minneapolis, Minn. 55402
McCarthy, James L.	6429 W. North Ave.	Oak Park, Ill. 60302
McCarthy, John A.	1800 N. Federal Hwy.	Pompano Beach, Fla. 33062
McCarty, Ben	Med. Arts Bldg.	Jackson, Miss. 39201
McCarty, Wm. M.	2312 15th St.	Troy, N. Y. 12180
McCaslin, Murray F.	550 Grant St.	Pittsburgh, Pa. 15219
McClanahan, Robert	63 E. 78th St.	New York, N. Y. 10021
McClanahan, Wm. S.	477 S. Broad St.	Meriden, Conn. 06450
McClelland, Randall J.	1124 Broadway	Quincy, Ill. 62301
McClure, Coye W.	415 N.W. 11th St.	Oklahoma City, Okla. 73103
McClure, G. David	629 S. First St.	Louisville, Ky. 40202
McClure, Hubert L.	6160 S. Yale	Tulsa, Okla. 74135
McCole, Cornelius E.	2799 W. Grande Blvd.	Detroit, Mich. 48202
McComiskey, James	1521 Delachaise St.	New Orleans, La. 70115
McConn, John D.	22507 Kent Ave.	Torrance, Cal. 90505
McCord, Clinton D.	1938 Peachtree Rd.	Atlanta, Ga. 30309
McCormick, G. L.	102 E. Main St.	Waukesha, Wisc. 53186

McCormick, Glen E.	10425 W. North Ave.	Milwaukee, Wisc. 53226
McCormick, Michael R. ...	102 E. Main St.	Waukesha, Wisc. 53186
McCormick, Wm. A.	75 N. Santa Anita Ave.	Arcadia, Cal. 91006
McCourt, James J.	4016 Hancock Dr.	Sacramento, Cal. 95821
McCoy, Carroll A.	1609 Glenmont Dr.	Glendale, Cal. 91207
McCoy, C. T.	312 Wolcott Bldg.	Hutchinson, Kans. 67501
McCoy, David A.	Woodward Bldg.	Birmingham, Ala. 35203
McCoy, Wallace W.	1122 N. Brand Blvd.	Glendale, Cal. 91202
McCoy, William J., III	600 W. Main Ave.	Knoxville, Tenn. 37902
McCrary, John A., III	Baylor College of Med., 1200 Morsund Ave.	Houston, Tex. 77025
McCrory, Charles F.	111 W. Adams St.	Jacksonville, Fla. 32202
McCrory, Thomas M.	2811 Lemmon Ave. E.	Dallas, Texas 75204
McCroskey, David L.	611 Washington Ave.	Maryville, Tenn. 37801
McCullough, Clarence J. ...	Washington Trust Bldg.	Washington, Pa. 15301
McCullough, Francis E.	955 N. State St.	Jackson, Miss. 39201
McCullough, Lester E.	David Whitney Bldg.	Detroit, Mich. 48226
McCurdy, Marion W.	1034 Nix Professional Bldg.	San Antonio, Tex. 78205
McCusker, W. D.	315 Main St.	Penn Yan, N. Y. 14527
McDaniel, David S.	404 Washington St.	The Dalles, Ore. 97058
McDaniel, Donald W.	404 Washington St.	The Dalles, Ore. 97058
McDaniel, R. L.	1500 Oak St.	Jacksonville, Fla. 32204
McDermott, John J.	689 W. Foothill Blvd.	Claremont, Cal. 91711
McDonald, Dorothy	Kaiser Permanente Clinic.	Redwood City, Cal. 94062
McDonald, Duncan K.	107 S. 9th E.	Salt Lake City, Utah 84102
McDonald, George	177 E. 75th St.	New York, N. Y. 10021
McDonald, Henry H.	65 N. Madison Ave.	Pasadena, Cal. 91101
McDonald, James E.	1046 Chicago Ave.	Oak Park, Ill. 60302
McDonald, P. Robb	Lankenau Med. Bldg.	Philadelphia, Pa. 19151
McDonald, Robert J.	4200 N. Woodward Ave.	Royal Oak, Mich. 48072
McDowell, Charles W.	542 Church St.	Decatur, Ga. 30030
McEntyre, James M.	606 The Rialto	Venice, Fla. 33595
McEvoy, Joseph P.	200 15th Ave., E.	Seattle, Wash. 98102
McEwen, James W.	670 Cherry St.	Terre Haute, Ind. 47801
McEwen, Stanley R.	1214 N. B St.	Fort Smith, Ark. 72901
McFadden, William M.	Hitchcock Clinic	Hanover, N. H. 03755
McFarland, Corley B.	211 N. Eddy & Colfax	South Bend, Ind. 46617
McFarland, Kenneth T. H. .	Jenkins Arcade	Pittsburgh, Pa. 15222
McFarland, Paul E.	550 W. Thomas Rd.	Phoenix, Ariz. 85013
McFarland, Joe R., Jr.	Nix Professional Bldg.	San Antonio, Tex. 78205
McGannon, William J.	14597 Madison Ave.	Lakewood, O. 44107
McGarry, H. Isabelle	636 Church St.	Evanston, Ill. 60201
McGarvey, William E.	City Bank Bldg.	Jackson, Mich. 49201
McGavic, John S.	1104 Montgomery Ave.	Rosemont, Pa. 19010
McGee, Harry B.	101 W. John	Bay City, Mich. 48706
McGee, Hugh E.	5 Pangborn Pl.	Hackensack, N. J. 07601
McGlynn, Lynn D.	2517 7th Ave. S.	Great Falls, Mont. 59401
McGowan, Bernard L.	198 Union Ave.	Framingham, Mass. 01701
McGowan, Thomas J. P. ...	164 E. Main St.	Huntington, N. Y. 11743
McGowan, William L.	5 W. 4th St.	Cincinnati, O. 45202
McGraw, James L.	109 S. Warren St.	Syracuse, N. Y. 13202
McGrew, Jerry C.	304 S. Cottonwood	Richardson, Tex. 75080
McGuckin, James T.	303 Mulberry, N.E.	Albuquerque, N. M. 87106
McGuire, Stuart W.	131 State St.	Portland, Me. 04101
McGuire, William P.	105 N. Braddock St.	Winchester, Va. 22601
McHenry, D. J.	940 S. Queen St.	York, Pa. 17403

McIntire, Waldean C.	3610 Dodge St.	Omaha, Nebr. 68131
McIntyre, David J.	1300 116th N. E.	Bellevue, Wash. 98004
McIver, John M.	351 The Southern Artery	Quincy, Mass. 02169
McKaig, Calvin N.	1001 N. Cooper	Arlington, Tex. 76012
McKay, David J.	2515 7th Ave. S.	Great Falls, Mont. 59401
McKay, Richard A.	847 W. Fourth St.	Waterloo, Ia. 50702
McKee, Bobby E.	505 E. Matthews	Jonesboro, Ark. 72401
McKee, Thomas L.	918 N.E. 26th Ave.	Ft. Lauderdale, Fla. 33304
McKee, Thomas P.	207 E. Watauga Ave.	Johnson City, Tenn. 37601
McKee, William F., Jr.	1600 Lakeland Hills Blvd.	Lakeland, Fla. 33802
McKendall, H. Raymond	295 Angell St.	Providence, R. I. 02906
McKenna, John F.	Box 94	Weems, Va. 22576
McKenna, Thomas J.	U.S. Bank Bldg.	Johnstown, Pa. 15901
McKenney, Marvin J.	1200 Michigan Ave.	E. Lansing, Mich. 48823
McKenzie, Keith S.	550 Water St., Bldg. B.	Santa Cruz, Cal. 95060
McKenzie, Walten H.	800 S. Lake St.	Ft. Worth, Tex. 76104
McKinney, J. Wesley	Exchange Bldg.	Memphis, Tenn. 38103
McKinney, Worthy W.	Prof. Park	Beckley, W. Va. 25801
McKinzie, James W.	3170 Loma Vista Rd.	Ventura, Cal. 93003
McKnew, Hector C.	843 N. 21st St.	Newark, O. 43055
McLaughlin, Brian C.	2266 N. Prospect Ave.	Milwaukee, Wisc. 53202
McLaughlin, Ralph S.	301 Belvedere Ct.	Punta Gorda, Fla. 33950
McLean, Edward N.	421 High St.	Oregon City, Ore. 97045
McLean, Richard K.	916 Louise St.	Santa Ana, Cal. 92703
McLellan, Thomas G., Jr.	323 Breakneck Rd.	Connellsville, Pa. 15425
McMackin, John V.	13105 Ixora Ct.	N. Miami, Fla. 33161
McMath, William B.	142 S. Jackson St.	Americus, Ga. 31709
McMeel, J. Wallace	100 Charles Rivers Plaza	Boston, Mass. 02114
McNair, Joel N.	1125 E. 17th St.	Santa Ana, Cal. 92701
McNamara, Thomas B.	Exchange Bldg.	La Crosse, Wisc. 54601
McNeer, Keith W.	5700 W. Grace St.	Richmond, Va. 23226
McNeil, David L.	Maison Blanche Bldg.	New Orleans, La. 70112
McNeil, John A.	1979 Summit Ave.	St. Paul, Minn. 55105
McNichols, William A., Jr.	101 First St.	Dixon, Ill. 61021
McPherson, Alice R.	6436 Fannin	Houston, Tex. 77025
McPherson, Samuel D., Jr.	1110 W. Main St.	Durham, N. C. 27701
McReynolds, William U.	1101 Maine St.	Quincy, Ill. 62301
McTigue, William N.	1812 K St. N. W.	Washington, D. C. 20006
McVay, William J.	4627 Fifth Ave.	Pittsburgh, Pa. 15213
McWilliams, John R.	First National Bldg.	Ann Arbor, Mich. 48108
Meacham, Charles T.	1911 Summer St.	Stamford, Conn. 06905
Meador, James C., Jr.	Naval Hospital	Charleston, S. C. 29408
Meckley, Arnold H.	1909 W. Wall St.	Midland, Tex. 79701
Medine, Meyer M.	28 E. 10th St.	New York, N. Y. 10003
Meek, Raymond E.	The North House	Stephentown, N. Y. 12168
Meger, Gene E.	Merchants Nat'l Bk. Bldg.	Cedar Rapids, Ia. 52401
Megus, Eugenia	10660 White Oak Ave.	Granada Hills, Cal. 91344
Mehney, Gayle H.	245 State S.E.	Grand Rapids, Mich. 49502
Mehri, Parviz B.	1 Padanaram Rd.	Danbury, Conn. 06810
Meinberg, William H.	906 Olive St.	St. Louis, Mo. 63101
Meisekothen, W. E.	5113 Monona Dr.	Madison, Wisc. 53716
Meisels, Alfred A.	Univ. Hosp.	Baltimore, Md. 21201
Meisenbach, Albert E.	712 N. Washington St.	Dallas, Tex. 75246
Meissner, Richard H.	Doctors Bldg.	Omaha, Nebr. 68131
Mellicker, Martin C.	129 S. Munn Ave.	East Orange, N. J. 07018
Meltzer, Murray A.	45 E. 68th St.	New York, N.Y. 10021

Menaker, Joseph T.	12692 Palm St.	Garden Grove, Cal. 92640
Mendelblatt, Frank I.	534 6th Ave.	St. Petersburg, Fla. 33701
Mennin, Gerald S.	27 Ludlow St.	Yonkers, N. Y. 10705
Mensher, Ira W.	50 Plaza St.	Brooklyn, N. Y. 11238
Merchant, Robert F.	909 Hyde St.	San Francisco, Cal. 94109
Meredith, Arch F., Jr.	Medico-Dental Bldg.	Stockton, Cal. 95202
Merideth, H. W.	3912 Anderson Ave., S.E.	Albuquerque, N.M. 87108
Merkel, Emil E.	610 N. Central Ave.	Glendale, Cal. 91203
Mermell, Lester	119 Highland Ave.	Middletown, N. Y. 10940
Merriam, George R., Jr.	635 W. 165th St.	New York, N. Y. 10032
Merrick, John R.	139 Sandwich St.	Plymouth, Mass. 02360
Merrill, H. Ross	3251 Fourth Ave.	San Diego, Cal. 92103
Merrill, Rowland H.	508 E. S. Temple	Salt Lake City, Utah 84102
Mertz, Robert D.	Med Art Clinic	Corsicana, Tex. 75110
Merz, Arthur E.	520 Franklin Ave.	Garden City, N. Y. 11530
Merz, Earl H.	700 N. Michigan Ave.	Chicago, Ill. 60611
Mesaros, Michael P.	222 N. Saginaw Rd.	Midland, Mich. 48640
Messenger, Harry K.	140 Marlborough St.	Boston, Mass. 02116
Messier, Paul E.	1010 Cass St.	Monterey, Cal. 93940
Mettier, Stacy R.	490 Post St.	San Francisco, Cal. 94108
Metz, Henry S.	2340 Clay St.	San Francisco, Cal. 94115
Metz, Paul	2844 Ocean Pkwy.	Brooklyn, N. Y. 11235
Meyer, David	1331 Union Ave.	Memphis, Tenn. 38104
Meyer, Dexter, Jr.	722 Scott St.	Covington, Ky. 41011
Meyer, Ernst J.	1696 Massachusetts Ave.	Cambridge, Mass. 02138
Meyer, Richard E.	1416 Maine St.	Quincy, Ill. 62301
Meyer, Roger A.	217 Manatee Ave., E.	Bradenton, Fla. 33505
Meyer, Samuel J.	111 N. Wabash Ave.	Chicago, Ill. 60602
Meyer, Sam L.	3181 S. W. Sam Jackson Pk. Rd.	Portland, Ore. 97201
Meyer, Saul N.	10401 Balboa Blvd.	Granada Hills, Cal. 91344
Meyer, Theodore O.	347 W. Berry St.	Ft. Wayne, Ind. 46802
Meyers, Marina P.	150 Forest Ave.	Glen Cove, N. Y. 11542
Michael, Michael J.	15901 W. Nine Mile Rd.	Southfield, Mich. 48075
Michaels, David D.	1350 W. 7th St.	San Pedro, Cal. 90732
Michaelson, Jesse J.	165 N. Village Ave.	Rockville Centre, N. Y. 11570
Michaile, Kenneth I.	1930 Chestnut St.	Philadelphia, Pa. 19103
Michie, James L.	Tripler General Hosp.	APO San Francisco, Cal. 96438
Michler, Raymond R.	426 Webber St.	Napa, Cal. 94558
Mickatavage, Rober C.	66 Milton Rd.	Rye, N. Y. 10580
Middleton, William H.	307 Henry St.	Alton, Ill. 62002
Milam, D. Franklin Jr.	1300 116th Ave. N.E.	Bellevue, Wash. 98004
Milauskas, Albert T.	1695 N. Sunrise Way	Palm Springs, Cal. 92262
Milburn, Graham B.	Nix Prof. Bldg.	San Antonio, Tex. 78205
Milder, Benjamin	211 N. Meramec Ave.	Clayton, Mo. 63105
Miles, Donald R.	555 W. Catalina Dr.	Phoenix, Ariz. 85013
Miles, N. E.	900 S. 19th St.	Birmingham, Ala. 35205
Miles, Paul W.	2821 N. Ballas Rd.	St. Louis, Mo. 63131
Milewski, Stanislaw A.	191 Main St.	Manchester, Conn. 06040
Milkie, C. Frederick	Deaconess Hospital	Buffalo, N. Y. 14208
Miller, Claude K.	P. O. Box 1627	Wenatchee, Wash. 98801
Miller, David	3 Hawthorne Pl.	Boston, Mass.
Miller, David F.	745 Kenney Ave.	Eau Claire, Wisc. 54701
Miller, David H.	303 Washington St.	Cumberland, Md. 21502
Miller, Edwin M.	81 Main St.	Newton, N.J. 07860

Miller, Gerald A.	St. Agnes Medical Center	Baltimore, Md. 21229
Miller, George E.	745 Kenney Ave.	Eau Claire, Wisc. 54701
Miller, Gordon R.	1688 Meridian Ave.	Miami Beach, Fla. 33139
Miller, J. Stanley	330 S. Fifth	Enid, Okla. 73701
Miller, James E.	Washington University School of Medicine	St. Louis, Mo. 63110
Miller, Jay F.	Agnew State Hosp.	San Jose, Cal. 95114
Miller, John R.	3780 12th St.	Riverside, Cal. 92501
Miller, Lowell C.	1101 Welch Rd.	Palo Alto, Cal. 94304
Miller, Marilyn T.	1046 Chicago Ave.	Oak Park, Ill. 60302
Miller, Michael M.	307 Victory Blvd.	Staten Island, N. Y. 10301
Miller, Milton A.	1175 E. Arrow Hwy.	Upland, Cal. 91786
Miller, Miriam	450 Sutter St.	San Francisco, Cal. 94108
Miller, Nathan H.	3761 Stocker St.	Los Angeles, Cal. 90008
Miller, Philip M.	211 Irvington Ave.	S. Orange, N. J. 07079
Miller, Ralph K.	909 W. John St.	Champaign, Ill. 61820
Miller, Richard A.	1331 Union Ave.	Memphis, Tenn. 38104
Miller, Richard R.	109 E. 14th St.	San Leandro, Cal. 94577
Miller, Robert G.	251 E. Chicago Ave.	Chicago, Ill. 60611
Miller, Robert J.	2500 Hospital Dr., Bldg. 11	Mt. View, Cal. 94040
Miller, Saul	1016 Fifth Ave.	New York, N. Y. 10028
Miller, Sidney N.	113 Hooker Ave.	Poughkeepsie, N. Y. 12601
Miller, T. Jerome	1230 N. 30th St.	Billings, Mont. 59101
Miller, William W.	4141 Geary Blvd.	San Francisco, Cal. 94118
Millett, Fay E., Jr.	1900 N. Oregon	El Paso, Tex. 79902
Mills, Charles K.	314 E. Main St.	Gainesville, Tex. 76240
Mills, Dawson A.	National Highway Safety Bureau	Washington, D. C. 20591
Mills, Henry P., Jr.	Med. Tower	Jackson, Miss. 39216
Mills, James B.	1211 Shartel	Oklahoma City, Okla. 73103
Milster, Clyde R.	906 Olive	St. Louis, Mo. 63101
Mims, James L., Jr.	730 N. Main	San Antonio, Tex. 78205
Minas, Thomas F.	2021 N. Central Ave.	Phoenix, Ariz. 85004
Minasian, Edmond V.	2600 Capitol Ave.	Sacramento, Cal. 95816
Mindel, Joel S.	4865 Far Hills Ave.	Kettering, O. 45429
Mings, Dwain E.	1515 Tenth Ave.	Monroe, Wisc. 53566
Minor, R. Hugh	40th & Hoyt	Everett, Wash. 98201
Minsky, Arthur	8601 Homelawn St.	Jamaica, N. Y. 11432
Minton, Lee R.	121 21st Ave. N.	Nashville, Tenn. 37203
Mintz, Maxwell A.	497 Glen St.	Glens Falls, N. Y. 12801
Mintz, Morris J.	17563 Greenfield	Detroit, Mich. 48235
Mirabile, Thomas J.	59 Burnside Ave.	E. Hartford, Conn. 06108
Miranda, Manuel N.	720 Ponce de Leon Ave.	Hato Rey, P.R. 00918
Mishler, Jay E.	1616 Pacific Ave.	Atlantic City, N. J. 08401
Mitchell, Arnold M.	5 Severance Cir.	Cleveland, O. 44118
Mitchell, Calvin H.	3000 W. Buffalo Ave.	Tampa, Fla. 33607
Mitchell, Claude W.	2300 California St.	San Francisco. Cal. 94115
Mitchell, Gatlin	800 Fifth Ave.	Fort Worth, Tex. 76104
Mitchell, Robert H.	131-E E. Marion Ave.	Punta Gorda, Fla. 33950
Mitnick, Nathan	20 E. Clinton St.	New Bedford, Mass. 02740
Mittica, Nicholas M.	708 N. Jefferson St.	New Castle, Pa. 16101
Moak, Wilson E.	Madigan General Hospital	Tacoma, Wash. 98431
Mock, Ernest L.	4212 29th St.	Mt. Rainier, Md. 20822
Mohney, Glenn E.	1131 Erie St.	Port Huron, Mich. 48060
Mohr, David P.	10 E. Chase St.	Baltimore, Md. 21202
Mohr, Selby	450 Sutter St.	San Francisco, Cal. 94108
Molsberry, Jasper M.	625 N. Milwaukee St.	Milwaukee, Wisc. 53202

Monaco, Louis	704 E. Grand Ave.	Escondido, Cal. 92025
Monahan, Robert H.	1573 University Ave.	St. Paul, Minn. 55104
Moncreiff, William F.	30 N. Michigan Ave.	Chicago, Ill. 60602
Monestere, Charles J.	21 Matilda Ct.	Bayport, N. Y. 11705
Monroe, Albert	Wynnewood Prof. Bldg.	Dallas, Tex. 75224
Monroe, Charles A.	5710 MacArthur Blvd.	New Orleans, La. 70114
Monsees, Wayne E.	403 Via Del Norte	La Jolla, Cal. 92037
Monstavicius, Barbara S.	450 Sutter St.	San Francisco, Cal. 94108
Montalvo, Andres	Prof. Bldg.	Santurce, P. R. 00908
Montana, Jerome A.	949 W. State St.	Trenton, N. J. 08618
Montano, Rocco A.	316 G St.	Marysville, Cal. 95901
Monte, Thomas D.	213 Park St.	Montclair, N. J. 07042
Montgomery, Charles J.	848 First Ave. N.	Naples, Fla. 33940
Montgomery, John L.	521 Congress Pkwy.	Athens, Tenn. 37303
Montgomery, John L. Jr.	402 Medical Arts Bldg.	Knoxville, Tenn. 37902
Montross, Henry E.	4223 W. Redondo Beach Blvd.	Lawndale, Cal. 90260
Moore, Conard D.	1200 Moursund Ave.	Houston, Tex. 77025
Moore, Daniel H., Jr.	1303 25th Ave.	Meridian, Miss. 39301
Moore, Donald E.	1100 Euclid Ave.	Syracuse, N. Y. 13210
Moore, Edward E.	3 Doctors Pk.	Asheville, N. C. 28801
Moore, E. Lowry	1303 25th Ave.	Meridian, Miss. 39301
Moore, Francis G.	1748 N. Highland Rd.	Pittsburgh, Pa. 15241
Moore, James I.	11 E. Chase St.	Baltimore, Md. 21202
Moore, Loran P.	1001 Center St.	Owensboro, Ky. 42301
Moore, Richard T.	975 Ryland St.	Reno, Nev. 89502
Moore, Thomas E.	45 Castro St.	San Francisco, Cal. 94114
Moore, T. Scott	24 N. St. Joseph Ave.	Niles, Mich. 49120
Moorman, John D.	Med. Arts Bldg.	Huntsville, Ala. 35801
Moorman, Lemuel T.	2045 Franklin St.	Denver, Colo. 80205
Moorman, Robert S., Jr.	409 St. Clair Ave. S. W.	Huntsville, Ala. 35801
Moraitis, Constantine Z.	4101 Brownsville Rd.	Pittsburgh, Pa. 15227
Morales, Luis A.	Fullana Bldg.	Ponce, P. R. 00731
Moran, Charles T.	Med. Arts Bldg.	Louisville, Ky. 40217
Moran, David D.	42 Main St.	Park Ridge, Ill. 60068
Moran, Frank J.	16311 Middlebelt Rd.	Livonia, Mich. 48154
Moreland, Joseph I.	645 Medical Center Dr. N. E.	Salem, Ore. 97301
Morgan, George E.	960 E. Green St.	Pasadena, Cal. 91101
Morgan, Irving J.	Jenkins Arcade	Pittsburgh, Pa. 15222
Morgan, Loran B.	110 W. 22nd Ave.	Torrington, Wyo. 82240
Morgan, Morton B.	1680 Meridian Ave.	Miami Beach, Fla. 33139
Morgan, Owen K.	Johnstown Bank & Trust Bldg.	Johnstown, Pa. 15901
Morgan, Paul W.	1 North High St.	West Chester, Pa. 19380
Morgan, Stephan S.	16 Hampton Village Plaza	St. Louis, Mo. 63109
Morgan, Walter E., III	408 S. Sycamore St.	Petersburg, Va. 23803
Morgana, Dante J.	Bewley Bldg.	Lockport, N. Y. 14094
Morimoto, Paul K.	58 E. Clinton St.	Joliet, Ill. 60431
Morledge, Charles C.	Hart Albin Bldg.	Billings, Mont. 59101
Morledge, Thomas E.	Hart Albin Bldg.	Billings, Mont. 59101
Morosco, Samuel G.	355 Prospect Rd.	Ashtabula, O. 44004
Morris, Donald A.	30 E. 40th St.	New York, N. Y. 10016
Morris, Felix R.	953 E. Main St.	Bridgeport, Conn. 06608
Morris, Hugh L.	1700 Brooklyn Ave.	Los Angeles, Cal. 90033
Morris, Jean W.	Johnson Bldg.	Muncie, Ind. 47304
Morris, Sheldon L.	2200 Providence Ave.	Chester, Pa. 19013
Morris, Walter R.	Med. Arts Bldg.	Louisville, Ky. 40217
Morrison, Frank D.	5455 E. Second St.	Tucson, Ariz. 85711

Morrison, George S.	113 S. Kentucky	Roswell, N. M. 88201
Morrison, George W.	2033 Park Ave.	Detroit, Mich. 48226
Morrison, H. Maxwell, Jr. ..	Pinehurst Med. Ctr.	Pinehurst, N. C. 28374
Morrison, James D.	1241 N. 28th St.	Billings, Mont. 59103
Morrison, Jos. F.	Wyoming Nat'l, Bk. Bldg.	Wilkes-Barre, Pa. 18701
Morrison, W. Howard	Doctors Bldg.	Omaha, Nebr. 68131
Morrissey, Arthur M.	24 Rural Ave.	Medford, Mass. 02155
Morrow, Kenneth A.	1001 Second St. W.	Ashland, Wisc. 54806
Morrow, W. Grady, Jr.	1812 N. Oregon	El Paso, Tex. 79902
Mortensen, Andreas V. N., .	120 Louiselle St.	Mobile, Ala. 36607
Moses, Jacob	150 E. Broad St.	Columbus, O. 43215
Moses, Lyle	11811 Shaker Blvd.	Cleveland, O. 44120
Moses, Robert A.	660 S. Euclid	St. Louis, Mo. 63110
Mosher, Henry A.	266 Beacon St.	Boston, Mass. 02116
Moskovitz, Mayer	225 W. Madison Ave.	El Cajon, Cal. 92020
Moskowitz, Herbert L.	116 Millburn Ave.	Millburn, N. J. 07041
Mosrie, A. J.	503 E. Market St.	Kingsport, Tenn. 37660
Moss, Ennis E., Jr.	4020 21st St.	Lubbock, Tex. 79410
Moss, Hugh M.	430 Union St.	Hackensack, N. J. 07601
Moss, L. Conner	1705 Rhode Island Ave.	Washington, D. C. 20006
Motley, Reid E.	930 Merchants Bank Bldg.	Cedar Rapids, Ia. 52401
Mott, Frederick E.	38 Trumbull St.	New Haven, Conn. 06510
Mott, Walter C.	75 Willett St.	Albany, N. Y. 12210
Mould, Ward L.	520 Franklin Ave.	Garden City, N. Y. 11530
Moulton, Everett C., Jr. ...	1214 North B. St.	Fort Smith, Ark, 72901
Moulton, Gardner N.	5 Grove St.	Bangor, Me. 04401
Moulton, Olin C.	130 N. Virginia St.	Reno, Nev. 89501
Mousel, Donald K.	975 Ryland St.	Reno, Nev. 89502
Mueller, Emma C.	9985 Sierra Ave	Fontana, Cal. 92335
Mueller, Julius H.	140 E. Granger Ave.	Modesto, Cal. 95350
Muenzler, W. Stanley	430 N. W. 12th St.	Oklahoma City, Okla. 73103
Muenzner, Richard J., Jr. ..	Bankers Bldg.	Milwaukee, Wisc. 53202
Muir, Everett B.	9 Exchange Pl.	Salt Lake City, Utah 84111
Muirhead, J. Fraser	450 Sutter St.	San Francisco, Cal. 94108
Mulberger, Robert D.	1930 Chestnut St.	Philadelphia, Pa. 19103
Mullen, Clifford J., Sr.	1409 Minnesota Ave.	Kansas City, Kans. 66102
Mullen, Raymond S.	3780 12th St.	Riverside, Cal. 92501
Mullenix, Charles W.	1775 Glenview Rd.	Glenview, Ill. 60025
Muller, Paul P. M.	118 E. 93rd St.	New York, N. Y. 10028
Mulligan, William P.	4615 35th Ave. S. W.	Seattle, Wash. 98126
Munday, Perry L.	249 E. Main St.	Newark, Dela. 19711
Mundt, G. Henry, Jr.	4020 Grand	Western Springs, Ill. 60558
Munion, Lucille M.	230 Hilton Ave.	Hempstead, N. Y. 11550
Munro, Dugald H.	159 Waterman St.	Providence, R. I. 02906
Murphy, Edward U.	24 N. W. Fourth St.	Evansville, Ind. 47708
Murphy, Leo J.	107 N. Clinton St.	Olean, N. Y. 14760
Murhphy, Robert H.	4753 N. Broadway	Chicago, Ill. 60640
Murphy, Weldon O.	2300 W. 7th Ave.	Amarillo, Tex. 79106
Murrah, William F. Jr.	1331 Union Ave.	Memphis, Tenn. 38104
Murray, Austin P.	1930 Chestnut St.	Philadelphia, Pa. 19103
Murray, Richard A.	2701 Eye St.	Sacramento, Cal. 95816
Murto, Robert E.	433 Bellevue Ave.	Trenton, N. J. 08618
Muscarella, Michael S.	1005 N.E. 125th St.	N. Miami, Fla. 33161
Myers, Frank L.	1025 Regent St.	Madison, Wisc. 53715
Myers, Roland H.	1331 Union	Memphis, Tenn. 38104
Myers, Spencer W., Jr.	501 E. Romie Ln.	Salinas, Cal. 93901

Nachazel, Delbert P., Jr. . . .	3800 Woodward Ave.	Detroit, Mich. 48201
Nachman, E. A.	417 E. Washington Ave.	Council Bluffs, Ia. 51501
Machman, Lisso	501 Fourth St.	Alexandria, La. 71301
Nachod, Grace R.	5501 Greene St.	Philadelphia, Pa. 19144
Nadbath, Rudolph P.	The Permanente Medical Group .	Hayward, Cal. 94545
Nadeau, Emile G.	923 Eliza St.	Green Bay, Wisc. 54301
Nadeau, George E.	128 E. Walnut St.	Green Bay, Wisc. 54301
Nadel, Alfred J.	440 E. 57th St.	New York, N. Y. 10022
Nagle, Baker Gerald	822 Second Ave. N.	Columbus, Miss. 39701
Nagle, Frank O.	37 S. 20th St.	Philadelphia, Pa. 19103
Nahn, Charles E.	1313 Fish Hatchery Rd.	Madison, Wisc. 53715
Naidoff, David	3500 Tudor St.	Philadelphia, Pa. 19136
Nail, James B.	1308 9th	Wichita Falls, Tex. 76301
Najac, Harold	400 Ocean Ave.	Brooklyn, N. Y. 11226
Nantz, Frank A.	Doctors Bldg.	Cincinnati, O. 45202
Naples, Carmon R.	711 Wayne Ave.	Silver Spring, Md. 20910
Naquin, Howard A.	14 W. Mt. Vernon Pl.	Baltimore, Md. 21201
Nase, Paul Kenneth	206 S. Sixth Ave.	W. Reading, Pa. 19602
Nassar, Jamil G.	1151 N. State St.	Jackson, Miss. 39201
Naugle, Thomas C.	150 Barrone St.	New Orleans, La. 70112
Nauheim, J. S.	2025 Merrick Ave.	Merrick, N. Y. 11566
Neal, Dean E.	11104 S. E. Stark St.	Portland, Ore. 97233
Neals, Henry J.	234 Bryn Mawr Ave.	Bryn Mawr, Pa. 19010
Neault, Roger W.	200 First St., S. W.	Rochester, Minn. 55901
Neeb, Walter G.	16840 E. Warren Ave.	Detroit, Mich. 48224
Neely, Robert A.	24 N. Bell	Bellville, Tex. 77418
Neely, Wanda	15955 Samaritan Dr.	San Jose, Cal. 95124
Nees, Oliver R.	805 Pacific Ave.	Long Beach, Cal. 90813
Nees, Oliver R., Jr.	2700 Bellflower Blvd.	Long Beach, Cal. 90815
Nehrenberg, Ted R.	307 Placentia	Newport Beach, Cal. 92660
Neidlinger, Robert W.	6120 Brandon Ave	Springfield, Va. 22150
Nelson, Donald G.	1701 26th St.	Bakersfield, Cal. 93301
Nelson, Elliot S.	4910 15th Ave.	Brooklyn, N. Y. 11219
Nelson, Hommer S.	626 First St.	Macon, Ga. 31201
Nelson, John H.	402 10th St.	Tuscaloosa, Ala. 35401
Nelson, Nathaniel F.	4910 15th Ave.	Brooklyn, N. Y. 11219
Nelson, Orville N.	2060 5th Ave., N.	St. Petersburg, Fla. 33713
Nelson, Robert C.	762 Altos Oaks Dr.	Los Altos, Cal. 94022
Nelson, William R.	1301 K St.	Modesto, Cal. 95354
Nemerson, Nathan.	2 High St.	Monticello, N. Y. 12701
Nerbonne, Joseph J.	231 Main St.	Brockton, Mass. 02401
Nerenberg, Sidney.	Med. Arts Bldg.	Minneapolis, Minn. 55402
Nesbit, Mark E.	1 S. Pinckney	Madison, Wisc. 53703
Nesbitt, Leslie B.	1000 W. La Veta Ave.	Orange, Cal. 92668
Nesburn, Anthony B.	272 S. Lake St.	Los Angeles, Cal. 90057
Nesburn, Henry R.	620 S. San Vicente Blvd.	Los Angeles, Cal. 90048
Nethercut, Glenway W.	321 Terrace Dr.	Marshall, Mich. 49068
Netzel, Robert J.	675 Orchard Lake Ave.	Pontiac, Mich. 48053
Neumayr, Thomas G.	115 St. Matthews	San Mateo, Cal. 94401
Nevill, Bobby D.	5055 N. Greeley	Portland, Ore. 97034
Nevyas, Herbert J.	1930 Chestnut St.	Philadelphia, Pa. 19103
Newburg, Jay A.	425 Sinclair St.	McKeesport, Pa. 15132
Newby, Kenneth G.	59 Racine St.	Menasha, Wisc. 54952
Newby, William E.	USPHS Hosp.	Baltimore, Md. 21211
Newel, J. Michael.	1045 'S' St.	Fresno, Cal. 23721
Newell, Frank W.	950 E. 59th St.	Chicago, Ill. 60637

Newhouse, Robert P.	30 W. 60th St.	New York, N. Y. 10023
Newman, Erwin W.	220 19th St. N. E.	Cedar Rapids, Ia. 52402
Newman, Matthew	100 N. Euclid	St. Louis, Mo. 63108
Newman, Ted B.	1288 N. Irwin	Hanford, Cal. 93230
Newsom, Samuel R.	1514 Jefferson Hwy.	New Orleans, La. 70121
Newton, Dana S.	200 15th Ave. E.	Seattle, Wash. 98102
Newton, Frank H.	2217 Cedar Springs Rd.	Dallas, Tex. 75201
Newton, James C.	815 Fifth Ave.	New York, N. Y. 10021
Newton, Norris L.	602 Main St.	Texarkana, Tex. 75501
Newton, Ray E.	1010 Harris Bldg.	Jackson, Mich. 49201
Ney, James E.	7635 W. Oklahoma Ave	Milwaukee, Wisc. 53219
Nicastro, Norman J.	2590 Nottingham Way	Trenton, N. J. 08619
Nicely, Alfred L.	Second Nat'l. Bldg.	Akron, O. 44308
Nicholas, John P.	10720 S. Paramount Blvd.	Downey, Cal. 90241
Nicholl, Russell J.	10515 Carnegie Ave.	Cleveland, O. 44106
Nichols, Robin R.	164 E. 8th Ave.	Chico, Cal. 95926
Nicholson, F. Peter	795 Front St.	Butte, Mont. 59701
Nickeson, Robert W.	550 Grant St., Carlton House	Pittsburgh, Pa. 15219
Nied, Walter S.	1524 W. Erie Ave.	Philadelphia, Pa. 19140
Niffenegger, James A.	800 McKinley Ave. N. W.	Canton, O. 44703
Nilsen, John A.	4450 W. 76th St.	Minneapolis, Minn. 55435
Nippe, Leonard	316 Michigan St.	Toledo, O. 43624
Nisbet, Alfred A.	726 McCullough Ave.	San Antonio, Tex. 78215
Nitz, George K., Jr.	426 17th St.	Oakland, Cal. 94612
Nodelman, Jacob	26 Elm St.	New Haven, Conn. 06510
Noel, George T.	Raleigh Bldg.	Kannapolis, N. C. 28081
Nofles, James W.	2715 Union Blvd.	St. Louis, Mo. 63113
Noguchi, Henry T.	321 E. Second St.	Los Angeles, Cal. 90012
Nolan, Edwin W.	3101 Breckenridge Ln.	Louisville, Ky. 40220
Norene, Robert A.	3701 Stocker St.	Los Angeles, Cal. 90008
Norman, Mark L.	Med. Arts Bldg.	Minneapolis, Minn. 55402
Norment, Robert L.	820 N. Stafford St.	Arlington, Va. 2203
Norris, Robert M.	1215 N. Alpine Rd.	Rockford, Ill. 61107
North, Alvin W.	490 Peachtree St. N. E.	Atlanta, Ga. 30308
Norton, Edward W. D.	1638 N.W. 10th Ave.	Miami, Fla. 33136
Norton, Herman J.	797 Elmwood Ave.	Rochester, N. Y. 14620
Nousek, James E., Jr.	2020 E. 93rd St.	Cleveland, O. 44106
Novak, Edward A., Jr.	162 Clinton St.	Redwood City, Cal. 94062
Novak, Joseph F.	Med. Arts Bldg.	Pittsburgh, Pa. 15213
Nowell, John F.	Annandale Doctors' Bldg.	Annandale, Va. 22003
Nowicki, Norbert J.	130 E. Randolph St.	Chicago, Ill. 60601
Noyes, Philip P.	420 Estudillo Ave.	San Leandro, Cal. 94577
Nozik, Robert A.	931 W. San Bruno Ave.	San Bruno, Cal. 94066
Nugent, Maurice W.	1127 Wilshire Blvd.	Los Angeles, Cal. 90017
Nugent, Milton E.	16th at Eoff	Wheeling, W. Va. 26003
Nunn, Robert F.	511 8th St.	Ocean City, N. J. 08226
Nursall, John F.	2163 Torrance Blvd.	Torrance, Cal. 90501
Nutting, Raymond J.	411 30th St.	Oakland, Cal. 94609
Nye, William F.	630 N. Cotner Blvd.	Lincoln, Nebr. 68505
Nystrom, Robert E.	262 S. Leggett Dr.	Abilene, Tex. 79605
Oakes, Milton C.	283 Park Ave., W.	Mansfield, O. 44902
Oakley, Kenneth H.	164 Hawthorne Ave.	Bend, Ore. 97701
Oaks, L. Weston	33 E. 2nd S.	Provo, Utah, 84601
Oaks, Merrill C.	930 N. 500 W.	Provo, Utah, 84601
Obear, Margaret F.	490 Post St., #650	San Francisco, Cal. 94102
Oberhoff, Peter	1515 Chain Bridge Rd.	McLean, Va. 22101

Oberlander, O. W., Jr.	600 E. Genesee St.	Syracuse, N. Y. 13202
Oberman, Arthur E.	9209 Colima Rd.	Whittier, Cal. 90605
O'Brien, C. S.	Rte. 6, Box 28	Tucson, Ariz. 85704
O'Brien, J. Miles	1461 State St.	El Centro, Cal. 92243
O'Brien, John D.	375 E. Main St.	Bay Shore, N. Y. 11706
O'Brien, Thomas P.	1415 Third St.	Corpus Christi, Tex. 78404
O'Bryne, Alvaro	1430 Tulane Ave.	New Orleans, La. 70112
Ocasio Canabas, Kermell ...	Ashford Med. Ctr.	Santurce, P. R. 00907
O'Connell, John D.	Woodland Medical Center, 140 Woodland St.	Hartford, Conn. 06105
O'Connor, C. Addison	433 Humboldt	Santa Rosa, Cal. 95403
O'Connor, Edward F.	1 Chicago Ave.	Oak Park, Ill. 60302
O'Connor, G. Richard	95 Kirkham St.	San Francisco, Cal. 94122
O'Connor, John W.	1861 Wadsworth Blvd.	Lakewood, Colo. 80215
O'Connor, Patrick R.	301 E. Walnut St.	Louisville, Ky. 40202
O'Connor, Robert E.	1306 Kanawha Blvd., E.	Charleston, W. Va. 25301
O'Dair, Robert B.	303 E. Town St.	Columbus, O. 43215
Odom, Robert E.	99 Evelyn Pl.	Asheville, N. C. 28801
Oeljen, Siegfried C. G.	329 N. State St.	Waseca, Minn. 56093
Offenbach, Bertha	51 Homer St.	Newton Center, Mass. 02159
Offutt, William N., III	177 N. Upper St.	Lexington, Ky. 40507
O'Gawa, Gilbert M.	Henry Ford Hosp.	Detroit, Mich. 48202
Oglesby, Claude D.	910 Madison Ave.	Memphis, Tenn. 38103
Oglesby, Richard B.	950 Francis Pl.	Clayton, Mo. 63105
O'Grady, Richard B.	1775 Glenview Rd.	Glenview, Ill. 60025
O'Gwynn, John Coleman III	1565 Dauphin St.	Mobile, Ala 36604
Ohmart, Walter A.	631 Monroe St.	Denver, Colo. 80206
Ohta, Victor M.	550 Water St.	Santa Cruz, Cal. 95060
Ojers, Gaylord W.	35 E. Elizabeth Ave.	Bethlehem, Pa. 18018
Ojha, Brij B.	303 S. Nappanee St.	Elkhart, Ind. 46514
Okamura, Ichiro D.	100 Charles River Plaza	Boston, Mass. 02114
O'Kane, Thomas W.	Central Medical Bldg.	St. Paul, Minn. 55104
O'Keefe, N. Thomas	Burn's Clinic	Petoskey, Mich. 49770
O'Keeffe, Edward R., Jr. ..	1304 Grand Blvd.	Schenectady, N. Y. 12308
Okie, Theodore B.	2665 Walnut St.	Huntington Park, Cal. 90255
Okun, Edward	4989 Barnes Hosp. Plaza	St. Louis, Mo. 63110
Old, William F.	4545 Fanuel	San Diego, Cal. 92109
Oleari, Valdo P.	1492 N. Main St.	Wheaton, Ill. 60187
Oleksy, Stanley P.	744 W. Michigan Ave.	Jackson, Mich. 49201
Olenick, Everett J.	1389 D St.	San Bernardino, Cal. 92405
Olive, George M., Jr.	18 Moore St.	Belmont, Mass. 02178
Oliver, Dalton S.	4848 North Blvd.	Baton Rouge, La. 70806
Oliver, Samuel H.	1010 Cass St.	Monterey, Cal. 93940
Olkon, Dora B.	510 S. Burnside	Los Angeles, Cal. 90036
Ollendorff, Ulrich	715 W. 175 th. St.	New York, N. Y. 10033
Olmsted, K. Elizabeth P. ...	568 Lafayette Ave.	Buffalo, N. Y. 14222
Olsen, Oluf E.	2108 N. Orange Ave.	Orlando, Fla. 32804
Olson, Burton G.	315 S. Main St.	Minot, N. D. 58701
Olson, Clyde L.	701 Abercorn	Savannah, Ga. 31401
Olson, Elbert R.	Box O, Gorgas Hosp.	Balboa Heights, C.Z.
Olson, James A.	17000 W. Eight Mile Rd.	Southfield, Mich, 48075
Olson, Nelse O.	423 Pacific Ave.	Bremerton, Wash. 98310
Olson, Richard S.	1495 Morse Rd.	Columbus, O. 43229
Olson, Richard T.	East Range Clinic	Virginia, Minn. 55792
O'Malley, Conor	220 Meridian Ave.	San Jose, Cal. 95126
O'Malley, Patrick F.	525 Sherland Bldg.	South Bend, Ind. 46601

O'Malley, Thomas P.	2501 Main St.	Stevens Point, Wisc. 54481
O'Neill, Charles L., Jr.	671 Broad St.	Newark, N. J. 07102
O'Neill, James F.	2801 1st Ave. N.	St. Petersburg, Fla. 33713
O'Neill, John C.	205 W. 2nd St.	Duluth, Minn. 55802
O'Neill, John F.	1605 22nd St., N.W.	Washington, D. C. 20008
Oosterhous, George E.	20 S. Park St.	Madison, Wisc. 53715
O'Roark, James F.	2320 Bath St.	Santa Barbara, Cal. 93105
Oropallo, Anthony J.	115 Gloucester Pike	Barrington, N. K. 08007
O'Rourke, J.	2 Holcombe St.	Hartford, Conn. 06112
O'Rourke, James F. X.	99 Park Ave.	Yonkers, N. Y. 10703
Ortiz-Gordils, Edgardo	Fullana Bldg.	Ponce, P. R. 00731
Osher, Morris S.	8040 Reading Rd.	Cincinnati, O. 45237
Osler, Jay K.	74 Birch St.	Bangor, Me. 04401
Ostler, H. Bruce	Univ. Cal Medical Center	San Francisco, Cal. 94122
Ostriker, Marilyn	144 Morgan St.	Stamford, Conn. 06905
Ostriker, Paul J.	144 Morgan St.	Stamford, Conn. 06905
Ostrom, William C.	1350 Union St.	Schenectady, N. Y. 12308
Ostrov, Charles S.	Doctors' Bldg.	Minneapolis, Minn. 55402
O'Toole, John J.	133 E. Napier Ave.	Benton Harbor, Mich. 49022
Otten, Donald E.	Box A	Pendleton, Ore. 98901
Ottum, John A.	417 S. Monroe Ave.	Green Bay, Wisc. 54301
Overmyer, Jay W.	58 N. 13th St.	San Jose, Cal. 95112
Overton, Jesse W.	229 Liberty St.	Newburgh, N. Y. 12550
Owens, Andrew J.	4441 W. Fond du Lac Ave.	Milwaukee, Wisc. 53216
Owens, Ella U.	Bushkill Dr., R. D. 2	Easton, Pa. 18042
Owens, Wm. C.	Bushkill Dr., R. D. 2	Easton, Pa. 18042
Owensby, Lindell C.	222½ W. 6th St.	Concordia, Kans. 66901
Ozment, Thomas L.	823 Warren Prof. Bldg.	Tulsa, Okla. 74135
Pace, Clinton A.	404 Sunrise Ave.	Roseville, Cal. 95698
Pachtman, Isadore	8075 Jenkins Arcade	Pittsburgh, Pa. 15222
Packer, Robert C.	315 W. Clay Ave.	Muskegon, Mich. 49440
Padfield, Earl G.	4320 Wornall Rd.	Kansas City, Mo. 64111
Page, David A.	325 Park Ave.	Huntington, L. I., N. Y. 11743
Page, Robert N., Jr.	232 N. E. Lincoln St.	Hillsboro, Ore. 97123
Page, Robert O.	National Bk. Bldg.	Lima, O. 45801
Page, Vernon	6 N. Michigan	Chicago, Ill. 60602
Pailet, Sanford L.	3814 Veterans Hwy.	Metairie, La. 70002
Palmberg, Karl J.	21675 Redwood Rd.	Castro Valley, Cal. 94546
Palmer, Marvin G.	2427 W. Falls	Kennewick, Wash. 99336
Palmer, Milton A.	18 Park Blvd.	Lancaster, N. Y. 14086
Palmer, Robert H., Jr.	1950 Arlington St.	Sarasota, Fla. 33579
Palmerton, Ernest S.	628½ 6th St.	Rapid City, S.D. 57701
Pannabecker, Charles L. ...	Jefferson Bldg.	Peoria, Ill. 61602
Panter, Edward G.	1245 E. Colfax Ave.	Denver, Colo. 80218
Panton, John H.	1 Madison St.	Oak Park, Ill. 60302
Pappas, Stephen S.	5185 MacArthur Blvd. N. W. ...	Washington, D. C. 20016
Paradis, Andre J.	130 Parker St.	Lawrence. Mass. 01843
Parelman, Allen G.	601 E. 63rd St.	Kansas City, Mo. 64110
Parisi, Peter J.	25 N. 14th St.	San Jose, Cal. 95112
Park, M. Benjamin	264 Andalusia Ave.	Coral Gables, Fla. 33134
Park, O. J.	444 Glen St.	Glen Falls, N.Y. 12801
Park, William F.	Wheeling Clinic	Wheeling, W. Va. 26003
Parke, David W.	477 S. Broad St.	Meriden, Conn. 06450
Parker, Bruce W.	7000 Cutler N. E.	Albuquerque, N. M. 87110
Parker, Camille K.	2500 E. Broadway	Logansport, Ind. 46947

Parker, Chas O., Jr.	207 E. Watauga Ave.	Johnson City, Tenn. 37601
Parker, Francis W., Jr.	2500 E. Broadway	Logansport, Ind. 46947
Parker, James H.	1500 Penn Ave.	Wyomissing, Pa. 19610
Parker, John T.	Box 87	Farmington, N. M. 87401
Parkerson, Walter T.	225 Hawthorne Ln.	Charlotte, N. C. 28204
Parks, Marshall M.	3400 Mass. Ave. N.W.	Washington, D. C. 20007
Parks, Wm. Carson	3660 N. Teutonia Ave.	Milwaukee, Wisc. 53206
Parrish, Richard K.	238 S. Second St.	Decatur, Ind. 46733
Parry, Thayer L.	175 S. Main St.	Akron, O. 44308
Parsons, Hugh E.	613 Magnolia	Tampa, Fla. 33606
Partridge, Eugene T.	2769 S. Park Ave.	Lackawanna, N. Y. 14218
Pasek, Edward A.	1312 S. Spring Ave.	Sioux Falls, S. D. 57105
Pass, Sheldon	7510 Fourth Ave.	Brooklyn, N. Y. 11209
Passmore, Jack W.	5565 Grossmont Center Dr.	La Mesa, Cal. 92042
Paston, Philip	518 N. Federal Hwy.	Lake Worth, Fla. 33460
Pachett, Orval W.	2415 W. Falls Ave.	Kennewick, Wash. 99336
Pate, John W.	55 Clinic Dr.	Madisonville, Ky. 42431
Patience, Hansi R.	1775 Glenview Rd.	Glenview, Ill. 60025
Paton, David	Johns Hopkins Hospital	Baltimore, Md. 21205
Paton, R. Townley	186 Old Town Road	Southampton, N. Y. 11968
Patrick, Kirk A., Jr.	1260 Main St.	Baton Rouge, La. 70802
Patterson, Harold C.	93 West St.	Danbury, Conn. 06810
Patterson, Harold L.	Box 7	Larned, Kans. 67550
Patterson, Reese W.	600 W. Main St.	Knoxville, Tenn. 37902
Patterson, Sam H.	402 N. University St.	Murfreesboro, Tenn. 37130
Patterson, Walter	2000 Mass. Ave., N.W.	Washington, D. C. 20036
Patti, Joseph C.	50 Union Ave.	Irvington, N. J. 07111
Patton, James R., Jr.	2210 Washington	Waco, Tex. 76702
Patz, Arnall	4419 Falls Rd.	Baltimore, Md. 21211
Paul, Thomas O.	1711 9th Ave. S.	Birmingham, Ala. 35205
Paulk, James R.	1303 Fourth St. S. W.	Moultrie, Ga. 31768
Paulson, Hubert O.	Sharp Bldg.	Lincoln, Nebr. 68508
Pavilack, Sidney	3419 Johnson St.	Hollywood, Fla. 33021
Pavlick, Theodore J.	1001 Walnut St.	Evansville, Ind. 47708
Pavlis, Robert J.	1099 Ohio River Blvd.	Sewickley, Pa. 15143
Pavlo, Irving L.	330 Dartmouth St.	Boston, Mass. 02116
Payne, Brittain F.	17 E. 72nd St.	New York, N.,Y. 10021
Payne, Frank	57 High St.	Berlin, N. H. 03570
Payne, John W.	14 W. Mount Vernon Pl.	Baltimore, Md. 21201
Payton, Calvin W.	309 E. Methvin	Longview, Tex. 75601
Peabody, Cary S.	16 Wick Ave.	Youngstown, O. 44503
Peabody, Robert R.	2222 N St.	Sacramento, Cal. 95816
Pearlman, Edwin	7312 Granby St.	Norfolk, Va. 23505
Pearlman, Jerome T.	UCLA Medical Center	Los Angeles, Cal. 90024
Pearlman, Maurice D.	2300 S. Rancho Dr.	Las Vegas, Nev. 89102
Pearlson, Harrison R.	720 Harrison Ave.	Boston, Mass. 02118
Pearlstone, Arnold D.	1700 Post Rd.	Fairfield, Conn. 06430
Pearson, Don C.	45 Allenmore Medical Center ...	Tacoma, Wash. 98405
Pearson, Ovid	101 Brunswick St.	Rochester, N. Y. 14607
Pearson, Robert S.	801 Princeton Ave. S. W.	Birmingham, Ala. 35211
Peartree, S. Patrick	Med. Arts Bldg.	Omaha, Nebr. 68102
Pease, Paul J.	814 Third National Bldg.	Dayton, O. 45402
Pechous, Paul G.	334 Fischer Bldg.	Dubuque, Ia. 52001
Peck, Howard B.	303-B Mulberry, N. E.	Albuquerque, N. M. 87106
Peebles, Charles H., Jr.	1673 Brabham Ave.	Columbia, S. C. 29204
Peebles, Jonathan B.	R. F. D. #3	Buchanan, Tenn. 38222

Pelletier, René W.	234 Lowry Medical Arts	St. Paul, Minn. 55101
Pellicane, Arthur O.	143-25 41st Ave.	Flushing, N. Y. 11355
Pember, Aubrey H.	Box 522	Lake Wales, Fla. 33853
Pember, John F.	508 W. Milwaukee St.	Janesville, Wisc. 53545
Pemberton, John W.	8601 W. Dodge Rd.	Omaha, Nebr. 68114
Pendergrast, David H.	1920 Irving St. N. E.	Washington, D. C. 20018
Pendexter, Sidney E., Jr.	299 S. Harrison St.	East Orange, N. J. 07018
Penn, Robert F.	1132 Waukegan Rd.	Glenview, Ill. 60025
Penn, Sidney W.	3485 Linden Ave.	Long Beach, Cal. 90807
Penner, Robert	685 3rd Ave.	Chula Vista, Cal. 92010
Pentecost, Gordon J.	Box 108	Kresgeville, Pa. 18333
Perera, Charles A.	70 E. 66th St.	New York, N. Y. 10021
Peretz, Jack	11717 Euclid Ave.	Cleveland, O. 44106
Peretz, Walter L.	140 E. 54th St.	New York, N. Y. 10022
Perez, J. Edward	2828 H St.	Bakersfield, Cal. 93301
Perez, Luis F.	L.S.U. School of Medicine	New Orleans, La. 70112
Perina, Anson	77 Maple Ave.	Morristown, N. J. 07960
Perkins, Edward W.	300 W. Franklin St.	Richmond, Va. 23220
Perkins, Henry R.	1445 Harper St.	Augusta, Ga. 30902
Perkins, Osborn P.	121 E. 60th St.	New York, N. Y. 10022
Perkinson, Raymond H.	1014 San Juan	Exeter, Cal. 93221
Perley, Edward P.	140 E. 54th St.	New York, N. Y. 10022
Perlman, Arnold R.	4560 Admiralty Way	Marina Del Rey, Cal. 90291
Perlmutter, Harold S.	R. D. 1, Box 473-D	Newton, N.J. 07860
Pernoud, Flavius G.	634 N. Grand	St. Louis, Mo. 63103
Pernoud, Michael F.	634 N. Grand	St. Louis, Mo. 63103
Perraut, L. Edward	1302 18th St., N. W.	Washington, D. C. 20036
Perreten, Frank A.	1801 High	Denver, Colo. 80218
Perritt, Richard A.	30 N. Michigan Ave.	Chicago, Ill. 60602
Perry, Claude S.	1275 Olentangy River Rd.	Columbus, O. 43212
Perry, Judith V.	550 N. Monroe St.	Hinsdale, Ill. 60521
Perry, Robert S.	114½ W. Buffalo St.	Ithaca, N. Y. 14850
Persing, Harry M., Jr.	2508 Broad Ave.	Altoona, Pa. 16601
Persky, Nathan	2025 Kings Hwy.	Brooklyn, N. Y. 11229
Perzia, Anthony P.	610 Florida Ave.	Tampa, Fla. 33602
Peter, A. L.	656 W. Market St.	Akron, O. 44303
Peter, Philip A.	1019 Madison	Seattle, Wash. 98104
Peters, Albert G.	9300 Ashland Ave.	Chicago, Ill. 60643
Petersen, Robert A.	300 Longwood Ave.	Boston, Mass. 02115
Petersen, Walter C.	1601 16th Ave.	Seattle, Wash. 98122
Peterson, Donald A.	20 S. Park St.	Madison, Wisc. 53715
Peterson, H. R.	1612 Tremont St.	Denver, Colo. 80202
Peterson, John H.	Medical Arts Bldg.	Duluth, Minn. 55802
Peterson, John W.	706 W. Main	Carbondale, Ill. 62901
Peterson, Lewis A.	164 E. 5900 South	Murray, Utah 84107
Peterson, Norman D.	362 Third St.	Laguna Beach, Cal. 92651
Petix, D. G.	2615 Grand Concourse	New York, N. Y. 10468
Petrauskas, Raymond R.	Malcolm Grow Hospital	Andrews AFB, Md. 20331
Petravice, Peter P.	1333 Orchard St.	Chicago Hgts., Ill. 60411
Pettis, J. Leighton	420 Magazine St.	Tupelo, Miss. 38801
Pettit, Paul H.	511 8th St.	Ocean City, N. J. 08226
Pettit, Thomas H.	Jules Stein Eye Inst.	Los Angeles, Cal. 90024
Pettit, William A.	1620 Marengo Ave.	South Pasadena, Cal. 91030
Pettit, William A., Jr.	595 E. Colorado St.	Pasadena, Cal. 90057
Petty, Robert W.	930 N. 500 W.	Provo, Utah 84601
Petzinger, Alexander F.	800 3rd St.	Marysville, Cal. 95901

Pfahl, S. Baird, Jr.	740 E. Park St.	Sandusky, O. 44870
Pfeifer, Robert H.	2540 N. E. 9th St.	Ft. Lauderdale, Fla. 33316
Pfeiffer, Raymond L.	330 Elm St.	New Canaan, Conn. 06840
Pfingst, Harry A.	1169 Eastern Pkwy.	Louisville, Ky. 40217
Pfister, Roswell R.	20 Staniford St.	Boston, Mass. 02114
Phelps, Gardner D.	844 W. Fourth St.	Waterloo, Ia. 50702
Phelps, G. Gustave	165 Green Bay Rd.	Wilmette, Ill. 60091
Phelps, Herschel R., Jr.	1500 16th Ave. Ct.	Greeley, Colo. 80631
Phelps, William L.	10611 Garland Rd.	Dallas, Tex. 75218
Philbrook, Seth S.	705 Harrison St.	La Porte, Ind. 46530
Phillips, Carlton C.	2 Church St. S.	New Haven, Conn. 06519
Phillips, Don M.	6465 S. Yale	Tulsa, Okla. 74135
Phillips, Donald C.	1501 Stubbs Ave.	Monroe, La. 71201
Phillips, James R.	641 Winn Ave.	Baton Rouge, La. 70806
Phillips, James W.	316 Main St.	Newport News, Va. 23601
Phillips, Roland L.	Matthews Bldg.	Owosso, Mich. 48867
Phillips, Warren C.	801 N. 2nd St.	Harrisburg, Pa. 17102
Pica, Vincent B.	3105 Nottingham Way	Trenton, N. J. 08619
Picetti, Benjamin M.	2233 Post St.	San Francisco, Cal. 94115
Pickel, Willis W.	3401 Folsom Blvd.	Sacramento, Cal. 95816
Pickett, William E.	644 Madison Ave.	Albany, N. Y. 12208
Pico, Guillermo	1475 Wilson Ave.	Santurce, P. R. 00907
Pierce, Charles W.	359 E. Main St.	Mt. Kisco, N. Y. 10549
Pierce, Gerald G.	17 E. 72nd St.	New York, N. Y. 10021
Pierce, L. Harrell	700 Cathedral St.	Baltimore, Md. 21201
Pierce, Patrick L.	711 Pass Rd.	Gulfport, Miss. 39501
Pierson, Max J.	17725 Manderson Rd.	Detroit, Mich. 48203
Pignolet, Wesley J.	36001 Euclid Ave.	Willoughby, O. 44094
Pike, Melvin H.	224 E. Larkin St.	Midland, Mich. 48640
Pilaro, Joseph Peter	112 Summer St.	Springfield, Vt. 05156
Pilger, Irvin S.	2865 Atlantic Ave.	Long Beach, Cal. 90806
Pikerton, A. Raymond, Jr.	3800 Reservoir Rd. N. W.	Washington, D. C. 20007
Pincus, Jack H.	91 School St.	Springfield, Mass. 01105
Pincus, Morris H.	881 Washington Ave.	Brooklyn, N. Y. 11225
Pinerman, Robert B.	539 W. State St.	Trenton, N. J. 08618
Pingree, George C.	164 E. 5900 South	Salt Lake City, Utah 84107
Pinkham, Ray A.	611 Whitcomb St.	Kalamazoo, Mich. 49001
Pinkoson, Charles	618 S.W. 4th Ave.	Gainesville, Fla. 32601
Pinnas, Gerald	7400 N. Kendall Dr.	Miami, Fla. 33156
Pino, Ralph H.	28 W. Adams	Detroit, Mich. 48226
Pinschmidt, Norman W.	1514 Jefferson Hwy.	New Orleans, La. 70121
Piper, Caesar B.	3850 W. Santa Barbara Ave.	Los Angeles, Cal. 90008
Pippitt, Richard B.	Memorial Hosp.	North Conway, N.H. 03860
Pirundini, Anthony P.	799 Carroll St.	Brooklyn, N.Y. 11225
Pischel, Dohrmann K.	490 Post St.	San Francisco, Cal. 94102
Piser, Alfred L.	2190 Carillo Rd.	Palm Springs, Cal. 92262
Pistolas, Nicholas G.	8811 Colesville Rd.	Silver Spring, Md. 20910
Pittman, Cole D.	520 E. Frank Phillips Blvd.	Bartlesville, Okla. 74003
Pittman, John E.	David Whitney Bldg.	Detroit, Mich. 48226
Place, E. Clifford	59 Livingston St.	Brooklyn, N. Y. 11201
Plain, Irving H.	31 Lincoln Pk.	Newark, N. J. 07102
Plainer, Truman D.	2525 Rural Rd.	Tempe, Ariz. 85281
Plant, John F.	2909 E. Grand River	Lansing, Mich. 48912
Platt, Donald R.	1010 W. Lake St.	Oak Park, Ill. 60301
Platt, Edward S.	706A Fleming St.	Hendersonville, N.C. 28739
Platt, George A.	1360 Mt. Hope Ave.	Rochester, N. Y. 14620

Platt, Walter M., Jr.	100 8th St.	New Bedford, Mass. 02740
Platt, William K.	711 N. McKinley Rd.	Lake Forest, Ill. 60045
Pliskow, Harold	15901 W. Nine Mile Rd.	Southfield, Mich. 48075
Pliss, Aaron	1275 Delaware Ave.	Buffalo, N. Y. 14209
Plotke, Harry L.	168 Aurora Ave.	St. Paul, Minn. 55103
Plotkin, Jack	1020 Huron Rd.	Cleveland, O. 44115
Podboy, August J.	28 S. Queen St.	York. Pa. 17403
Podell, David L.	67 E. 78th St.	New York, N.Y. 10021
Podos, Steven M.	Washington University School of Medicine	St. Louis, Mo. 63110
Pointer, Robert W.	1720 N. 8th St.	Sheboygan, Wisc. 53081
Polack, Frank M.	J. Hillis Miller Health Center, University of Florida	Gainesville, Fla. 32601
Polan, Charles M.	1611 13th Ave.	Huntington, W. Va. 25717
Pole, Samiel B. III	1 East Ave.	Bridgeton, N.J. 08302
Poley, Brooks J.	Doctors' Bldg.	Minneapolis, Minn. 55402
Polisner, Saul R.	143 Vaughan St.	Portland, Me. 04102
Pollack, Irvin P.	4419 Falls Rd.	Baltimore, Md. 21211
Pollack, Samuel	1107 Howard St.	Evanston, Ill. 60202
Pollard, Joel B.	921 Canal St.	New Orleans, La. 70112
Pollen, Abraham	636 Beacon St.	Boston, Mass. 02115
Pollock, Franklyn J.	3380 Manning Ct.	Los Angeles, Cal. 90064
Poon, James	8363 Vine St.	Cincinnati, O. 45216
Poore, John C.	1101 Welch Rd.	Palo Alto, Cal. 94304
Pope, James G.	177 N. Upper St.	Lexington, Ky. 40507
Pophal, Charles J.	5231 Mayfield Rd.	Lyndhurst, O. 44124
Popkin, Arnold B.	U. S. Highway No. 130	Hightstown, N. J. 08520
Popovich, Stephen J.	1915 Wilshire	Los Angeles, Cal. 90057
Portenar, Myron A.	1217 Madison Ave.	Lakewood, N. J. 08701
Porter, LeRoy G.	602 W. University Ave.	Urbana, Ill. 61801
Porter, Whitney C.	1570 Humboldt St.	Denver, Colo. 80218
Portfolio, Almerindo G.	20 Wilsey Sq.	Ridgewood, N. J. 07450
Portney, Gerald L.	Stanford Medical Center	Stanford, Cal. 94305
Posner, Adolph	667 Madison Ave.	New York, N. Y. 10021
Posner, Irvin L.	DePaul Medical Bldg.	Norfolk, Va. 23505
Posner, Leonard	20 Plaza St.	Brooklyn, N. Y. 11238
Posner, Marvin	1011 Madison Ave.	Albany, N. Y. 12208
Posner, Ronald E.	150 Mentor Ave.	Painesville, O. 44077
Post, Jarvis H.	500 Swank Bldg.	Johnstown, Pa. 15901
Post, Lawrence T.	211 N. Meramec Ave.	Clayton, Mo. 63105
Post, Winfred L.	2401 Jackson Ave.	Joplin, Mo. 64801
Potasz, Thos. M.	8203 Crenshaw Dr.	Inglewood, Cal. 90305
Potter, William B.	1801 Broadway	Galveston, Tex. 77550
Potts, Albert M.	950 E. 59th St.	Chicago, Ill. 60637
Potts, Charles R.	1010 Louisiana	Houston, Tex. 77002
Pougiales, Mary L. P.	915 3rd Ave. S. E.	Rochester, Minn. 55901
Poweleit, Alvin C.	802 Scott St.	Covington, Ky. 41011
Poweleit, Alvin D.	802 Scott St.	Covington, Ky. 41011
Powell, James R.	1610 N. El Dorado	Stockton, Cal. 95204
Powell, Louis F.	314 S. Missouri Ave.	Clearwater, Fla. 33516
Powell, Lyle S., Jr.	1855 San Miguel Dr.	Walnut Creek, Cal. 94596
Powell, Roy R.	3315 Country St.	Portsmouth, Va. 23707
Power, John E.	1017 E. First St.	Duluth, Minn. 55805
Power, John L.	2001 Fourth Ave.	San Diego, Cal. 92101
Powers, Douglas K.	1350 Tulip St.	Longmont, Colo. 80501
Powers, Thomas H.	4966 Glenway Ave.	Cincinnati, O. 45238

Pozelnik, Louis S.	Munson Army Hospital	Ft. Leavenworth, Kans. 66027
Praeger, Donald L.	9 Fulton Ave.	Poughkeepsie, N. Y. 12603
Pranikoff, M. Leo	159 Waterman St.	Providence, R. I. 02906
Prater, Bill G.	Professional Bldg.	Springfield, Mo. 65806
Pratt, Fred J.	63 S. 9th St.	Minneapolis, Minn. 55402
Pratt, Mary Van Horn	171 Harrison Ave.	Boston, Mass. 02111
Pratum, Rolf H.	'C' and Girard Sts.	Bellingham, Wash. 98225
Preefer, Charles J.	20 Bulson Rd.	Rockville Centre, N. Y. 11570
Preefer, Raymond R.	2601 N. Flagler Dr.	West Palm Beach, Fla. 33407
Prenner, Edward J.	109-33 71 Rd.	Forest Hills, N. Y. 11375
Presberg, Max H.	1675 Monroe Ave.	Rochester, N. Y. 14618
Presberg, Saul L.	1675 Monroe Ave.	Rochester, N. Y. 14618
Presley, George D.	613 Magnolia Ave.	Tampa, Fla. 33606
Preston, Frank R.	Naval Hosp.	San Diego, Cal. 92134
Preston, Helen E.	15421 Sixth St.	Victorville, Cal. 92392
Preston, Richard A.	520 W. 17th St.	Santa Ana, Cal. 92706
Preston, Robert W.	1031 S. Main St.	Harrisonburg, Va. 22801
Preston, W. O.	1220 S. Broadway	Lexington, Ky. 40504
Price, F. Raymond	103 Rutledge Ave.	Charleston, S. C. 29401
Price, James	Donner Lab., University of California	Berkeley, Cal. 94620
Price, James A.	680 W. Forest	Jackson, Tenn. 38301
Price, Will J., III	Lewis Bay Rd.	Hyannis, Mass. 02601
Prickman, William E.	825 S. 8th St.	Minneapolis, Minn. 55402
Priddy, Hames S.	827 Margaret Pl.	Shreveport, La. 71101
Priestley, Bruno S.	713 E. 13th St.	Little Rock, Ark. 72202
Primbs, George B.	515 E. Micheltorena St.	Santa Barbara, Cal. 93103
Prindle, Ronald E.	70 Mason St.	Geneva, N. Y. 14456
Pringle, Richard W.	308 High St.	Burlington, N. J. 08016
Pritchard, Dale B.	114½ W. Buffalo St.	Ithaca, N. Y. 14850
Pritikin, Roland I.	Talcott Bldg.	Rockford, Ill. 61101
Privett, John R.	1739 Foothill Blvd.	La Canada, Cal. 91011
Prochaska, Leonard J.	517 First National Bank Bldg. ..	Grand Forks, N. D. 58201
Proctor, Malvin	1865 Amsterdam Ave.	New York, N. Y. 10031
Proffitt, Jonas A.	704 W. Koenig	Grand Island, Nebr. 68801
Prokop, Bradford S.	918 W. 10th	Topeka, Kans. 66604
Prough, Wendell A.	303 S. Main St.	Bluffton, Ind. 46714
Pruett, Ronald C.	Retina Associates, 100 Charles River Plaza	Boston, Mass. 02114
Pruitt, Thomas D., Jr.	Daniel Boone Clinic	Harlan, Ky. 40831
Pryor, Boyce B., Jr.	1780 Dellwood	Memphis, Tenn. 38127
Pryor, Chester C., II	2828 Highland Ave.	Cincinnati, O. 45219
Pryor, Will R.	Heyburn Bldg.	Louisville, Ky. 40202
Pugh, George B.	420 Oak Hill	Youngstown, O. 44502
Pugh, Howard C.	David Whitney Bldg.	Detroit, Mich. 48226
Pugliese, Joseph F.	Narrows Mall Shopping Center ..	Kingston, Pa. 18704
Pugmire, Ralph, W.	2404 Washington Blvd.	Ogden, Utah 84401
Puk, John A.	1953 1st Ave. S. E.	Cedar Rapids, Ia. 52402
Pumphrey, Gordon H.	100 N. Main St.	Mt. Vernon, O. 43050
Puntenney, Irving	720 N. Michigan Ave.	Chicago, Ill. 60611
Purcell, Edward F.	2241 Central Ave.	Alameda, Cal. 94501
Purcell, Hal C.	1025 Pacific St.	San Luis Obispo, Cal. 93401
Purnell, Edward W.	2065 Adelbert Rd.	Cleveland, O. 44106
Purnell, James E.	927 Park Ave.	New York, N. Y. 10028
Puryear, G. Porter	211 S. Saratoga	New Orleans, La. 70112

Pushkin, Edward A.	122 S. Michigan	Chicago, Ill. 60603
Pyle, Gilbert C., Jr.	1501 E. Red River	Victoria, Tex. 77902
Quaglio, Nannette D.	W. State and Porter Sts.	Sharon, Pa. 16146
Quereau, James V. D.	138 N. 5th St.	Reading, Pa. 19601
Quickert, Marvin H.	220 Meridian Ave.	San Jose, Cal. 95126
Quinlan, Joseph D.	44 Prichard St.	Fitchburg, Mass. 01420
Quinn, Frank M.	Box 27, 2nd Gen. Hosp., APO	New York, N. Y. 09180
Quinn, James H.	Boston Bldg.	Salt Lake City, Utah 84111
Quinn, James R.	880 Woodwark	Pontiac, Mich. 48053
Quinn, Lester H.	2811 Lemmon Ave. E.	Dallas, Tex. 75204
Quinn, Robert E.	30 N. Walnut	Chillicothe, O. 45601
Quint, J. Harley	4545 Fanuel St.	San Diego, Cal. 92109
Quinto, Eugene L.	233 Main St.	New Britain, Conn.
Raab, Edward L.	Mt. Sinai School of Med., Fifth Ave. & 100th St.	New York, N. Y. 10029
Raab, George H.	1000 W. LaVeta	Orange, Cal. 92668
Raban, Reginald J.	99 W. Gate Dr.	Cherry Hill, N. J. 08034
Rabb, Maurice F.	55 E. Washington St.	Chicago, Ill. 60602
Rachlin, Maxwell	211 N. Meramec	Clayton, Mo. 63105
Rackwitz, George	200 E. Broadway	New York, N. Y. 10002
Radbill, Sidney G.	1919 Chestnut St.	Philadelphia, Pa. 19151
Radewan, M. G.	P. O. Box 1627	Wenatchee, Wash. 98801
Radl, Cyril J.	Wood Block	Manitowoc, Wisc. 54220
Rados, Berta D.	631 Nye Ave.	Irvington, N.J. 07111
Rados, Walter T.	631 Nye Ave.	Irvington, N.J. 07111
Radulovic, Michael	3611 Branch Ave.	Hillcrest Heights, Md. 20031
Radzimski, Eugene H.	333 Linwood Ave.	Buffalo, N. Y. 14209
Rahn, Elsa K.		Rockville Centre, N. Y. 11570
Raiford, Morgan B.	705 Juniper St. N.E.	Atlanta, Ga. 30308
Raine, Alan Charles	136-52 Cantara St.	Panorama City, Cal. 91402
Ralph, Fenn T.	551 Post Rd.	Darien, Conn. 06820
Ralston, Lewis A.	Eye & Ear Hospital, Box 1627	Wenatchee, Wash. 98801
Ralston, Marc A.	2600 Greenbush St.	Lafayette, Ind. 47902
Ramer, Philip	7441 W. Ridgewood Dr.	Parma, O. 44129
Ramm, Cerl H.	144 1st Ave. S.	St. Petersburg, Fla. 33733
Randall, Harry G.	1020 St. Paul St.	Baltimore, Md. 21202
Randolph, M. Elliott	1020 St. Paul St.	Baltimore, Md. 21202
Randolph, Robert C.	1119 Marshall St.	Manitowoc, Wisc. 54220
Ranker, Emery R.	2700 E. 14th St.	Oakland, Cal. 94601
Rankin, Charles A.	Ludlow & Heather Rd.	Upper Darby, Pa. 19082
Rankin, Richard B.	Post Office Box 3295	Concord, N. C. 28025
Raphael, Sylvan	2457 Grove Way	Hayward, Cal. 94546
Rasberry, James N.	1529 N. 25th St.	Birmingham, Ala. 35234
Rasgorshek, Robert H.	430 Aquila Ct.	Omaha, Nebr. 68102
Rasic, Philip J.	700 Broadway	Seattle, Wash. 98122
Raskind, Richard H.	111 E. 65th St.	New York, N. Y. 10021
Rath, William F.	Professional Bldg.	Wilmington, Dela. 19803
Rathgeber, Van D.	610 W. 10th St.	Ft. Worth, Tex. 76102
Rathkey, Arthur S.	130 W. 6th St.	McMinnville, Ore. 97128
Ravdin, Emile M.	8920 Wilshire Blvd.	Beverly Hills, Cal. 90211
Ravin, Louis C.	3100 W. Central Ave.	Toledo, O. 43606
Ravin, Oscar G.	2850 Sixth Ave.	San Diego, Cal. 92103
Ray, George H.	1835 Eye St., N.W.	Washington, D.C. 2006
Ray, G. Stewart	351 Myrtle Ave.	Albany, N. Y. 12208
Ray, Harold E.	23½ W. Main St.	Xenia, O. 45385

Rayfield, R. Clifton	696 E. Santa Clara St.	San Jose, Cal. 95112
Raymond, Larry A.	616 Medical Towers	Louisville, Ky. 40202
Reagan, Daniel J.	507 Main St.	Worcester, Mass. 01608
Reardon, Robert M.	4 Northcrest Ct.	Bloomington, Ill. 61701
Reasoner, Billy E.	1125 E. 17th St.	Santa Ana, Cal. 92701
Reaves, John E.	1029 Christine Ave.	Anniston, Ala. 36201
Reber, Jacob	1706 Pine St.	Philadelphia, Pa. 19103
Records, Raymond E.	4200 E. 9th Ave.	Denver, Colo. 80220
Reddoch, J. William, Jr. ...	2701 Napoleon Ave.	New Orleans, La. 70115
Reed, Charles L.	Jenkins Bldg.	Pittsburgh, Pa. 15222
Reed, James S.	650 Royal Ave.	Medford, Ore. 97501
Reed, John H.	1128 Vine St.	Gainesville, Ga. 30501
Reed, John W.	Duke University Medical Center .	Durham, N. C. 01742
Reed, Paul H.	727 W. 7th St.	Los Angeles, Cal. 90017
Reeder, James E., Jr.	430 Davidson Bldg.	Sioux City, Ia. 51101
Reeh, Merrill J.	919 S. W. Taylor St.	Portland, Ore. 97205
Reel, Charles M.	362 Freeport St.	New Kensington, Pa. 15068
Rees, Robert L.	107 S. 9th E.	Salt Lake City, Utah 84102
Reese, Algernon B.	73 E. 71st St.	New York, N. Y. 10021
Reese, Gilbert A.	1806 Professional Dr.	Sacramento, Cal. 95825
Reese, Warren S.	2118 Locust St.	Philadelphia, Pa. 19103
Reeves, J. Lane	701 Abercorn St.	Savannah, Ga. 31402
Reeves, John A.	722 Scott St.	Covington, Ky. 41011
Regal, Nathan	105 E. 63rd St.	New York, N. Y. 10021
Regan, Charles D. J.	243 Charles St.	Boston, Mass. 02114
Regan, Ellen F.	1 E. 71st St.	New York, N. Y. 10021
Regan, John E.	28 Harrison St.	Taunton, Mass. 02780
Regan, William F., Jr.	421 Huguenot St.	New Rochelle, N.Y. 10801
Register, Samuel T.	906 S. Ft. Harrison Ave.	Clearwater, Fla. 33516
Regnier, Edme	8 Broad St.	Salem, Mass. 01970
Reichel, John, Jr.	958 County Line Rd.	Bryn Mawr, Pa. 19010
Reichert, Clifford F.	475 Franklin St.	Framingham, Mass. 01701
Reichert, Donald J.	24 W. Villard St.	Dickinson, N. D. 58601
Reid, Frederick K.	310 E. Chestnut St.	Rome, N. Y. 13440
Reid, James D.	Professional Arts Ctr.	Marion, Ind. 46952
Reid, Wesley G.	34186 Spring Valley Dr.	Westland, Mich. 48185
Reik, Louis	9 W. 8th	Covington, Ky. 41011
Reiling, Paul J.	490 N. Alvernon	Tucson, Ariz. 85711
Reilly, Wm. M., Jr.	7 W. Wheeling St.	Washington, Pa. 15301
Rein, Walter J.	501 E. Franklin St.	Richmond, Va. 23219
Reinecke, Robert D.	Albany Medical College	Albany, N. Y. 12208
Reingold, Herbert J.	12139 Riverside Dr.	North Hollywood, Cal. 91607
Reinhardt, Paul H.	300 Homer	Palo Alto, Cal. 94301
Reinhorn, Abraham J.	597 E. 27th St.	Paterson, N. J. 07504
Reisig, Robert O.	20867 Mack Ave.	Grosse Pointe Woods, Mich. 48236
Reiter, Carl	4900 Sunset Blvd.	Los Angeles, Cal. 90027
Reitz, Herbert R.	446 Linwood Ave.	Buffalo, N. Y. 14209
Reitz, Russell E.	1705 Genesee St.	Utica, N. Y. 13501
Relihan, Donald A.	3333 E. Central	Wichita, Kans. 67206
Relyea, Richard L.	5700 Old Richmond Rd.	Richmond, Va. 23226
Rencher, Daniel M., III	1563 Springhill Ave.	Mobile, Ala. 36604
Rengel, Ricardo E.	1822 Ponce de Leon Ave.	Santurce, P. R. 00909
Retzlatt, John A.	17 Myrtle St.	Medford, Ore. 97501
Reuling, Frank H., Jr.	19 N. Washington St.	Winchester, Va. 22601

Reuter, Carl Henry	8 W. Main St.	Springfield, O. 45502
Reuter, John W.	U. S. Highway 50 E., R. R. 6	Bedford, Ind. 47421
Revels, Harry, III	802 N. Kingshighway Blvd.	St. Louis, Mo. 63108
Rex, Earl G.	420 S. Glendora Ave.	West Covina, Cal. 91790
Reynolds, Arthur M., Jr.	1515 Chain Bridge Rd.	McLean, Va. 22101
Reynolds, D. Richard	384 Post St.	San Francisco, Cal. 94108
Rhein, Leroy W.	3240 Main St.	Lemon Grove, Cal. 92045
Rhoades, A. L.	3134 N. 7th St.	Phoenix, Ariz. 85014
Rhodes, David H., Jr.	1 Oliver Plaza, 6th Ave. & Wood St.	Pittsburgh, Pa. 15222
Rice, Alan K.	2008 Robert T. Longway Blvd.	Flint, Mich. 48503
Rice, Jacob	99 Waltham St.	Lexington, Mass. 02173
Rice, John R.	Med. Arts Bldg.	Nashville, Tenn. 37212
Rice, Lee E.	2603 Broadway	Boulder, Colo. 80302
Rice, M. Hobson	542 Church St.	Decatur, Ga. 30030
Rice, Theodore A.	3134 N. 7th St.	Phoenix, Ariz. 85014
Rice, Willard G.	295 Lincoln St.	Worcester, Mass. 01605
Rich, Richard B.	1810 E. 62nd St.	Indianapolis, Ind. 46220
Richards, George M.	1837 El Camino de la Luz	Santa Barbara, Cal. 93105
Richards, John M.	1919 State St.	Santa Barbara, Cal. 93101
Richards, Oliver L., Jr.	2955 Harrison Blvd.	Ogden, Utah 84403
Richards, Richard D.	Univ. of Md. Hosp.	Baltimore, Md. 21201
Richards, William W.	USPHS Hosp.	San Francisco, Cal. 94118
Richards, Winn L.	2773 Madison Ave.	Ogden, Utah 84403
Richardson, Eric C.	140 E. 54th. St.	New York, N. Y. 10022
Richardson, James M., Jr.	4912 Woodlawn Ave.	Chicago, Ill. 60615
Richardson, Kenneth T.	University of Pittsburgh School of Medicine	Pittsburgh, Pa. 15213
Richburg, Frederick A.	2912 Fresno St.	Fresno, Cal. 93721
Richlin, Jay J.	405 N. Bedford Dr.	Beverly Hills, Cal. 90210
Richman, Donald W.	Box 2128	Martinsville, Va. 24112
Richman, Gary O.	384 Peachtree St. N. E.	Atlanta, Ga. 30308
Richman, Marc W.	720 Harrison Ave.	Boston, Mass. 02118
Richman, Morton W.	245 N. Broad St.	Philadelphia, Pa. 19107
Richmond, Richard D.	Box 1029	Beckley, W. Va. 25801
Richter, William C.	S. 427 Bernard	Spokane, Wash. 99204
Ricks, Robert M.	1175 E. Arrow Hwy.	Upland, Cal. 91786
Riddle, Ransford J.		Neavitt, Md. 21652
Rider, Mitchell B.	3535 Cherry Creek N. Dr.	Denver, Colo. 80209
Ridgeway, William G.	6651 Chippewa	St. Louis, Mo. 63109
Ridgway, William L.	490 Post St.	San Francisco, Cal. 94102
Ridley, John E.	2510 W. Capitol Dr.	Milwaukee, Wisc. 53206
Ridley, Robert W.	Guthrie Clinic	Sayre, Pa. 18840
Riechers, Robert J.	8 Medical Plaza	Glen Cove, N. Y. 11542
Riemer, Karl	403 Commonwealth Ave.	Boston, Mass. 02215
Rife, Charles J.	2003 Market St.	Camp Hill, Pa. 17011
Riffenburgh, Ralph S.	595 E. Colorado Blvd.	Pasadena, Cal. 91101
Rigg, James P.	2323 N. 7th St.	Grand Junction, Colo. 81501
Rigg, Robert W.	2323 N. Seventh St.	Grand Junction, Colo. 81501
Riker, Aaron D.	Riker Bldg.	Pontiac, Mich. 48058
Riker, J. L.	601 N. Second Ave.	Alpena, Mich. 49707
Riley, Bennet J.	2299 Bacon St.	Concord, Cal. 94520
Riley, Fenwick C.	200 1st St. S. W.	Rochester, Minn. 55901
Riley, John D.	324 Apache Medical Bldg.	Minneapolis, Minn. 55421

Ring, Henry G.	169 E. Flagler St.	Miami, Fla. 33131
Ring, Joseph A.	5370 Pearl Rd.	Parma, O. 44129
Ripple, Paul H.	558 N. Duke St.	Lancaster, Pa. 17602
Ritch, Joseph G., Jr.	2815 First Ave. N.	St. Petersburg, Gla. 33713
Ritchey, Chas L.	1638 B. St.	Hayward, Cal. 94541
Ritso, Olga	11 Webster St.	N. Tonawanda, N. Y. 14120
Riwchun, Meyer H.	191 North St.	Buffalo, N. Y. 14201
Rixey, Chas O.	Geisinger Med. Ctr.	Danville, Pa. 17821
Rizzuti, A. Benedict	160 Henry St.	Brooklyn, N. Y. 11201
Roach, Charles A.	393 N. Dunlap	St. Paul, Minn. 55104
Robb, Richard M.	300 Longwood Ave.	Boston, Mass. 02115
Robbin, David S.	454 Pennsylvania	Glen Ellyn, Ill. 60137
Robbins, James E.	620 S.W. 4th Ave.	Gainesville, Fla. 32601
Robbins, Jos. M.	628 S. San Vicente Blvd.	Los Angeles, Cal. 90048
Roberts, A. Warren	209 Pine St.	Texarkana, Tex. 75501
Roberts, Bernard A.	369 W. Blackwell St.	Dover, N. J. 07801
Roberts, C. Reid	25 Oak Ave.	Worcester, Mass. 01605
Roberts, James E.	645 W. Harding Way	Stockton, Cal. 95204
Roberts, Leo J.	40 S. Clay	Hinsdale, Ill. 60521
Roberts, N. Craig	255 Third Ave.	Long Branch, N.J. 07740
Roberts, Rufus A., Jr.	1201 W. Presidio	Ft. Worth, Tex. 76102
Roberts, R. Winston	Bowman Gray Med. Ctr.	Winston-Salem, N. C. 27107
Roberts, Shaler S., Jr.	416 N. Seminary St.	Florence, Ala. 35630
Roberts, Walter L.	2010 Wilshire Blvd.	Los Angeles, Calif. 90057
Roberts, William H.	2400 E. Mitchell St.	Humboldt, Tenn. 38343
Robertson, Dennis M.	200 1st St. S. W.	Rochester, Minn. 55901
Robertson, E. Norris, Jr.	1211 N. Shartel	Oklahoma City, Okla. 73103
Robertson, Gaynelle	U. of Texas Medical Branch	Galveston, Tex. 77550
Robertson, Wm. C.	Citizens Trust Bldg.	Portsmouth, Va. 23704
Robertson, Wm. Craig	228 S. Sixth St.	Gadsden, Ala. 35901
Robinson, Benjamin E.	602 W. University Ave.	Urbana, Ill. 61801
Robinson, Howard D.	2900 Whipple Ave.	Redwood City, Cal. 94062
Robinson, John P.	850 Margaret Pl.	Shreveport, La. 71101
Robinson, Nathaniel D.	265 Waterman St.	Providence, R. I. 02906
Robinson, Paul J.	2330 N. W. Flanders St.	Portland, Ore. 97210
Robinson, Wm. P.	4101 Tyson Ave.	Philadelphia, Pa. 19135
Robinson, James T.	4620 J. C. Nichols Pkwy.	Kansas City, Mo. 64112
Roca, Primitivo D.	277 Alexander St.	Rochester, N.Y. 14607
Roch, L. Marshall	406 White River Blvd.	Muncie, Ind. 47303
Roche, John R.	1554 Northern Blvd.	Manhasset, N. Y. 11030
Rock, Frederick	628 Washington Rd.	Pittsburgh, Pa. 15228
Rock, Robert L.	910 W. 19th	Austin, Tex. 78701
Rockey, Dean M.	724 12th S.E.	Auburn, Wash. 98002
Rocknem, Robert E.	110 S. 10th St.	Minneapolis, Minn. 55403
Rockwell, Paul A.	4425 Gollihar Rd.	Corpus Christi, Tex. 78411
Rodin, Frank H.	2233 Post St.	San Francisco, Cal. 94115
Rodin, Max	8618 Sepulveda Blvd.	Los Angeles, Cal. 90045
Rodman, Harold I.	1003 Spring St.	Silver Spring, Md. 20910
Roe, Chester T.	Professional Bldg.	Rockford, Ill. 61108
Roebuck, Jerome B.	408 S. Sycamore St.	Petersburg, Va. 23803
Rogers, J. William	Forsyth Medical Park	Winston-Salem, N. C. 27103
Rogers, John B.	1401 S. Hope St.	Los Angeles, Cal. 90015
Rogers, Jos. B.	512 Van Buren Ave.	Oxford, Miss. 38655
Rogers, Lee H.	420 W. Main	Tupelo, Miss. 38801
Rogers, Stephen H.	654 Madison Ave.	New York, N. Y. 10021
Rohm, Robert F.	1501 Locust St.	Pittsburgh, Pa. 15219

Rojas, Aurelio	6013 Cermak Rd.	Cicero, Ill. 60650
Rolett, Daniel M.	171 E. Post Rd.	White Plains, N. Y. 10601
Rolf, David E.	2740 Carnegie Ave.	Cleveland, O. 44115
Rolfes, H. F.	2112 16th St. N.	St. Petersburg, Fla. 33704
Roling, Edward A.		Lake Villa, Ill. 60046
Roll, Harold	1401 Reisterstown Rd.	Baltimore, Md. 21208
Rollins, Hal J., Jr.	348 N. Elm St.	Greensboro, N. C. 27401
Roloff, Louis W.	1101 Welch Rd.	Palo Alto, Cal. 94304
Romaine, Charles N., IV.	5700 W. Grace St.	Richmond, Va. 23226
Roman, Stanley J.	15020 Michigan Ave.	Dearborn, Mich. 48126
Romano, Paul E.	2300 Children's Plaza	Chicago, Ill. 60614
Romayananda, Nongnart C.	Johns Hopkins Hosp.	Baltimore, Md. 21205
Rome, Albert	309 N. Logan Ave.	Danville, Ill. 61832
Rome, Sol	1515 N. Vermont	Los Angeles, Cal. 90027
Romejko, Walter J.	1234 19th St. N. W.	Washington, D. C. 20036
Romig, John E.	209 State St.	Harrisburg, Pa. 17101
Roncke, George J.	1225 W. Mitchell St.	Milwaukee, Wisc. 53204
Rones, Benjamin	1302 18th St., N.W.	Washington, D. C. 20036
Root, Amos B.	3315 4th Ave.	San Diego, Cal. 92103
Roper, Kenneth L.	Prudential Plaza	Chicago, Ill. 60601
Rosa, Elias R.	El Monte Mall	Hato Rey, P.R. 00918
Rosborough, James F., Jr.	Naval Hosp.	Oakland, Cal. 94627
Rose, A. Lawrence	7400 N. Kendall Dr.	Miami, Fla. 33156
Rose, Arnold L.	120 Summit Ave.	Summit, N. J. 07901
Rose, Howard N.	1550 Riverside Ave.	Jacksonville, Fla. 32204
Rose, Lawrence	2200 O'Farrell St.	San Francisco, Cal. 94115
Rose, Turpin H.	432 Main St.	Danbury, Conn. 06810
Rosehill, David B.	15240 Piedmont Rd.	Saratoga, Cal. 95070
Rosen, Emanuel D.	112 Main St.	Allenhurst, N. J. 07711
Rosen, Morris	1239 Glenview St.	Philadelphia, Pa. 19111
Rosenbaum, Harry D.	4511 Forest Park Blvd.	St. Louis, Mo. 63108
Rosenbaum, J. Geo.	2460 Fairmount Blvd.	Cleveland, O. 44106
Rosenbaum, Louis J.	777 E. Brill St.	Phoenix, Ariz. 85006
Rosenberg, A. S.	142 Joralemon St.	Brooklyn, N. Y. 11201
Rosenberg, Alan J.	384 Post St.	San Francisco, Cal. 94108
Rosenberg, Elliot	16260 Ventura Blvd.	Encino, Cal. 91316
Rosenberg, Seligman	1331 Anderson Ave.	Ft. Lee, N. J. 07024
Rosenberg, Wm.	130 E. Randolph Dr.	Chicago, Ill. 60601
Rosenblatt, Monroe N.	140 Lockwood Ave.	New Rochelle, N. Y. 10801
Rosenbluth, Joseph C.	4277 Hempstead Tnpk.	Bethpage, N. Y. 11714
Rosenfeld, Cecelia	15247 Sunset Blvd.	Pacific Palisades, Cal. 90272
Rosenfeld, Robert A.	218-07 Peck Ave.	Queens Village, N. Y. 11427
Rosenthal, A. Ralph	4420 Rosedale Ave.	Bethesda, Md. 20014
Rosenthal, Benjamin C.	41 Eastern Pkwy.	Brooklyn, N. Y. 11238
Rosenthal, Gerald C.	41 Eastern Pkwy.	Brooklyn, N. Y. 11238
Rosenthal, J. Robert	41 Eastern Pkwy.	Brooklyn, N.Y. 11238
Rosenthal, J. Wm.	1419 Delachaise St.	New Orleans, La. 70115
Rosenthal, Morton L.	20 E. 9th St.	New York, N. Y. 10003
Rosenthal, Perry	33 Pond Ave.	Brookline, Mass. 02146
Rosenthal, Stephen A.	175 Jericho Turnpike	Syosset, N. Y. 11791
Rosenthal, Stuart A.	50 Samsondale Plaza	W. Haverstraw, N. Y. 10993
Rosner, Robert S.	20119 Van Aken Blvd.	Cleveland, O. 44122
Ross, Jerome	3455 Wilkens Ave.	Baltimore, Md. 21229
Ross, John D.	415 11th Ave. S.	Nampa, Ida. 83651
Ross, Joseph V. M.	321 E. Front St.	Berwick, Pa. 18603
Ross, Milton G.	V. A. Hosp.	Northampton, Mass. 01060

Ross, Perry W.	5426 N. Sheridan Rd.	Chicago, Ill. 60640
Roszell, Leo H.	309 Second National Bldg.	Akron, O. 44308
Roth, B. Paul	1022 W. Ivy	Moses Lake, Wash. 98837
Roth, F. Dale	490 Post St.	San Francisco, Cal. 94102
Roth, Malcolm S.	100 Constitution Plaza	Hartford, Conn. 06103
Roth, Nathan H.	1437 San Marino Ave.	San Marino, Cal. 91108
Rothberg, Maurice	347 W. Berry St.	Fort Wayne, Ind. 46802
Rothen, Robert M.	1301 W. 38th St.	Austin, Tex. 78705
Rothfeder, Howard L.	13362 Newport Ave.	Tustin, Cal. 92680
Rothman, Harold	2911 Kings Hwy.	Brooklyn, N. Y. 11229
Rouen, Robert L.	1209 Harrison	Elkhart, Ind. 46514
Rouse, David M.	212 E. Monroe St.	Mexico, Mo. 65265
Rouse, Hillrie K.	Box 1018	Gulfport, Miss. 39501
Row, D. Hamilton	23 E. Ohio St.	Indianapolis, Ind. 46204
Rowan, Ivan R.	13654 Cantara	Panorama City, Cal. 91324
Rowe, Fred A.	508 Mid State Medical Center	Nashville, Tenn. 37203
Rowe, Kenneth W., Jr.	Holmes Hospital, Eden & Bethesda Aves.	Cincinnati, O. 45219
Rowell, Peter P.	1309 Liberty St. S. E.	Salem, Ore. 97302
Rowel, Roger R.	542 Church St.	Decatur, Ga. 30030
Rowen, Gerald E.	2000 Clark	Miles City, Mont. 59301
Rowland, Ivo E.	222 Madison St.	Joliet, Ill. 60435
Rowland, Robert C.	602 S. Abe	San Angelo, Tex. 76901
Rowlett, William M.	1611 S. Main St.	Hopkinsville, Ky. 42240
Roy, Frederick H.	4301 E. Markham	Little Rock, Ark. 72201
Royals, Walter C.		San Antonio, Tex. 78209
Royce, Emery E.	601 N. Wilmot Rd.	Tucson, Ariz. 85711
Royer, Charles A.	430 N.W. 12 St.	Oklahoma City, Okla. 73103
Rozanksi, Thomas I.	10 Lavenham Ct.	Cherry Hill. N. J. 08034
Rozansky, Norman M.	306 Hawthorn St.	San Diego, Cal. 92101
Rubenstein, Robert A.	6505 Alvarado Rd.	San Diego, Cal. 92120
Rubin, Gerald S.	7000 Cutler Ave. N. E.	Albuquerque, N.M. 87110
Rubin, Herbert S.	1030 President Ave.	Fall River, Mass. 02720
Rubin, I. Edward	255 S. 17th St.	Philadelphia, Pa. 19131
Rubin, Laurence E.	9801 Georgia Ave.	Silver Spring, Md. 20902
Rubin, M. Harvey	1311 N. Elm St.	Greensboro, N. C. 27401
Rubin, Melvin L.	Univ. of Fla. Med. Ctr.	Gainesville, Fla. 32601
Rubin, Milton R.	1331 Wishon Ave.	Fresno, Cal. 93728
Rubin, Nathan S.	1401 N. Palafox St.	Pensacola, Fla. 32501
Rubin, William	184 Livingston Ave.	New Brunswick, N. J. 08902
Rucker, C. Wilbur	Mayo Clinic	Rochester, Minn. 55901
Rucker, Thomas K.	6533 Drew Ave. S.	Minneapolis, Minn. 55435
Rudens, Maurice C.	433 N. 4th St.	Montebello, Cal. 90640
Rudolph, Carl J.	110 W. Barlett St.	South Bend, Ind. 46601
Rudolph, Edward A.	Midwest Bldg.	Aberdeen, S. D. 57401
Rudolph, Kenneth J.	3700 Bellemeade Ave.	Evansville, Ind. 47715
Ruedemann, Albert D.	David Whitney Bldg.	Detroit, Mich. 48226
Ruedemann, Albert D., Jr.	David Whitney Bldg.	Detroit, Mich. 48226
Rufé, John R.	1102 Grand Ave.	Kansas City, Mo. 64106
Ruggeri, Charles	Boston Bldg.	Salt Lake City, Utah 84111
Ruiz, Richard S.	Hermann Prof. Bldg.	Houston, Tex. 77025
Rumage, Jos P.	Audubon Bldg.	New Orleans, La. 70112
Rummel, W. David	1003 Division St.	Prescott, Ariz. 86301
Rundle, Herman L.	400 Newport Center Dr.	Newport Beach, Cal. 92660
Rundles, Walter Z., Jr.	500 S. Grand Traverse	Flint, Mich. 48503
Runge, Paul M.	47 W. Elm St.	Brockton, Mass. 02401

Runyan, Thomas E.	Box 304, Fitzsimons General Hosp.	Aurora, Colo. 80240
Rup, Edmund C.	21 Woodland St.	Hartford, Conn. 06105
Rupple, James H.	80 Sheboygan St.	Fon Du Lac, Wisc. 54935
Rush, Calvin C.	106 W. Greene St.	Waynesburg, Pa. 15370
Rusher, Wm. D.	3500 Kensington Ave.	Richmond, Va. 23221
Rusk, Harvey S.	131 Colorado Ave.	Pueblo, Colo. 81005
Russell, Daniel A., Jr.	730 N. Main	San Antonio, Tex. 78205
Russell, James S.	528 Nautilus St.	La Jolla, Cal. 92037
Russell, Roland D.	317 E. Chicago St.	Elgin, Ill. 60120
Russman, Burton A.	30 N. Michigan Ave.	Chicago, Ill. 60602
Russo, Charles E.	Hermenna Professional Bldg.	Houston, Tex. 77025
Ruth, Paul E.	4223 Oak Knoll Dr.	Youngstown, O. 44512
Ryan, Edward P.	66 Park St.	Glens Falls, N. Y. 12801
Ryan, Emmett J. L.	102 Nahant St.	Lynn, Mass. 01902
Ryan, Gerald S.	200 S. Broadway	Tarrytown, N. Y. 10591
Ryan, John J.	Medical Towers Bldg. N.	Louisville, Ky. 40202
Ryan, Ralph W.	158 High St.	Morgantown, W. Va. 26505
Ryan, Stephen J.	403 Commonwealth Ave.	Boston, Mass. 02115
Ryan, Terry D.	780 Chestnut St.	Springfield, Mass. 01107
Ryan, Wm. F.	761 Washington St.	Norwood, Mass. 02062
Ryan, Wm. H.	1700 McHenry Village Way	Modesto, Cal. 95350
Ryerson F. Stuart	1774 Alameda	Pomona, Cal. 91767
Sabates, Felix N.	6700 Troost	Kansas City, Mo. 64131
Sabin, Fred C.	1414 W. Fair Ave.	Marquette, Mich. 49855
Sachs, Baruch J.	636 Beacon St.	Boston, Mass. 02215
Sachs, David D.	2320 Sutter St.	San Francsico, Cal. 94115
Sachs, James W.	251 E. Baltimore St.	Hagerstown, Md. 21740
Sacks, Joel G.	303 E. Chicago Ave.	Chicago, Ill. 60611
Sacks, Norman J.	2140 Scottwood	Toledo, O. 43620
Sacks-Wolner, Erwin P.	333 W. State St.	Trenton, N. J. 08618
Safir, Aran	The Mount Sinai Hospital, 100th St. & 5th Ave.	New York, N. Y. 10029
Sage, Harry M.	3545 Olentangy River Rd.	Columbus, O. 43214
Sage, Harry M., Jr.	3545 Olentangy River Rd.	Columbus, O. 43214
Sage, Webster LeG., Jr.	555 W. Catalina	Phoenix, Ariz. 85013
St. Clair, Robert T.	113 N. Church	Visalia, Cal. 93277
St. Dizier, Roger V., Jr.	500 St. Landry	Lafayette, La. 70501
Saint-Germain, Ellis L.	209 Pigford Bldg.	Meridian, Miss. 39301
St. Louis, Joseph A., Jr.	275 Carpenter Dr. N. E.	Atlanta, Ga. 30328
Sakler, Allen M.	Lincoln Federal Bldg.	Louisville, Ky. 40202
Sakler, Barnet R.	19 Garfield Pl.	Cincinnati, O. 45202
Salasky, Milton	Med. Tower Bldg.	Norfolk, Va. 23507
Salatino, Ralph N.	210 E. 15th St.	New York, N. Y. 10003
Sallee, Wm. T.	17000 W. Eight Mile Rd.	Southfield, Mich. 48075
Salmon, Louis R.	Applebrook Farm Rd. & Hwy. 35	Middletown, N. J. 07748
Salmon, Mickey L.	3944 Ritz Center	St. Louis, Mo. 63125
Salomon, Maurice S.	2300 Sutter St.	San Francisco, Cal. 94115
Saltzman, Samuel L.	334 W. 86th St.	New York, N. Y. 10024
Sambursky, José S.	42 Riverside Dr.	Binghamton, N. Y. 13905
Sampson, John J.	2810 E. Pikes Peak Ave.	Colorado Springs, Colo. 80909
Sampson, Whitney G.	530 W. 20th St.	Houston, Tex. 77008
Samson, C. L. M.	150 Baronne St.	New Orleans, La. 70112
Samson, Cesar R.	Colfax Manor Gardens, Roselle & W. Colfax Ave.	Roselle Park, N. J. 07024

Samuel, Jerome	2000 Kings Hwy.	Brooklyn, N. Y. 11229
Samuels, S. Lawrence	1111 Park Ave.	Plainfield, N. J. 07060
Sanacore, Jos. A.	297 Graham Ave.	Brooklyn, N. Y. 11211
Sand, Bruce J.	6360 Wilshire Blvd.	Los Angeles, Cal. 90048
Sandall, Gary S.	611 Church St.	Ann Arbor, Mich. 48104
Sanderlin, Joseph M.	3rd Marine Division, FPO	San Francisco, Cal. 96602
Sanders, Gerald S.	5363 Balboa Blvd.	Encino, Cal. 91316
Sanders, Harmon U.	2246 Rhode Island	Lawrence, Kans. 66044
Sanders, Harold J.	8121 Van Nuys Blvd.	Panorama City, Cal. 91402
Sanders, Norman	1100 N.E. 163rd St.	Miami Beach, Fla. 33162
Sanders, T. E.	100 N. Euclid Ave.	St. Louis, Mo. 63108
Sanders, Wallace R.	1502 8th St.	Wichita Falls, Tex. 76301
Sandler, Robert	Med. Arts Bldg.	Baltimore, Md. 21201
Sands, Abraham M.	874 Carroll St.	Brooklyn, N. Y. 11215
Sandt, Karl E.	7809 Herschel Ave.	La Jolla, Cal. 92037
Sanfacon, Thomas A.	340 Park Ave.	Paterson, N. J. 07504
Sanger, Welborn W.	1111 N. Lee	Oklahoma City, Okla. 73103
Sannella, Lee S.	215 Valley View Dr.	Petaluma, Cal. 94952
Santos, George P.	418 Washington St.	Brighton, Mass. 02135
Sappenfield, Luther C., Jr.	1629 Owen Dr.	Fayetteville, N. C. 28304
Saradarian, Albert V.	921 Bergen Ave.	Jersey City, N.J. 07306
Saradarian, Edward V.	26 Madison Ave.	Morristown, N. J. 07960
Saran, Nirmal	San Joaquin Gen. Hosp.	Stockton, Cal. 95201
Sargent, Chas A.	3838 Hillcroft	Houston, Tex. 77027
Sargent, Willard S.	233 A. St.	San Diego, Cal. 92101
Sarin, Lov K.	Lankenau Med. Bldg.	Philadelphia, Pa. 19151
Sarnat, Leonard A.	1950 Sheridan Rd.	Highland Park, Ill. 60035
Sarrail, J. Albert	450 Sutter St.	San Francisco, Cal. 94108
Sarro, Louis J.	1334 Med-Dent. Bldg.	Seattle, Wash. 98101
Saskin, Edward	34 Plaza St.	Brooklyn, N. Y. 11238
Sass, Wm. O.	515 3rd St.	Niagara Falls, N. Y. 14301
Sassaman, Franklin W.	301 Bronson Medical Center	Kalamazoo, Mich. 49006
Sauer, John	30 E. 40th St.	New York, N. Y. 10016
Saul, Robert W.	Medical Arts Bldg.	Pittsburgh, Pa. 15213
Saunders, James A.	11104 S. E. Stark St.	Portland, Ore. 97216
Saunders, Joseph H.	288 S. Limestone St.	Lexington, Ky. 40508
Saunders, Meredith R.	1422 Woodland Ave.	Des Moines, Ia. 50309
Sauter, Frederick	1 Hanson Pl.	Brooklyn, N. Y. 11217
Sawyer, Norman M	Johnson City Eye Hospital	Johnson City, Tenn. 37601
Sawyer, Thomas R.	811 E. Wisconsin Ave.	Milwaukee, Wisc. 53202
Saxe, Julian S.	230 Fifth Ave.	Indialantic, Fla. 32901
Sayad, Wm. Y.	1515 N. Flagler Dr.	West Palm Beach, Fla. 33401
Scanlon, John E.	161 Clinton St.	Watertown, N. Y. 13601
Scanlon, William A.	1870 W. Galena Blvd.	Aurora, Ill. 60506
Scarney, Herman D.	William Beaumont Medical Bldg.	Royal Oak, Mich. 48072
Schachat, Walter S.	799 Park Ave.	New York, N. Y. 10021
Schachne, Lewis	150 E. 56th St.	New York, N. Y. 10022
Schaefer, Arthur J.	4766 Main St.	Buffalo, N. Y. 14226
Schaeffer, Alexander J.	6317 Wilshire Blvd.	Los Angeles, Cal. 90048
Schaeffer, Edward M.	600 S. Glenstone Blvd.	Springfield, Mo. 65801
Schaeffer, Robert S.	200 S. Broadway	Tarrytown, N. Y. 10591
Schafer, David L.	2401 Pennsylvania Ave.	Wilmington, Dela. 19806
Schaffer, David B.	1740 Bainbridge St.	Philadelphia, Pa. 19146
Schafrank, Michael S.	72-35 112 St.	Forest Hills, N. Y. 11375
Schall, Samuel M.	30 N. Michigan Ave.	Chicago, Ill. 60602

Schalmo, E. H.	3615 W. Oklahoma Ave.	Milwaukee, Wisc. 53215
Schane, David	20211 Greenfield	Detroit, Mich. 48235
Schapero, Dorothea S.	7301 Sepulveda Blvd.	Van Nuys, Cal. 91405
Schardt, Walter M.	191 Main St.	Manchester, Conn. 06040
Schechtman, Charles T.	Cedar Lake Medical Center	New Britain, Conn. 06052
Scheffler, Milton M.	55 E. Washington St.	Chicago, Ill. 60602
Scheidt, John E.	301 W. Bastanchury Rd.	Fullerton, Cal. 92632
Scheie, Harold G.	3400 Spruce St.	Philadelphia, Pa. 19104
Scheiner, Stanley A.	1990 N. E. 163rd St.	N. Miami Beach, Fla. 33162
Schepens, Charles L.	100 Charles River Plaza	Boston, Mass. 02114
Scher, David	Medical Towers	Houston, Tex. 77025
Scheribel, Karl J.	55 E. Washington St.	Chicago, Ill. 60602
Schertz, Truman B.	2022 Swift	North Kansas City, Mo. 64116
Schiff, Frank S.	206 E. Las Tunas Dr.	San Gabriel, Cal. 91776
Schiller, Shedon B.	Heyburn Bldg.	Louisville, Ky. 40202
Schimek, Robert A.	1514 Jefferson Hwy.	New Orleans, La. 70121
Schlaegel, T. F., Jr.	Indiana University Medical Center	Indianapolis, Ind. 46202
Schloss, Morton	7400 N. Kendall Dr.	Miami, Fla. 33156
Schlossman, Abraham	667 Madison Ave.	New York, N. Y. 10021
Schmetz, Frank J., Jr.	Naval Hosp.	Oakland, Cal. 94627
Schmidt, Carl F.	1836 South Ave.	Lacrosse, Wisc. 54601
Schmidt, David W.	1230 N. Maple Rd.	Ann. Arbor. Mich. 48103
Schmidt, Herbert	250 Patchogue-Yaphank Rd.	E. Patchogue, N. Y. 11772
Schmidt, Herbert G.	1714 E. Capitol Dr.	Milwaukee, Wisc. 53211
Schmidt, Paul J.	7939 S. Western	Chicago, Ill. 60620
Schmidtke, Reinhardt L.	Univ. of Minnesota, Health Service	Minneapolis, Minn. 55455
Schmoll, Robert J.	521 W. Wayne	Ft. Wayne, Ind. 46802
Schnebly, John T.	9801 Georgia Ave.	Silver Spring, Md. 20902
Schneider, Bernard	2301 S. Broad St.	Philadelphia, Pa. 19148
Schneider, Howard J.	9 E. 91st St.	New York, N. Y. 10028
Schneider, Howard R.	2084 Bedford Avenue	Bellmore, N. Y. 11710
Schneider, Julius	178 E. 71st St.	New York, N. Y. 10021
Schnell, Edward W.	Great Northern Med. Ctr.	North Olmsted, O. 44070
Schnellmann, Donald C.	500 Northwest Plaza	St. Ann, Mo. 63074
Schnoor, Thomas G.	526 Soquel Ave	Santa Cruz, Cal. 95060
Schocket, Stanley S.	22 S. Green St.	Baltimore, Md. 21202
Schoel, Robert E.	211 S. Saratoga St.	New Orleans, La. 70112
Schoenberg, Max	1749 Grand Concourse	Bronx, N. Y. 10453
Schoenfeld, Jay B.	520 Westfield Ave.	Elizabeth, N. J. 07208
Scholz, Roy O.	11 E. Chase St.	Baltimore, Md. 21202
Schonberg, Albert L.	801 Encino Pl., N.E.	Albuquerque, N. M. 87106
Schonberg, Stephen S.	2220 Lynn Rd.	Thousand Oaks, Cal. 91360
Schoon, Doris V.	925 S. Gilbert	Ansheim, Cal. 92804
Schopp, Robert C.	49 Linwood Ave.	Buffalo, N. Y. 14209
Schott, Edward C.	656 W. Market St.	Akron, O. 44303
Schott, Edward G.	1011 N. 8th St.	Sheboygan, Wisc. 53081
Schrimpf, Cyril E.	180 W. McMillan St.	Cincinnati, O. 45219
Schub, Martin	245 Engle St.	Englewood, N. J. 07631
Schubert, Thomas W.	245 4th St. Bldg.	Bremerton, Wash. 98310
Schuler, Roger W.	2111 N. Wood Ave.	Linden, N.J. 07036
Schulsinger, Samuel	80 Clinton Ave.	Newark, N.J. 07114
Schultz, Abraham	7190 W. Grand Ave.	Chicago, Ill. 60635
Schultz, Alfred G.	237 E. State St.	Jacksonville, Ill. 62650
Schultz, Arthur E.	241 E. Saginaw	E. Lansing, Mich. 48823

Schultz, Cleon L.	113 S. Kentucky	Roswell, N. M. 88201
Schultz, Don L.	31 Royal Palm Blvd.	Vero Beach, Fla. 32960
Schultz, Gerald R.	340 Main St.	Worcester, Mass. 01608
Schultz, Jacob F.	1010 Louisiana St.	Houston, Tex. 77002
Schultz, Richard O.	8700 W. Wisconsin Ave.	Milwaukee, Wisc. 53226
Schulz, Harold P.	909 Hyde St.	San Francisco, Cal. 94109
Schulz, Kurt J.	4645 Broadway	Gary, Ind. 46409
Schulze, Richard R.	Paulsen at 67th	Savannah, Ga. 31404
Schumacher, James C.	11 W. Monument Bldg.	Dayton, O. 45402
Schuman, Irving	10808 Washington Blvd.	Culver City, Cal. 90230
Schunk, Peter A.	1317 N. Academy Blvd.	Colorado Springs, Colo. 80909
Schuster, Harvey S.	U.S.A.F. Regional Hospital, Maxwell Air Force Base	Montgomery, Ala. 36113
Schuster, Stephen A.	El Paso Nat'l Bank Bldg.	El Paso, Tex. 79901
Schut, Almon L.	252 E. Lovell St.	Kalamazoo, Mich. 49006
Schutz, Joseph A.	2804 Main St.	Buffalo, N. Y. 14214
Schutz, Sigmund	150 W. 55th St.	New York, N. Y. 10019
Schutz, Wm. J.	Medical Towers Bldg., N.	Louisville, Ky. 40202
Schwab, Gerald J.	416 St. Mark Ct.	Peoria, Ill. 61603
Schwade, Irwin	255 W. 23rd St.	New York, N. Y. 10011
Schwarting, Bland H.	Med. Prof. Bldg.	San Antonio, Tex. 78212
Schwartz, Ariah	1515 Trousdale Dr.	Burlingame, Cal. 94010
Schwartz, Bernard	171 Harrison Ave.	Boston, Mass. 02111
Schwartz, Edward	112 E. 9th St.	Chester, Pa. 19013
Schwartz, Frank E.	1306 W. Ave. J.	Lancaster, Cal. 93534
Schwartz, Frederick O.	508 N. Grand Blvd.	St. Louis, Mo. 63103
Schwartz, Herbert N.	60 Gillett St.	Hartford, Conn. 06105
Schwartz, John T.	1609 Ladd St.	Silver Spring, Md. 20902
Schwartz, Jules L.	1777 Grand Concourse	Bronx, N. Y. 10453
Schwartz, Leo H.	749 Central Ave.	Dover, N.H. 03820
Schwartzman, Harry	501 Washington St.	Boston, Mass. 02111
Schwartzman, Joseph D.	37-19 73rd St.	Jackson Heights, N. Y. 11372
Schwarz, Robert J.	317 W. C St.	Ontario, Cal. 91761
Schwarzkopf, Geo. C.	5900 Atlantic Ave.	Ventnor, N. J. 08406
Schweitzer, L. Fernando	7812A Fulton	Houston, Tex. 77022
Schwerdt, Richard F.	104 W. Clark St.	Champaign, Ill. 61820
Schwilk, Norman F., Jr.	3701 J. St.	Scramento, Cal. 95816
Sciarrino, John F.	4760 Sunrise Hwy.	Massapequa Park, N. Y. 11762
Scilleri, John	660 Broadway	Paterson, N. J. 07514
Scimeca, Anthony A.	490 Atlantic Ave.	East Rockaway, N. Y. 11518
Scimeca, Henry A.	33 Cypress Ln.	Willingboro, N. J. 08046
Scott, Alan B.	3905 Sacramento St.	San Fransisco, Cal. 94118
Scott, Alfred W.	7 Bay State Rd.	Boston, Mass. 02215
Scott, David H.	7 Thorndike St.	Beverly, Mass. 01915
Scott, Joseph M.	1320 Linden Ave.	Memphis, Tenn. 38104
Scott, Pierre B.	3541 W. Braddock Rd.	Alexandria, Va. 22302
Scott, Robert K.	126 Main St.	Logan, W. Va. 25601
Scovis, John	749 S. Garland Ave.	Los Angeles, Cal. 90017
Scruggs, James H.	2223 Austin Ave.	Waco, Tex. 76701
Scuderi, Richard A.	68-63 Fresh Pond Rd.	Queens, N. Y. 11227
Scurti, Bernard V.	43-15 159th St.	Flushing, N. Y. 11358
Seale, Earl S.	126 Bay State Rd.	Boston, Mass. 02215
Seale, Hubert J.	1325 Hickory St.	Abilene, Tex. 79601

Seaman, David	407 Professional Arts Bldg.	Aberdeen, S. D. 57401
Sears, James L.	12165 Pastoral Rd.	San Diego, Cal. 92128
Sears, Marvin L.	333 Cedar St.	New Haven, Conn. 06510
Seaton, Lewis H.	Eye Clinic, Naval Hospital	Jacksonville, Fla. 32214
Sebastian, Eugene F.	207 State St.	Harrisburg, Pa. 17101
Sebestyen, John G.	636 Beacon St.	Boston, Mass. 02215
Seeger, Frank L.	1609 Pasadena Ave. S.	St. Petersburg, Fla. 33707
Seeger, Jos G.	277 Alexander St.	Rochester, N. Y. 14607
Seelenfreund, Morton H. ..	20 E. 68th St.	New York, N. Y. 10021
Seidel, Jerry G.	120 Main St.	Park Ridge, Ill. 60068
Seidenberg, Boyd H.	4 Wilsey Square	Ridgewood, N. J. 07450
Seiff, Stephen S.	435 N. Roxbury Dr.	Beverly Hills, Cal. 90210
Seiller, Barry L.	1800 Grand Ave.	Waukegan, Ill. 60085
Selby, George D.	1835 Eye St., N.W.	Washington, D. C. 20006
Seligson, Alvin	28-05 Fair Lawn Ave.	Fair Lawn, N. J. 07410
Seligstein, Milton B.	Planters Nat. Bk. Bldg.	Memphis, Tenn. 38103
Selinger, Samuel	109-6th St.	Hackettstown, N. J. 07840
Sella, John L.	6114 W. Capitol Dr.	Milwaukee, Wisc. 53216
Sellitto, Anthony M.	115 Connett Pl.	South Orange, N. J. 07079
Sellyei, Louis F., Jr.	731 12th St. N.	St. Petersburg, Fla. 33705
Seltzer, Sidney M.	315 Calhoun St.	Charleston, S. C. 29401
Semple, Henry C.	1359 Springhill Ave.	Mobile, Ala. 36604
Senita, G. Robt.	198 Lincoln Ave.	Pittsburgh, Pa. 15202
Seretan, Edward L.	111-32 76th Ave.	Forest Hills, N. Y. 11375
Sergis, Mooshy	127 E. Acacia	Stockton, Cal. 95202
Settembrini, Chas L.	699 Gramatan Ave.	Mt. Vernon, N. Y. 10552
Settler, Sheridan H., Jr. ...	Andrew Mem. Hosp.	Tuskegee, Ala. 36088
Sever, Raymond J.	3000 Medical Park Dr.	Tampa, Fla. 33612
Severin, Sanford L.	6500 Fairmount Ave.	El Cerrito, Cal. 94530
Seward, William H.	5225 Connecticut Ave. N. W. ...	Washington, D. C. 20015
Sexton, Robt. R.	5323 Harry Hines Blvd.	Dallas, Tex. 75235
Shaad, Dorothy J.	Univ. of Kansas Medical Center .	Kansas City, Kans. 66103
Shafer, Donald M.	140 E. 54th St.	New York, N. Y. 10022
Shaffer, Robert N.	490 Post St.	San Francisco, Cal. 94102
Shahan, Philip T.	211 N. Meramec Ave.	St. Louis, Mo. 63105
Shahidi, Massoud M.	1200 Douglas Ave.	Ames, Ia. 50010
Shainhouse, Arthur	1217 48th St.	Brooklyn, N. Y. 11219
Shakib, Manoucher	737 Park Ave.	New York, N. Y. 10021
Shaklan, Barry N.	USAF Regional Hospital	Eglin AFB, Fla. 35242
Shanedling, Philip D.	6333 Wilshire Blvd.	Los Angeles, Cal. 90048
Shaner, Harold J.	1017 E. Robinson St.	Orlando, Fla. 32801
Shankel, Harry W.	Republic Bldg.	Denver, Colo. 80202
Shannon, C. Richard	5301 F St.	Sacramento, Cal. 95819
Shannon, Gerard M.	8118 Bustleton Ave.	Philadelphia, Pa. 19152
Shapira, Theodore M.	111 N. Wabash Ave.	Chicago, Ill. 60602
Shapiro, Burton J.	3620 N. Meridian	Indianapolis, Ind. 46208
Shapiro, Irving	Medical Arts Bldg.	Minneapolis, Minn. 55402
Shapiro, Leonard Z.	300 N. Main St.	Spring Valley, N. Y. 10977
Shapiro, Manuel A.	10605 Chester Ave.	Cleveland, O. 44106
Shapiro, Martin L.	Cinnaminson Med. Ctr.	Cinnaminson, N. J. 08077
Shapiro, Robert S.	900 Madison Ave.	Plainfield, N. J. 07060
Shapley, Albert	1148 Fourth St.	Santa Monica, Cal. 90403
Sharbaugh, Geo. B.	25 Prospect St.	Trenton, N. J. 08168
Sharp, James F.	465 N. Roxbury Dr.	Beverly Hills, Cal. 90210
Sharrer, Margaret C.	Jenkins Bldg.	Pittsburgh, Pa. 15222
Sharvelle, Derek J.	204 W. Hill Ave.	Gallup, N. M. 87301

Shaver, Robert P.	5700 N.W. Grand Blvd.	Oklahoma City, Okla. 73103
Shaw, Elmer A.	520 Commonwealth Ave.	Boston, Mass. 02215
Shaw, Frederick C.	203 Elm St.	Westfield, N. J. 07090
Shaw, Harry E.	Jenkins Arcade	Pittsburgh, Pa. 15222
Shaw, Howard A.	6533 Drew Ave., S.	Minneapolis, Minn. 55435
Shaw, Jules H.	510 Commonwealth Ave.	Boston, Mass. 02215
Shaw, Ned.	526 Penn St.	Camden, N. J. 08102
Shea, Thomas R.	Medical Arts Clinic	Sherman, Tex. 75090
Shearer, Robt. V.	Loma Linda Univ. Hosp.	Loma Linda, Cal. 92354
Shearin, William A.	1300 St. Mary's St.	Raleigh, N. C. 27605
Sheehy, James E.	120 E. Washington St.	Syracuse, N. Y. 13207
Sheets, John H.	1173 E. 42nd St.	Odessa, Tex. 79760
Shegedyn, Taras	19 Holly St.	Cranford, N. J. 07016
Shekter, William B.	2200 O'Farrell St.	San Francisco, Cal. 94115
Shelton, Philip A.	85 Jefferson St.	Hartford, Conn. 06106
Shenon, Peter W.	1855 San Miguel Dr.	Walnut Creek, Cal. 94596
Shepard, Dennis D.	1414 S. Miller St.	Santa Maria, Cal. 93454
Shepherd, Edwin M.	1306 Kanawha Blvd. E.	Charleston, W. Va. 25301
Shepherd, John R.	3196 Maryland Pkwy.	La Vegas, Nev. 89109
Shepherd, Virgil J.	Wilford-Hall Hosp.	Lackland AFB, Tex. 78236
Sheppard, E. A. W.	5185 MacArthur Blvd. N.W.	Washington, D. C. 20016
Sheppard, Louis B.	Med. Arts Bldg.	Richmond, Va. 23219
Sherbin, Herbert D.	12500 Twelve Mile Rd.	Warren, Mich. 48093
Sherman, A. R.	Harwood Mem. Hosp., Christiansted	St. Croix. V.I. 00821
Sherman, Alfred, G.	1602 W. Fountain St.	Albert Lea, Minn. 56007
Sherman, Arthur E.	144 S. Harrison St.	East Orange, N. J. 07018
Sherman, Harry	11 Fifth Ave.	New York, N. Y. 10003
Sherman, Maurice E.	57 W. 57th St.	New York, N. Y. 10019
Sherman, Oscar R.	2334 N.E. 53rd St.	Ft. Lauderdale, Fla. 33308
Sherman, Spencer E.	166 E. 63rd St.	New York, N. Y. 10021
Sherrill, Richard W.	523 First Union Bank Bldg.	Winston-Salem, N. C. 27101
Sherwood, Robt. O.	115 St. Matthews Ave.	San Mateo, Cal. 94401
Shiach, John M.	Cobb Med. Ctr.	Seattle, Wash. 98101
Shields, Herbert B., Jr.	Broadway Tower	Enid, Okla. 73701
Shier, Julius M.	520 Passaic Ave.	Passaic, N. J. 07055
Shilling, Raymond L.	621 E. River St.	Elyria, O. 44035
Shinkawa, Shigeo	V. A. Hosp.	Temple, Tex. 76501
Shipley, John L.	508 E. Main St.	Elizabeth City, N. C. 27909
Shirley, Louis A.	USAF Reg. Hospital SAFB	Wichita Falls, Tex. 76311
Shoch, David E.	303 E. Chicago Ave.	Chicago, Ill. 60611
Shockley, Leo S.	20800 Westgate Ctr.	Cleveland, O. 44126
Shoemaker, Robt. E.	1248 Hamilton St.	Allentown, Pa. 18102
Shoff, Mahlon J.	207 E. Northern Lights Blvd. ...	Anchorage, Alaska 99503
Shope, E. Pierce	Wilson Bldg.	Camden, N. J. 08102
Shortridge, Charles M.	711 S. Jefferson St.	Roanoke, Va. 24008
Shoss, Samuel	603 Medical Towers	Houston, Tex. 77025
Shrader, Edward C.	Heyburn Bldg.	Louisville, Ky. 40202
Shreck, Horace W.	422 N. Hastings Ave.	Hastings, Nebr. 68901
Shulman, Albert G.	88 Walnut St.	Binghamton, N. Y. 13905
Shulruff, Harry	3701 Main St.	East Chicago, Ind. 46312
Shultz, David M.	9535 Reseda Blvd.	Northridge, Cal. 91324
Shum, Lule M.	4900 Sunset Blvd.	Los Angeles, Cal. 90027
Shumate, Robert E. L.	613 Talbotton Rd.	Columbus, Ga. 31904
Shupala, Edward	2100 Dudley Ave.	Parkersburg, W. Va. 26101
Shurmer, Richard A.	1908 Glen Springs Dr.	Fremont, O. 43420

Sibbett, Wm. A.	3701 Stocker St.	Los Angeles, Cal. 90008
Sibley, Wixom S.	162 Clinton St.	Redwood City, Cal. 94062
Sichi, Wm. T.	Med. Prof. Bldg.	San Antonio, Tex. 78212
Sidrys, Rimvydas	111 Westgate Plaza	Streator, Ill. 61364
Siegel, Howard S.	2475 E. 22nd St.	Cleveland, O. 44115
Siegel, Ralph E.	121 Market St.	Perth Amboy, N. J. 08861
Siegel, Richard C.	4277 Hempstead Turnpike	Bethpage, N. Y. 11714
Siemon, Glenn	2020 Truxtun Ave.	Bakersfield, Cal. 93301
Siewer, Otto L.	1870 W. Galena Blvd.	Aurora, Ill. 60506
Sifri, David G.	2745 Anderson Ferry Rd.	Cincinnati, O. 45238
Sigband, Michael H.	202 Hospital Cir.	Westminster, Cal. 92683
Silis, Stephen J.	301 S. Allen St.	Albany, N. Y. 12208
Silodor, Carl J.	1341 Hamburg Tnpk.	Wayne, N. J. 07470
Silver, Bernd	211 N. Meramec Ave.	St. Louis, Mo. 63105
Silver, David	200 W. 57th St.	New York, N. Y. 10019
Silver, Robert A.	572 Park Ave.	New York, N. Y. 10021
Silverberg, Joseph D.	1295 Portland Ave.	Rochester, N. Y. 14621
Silverman, Jay J.	9201 Sunset Blvd.	Los Angeles, Cal. 90069
Silverman, Sheppy J.	5319 Dashwood	Bellaire, Tex. 77401
Silverman, Stanley	153 N. Auten Ave.	Somerville, N. J. 08876
Silverstein, Arthur L.	16 Crescent Ave.	Passaic, N. J. 07055
Silverstein, Murray H.	509 W. Merrick Rd.	Valley Stream, N.Y. 11580
Simcoe, C. William	3233 E. 31st St.	Tulsa, Okla. 74105
Sime, David W.	550 Brickell Ave.	Miami, Fla. 33131
Simel, Paul J.	111 W. Wendover Ave.	Greensboro, N. C. 27401
Simkus, Aldona B.	15542 Cicero Ave.	Oak Forest, Ill. 60452
Simmonds, Noel T.	1300 Jackson St.	Alexandria, La. 71301
Simmons, John R.	Brooke Gen. Hosp.	Ft. Sam Houston, Tex. 78234
Simmons, Richard E.	363 E. Town St.	Columbus, O. 43215
Simmons, Richard J.	5 Bay State Rd.	Boston, Mass. 02215
Simon, Kenneth A.	8218 Wisconsin Ave.	Bethesda, Md. 20014
Simons, Edward J.	9735 Wilshire Blvd.	Beverly Hills, Cal. 90212
Simons, Leander T.	Lowry Med. Arts Bldg.	St. Paul, Minn. 55102
Simons, Stanley J., Jr.	1100 Southgate	Pendleton, Ore. 97801
Simonton, John T.	66 Milton Rd.	Rye, N. Y. 10580
Simpson, G. Victor	1330 New Hampshire Ave. N.W.	Washington, D. C. 20036
Sims, C. Norton	2665 Cleveland Ave.	Fort Myers, Fla. 33901
Simses, John P.	1151 Park Ave.	Bridgeport, Conn. 06604
Sinclair, Stephen G.	205 W. 6th St.	East Liverpool, O. 43920
Singer, Bernard	104 East Ave.	Norwalk, Conn. 06851
Singer, David J.	1160 Kane Concourse, Bay Harbor Islands	Miami Beach, Fla. 33154
Singer, Joseph A.	Ehrling Bergquist, USAF Hospital	Offutt AFB, Nebr.
Singer, Max	21 E. 79th St.	New York, N. Y. 10021
Singer, Milton	2310 N. W. Irving St.	Portland, Ore. 97210
Singer, Robert L.	2147 Mowry Ave.	Fremont, Cal. 94536
Singer, Roy R.	27 Elm St.	Worcester, Mass. 01608
Siniscal, Arthur A.	3720 Washington Blvd.	St. Louis, Mo. 63108
Sinskey, Robt. M.	2222 Santa Monica Blvd.	Santa Monica, Cal. 90404
Sisler, Hampson A.	13 W. 13th St.	New York, N. Y. 10011
Sison, Manuel A.	11633 S. Hawthorne Blvd.	Hawthorne, Cal. 90250
Sitney, J. Jay	4155 Moorpark Ave.	San Jose, Cal. 95117
Sivulich, Michael J.	406 Main St.	Johnstown, Pa. 15901
Skala, Michael J.	6620 Coyle Ave.	Carmichael, Cal. 95608
Skeehan, Raymond A.	1633 Fillmore	Denver, Colo. 80206

Skemp, Samuel.J.	815 S. 10th St.	La Crosse, Wisc. 54601
Skilling, Francis C.	Ingraham Bldg.	Miami, Fla. 33131
Skinner, Scott W.	70 Mason St.	Geneva, N. Y. 14456
Skirball, Jos. J.	353 Commonwealth Ave.	Boston, Mass. 02115
Skov, Peter T.	105 Contempo Ave.	West Monroe, La. 71291
Skow, John D.	4235 Sector Rd.	Toledo, O.
Skowron, John J.	5936 N. Milwaukee Ave.	Chicago, Ill. 60646
Skowron, Ralph A.	S. Jersey Med. Ctr.	Cherry Hill, N. J. 08034
Slabaugh, Carlyle B.	3154 Reid Dr.	Corpus Christi, Tex. 78404
Slack, Wm. J.	205 W. Second St.	Duluth, Minn. 55802
Slansky, Harvey H.	99 Waltham St.	Lexington, Mass. 02173
Slater, Iris R.	127 A E. 71st St.	New York, N. Y. 10021
Slatin, Louis	151 E. Decatur	Decatur, Ill. 62521
Slaughter, Howard C.	1001 Walnut St.	Evansville, Ind. 47708
Sleight, Justin L.	2909 E. Grand River Ave.	Lansing, Mich. 48912
Slight, J. Rigby	530 Lomas Santa Fe Dr.	Solana Beach, Cal. 92075
Sloan, David B. Jr.	905 Murchison Bldg.	Wilmington, N. C. 28401
Sloan, Henry L., Jr.	1600 E. 3rd St.	Charlotte, N. C. 28204
Sloan, Malachi W., II	5335 Far Hills Ave.	Dayton, O. 45429
Sloane, Albert E.	416 Marlborough St.	Boston, Mass. 02215
Sloane, Henry O.	23 S. Hillside Ave.	Ventnor City, N. J. 08406
Slomka, Edwin B.	126 W. End Ave.	Somerville, N. J. 08876
Slomka, Sol	40 W. 86th St.	New York, N. Y. 10024
Small, Bernard L.	999 Central Ave.	Woodmere, N. Y. 11598
Small, David	3581 N. Federal Hwy.	Pompano Beach, Fla. 33064
Small, Mary Louise	16 W. Read St.	Baltimore, Md. 21201
Small, Robert G.	2817 Parklawn Dr.	Midwest City, Okla 73110
Smallman, Robert A.	675 Delaware Ave.	Buffalo, N. Y. 14202
Smart, Don M.	10611 Garland Rd.	Dallas, Tex. 75218
Smedal, Erling A.	456 W. Park Ave.	Mansfield, O. 44906
Smelley, James A.	1717 North Loop W.	Houston, Tex. 77008
Smiley, Sheldon S.	121 Wakelee Ave.	Ansonia, Conn. 06401
Smillie, John W.	326 N. Ingalls St.	Ann. Arbor, Mich 48104
Smith, Alfred G., II	6601 S.W. 80th St.	South Miami, Fla. 33143
Smith, Alma C.	71 San Miguel Dr.	Chula Vista, Cal 92011
Smith, Alvin H.	33 Stonybrook Dr. S.	Levittown, Pa. 19055
Smith, Arthur C., Jr.	410 W. Church St.	Elmira, N. Y. 14901
Smith, Barry F.	521 Park Ave.	New York, N. Y. 10021
Smith, Bryant P.	616 Monrovia St.	Shreveport, La. 71106
Smith, Byron	722 Park Ave.	New York, N. Y. 10021
Smith, Carlie S.	1223 S. Kentwood	Springfield, Mo. 65804
Smith, Clarence G.	1422 Euclid Ave.	Cleveland, O. 44115
Smith, Clifford E.	261 E. Lincoln Hwy.	Dekalb, Ill. 60115
Smith, Cody L.	255 W. Madison	El Cajon, Cal. 92020
Smith, Corwin M.	7777 Montgomery Rd.	Cincinnati, O. 45236
Smith, Dale C.	3700 W. 83rd	Shawnee Mission, Kans. 66208
Smith, Darrell F.	1300 S. Eliseo Dr.	Greenbrae, Cal. 94094
Smith, David M.	Cobb. Med. Ctr.	Seattle, Wash. 98101
Smith, David R.	80 Troy Rd. Ctr.	Delaware, O. 43015
Smith, Dennis V.	4020 Cadillac Dr.	Farwell, Mich. 48104
Smith, Edward W.	421 Huguenot St.	New Rochelle, N. Y. 10801
Smith, Eugene C.	606 Stevens St.	Flint, Mich. 48503
Smith, Glenn H.	1119 Pajaro St.	Salinas, Cal. 93901
Smith, Henry C.	1211 Twenty-First Ave. S.	Nashville, Ten.. 37212
Smith, Henry I.	Bassett Army Hospital, APO	Seattle, Wash. 98731
Smith, Herschel S.	316 E. 4th St.	Bloomington, Ind. 47401

Smith, Homer E.	70 S. 9th East	Salt Lake City, Utah 84102
Smith, J. Lawton	1638 N.W. 10th Ave.	Miami, Fla. 33136
Smith, J. William	2309 Austin Ave.	Waco, Tex. 76701
Smith, James L.	623 Woodlane	Little Rock, Ark. 72201
Smith, Jaroud B.	317 Juana Ave.	San Leandro, Cal. 94577
Smith, Jean B.	521 Park Ave.	New York, N. Y. 10021
Smith, Joe R.	1504 E. Broadway	Columbia, Mo. 65201
Smith, John R.	2010 Church St.	Nashville, Ten. 37203
Smith, Joseph G.	730 7th St.	Eureka, Cal. 95501
Smith, Keith B.	633 Washington Rd.	Pittsburgh, Pa. 15228
Smith, Laurence W.	1288 N. Irwin	Hanford, Cal. 93230
Smith, Mason	2035 Monument Ave.	Richmond, Va. 23220
Smith M. Dale	313 S. 5th St.	Gadsden, Ala. 35902
Smith, Morton E.	Washington Univ. Sch. Med.	St. Louis, Mo. 63110
Smith, Oren R., Jr.	Box 4032, 48th TAC Hosp., APO	New York 09179
Smith, Paul B., Jr.	Med. Arts Bldg.	Tacoma, Wash. 98402
Smith, Richard O.	73 Third St., N.W.	Pulaski, Va. 24301
Smith, Richard S.	Albany Med. College	Albany, N. Y. 12208
Smith, Robb. V.	261 E. Lincoln Hwy.	Dekalb, Ill. 60115
Smith, Ronald P.	7 N. Catherine St.	Plattsburgh, N. Y. 12901
Smith, Ruby A.	14 W. Mt. Vernon Pl.	Baltimore, Md. 21201
Smith, Taylor	706 D St.	San Rafael, Cal. 94901
Smith, Taylor R.	10 Hawthorne Pl.	Boston, Mass. 02114
Smith, Theodore N.	603 State Tower	Syracuse, N. Y. 13202
Smith, Thomas A.	1310 Wisconsin	Grand Haven, Mich. 49417
Smith, Vernon L.	1750 N. Palafox	Pensacola, Fla. 32502
Smith, Wallace B.	10901 Winner Rd.	Independence, Mo. 64052
Smith, Warren F.	414 S. Oak Park Ave.	Oak Park, Ill. 60302
Smith, Wm. A.	3393 Peachtree Rd., N.E.	Atlanta, Ga. 30326
Smith, Wm. L.	P. O. Box 110	Tampa, Fla. 33601
Smithson, Robt. A.	1530 Arizona Ave.	Santa Monica, Cal. 90404
Smoleroff, Jules W.	565 Park Ave.	New York, N. Y. 10021
Smolin, Gilbert	931 W. San Bruno Ave.	San Bruno, Cal. 94066
Smoller, Arnold J.	2200 O'Frarrell Blvd.	San Francisco, Cal. 94115
Sneed, Robert J.	1001 Second St. W.	Ashland, Wisc. 58406
Snell, Albert C.	260 Crittenden Blvd.	Rochester, N.,Y. 14620
Snell, Melvil N.	8930 S. Sepulveda Blvd.	Los Angeles, Cal. 90045
Snider, Louis R.	950 25th St., Suite E-18	Ogden, Utah 84401
Snider, Ned L.	Physicians & Surgeons Clinic, 1101 Maine St.	Quincy, Ill. 62301
Snip, Russell T.	505 Howard St.	San Antonio, Tex. 78212
Snow, Harold L.	53 Jefferson Ln.	Palo Alto, Calif. 94303
Snow, Virgil C.	1053 R St.	Fresno, Cal. 93721
Snowhite, Arthur B.	Professional Arts Center	Marion, Ind. 46952
Snydacker, Daniel	111 N. Wabash Ave.	Chicago, Ill. 60602
Snyder, Alan A.	206 E. Las Tunas Dr.	San Gabriel, Cal. 91776
Snyder, Harry D.	1120 N. Easton Rd.	Willow Grove, Pa. 19090
Snyder, M. Wilson	32 Jefferson Ave.	Sharon, Pa. 16146
Snyder, Stuart S.	136 E. 64th St.	New York, N. Y. 10021
Snyder, William B.	Univ. Hosp.	Iowa City, Ia. 75235
Soderstrom, John F.	1207 Fairchild Ct.	Woodland, Cal. 95695
Sogg, Richard L.	281 E. Hamilton Ave.	Campbell, Cal. 95008
Soll, David B.	5001 Frankford Ave.	Philadelphia, Pa. 19124
Soll, Raphael I.	223 Old Hook Rd.	Westwood, N. J. 07675
Solomon, O. David	1020 Huron Rd.	Cleveland, O. 44115
Solomon, Yale	375 E. Main St.	Bay Shore, N. Y. 11706

Somers, Kenneth	2115 Salisbury Rd.	Silver Spring, Md. 20910
Sonnier, Earl J.	913 Ave. C.	Marrero, La. 70072
Sonnier, Wm., Jr.	1458 S. College Rd.	Lafayette, La. 70501
Sonntag, Richard W.	465 E. South Temple St.	Salt Lake City, Utah 84111
Sonntag, Walter M.	7668 Skyway	Paradise, Cal. 95969
Soper, Gail R.	636 Church St.	Evanston, Ill. 60201
Sophocleus, Gregory J.	Investment Bldg., 1 Investment Pl.	Townson, Md. 21204
Sorenson, James M.	1714 E. Capitol Dr.	Milwaukee, Wisc. 53211
Sorenson, Lionel W.	2320 Channing Way	Berkeley, Cal. 94704
Sorenson, Roger W.	2080 Century Park E.	Los Angeles, Cal. 90067
Sornson, E. T.	2455 Grear St. N.E.	Salem, Ore. 97301
Sorrel, Sydney M.	741 Broadway	Somerville, Mass. 02144
Sotoodeh, Bagher	105 E. Laurel St.	San Antonio, Tex. 78212
Souders, Benj. F.	424 Walnut St.	Reading, Pa. 19601
Southgate, Paul T.	Professional Bldg.	Long Beach, Cal. 90813
Sovik, Wm. E.	Mahoning Bank Bldg.	Youngstown, O. 44503
Sowa, Elizabeth C.	1550 S. Plaza Dr.	Evansville, Ind. 47715
Sozanski, J. C.	542 Eastern Ave.	Lynn, Mass. 01902
Spaeth, Edmund B.	1930 Chestnut St.	Philadelphia, Pa. 19103
Spaeth, George I.	1601 Spring Garden St.	Philadelphia, Pa. 19118
Spaeth, Philip G.	1930 Chestnut St.	Philadelphia, Pa. 19103
Spalding, David L.	Professional Bldg.	Springfield, Mo. 65806
Spalter, Harold F.	635 W. 165th St.	New York, N. Y. 10032
Spangler, William E.	Elmerdorf USAF Hospital, Anchorage, Alaska	APO, Seattle 98742
Spanierman, Greta	201 E. 77th St.	New York, N. Y. 10021
Sparber, Herman	4701 15th Ave.	Brooklyn, N. Y. 11219
Sparks, George M.	Marshfield Clinic	Marshfield, Wisc. 54449
Spaulding, Abbot G.	6131 Campus Lane	Cincinnati, O. 45230
Spauling, William L.	Med. Arts Bldg.	Tacoma, Wash. 98402
Speaker, Other F.	1950 Court St.	Redding, Cal. 96001
Spear, Dean	107 S. Ninth E.	Salt Lake City, Utah 84102
Spence, George D.	1005 E. High St.	Charlottesville, Va. 22901
Spencer, Norman A.	....	Amherst, Mass. 01002
Spencer, Robert W.	2021 S. Lewis	Tulsa, Okla. 74104
Spencer, William H.	University of California Hosp. ..	San Francisco, Cal.
Sperling, Adelle B.	1033 S. 17th St.	Birmingham, Ala. 35205
Sperrazza, Augustine J.	406 Fulton St.	Troy, N. Y. 12180
Spiegleman, Arthur M.	526 Penn St.	Camden, N. J. 08102
Spielman, Ronald L.	1688 Meridian Ave.	Miami Beach, Fla. 33139
Spielman, Stanley L.	495 Biltmore Way	Coral Gables, Fla. 33134
Spiller, Arthur E.	945 Great Plain Ave.	Needham, Mass. 02192
Spirito, Anthony M.	411 Morris Ave.	Elizabeth, N. J. 07208
Spiro, Barbara	1832 E. 87th St.	Chicago, Ill. 60617
Spiro, Henry	26789 Woodward	Huntington Woods, Mich. 48070
Spitalny, Lawrence A.	52 E. Monterey Way	Phoenix, Ariz. 85012
Spitzer, Kenneth H.	State Tower Bldg.	Syracuse, N. Y. 13202
Spivack, Isaac D.	P. O. Box 45	Liberty, N.Y. 12754
Spivey, Bruce E.	Dept. Ophthal. fac. Med. Ctr. P.O. Box 7999	San Francisco, Cal. 94120
Spizziri, Louis J.	350 Franklin Ave.	Wyckoff, N. J. 07481
Sponaugle, H. Dale	3315 Country St.	Portsmouth, Va. 23707
Spradling, Richard L.	530 N.W. 27th	Corvallis, Ore. 97330
Sprogis, Ivars	7 Fox St.	Poughkeepsie, N. Y. 12601

Sproule, Ralph T.	1024 E. State St.	Milwaukee, Wisc. 53202
Sprunt, C. Worth	1150 Conn. Ave., N.W.	Washington, D. C. 20036
Spurgeon, Frederick C.	927 Deep Valley Dr.	Palos Verdes Peninsula, Cal. 90274
Spurney, Robert V.	20620 N. Park Blvd.	Shaker Heights, O. 44122
Stadnik, Louis J.	American Nat'l Bank Bldg.	Cheyenne, Wyo. 82001
Stafford, Thomas J.	636 Church St.	Evanston, Ill. 60201
Stafford, Walter R.	141 N. Meramec Ave.	Clayton, Mo. 63105
Stager, David R.	8226 Douglas Ave.	Dallas, Tex. 75225
Stahl, Norman O.	201 Eastern Pkwy.	Brooklyn, N. Y. 11238
Staley, Irving T.	652 Church St.	Marietta, Ga. 30060
Stallings, Lelan E.	422 W. Jackson	Carbondale, Ill. 62901
Stam, Jacob J.	One Hanson Pl.	Brooklyn, N. Y. 11217
Stambaugh, James L., Jr.	1221 S. Broadway	Lexington, Ky. 40504
Stambaugh, N. F., Jr.	60 Wyoming St.	Dayton, O. 45409
Stambaugh, Reginald J.	2707 N. Flagler Dr.	W. Palm Beach, Fla. 33407
Stamm, Thomas J.	7546 W. North Ave.	Elmwood Park, Ill. 60635
Stanfield, Thomas F.	P.O. Box 1226	Anderson, S. C. 29621
Stanford, Gary B.	333 S. 9th St. East.	Salt Lake City, Utah 84102
Stanley, John A.	Bowman Gray School of Medicine	Winston-Salem, N. C. 27103
Stansbury, John R.	3085 Loma Vista Rd.	Ventura, Cal. 93003
Stark, Arthur G.	1612 Tremont Pl.	Denver, Colo. 80202
Stark, Jesse B.	900 Fifth Ave.	New York, N. Y. 10021
Starr, Henry J.	6201 Riverdale Rd.	Riverdale, Md. 20840
Starr, Wilson C.	635 W. 165th St.	New York, N. Y. 10032
Stasior, Orkan G.	668 Madison Ave.	Albany, N. Y. 12208
Staton, Younger A.	1411 N. Flagler Dr.	West Palm Beach, Fla. 33401
Statti, Louis W.	Jenkins Arcade	Pittsburgh, Pa. 15222
Statton, Roy F.	Sharp Bldg.	Lincoln, Nebr. 68508
Stavola, Frances P.	123 E. 61st St.	New York 21, N. Y. 10021
Stealey, Robert L.	626 S. Main St.	Findlay, O. 45840
Steele, Edward F.	630 W. Water St.	Elmira, N. Y. 14905
Steele, Willard H., Jr.	744 McCallie Ave.	Chattanooga, Ten.. 37402
Steffens, Lincoln F.	1200 Main	Dubuque, Ia. 52001
Steiman, Solomon E.	45 Lewis St.	Lynn, Mass. 01902
Stein, Lester	226 N. Fourth St.	Steubenville, O. 43952
Steinbach, Louis	555 Kappock St.	New York, N. Y. 10463
Steinberg, Abraam	3700 Fifth Ave.	Pittsburgh, Pa. 15213
Steinberg, Theodore	155 Thesta St.	Fresno, Cal. 93701
Steiner, Albert A.	2299 Post St.	San Francisco, Cal. 94115
Steinfeld, Richard G.	579 Main St.	Metuchen, N. J. 08840
Steinmetz, Arthur F.	1237 B St.	Hayward, Cal. 94541
Steinmetz, Charles G., III	4606 Spruce St.	Philadelphia, Pa. 19139
Steinmetz, John R.	109 E. 14th St.	San Leandro, Ca. 94577
Steinmetz, Rodney D.	4600 N. Habana Ave.	Tampa, Fla. 33614
Steinvurzel, Bernardo	34 Livingston St.	Poughkeepsie, N. Y. 12601
Stella, Salvatore L.	207 Walnut Ave.	San Diego, Cal. 97103
Stenerodden, Sidney C.	809 Oak St. S. E.	Salem, Ore. 97301
Stephan, John D.	501 W. Broadway	Missoula, Mont. 59801
Stephan, Lewis B.	18 Robin Pk. Blvd.	Oberlin, O. 44074
Stephens, Bruce M.	2241 Central Ave.	Alameda, Cal. 94501
Stephens, Cole P.	990 Sonoma Ave.	Santa Rosa, Cal. 95405
Stephens, H. Frederick	110 Lockwood St.	Providence, R. I. 02903
Stephens, Karl F.	110 Lockwood St.	Providence, R. I. 02903
Stephens, Ralph W.	505 N. Arlington	Reno, Nev. 89503
Stephens, Stuart B.	2241 Central Ave.	Alameda, Cal. 94501

Stephens, Vernon D.	3545 Olentangy River Rd.	Columbus, O. 43214
Stephenson, Harry C.	97th U. S. Army Hospital, APO .	New York 09757
Stephenson, Wm. V.	Bell Bldg.	Toledo, O. 43624
Stern, Charles	59 Gelston Ave.	Brooklyn, N. Y. 11209
Stern, Charles	Med. Arts Bldg.	Natchez, Miss. 39120
Stern, Earl L.	1496 Portola Dr.	San Francisco, Cal. 94127
Stern, Henry	350 Central Park W.	New York, N. Y. 10025
Stern, Richard U.	188 Clinton Ave.	Newark, N. J. 07108
Stern, Sheldon D.	28 W. Adams	Detroit, Mich. 48226
Stern, Sidney G.	3840 Woodruff Ave.	Long Beach, Cal. 90808
Sternberg, Paul	111 N. Wabash Ave.	Chicago, Ill. 60602
Sterner, Donald C.	Lowry Med. Arts Bldg.	St. Paul, Minn. 55102
Stertzbach, C. W.	3610 Market St.	Youngstown, O. 44507
Stevens, Jason H.	1500 E. Katella Ave.	Orange, Cal. 92667
Stevens, Norman D.	806 Central Ave.	Woodmere, N. Y. 11598
Stevens, Ralph W.	8 S. Second St.	Walla Walla, Wash. 99362
Stevens, Rosemary	83-80 118th St.	Kew Gardens, N. Y. 11415
Stevenson, Roger	Bureau of Medicine and Surgery, Navy Department	Washington, D. C. 20390
Stevenson, Thomas C.	630 Menlo Ave.	Menlo Park, Cal. 94025
Stevenson, Walter D., Jr.	1124 Broadway	Quincy, Ill. 62301
Stewart, Angus B.	2414 Buhne St.	Eureka, Cal. 95501
Stewart, C. Thomas	801 Broadway	Seattle, Wash. 98122
Stewart, Landis C.	750 High St.	Adrian, Mich. 49221
Stewart, Robt. B.	600 S. Glenstone	Springfield, Mo. 63804
Stewart, Robert H.	1121 Hermann Prof. Bldg.	Houston, Tex. 77025
Stewart, Roy A.	427 N. Main Ave.	Newton, N. C. 28658
Stewart, Walter E.	2130 S. Center St.	Terre Haute, Ind. 47802
Stickle, Arthur W.	135 W. Adams	St. Louis, Mo. 63122
Stiernberg, Douglas D.	702 9th St. N.	Texas City, Tex. 77590
Stillerman, Manuel L.	111 N. Wabash Ave.	Chicago, Ill. 60602
Stine, George T.	303 E. Town St.	Columbus, O. 43215
Stiny, C. Peter	40300 Date St.	Hemet, Cal. 92343
Stivrins, Kazimir	3145 'O' St.	Lincoln, Nebr. 68501
Stock, Karl W.	1710 W. 10th	Topeka, Kans. 66604
Strocker, Frederick W.	1110 W. Main St.	Durham, N. C. 27701
Stocker, Lawrence L.	7310 W. Seven Mile Rd.	Detroit, Mich. 48221
Stodd, Russell T.	11104 S. E. Stark St.	Portland, Ore. 97216
Stohlman, George C.	10549 Florida Ave.	Tampa, Fla. 33612
Stokes, Hunter R.	161 W. Cheves St.	Florence, S. C. 29501
Stokes, James A.	1021 E. Robinson Ave.	Orlando, Fa. 32801
Stokes, J. Howard	161 W. Cheves St.	Florence, S.C. 29501
Stokes, J. J.	478 Peachtree St., N.E.	Atlanta, Ga. 30308
Stoll, Kennard O.	1741 W. Avenue J.	Lancaster, Cal. 93534
Stolzar, Irwin H.	Bramlette Bldg.	Longview, Tex. 75601
Stone, Howard H.	2080 Century Park E.	Los Angeles, Cal. 90067
Stone, Sidney L.	22790 Kelly Rd.	E. Detroit, Mich. 48021
Stone, Vean M.	4440 Brockton Ave.	Riverside, Cal. 92501
Stone, W. Conrad	1138 Second St., S.W.	Roanoke, Va. 24016
Stone, William, Jr.	405 N. Bedford Dr.	Beverly Hills, Cal. 90212
Stonecypher, David D.	5565 Grossmont Ctr. Dr.	La Mesa, Cal. 92041
Stonehill, Alfred A.	6 N. Michigan Ave.	Chicago, Ill. 60602
Stoner, Cyrus H.	340 Boulevard, N.E.	Atlanta, Ga. 30312
Stough, John T.	5000 Montross	Houston, Tex. 77006
Stow, M. Noel	3900 Wisconsin Ave, N. W.	Washington, D. C. 20016
Straatsma, Bradley R.	Jules Stein Eye Inst.	Los Angeles, Cal. 90024

Strassman, Martin L.	c/o Aaron Levy, M.D., 145 E. 50th St.	New York, N. Y. 10022
Stratford, Thos. P.	Med. Arts Bldg.	Richmond, Va. 23219
Stratton, J. David	1012 Kings Dr.	Charlotte, N. C. 28207
Strause, Harold L., Sr.	244 N. 5th St.	Reading, Pa. 19601
Strause, Harold L., Jr.	244 N. 5th St.	Reading, Pa. 19601
Strauss, Albert	2920 Broadway	West Palm Beach, Fla. 33407
Strawn, Robert L.	722 Scott St.	Covington, Ky. 41011
Street, Herbert S.	1204 13th Ave., S.E.	Decatur, Ala. 35601
Streeten, Barbara W.	334 Berkeley Dr.	Syracuse, N. Y. 13210
Streicher, Carl J.	Medical Bldg.	Ashtabula, O. 44004
Strick, Arthur	351 Hospital Rd.	Newport Beach, Cal. 92660
Strong, James C., Jr.	Republic Bldg.	Denver, Colo. 80202
Strong, Leroy F.	515 Lakeside Dr., S.E.	Grand Rapids, Mich. 49506
Stroud, S. K.	3154 Reid Dr.	Corpus Christi, Tex. 78404
Strow, Wallace F.	411 S. Seventh St.	Springfield, Ill. 62701
Struble, Gilbert C.	10782 Weyburn Ave	Los Angeles, Cal. 90024
Struve, Clemens A.	3166 Reid Dr.	Corpus Christi, Tex. 78404
Stuard, Chas. G.	Utica Sq. Med. Ctr.	Tulsa, Okla. 74114
Stuart, James A.	4701 N. Federal Hwy.	Ft. Lauderdale, Fla. 33308
Stuart, Robert L.	1005 Adams Ave.	La Grande, Ore. 97850
Stubbs, Joseph T., Jr.	720 E. 71st. St.	Savannah, Ga. 31405
Student, Richard E.	Apache Med. Bldg.	Minneapolis, Minn. 55421
Stump, Robert B.	P. O. Box 407	Cheyenne, Wyo. 82001
Sturm, Rodney J.	1025 Regent St.	Madison, Wisc. 53715
Sturman, Robert M.	8 E. 84th St.	New York, N. Y. 10028
Sturman, Wm. A.	299 S. Harrison St	East Orange, N. J. 07018
Suares, John C.	344 Arnold Ave.	Greenville, Miss. 38701
Suarez, Alfred F.	10090 Main St.	Fairfax, Va. 22030
Sudarsky, R. David	178 E. 71st St.	New York, N. Y. 10021
Sudranksi, Herbert F.	Veterans Administration Hosp.	Salem, Va. 24153
Sugar, H. Saul	Fisher Bldg.	Detroit, Mich. 48202
Suitor, Jesse H.	Marine Corps Recruit Depot	San Diego, Cal. 92134
Sullivan, Charles T.	2255 Clinton Ave. S.	Rochester, N. Y. 14618
Sullivan, Clifford P.	2800 W. 87th St.	Chicago, Ill. 60652
Sullivan, Edmund H.	701 S. Acadian Thruway	Baton Rouge, La. 70806
Sullivan, Garrett L.	275 Charles St.	Boston, Mass. 02114
Sullivan, John E., Jr.	845 Kearny Ave.	Arlington, N. J. 07032
Sullivan, John J.	989 James St.	Syracuse, N. Y. 13203
Sullivan, John V.	715 Mills Bldg.	Topeka, Kans. 66612
Sullivan, Paul B.	Hitchcock Clinic	Hanover, N. H. 03755
Sullivan, T. Ward	751 Teaneck Rd.	Teaneck, N. J. 07666
Sullivan, Wm., B.	2800 W. 87th St.	Chicago, Ill. 60652
Sultan, Burton S.	131 Fulton Ave.	Hempstead, N. Y. 11550
Sulzman, John H.	1831 Fifth Ave.	Troy, N. Y. 12180
Sun, K. S.	Box 451	Ames, Ia. 50010
Sunderhaus, Earl	417 Biltmore Ave.	Asheville, N. C. 28801
Surratt, Mary N.	1010 E. 86th St.	Indianapolis, Ind. 46240
Suson, Elieser B.	8700 W. Wisconsin Ave.	Milwaukee, Wisc. 53226
Susskind, Bernard	501 Main St.	Toms River, N. J. 08753
Sussman, John D.	200 S. Broadway	Tarrytown, N. Y. 10591
Sussman, Walter	2025 Merrick Ave.	Merrick, N. Y. 11566
Sutliff, Frederick P.	3701 N. Broad St.	Philadelphia, Pa. 19140
Sutton, James C.	7705 S. E. Division St.	Portland, Ore. 97215
Svoboda, Joseph R.	5700 Old Richmond Ave.	Richmond, Va. 23226
Swab, Charles M.	812 Medical Arts Bldg.	Omaha, Nebr. 68102

Swab, Elizabeth M.	Medical Arts Bldg.	Omaha, Nebr. 68102
Swan, Jerome W.	Med. Arts Bldg.	Grand Rapids, Mich. 49502
Swan, Kenneth C.	3181 S.W. Sam Jackson Pk. Rd. .	Portland, Ore. 97201
Swanson, Clifford A.	4200 Cathedral Ave. N.W.	Washington, D. C. 20016
Swanson, Eldon C.	215 N. Magnolia Ave.	Green Cove Springs, Fla. 32043
Swanson, Eric M.	1712 Central Ave.	Ft. Dodge, Ia. 50501
Swartz, Gerald	5555 Main St.	Buffalo, N. Y. 14221
Sweeney, John T.	21724 Lorain Rd.	Fairview Park, O. 44126
Sweterlitsch, Louis H.	65 E. Elizabeth Ave.	Bethlehem, Pa. 18018
Swets, Edward J.	5055 E. Kentucky Ave.	Denver, Colo. 80222
Wett, Wilber F.	18 Sixth Ave.	San Francisco, Cal. 94118
Swick, David A.	41 Center Pl.	Staten Island, N. Y. 10306
Swift, John E.	6601 S. W. 80th St., S	Miami, Fla. 33143
Swigert, J. Leonard	1570 Humboldt St.	Denver, Colo. 80218
Swiontkowski, Stanley D. ..	6132 S. Kedzie Ave.	Chicago, Ill. 60629
Switzer, Fred D.	McAlester Cl.	McAlester, Okla. 74501
Swords, Collins W.	2424 Coral Way	Miami, Fla. 33145
Sykes, John H. J.	428 Baltimore	San Antonio, Tex. 78215
Sykowski, Peter S.	101 E. 4th St.	Scottsdale, Ariz. 85251
Syracuse, Victor R.	29 Washington Sq. W.	New York, N. Y. 10011
Szewczyk, Edward J.	402 N. 9th St.	East St. Louis, Ill. 62201
Szewczyk, Thaddeus S.	402 N. 9th St.	East St. Louis, Ill. 62201
Szuter, Carl F.	U.S.P.H.S. Indian Hospital	Phoenix, Ariz. 85014
Taake, Wm. H.	3085 Loma Vista Rd.	Ventura, Cal. 93003
Tabankin, Alvin	191 North St.	Buffalo, N. Y. 14201
Tabb, W. Granville, Jr.	1938 Peachtree Rd., N.W.	Atlanta, Ga. 30309
Tabor, George L.	625 Broadway	San Diego, Cal. 92101
Tacke, Arthur W.	400 W. Silver Spring Dr.	Milwaukee, Wisc. 53217
Taffet, Simeon	105 Stevens Ave.	Mt. Vernon, N. Y. 10550
Taggart, Geo. W.	2 E. Broad St.	Hazleton, Pa. 18201
Taiara, Camilo	3620 Army St.	San Francisco, Cal. 94110
Tait, Edwin C.	1324 W. Main	Norristown, Pa. 19401
Takach, Robert J.	325 Kennedy Memorial Dr.	Waterville, Me. 04901
Talbot, Thos. E.	2330 N.W. Flanders St.	Portland, Ore. 97210
Tallman, Carter B.	130 Parker St.	Lawrence, Mass. 01842
Tamler,Edward	Pacific Medical Center	San Francisco, Cal. 94115
Tananis, Leonard J.	610 W. Market St.	Pottsville, Pa. 17901
Tandy, Wm.	2313 Bagley Ave.	Los Angeles, Cal. 90034
Tani, Geo. T.	Lowry Med. Arts Bldg.	St. Paul, Minn. 55102
Tannenbaum, Chas. S.	612 W. Duarte Rd.	Arcadia, Cal. 91007
Tannenbaum, Maurice	50 S. Highland Ave.	Ossining, N. Y. 10562
Tanner, K. Nolen	900 N. W. Joy St.	Portland, Ore. 97229
Tanner, Owen R.	300 Homer Ave.	Palo Alto, Cal. 94301
Tantillo, Nicholas P.	One Hanson Pl.	Brooklyn, N. Y. 11217
Tanton, John H.	Burns Clinic	Petoskey, Mich. 49770
Tarter, Robert C.	345 Terracina Blvd.	Redlands, Cal. 92373
Tashma, Albert	7080 Hollywood Blvd.	Los Angeles, Cal. 90028
Tasker, Mary B.	2701 Eye St.	Sacramento, Cal. 95816
Tasman, William S.	187 E. Evergreen Ave.	Philadelphia, Pa. 19118
Tatar, Jos	1893 Sheridan Rd.	Highland Park, Ill. 60035
Taterka, Harvey B.	140 E. 83rd. St.	New York, N. Y. 10028
Taub, Robt.	6 N. Michigan Ave.	Chicago, Ill. 60602
Taube, Jack I.	Hume Mansur Bldg.	Indianapolis, Ind. 46204
Taylor, Coleman	2300 W. 7th Ave.	Amarillo, Tex. 79106
Taylor, Daniel M.	300 Kensington Ave.	New Britain, Conn. 06050

Taylor, E. Merle	1020 S. W. Taylor St.	Portland, Ore. 97205
Taylor, Frank W.	2060 Glendale Ave.	Toledo, O. 43614
Taylor, Harry B., Jr.	508 Medical Tower	Norfolk, Va. 23507
Taylor, Irvin S.	Harwood Bldg.	Scarsdale, N.Y. 10583
Taylor, Joseph W., Jr.	4600 N. Habana Ave.	Tampa, Fla. 33614
Taylor, Kim Y.	857 E. 2nd South	Salt Lake City, Utah 84102
Taylor, Michael A.	12th Ave. at Spruce	Yakima, Wash. 98902
Taylor, Robert P.	615 Roswell St.	Marietta, Ga. 30060
Taylor, Shahane R., Jr.	348 N. Elm St.	Greensboro, N. C. 27401
Taylor, W. Wickham	Medical Tower	Norfolk, Va. 23507
Taylor, William H.	1004 Beverly Dr.	Rockledge, Fla. 32955
Tchao, Jou S.	181 Russell St.	Lewiston, Me. 04240
Teasdale, L. R.	1411 N. Flagler Dr.	West Palm Beach, Fla. 33401
Tebbet, Royce D.	202 E. 2nd St.	Casper, Wyo. 82601
Tedesco, Joseph A.	E. 12122 Cataldo	Spokane, Wash. 99206
Tedford, John H.	Thomas Davis Clinic, 5th & Alvernon	Tucson, Ariz. 85702
Teeling, Brendan J.	8 Thorndike St.	Beverly, Mass. 01915
Teitelbaum, Marvin J.	2901 Wilshire Blvd.	Santa Monica, Cal. 90403
Teitgen, Ralph E.	1684 N. Prospect Ave.	Milwaukee, Wis. 53202
Teixler, Victor A.	Hume Mansur Bldg.	Indianapolis, Ind. 46204
Teknipp, William J.	21100 Southgate Park Blvd.	Maple Hts., O. 44137
Teyler, Richard M.	1306 W. Avenue J.	Lancaster, Cal. 93534
Tennant, Jerald L.	122 W. Colorado Blvd.	Dallas, Tex. 75208
Tennenbaum, Albert E.	1812 N. Broadway	Melrose Park, Ill. 60160
Tenney, Alonzo C.	5200 Gibson Blvd S. E.	Alburquerque, N. M. 87108
Tenzel, Richard R.	1110 N.E. 163rd St.	N. Miami Beach, Fla. 33162
Tepper, Norman N.	25 E. Washington St.	Chicago, Ill. 60602
ter Kuile, Reinold W.	88 W. Ridgewood Ave.	Ridgewood, N. J. 07450
Terman, Gerald A.	2244 Lloyd Ctr.	Portland, Ore. 97232
Terner, Irwin S.	527 Broad St.	Sewickley, Pa. 15143
Terraciano, Pasqual A.	2241 Esplanade	Bronx, N. Y. 10469
Terrero, Angel R.	State Tower Bldg.	Syracuse, N. Y. 13202
Terrill, Richard W.	446 W. Pontiac St.	Fort Wayne, Ind. 46807
Terris, Gerald	4900 Sunset Blvd.	Los Angeles, Cal. 90027
Tesar, Charles E.	2001 S. Seventh St.	Rapid City, S. D. 57701
Teschner, Bernard M.	56 Doyer Ave.	White Plains, N. Y. 10605
Teska, Byron A.	Medical Arts Bldg.	Minneapolis, Minn. 55402
Tess, Allen F.	1245 Graham Rd.	St. Louis, Mo. 63031
Tetlie, James P.	Medical Arts Bldg.	Duiuth, Minn. 55802
Texada, Donald E.	2515 Line	Shreveport, La. 71104
Tharp, Donald W.	2923 W. Jackson St.	Muncie, Ind. 47304
Theis, Franklyn B.	209 S. Broadway	Nyack, N. Y. 10960
Thel, Henry C., Jr.	1404 Brodhead Rd.	Aliquippa, Pa. 15001
Theodore, Frederick H.	625 Park Ave.	New York, N. Y. 10021
Thoeny, Oscar W.	1313 N. Second St.	Phoenix, Ariz. 85004
Thoft, Richard A.	285 Washington St.	Marblehead, Mass. 01945
Thomas, Charles I.	2065 Adelbert Rd.	Cleveland, O. 44106
Thomas, Edward R	60 Wyoming St.	Dayton, O. 45409
Thomans, Edward R., Jr.	60 Wyoming St.	Dayton, O. 45409
Thomas, Edwin B.	121 Walpole St.	Norwoord, Mass. 02062
Thomas, Francis T.	77 Ponfield Rd.	Bronxville, N. Y. 10708
Thomas, Jas. A.	390 E. Chicago St.	Coldwater, Mich. 49036
Thomas, John H.	1621 E. Market St.	Warren, O. 44483
Thomas, Richard L.	Medical Village, 48th & A St.	Lincoln, Nebr. 68510
Thomas, Robert M., Jr.	550 Washington St.	San Diego, Cal. 92103

Thomas, Robert P.	905 G 15th St.	Augusta, Ga. 30901
Thomas, W. Maxwell	2811 Lemmon Ave. E.	Dallas, Tex. 75204
Thomas, Weldon L.	1492 N. Main St.	Wheaton, Ill. 60187
Thomas, Wendell C.	Naval Hospital	Camp. Pendleton, Cal. 92055
Thompson, Chas. R., Jr.	1415 N.E. 45th St.	Seattle, Wash. 98105
Thompson, Frank B.	206 E. Las Tunas Dr.	San Gabriel, Cal. 91776
Thompson, Hardy E., Jr.	910 W. 19th	Austin, Tex. 78701
Thompson, H. Stanley	Univ. of Iowa	Iowa City, Ia. 52240
Thompson, James P.	S. 12th Ave. at Spruce	Yakima, Wash. 98902
Thompson, James P.	129 N. Washington St.	Easton, Md. 21601
Thompson, James R.	The Bemidji Clinic	Bemidji, Minn. 56601
Thompson, John M.	Sherland Bldg.	South Bend, Ind. 46601
Thompson, John R.	327 E. State St.	Columbus, O. 43215
Thompson, Marguerite E.	Pikeville Medical Bldg.	Pikeville, Ky. 41501
Thompson, O. H., Jr.	604 Camden Ave.	Salisbury, Md. 21801
Thompson, Paul D.	Hume Mansur Bldg.	Indianapolis, Ind. 46204
Thompson, Robert E.	900 Second National Bldg.	Akron, O. 44308
Thompson, Roger T.	1507 Tower Ave.	Superior, Wisc. 54880
Thompson, Rollin L.	3535 Cherry Creek N. Dr.	Denver, Colo. 80209
Thompson, Samuel R.	Prof. Arts Ctr.	Marion, Ind. 46952
Thompson, Wm. E.	3244 E. Douglas	Wichita, Kans. 67208
Thomson, Richard J.	807 W. Sterling	Baytown, Tex. 77520
Thoreson, H. Theodore	2402 W. Jefferson	Boise, Ida. 83702
Thorlakson, Neil F.	416 Cobb Medical Center	Seattle, Wash. 98004
Thorn, James, I.	P. O. Box 1627	Wenatchee, Wash. 98801
Thornburgh, Robt. G.	1066 Atlantic Ave.	Long Beach, Cal. 90813
Thornfeldt, Paul R.	919 Taylor St.	Portland, Ore. 97205
Thornhill, Geo. T., Jr.	720 W. Jones St.	Raleigh, N.,C. 27603
Thornton, Spencer P.	2010 Church St.	Nashville, Tenn. 37203
Thorpe, Harvey E.	3600 Forbes Ave.	Pittsburgh, Pa. 15213
Thorpe, Richard M.	220 Meyran Ave.	Pittsburgh, Pa. 15213
Thorson, John A.	700 Locust St.	Dubuque, Ia. 52001
Thorson, Jon C.	2500 Hospital Dr.	Mt. View, Cal. 94040
Thrasher, Barrie H., Jr.	490 Peachtree St.	Atlanta, Ga. 30318
Thumim, Mark	760 Saybrook Rd.	Middletown, Conn. 06457
Thurmond, Jack A.	Mid Valley Med. Arts Bldg.	Weslaco, Tex. 78596
Thygeson, Phillips	Univ. of Cal. Med. Ctr.	San Francisco, Cal. 94122
Tibbens, Geo. F.	Wash. Trust Bldg.	Washington, Pa. 15301
Tibbetts, Otis B.	181 Gamage Ave.	Auburn, Me. 04210
Ticho, Karl E.	8625 S. Cicero Ave.	Chicago, Ill. 60652
Tiedke, Gunther E.	120 N. Michigan Ave.	Saginaw, Mich. 48602
Tieman, Lorne S.	18 Roberts St.	Middletown, N. Y. 10940
Tierney, Jon P.	920 Medical Arts Bldg.	Minneapolis, Minn. 55402
Tignor, Richard F.	520 W. Fourth St.	Williamsport, Pa. 17701
Tilghman, Walter W.	210 N. Central	Glendale, Cal. 91203
Till, Bruce L.	1100 Southgate	Pendleton, Ore. 97801
Tillett, Chas. W.	2200 E. 7th St.	Charlotte, N. C. 28204
Tillett, Grace M.	2200 E. 7th St.	Charlotte, N. C. 28204
Tillman, Jos. M., Jr.	434 W. Lindley Ave.	Philadelphia, Pa. 19120
Tindall, Harry C.	1938 Peachtree Rd., N.W.	Atlanta, Ga. 30309
Tinkess, Donald E.	Ituri Towers	Greenwich, Conn. 06830
Tipshus, Alfons F.	900 Kiely Blvd.	Santa Clara, Cal. 95051
Tirico, Jos G.	1000 W. La Veta	Orange, Cal. 92668
Tirrill, Willard O., III	218 20th Ave. N.	Nashville, Tenn. 37203
Tisher, Paul W.	99 W. Main St.	New Britain, Conn. 06050

Title, Mitchel	50 Samsondale Plaza	W. Haverstraw, N. Y. 10993
Titone, Charles S.	37-42 73rd St.	Jackson Heights, N. Y. 11372
Titus, Charles O.	5500 Prospect Pl.	Chevy Chase, Md. 20015
Tobin, Henry L.	84 Front St.	Binghamton, N. Y. 13905
Todoro, Jos. C.	229 Main St.	Hamburg, N. Y. 14075
Todtfeld, Paul	80 Maple Ave.	Smithtown, N. Y. 11787
Tokar, V. Raymond	28 S. Mountain Ave.	Montclair, N. J. 07042
Toland, Joseph C.	5927 N. Fifth St.	Philadelphia, Pa. 19120
Toland, Virgil A.	550 W. Thomas Rd.	Phoenix, Ariz. 85013
Toll, Wm. G.	750 Park Ave.	New York, N. Y. 10021
Tomarelli, Raymond C.	Empire Bldg.	Pittsburgh, Pa. 15222
Tomas, Teofilo	909 Riverside Dr.	Milledgeville, Ga. 31034
Tomassene, Raymond A.	Box 728	Wheeling, W. Va. 26003
Tomlinson, J. Wesley	900 Chester Pike	Sharon Hill, Pa. 19079
Tomlinson, John W.	1515 Pacific	Everett, Wash. 98201
Topilow, Arnold	796 Ave. C.	Bayonne, N. J. 07002
Topinka, Walter A.	Ambaum Blvd. at S.W. 142nd	Seattle, Wash. 98166
Torchia, Richard T.	4235 Secor	Toledo, O. 43623
Torres, Alberto F.	1010 W. Wall	Midland, Tex. 79701
Totino, Jos. A.	1443 Upland St.	Chester, Pa. 19013
Touma, Alfred	26789 Woodward Ave.	Huntington Woods, Mich. 48070
Tour, Robert L.	384 Post St.	San Francisco, Cal. 94108
Townes, C. Dwight	1169 Eastern Pkwy.	Louisville, Ky. 40217
Toyama, Roy	Hagadone Bldg.	Coeur d'Alene, Ida. 83814
Trachtenberg, Lee H.	513 Ridge Rd.	Munster, Ind. 46321
Traganza, Robt. W.	302 Marlton Pike	Cherry Hill, N. J. 08034
Trant, John H. III	1720 Sir Wm. Osler Dr.	Virginia Beach, Va. 23454
Trantham, Harry E.	407 Vardry St.	Greenville, S.C. 29601
Trapp, Claude W.	147 N. Upper St.	Lexington, Ky. 40507
Traul, Robt. E.	1909 S. Main St.	Findlay, O. 45840
Trautmann, James C.	200 First St. S. W.	Rochester, Minn. 55901
Travis, Willis E.	90 S. Hamilton St.	Poughkeepsie, N. Y. 12603
Traykovski, Alexander	46 W. 86th St.	New York, N. Y. 10024
Trayner, Edwin M.	111 Dean Dr.	Tenafly, N. J. 07670
Tredennick, C. Nicholas	110 E. Diamond St.	Butler, Pa. 16001
Tredennick, John T.	329 Main St.	Johnstown, Pa. 15905
Tredici, Thos. J.	School of Aerospace Med.	Brooks AFB, Tex. 78235
Trenberth, Sterling M.	474 S. Swall Dr.	Beverly Hills, Cal. 90211
Trent, Robt. I.	Pasteur Med. Bldg.	Oklahoma City, Okla. 73103
Tresley, Jack	25 E. Washington St.	Chicago, Ill. 60602
Trichter, Benj.	515 Ocean Ave.	Brooklyn, N. Y. 11226
Trimble, John G.	116 S. Buckeye St.	Kokomo, Ind. 46901
Troia, Carl J.	2605 S. 84th St.	Omaha, Nebr. 68124
Trokel, Stephen L.	635 W. 165th St.	New York, N. Y. 10032
Trolan, Howard	515 Soquel Ave	Santa Cruz, Cal. 95060
Trotta, Nicholas C.	51 Chestnut St.	Ridgewood, N. J. 07450
Trotter, Robt. R.	West Va. Univ. Med. Ctr.	Morgantown, W. Va. 26506
Troubalos, Stephen	6 Rockwood Terr.	Jamaica Plain, Mass. 02130
Troup, Wilson J.	123 N. Military Ave.	Green Bay, Wisc. 54303
Troutman, Richard C.	115 E. 64th St.	New York, N. Y. 10021
Trowbridge, Dwight H.	2912 Fresno St.	Fresno, Cal. 93721
Troyer, Dana O.	201 E. Clinton	Goshen, Ind. 46526
True, William R.	1010 Cass St.	Monterey, Cal. 93940
Trueman, Robt. H.	2101 Chestnut St.	Philadelphia, Pa. 19103

Truhlsen, Stanley M.	Doctors Bldg.	Omaha, Nebr. 68131
Tschetter, Richard T.	1200 S. Euclid St.	Sioux Falls, S. D. 57105
Ts'o, Mark O. M.	Armed Forces Institute of Pathology	Washington, D. C. 20305
Tsujimura, James K.	2218 Lloyd Center	Portland, Ore. 97232
Tuck, Herbert A.	50 Oliver St.	Fitchburg, Mass. 01420
Tuck, Kenneth D.	1138 Second St.	Roanoke, Va. 24016
Tucker, Donald P.	277 Alexander St.	Rochester, N. Y. 14607
Tucker, Jas. L., Jr.	1818 Pine St.	Abilene, Tex. 79601
Tucker, Leonard C.	2177 S. Taylor Rd.	University Heights, O. 44118
Tudor, Robert C.	405 W. 6th St.	Ontario, Cal. 91762
Tukel, Floyd S.	1922 Monroe	Dearborn, Mich. 48124
Tulevech, Chas. B., Jr.	635 Belle Terre Rd.	Port Jefferson, N. Y. 11777
Tulloch, George M.	1212 N. Hudson	Oklahoma City, Okla. 73103
Turkel, Henry W.	850 Bryant St.	San Francisco, Cal. 94103
Turnbull, Don C.	Woodward Bldg.	Birmingham, Ala. 35203
Turner, David H.	1010 E. Third St.	Chattanooga, Tenn. 37403
Turner, Larry	1110 W. Main St.	Durham, N. C. 27701
Turtz, Arnold I.	525 Park Ave.	New York, N. Y. 10021
Tusak, Ervin A.	115 E. 90th St.	New York, N. Y. 10028
Tuttle, William S.	902 Frostwood	Houston, Tex. 77024
Tuveson, Gerry R.	1070 Warrington Rd.	Deerfield, Ill. 60015
Tweedy, Franklin V.	719 Church St.	Lynchburg, Va. 24504
Twitchell, M. Coleman	217 S. Union St.	Burlington, Vt. 05401
Tyler, J. Wayne	425 W. Bannock St.	Boise, Ida. 83702
Tyler, Lockland V., Jr.	Medical Center Clinic	Pensacola, Fla. 32502
Tyner, Geo. S.	Univ. of Colo. Med. Ctr.	Denver, Colo. 80220
Tyner, Harlan H.	3202 N. Meridian St.	Indianapolis, Ind. 46208
Ulanday, Ted B.	509 E. Santa Clara St.	San Jose, Cal. 95112
Underriner, Richard J.	4753 Broadway	Chicago, Ill. 60640
Underwood, Dick H.	6700 Troost	Kansas City, Mo. 64131
Underwood, Ernest A.	410 E. 20th St.	Vancouver, Wash. 98663
Unruh, John W.	1165 W. Harvard Ave.	Roseburg, Ore. 97470
Unsworth, Arthur C.	85 Jefferson St.	Hartford, Conn. 06106
Updegraff, Ambrose G.	1607 9th St. N.	St. Petersburg, Fla. 33704
Urban, Eva A.	241 E. Saginaw	E. Lansing, Mich. 48823
U'Ren, Harold M.	2307 N.W. Overton St.	Portland, Ore. 97210
Uribe, Luis E.	9 E. 91st. St.	New York, N. Y. 10028
Urist, Martin J.	Route 5, Box 338	South Haven, Mich. 49090
Urweider, Herbert A.	3900 Wisconsin Ave. N. W.	Washington, D. C. 20016
Utens, Max	10092 Chapman Ave.	Garden Grove, Cal. 92640
Vaccaro, Eugene A.	1320 Linden Ave.	Memphis, Tenn. 38104
Vaiser, Albert	Medical Arts Bldg.	Dallas, Tex. 75201
Valdivieso, Jorge R.	U. S. Naval Hospital	Portsmouth, Va. 23708
Vallotton, Wm. W.	Medical University Hosp.	Charleston, S. C. 29401
Valone, Richard J.	3 Parkside Ct.	Utica, N. Y. 13501
Van Arnam, Carl E.	1208 N.W. 6th St.	Gainesville, Fla. 32601
Van Arsdall, Jas. R.	Bradley Med. Ctr.	Cleveland, Tenn. 37311
Van Atta, Roger A.	628 Columbus St.	Ottawa, Ill. 61350
Van Bergen, Thos. M.	Republic Bldg.	Denver, Colo. 80202
Van Buren, John J.	88-49 163rd St.	Jamaica, N. Y. 11432
Van Buskirk, Edmund L.	2600 Greenbush St.	Lafayette, Ind. 47902
Vancil, Gordon Q.	164 Division St.	Elgin, Ill. 60120
Vanderbeek, Frank B.	683 E. 27 St.	Paterson, N. J. 07504
Van Donge, Norman W.	1805 State St.	Santa Barbara, Cal. 93101

Van Dyk, Henry J. L.	Univ. of Utah, College of Medicine	Salt Lake City, Utah 84112
VanDyke, Don P.	607 E. Main	Kent, O. 44240
Van Fossen, Albert W.	303 E. Town St.	Columbus, O. 43215
van Herick, Wm.	595 Buckingham Way	San Francisco, O. 43215
van Heuven, Wichard A. J.	Albany Med. Coll.	Albany, N. Y. 12208
Van Lonkhuyzen, Maurice	131 State St.	Portland, Me. 04101
Van Nostrand, Donald S.	115 E. 61st St.	New York, N. Y. 10021
Van Portfliet, Paul	245 State St., S.E.	Grand Rapids, Mich. 49502
Van Riesen, Milton H.	633 N. Central Ave.	Glendale, Cal. 91203
Van Riet, Lieven J.	2000 Crawford St.	Houston, Tex. 77002
Van Sandt, Jean F.	600 E. Main St.	Olney, Ill. 62450
Vanzant, Thos. J.	Hermann Prof. Bldg.	Houston, Tex. 77025
Varbedian, Thos. G.	195 W. Brown St.	Birmingham, Mich. 48011
Vaughan, Daniel G.	220 Meridian Ave.	San Jose, Cal. 95126
Vaughan, James B.	129 Delaware Rd.	Kenmore, N. Y. 14217
Vaughn, Arthur R., Jr.	5329 Rising Sun Ave.	Philadelphia, Pa. 19120
Veenis, C. Y.	121 University Pl.	Pittsburgh, Pa. 15213
Vegliante, Michael E.	174 Bradley St.	New Haven, Conn. 06511
Veirs, Everett R.	Scott & White Clinic	Temple, Tex. 76501
Venable, H. Philip	2841 N. Union Blvd.	St. Louis, Mo. 63115
Verity, Alden M.	12456 E. Washington Blvd.	Whittier, Cal. 90602
VerLee, David L.	606 Mott Foundation Bldg.	Flint, Mich. 48502
Vernlund, Robert J.	85 Jefferson St.	Hartford, Conn. 06106
Véronneau-Troutman, Suzanne	755 Park Ave.	New York, N. Y. 10021
Versic, Thomas C.	7424 Paddock Rd.	Cincinnati, O. 45216
Vertuno, John W.	231 W. Washington St.	Chicago, Ill. 60606
Vesey, Frank A.	200 E. 64th St.	New York, N. Y. 10021
Vetromile, Gerard A.	800 S. El Camino Real	San Clemente, Cal. 92672
Vey, E. Kenneth	1529 Park Bldg.	Pittsburgh, Pa. 15222
Vickery, Robt. D.	Doctors Bldg.	Omaha, Nebr. 68131
Vidal, Fred L.	6075 Roswell Rd. N. E.	Atlanta, Ga. 30328
Vidal, Jose H.	2300 Rancho Dr.	Las Vegas, Nev. 89102
Villadolid, Victor F.	520 Franklin Ave.	Garden City, N. Y. 11530
Villani, Patrick A.	20811 Kelly Rd.	E. Detroit, Mich. 48021
Vincent, Bayard R.	1711 Woodlawn Ave.	Wilmington, Dela. 19806
Vincent, Nicholas J.	5333 Hollister Ave.	Santa Barbara, Cal. 93105
Vine, H. Jean S.	36 Crossroads	Rochester, Minn. 55901
Violé, Armand	1930 Wilshire Blvd.	Los Angeles, Cal. 90057
Vittone, Ronald B.	811 Ligonier St.	Latrobe, Pa. 15650
Vlachos, George	1882 Grand Concourse	Bronx, N. Y.
Vogel, Adolph W.	Plymouth Rd.	Cwynedd Valley, Pa. 19004
Vogel, Herbert P.	1695 Grand Concourse	Bronx, N. Y. 10453
Volk, David	2460 Fairmount Blvd.	Cleveland Heights, O. 44106
Volk, Myron	18599 Lake Shore Blvd.	Cleveland, O. 44119
Voltz, Vernon C.	2500 N. Rockton Ave.	Rockford, Ill. 61103
von Glahn, Noel A.	19075 Middlebelt Rd.	Livonia, Mich. 48152
von Noorden, Gunter K.	Johns Hopkins Hospital	Baltimore, Md. 21205
von Sallmann, Ludwig	5506 Huntington Parkway	Bethesda, Md. 20014
Voorhees, Chas. H.	308 College Ave.	Elmira, N. Y. 14901
Vorenkamp, Richard J.	1120 W. Spruce St.	Yakima, Wash. 98902
Vorisek, Elmer A.	6205 Woodland Rd.	Des Moines, Ia. 50312
Vossler, Albert E.	David Whitney Bldg.	Detroit, Mich. 48226
Vrooman, Carl O.	55 Claremont Ave.	Mt. Vernon, N. Y. 10550
Vucicevic, Zarko M.	3400 Spruce	Philadelphia, Pa. 19104

Vygantas, Charles M.	30 N. Michigan Ave.	Chicago, Ill. 60602
Wachtel, Daniel L.	515 Church St.	Bound Brooks, N. J. 08805
Wachtel, Joel G.	303 E. Town St.	Columbus, O. 43215
Waddell, Marion C.	Med. Arts Bldg.	Richmond, Va. 23219
Wade, Frederick E.	1103 Grand Ave.	Kansas City, Mo. 64106
Wadsworth, Gerald E.	478 Peachtree St., N.E.	Atlanta, Ga. 30305
Wadsworth, Jos. A. C.	Duke Med. Ctr.	Durham, N. C. 27706
Wagenaar, Philip	334 N. E. Northgate Way	Seattle, Wash. 98125
Wager, Harol E.	1109 Harrison Ave.	Panama City, Fla. 32401
Wagman, Ora H.	45 Bay State Rd.	Boston, Mass. 02215
Wagner, Alfred W.	2615 Eye St.	Sacramento, Cal. 95816
Wagner, Wm. F.	3490 Linden Ave.	Long Beach, Cal. 90807
Wahl, Jos. W.	1836 South Ave.	LaCrosse, Wisc. 54601
Wahlen, Henry E.	6624 Fannin St.	Houston, Tex. 77025
Wahlig, Alexander F., Jr. ..	Lakeview Medical Bldg.	Bath, N. Y. 14810
Wainstock, Michael A.	David Whitney Bldg.	Detroit, Mich. 48226
Waldie, Robert H.	2025 Morse Ave.	Sacramento, Cal. 95825
Waldman, Jos.	1930 Chestnut St.	Philadelphia, Pa. 19103
Walker, Glenn L.	Med. Arts Bldg.	Burlington, Ia. 52601
Wall, Walton	320 N. Magnolia Ave.	Orlando, Fla. 32801
Wallace, Fred C.	1320 Linden	Memphis, Tenn. 38104
Wallace, Grady M.	3801 W. 19 St.	Lubbock, Tex. 79410
Walber, Fred E.	740 Oxford Ave.	Idaho Falls, Ida. 83401
Walma, Daniel	26 Sheldon S.E.	Grand Rapids, Mich. 49502
Walsh, Alton L.	240 Meridian Rd.	San Jose, Cal. 95126
Walsh, Frank B.	Johns Hopkins Hospital	Baltimore, Md. 21205
Walsh, Michael	1101 S. 2nd St.	Springfield, Ill. 62704
Walsh, Rita	1008 N. Main	Bloomington, Ill. 61701
Walsh, Thomas J.	1100 Bedford St.	Stamford, Conn. 06905
Walter, William L.	135 W. Adams St.	Kirkwood, Mo. 63122
Walters, Florence A.	5354 Milwaukee Ave.	Chicago, Ill. 60630
Walters, Phil V.	207 E. Watauga Ave.	Johnson City, Tenn. 37601
Waltman, Stephen R.	3003 Van Ness St. N. W.	Washington, D. C. 20008
Walton, David S.	300 Longwood Ave.	Boston, Mass. 02115
Wan, P. C.	4225 Saviers Rd.	Oxnard, Cal. 93030
Wapner, John M.	202 N. 17th St.	Allentown, Pa. 18104
Ward, Clarence V.	Lehmann Bldg.	Peoria, Ill. 61602
Ward, Harold J.	75 N. Santa Anita Ave.	Arcadia, Cal. 91006
Ward, Harold W.	1225 Miccosukee Rd.	Tallahassee, Fla. 32303
Ward, Jas. F.	1215 S. 12th St.	Tacoma, Wash. 98405
Ward, James V.	2015 Fairfield Ave.	Shreveport, La. 71104
Ward, Robert H.	11 N. Loudon Heights	Albany, N. Y. 12211
Warner, Raymond C.	1684 N. Prospect Ave.	Milwaukee, Wisc. 53202
Warren, Jeffrey L.	103 W. College Ave.	Appleton, Wisc. 54911
Warren, Lloyd P.	5205 E. 21st St.	Wichita, Kans. 67208
Wasmund, Clarence W.	Interstate Medical Center	Red Wing, Minn. 55066
Wass, Harold E.	333 Linwood Ave.	Buffalo, N. Y. 14209
Wass, Richard A.	3815 Pelham Rd.	Dearborn, Mich. 48124
Wasson, Paul E.	800 McKinley Ave. N. W.	Canton, O. 44703
Watkins, John G.	Donaghey Bldg.	Little Rock, Ark. 72201
Watkins, John O.	359 Pine St.	Spartanburg, S. C. 29302
Watson, J. Edwin	18524 Grand River	Detroit, Mich. 48223
Watson, John W.	607 N. Central Ave.	Glendale, Cal. 91203
Watson, Leo G.	3433 S. Lafountain	Kokomo, Ind. 46901
Watson, Pearl A.	6217 16th St. N.W.	Washington, D. C. 20011

Watson, Richard E.	USVA Out-patient Clinic, Bldg. 18	St. Paul, Minn. 55111
Watson, Thomas Y.	640 N. Woodward	Birmingham, Mich. 48011
Watt, Russell H.	309 E. Church St.	Marshalltown, Ia. 50158
Watzke, Robt. C.	Univ. Hospitals	Iowa City, Ia. 52240
Waugh, David	New St.	Sharon, Conn. 06069
Waugh, Richey L., Jr.	33 Mulberry St.	Springfield, Mass. 01105
Way, James A.	2315 E. Third St.	Bloomington, Ind. 47401
Weatherall, Richard H.	3155 Stagg Dr.	Beaumont, Tex. 77701
Weaver, Emerson M. F.	727 W. 7th St.	Los Angeles, Cal. 90017
Weaver, Harry S., Jr.	1930 Chestnut St.	Philadelphia, Pa. 19103
Weaver, Jack D.	959 N. Emporia	Wichita, Kans. 67214
Weaver, Rex W.	500 W. 10th Pl.	Mesa, Ariz. 85201
Weaver, Richard G.	N. C. Baptist Hospital	Winston-Salem, N. C. 27103
Weaver, Robert P.	8 Medical Plaza	Glen Cove, N. Y. 11542
Webb, Edw. F.	5112 Oakton St.	Skokie, Ill. 60076
Webb, James J.	520 W. Main St.	Blytheville, Ark. 72315
Webb, James W.	920 S. Main St.	Jonesboro, Ark. 72401
Webb, Paul B., Jr.	6651 Chippewa	St. Louis, Mo. 63109
Webb, Robt. B., Jr.	408 S. Sycamore St.	Petersburg, Va. 23803
Weber, Murry K.	23101 Sherman Way	Canoga Park, Cal. 91304
Webster, Franklin R.	State Tower Bldg.	Syracuse, N. Y. 13202
Webster, Robert G., Jr.	2400 Clay St.	San Francisco, Cal. 94115
Weed, Chester A.	1005-B Farmington Ave.	West Hartford, Conn. 06107
Weekley, Robt. D.	5370 Pearl Rd.	Parma, O. 44129
Weeks, Carrol L.	1930 Wilshire Blvd.	Los Angeles, Cal. 90057
Weene, Lawrence E.	599 Pleasant St.	Brockton, Mass. 02401
Wehr, Maurice B.	2355 Fort St.	Lincoln Park, Mich. 48146
Weidenthal, Daniel T.	11811 Shaker Blvd.	Cleveland, O. 44120
Weih, Jack E.	1105 E. Front	Traverse City, Mich. 49684
Weil, Sidney	1840 Grand Concourse	New York, N. Y. 10457
Weil, Victor J.	750 Broadway	Paterson, N. J. 07514
Weiler, David L.	485 Kinderkamack Rd.	Oradell, N. J. 07649
Weimer, John R.	1028 Connecticut Ave. N.W.	Washington, D. C. 20036
Weinberg, Herman C.	2177 S. Taylor Rd.	University Heights, O. 44118
Weinberg, Joel K.	Brewster-Carmel Prof. Bldg.	Brewster, N. Y. 10509
Weiner, Alvin	2100 Baynard Blvd.	Wilmington, Dela. 19802
Weiner, Harry I.	1812 Sumner Ave.	Aberdeen, Wash. 98520
Weiner, Herman L.	1900 J. F. K. Blvd.	Philadelphia, Pa. 19103
Weiner, Peter G.	2705 Loma Vista Rd.	Ventura, Cal. 93003
Weiner, Robert L.	2121 E. 18th Ave.	Denver, Colo. 80206
Weingarten, Joel E.	28 W. Adams	Detroit, Mich. 48226
Weingeist, Samson	30-74 36th St.	Long Island City, N. Y. 11103
Weinman, Edward B.	401 Market St.	Steubenville, O. 43952
Weinstein, Albert	340 Capitol Ave.	Bridgeport, Conn. 06606
Weinstein, George W.	Johns Hopkins Hospital	Baltimore, Md. 21205
Weinstein, Irvine	2845 University Ave.	New York, N. Y. 14068
Weinstock, Frank J.	214 Dartmouth Ave. S.W.	Canton, O. 44710
Weintraub, Alfred	115 E. 82nd St.	New York, N. Y. 10028
Weir, Robert Kiley	4240 Blue Ridge Blvd.	Kansas City, Mo. 64133
Weis, Donald R.	636 Beacon St.	Boston, Mass. 02215
Weisbach, Philip T., Jr.	3155 Stagg Dr.	Beaumont, Tex. 77701
Weisbaum, M. Byron	520 E. Allen St.	Springfield, Ill. 62703
Weisberg, Howard K.	1095 Park Ave.	New York, N. Y. 10028
Weisel, John T.	17 Myrtle St.	Medford, Ore. 97501
Weisenheimer, E. J.	3640 Lomita Blvd.	Torrance, Cal. 90503

Weiser, Albert	390 Pine St.	Fall River, Mass. 02720
Weiskopf, Henry S.	504 Broadway	Gary, Ind. 46402
Weisman, Frederick L.	9535 Reseda Blvd.	Northridge, Cal. 91324
Weiss, Daniel I.	3755 Henry Hudson Pkwy.	Riverdale, N. Y. 10463
Weiss, Edward C.	95 Northfield Ave.	West Orange, N. J. 07052
Weiss, Harry	37-21 Parsons Blvd.	Flushing, N. Y. 11354
Weiss, Herman	465 N. Roxbury Dr.	Beverly Hills, Cal. 90210
Weiss, Joseph F.	2400 S. W. Vermont St.	Portland, Ore 97219
Weiss, Larry L.	751 Bethesda Rd.	Winston-Salem, N. C. 27103
Weiss, Leon M.	9 Mayflower Rd.	Scarsdale, N. Y. 10583
Weiss, Sidney	2037 Locust St.	Philadelphia, Pa. 19103
Weisser, C. Wm.	Grant Bldg.	Pittsburgh, Pa. 15219
Weitzner, Walter B.	630 Ocean Ave.	Brooklyn, N. Y. 11226
Weixel, Francis X.	Nix. Prof. Bldg.	San Antonio, Tex. 78205
Weizenblatt, Sprinza	29 N. Market St.	Asheville, N. C. 28801
Welch, James W., Jr.	4300 Parliament Dr.	Alexandria, La. 71301
Welch, Robt. B.	14 W. Mt. Vernon Pl.	Baltimore, Md. 21201
Wellman, Paul K.	4122 Shelbyville Rd.	Louisville, Ky. 40207
Wells, August H.	549 Frederick St.	Santa Cruz, Cal. 95060
Wells, Francis B.	147 N. Upper St.	Lexington, Ky. 40507
Wells, Wm. C.	411 Happy Valley Rd.	Glasgow, Ky. 42141
Welo, Bob L.	Wyoming Bldg.	Casper, Wyo, 82601
Welt, Milton	401 Park Blvd.	Massapequa Pk., N. Y. 11762
Wenaas, Elmer J.	420 Oak Hill Ave.	Youngstown, O. 44502
Wendell, Franklyn R.	918 S. Fairmont Ave	Lodi, Cal. 95240
Wendland, John P	6533 Drew Ave. S.	Minneapolis, Minn. 55435
Wenger, Samuel	42-27 Union St.	Flushing, N. Y. 11358
Wenner, Waldemar T.	303 Physicians & Surgeons Bldg.	St. Cloud, Minn. 56301
Wenzel, Paul A.	3191 S. Broadway	Englewood, Colo. 80110
Wegeland, Floyd L., Jr.	Letterman Gen. Hosp.	San Francisco, Cal. 94129
Werner, Chas. W.	8207 E. 3rd St.	Downey, Cal. 90240
Werner, Geo. B.	42 Riverside Dr.	Binghamton, N. Y. 13905
Wesberry, Jesse M.	2900 S. Perkins Rd.	Memphis, Tenn. 38118
Weseley, Alan C.	600 E. 18th St.	Brooklyn, N. Y. 11226
Wesson, Thos. W.	Box 257	Tupelo, Miss. 38801
West, Francis J.	195 Ashmont St.	Dorchester, Mass. 02124
Weston, Chas. L.	120 N. Dudley St.	Macomb, Ill. 61455
Weston, Horace L.	15901 W. 9 Mile Rd.	Southfield, Mich. 48075
Westsmith, Richard A.	Main St.	Lakeville, Conn. 06039
Wetterholm, Dennis H.	2007 17th St.	Bakersfield, Cal. 93301
Wetzel, John O.	700 Intracoastal Dr.	Ft. Lauderdale, Fa. 33304
Wetzig, Paul C.	Box 2170	Colorado Springs, Colo. 80901
Wexler, David	103 E. 86th St.	New York, N. Y. 10028
Weyand, Geo. M.	2007 17th St.	Bakersfield, Cal. 93301
Wheatly, Wm. K.	324 N. Duke St.	Lancaster, Pa. 17602
Wheeler, Maynard C.	815 Park Ave.	New York, N. Y. 10021
Wheeler, Wm. J.	910 N. 4th St.	Wilmington, N. C. 28401
Whelchel, Merritt C.	905 15th St.	Augusta, Ga. 30902
Wheliss, John A.	1300 St. Mary's St.	Raleigh, N. C. 27605
Wherley, Harold F.	Blvd. Med. Bldg.	Dover, O. 44622
Whinery, Robt. D.	2409 Towncrest Dr.	Iowa City, Ia. 52240
Whisnant, Robert A., Jr.	2255 Langhorne Rd.	Lynchburg, Va. 24501
White, Carl H.	106 River St.	Fenton, Mich. 48436
White, David W.	506 Church St.	Lynchburg, Va. 24504
White, Donald E.	360 E. Seventh St.	Upland, Cal. 91786

Name	Address	City/State/ZIP
White, Fred D.	Bluefield Sanitarium Cl.	Bluefield, W. Va. 24701
White, Frederick C.	120 Broadway	Richmond, Cal. 94804
White, J. Henry	173 W. Oak St.	Basking Ridge, N. J. 07920
White, John J.	653 N. State St.	Jackson, Miss. 39201
White, John J., Jr.	668 Forsyth Medical Park	Winston-Salem, N. C. 27103
White M. Jeffrey	5400 W. Gray St.	Tampa, Fla. 33609
White, Orson W.	Med. Arts Bldg.	Salt Lake City, Utha 84111
White, Stephen V.	3838 Hillcroft	Houston, Tex. 77027
White, Steven M.	Route #2, Stantonsburg, Rd. Extension	Greenville, N. C. 27834
White, Thos. P.	42 Weston St.	Waltham, Mass. 02154
White, William O.	1349 Druid Park Ave.	Augusta, Ga. 30904
Whitehead, Craig A.	706 Franklin	Tampa, Fla. 33602
Whitehead, David C.	Medical Tower	Norfolk, Va. 23507
Whitelock, Leland D., Jr.	U.S.P.H.S. Hospital	Norfolk, Va. 23508
Whitham, Elmer L.	345 Union St.	New Bedford, Mass. 02740
Whitham, Lloyd B.	Box 6734	Towson, Md. 21204
Whitmer, Kenneth S.	550 Brickell Ave.	Miami, Fla. 33131
Whitney, J. B.	412 Country St.	New Bedford, Mass. 02790
Whitney, Percy T.	R. D. #3, Surry Rd.	Ellsworth, Me. 04605
Whitsell, David C.	126 W. First St.	Hinsdale, Ill. 60521
Whitsell, Fay M.	2441 W. 79th St.	Chicago, Ill. 60652
Whitten, Richard H.	2916 Fresno St.	Fresno, Cal. 93721
Whitworth, Claiborne G.	1005 E. High St.	Charlottesville, Va. 22901
Wholihan, John W.	604 W. Michigan Ave.	Jackson, Mich. 49201
Wible, Clair E.	1176 S. Queen	York, Pa. 17403
Wick, Alfred A.	2120 Carew St.	Ft. Wayne, Ind. 46805
Wick, H. Ward	858 Fourth St.	Santa Rosa, Cal. 95403
Wicker, Henry S.	6218 Georgia Ave., N.W.	Washington, D. C. 20011
Wickerham, Earl P., Jr.	402 Jenkins Bldg.	Pittsburgh, Pa. 15222
Wickliffe, Robt. C. M.	1211 E. Pennsylvania Ave.	Escondido, Cal. 92025
Widener, Geo. H.	1903 Broadway	Paducah, Ky. 42001
Widner, Russell R.	309 E. Church St.	Marshalltown, Ia. 50158
Wiedman, Michael S.	452 Pleasant St.	Malden, Mass. 02148
Wiegmann, O. A.	1700 W. Wisconsin Ave.	Milwaukee, Wisc. 53233
Wies, Frederick A.	690 Howard Ave.	New Haven, Conn. 06519
Wiener, Frederick A.	285 Central Ave.	Lawrence, N. Y. 11559
Wieselthier, Maurice L.	222 E. 17th St.	Brooklyn, N. Y. 11226
Wiesen, Arnold M.	30 Central Park S.	New York, N. Y. 10019
Wiesinger, Herbert	2015 Monument Ave.	Richmond, Va. 23220
Wigdor, Aaron	Stony Brook Prof. Bldg.	Lake Grove, N. Y. 11755
Wiggs, Eugene O.	303 Josephine	Denver, Colo. 80206
Wike, Sidney	3-L Doctors' Bldg.	Bristol, Tenn. 37620
Wikler, Irving	3343 Fourth Ave.	San Diego, Cal. 92103
Wilber, Inez E.	1150 Connecticut Ave. N.W.	Washington, D. C. 20036
Wilbrandt, Hans R.	5324 W. 16th St.	Indianapolis, Ind. 46224
Wilbur, Ronald E.	2540 N.E. 9th St.	Ft. Lauderdale, Fla. 33304
Wilcox, Lloyd M.	124 Main St.	Bristol, Conn. 06010
Wild, John J.	1645 N. Alvernon	Tucson, Ariz. 85716
Wilder, Howard L.	30 N. Michigan Ave.	Chicago, Ill. 60602
Wilder, Lowell W.	3333 E. Central	Wichita, Kans. 67208
Wilder, William W.	4623 Poplar Ave.	Memphis, Tenn. 38117
Wildgen, Bernard C.	Med. Arts Ctr.	Muskegon, Mich. 49440
Wilensky, M. Carl	Maison Blanche Bldg.	New Orleans, La. 70112
Wiley, Jason L.	501 Metcalf Bldg.	Auburn, N. Y. 13021
Wilhelm, Daniel A.	303 S.E. 17th St.	Fort Lauderdale, Fla. 33316
Wilhelm, Harry W.	U.S. Naval Hospital, FPO	New York, N. Y. 09521

Wilkes, J. W.	Jones Bldg.	Columbia, Tenn. 38401
Wilkins, Paul C.	2307 N.W. Overton St.	Portland, Ore. 97210
Wilkins, Robert B.	1121 Hermann Professional Bldg..	Houston, Tex. 77025
Wilkinson, Arthur P.	880 S. Woodward Ave.	Pontiac, Mich. 48053
Wilkinson, Joel A.	Petroleum Tower	Shreveport, La. 71101
Wilkinson, William C.	880 Woodward	Pontiac, Mich. 48053
Willard, Donald E.	450 Clarkson Ave.	Brooklyn, N. Y. 11203
Willard, Robert L.	3626 Monroe St.	Toledo, O. 43606
Willcockson, T. H.	415 W. 3rd	Yankton, S.D. 57078
Willey, Loys W., Jr.	1311 Cleveland Ave.	Atlanta, Ga. 30344
Williams, Barney K., Jr. ...	961 Water St.	Kerrville, Tex. 78028
Williams, Brian H.	750 Las Gallinas Ave.	San Rafael, Cal. 94901
Williams, Frank M.	Bascom Palmer Eye Institute ...	Miami, Fla. 33136
Williams, Fred C.	45 Castro St.	San Francisco, Cal. 94127
Williams, Frederick D.	1 Atlantic St.	Stamford, Conn. 06901
Williams, Jas. K.	Med. Arts Ctr.	Pascagoula, Miss. 39567
Williams, Mervyn M.	Main St.	Gouldsboro, Pa. 18424
Williams, Neil S.	1702 S. Univ. Dr.	Fargo, N. D. 58102
Williams, Philips D., Jr.	9150 Perry Hwy.	Pittsburgh, Pa. 15237
Williams, Richard K.	2015 Monument Ave.	Richmond, Va. 23220
Williams, Van R.	210 State St.	New Orleans, La. 70118
Williams, Walton H.	303 Curryer Rd.	Middletown, O. 45042
Willamson, Douglas E.	950 Cooper St.	Venice, Fla. 33595
Willner, Stuart N.	1355 Orange Ave.	Winter Park, Fla. 32789
Willoughby, Jas. O.	727 Laurel Ave.	Bowling Green, Ky. 42101
Willoughby, Wm. A.	Fisher Bldg.	Detroit, Mich. 48202
Wills, Theodore E.	2354 50th Ave.	Greeley, Colo. 80631
Wilsey, John D.	1900 S. Hawthorne Rd.	Winston-Salem, N. C. 27103
Wilson, Alfred	2910 W. St. S. E.	Washington, D. C. 20020
Wilson, Arthur H.	14031 Ambaum Blvd.	Seattle, Wash. 98166
Wilson, Chas. F.	Pikeville Med. Bldg.	Pikeville, Ky. 41501
Wilson, Clinton A.	3875 Wilshire Blvd.	Los Angeles, Cal. 90005
Wilson, Frances C.	1700 S. MacDill Ave.	Tampa, Fla. 33609
Wilson, Fred M.	1100 W. Michigan St.	Indianapolis, Ind. 46202
Wilson, Henry B.	6 E. Eager St.	Baltimore, Md. 21202
Wilson, Jas. E.	14 N. Camilla St.	Memphis, Tenn. 38104
Wilson, Jas. R.	321 N. Larchmont Blvd.	Los Angeles, Cal. 90004
Wilson, John M.	207 E. Watauga Ave.	Johnson City, Tenn. 37601
Wilson, Louis A.	Med. College of Ga.	Augusta, Ga. 30902
Wilson, Paul E.	1724 Memorial Dr.	Clarksville, Tenn. 37040
Wilson, R. Sloan	4301 W. Markham	Little Rock, Ark. 72201
Wilson, W. Webb	135 Monte Vista	Watsonville, Cal. 95076
Wilson, Warren A.	1127 Wilshire Blvd.	Los Angeles, Cal. 90017
Wilson, Wayne R., Jr.	Naval Supp. Act., Box 19, FPO .	N. Y. 09521
Windsor, C. E.	4511 Forest Park	St. Louis, Mo. 63108
Winger, Ira B.	709 Madison	Toledo, O. 43624
Winn, Thos. M.	157 N. Maple Ave.	Covington, Va. 24426
Winn, William E., Jr.	4 G St.	San Rafael, Cal. 94901
Winograd, Lawrence A.	1701 S. Federal Blvd.	Denver, Colo. 80219
Winstanley, Robert A.	500 Swank Bldg.	Johnstown, Pa. 15901
Winston, Richard K.	Doctors Bldg.	Valdosta, Ga. 31601
Winter, Abraham T.	86-35 Queens Blvd.	Elmhurst, N. Y. 11373
Winter, Frank C.	1101 Welch Rd.	Palo Alto, Cal. 94304
Winters, David M.	19231 Victory Blvd.	Reseda, Cal. 91335
Wintrich, H. Peter	1177 N.E. 8th St.	Delray Beach, Fla. 33444
Wippermann, Frederich F. .	110 S. 10th St.	Minneapolis, Minn. 55403

Wirostko, Emil	635 W. 165th St.	New York, N. Y. 10032
Wirth, Norman V.	545 N.E. 47th	Portland, Ore. 97213
Wirtschafter, Jonathan D.	University of Kentucky Medical Center	Lexington, Ky. 40506
Wise, Arthur C.	2409 Towncrest Dr.	Iowa City, Ia. 52240
Wise, Geo. N.	30 W. 59th St.	New York, N. Y. 10019
Wise, James B.	800 N. E. 13th	Oklahoma City, Okla. 73104
Wishbow, Alexander J.	10 Pine St.	Morristown, N. J. 07960
Wissner, Ulrich C.	1401 S. Hope St.	Los Angeles, Cal. 90015
Witt, John E.	2020 Truxtun Ave.	Bakersfield, Cal. 93301
Wittchow, Allen W.	710 E. Grand Ave.	Wisconsin Rapids, Wisc. 54494
Witter, Gordon L.	2 W. Fern.	Redlands, Cal. 92373
Witter, Stanton L.	5700 N.W. Grand Blvd.	Oklahoma City, Okla. 73112
Wixted, Julia L.	919 E. Jefferson Blvd.	South Bend, Ind. 46617
Wohlrabe, Robert G.	4450 W. 76th St.	Minneapolis, Minn. 55435
Wold Keith C.	2737 E. Oakland Pk. Blvd.	Ft. Lauderdale, Fla. 33306
Wolf, Lewis R.	3474 Frankford Ave.	Philadelphia, Pa. 19134
Wolfe, Richard L.	14 W. Mt. Vernon Pl.	Baltimore, Md. 21201
Wolff, Jerome M.	935 Park Ave.	Plainfield, N. J. 07060
Wolff, Joachim B.	119-30 80 Rd.	Kew Gardens, N. Y. 11415
Wolff, Paul G.	1819 Broadway	Cape Girardeau, Mo. 63701
Wolff, Stewart M.	803 Cathedral St.	Baltimore, Md. 21201
Wolkowicz, Michael I.	2022 Spruce St.	Philadelphia, Pa. 19103
Wollin, Nathaniel C.	1 N. Main St.	Cortland, N. Y. 13045
Wolper, Jack	1151 Hancock St.	Quincy, Mass. 02169
Wolstan, S. David	11860 Wilshire Blvd.	Los Angeles, Cal. 90025
Wolston, Edward C.	Laconia C1.	Laconia, N.H. 03246
Wolter, J. Reimer	University Hospital	Ann Arbor, Mich. 48104
Womack, William T.	Medical Arts Bldg.	San Angelo, Tex. 76901
Wones, Edward M.	2634 Grand Ave.	Waukegan, Ill. 60085
Wong, Andrew S.	2 Church St. S.	New Haven, Conn. 06519
Wong, Guy Y.	900 Kiely Blvd.	Santa Clara, Cal. 95051
Wong, Mitchel	3-B Medical Arts Square	Austin, Tex. 78705
Wong, Vernon G.	10N311 National Eye Institute	Bethesda, Md. 20014
Wood, B. Jean	Oakwood Shopping Center	Gretna, La. 70053
Wood, Christopher	1218 Kings Hwy. N.	Myrtle Beach, S. C. 29577
Wood, Edwin S.	1004 Main St.	M. Vernon, Ill. 62864
Wood, Everet H.	4800 Gibson Blvd. S. E.	Albuquerque, N. M. 87108
Wood, Maynard A.	3145 'O' St.	Lincoln, Nebr. 68500
Wood, Thos. P., Jr.	5925 Forest Ln.	Dallas, Tex. 75230
Wood, T. Rodman	272 S. Lake St.	Los Angeles, Cal. 90057
Woodard, M. Wayne	Fatiron Bldg.	Asheville, N. C. 28801
Woodbury, George R.	4646 Poplar Ave.	Memphis, Tenn. 38117
Woodfin, M. Clarke, Jr.	750 Washington Ave.	Montgomery, Ala. 36104
Woodson, W. Burbank	103 E. Central Ave.	Temple, Tex. 76501
Woodward, James M., Jr.	Republic Bldg.	Denver, Colo. 80202
Woodward, Paul M., Jr.	500 S. Breiel Blvd.	Middletown, O. 49042
Woody, Joe H.	Doctors Bldg.	Charlotte, N.C. 28207
Woolmington, Merrill H.	200 Eagle Rd.	Wayne, Pa. 19087
Woolworth, Jos. D.	243 Columbia Ave.	Shreveport, La. 71101
Wootton, Jas. C.	425 W. 5th Pl.	Mesa, Ariz. 85201
Workman, Jos. B., Jr.	1673 Brabham Ave.	Columbia, S. C. 29204
Worlton, Jas. T.	801 N. Cascade Ave.	Colorado Springs, Colo. 80903
Wortham, Edwin	1300 Bancroft Ave.	San Leandro, Cal. 94577

Worthen, David M.	University of Florida Medical Center	Gainesville, Fla. 32601
Wotring, John M.	220 N. 6th St.	Reading, Pa. 19601
Wright, C. Larry	USPHS Hospital	Seattle, Wash. 98114
Wright, Edwin S.	10614 Riverside Dr.	North Hollywood, Cal. 91602
Wright, Harvey B.	1203 Jefferson St.	Laurel, Miss. 39440
Wright, Harvey D.	303 E. Town St.	Columbus, O. 43215
Wright, Jas. C.	2339 Virginia Beach Blvd.	Virginia Beach, Va. 23454
Wright, J. R.	301 Northside Dr. N. W.	Gainesville, Ga. 30501
Wright, John	USAF Hosp. Tachikawa, APO ..	San Francisco, Cal. 96323
Wright, L. David	1546 S. Brownlee Blvd.	Corpus Christi, Tex. 78404
Wright, Robt. L.	860 E. Broad St.	Elyria, O. 44035
Wuerschmidt, Marcus A. ...	214 W. 1st. St.	Oswego, N. Y. 13126
Wuest, Frederick C.	250 N. Central Ave.	Wayzata, Minn. 55391
Wyatt, Davis B.	300 W. Franklin St.	Richmond, Va. 23220
Wyble, Merrick J.	526 Prudhomme Ln.	Opelousas, La. 70570
Wyman, Geo. J.	1200 Hamilton Blvd.	Peoria, Ill. 61606
Wynsen, Robert C.	1120 W. LaPalma	Anaheim, Cal. 92801
Yacht, Donn L.	900 Kiely Blvd.	Santa Clara, Cal. 95051
Yancey, William A.	550 Washington St.	San Diego, Cal. 92103
Yannuzzi, Lawrence A.	525 Park Ave.	New York, N. Y. 10021
Yanoff, Myron	1930 Chestnut St.	Philadelphia, Pa. 19103
Yarbrough, Jos. C., Jr.	1530 N. Fant St.	Anderson, S. C. 29621
Yassin, John G.	Malcolm Grow Medical Center, Andrews AFB	Washington, D. C. 20331
Yasuna, Elton R.	130 Elm. St.	Worcester, Mass. 01609
Yatzkan, David N.	1803 West St.	Homestead, Pa. 15120
Yazujian, Levon D.	419 W. State St.	Trenton, N. J. 08618
Yingling, Paul V.	....	Bisbee, Ariz. 85603
Yockey, Robt. H.	150 N. Jefferson St.	Kittanning, Pa. 16201
Yockey, Robert L.	7700 E. Indian School Rd.	Scottsdale, Ariz. 85251
Yocum, Paul S.	504 Broadway	Gary, Ind. 46402
Yoder, Dewey D.	R. R. #1	Pierceton, Ind. 46562
Yoe, Lionel M.	109 Doctors Bldg.	Columbus, Ga. 31901
Yood, Julian M.	5900 Building Eastgate Center ..	Chattanooga, Tenn. 37411
York, Albert T.	National Eye Institute, Bldg. 31, 6A-52	Bethesda, Md. 20014
Youakim, Maurice I.	155 Bay St.	Glens Falls, N. Y. 12801
Youens, H. T., Jr.	1221 Bowie	Columbus, Tex. 78934
Young, Arnold I.	193 N. Harrison St.	Princeton, N. J. 08540
Young, Bryce J.	900 Sunset Dr.	La Grande, Ore. 97850
Young, Chas. A., Jr.	122 Mountain Ave. S.W.	Roanoke, Va. 24016
Young, Frank C., Jr.	Womack Army Hospital	Ft. Bragg, N. C. 28307
Young, John A.	1600 E. Third St.	Charlotte, N. C. 28204
Young, Jos. O.	251 Cajon St.	Redlands, Cal. 92373
Young, Lawrence L.	825 W. Market St.	Lima, O. 45805
Young, Lois A.	Univ. of Maryland Hospital	Baltimore, Md. 21201
Young, Morris N.	170 Broadway	New York, N. Y. 10038
Young, Robt. L.	504 Broadway	Gary, Ind. 46402
Yourish, Norman B.	400 N. Broadway	Jericho, N. Y. 11753
Yudell, Robert B.	120 Cottage Pl.	Charlotte, N. C. 28207
Yukins, Richard E.	B7 Medical Plaza, 1101 Welch Rd.	Palo Alto, Cal.
Yung, Donald J.	2567 Sheridan Dr.	Tonawanda, N. Y. 14150
Zagranisiki, Raymond J. ...	1497 Chapel St.	New Haven, Conn. 06511
Zamora, Pablo J.	Fitzsimons General Hospital	Denver, Colo. 80240

Zane, Ernest S.	23315 Washington	Colton, Cal. 92324
Zanek, Otto L.	Medical Towers	Houston, Tex. 77025
Zankan, Leo	19231 Victory Blvd.	Reseda, Cal. 91335
Zaret, Milton M.	910 Fifth Ave.	New York, N.Y. 10021
Zeavin, Bernard H.	312 S. Washington St.	Alexandria, Va. 22314
Zehl, Donald N.	260 Crittenden Blvd.	Rochester, N. Y. 14620
Zeiger, Burton	1750 E. 87th St.	Chicago, Ill. 60617
Zeiss, Edward J.	1620 N. Meade St.	Appleton, Wisc. 54911
Zeiss, John C.	1620 N. Meade St.	Appleton, Wisc. 54911
Zieter, Henry J.	807 N. San Joaquin St.	Stockton, Cal. 95202
Zekman, Theodore N.	111 N. Wabash Ave.	Chicago, Ill. 60602
Zeller, Robt. W.	1115 S. W. Taylor St.	Portland, Ore. 97205
Zeman, Theodore C.	2600 H St.	Sacramento, Cal. 95816
Zemer, Edw. A.	3305 Grove Ave.	Berwyn, Ill. 60403
Zepp, Charles E.	673 East River	Elyria, O. 44035
Zilka, Nadim	212 Jackson Ave.	Syosset, N. Y. 11791
Zimmermann, Albert W., Jr..	635 Germantown Pike	Norristown, Pa. 19401
Zimmerman, Alvin	1062 Murrieta Blvd.	Livermore, Cal. 94550
Zimmerman, Ernest M.	1800 Eye St. N. W.	Washington, D. C. 20006
Zimmerman, Leon W.	664 Farmington Ave.	Hartford, Conn. 06105
Zimmerman, Mervin H.	1801 Eye St. N.W.	Washington, D. C. 20006
Zimmerman, William G.	435 Cherry St. S. E.	Grand Rapids, Mich. 49502
Zingaro, Frank F.	111 Centre St.	Nutley, N. J. 07110
Zinn, Sheldon	555 W. Catalina Dr.	Phoenix, Ariz. 85013
Ziskin, Daniel E.	6317 Wilshire Blvd.	Los Angeles, Cal. 90048
Zopf, Delvin L.	8790 W. Colfax Ave.	Lakewood, Colo. 80215
Zescheile, F. Paul, III	1207 Fairchild Ct.	Woodland, Cal. 95695
Zubero, Jose L.	2505 Riverside Ave.	Jacksonville, Fla. 32204
Zucker, Leon	29 Central Ave.	Waterbury, Conn. 06702
Zuckerman, Bernard D.	2 Church St. S.	New Haven, Conn. 06519
Zuckerman, Joshua E.	875 Park Ave.	New York, N. Y. 10021
Zugsmith, Geo. S.	1350 W. 7th St.	San Pedro, Cal. 90732
Zullo, Jas. E.	104 Kingsboro Ave.	Gloversville, N. Y. 12078
Zweifach, Philip H.	40 E. 66th St.	New York, N. Y. 10021
Zweng, H. Christian	300 Homer Ave.	Palo Alto, Cal. 94301

Supplementum

Aaron, Stuart D.	251 Riverside Ave.	Westport, Conn. 06880
Aggarwal, Saroj	9119 Miles Ave.	Cleveland, Ohio 44105
Aiello, Michal V.	7801 - 4th Ave.	Brooklyn, New York 11209
Aiken, Jerry H.	9985 Sierra Ave.	Fontana, Calif. 92335
Akashi, Ronald H.	823 S. Atlantic Blvd.	Monterey Park, Calif. 91754
Alford, W. Eugene	902 Frostwood	Houston, Texas 77024
Alley, Albert A.	12th & Oak Streets	Lebanon, Penna. 17042
Allie, Allen J.	2299 Bacon St.	Concord, Calif. 94520
Alloway, W. Lyle	6019 N. Campbell	Chicago, Illinois 60659
Almquist, Howard T.	Walter Reed General Hospital	Wash., D.C. 20012
Amalong, Ronald J.	600 South Orlando Ave.	Maitland, Fla. 32751
Amin, Navinkumar J.	607 N. Grand	St. Louis, Mo. 63119
Anderson, Rodney A.	1805 E. 19th St.	Cheyenne, Wyoming 82001
Antonucci, Louis	2495 Kensington Ave.	Snyder, New York 14226
Apostol, John G.	815 E. Main St.	Medford, Oregon 97501

Appleby, Reid S., Jr. ..... 552 Toll Gate Rd. .... Warwick, Rhode Island 02886
Applegate, Francis R. ..... 1010 Downing Ave. .... Hays, Kansas 67601
Arny, Peter D. .... 451 North Dunlap .... St. Paul, Minn. 55104
Ashley, John D. .... 401 East 'C' St. .... North Platte, Nebraska 69101

Askew, Wallace A. .... 2916 North Third St. .... Phoenix, Arizona 85012
Asseff, Carl F. .... 2475 East 22nd St. .... Cleveland, Ohio 44115
Atkinson, Stewart .... 705 Juniper St., N.E. .... Atlanta, Georgia 30308
Awan, Khalid J. .... 218 - 13th St. .... Norton, Virginia 24273
Azar, George J. Jr. .... 4731 North Blvd. .... Baton Rouge, Louisiana 70806

Bachner, Irving N. .... 9 Central St. .... Lowell, Mass. 01852
Baise, George R. .... 288 Main St. .... Winchester, Mass. 01890
Baker, Walter J. .... 633 Washington Rd. .... Pittsburgh, Penna. 15228
Baker, William L. .... 1515 - 10th St. .... Monroe, Wisconsin 53566
Ballou, Gordon S. .... 939 E. Emerald Ave. .... Knoxville, Tenn. 37917
Banholzer, John A. .... 419 6th St. .... Juneau, Alaska 99801
Barbee, John Y., Jr. ..,... 1919 State St. .... New Albany, Indiana 47150
Barnett, James M. .... 2416 Peck St. .... Muskegon Hts., Michigan 49444

Barnwell, William L. ...... 1217 Memorial Dr. .... Dalton, Georgia 30720
Barr, Daniel R. .... 1025 David Whitney Bldg. ..... Detroit, Michigan 48226
Barron, Arnold .... 9400 East Rosecrans .... Bellflower, Calif. 90706
Basinski, Jerome V. ...... 301 West Lincoln .... Belleville, Illinois 62221
Bass, Walter R. .... 9503 East 63rd .... Raytown, Missouri 64133
Beams, Ronald N. .... 5506 E. 16th St. .... Indianapolis, Indiana 46218
Bedell, R. Bruce .... 501 Insurance Exchange Bldg. .. Sioux City, Iowa 51101
Bedotto, Carmine .... 120 West Palmetto Park Rd. .... Boca Raton, Florida 33432
Behrendt, Thomas .... 1025 Walnut St. .... Philadelphia, Penna. 19107
Behrens, Myles M. .... 635 W. 165th St. .... New York, New York 10032
Beighle, Richard W. ...... 1903 Bancroft .... Missoula, Montana 59801
Beisner, Donald H. .... 600 So. Glenstone Blvd. .... Springfield, Missouri 65802
Belkowitz, Martin J. ...... 7 Walker .... Fort Leavenworth, Kansas 66027

Bell, Randall W. .... 200 Eagle Rd. ....:.... Wayne, Penna. 19087
Beltran, Rafael .... 910 Grand Concourse .... Bronx, New York 10451
Bercovici, Edwin B. ...... 9001 North 76th St. .... Milwaukee, Wisc. 53223
Bergsma, Donald R. ...... National Eye Institute .... Bethesda, Maryland 20014
Bergstrom, Terry J. .... USAF Regional Hosp. .... March AFB, Calif. 92508
Berman, M. Jay .... 4545 Fanuel .... San Diego, Calif. 92109
Bersier, Andre M. .... 2660 Main St. .... Bridgeport, Conn. 06606
Bertuch, A. William ...... U.S. Naval Hospital .... Philadelphia, Penna. 19145
Bigger, John F., Jr. .... 4901 Barnes Hospital Plaza ..... St. Louis, Missouri 63110
Billman, Herbert R. ...... Medical Arts Bldg. .... Minneapolis, Minn. 55402
Black, Thomas C., Jr. ..... 601 East 63rd .... Kansas City, Missouri 64110
Blahnik, C. L. .... 417 Monroe .... Green Bay, Wisconsin 54301
Blankenship, George W. ... 15th & Lake St. .... San Francisco, Calif. 94114
Blitzer, Ronald J. .... 546 St. Georges Ave. .... Rahway, New Jersey 07065
Bobo, Charles B. .... 1184 Edgefield St. .... Greenwood, South Carolina 29646

Bohigian, George M. ...... U.S. Naval Hospital .... Camp Lejeune, North Carolina 28542

Bosland, Jon H. .... 1051 116th N.E. .... Bellevue, Washington 98004
Bowe, Richard G. .... Allenmore Medical Ctr. .... Tacoma, Washington 98405
Bowers, Robert G., Jr. .... Scott & White Clinic .... Temple, Tex. 76501

Bowman, David H.	501 Howard Ave.	Altoona, Penna. 16635
Brachvogel, Max W.	Allenmore Medical Center	Tacoma, Wash. 98405
Bradley, Charles K.	1128 Vine St.	Gainesville, Ga. 30501
Brandenberg, Karl B.	1550 West Rosedale	Fort Worth, Tex. 76104
Brandt, David E.	3825 West 9th St.	Waterloo, Iowa 50702
Brandt, Eugene M.	7080 Hollywood Blvd.	Los Angeles, Calif. 90028
Brar, B. S.	24 Baldwin Ave.	Jersey City, N.J. 07304
Brar, G. K.	2374 Steuben St.	Union, N.J. 07083
Brayton, John R., Jr.	1750 N. Palafox St.	Pensacola, Fla. 32502
Brenner, R. Larry	3320 Plainview	Pasadena, Tex. 77504
Bresky, Roy H.	950 N. Federal Highway	Pompano Beach, Fla. 33062
Briska, Philip T.	USN Hospital	Camp Pendleton, Calif. 92055
Brose, Brenda R.	636 Church St.	Evanston, Ill. 60201
Brounley, David W.	920 Atlantic Ave.	Long Beach, Calif. 90813
Brown, Bernice Z.	1155 No. Vermont Ave.	Los Angeles, Calif. 90029
Brown, David C.	2150 West First St.	Ft. Myers, Fla. 33901
Brown, Harry S.	515 E. Micheltorena	Santa Barbara, Calif. 93103
Brown, Richard M.	680 Church St. N.E.	Marietta, Ga. 30060
Brown, Robert H.	215 East 64th St.	New York, N.Y. 10021
Bruckner, Howard L.	1911 Valley Spring Rd.	Augusta, Ga. 30904
Bryan, Albert H.	Medical Center	Yakima, Washington 98902
Bryant, John A.	975 Ryland St.	Reno, Nevada 89502
Buckley, Theresa L. R.	1160 West Howard Ave.	Biloxi, Miss. 39530
Buerk, Gerald S.	530 Main St.	Hamilton, Ohio 45013
Burns, Frank M.	509 W. Main St.	Dothan, Ala. 36301
Burns, Stanley B.	108 East 66th St.	New York, N.Y. 10021
Burress, Donald A.	Gresham Community Hospital ..	Gresham, Ore. 97030
Bystrom, John T.	1350 So. Eliseo Dr.	Greenbrae, Calif. 94904
Caldwell, John B. H.	301 Medical Arts Bldg.	Richmond, Va. 23219
Calhoun, J. Bryant	333 N. San Mateo Dr.	San Mateo, Calif. 94401
Calhoun, Joseph H.	2600 N. Lawrence St.	Philadelphia, Pa. 19130
Calogeris, Constance M. ...	9400 East Rosecrans	Bellflower, Calif. 90706
Cameron, Robert W.	50 S. Ninth East	Salt Lake City, Utah 84102
Campbell, Mearl L.	2165 Fourth St.	Livermore, Calif. 94550
Campbell, William H.	1411 West 4th St.	Coffeyville, Kansas 67337
Cantolino, S. J.	801 Manatee Ave. W.	Bradenton, Fla. 33505
Carlson, Clifford A.	3366 Oakdale Ave. N.	Robbinsdale, Minn. 55422
Carothers, Gary G.	Womack Army Hospital	Fort Bragg, N.C. 28307
Carpentieri, Joseph C.	21 Woodland St.	Hartford, Conn. 06105
Carreno, Octavio B.	5522 S.W. 8th St.	Miami, Fla. 33134
Carroll, Robert McH.	246 E. State St.	Westport, Conn. 06880
Carrozza, Harry D.	5735 Ridge Ave.	Philadelphia, Pa. 19128
Carson, Stanley	1155 N. Vermont Ave.	Los Angeles, Calif. 90029
Casebeer, J. Charles	1355 North Beaver St.	Flagstaff, Arizona 86001
Caspar, George H.	11104 S.E. Stark St.	Portland, Ore. 97216
Catullo, D. Lawrence	22 Hamilton Ave.	Yonkers, N.Y. 10705
Cerasoli, James R.	Denver General Hospital	Denver, Colo. 80204
Chan, Anne K.	1601 Spring Garden St.	Philadelphia, Pa. 19130
Chandler, Billy M.	406 W. Pershing Blvd.	North Little Rock, Ark. 72114
Chapin, Leverett L.	1500 16th Ave. Court	Greeley, Colo. 80631
Charles, Norman C.	30 Central Park So.	New York, N.Y. 10019
Chaudhry, M. Anwar	163 Engle St.	Englewood, N.J. 07631
Chen, Vivian	2 Hillwood Rd.	East Brunswick N.J. 08816
Cherubini, Thomas D.	103 East 84th St.	New York, N.Y. 10028

Chishti, Muhammad I.	550 First Ave.	New York, N.Y. 10016
Choi, Chung S.	Daniel Boone Clinic	Harlan, Kentucky 40831
Chowchuvech, Endliam ...	1249 Fifth Ave.	New York, N.Y. 10029
Chylack, Leo T., Jr.	721 Huntington Ave.	Boston, Mass. 02115
Cignetti, Franklin E.	95 Kirkham St.	San Francisco, Calif. 94122
Citron, George B.	556 Main St.	Waltham, Mass. 02154
Civitella, Thomas R.	Naval Submarine Medical Center .	Groton, Conn. 06340
Clark, Gerald	Trover Clinic	Madisonville, Ky. 42431
Clark, Robert L.	207 E. Watauga Ave.	Johnson City, Tenn. 37601
Cofield, D. Dean	351 S. Lincoln	Bloomington, Ind. 47401
Cohen, David N.	National Naval Medical Center ..	Bethesda, Maryland 20014
Cohen, Mark M.	280 W. MacArthur Blvd.	Oakland, Calif. 94611
Cole, Rosser R.	119 N. Locke	Farmington, New Mex. 87401
Coleman, Ernest H., Jr.	4000 Market St.	Camp Hill, Pa. 17011
Coles, William H.	80 Barre St.	Charleston, S.C. 29401
Compton, John D. Jr.	1184, Edgefield St.	Greenwood, S.C. 29646
Condon, Thomas J.	390 Main St.	Worcester, Mass. 01608
Connell, Milton M.	1430 North 5th St.	Phoenix, Ariz. 85004
Connelly, Michael W.	120 First Capitol Dr.	St. Charles, Mo. 63301
Cook, Jerry W.	7010 North Cherry	Kansas City, Mo. 64118
Cooper, Jack M.	1224 Lowry Medical Arts Bldg. .	St. Paul, Minn. 55102
Coover, Richard B.	9611 Champion Court	Manassas, Va. 22110
Corbett, Dennis F.	650 Franklin St.	Schenectady, N.Y. 12305
Cotten, Milam S.	705 Hall Avenue	Hattiesburg. Miss. 39401
Cottingham, Andrew J., Jr. .	Eye Clinic, 130th Station Hospital, APO	N.Y. 09102
Cowden, John W.	130th General Hospital APO ...	N.Y. 09696
Cox, William V.	189 Jefferson Ave.	Salem, Mass. 01970
Craig, Elson L.	466 W. Tenth Ave.	Columbus, Ohio 43210
Crary, Ely J.	4730 Austell Rd.	Austell, Ga. 30001
Crawford, John R.	Ketner Center	Salisbury, N.C. 28144
Crawford, John R., III	1610 Vaughn Rd.	Burlington, N.C. 27215
Creasman, John P, ...	500 West 10th Place	Mesa, Arizona 85201
Crotty, Garrett J.	2100 N. Orange Ave.	Orlando, Fla. 32804
Crowder, Benjamin M.	560 Ave. K, S.E.	Winter Haven, Fla. 33880
Cunin, Burton M.	100 Constitution Plaza	Hartford, Conn. 06103
Cupples, Howard P.	U.S. Naval Hospital	Newport, R.I. 02840
Currie, Hugh B.	15 Medical Dr.	Amarillo, Tex. 79106
Custer, Allen L.	6226 196th S.W.	Lynnwood, Wash. 98036
Dahl, Andrew A.	140 Main St.	Fishkill, N.Y. 12524
Dankmyer, Frederick L. ...	300 S. Centre St.	Pottsville, Pa. 17901
Davidorf, Frederick H.	320 West Tenth Ave.	Columbus, Ohio 43210
Davidson, A. Dale	1017 E. First St.	Duluth, Minn. 55805
Davidson, J. David	1720 8th Ave., So.	Birmingham, Ala 35233
Davis, Floyd L. O.	So. Fulton Professional Plaza ...	East Point, Ga. 30344
Davis, Wilkes H., Jr.	Vanderbilt Univ. Hospital	Nashville, Tenn. 37232
Davisson, Walter F., Jr.	913 Leslie Blvd.	Jefferson City, Mo. 65101
Deligeorges, John	7010 N. Cherry	Kansas City, Mo. 64118
Denler, Loren L.	Loma Linda University Medical Center	Loma Linda, Calif. 92354
Dephouse, Don A.	30 E. Ninth St.	Holland, Mich. 49423
Dieruf, William J.	3080 Ackerman Blvd.	Kettering, Ohio 45429
Diller, Duane A.	5055 N. Greeley Ave.	Portland, Ore. 97217
DiMarco, Joseph C.	78 So. Main St.	Phillipsburg, N.J. 08865
Dinter, George	1602 A East Ocean Blvd.	Stuart, Fla. 33494

Dixon, Thomas M.	521 Third Street West	Sonoma, Calif. 95476
Dorn, Paul A.	4302 St. Barnabas Rd.	Marlow Hts., Md. 20031
Doty, John W.	1001 Second St., West	Ashland, Wisc. 54806
Dreher, Robert J.	11 Maple St.	Rockland, Maine 04841
Dreyer, David J.	7 Wentworth St.	Rochester, N.H. 03867
Dunn, Francis C., Jr.	1725 South St.	Geneva, Ill. 60134
Dunn, Michael W.	1077 North Ave.	New Rochelle, N.Y. 10804
DuPont, George Z.	3325 No. Broadway	Los Angeles, Calif. 90031
Dvorak, David G.	212 Bronson Medical Center	Kalamazoo, Mich. 49006
Ebersole, Carl M.	1760 Gold St.	Redding, Calif. 96001
Edelstein, Arthur J.	3637 Century Blvd.	Lynwood, Calif. 90262
Ederington, John B.	1301 Washington St.	Vicksburg, Miss. 39180
Edwards, David A., Jr.	16870 W. Bernardo Dr.	San Diego, Calif. 92127
Ehrhardt, Alan A.	130 Warren St.	Beaver Dam. Wisc. 53916
Eichler, Philip N.	50 Newark Ave.	Belleville, N.J. 07109
Ellingsen, Bruce A.	S 427 Bernard	Spokane, Wash. 99204
Emery, Jared M.	Baylor College of Medicine	Houston, Tex. 77025
Eriksen, David E.	1614 S. Byrne Rd.	Toledo, Ohio 43614
Errico, J. M.	319 Westwood Ave.	High Point, N.C. 27262
Everett, Charles J.	428 Decatur St.	Sandusky, Ohio 44870
Fagelman, Jerry S.	28043 Hoover	Warren, Michigan 48093
Farber, Joseph M.	420 Estudillo Ave.	San Leandro, Calif. 94577
Fargason, Crayton A.	U.S. Naval Hospital	Camp Lejeune, N.C. 28542
Farrell, Thomas A.	Mary Imogene Bassett Hospital	Cooperstown, N.Y. 13326
Faulkner, H. Wade	1359 Springhill Ave.	Mobile, Alabama 36604
Favata, John	1389 West Main St.	Waterbury, Conn. 06708
Federman, Jay L.	Lankenau Hospital	Philadelphia, Penna. 19151
Fetkenhour, Carl L.	303 E. Chicago Ave.	Chicago, Ill. 60611
Fezza, Andrew J.	2447 Whitney Ave.	Hamden, Conn. 06518
Fine, I. Howard	Eugene Medical Center	Eugene, Oregon 97401
Fiore, John V., Jr.	12892 Palm St.	Garden Grove, Calif. 92640
Fischbein, Fredric I.	80 South Main St.	Middletown, Conn. 06457
Fitzgerald, Constance R.	University of Florida	Gainesville, Fla. 32601
FitzGerald, James L., Jr.	322 Dewey St.	Bennington, Vt. 05201
Fivian, Gerald J.	1035 Bellevue Ave.	St. Louis, Mo. 63117
Flaxel, John T.	Medical Center Bldg.	North Bend, Ore. 97459
Flickinger, Roger R., Jr.	102 E. Main St.	Waukesha, Wisc. 53186
Floerchinger, James S.	1612 Tremont	Denver, Colo. 80202
Ford, Charles R.	1305 N. West St.	Wichita, Kans. 67203
Forster, Richard K.	1638 N.W. 10th Ave.	Miami, Fla. 33152
Framm, Daniel H.	1515 Chain Bridge Rd.	McLean, Va. 22101
France, Thomas D.	University Hospitals	Madison, Wisc. 53706
Frank, Marvin G.	744 Galloping Hill Rd.	Roselle Park, N.J. 07204
Franklin, Stephen H.	1303 Delaware Ave.	Wilmington, Del. 19806
Frederiksen, Michael J.	USPHS Hospital	Fort Defiance, Ariz. 86504
Freeman, Melvin I.	1118-9th Ave.	Seattle, Wash. 98101
Freshman, Michael E.	2400 21st St.	Troy, N.Y. 12180
Friedman, Alan H.	111 East 210th St.	Bronx, New York 10467
Frueh, Bartley R.	909 University Ave.	Columbia, Mo. 65201
Fulhorst, H. William	Tripler Army Medical Center, Box 192, APO	San Francisco 96438
Fulwyler, R. L.	U.S. Naval Hospital – Boston	Chelsea, Mass. 02150
Gaasterland, Douglas E.	National Institute of Health, National Eye Institute	Bethesda, Md. 20014
Gabriels, F. Forrest	808 B Madison Ave.	Albany, N.Y. 12208
Gardner, Philip L.	2241 Central Ave.	Alameda, Calif. 94501

Gardner, Richard E.	17 Terry Court	Staunton, Va. 24401
Gartner, Joseph F.	1249 Savannah Highway	Charleston, S.C. 29407
Gaudio, Alexander R.	85 Jefferson St.	Hartford, Conn. 06106
Geiger, Gerald F.	422 North Hastings Ave.	Hastings, Nebraska 68901
George, Donald E.	2 South Street	Auburn, N.Y. 13021
Gerber, Melvin	5200 Braeburn Dr.	Bellaire, Tex. 77401
Gerkin, David G.	1928 Alcoa Highway	Knoxville, Tenn. 37920
Gieser, Richard G.	1492 N. Main St.	Wheaton, Ill. 60187
Gillett, Robert B.	10 Oakdale	Houston, Tex. 77006
Gilman, Michael	91 School St.	Springfield, Mass. 01105
Ginsberg, Stephen P.	1812 K St. N.W.	Washington, D.C. 20006
Gleason, John R.	1712 Heyburn Bldg.	Louisville, Ky. 40202
Gleaton, Hugh E., Jr.	800 N. Fleming St.	Hendersonville, N.C. 28739
Glenn, John S.	24 Church St.	Torrington, Conn. 06790
Glodek, John F.	20 Lakeside Dr. West	Levittown, Penna, 19053
Gold, Daniel H.	Walter Reed Army Medical Center	Washington, D.C. 20012
Goldbaum, Michael H.	525 East 68th St.	New York, N.Y. 10021
Goldberg, Darryl T.	26789 Woodward	Huntington Woods, Mich. 48070
Goldman, Ronald J.	311 Del Mar Ave.	Chula Vista, Calif. 92010
Goldwyn, Robert H.	7400 North Kendall Dr.	Miami, Fla. 33156
Gombos, George M.	450 Clarkson Ave.	Brooklyn, N.Y. 11203
Goode, Fietcher H.	7994 Wilkinsville	Millington, Tenn. 38053
Goode, Michael I.	16260 Ventura Blvd.	Encino, Calif. 91316
Gordon, Joel S.	4715 Chestnut St.	Bethesda, Md. 20014
Gormley, Robert J.	723 Main St.	Niagara Falls, N.Y. 14092
Gorn, Robert A.	53 Pond Ave.	Brookline, Mass. 02146
Grady, Frank J.	USPHS Hospital	Galveston, Tex. 77550
Graham, James L., Jr.	231 Lexington Medical Mall	West Columbia, S.C. 29169
Grant, Frederick J.	100 Casa St.	San Luis Obispo, Calif. 93401
Greenfield, Val S.	5001 Frankford Ave.	Philadelphia, Pa. 19124
Greenspan, Irwin	23-91 Bell Blvd.	Bayside, N.Y. 11360
Gregory, Conrad	3958 Convention St.	Baton Rouge, La. 70815
Griffiths, John D.	8601 West Dodge Rd.	Omaha, Neb. 68114
Grover, Norman R.	Raymond W. Bliss Army Hospital	Fort Huachuca, Ariz. 85613
Gudas, Peter P., Jr.	77 Warren St.	Brighton, Mass. 02135
Guyton, William F.	1208 N.W. 6th St.	Gainesville, Fla. 32601
Guzak, Steven V., Jr.	1115 Republic Bldg.	Denver, Colo. 80202
Haas, Howard J.	315 Alberta Dr.	Amherst, N.Y. 14226
Hackett, John N.	507 S. LaGrange Rd.	LaGrange, Ill. 60525
Haddad, N. J.	16 Murray Ave.	Annapolis, Md. 21401
Hagadus, Ronald J.	410 Bedford Rd.	Bedford Hills, N.Y. 10507
Hall, Marvin K., Jr.	401 Pinecrest Dr. E.	Marshall, Tex. 75670
Hall, Robert E.	Blount Prof. Bldg.	Knoxville, Tenn. 37920
Harper, David G.	205 West 2nd St.	Duluth, Minn. 55803
Harrell, Wade W.	319 Westwood Ave.	High Point, N.C. 27262
Harris, Gilbert W.	309 E. Church	Marshalltown, Iowa 50158
Harris, Laurence S.	1249 Fifth Ave.	New York, N.Y. 10029
Harris, William K.	3325 N. Interstate Ave.	Portland, Ore. 97210
Hartman, Joseph	3994 Park Blvd.	San Diego, Calif. 92103
Hattenhauer, John M.	614 1st St.	Wausau, Wisc. 54401
Hehn, Richard W.	2nd St. & Sherman Ave.	Coeur d'Alene, Idaho 83814
Hein, Herbert F.	50 Park Pl.	Newark, N.J. 07101
Heiss, Robert E.	1900 W. Littleton Blvd.	Littleton, Colo. 80120
Hermundstad, Orin A.	1520 Vernon St.	Stoughton, Wisc. 53589

Herring, H. J.	Hammondsport Rd.	Bath, N.Y. 14810
Heyner, Gregory J.	6740 Forest Hill Ave.	Richmond, Va. 23225
Hicks, Edward L.	U.S. Naval Hospital	Great Lakes, Ill. 60088
Hillman, Milton H.	7080 Hollywood Blvd.	Los Angeles, Calif. 90028
Himelstein, Samuel C.	810 Enfield St.	Enfield, Conn. 06082
Hirose, Tatsuo	100 Charles River Plaza	Boston, Mass. 02114
Ho, Samuel S.	423 Main St.	Laconia, N.H. 03246
Hodes, Barton L.	701 Deerfield Rd.	Deerfield, Ill. 60015
Hofmann, Ronald J.	512 Davenport Bank Bldg.	Davenport, Iowa 52801
Hofmann, William B.	512 Davenport Bank Bldg.	Davenport, Iowa 52801
Holmstrom, Robert D.	1720 N. 8th St.	Sheboygan, Wisc. 53081
Horowitz, Philip	Barclay Pavilion, Rte. 70	Cherry Hill, N.J. 08034
Householder, John A.	22775 Pacific Coast Hwy.	Malibu, Calif. 90265
Houser, Ben P., Jr.	458 E. Broad St.	Tamaqua, Pa. 18252
Huberman, Jean Pierre	USAH	Ft. Carson, Colo. 80907
Huberman, Richard	4660 Kenmore Ave.	Alexandria, Va. 22304
Huerter, Quentin C.	771 New Brotherhood Bldg.	Kansas City, Kan. 66101
Hughes, Ronald M.	1365 Clifton Rd.	Atlanta, Ga. 30322
Hulbert, James E.	1329 Broadway	Longview, Wash. 98632
Hull, William M., Jr.	1355 Ebenezer Rd.	Rock Hill, S.C. 27930
Humphrey, William T.	243 Charles St.	Boston, Mass. 02114
Hunt, E. Woodrow, Jr.	Box 64, Naval Hospital, M.C.B.	Camp Pendleton, Calif. 92055
Hunter, David M.	Wilford Hall Hospital, Lackland A.F.B.	San Antonio, Tex. 78236
Hunter, Lawrence H.	61 Eastern Parkway	Brooklyn, N.Y. 11238
Hutson, Rodney K.	6200 Hillcroft	Houston, Tex. 77036
Hutt, Alfred	10 Hospital Dr.	Holyoke, Mass. 01040
Hutton, John E.	232 Baltimore St.	Hanover, Pa. 17331
Hutton, William L.	Bascom-Palmer Eye Institute	Miami, Fla. 33152
Hyman, Barry N.	Baylor University	Houston, Tex. 77025
Irish, Ann	5500 Ridge Rd.	Cleveland, Ohio 44129
Jackson, Stephen M.	30th Field Hospital, APO	New York 09178
Jacobs, Ivan R.	6200 Wilshire Blvd.	Los Angeles, Calif. 90048
Jarudi, Nabil I.	University Hospital	Iowa City, Iowa 52240
Johnson, Alvin	1761 Gordon Rd. S.W.	Atlanta, Ga. 30310
Johnson, Darryl L.	3433 So. La Fountain	Kokomo, Ind. 46901
Johnson, Frank D.	1406 W. High	Mt. Pleasant, Mich. 48858
Johnson, Jeff	1903 Broadway	Paducah, Ky. 42001
Jones, Charles E.	2918 Hamilton Blvd.	Sioux City, Iowa 51104
Jones, Dan B.	Baylor College of Medicine	Houston, Tex. 77025
Jones, David G.	501 N. 17th St	Allentown, Pa. 18104
Jones, Frank L.	USAF Medical Center	Wright-Patterson AFB Ohio 45433
Jones, John D.	1312 Main St.	Lubbock, Tex. 79401
Jones, Robert N.	224 West Evergreen	San Antonio, Tex. 78212
Jones, Wirt A.	478 Peachtree St. N.E.	Atlanta, Ga. 30308
Jordan, Herman C.	136th St. and Lenox Ave., Harlem Hospital Center	New York, New York 10037
Jorgensen, Roger L.	1350 Tulip	Longmont, Colo. 80501
Judge, James W.	607 Carey Ave.	Wilkes Barre, Pa. 18702
Jurtshuk, Tania	30 Fifth Ave.	New York, N.Y. 10011
Kaplan, Martin B.	4450 West 76th St.	Edina, Minn. 55435
Kaplan, Rosalind P.	55 Seacord Rd.	New Rochelle, N.Y. 10804
Karlsberg, Robert C.	4528 Central Ave.	St. Petersburg, Fla. 33711
Kassoff, Aaron	980 Western Ave.	Albany, N.Y. 12203

Katzen, Leeds E.	301 St. Paul Place.	Baltimore, Md. 21202
Katzin, Dick	230 Lothrop St.	Pittsburgh, Pa. 15213
Kaur, Surinder	301 St. Paul Place	Baltimore, Md. 21202
Kearney, John J.	243 Charles St.	Boston, Mass. 02114
Keatts, James G.	1010 Federal Rd.	Houston, Tex. 77015
Kelertas, Algimantas	Veterans Administration Hospital	Hines, Ill. 60141
Kelly, Gordon R.	121 West St.	Rutland, Vt. 05701
Kelly, Thomas L.	9 Central Street, Lowell	Massachusetts 01852
Kenny, Geves S.	1961 Fourth Ave.	San Diego Calif. 92101
Kim, Yong J.	2230 Lynn Rd.	Thousand Oaks, Calif. 91360
King, Yum Y.	1008 West 11th	Pine Bluff, Ark. 71601
Kingham, James D.	8700 W. Wisconsin	Milwaukee, Wisc. 53233
Kini, Mohandas M.	750 Harrison Ave.	Boston, Mass. 02118
Kirby, Charles G.	305-67th St. W.	Bradenton, Fla. 33505
Knapp, Don B., II	3639 Central Avenue	St. Petersburg, Fla. 33713
Knutzen, John H.	260 Cohasset Lane	Chico, Calif. 95926
Koerner, Alan	4900 Sunset Blvd.	Los Angeles, Calif. 90027
Kohlhepp, Paul A.	300 Hospital Dr.	Glen Burnie, Md. 21061
Kolder, Hansjoerg EJW	University Hospital	Iowa City, Iowa 52240
Koller, Harold P.	Barclay Pavilion – East	Cherry Hill, N.J. 08034
Kontra, Dennis J.	5200 Washington Ave.	Racine, Wisc. 53406
Kozart, David M.	1930 Chestnut St.	Philadelphia, Pa. 19103
Krachmer, Jay H.	210 State St.	New Orleans, La. 70118
Kraft, William E.	7906 Buffalo Ave.	Niagara Falls, N.Y. 14304
Kramer, Steven G.	Madigan General Hospital, Box 111	Tacoma, Wash. 98431
Krinzman, Edward A.	2100 E. Hallandale Beach Blvd. .	Hallandale, Fla. 33009
Krug, James A.	32238 Schoolcraft	Livonia, Mich. 48150
Kulvin, Stephen M.	1688 Meridian Ave.	Miami Beach, Fla. 33139
Kurland, Louis R.	3419 Johnson St.	Hollywood, Fla. 33021
Kut, Leonard J.	8625 So. Cicero	Chicago Ill. 60652
Kutner, Stephen S.	Baptist Professional Bldg.	Atlanta, Ga. 30312
Kwedar, Stephen	1025 S. 7th St.	Springfield, Ill. 62703
Lafluer, Kenneth C.	P.O. Box 1090	Opelousas, La. 70570
Lagomarsino, William E. ...	Medical Arts Clinic.	Corsicana, Tex. 75110
Laino, Peter L.	525 E. 68th	New York, N.Y. 10021
LaMarche, Donald E.	93 Washington St.	Taunton, Mass. 02780
Lambert, Brent W.	HMR Box 1845, Keesler AFB ...	Biloxi, Miss. 39534
Lambert, Joseph N.	1401 Avocado Ave.	Newport Beach, Calif. 92660
Lamm, Ronald M.	1720 North 'E' St.	Pensacola, Fla. 32501
Lanard, Margaret S.	3637 Century Blvd.	Lynwood, Calif. 90262
Langerman, David W.	1 Prel Plaza	Orangeburg, N.Y. 10962
Langston, Deborah P.	243 Charles St.	Boston, Mass. 02114
Lanter, David L.	1515 Chain Bridge Rd.	McLean, Va. 22101
LaPiana, Francis G.	Walter Reed General Hospital ...	Washington, D.C. 20012
Larson, Allen K.	3939 W. 50th St.	Edina, Minn. 55424
Lashier, Harvey M.	607 N. Central Ave.	Glendale, Calif 91203
Lauring, Lewis M.	Letterman General Hospital	San Francisco, Calif. 94129
Layden, William E.	301 E. Walnut St.	Louisville, Ky. 40202
Layer, James M.	3939 W. 50th St.	Minneapolis, Minn. 55424
Lazenby, G. William	4312 U.S. Highway 19 No.	Tarpon Springs, Fla. 33589
Lederman, Martin E.	1515 Chain Bridge Rd.	McLean, Va. 22101
Lee, Rory T. Y.	Veterans Administration Hospital	Oteen, N.C. 28805
Lees, John	2715 Willetta St.	Albany, Ore. 97321
Leffler, Martha B.	4790 Montgomery Rd.	Ellicott City, Md. 21043
Lefler, W. Hampton	110 East A St.	Newton, N.C. 28658

Lenartz, Bruce J.	640 E. Grand Ave.	Escondido, Calif. 92025
Leonard, Richard B.	1185 Dundee Ave.	Elgin, Ill. 60120
Lernor, Richard E.	2040 W. Wisconsin Ave.	Milwaukee, Wisc. 53233
Leslie, C. Doyle	1301 West 38th St.	Austin, Tex. 78705
Levenson, Ernest	3126 So. 27th St.	Milwaukee, Wisc. 53215
Levin, Jules S.	Professional Bldg., Augustine Cut Off	Wilmington, Del. 19803
Levine, Joel R.	61 Camino Alto	Mill Valley, Calif. 94941
Levy, Robert M.	301 Ebbtide Dr.	North Palm Beach, Fla. 33408
Le Win, Donald P.	Doctors Bldg.	Minneapolis, Minn. 55402
Lewis, Jeffrey	605 Park Ave.	New York, N.Y. 10021
Lewis, Leon V.	5727 Main St.	Williamsville, N.Y. 14221
Lewis, Norman G., Jr.	528 Nautilus St.	La Jolla, Calif. 92037
Lichtig, Michael L.	279 Third Ave.	Long Branch, N.J. 07740
Linabery, Linferd G.	200 E. Main	Midland, Mich. 48640
Lindblad, Randolph M.	600 Meridian S.	Puyallup, Wash. 98371
Lindner, Milton J.	1014 Medical Arts Bldg.	San Antonio, Texas 78205
Linwong, Meth	1492 N. Main St.	Wheaton, Ill. 60187
Lippman, Jay I.	130 E. 18th St.	New York, N.Y. 10003
Lipson, Martin L.	516 Trail Ave.	Frederick, Md. 21701
Liu, Edward T.	Box 50, Stanaford Rd.	Beckley, West Va. 25801
Locke, Clyde R.	38-04 28th Ave.	Long Island City, N.Y. 11103
Logan, Neal J.	58 Davis Rd.	Westover AFB, Mass. 01022
Loree, Paul J.	1914 Colvin Blvd.	Tonawanda, New York 14150
Loreti, Michael R.	124 Gregory Ave.	Passaic, N.J. 07055
Lovell, Richard K.	P.O. Box 846	Russellville, Ark. 72801
Luber, Robert J.	1500 Shermer Rd.	Northbrook, Ill. 60062
Lucier, Alfred C.	30 Hampden Rd.	Upper Darby, Penna. 19082
McCaffery, Patrick G.	11411 Brookshire	Downey, Calif. 90241
McCaleb, William E., III	609 W. 32nd	Austin, Tex. 78705
McElroy, Wilbur J.	1616 West 8th	Topeka, Kan. 66606
McGee, Hugh E., Jr.	5 Pangborn Place	Hackensack, N.J. 07601
McGee, James P.	1716 Locust	Sterling, Ill. 61081
McGroarty, John J.	10614 Riverside Dr.	North Hollywood, Calif. 91602
McIsaac, Malcolm C.	154 Cazenovia St.	Buffalo, N.Y. 14210
McKendell, Lawrence V.	3505 Broadway	Oakland, Calif. 94611
McKinnon, Thomas D.	1717 - 11th Ave. So	Birmingham, Ala. 35205
McManus, Michael D.	1100 Sixth St.	Traverse City, Mich. 49684
McNeer, Paul R.	501 East Franklin St.	Richmond, Va. 23219
MacCarthy, Charles F.	614 First St.	Wausau, Wisc. 54401
Machanic, P. Brian	220 No. Washington St.	Rome, N.Y. 13440
Macias, Lambert C.	3411 N. 5th Ave.	Phoenix, Ariz. 85013
MacMillan, David W.	501 E. Franklin St.	Richmond, Va. 23219
Macoul, Kenneth L.	101 Amesbury St.	Lawrence, Mass. 01840
Mahar, Paul J.	Hitchcock Medical Center, Rt. 224	Yongstown, Ohio
Mahoney, Charles F., Jr.	514 Brick Blvd.	Brick Town, N.J. 08723
Malek, R. W.	43 Austin St.	Portsmouth, N.H. 03801
Mandel, Harvey J.	3725 Henry Hudson Parkway	Riverdale, New York 10463
Manguikian, Dertad	2150 Pennsylvania Ave. N.W.	Washington, D.C. 20037
Manning, Odeen	22554 Ventura Blvd.	Woodland Hills, Calif. 91364
Marak, George E. Jr.	1451 Belle Haven Rd.	Alexandria, Va. 22307

Maravalli, Camille J.	406 Main St.	Johnstown, Pa. 15901
Margherio, Raymond R.	3800 Woodward	Detroit, Mich. 48024
Markovits, Andrew S.	7512 Soquel Dr.	Aptos, Calif. 95003
Markowitz, Martin A.	5 Severance Circle	Cleveland Hts., Ohio 44118
Marquis, Malcolm M.	2209 Lloyd Center	Portland, Ore. 97232
Mase, Darrel J. Jr.	243 Sevilla Ave.	Coral Gables, Fla. 33134
Matas, Brian R.	2200 O'Farrell St.	San Francisco, Calif. 94105
Matusow, Gene R.	441 East 68th St.	New York, N.Y. 10021
Matusow, Paul D.	56 Doyer Ave.	White Plains, N.Y. 10605
May, Robert O.	USAF Medical Center, Keesler AFB	Biloxi, Miss. 39534
Melluish, James W.	350 S. Burdick Mall	Kalamazoo, Mich. 49006
Meltzer, Gerald E.	1666 Elmira St.	Aurora, Colo. 80010
Meltzer, Glenn A.	116 Belmont St.	Worcester, Mass 01605
Meltzer, Joseph F.	764 Park Ave.	New York, N.Y. 10021
Merey, John H.	235 East 2nd St.	New York, N.Y. 10010
Meshel, Leroy G.	2340 Clay St.	San Francisco, Calif. 94115
Meyer, Melvin E.	4424 Hampton Ave.	St. Louis, Mo. 63109
Meyer, Russell	1408 Hickman Dr.	Virginia Beach, Va. 23454
Michon, Joseph, Jr.	Eye Clinic, U.S. Army Hospital	Ft. Devens, Mass. 01433
Mielcarek, Leon M., Jr.	36 East Baltimore Pike	Media, Pa. 19063
Miller, Edward D.	3030 Lake Ave.	Fort Wayne, Ind. 46805
Miller, George L.	16542 Ventura Blvd.	Encino, Calif. 91316
Miller, George S.	303 George St.	New Brunswick, N.J. 08901
Miller, James B.	1127 Wilshire Blvd.	Los Angeles, Calif. 90017
Miller, Paul R.	Box 18, 97th General Hospital, APO	New York 09757
Mills, John E.	123 Congress St.	Pasadena, Calif. 91105
Milne, Milton J.	1111 Spring St.	Silver Spring, Md. 20910
Milt, Stephen C.	Eel River Circle #4	Plymouth, Mass. 02360
Minaya, Jose	947 West 8th St.	Los Angeles, Calif. 90017
Mineo, Cyrus L.	286 Griffen St.	Phoenixville, Pa. 19460
Miura, Calvin M.	US Army Hospital, Camp Zama, Japan, APO	San Francisco 96343
Mixon, William A.	1901 Oak Park Blvd.	Lake Charles, La. 70601
Moeller, Raymond H.	4340 West 95th St.	Oak Lawn, Ill. 60453
Mohr, Armin A. A.	1840 Skagit Village	Burlington, Wash. 98233
Monroe, William M.	Route 8, Box 376	Greenville, North Carolina 27834
Monterastelli, Albert N.	1708 N. Garey	Pomona, Calif. 91767
Moody, Everett A.	2105 W. Carpenter Fwy. West	Irving, Tex. 75062
Moody, Jackson C.	505 E. Pearl St.	Harrisonville, Mo. 64701
Moore, Gregory C.	Sea Girt Professional Bldg.	Sea Girt, New Jersey 08750
Moore, Lawrence W., Jr.	1110 W. Main St.	Durham, N.C. 27701
Morabito, Carmine D.	375 E. Main St.	Bayshore, N.Y. 11706
Morris, William R.	4230 Highway 51, S.	Memphis, Tenn. 38116
Morrison, David P.	106 E. State St.	Doylestown, Pa. 18901
Morse, Peter H.	3400 Spruce St.	Philadelphia, Pa. 19104
Moura, Roberto A.	6436 Fannin St.	Houston, Tex. 77025
Muldoon, Thomas O.	815 Fifth Ave.	New York, N.Y. 10023
Mumma, John V.	409 Camden St.	San Antonio, Tex. 78215
Mund, Michael L.	10 N.D. Perlman Pl.	New York, N.Y. 10003
Murphy, Edward B., Jr.	720 Harrison Ave.	Boston, Mass. 02165
Murray, W. Lee	11201 Colorado	Kansas City, Mo. 64137
Musson, Kenneth H.	1105 E. Front St.	Traverse City, Mich. 49684
Nagy, Frank M.	1755 Coburg Rd.	Eugene, Ore. 97401

Naidoff, Michael A.	3 D Hamill Rd.	Baltimore, Md. 21210
Nakanishi, Alan S.	McDonald Army Hospital	Fort Eustis, Va. 23604
Nasser, Robert E.	3549 Meadowbrook Dr.	Napa, Calif. 94558
Nathenson, Aeron L.	106-W Meadowbrook Bldg.	St. Louis Park, Minn. 55416
Nelson, Robert A.	2045 Jefferson St.	Napa, Calif. 94558
Nevins, Robert C., Jr.	705 N. Olive Ave.	West Palm Beach, Fla. 33401
Newman, Gordon H.	6011 Harry Hines Blvd.	Dallas, Tex. 75235
Newmark, Emanuel	Brooke Army Medical Center, Fort Sam	Houston, Tex. 78234
Newsom, William A.	620 SW 4th Ave.	Gainesville, Fla. 32601
Newton, Clyde A.	9 Belmont Ave.	Brattleboro, Vt. 05301
Nichols, Charles W.	3400 Spruce St.	Philadelphia, Pa. 19104
Nicklas, Thomas O.	814 South Walnut	Stillwater, Okla. 74074
Noah, Van B.	3821 Merton Dr.	Raleigh, N.C. 27609
Noorthoek, David J.	500 Grand Ave., So.	San Francisco, Calif. 94080
Norris, John L.	13222 Via Grande Ct.	Saratoga, Calif. 95070
Nosce, Luis V., Jr.	84 Burnham Rd.	West Hartford, Conn. 06110
Odrcic, Kazimir J.	211 N. Eddy	South Bend, Indiana 46617
Olsen, Gerald M.	1017 Robertson	Ft. Collins, Colorado 80521
Ott, F. Thomas	135 W. Adams Ave.	Kirkwood, Mo. 63122
Ottis, M. Larry	130 N.E. Manzanita Ave.	Grants Pass, Ore. 97526
Page, John A.	800 1st St.	Macon, Ga. 31201
Palena, Peter V.	Media Clinic.	Media, Penna. 19063
Palmer, Edward	100 Casals Place	Bronx, New York 10475
Palmer, Steven S.	515 Lakeside Drive, S. E.	Grand Rapids, Michigan 49506
Pangilinan, Rizal V.	Wheeling Clinic	Wheeling, West Va. 26003
Panichella, Thomas J.	124 Main St.	Huntington, New York 11743
Paris, George L.	1300 Grane St.	Menlo Park, Calif. 94025
Parisi, James A.	3245 Nostrand Ave.	Brooklyn, New York 11229
Patel, Dilipkumar J.	Albany Medical Center	Albany, N.Y. 12208
Pawlowski, Gene J.	13652 Cantara St.	Panorama City, Calif. 91402
Pearah, J. David	25 Stevens Ave.	West Lawn, Pa. 19609
Perkins, Donald F.	Greenfields Professional Bldg., Rt 45 & Griscom Rd.	Woodbury, N.J. 08096
Person, Donald H.	20420 Lake Chabot Rd.	Castro Valley, Calif. 94546
Phelps, Charles D.	University Hospitals	Iowa City, Iowa 52240
Piepergerdes, Larry G.	4240 Blue Ridge Blvd.	Kansas City, Mo. 64133
Pierce, Robert D.	405 West 15th St.	Pueblo, Collo. 81003
Pieroni, D. W.	1111 S. Raleigh Ave.	Sheffield, Alabama 35660
Pinto, Peter J.	140 E. 54th St.	New York, N.Y. 10022
Plager, Stephan D.	USAF Medical Center Scott	Belleville, Ill. 62225
Plummer, Leo J.	1040 4th St.	Des Moines, Iowa 50314
Poor, Stephen, J., III	349 Great Plain Ave.	Needham, Mass. 02192
Porter, Joel	Temple University Hospital	Philadelphia, Penna. 19140
Pratt, Jordan C.	2340 Eastern Blvd.	York, Pa. 17402
Prawak, Theodore P.	2645 Sheridan Dr.	Tonawanda, N.Y. 14150
Price, Ronald L.	2020 E. 93rd St.	Cleveland, Ohio 44106
Pryor, James G.	1110 Arnold Ave.	Point Pleasant, N.J. 08742
Putterman, Allen M.	111 No. Wabash	Chicago, Ill. 60602
Pyron, William W.	1204 13th Ave., S.E.	Decatur, Alabama 35601
Rahman, Moududur	634 North Grand Blvd.	St. Louis, Mo. 63103
Ramey, Ralph, Jr.	USAF Hospital Wiesbaden, APO	New York 09220
Ramsell, John T.	4239 Farnam St.	Omaha, Nebraska 68131

Rappaport, Alexander A. ...	8555 Tidewater Dr.	Norfolk, Va. 23503
Rashid, Richard C.	424 Division St., S.	Charleston, West Va. 25309
Rathbun, J. Earl	858 Fourth St.	Santa Rosa, Calif. 95403
Rayner, James W.	512 Van Buren Ave.	Oxford, Miss. 38655
Read, Frank W.	9 Deering St.	Portland, Maine 04101
Read, Silas C., Jr.	759 Cobb St.	Athens, Ga. 30601
Redding, Marshall S.	1142 N. Road Street	Elizabeth City, N.C. 27909
Reed, Ralph E.	12394 S.W. 82nd Ave.	Miami, Fla. 33156
Reeser, Frederick H., Jr. ...	243 Charles St.	Boston, Mass. 02114
Reinstein, Ned M.	USAF Regional Hospital	Minot, No. Dakota 58701
Reitman, Howard S.	1419 Delachaise St.	New Orleans, La. 70115
Relland, Maureen A.	737 Park Ave.	New York, N.Y. 10021
Reves, M. William	440 Brockton Ave.	Riverside, Calif. 92501
Richards, Paul F.	303 East Town St.	Columbus, Ohio 43215
Rickards, Charles R.	Professional Bldg., Augustine Cutoff	Wilmington, Del. 19803
Riekhof, F. Tempel	50 North Medical Dr.	Salt Lake City, Utah 84112
Ringer, Jerry N.	1008 N. Main St.	Bloomington, Ill. 61701
Roberts, James M.	5800 Monroe	Sylvania, Ohio 43560
Robison, Horace C., Jr.	923 Fir St.	Longview, Washington 98632
Rosenberg, Lewis	3485 Linden Ave.	Long Beach, Calif. 90807
Rosenberg, Richard S.	3660 Arlington Ave.	Riverside, Calif. 92506
Rosenberg, Sidney	355 East 72nd St.	New York, N.Y. 10021
Rosenthal, Sanford I.	5105 Paulsen St.	Savannah, Ga. 31405
Roth, Alan M.	Jules Stein Eye Institute	Los Angeles, Calif. 90024
Roty, Harry	1025 Regent St.	Madison, Wisc. 53715
Roy, Donald E.	Naval Hospital Philadelphia	Philadelphia, Pa. 19145
Royo, Paris E.	1355 Florin Rd.	Sacramento, Calif. 95822
Rucker, George D.	1035 Creswell St.	Shreveport, La. 71101
Rule, Jack A.	Ft. Sanders Professional Bldg. ...	Knoxville, Tenn. 37916
Rundle, John P.	3200 Main	Vancouver, Wash. 98662
Rundle, T. J.	1142 N. Road St.	Elizabeth City, N.C. 27909
Rutkowski, Paul C.	229 East 29th St.	New York, N.Y. 10016
Ryan, Stephen J., Jr.	Johns Hopkins Hospital	Baltimore, Md. 21205
Sable, Richard S.	57 Union St.	Marlboro, Mass. 01752
Salz, James J.	193 N. Robertson	Beverly Hills, Calif. 90211
Sanders, Calvin D.	210 State St.	New Orleans, La. 70118
Sargent, Robert A.	1601 Spring Garden St.	Philadelphia, Pa. 19130
Sauer, David W.	850 Middlefield Rd.	Palo Alto, Calif. 94301
Scafidi, Arnauld F.	501 North Main St.	Suffolk, Va. 23434
Scanlan, Joseph M.	750 Washington Ave.	Montgomery, Alabama 36104
Schatz, Howard	2340 Clay St.	San Francisco, Calif. 94115
Scher, Robert A. .....;...	158 Main St.	Huntington, N.Y. 11743
Schlussel, Herschel L.	1812 Middle Belt Rd.	Garden City, Mich. 48135
Schonder, A. A.	193 N. Robertson Blvd.	Beverly Hills, Calif. 90211
Schuster, Stephen A. D. ...	El Paso National Bank Bldg.	El Paso, Tex. 79901
Scott, Dorothy C.	625 Highland Bldg. So. Highland Mall	Pittsburgh, Pa. 15206
Scott, William E.	University Hospitals	Iowa City, Iowa 52240
Scudder, Marilyn J.	University of Minnesota Hospitals	Minneapolis, Minn. 55455
Seeley, Ronald L.	3000 W. Buffalo Ave	Tampa, Florida 33607
Sehgal, V. N.	178 E. 71st St.	New York, N.Y. 10021
Seibold, William R.	39th & Colby Ave.	Everett, Wash. 98201
Serros, Robert N.	95 W. Columbia St.	Orlando, Fla. 32806

Shacklett, David E.	School of Aerospace Medicine ..	Brooks AFB, Texas 78235
Shafer, James W.	4212 N. 16th St.	Phoenix, Ariz. 85016
Shalev, Joseph	Rose de Lima Hospital	Henderson, Nevada 89015
Shapiro, James S.	400 29th St.	Oakland, Calif. 94609
Shapiro, Mitchell	1400 S. Orlando Ave.	Winter Park, Florida 32789
Shapiro, Richard D.	3893 E. Market St.	Warren, Ohio 44484
Sheehey, William R.	2259 Clinton Ave. So	Rochester, New York 14618
Sheinberg, Philip	1212 W. Presidio	Ft. Worth, Tex. 76102
Sheridan, Edward J.	HSSE, USAF Medical Center ...	Wright-Patterson AFB, Ohio 45433
Sherins, Robert S.	2200 Santa Monica Blvd.	Santa Monica, Calif. 90404
Sherrill, James W., Jr.	405 Via del Norte	La Jolla, Calif. 92037
Shields, Jerry A.	1601 Spring Garden St.	Philadelphia, Penna, 19130
Shock, John P.	Box 18, Letterman General Hospital	San Francisco, Calif. 94129
Shugarman, Richard G.	1119 S. Flagler Dr.	W. Palm Beach, Fla. 33401
Sigband, Daniel J.	18700 Main St.	Huntington Beach, Calif. 92648
Sigmund, Charles A.	500 Northwest Plaza	St. Louis, Mo. 63074
Siliquini, John J.	3448 Guilford St.	Philadelphia, Pa. 19136
Silver, Allen E.	1916 Belair Rd.	Fallston, Md. 21047
Silverberg, Harvey H.	10137 Riverside Dr.	North Hollywood, Calif. 91602
Silverman, Joel P.	789 Howard Ave.	New Haven, Conn. 06510
Simons, Herbert J.	Naval Hospital	St. Albans, N.Y. 11425
Sinchai, Pravit	1430 Tulane Ave.	New Orleans, La. 70112
Sing, James F.	2200 O'Farrell St.	San Francisco, Calif. 94115
Singal, Sheldon	Box 1609 USAF Hospital Lakenheath, APO	New York 09179
Skalka, Harold W.	USAF Regional Hospital	Maxwell AFB, Alabama 36113
Skille, Boyd A.	2307 E. 38th Ave.	Anchorage, Alaska 99504
Slaney, John D.	345 Terracina Blvd.	Redlands, Calif. 92373
Slaughter, Frederick D.	245 Midway St.	Bristol, Tenn. 37620
Slavens, Robert L.	603 State Tower Bldg.	Syracuse, N.Y. 13202
Sloan, Matthew	2865 Atlantic Ave.	Long Beach, Calif. 90806
Sloan, Sherwin H.	2080 Century Park East	Los Angeles, Calif. 90067
Slusher, M. Madison	85 Main St.	North Adams, Mass. 01247
Smith, Charles L.	351 East Boundary	Perrysburg, Ohio 43551
Smith, David E.	1600 East Third St.	Charlotte, N.C. 28204
Smith, Donald L.	1206 E. Silver Spring Blvd.	Ocala, Florida 32670
Smith, Joe E.	Veterans Administration Hospital	Tuskegee, Ala. 36083
Smith, Richard D.	3600-1st Ave. No.	St. Petersburg, Fla. 33713
Smith, Robert W.	824 Pine St.	Texarkana, Tex. 75501
Smith, William E.	1701 S. Federal Blvd.	Denver, Colo. 80219
Snyder, Joseph	1109 Spring St.	Silver Spring, Md. 20910
Sohocki, John B., II	2558 Morgan Ave.	Corpus Christi, Tex. 78413
Sollie, Stanley C.	97th General Hospital, APO	New York 09757
Souders, Thomas B.	424 Walnut St.	Reading, Pa. 19601
Spencer, Louis M.	1100 N. Ventura Rd.	Oxnard, Calif. 93030
Sperduto, Robert D.	12840 Riverside Dr.	N. Hollywood, Calif. 91607
Stadwiser, J. Bruce	7126 N. Third St.	Phoenix, Ariz. 85020
Standefer, James E.	4450 West 76th	Minneapolis, Minn. 55435
Starer, Larry J.	Chester Pike & Sellers Ave	Ridley Park, Pa. 19078
Stein, Mervyn R.	750 Las Gallinas Ave	San Rafael, Calif. 94903
Steinbaum, Norman F.	595 Chestnut Ridge Rd.	Woodcliff Lake, N.J. 07675
Stewart, H. Lee	350 Parnassus	San Francisco, Calif. 94122

Stewart, John J., Jr.	1012 W. Bay Dr.	Largo, Fla. 33540
Stiles, Steven P.	6317 Wilshire Blvd.	Los Angeles, Calif, 90048
Stinchcomb, David E.	1701 Moon St. N.E.	Albuquerque, New Mex. 87112
Stong, Fred V.	750 Swift Blvd.	Richland, Wash. 99352
Stram, Thomas W.	Marshfield Clinic	Marshfield, Wisc. 54449
Strome, Robert R.	181 Main St.	Huntington, N.Y. 11743
Strum, Donald H.	Box 27, 2nd General Hospital, APO	New York 09180
Sullivan, Gerald E.	730 Fairview Ave	Bowling Green, Kentucky 42101
Sullivan, Tim, Jr.	1716 Locust St.	Sterling, Ill. 61081
Susel, Richard M.	3455 Wilkens Ave.	Baltimore, Md. 21229
Swarr, James H.	825 L Street	Anchorage, Alaska 99501
Swinton, Stanley D.	2830 E. Oakland Park Blvd.	Fort Lauderdale, Fla. 33306
Sylvester, Roland J.	165 Duperier Ave.	New Iberia, La. 70560
Taleff, Michael	1303 25th Ave.	Meridian, Miss. 39301
Tan, Ben Gee	1212 So. 11th	Tacoma, Wash. 98405
Tanne, Emanuel	1255 Whispering Pines	St. Louis, Mo. 63141
Tate, H. Randolph	1120 First Colonial Rd.	Virginia Beach, Va. 23454
Taugher, Philip J.	6080 South 108 St.	Hales Corners, Wisc. 53130
Taylor, J. Elliot	Old Main Road	Falmouth, Mass. 02574
Taylor, Waller L., Jr.	414 25th St.	Virginia Beach, Va. 23451
Thatcher, Daniel B.	Colorado Springs Eye Clinic	Colorado Springs, Colo. 80901
Thorp, T. Ramsey	Stenton Ave. and Mermaid Lane .	Philadelphia, Pa. 19118
Thrasher, Helen R.	7714 Second Ave. So	Birmingham, Ala. 35206
Tibble, Dennis M.	1203 N. Michigan Ave.	Saginaw, Mich. 48602
Tongue, Andrea C.	3181 SW Sam Jackson Park Rd. . .	Portland, Ore. 97201
Townes, David E.	1169 Eastern Parkway	Louisville, Ky. 40217
Townsend, William M.	4 Primrose St.	Chevy Chase, Md. 20015
Tragakis, Michael P.	525 East 68th St.	New York, N.Y. 10021
Trattler, Henry L.	1516 Venera Ave.	Coral Gables, Fla. 33146
Trimber, Connell J.	121 N. Washington St.	Alexandria, Va. 22314
Troup, Elliott V.	2233 Hamline Ave. North	St. Paul, Minnesota 55113
Tull, John W.	3100 Wyman Park Dr.	Baltimore, Md. 21211
Tunnell, LeRoy	656 W. Market St.	Akron, Ohio 44303
Upton, Henry Y.	202 Auburn Ave.	Auburn, Wash. 98002
Utley, Phillip M.	920 S. Main St.	Jonesboro, Ark, 72401
Vaughan, Elizabeth R.	2811 Lemmon Ave. E.	Dallas, Tex. 75204
Viggiano, Louis X.	410 Township Line	Havertown, Pa. 19080
Villaseñor, Richard A.	14935 Rinaldi	Mission Hills, Calif. 91340
Vinger, Paul F.	99 Waltham St.	Lexington, Mass. 02173
Vogel, Alexander S.	33 Davis Ave.	White Plains, N.Y. 10605
Vozeolas, Spero	16 Ross Ave.	Staten Island, N.Y. 10306
Wadina, Gerald W.	3445 E. Plankinton Ave.	Cudahy, Wisc. 53110
Wagner, R. Paul	201 Carson Ave.	Alamosa, Colo. 81101
Wainwright, Neil D.	830 W. Abriendo Ave.	Pueblo, Colo. 81005
Waldman, Harold L.	77 Prospect Ave.	Hackensack, N.J. 07601
Waller, John P.	32238 Schoolcraft	Livonia, Mich. 48150
Waller, Robert R.	Mayo Clinic	Rochester, Minn. 55901
Wamsley, Tamara C.	511 Petaluma Ave.	Sebastopol, Calif. 95472
Wasserman, Robert L.	1355 Roanoke Ave.	Riverhead, N.Y. 11901
Watanabe, Haruki	1919 7th Ave. South	Birmingham, Ala. 35233
Watson, David S.	1000 Ryland St.	Reno, Nevada 89502
Waxler, Paul	800 Islington St.	Portsmouth, N.H. 03801

Wayman, R. Douglas	1154 Montgomery Dr.	Santa Rosa, Calif. 95405
Weaver, Harold L.	2556 Morgan	Corpus Christi, Texas 78405
Webb, Robert W.	1312 West Delmar	Godfrey, Ill. 62035
Weber, A. Alan	1300 South Eliseo Dr.	Greenbrae, Calif. 94904
Weeks, Ralph H.	9400 East Rosecrans	Bellflower, Calif. 90706
Weichsel, Ruth H.	67 East 78th St.	New York, N.Y. 10021
Weintraub, Joel	50 Hempstead Ave.	Lynbrook, N.Y. 11563
Weiss, Irwin S.	4900 Sunset Blvd.	Los Angeles, Calif. 90027
Weissman, Jerry	3301 William Penn Highway	Pittsburgh, Pa. 15235
Wells, John A.	1516 Gregg St.	Columbia, S.C. 29201
Wells, Robert N.	1045 'S'	Fresno, Calif. 93721
West, Carole E.	Illinois Eye & Ear Infirmary	Chicago, Ill. 60612
Westbrook, Kenneth L.	2824 West Main St.	Visalia, Calif. 93277
Westfall, F. Franklin, Jr.	6000 Wisconsin Ave.	Chevy Chase, Md. 20015
Wherley, Benjamin J.	Boulevard Medical Bldg.	Dover, Ohio 44622
White, Robert H. Jr.	8118 Bustleton Ave.	Philadelphia, Pa. 19152
White, Stewart A.	50 Montgomery Dr.	Santa Rosa, California 95404
Wilkerson, E. Randolph, Jr.	1012 Kings Dr.	Charlotte, North Carolina 28207
Wilkinson, Charles P.	210 Pasteur Bldg.	Oklahoma City, Okla. 73103
Wilson, Jack W.	401 Lowell Dr.	Huntsville, Ala. 35801
Winchester, Jane A.	Box 151	Turners Falls, Mass. 01301
Wind, Chiel A.	University Hospital	Jacksonville, Fla. 32209
Winkler, Martin	9909 Frankstown Rd.	Pittsburgh, Pa. 15235
Winkler, Moseley H.	1306 Kanawha Blvd. East	Charleston, West Va. 25301
Winn, Samuel M.	3816 Hollywood Blvd.	Hollywood, Fla, 33021
Wittke, Paul E.	USAF Regional Hospital	Fairchild AFB, Washington 99011
Wobig, John L.	Medical Arts Bldg.	Portland, Ore. 97205
Wood, John W.	1309 Liberty Street, S.E.	Salem, Ore. 97302
Wood, Larry W.	1307 Crestdale Rd.	Lincoln, Nebraska 68510
Wood, Thomas O.	858 Madison Ave.	Memphis, Tenn, 38103
Wunsh, Stuart E.	1030 Clifton Ave.	Clifton, N.J. 07013
Wurster, Jerry B.	4320 Wornall Rd.	Kansas City, Mo. 64111
Yeargan, Wilfred W., Jr.	577 Seventeenth St.	Tuscaloosa, Ala. 35401
Young, N. William, Jr.	Home Savings & Loan Bldg.	Durham, N.C. 27701
Youssefi, Bijan	V.A. Center, 1601 Kirkwood Highway	Wilmington, Del. 19805
Zaffuto, Stephen F.	988 Fifth Ave.	New York, N.Y. 10021
Zappia, Robert J.	2 West Fern Ave.	Redlands, Calif. 92373
Zinn, Keith M.	Mt. Sinai Hospital, 100th St. & Fifth Ave.	New York, N.Y. 10029
Zipf, Richard F.	2921 El Camino Ave.	Sacramento, Calif. 95821

NOSOCOMIA QUIBUS OCULIS AEGRI CURANTUR

Residency programs in the following hospitals have been approved by the Council on Medical Education and the American Board of Ophthalmology through the Residency Review Committee for Ophthalmology, for three or more years of acceptable training in the specialty.

	Chief of Service or Program Director	Annual Admissions

UNITED STATES AIR FORCE

District of Columbia
Walter Reed General, Washington ....   B. Appleton   900

Texas
Wilford Hall U.S.A.F. Medical Center, San
     Antonio ....   V. J. Shepherd   564
Brooke General, San Antonio ....   J. R. Simmons   452

UNITED STATES ARMY
California
Letterman General, San Francisco ....   F. L. Wergeland, Jr.   328

Colorado
Fitzsimons General, Denver ....   W. W. Mears   370

UNITED STATES NAVY
California
Naval, Oakland ....   F. J. Schmetz   218
Naval, San Diego ....   D. G. Boyden   714

Maryland
Naval, Bethesda ....   L. M. King, Jr.   472

Pennsylvania
Naval, Philadelphia ....   W. R. Wilson, Jr.   193

UNITED STATES PUBLIC HEALTH SERVICE

California
U.S. Public Health Service, San Francisco ....   W. W. Richards   175

Louisiana
U.S. Public Health Service, New Orleans .....   C. D. Sanders   197

Maryland
U.S. Public Health Service, Baltimore ....   H. G. Randall   247

New York
U.S. Public Health Service (Staten Island), New
     York City ....   H. L. Trattler   259

Washington
U.S. Public Health Service, Seattle ....   See Univ. of Washington Affi-
     liated Hospitals, Seattle Wash.

DEPARTMENT OF HEALTH, EDUCATION, AND WELFARE
Washington
St. Elizabeths, Washington ....   See George Washington Univ. Affil.
     Hosps., Washington, D.C.

	Chief of Service or Program Director	Annual Admissions
OTHER FEDERAL		
Canal Zone		
Gorgas, Balboa Heights	R. H. Rupp	170

NONFEDERAL AND VETERANS ADMINISTRATION

Alabama		
Birmingham:		
Eye Foundation	J. D. Davidson	2.204
University of Alabama Medical Center	S. J. Kelly	...
University of Alabama Hospitals and Clinics ..	....	557
Children's	....	
Veterans Admin.	....	206
Tuskegee:		
Veterans Admin.	S. H. Settler, Jr.	152
Arkansas		
Little Rock:		
University of Arkansas Medical Center	F. T. Fraunfelder	...
Arkansas Baptist Medical Center	....	766
University	....	697
Veterans Admin. Consolidated	....	322
California		
Bakersfield:		
Kern County General	D. H. Wetterholm	57
Davis:		
University of California (Davis) Affiliated Hos-		
pitals	G. L. Portney	...
Sacramento Medical Center (Sacramento)	....	149
Fresno:		
Valley Medical Center of Fresno	F. D. Berry	159
Irvine:		
University of California (Irvine) Affiliated Hos-		
pitals Orange County Medical Center		
(Orange)	J. G. Tirico	314
Loma Linda:		
Loma Linda University	R. V. Shearer	519
Long Beach:		
Veterans Admin.	T. L. Balding	441
Los Angeles:		
Cedars-Sinai Medical Center Cedars of Lebanon		
Hospital Division	....	...
Mount Sinai Hospital Division	....	...
Hollywood Presbyterian	S. Rome	1,217
Los Angeles County-U.S.C. Medical Center ...	A. E. Oberman	874
U.C.L.A.	B. R. Straatsma	1,703
Veterans Admin. Center-Wadsworth	R. E. Bartlett	574
White Memorial Medical Center	G. K. Kambara	351

	Chief of Service or Program Director	Annual Admissions
Oakland:		
Highland General	E. H. Brugge	119
Orange:		
Orange County Medical Center	See Univ. of California (Irvine) Aff. Hosps., Irvine	
Palc Alto:		
Veterans Admin.	See Stanford University Affiliated Hospitals, Stanford	
Sacramento:		
Sacramento Medical Center	See University of California (Davis) Affil. Hosps., Davis	
San Francisco:		
Pacific Medical Center – Presbyterian	B. E. Spivey	950
University of California Program	M. J. Hogan	...
H. C. Moffitt-University of California Hospitals.	M. J. Hogan	540
Veterans Admin.	D. D. Jesberg	232
San Jose:		
Santa Clara Valley Medical-Center	See Stanford University Affiliated Hospitals, Stanford	
San Mateo:		
Harold D. Chope Community	See Stanford University Affiliated Hospitals, Stanford	
Stanford:		
Stanford University Affiliated Hospitals	A. A. Dellaporta	....
Stanford University	A. A. Dellaporta	212
Veterans Admin. (Palo Alto)	A. A. Dellaporta	300
Santa Clara Valley Medical Center (San Jose) .	F. D. Berry	136
Harold D. Chope Community (San Mateo) ...	R. O. Sherwood	4,926
San Joaquin General (Stockton)	M. Sergis	101
Stockton:		
San Joaquin General	See Stanford University Affiliated Hospitals, Stanford	
Torrance:		
Los Angeles County Harbor General	A. E. Kreiger	369
Colorado		
Denver:		
Denver General	J. R. Cerasoli	168
University of Colorado Affiliated Hospitals ...	P. P. Ellis	...
University of Colorado Medical Center	P. P. Ellis	285
Veterans Admin.	C. Whistler	145
Connecticut		
Hartford:		
University of Connecticut Affiliated Hospitals .	J. O. Rourke	...
University of Connecticut Hospital-MC Cook Division	....	157
Hartford	W. B. Bremster	913
New Haven:		
Yale-New Haven Medical Center Yale-New Haven	M. L. Sears	837

	Chief of Service or Program Director	Annual Admissions
Delaware		
Wilmington:		
Veterans Admin.	See Jefferson Med. College Affil. Hosps., Philadelphia, PA.	
Wilmington Medical Center	See Jefferson Med. College Affil. Hosps., Philadelphia, PA.	
District of Columbia		
Washington:		
Freedmen's	C. L. Cowan	160
Georgetown University Affiliated Hospitals ...	P. Y. Evans	...
Georgetown University	M. A. Lemp	141
District of Columbia General	G. E. Marak, Jr.	216
Sibley Memorial	A. M. Reynolds, Jr.	652
Veterans Admin.	A. R. Pilkerton	174
George Washington University Affiliated Hospitals	M. F. Armaly	...
George Washington University	M. F. Armaly	525
Armed Forces Institute of Pathology	L. E. Zimmerman	...
Children's Hospital of the District of Columbia	D. Friendly, M. Parks	1,260
St. Elizabeths	H. S. Wicker	98
Washington Hospital Center	R. Day	1,815
Florida		
Gainesville:		
University of Miami Affiliated Hospitals	H. E. Kaufman	...
William A. Shands Teaching Hosp. and Clinics .	H. E. Kaufman	1,466
University Hospital of Jacksonville (Jacksonville)	H. E. Kaufman, C. A. Wind	340
Veterans Admin.	D. M. Worthen	494
Jacksonville:		
University Hospital of Jacksonville	See University of Florida Affiliated Hospitals, Gainesville	
Miami:		
University of Miami Affiliated Hospitals	E. W. Norton, G. O'Grady	...
Jackson Memorial	....	2,356
Veterans Admin.	....	316
Georgia		
Atlanta:	F. P. Calhoun, Jr.	...
Emory University Affiliated Hospitals	....	221
Emory University	....	497
Grady Memorial	....	314
Veterans Admin. (Decatur)		
Augusta:	R. P. Thomas	...
Medical College of Georgia Hospitals	....	414
Eugene Talmadge Memorial	....	452
University	....	85
Veterans Admin.		
Illinois		
Chicago:		
Cook County	M. Frenkel	522
Michael Reese Hospital and Medical Center ...	M. L. Stillerman	620
Northwestern University-MC Gaw Medical Center	D. E. Shoch	...

	Chief of Service or Program Director	Annual Admissions
Chicago Wesley Memorial	E. H. Merz	635
Children's Memorial	P. E. Romano	275
Passavant Memorial	D. E. Shoch	649
Veterans Admin. Research	D. E. Shoch	210
Presbyterian-St. Luke's	W. F. Hughes	600
University of Chicago Hospitals and Clinics ...	F. W. Newell	625
University of Illinois	M. F. Goldberg	853
Evanston:		
Evanston	C. V. Barrett	501
Hines:		
Veterans Admin.	See Loyola University Affiliated Hospitals,	
Maywood:	Maywood	
Loyola University Affiliated Hospitals	J. E. McDonald	...
Loyola University	J. E. McDonald	...
Veterans Admin. (Hines)	J. R. Fitzgerald	381

Indiana
Indianapolis:

Indiana University Medical Center	F. M. Wilson	...
Indiana University Hospitals	....	789
Marion County General	....	222
Veterans Admin.	....	153

Iowa
Iowa City:

University of Iowa Affiliated Hospitals	F. C. Blodi	...
University of Iowa Hospitals	F. C. Blodi	2,125
Veterans Admin.	T. Burton	232

Kansas
Kansas City:

University of Kansas Medical Center	A. N. Lemoine	835
St. Luke's (Kansas City, MO.)	....	...
Veterans Admin. (Kansas City, MO.)	L. L. Hyde	294

Kentucky
Lexington:

University of Kentucky Medical Center	J. D. Wirtschafter	
University	....	400
Veterans Admin.	....	123

Louisville:

University of Louisville Affiliated Hospitals ...	P. R. O'Connor	...
Louisville General	P. R. O'Connor	158
Children's	W. C. Edwards	831
Veterans Admin.	P. R. O'Connor	149

Louisiana
New Orleans:

Louisiana State University Affiliated Hospitals	....	...
Charity Hospital of Louisiana	G. M. Haik	463
Ochsner Foundation	R. A. Schimek	457

	Chief of Service or Program Director	Annual Admissions
Tulane University Affiliated Hospitals	M. G. Holland	...
Charity Hospital of Louisiana	M. G. Holland	650
Eye, Ear, Nose and Throat	M. G. Holland	1,827
Touro Infirmary	W. Diaz	248
Veterans Admin.	M. G. Holland	314

Shreveport:
| Confederate Memorial Medical Center .... | L. A. Breffeilh .... | 455 |

Maryland
Baltimore:
Greater Baltimore Medical Center	R. E. Hoover	1,594
Johns Hopkins	A. E. Maumenee	2,088
Maryland General	H. B. Wilson	1,006
Sinai Hospital of Baltimore	H. K. Goldberg	341
University of Maryland	E. D. Richards	617

Massachusetts
Boston:
Boston University Affiliated Hospitals	H. Leibowitz, S. Lessell	...
Boston City	S. Lessell	269
University	H. Leibowitz	350
Massachusetts Eye and Ear Infirmary	H. F. Allen	6,114
Tufts University Affiliated Hospitals	B. Schwartz	...
New England Medical Center Hospitals	B. Schwartz	145
Veterans Admin.	....	...

Michigan
Allen Park:
| Veterans Admin. .... | See Wayne State University Affiliated Hospitals, Detroit | |

Ann Arbor:
University of Michigan Affiliated Hospitals ...	J. W. Henderson	...
University	J. W. Henderson	1,613
Veterans Admin.	J. W. Henderson, J. Wolter	137
Wayne County General (Eloise)	J. W. Henderson	198

Detroit:
Grace	M. Croll	711
Harper	W. Davies	1,120
Henry Ford	J. S. Guyton	999
Sinai Hospital of Detroit	H. S. Sugar	799
Wayne State University Affiliated Hospitals ...	R. S. Jampel	...
Veterans Admin. (Allen Park)	....	84
Detroit General	....	...

Eloise:
| Wayne County General .... | See University of Michigan Affiliated Hospitals, Ann Arbor | |

Minnesota
Minneapolis:
University of Minnesota Affiliated Hospitals ..	J. E. Harris	...
Hennepin County General	H. A. Shaw	180
University of Minnesota Hospitals	J. E. Harris	1,049
Veterans Admin.	J. E. Harris	328

	Chief of Service or Program Director	Annual Admissions
St. Paul-Ramsey (St. Paul)	R. H. Monahan	126
Rochester:		
Mayo Graduate School of Medicine	J. W. Henderson	...
Rochester Methodist	....	897
St. Mary's	....	...
St. Paul:		
St. Paul-Ramsey	See Univ. of Minnesota Affiliated Hospitals, Minneapolis	
Mississippi		
Jackson:		
University of Mississippi Medical Center	S. B. Johnson	...
University	....	764
Veterans Admin. Center	....	157
Missouri		
Columbia:		
University of Missouri Medical Center	W. M. Hart	352
Kansas City:		
Kansas City General Hospital and Medical Center	F. N. Sabates	126
St. Luke's	See University of Kansas Medical Center, Kansas City, Kansas	
Veterans Admin.	See University of Kansas Medical Center, Kansas City, Kan.	
St. Louis:		
Homer G. Phillips	H. P. Venable	217
St. Louis University Group of Hospitals	R. D. Mattis	...
Cardinal Glennon Memorial Hospital for Children	H. R. Brady	311
Firmin Desloge General	....	...
Washington University Affiliated Hospitals ...	B. Becker	...
Barnes Hospital Group	B. Becker	3,196
Jewish Hospital of St. Louis	E. Berg	433
St. Louis City	A. E. Kolker	167
Veterans Admin.	B. Becker	300
Nebraska		
Omaha:		
University of Nebraska Affiliated Hospitals ...	R. E. Records	...
Douglas County	H. J. Gifford	...
University of Nebraska	R. E. Records	82
Veterans Admin.	R. E. Records	180
New Jersey		
East Orange:		
Veterans Admin.	See CMDNJ-New Jersey Medical School Aff. Hosps. Newark	
Jersey City:		
Jersey City Medical Center	See CMDNJ-New Jersey Medical School Aff. Hosps. Newark	
Newark:		
CMDNJ-New Jersey Medical School Affiliated Hospitals	A. A. Cinotti	...

	Chief of Service or Program Director	Annual Admissions
Jersey City Medical Center (Jersey City)	A. A. Cinotti	...
Martland	A. A. Cinotti	203
United Hospitals Medical Center – Newark Eye and Ear Infirmary	J. D. Burke	1,264
Veterans Admin. (East Orange)	J. L. Harris	200

New York
Albany:

Albany Medical Center Affiliated Hospitals ...	R. D. Reinecke	...
Albany Medical Center	....	680
Child's	....	836
Veterans Admin.	....	190

Buffalo:

Buffalo General	C. H. Addington	1,008
Deaconess Hospital of Buffalo	E. P. Olmsted	817
Edward J. Meyer Memorial	W. Y. Jones	186

East Meadow:

Nassau County Medical Center-Meadowsbrook Div.	E. K. Rahn................	317

Hanhasset:

North Shore	I. H. Kaufman	320

New Hyde Park:

Long Island Jewish-Hillside Medical Center Program	P. H. Ballen	...
Long Island Jewish-Hillside Medical Center ...	....	313
Queens Hospital Center (New York City)	....	229

New York City:

Albert Einstein College of Medicine Affiliated Hospitals	P. Henkind	...
Bronx Municipal Hospital Center	....	600
Hospital of the Albert Einstein College of Medicine	....	70
Montefiore Hospital and Medical Center	....	940
Beth Israel Medical Center	A. Barnert	476
Bronx-Lebanon Hospital Center	S. S. Epstein	...
Bronx Eye Infirmary	S. S. Epstein	1,571
Brooklyn Eye and Ear	M. A. Lasky	2,970
Catholic Medical Center of Brooklyn and Queens Hospital of the Holy Family	D. S. Martin	179
French and Polyclinic Medical School and Health Center	S. Schutz	362
Polyclinic Division	....	...
Jewish Hospital and Medical Center of Brooklyn	M. Lasky	284
Lenox Hill	J. Sauer	398
Manhattan Eye, Ear and Throat	F. H. Constantine	5,129
Montefiore Hospital and Medical Center	See Albert Einstein College of Medicine Affiliated Hospitals	
Mount Sinai Hospital Training Program	I. H. Leopold	...
Mount Sinai	I. H. Leopold	500
City Hospital Center at Elmhurst	A. Safik	229

	Chief of Service or Program Director	Annual Admissions
New York Eye and Ear Infirmary	J. G. Cole	5,464
New York	D. M. Shafer	1,158
New York Medical College-Metropolitan Hospital Center	M. A. Galin	....
Unit 1, Flower and Fifth Avenue Hospitals ...	L. Harris	1,436
Unit 2, Metropolitan Hospital Center	R. Cavero	433
Unit 3, Bird S. Coler Memorial Hospital and Home	M. Best	33
New York University Medical Center	G. M. Breinin	...
Bellevue Hospital Center	G. M. Breinin	327
University	G. M. Breinin	783
Veterans Admin. (Manhattan)	H. B. Taterka..............	351
Presbyterian (Institute of Ophthalmology) ...	A. G. de Voe	4,309
Veterans Admin. (Bronx)	I. H. Leopold	409
Queens Hospital Center	See Long Island Jewish Hosp. Training Program, New Hyde Park	
St. Clare's Hospital and Health Center	W. J. Maher	632
St. Luke's Hospital Center	I. C. Newton	346
St. Vincent's Hospital and Medical Center of New York	R. D' Amico	343
State University, Kings County Hospital Center	D. Willard	...
Brooklyn-Cumberland Medical Center	G. Gombos	311
Kings County Hospital Center	R. C. Troutman	460
Long Island College	A. I. Fink	352
Maimonides Medical Center	J. Goldstein	389
State University	D. Willard	124
Veterans Admin. (Brooklyn)	A. M. Levine	278
Rochester:		
St. Mary's	C. E. de Santis	718
Strong Memorial Hospital of the University of Rochester	A. C. Snell	297
Syracuse:		
S.U.N.Y. Upstate Medical Center	J. L. Mc Graw	750
Crouse Irving-Memorial	....	...
State University	....	121
Veterans Admin.	....	...
Valhalla:		
Grasslands	J. A. Duncan	90
North Carolina		
Chapel Hill:		
North Carolina Memorial Hospital Mc Pherson .	S. D. Mc Pherson, Jr.	...
North Carolina Memorial	....	300
Mc Pherson (Durham)	....	847
Durham:		
Duke University Affiliated Hospitals	J. Wadsworth	...
Duke University Medical Center	J. Wadsworth	857
Veterans Admin.	A. C. Chandler, Jr.	484
Mc Pherson Hospital, North Carolina Memorial Mc Pherson	S. D. Mc Pherson, Jr.	...
North Carolina Memorial (Chapelhill)	....	300
Mc Pherson	....	847

	Chief of Service or Program Director	Annual Admissions
Winston-Salem:		
Bowman Gray School of Medicine Affiliated Hospitals	....	...
North Carolina Baptist	W. Roberts	557
Ohio		
Akron:		
Akron City	D. W. Mathias	473
Cincinnati:		
University of Cincinnati Hospital Group	T. Asbury	...
Cincinnati General	....	271
Veterans Admin.	....	...
Cleveland:		
Case Western Reserve University Affiliated Hospitals	C. I. Thomas	...
Cleveland Metropolitan General	....	296
University Hospitals of Cleveland	....	872
Veterans Admin.	....	185
Cleveland Clinic	F. A. Gutman	281
St. Vincent Charity	H. S. Siegel	535
Mount Sinai Hospital of Cleveland	J. A. Gans	767
St. Luke's	R. J. Nicholl	...
Columbus:		
Ohio State University Hospitals	T. A. Makley, Jr.	10
Oklahoma		
Oklahoma City:		
University of Oklahoma Health Sciences Center	T. E. Acers	...
University of Oklahoma Hospitals	T. E. Acers	301
Veterans Admin.	R. G. Small	354
St. Anthony	T. E. Acers	1,338
Oregon		
Portland:		
Good Samaritan Hospital and Medical Center .	J. Goldman	1,612
University of Oregon Affiliated Hospitals	K. C. Swan	...
University of Oregon Medical School Hospitals and Clinics	....	573
Veterans Admin.	....	384
Pennsylvania		
Danville:		
Geisinger Medical Center	J. L. Curtis	779
Philadelphia:		
Hospital of the University of Pennsylvania	H. G. Scheie	1,485
Graduate Hospital of the University of Pennsylvania	R. H. Trueman	125
Children's Hospital of Philadelphia	H. G. Scheie, D. Schaffer	213
Philadelphia General	H. G. Scheie	1,391

	Chief of Service or Program Director	Annual Admissions
Presbyterian-University of Pennsylvania Medical Center	R. D. Mulberger	358
Veterans Admin.	H. G. Scheie	187
	A. H. Keeney	...
Thomas Jefferson University Affiliated Hospitals	T. D. Duane	...
Thomas Jefferson University	T. D. Duane	375
Lankenau	P. R. Mc Donald	516
Veterans Admin. (Wilmington, Del.)	T. D. Duane	38
Wilmington Medical Center (Wilmington, Del.) .	S. Franklin	583
Wills Eye Hospital-Temple University	A. H. Keeney	4,936
Wills Eye Hospital and Research Institute	A. H. Keeney	...
St. Christopher's Hospital for Children	A. H. Keeney, R. Harley	288
Pittsburgh;		
Hospitals of the University Health Center of Pittsburgh	K. T. Richardson	...
Allegheny General	P. F. Holl	148
Children's Hospital of Pittsburgh	D. A. Hiles	152
Eye and Ear Hospital of Pittsburgh	K. T. Richardson	4,103
Mercy	....	...
Veterans Admin.	R. N. Lehman	406
Hospitals of the University Health Center of Pittsburgh Montefiore	S. Goldberg	...
St. Francis General-Western	....	925
Pennsylvania Hospitals	C. W. Weisser.................	...
St. Francis General	C. W. Wiesser	570
Western Pennsylvania	....	...
Sayre:		
Robert Packer	E. Kulczycki	543
Puerto Rico		
San Juan:		
University of Puerto Rico Affiliated Hospitals .	G. Pico	...
Municipal Hospital Dr. Rafael Lopez Nussa ...	....	621
University District	....	271
Veterans Admin. Center	....	328
Rhode Island		
Providence:		
Rhode Island	H. F. Stephens	1,210
South Carolina		
Charleston:		
Medical University of South-Carolina Teaching Hospitals	W. W. Vallotton	...
Medical University of South Carolina	....	613
Charleston County	....	38
Veterans Admin.	....	168
Tennessee		
Chattanooga:		
S.E. Tennessee Medical Education Center	I. L. Arnold	...

	Chief of Service or Program Director	Annual Admissions
Baroness Erlanger	I. L. Arnold	1,109
T. C. Thompson Children's		...
Memphis:		
University of Tennessee Affiliated Hospitals	R. L. Hiatt	...
City of Memphis Hospitals	R. L. Hiatt	449
Methodist	J. M. Freeman, Jr.	1,883
Veterans Admin.	G. R. Woodbury	432
Nashville:		
George W. Hubbard Hospital of the Meharry Medical College	A. C. Hansen	73
Vanderbilt University Affiliated Hospitals	J. H. Elliott	...
Vanderbilt University	J. H. Elliott	907
Nashville Metropolitan General	J. L. Sawyers	87
Veterans Admin.	J. H. Elliott	266
Texas		
Dallas:		
University of Texas Southwestern Medical School Affiliated Hospitals		...
Parkland Memorial	J. R. Lynn	357
Veterans Admin.	S. B. Gostin	319
Galveston:		
University of Texas Medical Branch Hospitals	E. C. Ferguson, 3D	566
Houston:		
Baylor College of Medicine Affiliated Hospitals.	D. Paton	...
Ben Taub General		413
Methodist		1,569
Veterans Admin.		468
Hermann	R. S. Ruiz	1,763
San Antonio:		
University of Texas at San Antonio Teaching Hospitals		...
Bexar County Teaching	G. W. Weinstein	201
Temple:		
Scott and White Memorial	R. D. Cunningham	862
Utah		
Salt Lake City:		
University of Utah Affiliated Hospitals	H. J. L. Van Dyk	...
University		199
Veterans Admin.		...
Virginia		
Charlottesville:		
University of Virginia	M. K. Humphries, Jr.	548
Richmond:		
Veterans Admin.	E. W. Perkins	319
Virginia Commonwealth University M.C.V. Affiliated Hospitals		...
Medical College of Virginia Hospitals	D. Guerry, 3D	335

	Chief of Service or Program Director	Annual Admissions
Washington		
Seattle:		
University of Washington Affiliated Hospitals .	R. E. Kalina	...
University	R. E. Kalina	165
Harborview Medical Center	D. F. Milam	84
Children's Orthopedic Hospital and Medical		
Center	R. H. Johnson	237
U.S. Public Health Service	P. D. Kramar	106
Veterans Admin.	R. E. Kalina	129
West Virginia		
Morgantown:		
West Virginia University Medical Center	R. R. Trotter	231
Wisconsin		
Madison:		
University of Wisconsin Affiliated Hospitals ..	M. D. Davis, J. C. Allen	...
University Hospitals	M. D. Davis, J. C. Allen	1,244
Veterans Admin.	J. C. Allen	144
Milwaukee:		
Medical College of Wisconsin Affiliated Hospitals	R. O. Schultz	...
Milwaukee County General	R. O. Schultz	373
Lutheran Hospital of Milwaukee	A. C. Kissling	425
Milwaukee Children's	H. Giller	350
Veterans Admin. Center (Wood)	R. H. Lehman	475

INSTITUTA SCHOLAEQUE CAECIS DESTINATAE

No data received.

ARGENTINA

Consejo Argentino de Oftalmología

Presidente: Dr. Roger E. Zaldivar
Vice-Presidente: Dr. Florentino Pena
Secretario: Dr. Alberto O. Ciancia
Tesorero: Dr. José H. Segarra
Dirección postal: Av. España 888, Mendoza

Reune en su Consejo Directivo a representantes de todas las Cátedras — estatales y privadas — y todas las Sociedades de Oftalmología del país.

SOCIETATES OPHTHALMOLOGICAE

Nationalis

Sociedad Argentina de Oftalmología

Presidente: Dr. Enrique Malbran
Dir. postal: Viamonte 1464, 1° Piso, Dto. 2, Buenos Aires

Regionales

Sociedad de Oftalmología de Cordoba

Presidente: Dr. Carlos A. Remonda
Dir. postal: Colón 637, Córdoba

Sociedad de Oftalmología del Litoral

Presidente: Dr. Blas M. Gallo
Dir. postal: Italia 663, Rosario (Sta.Fe)

Sociedad de Oftalmología de La Plata

Presidente: Dr. Julio O. Priento Diaz
Dir. postal: Calle 11 N° 729, La Plata, Pcia. Buenos Aires

Sociedad de Oftalmología de Mar del Plata

Presidente: Dr. Carlos A. Gavio
Dir. postal: San Martín 2675, Mar del Plata, Pcia. Buenos Aires

Sociedad de Oftalmología de Tucumán

Presidente: Dr. Jorge Lischinsky
Dir. postal: Casilla Correo 54, Correo Central, S. M. de Tucumán

Sociedad de Oftalmología de Mendoza

Presidente: Dr. Reinaldo Lange
Dir. postal: Hospital Central, ler piso, ala oeste, Mendoza

NOMINA ET DOMICILIA MEDICORUM AB OCULIS

Abad, Angel	Córdoba 154	Bell Ville, Córdoba
Abadie, Horacio	Paysandú 25	Buenos Aires
Abate, Victor	Moldes 1163	Buenos Aires
Abdala, Alberto A.	Guemes 71	Santiago del Estero
Abduca, Ricardo	Dean Funes 7	Chivilcoy, Bs. As.
Aberastain, Tomás G.	Las Heras 2153	Buenos Aires
Abinzano Argañaraz, Fidel	29 de setiembre 2046-Dto. B.	Lanús, Bs. As.
Abramosky, Alberto	Sarmiento 73	San Martín, Bs. As.
Abrebanel, Víctor	Belgrano 1053	Salta
Acosta, Antonio	Rivadavia 337	Quilmes, Bs. As.
Acosta, Eduardo	Sdo. de la Independencia 755	Buenos Aires
Acosta, Jorge	Rivadavia 337	Quilmes, Bs. As.
Adiez, Magin	Callao 132–EP	Buenos Aires
Aguilar, Jorge	Italia 16, 1° P.	Lomas de Zamora, Bs. As.
Aguinaga, Luis	R. Ortega 644	Mendoza
Aguirre, Susana L. de	Brandsen 25	Bahía Blanca, Bs. As.
Agullo, Armando	Belgrano 775	San Pedro, Bs. As.
Aguzin, Cristóbal	Saavedra 580	Formosa
Aisemberg, Leopoldo	Alem 357	Monte Grande
Alazraki, Mario	Moreno 2524–2°	Mar del Plata
Albarracin, Pedro	Betveder 11	Villa Mercedes, S.L.
Albesi, Eduardo	Juncal 2507–1°	Buenos Aires
Albornoz, Roberto	Cabildo 559–9°	Buenos Aires
Alcalá Hernández, Jorge	Peña 2222–P.B.	Buenos Aires
Alcoba, José G.	Segundo Congreso 333	B° Maipú, Córdoba
Alesandria, Oscar	Calle 24 N° 888	La Plata
Alfano, Norberto	Fraga 64	Buenos Aires
Alfonso, Alfredo R.	Jujuy 1572	Tucumán
Alias, Arnaldo	San Juan 379	Córdoba
Allende, Arnaldo R.	4 de enero 3189	Santa Fe
Allezzandrini, Arturo	Ayacucho 307–1°	Buenos Aires
Alliani, Juan P.	Pte. Roca 1161	Rosario, Sta. Fe
Alliani, Juan P. (h)	Pte. Roca 1161	Rosario, Sta. Fe
Allperín, José	Viamonte 1481	Buenos Aires
Alsina, Antonio	Sarmiento 695	Mendoza
Alvarez, Arturo	Av. del Trabajo 5814	Buenos Aires
Alvarez Hiriburu, Anibal	Hipólito Irigoyen 4205	Buenos Aires
Alvarez Noque, Luciano	Mitre 898	Mendoza
Alvarez, Ramón	Bolivar 1288	Corrientes
Alvarez, Ricardo	12 de octubre 315	Quilmes, Bs. As.
Alza, Enrique	Calle 11 N° 729	La Plata
Alza, Miguel A.	Calle 10 N° 1043	La Plata
Alzaga, Carlos	Zelarrayan 610	Bahía Blanca
Anastasi, Federico	Superi 275	Rosario, Sta. Fe
Anauati, Ernesto	Malabia 320	Buenos Aires
Andrade, César	Urquiza 211	Lincoln, Bs. As.
Andrada, Ernesto	Sarmiento 730	Catamarca
Anelli, Juan	Libertad 181	Sgo. del Estero

Angel, Esteban	Av. Directorio 1719	Buenos Aires
Anglarill, Alberto	Bolivar 45	Salto, Bs. As.
Antonini, Carlos	Andrés Pasos 189	PaX́ana, Entre Rios
Aquila, Carlos	Av. Rolon 3185	Boulogne. Bs. As.
Aragon, Fernando	Escalada 782	Buenos Aires
Arce, Magdalena B.	Aráoz 2445–2°	Buenos Aires
Argento, Jorge	Luis M. Campos 1235–3° P. 'D' .	Buenos Aires
Arguelles, Eugenio	Moreno 2854	Santa Fe
Arguero, Patricio	Lib. San Martín 1177	San Fernando, Bs. As.
Arioli, Orestes	San Martín 3638	Mar del Plata
Arouh, Julio	Junin 917–5° 'D'	Buenos Aires
Arrechea, Alfonso	Callao 481–3ᵘ	Buenos Aires
Arrigoni, Hugo	Isabel La Católica 150	Mendoza
Arroche, Juan A.	Olavarria 607	Buenos Aires
Artigas, Enrique	Muñecas 387	Tucumán
Artigas, Marcelino	Muñecas 387	Tucumán
Arturi, Carlos S.	Calle 2 N° 919	La Plata
Arzuaga, Carlos	Bolivia 440	Buenos Aires
Ascani, Edmundo	Juramento 2010	Buenos Aires
Ase, Raú	Lamadrid 349	Jujuy
Ase, Salomón	Lamadrid 349	Jujuy
Asis, Josefa	España 25	La Rioja
Auzunbud, Jorge	San Luis 1490	Rosario, Sta. Fe
Avaro, Ricardo	La Salada	Santa Fe
Averboch, Alberto	Bartolomé Mitre 1985	Buenos Aires
Aycaguer, Onofre	Calle 6 N° 490	La Plata
Badía, José A.	Junin 1616	Buenos Aires
Badía, José (h)	Junin 1616	Buenos Aires
Bainttein, Natalio	Montevideo 1096	Paso de los Andes, Córdoba
Ballesteros, Omar	San Juan 3992	Buenos Aires
Balza, Jorge	Azcuénaga 1059	Buenos Aires
Balzaretti, Alejandro	Perú 857	Buenos Aires
Bambill, Aristóbulo	Urquiza 243	Punta Alta, Bs. As.
Bar, Jorge	Cangallo 2335 7° 'E'	Buenos Aires
Bara, Bernardo	V. Alsina 2263 2° 'A'	Valentín Alsina, Bs. As.
Baranda, Hernán C.	Av. Sarmiento 222	Resistencia, Chaco
Barcat, Jorge	Iritorco 2943	B° Ameghino, Córdoba
Barnetche, Juan	Calle 17 N° 578	Mercedes, Bs. As.
Barón Gofanovich, Héctor	Av. Gral. Paz 63	Ciudadela, Bs. As.
Baron Gofanovich, Jaime ..	Av. Gral. Paz 63	Ciudaldela, Bs. As.
Baron, Natalio	Belgrano 850	Salta
Barril, Luis P.	Rivadavia 330	Comodoro Rivadavia
Barrio, Enrique	Rivadavia 20–4°	Mendoza
Barros, Nora G. de	Calle 43 N° 745	La Plata
Bazet, Reńe E.	Alberdi 489	San Francisco, Cba.
Beckerman, Isaac	Av. Córdoba 4539	Buenos Aires
Belinky, Bernardo	V. Sarsfield 91	Concordia, E. Rios
Belinky, Silvia	Mendoza 474–6°	Rosario, Sta. Fe
Belloso, Waldoz	Guemes 4163–2°	Buenos Aires
Beltrami, Luis	Laprida 958–1°	Rosario, Sta. Fe
Beltrán Nuñez, Roberto ...	Callao 1026	Buenos Aires
Benedetti, Alejandro	Vedia 367	9 de Julio, Bs. As.
Benedetti, Edmundo	Vedia 367	9 de Julio, Bs. As.
Beney, Manuel	San Martín 3091	Santa Fe
Benito Gaete, Alfredo A. ..	Ayacucho 1518 10° 'A'	Buenos Aires
Benjamín, Alberto	Larrea 527	Buenos Aires

Berardo, Luis	Av. Nuñez 2900	Arguello, Córdoba
Berardo, Orlando	Faustino Allende 119	Bajo Palermo, Córdoba
Beraza, Héctor R.	Guemes 3738-6ᵛ	Buenos Aires
Bereilh, Armando	Drago 23-1°	Bahía Blanca
Bereilh, Armando (h)	L. M. Drago 23	Bahía Blanca
Bergaglio, Arnoldo	Av. Cobo 448	Rufino, Sta. Fe
Bergstein, Aida	Calle 61 N° 572	La Plata
Berhabe, Ana M. de	Videla 435	Quilmes, Bs. As.
Berman, Félix	San Lorenzo 341	Tucumán
Bertotto, Enrique (h)	Laprida 808--5°	Rosario, Sta. Fe
Besuschio, Edelmiro	Sta. Fe 3401-2°	Buenos Aires
Bianco, Benito	Entre Rios 842	Rosario, Sta. Fe
Bianco, Roberto	Entre Rios 842	Rosario, Sta. Fe
Bidegain, Mauricio	Burgos 739	Azul, Bs. As.
Billordo, Javier	Azcuenaga 663-8°	Buenos Aires
Bisceglia, Humberto	Gualeguaychu 3848	Buenos Aires
Blanco, Carlos	Laprida 1243	Rosario, Sta. Fe
Blanco, Juan	Canning 1693	Buenos Aires
Blasser, Juan C.	Avellaneda 459	Rio Gallegos, Sta. Cruz
Bochoeyer, Mauricio	Rivadavia 4370-3°	Buenos Aires
Boero, Carlos R.	Piedras 1715	Buenos Aires
Boero, Enrique	Lavalle 79	Avellaneda, Bs. As.
Boldú, Carlos A.	9 de Julio 767	Oberá, Misiones
Bolomo, Salomón	Tucumán 543	Catamarca
Bonasegna, Marcelo	Otamendi 425	Buenos Aires
Bordet, Domingo	Cnel. Diaz 1794	Buenos Aires
Bori, Juan C.	Calle 51 N° 772	La Plata
Boric, Julia	San Luis 666	Quilmes, Bs. As.
Borojovich, Jorge	Yatay 746-2°	Buenos Aires
Borovinsky, Moyos	Varela 879	Buenos Aires
Bortman, Baldomero	J. B. Justo 2639	Buenos Aires
Bottini, Ernesto	Araoz 2911	Buenos Aires
Bourrou Moulie, Horacio ..	Córdoba 1406-1°	Buenos Aires
Braccia, Mario	Moreno 341	Lavallol, Bs. As.
Braillard, Julio	Chacabuco 555	Pte. R.S. Peña, Chaco
Braslavsky, Néstor	Fgta. Sarmiento 1640-6° '28' ..	Buenos Aires
Braver, Héctor	Segurola 1557	Buenos Aires
Brignani, José	Moreno 184	Trenque Lauquen, Bs. As.
Brochard, Alberto	Acassuso 310	San Isidro, Bs. As.
Brodsky, Mauricio	Segurola 1188	Buenos Aires
Broin, Carlos	Dean Funes 873	Córdoba
Bruno, Angelina	V. Sarsfield 1039	Córdoba
Bruno, Jorge C.	V. Sarsfield 1039	Córdoba
Brunzini, Mario A.	Laprida 1307-'2'	Buenos Aires
Bruschtein, Fabio J.	Av. del Trabajo 3683	Buenos Aires
Bruzzo, Héctor A.	Drago 79	Bahía Blanca
Brzezinski, Jacobo	Córdoba 991-3°	Buenos Aires
Bublik, Armando A.	Anchorena 1463-8°	Buenos Aires
Bueno, Francisco	Belgrano 548	Galvez, Sta. Fe
Buffo, Alberto P.	Moreno 176	Balhía Blanca
Bugnone, Cristina C. de ...	Urquiza 636	Gualeguaychú, E. Rios
Bugnone, Ernesto	L. N. Palma yDiaz	Gualeguaychú, E. Rios
Burgos, Horacio	Miró 16	Buenos Aires
Busleisman, Mario	Sol de Mayo (S) 640-B° Sta. Ana	Córdoba
Bustos, Adelma	Andrés Ferreira 135	Caseros, Bs. As.
Butin, Eduardo	San Martín 3364	Olavarría, Bs. As.

Byrnes, Victor M.	Cabildo 2785	Buenos Aires
Cabral Mercado. Emilio ...	Estomba 1710	Buenos Aires
Cabrera. Miguel A.	Rivadavia 2643–8°	Buenos Aires
Cáceres Zorrilla, Gerardo ..	Ayacucho 372	Posadas, Misiones
Cadierno, Abel	Merced 56	Pergamino, Bs. As.
Cadiz, Mario	J. B. Alberdi 7091	Buenos Aires
Cagnacci, Alberto H.	San Juan 2767–PB	Buenos Aires
Cagnacci, Alberto	San Martín 304	Campana, Bs. As.
Cajal, Renee Dante	Rivadeo 1560	Córdoba
Calvo, Rafael Félix	J. B. Justo 151	Neuquén
Cambiaso, Raúl H.	Dean Funes 1649	Buenos Aires
Campayo, Carlos Hugo	Brandsen 123–'1'	Córdoba
Campuzano, Guillermo	Laprida 333	Huinca Renancó, Cba.
Canciello, Antonio	Iriarte 2198	Buenos Aires
Canese, Guillermo C.	Cabildo 689–1°	Buenos Aires
Cantoni, Osiris	Rivadavia 628 E.	San Juan
Cappello, Ernesto A.	Urquiza 834	Concordia, E. Rios
Carballo, Floreal	R. Falcón 2335	Buenos Aires
Carcano, Juan	Rosario 286–12°	Buenos Aires
Cárdenas, Alberto	Buenos Aires 10	Santiago del Estero
Cárdenas, Julio N.	San Martín 77	Santiago del Estero
Cardona, Jorge L.	Mitre 135	San Nicolás, Bs. As.
Caretti, Joaquín A.	Callao 132 E.P.	Buenos Aires
Caride Ceballos, Juan	Puevrredón 1337	Buenos Aires
Carreras, Rodolfo	Chacabuco 340	Tandil, Bs. As.
Carroll, Eduardo	Ciudad de la Paz 1933	Buenos Aires
Casabianca, Marcelo	Rivadavia 3233	Santa Fe
Casas, Rubén	Hilario Lagos 267	Sante Rosa
Cassara, Martín E.	San Martín 828	Gral. Pico, La Pampa
Castagnola, María M.	Ayacucho 1364–2°	Buenos Aires
Castiglione, José F.	Amenabar 884	Buenos Aires
Castillo, Jorge Luis	Mendoza 421	Tucumán
Castorina, Mario A.	Cabildo 1478–PB	Buenos Aires
Castro Rivadulla, Constantino	Calle 39–N° 384	La Plata
Castro, Juan Carlos	Belgrano 75–2° '2'	Córdoba
Castro, Osvaldo	9 de Julio 351	San Martín, Mendoza
Castro, Costa Aída	Hosp. Marcial Quiroga	Rivadavia, San Juan
Castro, Yolanda de	9 de Julio 351	San Martín, Mendoza
Catalan, Julio	Laprida 195–1° 'C'	Tucumán
Catalan, Mario	Laprida 195–1° 'C'	Tucumán
Cattani, Norberto A.	Roca 1741	Vicente López, Bs. As.
Catella, Mario	Obispo Salguero 223	Córdoba
Cavalari, Oscar	Mejico 3070	Buenos Aires
Cavalli, José	H. Irigoyen 840	Monteros, Córdoba
Cello Zambrano, Gerónimo .	San Martín 2877	Santa Fe
Ceraso, Marta	A. Carbone 3481	Santos Lugares, Bs. As.
Ceriani, Juan C.	Gallo 1463	Buenos Aires
Cernocky, Carlos M.	Laprida 1550	Godoy Cruz, Mendoza
Cerutti, Jorge	Mitre 228	San Nicolás, Bs. As.
Chara, Abraham	Libertad 1715	Córdoba
Charles, Daniel E.	San Martín 2675 3°	Mar del Plata
Chervin, Manuel	San Lorenzo 1050	Corrientes
Chianello, Miguel F.	Victorica 2445	Buenos Aires
Chianello, Miguel (h)	Blanco Encalada 5297	Buenos Aires
Chumacero Fernández, Ramón	Calle 3 N° 564	Cerro de Las Rosas, Córdoba

Ciancia, Alberto O.	Callao 1395–PB	Buenos Aires
Cianni, Edgardo	Colombres 1331	Buenos Aires
Ciapponi, Rogelio	Rivadavia 330	Villa Angela. Chaco
Cibils, Roberto	San Juan de Dios 345	Dorrego, Mendoza
Cienfuegos, María del Carmen	Calle 38 N° 401	La Plata
Cikotic, Antonio	Constitución 1981 1° 'D'	Buenos Aires
Ciocchi, Pedro	Laprida 165–3°	Lomas de Zamora, Bs. As.
Cios, José	Perú 2515	San Justo, Bs. As.
Claps, Leonardo	Diagonal 77 N° 212–2° 'E'	La Plata
Cocucci, Delia	Terrada 2655 'A'	Buenos Aires
Codo, Julio	San Martín 522 esq. Libertad	Carlos Paz, Córdoba
Colaneri, Nazario	Chacabuco 55	Pte. R.S. Peña, Chaco
Colella, Edgardo	Pueyrredón 68	Rosario, Sta. Fe
Columba, Guillermo	Arce 889	Buenos Aires
Conversano, Miguel	24 de noviembre 1085	Buenos Aires
Copello, Manuel	Sta. Rosa 408	Córdoba
Copello, Timar	Bolívar 557	Azul, Bs. As.
Cornejo Mosquera, Félix	9 de Julio 1196	Lanús, Bs. As.
Corradi, Juan	R. Falcón 5665	Wilde
Corradini, Osvaldo	Sarmiento 145	Cutral-Co, Neuquén
Correa, Carlos L.	Soldado Ruiz 1080	Córdoba
Corsellas, Agustín	Laprida 1727-PB	Buenos Aires
Cortínez, Sergio	Félix de Azara 730 1° 'D'	Rosario, Sta. Fe
Costa, Roberto	Sta. Fe 1592–5° 'J'	Buenos Aires
Costello, Federico	Rondeau 1862	Rosario, Sta. Fe
Cottonaro, Graciela	Buenos Aires 935	Córdoba
Courtis, Baudilio	Paraná 750	Buenos Aires
Courtis, José María	Paraguay 1949	Buenos Aires
Cramer, Federico	Paraná 830	Buenos Aires
Cremona, Eduardo	Juncal 1181–2°	Buenos Aires
Crisapulli, Antonio	Cosquín 750	Buenos Aires
Cubero, Andrés	Colón 555	Goya, Corrientes
Cura, Eduardo	Belgrano 1114–1°	Córdoba
Curuchet, Jorge T.	Estrada 251	Haedo, Bs. As.
Cuzzani, Tomás O.	Larrea 1058–PB–'B'	Buenos Aires
Cuzzani, Oscar E.	Larrea 1058	Buenos Aires
Czerweny, Hygo	Libertad 1548	Rosario, Sta. Fe
D'Alessandro, Angegela M.	Andonaegui 975	Buenos Aires
D'Alessandro, Pablo	Parera 164	Buenos Aires
Dalmagro, Juan	Corrientes 29–2°	Córdoba
Dalmagro, Norma P. de	Corrientes 29–2°	Córdoba
Damel, Angélica	Anchorena 1205–7°	Buenos Aires
Damonte, Edelmiro	Alem 463	Rafaela, Sta. Fe
Damonte, Juan C.	San Juan 1853–5°	Buenos Aires
Danel, Anibal	Calle 47 N° 830	La Plata
Daro, Julio H.	Caseros 3744-PB	Buenos Aires
Dasque, Pablo	Azcuénaga 1171–3°	Buenos Aires
Deferrari, Elda Rino de	Saavedra 222	Buenos Aires
De Francesco, Vicente	Billinghurst 1624	Buenos Aires
Delaloye, Nicanor F.	Rep. de Siria 4213	Santa Fe
Del Gener, María	Independencia 351	Sarandí
Dellacasa, Eduardo	Luro 2668–1° P.	Mar del Plata
Dellatorre, Carlos	Alvear 283	Martínez, Bs. As.
De Mauri, Pedro	Independencia 1658 1° 'D'	Mar del Plata
Denes Arduino, Enrique	Luis M. Drago 227	Buenos Aires

De Nicola, Roberto	Cangallo 1834	Buenos Aires
Dente, Horacio	Moreno 3268	Mar del Plata
Dente, Juan Carlos	Plaza España 163	La Plata
D'Eramo, Cayetano	Laprida 1450	Rosario, Sta. Fe
Derdoy, Jorge	Italia 1262	Rio Cuarto, Cba.
De Rosa, Pedro	V. López 1742–1° 'A'	Buenos Aires
Desio, Carlos A.	Urguiza 681	Paraná, E. Rios
Despontin, Leopoldo	San Martín de Tours 2980	Buenos Aires
De Vecchio, Hugo	Rioja 1145	Corrientes
Diaz, Carlos	Corrientes 1814–4°	Buenos Aires
Diaz, Miguel Angel	Córdoba 41	Luján de Cuyo, Mza.
Diez, Horacio	Lope de Vega 2016	Buenos Aires
Dilella, Edmundo	Belgrano 850	Salta
Di Marco, Juan C.	Uruguay 534	Beccar, Bs. As.
Di Pinto, Félix	Lima 90–1° P.	Córdoba
Di Sanso, José D.	Cuenca 3257–'C'	Buenos Aires
Dislacio, Elio	25 de mayo 716	Tucumán
Di Tullo, Eduardo	Vergara 2208	Florida, Bs. As.
Dodds, Ricardo A.	R. Peña 1386	Buenos Aires
Dolzani, Armando D.	Bvard. Oroño 908–18° P.	Rosario, Sta. Fe
Dolzani, Dante (h)	Guido 1724	Buenos Aires
Dolzani, Libertad A. de ...	Bvard. Oroño 908–18° P.	Rosario, Sta. Fe
Domingorena, Ernesto	Pavón 8848	Lomas de Zamora, Bs. As.
Dorucci, Luis	Guemes 3154	Buenos Aires
Dubin, Mauricio	Canning 310–1° P.	Buenos Aires
Duci, Arturo	Sarmiento 695	Mendoza
Echegaray, Julio	Gral. Paz 29 Oeste	San Juan
Echevarría, Héctor	Tupungato 1060	Rosario, Sta. Fe
Eguia, Roberto	España 356	Lomas de Zamora, Bs. As.
Elaskar, Santiago	Rivadavia 53–3° P.	Quilmes, Bs. As.
Elias, Alfredo	9 de Julio 1216	Rosario, Sta. Fe
Elicagaray, Ricardo	Rivadavia 770	Trelew, Chubut
Elisavetzky, Lázaro	Gral. Paz 1066	Rio Cuarto, Cba.
Elizalde, Francisco	Arroyo 959	Buenos Aires
Elizondo, Graciela	Sáenz Peña 1782	Godoy Cruz, Mza.
Elkin, Arnoldo	Arroyo 1061	Buenos Aires
Elkin, Benjamín	Santo Tomé 3235	Buenos Aires
Endrek Garzón, Mario	La Granja 69	Alto Verde, Cba.
Enriori, Juan J.	Rioja 1558	Monte Caseros, Corrientes
Erausquin, Héctor	Cangalo 1457–1° P.	Buenos Aires
Erbstein, Simón	Guemes 4028–4° P.	Buenos Aires
Esbry, Luis	Tucumán 213–2° P.	San Juan
Escariz, Benito H.	Rosales 1226	Adrogué, Bs. As.
Espósito, Roberto J.	Paraguay 2996	Buenos Aires
Esquivel, Arístides	Zeballos 1864	Rosario, Sta. Fe
Estape, D.	Paraguay 4158	Buenos Aires
Estupiñán Fazio, Carlos ...	Sta. Fe 2029–1° P.	Buenos Aires
Etchemendigaray, Arturo ..	9 de Julio 10	San Nicolás, Bs. As.
Faé, Nilda	Calle 42 N° 509 1/2	La Plata
Fanjul, Ricardo	C. Alvarez 722	Tucumán
Farack, Otilia	Sta. Fe 2590–2° P.	Buenos Aires
Farjat, Oscar	Caseros 876	Salta
Fassi, Alberto	Calle 9 N° 521	Cerro de las Rosas, Córdoba
Ferdrin, Juan C.	Rosetti 1825	Buenos Aires
Fernández, Hector	Gorriti 214	Bahía Blanca
Fernández Meijide, Roberto .	Rio Bamba 821–3° 'D'	Buenos Aires

Fernández Mendez, Casiano .	Jujuy 110–4° 'B'	Buenos Aires
Fernández Rabadán, Armando	Córdoba 1882–1° P.	Mar del Plata
Fernandez Sasso, David A. .	Avda. de Mayo 1437–2° P.	Buenos Aires
Ferraresi, Edgardo	Charlone 827	Avellaneda, Bs. As.
Ferraro, Fernando	Sarmiento 1402	San Miguel, Bs. As.
Ferreira, José	Obispo Trejo 1120	Córdoba
Ferrer, Arata Alberto	Rivadavia 1993	Buenos Aires
Ferrero, Dante	San Martín 2877	Santa Fe
Ferrero, Elmo	San Martín 339	Villa María, Cba.
Ferros, Susana	Monoblock 5–PB 'B' .,......	Barrio Autopista, Tapiales
Fichetti, Miguel A.	Cnel. Diaz 1781	Buenos Aires
Fidelio, Hugo	Hospital Centenario Urquiza 3100	Rosario, Sta. Fe
Figari, Jorge	Hosp. Pte. Alvear-B° Gral. Mosconi	Comodoro Rivadavia, Chubut
Filgueira, Eduardo	C. Alvarez 770	Tucumán
Filippi, Victor	Rivadavia 137–1° P.	Junín, Bs. As.
Fleschler, Osoas	Sta. Fe 3942–10° P. 'B'	Buenos Aires
Folador, Luisa	C.C. Vigil 732	Mendoza
Folco, Raúl	J. M. Moreno 218–2° 'D'	Buenos Aires
Fontenlos, Juan	España 185	Cipolletti, Rio Negro
Forcada, Victor	Olascoaga 435	San Rafael, Mza.
Fracchia, Alberto	Bmé. Mitre 256	Resistencia, Chaco
Fracchia, Américo	Bmé. Mitre 256	Resistencia, Chaco
Frasnedo, Carlos	Alberdi 326	Junín, Bs. As.
Freile, Carlos	San Martín 276	Comodoro Rivadavia, Chubut
Freire, Carlos A.	Esmeralda 949–5° P.	Buenos Aires
Fresco, M. Ortiz de	Dean Funes 490	Formosa
Frey, Hugo	1° de Mayo 1017	Marcos Juarez, Córdoba
Frias, Cornejo Pedro	Rivadavia 1902	Buenos Aires
Frigerio, Emilio	R. L. Falcón 1894–4°	Buenos Aires
Fugazzotto, Juan	San Martín 3316	Mendoza
Fulugonio, Arturo	Rio Bamba 1026	Buenos Aires
Furno, Sola Nino	Entre Rios 142	Rosario, Sta. Fe
Furrer, Amalia	Emilio Lamarca 3936	Buenos Aires
Gabrielli, Alejandro	Sobremonte 935	Rio Cuarto, Cba.
Gabrielli, Eduardo	Jujuy 253	Córdoba
Gaisiner, Pini D.	Paraguay 1398	Rosario, Sta. Fe
Galan, Francisco	Viamonte 1866	Buenos Aires
Galan, María M.	Calle 11 N° 729	La Plata
Galeotta, Augusto	Heredia 1490	Buenos Aires
Galletti, Angel	Libertad 1954–Dto. 4	Córdoba
Galli, Roberto	Sarmiento 162	Bell Ville, Cba.
Gallo, Blas María	Balcarce 798–5° 'C'	Rosario, Sta. Fe
Gallo, Carlos	Rioja 1770	Rosario, Sta. Fe
Gallo, Eduardo	Paraguay 40	Rosario, Sta. Fe
Galo, Miguel E.	24 de setiembre 1324	Tucumán, Concepción
Galperín, Abel	V. Alsina 3229	Valentín Alsina, Bs. As.
Galup, Alberto R.	Pje. Estrada 463	Adrogué, Bs. As.
Galup, Alberto (h)	Alte. Brown 3100	Temperley, Bs. As.
Galvan, Carlos I.	Calle 1 N° 1528 ..,........	La Plata, Bs. As.
Gambino, Mario	Alte. Brown 881–1° P.	Buenos Aires
Garcés, Alejandro ......:	C. Richieri 401	San Lorenzo, Sta. Fe
Garcete, María C.	A. Garzon 1570	Córdoba
Garcia, Angel M.	Azcuénaga 1793	Buenos Aires
Garcia, Dávila	Merlo 460	Moreno, Bs. As.

Garcia, Diego	Córdoba 41	Luján de Cuyo, Mendoza
García Bazarra, José	Mendoza 4301	Buenos Aires
García Centurion, Jorge L.	Junin 646	San Luis
García Duran, Elías	Belgrano 236	San Nicolás, Bs. As.
García, Guillermo	Pte. Alvear 320	Haedo, Bs. As.
García, Juan C.	España 10	Alta Gracia, Cba.
García Mogort, Luis	Viamonte 1464	Buenos Aires
García Nocito, Pedro	Córdoba 1300–6° P.	Buenos Aires
Garcia, Osvalo	Av. Hudson 324–1° Of. 6	Berazategui, Bs. As.
García Soto, Raúl	Cabildo 173	Buenos Aires
Garcia, Roberto P.	12 de octubre 219	Avellaneda, Bs. As.
Gardella, Manlio	Dorrego 1175	Comodoro Rivadavia, Chubut
Garfinkel, Cristina	Junin 1153–10° 'A'	Buenos Aires
Gartín, Cesar	Gral Venancio Flores 4031	Buenos Aires
Gastaldi, Magdalena Grassi de	Rivadavia 4977–1° P.	Buenos Aires
Gastaldi, Tomás	Rivadavia 4977–1° P.	Buenos Aires
Gavarini, Oscar	25 de mayo 742	Gualeguaychú, Entre Rios
Gavio, Carlos A.	San Martín 2675	Mar del Plata
Geddes, Oscar A.	Belgrano 206	Bahía Blanca
Geria, Roberto	Rodriguez Peña 1653 10° 'A'	Buenos Aires
Gerones, Martha S. de	Calle 51 N° 355–12°	La Plata
Gervasoni, Jorge	Roca 202	Neuquén
Giambruni, Juan I.	Calle 2 N° 609	La Plata
Giavai, Juan	Salta 1031	Jujuy
Gicolini, Dante E.	Pellegrini 278	San Rafael, Mza.
Gigena, Sánchez	Espora 645	Adrogué, Bs. As.
Gilabert, Norberto	J. B. Alberdi 5888	Buenos Aires
Gil, Estela L. de	Perito Moreno 175	Neuquén
Gil Fernández, Hugo	Perito Moreno 175	Neuquén
Giorgi, Angel A.	Mitre 1083	San Miguel, Bs. As.
Giqueaux, Roberto	Corrientes 832	Rosario, Sta. Fe
Gitelman, Clemenso	Canning 2356–9° 'A'	Buenos Aires
Giudici, Roberto	Ing. Arias 2350	Castelar, Bs. As.
Gjurkovic, Jorge	Pellegrini 789	Santa Rosa, La Pampa
Golda, Mauricio	Luro 3170	Mar del Plata
Golovin, Vladimiro	Independencia 825	Villa Ballester. Bs. As.
Gómez, L. Carmen	Pje. Lucio V. López 465	Tucumán
Gómez, Brunel J. A.	Córdoba 1258	Corrientes
Gómez, Néstor	Gurruchaga 818	Hurlingham, Bs. As.
Gómez Morales, Adolfo	Junín 1479	Buenos Aires
Gonella, Alejandro	Pueyrredón 442	Buenos Aires
Gonella, Juan A.	Pueyrredón 442–3° P.	Buenos Aires
Gonnella, José P.	Larrea 784–1° P.	Buenos Aires
González del Cerro, Manuel .	Bv. Argentino 8402	Rosario, Sta. Fe
González Mujica, Marcelo	Santa Fe 2245–3° 'B'	Buenos Aires
González Santos, Raúl	Av. Lincoln 3512	Buenos Aires
Gordillo, Carlos H.	Laprida 548	Tucumán
Gracia, José	H. Irigoyen 384	Córdoba
Gracia, José (h)	Oncativo 1736	Córdoba
Grammatico, Alfredo	Juncal 1612–1° P.	Buenos Aires
Granados, Eduardo	Tucumán 1601–7° P.	Rosario, Sta. Fe
Govi, Julio	Av. Maipú 2507	Olivos, Bs. As.
Grayeb, Elías	Arenales 1915	Martínez, Bs. As.
Grigera, Emilio	Maipú 821–1° 'F'	Vicente López, Bs. As.
Grimblat, Jorge	Rivadavia 5651–14°	Buenos Aires

Grinberg, José	H. Irigoyen 10877	Temperley, Bs. As.
Groba, Roberto	San Pedrito 185	Buenos Aires
Grondona, Jorge P.	Callao 500–PB	Buenos Aires
Groppa, Pedro	Zelarrayán 1155	Buenos Aires
Grossi, Roberto	J.M. Gutiérrez 2530 7° '28'	Buenos Aires
Grosvald, Abraham	Callao 531–2° 'B'	Buenos Aires
Guagnini, Pedro E.	Sánchez de Bustamante 1886	Buenos Aires
Gualdoni, Carlos	Calle 60 N° 645	La Plata
Guallart, Carlos A.	Calle 6 N° 1378 '2'	La Plata
Guallart, Mario F.	Merced 1262	Pergamino, Bs. As.
Guarnieri, José	Carril Sarmiento 1325	Maipú, Mendoza
Gueicamburu, Horacio J.	Calle 14 N° 633	Mercedes, Bs. As.
Guerrero, José	Rufino Ortega 68	Rivadavia, Mendoza
Guevara, Victor H.	Neuquén 590–PB 'F'	Buenos Aires
Guillet, Alfredo	Pedernera 333	Mercedes, San Luis
Guiñazu Lemos, Fernando	Lemos 37–1° '2'	Godoy Cruz, Mendoza
Guiñez, Pablo	Belgrano 684	Salta
Guisasola, Carlos	Sta. María 624–PB 'C'	Buenos Aires
Gunski, Miguel A.	Av. Sarmiento s/n	Apóstoles, Misiones
Gurovich, Lidia	Castex 3330–12° 'B'	Buenos Aires
Gutierrez, Alfredo	Tucumán 998	Gral. Roca, Rio Negro
Halac Martinoli, José M.	L. de la Torre 613	Santa Rosa, La Pampa
Hana, Julio C.	Juan F. Aranguren 548–5° 'D'	Buenos Aires
Hancevich, Santiago	Mendoza 1333	Rosario, Santa Fe
Hauvilier, Verónica	Hualfin 799	Buenos Aires
Hendlin, Félix E.	San Martín 59	Concordia, E. Rios
Hernández, Roberto	Rio de Janeiro 9 2° 'A'	Buenos Aires
Herran, Aida Tangeloff de	Austria 1754–5° '13'	Buenos Aires
Herrera Villafañe, Enrique	Gral. Belgrano y 501	Manuel Gonnet, Bs. As.
Hick, Jacobo	Moreno 329	San Martín, Bs. As.
Hidalgo, Carlos	Colón 783	Azul, Bs. As.
Hirsch, Mario	Granaderos 846–2°	Buenos Aires
Hocsman, Blanca	Urquiza 182	Basavilbaso, E. Rios
Holgado, Luis M.	Uriburu 1479	San Lorenzo, Sta. Fe
Huber, Enrique	Paraguay 160	Rosario, Sta. Fe
Huerta, Néstor	Julio Roca 1115	Pergamino, Bs. As.
Hulsbus, Ricardo	Fco. Lacroze 2336 8° 'A'	Buenos Aires
Igarteburu, Rodolfo	Moreno 593	Quilmes, Bs. As.
Ihlow, Conrado	Bvrd. Ballester 365	Villa Ballester, Bs. As.
Imbern, Salvador	Oroño 981	Rosario, Sta. Fe
Infantino, José	Del Valle 473	Pehuajó, Bs. As.
Iñiguez, Horacio	Calle 1 N° 1528	La Plata
Iribarren, Federico	Arenales 981 2°P.	Buenos Aires
Iribarren, Federico (h)	Arenales 981–2°P.	Buenos Aires
Iribarren, Fernando	Arenales 981–2°P.	Buenos Aires
Iribarren, Luis	Urquiza 784	Paraná, E. Rios
Iribarren, Rafael	Arenales 981–2° P.	Buenos Aires
Israel, Alberto	Virrey Loreto 2438 PB 'B'	Buenos Aires
Issa, José A.	Florida 349	Salta
Iudica, Juan	Colón 185–2° P.	Mendoza
Jairala, Felipe	Buenos Aires 261	Concordia, E. Rios
Jairala, Ignacio	Rioja 1791	Rosario, Sta. Fe
Jara, Juan Alberto	Ferrando Bayo 735	Rosario
Jimenez, Elsa S. de	Arturo M. Bas 70	Córdoba
Jofre, José L.	Jujuy 2980	Córdoba
Joisen, Marcos	Casilla Correo 145	Juarez, F.C.G.N.R.

Jolly, Carlos H.	Juncal 2275–3° 'H'	Buenos Aires
Jozami, Juan	Sarmiento 3520	Sante Fe
Juarez Beltrán, Claudio	Dean Funes 429	Córdoba
Juarez Beltrán, Claudio (h)	Av. Olmos 179–3°P.	Córdoba
Junod, Gabriel	Araoz 2814	Buenos Aires
Jure, Francisco	Guemes 677	Jujuy
Jure, Guillermo	Guemes 677	Jujuy
Jurgens, Eduardo	Sta. Fe 2245–3° 'B'	Buenos Aires
Just Tiscornia, Alberto B.	M.T. de Alvear 788–3°	Buenos Aires
Just Tiscornia, Benito	Charcas 788–3°P.	Buenos Aires
Kalaidjian, Rodolfo	José Bonifacio 2680	Buenos Aires
Kalejman, Héctor	Mendoza 612	San Juan
Kaplan, Miguel	Valentín Gómez 2904 4° '19'	Buenos Aires
Kasap, David	Teodoro Roosvelt 5281–1°	Buenos Aires
Katz, Celia	Arquitecto Thays 75	Córdoba
Kaufer, Gunther	Roca 1984	Florida, Bs. As.
Kettekhate Cramer, Federico	Paraná 830	Buenos Aires
Klein, Jorge	Suipacha 831	Buenos Aires
Kogan, Jorge	Cuenca 3720–2° '6'	Buenos Aires
Kohan de Lerner, Mabel E.	Anchorena 1463–6° 'B'	Buenos Aires
Korn, Enrique	Av. F. Amehino 911	Esquel, Chubut
Kostinowsky, Myriam B. de	San Martín 3138	Rosario, Sta. Fe
Kriscautzky, Raul	Rivadavia 205	La Banda, Santiago del Estero
Kurlat, Pedro	Corrientes 2215–1°P.	Buenos Aires
Kutys, Jorge	Igarteche 126	Concepción del Uruguay, Entre Rios
Labat, Juan C.	Mitre 1565	Mendoza
Lachman, Rodolfo	Lavalle 1735–1° 'A'	Buenos Aires
Lagos Olivari, Eduardo	Paraguay 1132–1°P.	Buenos Aires
Lagleyze, Julio	Laprida 1727	Buenos Aires
Lagunas, Enrique	San Martín 2576	Rosario, Sante Fe
Laje, Carlos E.	Av. Olmos 179–1°P.	Córdoba
Laje Weskamp, Carlos	Av. Olmos 179–1°P.	Córdoba
Laje Poviña, Luis	Av. Gral. Paz 186 5° 'B'	Galería London, Córdoba
Lamela, Norma A.	Rojas 377	Buenos Aires
Landaburu, Argentino J.	Pampa 4261	Buenos Aires
Landó, Mario	Callao 384–4°P.	Buenos Aires
Lange, Reynaldo	San Martín 1052–1°	Mendoza
La Palma, Carlos	Sarmiento 902	Concepción del Uruguay, Entre Rios
Larre, Rafael J.	Maipú 645–4° '10'	Buenos Aires
Larrea, Enrique	Gral. Acha 317 Sur	San Juan
Larrea, Pedro	Colón 33	Córdoba
Laszcs, Irene	Uriarte 2452	Buenos Aires
Lataza Casamello, Jorge	Pirovano 162	Resistencia, Chaco
Laterra, Enrique	Cramer 707	Bernal, Bs. As.
Lattanzio, Alberto	Costa Rica 6086	Buenos Aires
Lavin, José	Aranguren 458	Buenos Aires
Lazarte, Armando	Bja. Caseros 342	Córdoba
Lazzari, Juan C.	S. de la Independencia 1253	Buenos Aires
Leibar, Santos E.	Rivadavia 2868	Buenos Aires
Leiter, Salomón	H. Irigoyen 610	Quilmes, Bs. As.
Lemos, Olga A. de	Cnel. Sayos 2633	Lanús, Bs. As.
Lendino, Emilio	Calle 22N° 485	Mercedes, Bs. As.
Lenti, Joaquín	Carlos Pellegrini 128	San Martín, Bs. As.

Leon, Alberto	H. Irigoyen 2028	Florida, Bs. As.
Lerner, Adolfo	Charcas 2074–3° 'B'	Buenos Aires
Levatti, Rómulo	Av. Quintana 89–1°	Buenos Aires
Levit, Jorge	Laprida 1242–PB	Buenos Aires
Libedín, Lida G. de	Talcahuano 840	Buenos Aires
Libman, Elías	Paraná 1083	Buenos Aires
Lienau, Rodolfo	Echeverría 2336	Buenos Aires
Lima, Enrique J.	San Juan 2767	Buenos Aires
Lipko, Frida	Tres Arroyos 1002	Buenos Aires
Lischinsky, Jorge	Junín 692	Tucumán
Lista, Dalmiro	9 de Julio 171–1°P.	Córdoba
Livellara, Alejandro	Rioja 1263	Mendoza
Livinston, Roberto	Charcas 1577–1°P.	Buenos Aires
Locascio, Irma	Cabildo 1695–1°P.	Buenos Aires
Lombardi, Atilio	Guemes 3115–7° 'B'	Buenos Aires
Longobuco, Ricardo	Independencia 3523	Buenos Aires
Longoni, Rodolfo	Necochea 269	Resistencia, Chaco
López, Andrés	Aberastain 134 Sur	San Juan
López, Mario	O'Higgins 4525–11°	Buenos Aires
López, Mario E.	Calle 8 N° 1018	25 de Mayo, Bs. As.
López, Raúl	S. de Bustamante 2156–4° 'C'	Buenos Aires
López Suhette, José	Alte. Brown 2069	Lomas del Mirador. Bs. As.
Lorenzini, Francisco	Lavalle 3077	Olavarría, Bs. As.
Lorenzo, Cándida	Av. 9 de Julio 219 Oeste	San Juan
Lorenzo, Gustavo	Rodriguez Peña 797	Buenos Aires
Losada, Eugenio	Roca 1161	Rosario, Santa Fe
Lovrincevic, Juan	Chacabuco 958	Venado Tuerto, Sta. Fe
Lowe, Guillermo	Baigorria 2926	Buenos Aires
Luchelli, Luis B. Roberto	Quintino Bocayuva 240	Buenos Aires
Ludner, José	Santa Fe 778–8°P.	Rosario, Santa Fe
Luna Pinto, José	Colón 784	Córdoba
Luppi, Alberto	Calle 3 N° 1278	La Plata, Bs. As.
Luppi, Luis	Independencia 1166	Firmat, Santa Fe
Machiavello, Juan	Ayacucho 267	Buenos Aires
Mackevicius, Leiba	Corrientes 2775–9°	Buenos Aires
Maffrand, Roque	Caseros 10–1°P.	Córdoba
Maffrand, Roque A.	Hosp. Centenario	Rosario, Sta. Fe
Maffrand de Broin, Susana	Dean Funes 873–'D'	Córdoba
Maggi Zavalía, Juan Carlos	San Jerónimo 3370	Santa Fe
Magrini, Antonio	Villegas 246–1°P.	S.C. de Bariloche, Rio Negro
Magris, Alberto	Mendoza 1470	Villa María, Cba.
Mainoli, Martín	Guemes 435	Salta
Makowsky, Diana de	Entre Rios 74	Resistencia, Chaco
Malbrán, Enrique	Parera 164	Buenos Aires
Maltagliatti, Miguel	Calle 56 N° 1280	La Plata, Bs. As.
Manavella, Lorenzo	3 de febrero 1475	Rosario, Santa Fe
Manes, Eduardo	Tucumán 741, PB	Buenos Aires
Manguel, Edgardo	Ciudad de la Paz 1735 'D'	Buenos Aires
Maniero, Daniel	25 de mayo 1359	Mendoza
Manolakis, Mario	Tolosa 980	Berisso, Bs. As.
Manzi, Mario A.	Colón 441–8° 'A'	Córdoba
Manzione, Bartolo	H. Irigoyen 591	Tandil, Bs. As.
Manzitti, Edgardo	Santa Fe 2245	Buenos Aires
Marcantonio, Rosa	Calle 34 N° 690	La Plata
Marceillac, Eduardo Luis	Olazabal 2490	Buenos Aires
Marco, Alberto	Isabel La Católica 538 'H'	Córdoba

Marcone, Guillermo	Rivadavia 18210	Morón, Bs. As.
Marconi, Guillermo	Alvear 235	Martínez, Bs. As.
Marchevsky, Lydia	Ayacucho 623	Mendoza
Marchevsky, Moisés	Rioja 1138	Mendoza
Marengo, Ernesto	Charcas 4165–1° 'A'	Buenos Aires
Mariani, Alfredo	Santander 1817–'2'	Buenos Aires
Mariani, Victor	R. Falcón 2604	Buenos Aires
Marincovich, José	B. Mitre 178	Luján, Bs. As.
Marpegan, Humberto	Pueyrredón 70	Villa Ballester, Bs. As
Martín, Martín E.	Gral. Paz 1108	Córdoba
Martínez, Jorge	R. Peña 1398	Martínez, Bs. As.
Martínez, Juan J.	Consejal Peñaloza (S) 353	Córdoba
Martino, Alberto	Urquiza 1017–2°	Rosario, Sta. Fe
Marttinetti, Hugo	Balcarce 604	Tucumán
Mary, Rodolfo	Lamadrid 291	Quilmes, Bs. As.
Masih, Carlos	Belgrano 820	Córdoba
Massanisso, Jorge	Av. Córdoba 1886–2°	Buenos Aires
Massari, Oscar	San Martín 185	Corral de Bustos, Córdoba
Mayorga, Eugenia de	25 de mayo 257–1°	Morón, Bs. As.
Mayorga, Humberto	Pte. Quintana 719	Castelar, Bs. As.
Mazzuli, Héctor	Sarmiento 4612	Buenos Aires
Medina, Ricardo	H. Irigoyen 1020	Rio Cuarto, Córdoba
Melani, Heraldo	Chacabuco 125	Chascomús, Bs. As.
Melek, Nélida	Segurola 160–1°	Buenos Aires
Méndez, Raúl H.	Calle 11 N° 729	La Plata, Bs. As.
Méndez, Salvador	B. Irigoyen 918	Gral. Rodriguez, Bs. As.
Meroni, José A.	Calle 5 N° 1145	La Plata, Bs. As.
Meroni, Juan C.	Calle 5 N° 1145	La Plata, Bs. As.
Mertre, Carlos J.	Aizpurúa 2980	Buenos Aires
Meszen, Gregorio	Córdoba 2645–3°	Buenos Aires
Meyer, Walter	Colón 3399	Mar del Plata, Bs. As.
Michelini, Enrique	Sarmiento 579	Saladillo, Bs. As.
Mila, Teresa	Sarmiento 1402	San Miguel, Bs. As.
Milenckowicz, Dragan	Buenos Aires 160	Dolores, Bs. As.
Mileo José R.	Vte. López 1853–3°	Buenos Aires
Miller, Rosa	Av. Mitre 374–11°	Avellaneda, Bs. As.
Mindlin, Alberto	Av. Centenario 1107	San Isidro, Bs. As.
Miquelarena, Pablo	Av. Roca 822	Pergamino, Bs. As.
Misteli, Ivonne	San Martín 1430	Mendoza
Mitnik, Luis	9 de Julio 68–1°	Córdoba
Moccorrea, Héctor	Av. Quintana 89–1°	Buenos Aires
Mocorrea, Julio	Santa Fe 2079	Buenos Aires
Moguilner, Natalio	Cabildo 4283	Buenos Aires
Moguilner, Néstor	Cabildo 4283	Buenos Aires
Moisés, Bety	Magnasco 72	Rio Tercero, Córdoba
Molas Raggio, Armando ...	El Maestro 5	Buenos Aires
Molina, Miguel	Dean Funes 432	Córdoba
Momesso, Adriana	Aguero 777–2° '5'	Buenos Aires
Monczor, Eva R. de	Ferrer 423	Marmol, Bs. As.
Monlao, Carlos	Gral. Mosconi 3147	Buenos Aires
Montagna, Pascual	Avellaneda 207	Bernal, Bs. As.
Montagna, Pascual (h)	Bocusi 161	Florencio Varela, Bs. As.
Montanaro, Juan C.	Canning 3350–5°	Buenos Aires
Montani, Dalcio	Córdoba 1776.	Rosario, Santa Fe
Montani, Mario	Sgo. Cabral 147–2°	Rosario, Santa Fe
Monteagudo, Pedro	Oliden 176	Lomas de Zamora, Bs. As.

Monteoliva, Héctor	Calle 12 N° 67	La Plata, Bs. As.
Montes, Carlos G.	Calle 70–N° 939	La Plata, Bs. As.
Monti, Néstor H.	Necochea 3345	Santa Fe
Moraschi, José	Virrey Cevallos 184	Buenos Aires
Morcos, Nicolás	Salta 1728	Mendoza
Moreira de Pereyra, Antonia	3 de febrero 1561	Rosario, Santa Fe
Moreno, Pedro	Famailla 2772	Buenos Aires
Moris, Ernesto L.	Buenos Aires 159	Tucumán
Mosquera, José M.	Juncal 1177–2°	Buenos Aires
Movileswky, Rosalinda	Av. Rivadavia 4370 9° 'C'	Buenos Aires
Moyano, Roberto	Córdoba 111–3°	San Francisco, Cba.
Mulet, Elena M. de	9 de julio 2140	Mendoza
Murgo, Antonino	Roca 2739	Hurlingham, Bs. As.
Murillo, José	French 2727	Buenos Aires
Muro, Luciano	Montevideo 521	Berisso, Bs. As.
Muro Oñaderra, Gastón ...	Santa Fe 2363	Casilda, Santa Fe
Muzzio, Juan C.	Hosp. Prov. de Comunidad-Córdoba 4545	Mar del Plata
Nafarrate, José A.	Santa Fe 1555	Buenos Aires
Nahum, Lucio	Cabildo 3722	Buenos Aires
Nahum, Roberto	Cabildo 3722	Buenos Aires
Nallar, Lindor	Pueyrredón 1746	Buenos Aires
Nano, Héctor M.	Rivadavia 7047–3°	Buenos Aires
Nano, Hugo D.	Sarmiento 1402	San Miguel, Bs. As.
Navarrete, Edgardo	Cangallo 4281–8°	Buenos Aires
Navarro, Jorge	San Juan 845	Rosario, Santa Fe
Naveyra, Alberto	Calle 38 N° 876 1/2 Dto. 3	La Plata, Bs. As.
Naveyra, Susana de	Calle 38 N° 876	La Plata, Bs. As.
Nazar, Lemuel	Pueyrredón 1361–8° 'D'	Buenos Aires
Negri, Herminio P.	24 de noviembre 2273	Buenos Aires
Nemoy, Enrique	Justa L. de Atucha 150	Zárate, Bs. As.
Neumann, Paulina Satanowsky de	Juncal 685	Buenos Aires
Nícoli, Carlos	Boedo 1070	Buenos Aires
Nícoli, Carlos (h)	Boedo 1070	Buenos Aires
Nieto, Raúl	Paraguay 50	Alto Alberdi, Cba.
Nihoul, Jorge L.	Av. Olmos 380–5°	Córdoba
Niño de Guzmán Heredia, Luis	Esmeralda 1075–4°	Buenos Aires
Nocetti, Abel	Calle 11 N° 1288	La Plata
Noceti, Atilio	Juncal 1470–7°	Buenos Aires
Nocetti de la Torre, Jorge ..	Santa Fe 3694–1°	Buenos Aires
Norbis, Atilio L.	Las Heras 1946	Buenos Aires
Nores, Rodolfo	Cnel. Rauch 3243	Castelar, Bs. As.
Oblati, Enrique	Vélez Sarsfield 2929	Lanús, Bs. As.
Obregón Oliva, Roberto ...	Belgrano 54	Córdoba
Ocampo, Alberto	Cerrito 1265	Buenos Aires
O'Farrell, Gabriel	R. Peña 1386	Buenos Aires
Ojeda, Beatriz C. de	Brown 457	Rafaela, Santa Fe
Olivera, Alejandro	Lavalle 3584	Buenos Aires
Oliveri, Rubén	Yerbal 3020	Buenos Aires
Ollé, Rodolfo	Corrientes 1719	Buenos Aires
Olmos, Hugo	Caseros 876	Salta
Onnis, Roger	Pje. Fader 131	Córdoba
Olsak, Alberto	Bmé. Mitre 73	Ramos Rcjía, Bs. As.
Orfila, Enrique C.	Cerrito 330–2°	Buenos Aires

Ortega, Julio	9 de Julio 170	Rafaela, Santa Fe
Ortiz, Azucena U. de	Boedo 160	Bernal, Bs. As.
Ortiz Olmedo, Arturo	Av. 24 de setiembre 1041	Córdoba
Oyenard, Adolfo H.	Charcas 2346	Buenos Aires
Pacheco, Horacio	Libertador 2168	Buenos Aires
Páez Allende, Francisco	Bv. Pellegrini 3090	Santa Fe
Páez Allende, José	Laprida 5010-Mon. 2–10° 'D'	Santa Fe
Pagano, Roberto	José Bonifacio 2270	Buenos Aires
Pagniez, Arturo	Sarmiento 1714–6°	Buenos Aires
Pailhé, Pedro	Calle 59–N° 2335	Necochea, Bs. As.
Palazzo, Jorge	Medrano 172	Buenos Aires
Palermo, Néstor	Alte. Brown 137	Chacabuco, Bs. As.
Palioni, Juan	E. Lamarca 5186	Buenos Aires
Palma, Luis	España 818	Campana, Bs. As.
Palmier Pardo, J.	3 de Febrero 3017	Rosario, Santa Fe
Paniagua, Ramírez	Moreno y Córdoba	Mar del Plata, Bs. As
Panizza, Luis M.	Av. Colón 276–11°	Córdoba
Pantalone, Vicente	M. García 545	Buenos Aires
Pañavecino, Mario	Av. Moreno 622	Santiago del Estero
Paonessa, Fernando	Belgrano 1431–5°	Buenos Aires
Papale, Hugo	Araujo 1117	Buenos Aires
Pardo, Carlos E.	Independencia 90	Laboulaye, Córdoba
Pardo, José M.	San Martín 2877	Santa Fe
Pardo, Mario C.	Carballo 1620 (164)	Paisamar, Mar del Plata
Parodi, Jorge	Anatole France 2133	Lanús, Bs. As.
Parolin, Luis	Lisandro de la Torre 2757	Santa Fe
Pascual, José	Calle 45 N° 844	La Plata, Bs. As.
Pastor, Héctor	Sta. Fe 4990–8° 'E'	Buenos Aires
Paunessa, José	Barrientos 1566	Buenos Aires
Pelliza, Hugo (h)	9 de Julio 237	La Rioja
Pelliza, Hugo	La Noria 1273	Quinta Santa Ana, Córdoba
Pena, Florentino	San Martín 814	Mendoza
Peralta, Sofía P. de	Corrientes 567	Goya, Corrientes
Perea, Horacio	Pereyra Lucena 2516	Buenos Aires
Pereira, Carlos	Córdoba 1889	Buenos Aires
Pereira, Roberto	Calle 51 N° 756	La Plata, Bs. As.
Peretti, Rialdo	Cnel. Dorrego 475	Rojas, Bs. As.
Pereyra, Lorenzo	3 de Febrero 1561	Rosario, Santa Fe
Pérez, Anuar	Yatay 1047	Paso de los Libres, Corrientes
Pérez, Darío A.	Colón 491	Posadas, Misiones
Pérez, Genovese	Paraguay 1845–8°	Buenos Aires
Pérez, Humberto	Fco. Beiró 5254	Buenos Aires
Pérez, Mauro	Timbúes 851	Castelar, Bs. As.
Pérez Riso, María	San Jerónimo 1957	Santa Fe
Pérez, Trinidad	Agustín Gómez 277 Este	San Juan
Perie, Pedro	Kilómetro 9	El Dorado, Misiones
Perli, Mario	Alsina 168	Quilmes, Bs. As.
Peruzzo, Oscar	Cangallo 1821–5°	Buenos Aires
Pesce, Edmundo	Rivadavia 2031–2°	Buenos Aires
Petry, Carlos E.	Calle 56–N° 625	La Plata, Bs. As.
Peyret, Jorge A.	Santa Fe 995–3°	Buenos Aires
Peyret, Jorge M.	Santa Fe 995	Buenos Aires
Pfefferman, Abraham	Azcuénaga 248	Buenos Aires
Pianciola, Alberto	Rivadavia 2358	Buenos Aires
Piantoni, Carlos	Av. R. Nuñez 2946	Arguello, Córdoba

Piantoni, Guido	Granaderos 65	Buenos Aires
Piantoni, Gustavo	Pueyrredón 1959	Buenos Aires
Picardi, Roberto	Jujuy 253	Córdoba
Piccioni, Edmundo	S. de Bustamante 2184–2° 'F'	Buenos Aires
Pícoli, Héctor R.	Rio Bamba 434	Buenos Aires
Piselli, Néstor M.	Pasco 1050	Rosario, Santa Fe
Pistonesi, Héctor	Sarmiento 266	Bahía Blanca, Bs. As.
Pistorio Soler, J.	Calle 4 N° 1085	Barrio Crisol, Norte, Córdoba
Pizzi, Victor	Forest 804	Buenos Aires
Plotkin, Carlos	Saenz 1217	Buenos Aires
Polakon, Dimitri	Pueyrredón 443	Villa Ballester, Bs. As.
Pollola, Eugenio	Eduardo Acevedo 211–PR	Buenos Aires
Pomponio, Ariel	Betolaza 233	Tres Arroyos, Bs. As.
Ponce de León, F.	Casilla Correo 154	Córdoba
Ponce de León, J.	Lamadrid 665	Tucumán
Ponce de León, María de	Casilla Correo 154	Córdoba
Poppi, Mario	Paraguay 2465	Buenos Aires
Posak, Carlos	Rivadavia 3174–2°	Mar del Plata, Bs. As.
Posse, Ramón V.	Moldes 985	Buenos Aires
Possi, Fernando	Lavalle 1730	Buenos Aires
Potenza, Angel P.	Boyacá 332	Buenos Aires
Poverene, José	Chiclana 510	Bahía Blanca, Bs. As.
Prados, Fortunato	Sarmiento 83	Santiago del Estero
Priani, Pedro	Anchorena 1205–6°	Buenos Aires
Prieto Díaz, Julio	Calle 11 N° 729	La Plata, Bs. As.
Priolo, Juan R.	Somellera 721	Adrogué, Bs. As.
Prytula, Mabel	9 de Julio 54	Bernal, Bs. As.
Puente, Alicia Santillan de	Batalla del Pari 927–PR 'B'	Buenos Aires
Puente, Susana	Junín 1131–2°	Buenos Aires
Puentes, Ignacio	Dean Funes 1132	Córdoba
Pulido, Aldo R.	Zuviría 173	Salta
Puppo, Bernardo J.	Coronel Díaz 1711	Buenos Aires
Quaintenne, Enrique	Madero 1127	Olivos, Bs. As.
Quesada, Alfredo	Ntra. Sra. del Buen Viaje 535	Morón, Bs. As.
Quiles, Jorge R.	Santa Fe 307	Tucumán
Racedo, Lucas	Paraguay 630	Rosario, Santa Fe
Radziwilowsky, Luis	Junín 1140–8° 'B'	Buenos Aires
Raed, Héctor	Rivadavia 628 E.	San Juan
Raibon, Nélida	M. Rodriguez 1272	Buenos Aires
Rainaudi, José	Sarmiento 1714–6°	Buenos Aires
Raimondi, Juan P.	Av. Alvear 1807–1°	Buenos Aires
Ramirez, Guillermo	V. Sarsfield 5299	Munro, Bs. As.
Ramos, Julio A.	Murguiondo 4057–1°	Galería Lugano, Buenos Aires
Ramummo, Donato	Catamarca 1457	Mar del Plata, Bs. As.
Rapetti, Rinaldo	Rivadavia 2396–4°	Buenos Aires
Ratto, Roberto	Azcuénaga 1049	Buenos Aires
Ravetti, Eduardo	Constitución 971	Rio Cuarto, Córdoba
Ravinovich, Eduardo	Belgrano 608	Trelew, Chubut
Raycevich, Alejandro	Pringles 4140	Florida, Bs. As.
Ré, Benjamín E.	Av. Santa Fe 4963	Buenos Aires
Ré, Benjamín V.	Av. Santa Fe 4963	Buenos Aires
Rearte, Horacio	España 1310	Concepción, Tucumán
Reca, Arturo	Alem 29	Parána, Entre Rios
Reca, Martín	Arenales 3044–PB	Buenos Aires

Reca, Oscar	Alem 57	Paraná, Entre Rios
Reca, Osvaldo	Paraguay 1845	Buenos Aires
Recagno, Atilio	Larrea 832	Buenos Aires
Reinecke, Florencia	Rivera Indarte 422	Buenos Aires
Reissig, Anibal	Rivadavia 6368	Buenos Aires
Reissig, Héctor	Rivadavia 6368	Buenos Aires
Remedi, J.	Calle 15 N° 939	Miramar, Bs. As.
Remedi, Guillermo	Pampa 52	Córdoba
Remonda, Carlos	Av. Colón 33−2°	Córdoba
Remonda, Juan	Av. Colón 33−2°	Córdoba
Renard, Rafael	Sucre 2619	Buenos Aires
Rey, Hugo	Belgrano 2609	Mar del Plata, Bs. As.
Richarson, Jorge	Obispo Oro 138	Córdoba
Riera, Alfredo	San Martín esq. Loubet	Villa Belgrano, Córdoba
Rigo, Edmundo	L. de la Torre 234	Villa María, Córdoba
Rillo Cabanne, Germán	Luro 2668−1°	Mar del Plata, Bs. As.
Rinaldi, Teodoro	Viamonte 2759−'A'	Buenos Aires
Rios Velar, César	Callao 1052	Buenos Aires
Rios, Rodolfo	Otero 126	Jujuy
Rivas, Oscar	Alberdi 12	San Pedro de Jujuy, Jujuy
Rivera, Enrique	Calle 26 N° 857	Mercedes, Bs. As.
Rivera, Juan	Rivadavia 229	Junín, Bs. As.
Rizzolo, Juan	Davila 775	Buenos Aires
Roca, Félix	Corrientes 127	San Francisco, Cba.
Roca, Jorge Ivan	Urquiza 77	Mercedes, San Luis
Roccatagliata, Horacio F.	Independencia 2948	Buenos Aires
Rocco, Américo	Chacabuco 1215	Buenos Aires
Rocha Penteado, Renato	Urquiza 3100	Rosario, Santa Fe
Rodrigo, Alinda	Cañada Morón 282	Villa Tessey, Bs. As.
Rodriguez, Alejandro	Mancione 1	Añatuya, Santiago del Estero
Rodriguez, Carlos	Rondeau 85−2°	Córdoba
Rodriguez, Gerardo	Chacabuco 137	San Martín, Mendoza
Rojas, Carlos	Viamonte 1464−6°	Buenos Aires
Rojkind, Abraham	Rio de Janeiro 58	Buenos Aires
Rojo, Gregorio	24 de noviembre 1580	Buenos Aires
Román, Ernesto C.	Perú 1145	Buenos Aires
Román, Juan	Bolívar 111	Posadas, Misiones
Romero, Horacio V.	Pampa 5124	Buenos Aires
Romero Etchevarne, Alfredo	Guise 2065−4°	Buenos Aires
Roncoroni, Jorge	Chorroarín 17−1°	Buenos Aires
Ros, Fernando	Necochea 138	Resistencia, Chaco
Rosa, Roberto	Almafuerte 2980	San Justo, Bs. As.
Rosemberg, Isaac	José Hernández 1955−10° '42'	Buenos Aires
Rosenzuaig, León	San Martín 791−4°	Rosario, Santa Fe
Rosso Nano, Nélida	Austria 2123−3°	Buenos Aires
Rottgardt, Arturo	Gaona 2087−5° 'B'	Buenos Aires
Roulier, Mónica	R. S. Peña 725−3°	Buenos Aires
Roveda, José M.	Lezica 4472	Buenos Aires
Roveda, Carlos	Sarmiento 4151-30°	Buenos Aires
Rubil, Julio	Manzanares 1666	Buenos Aires
Rucando, José	Catilli 620	Venado Tuerto, Santa Fe
Ruderman, Ebert	9 de Julio 1184	Lanús, Bs. As.
Rudzinski, Nicolás	Rivadavia 1037	Oberá, Misiones
Ruffa, Raúl	Av. Colón 1951−'E'	Córdoba
Ruiz Moreira de Pereyra, Antonio	3 de Febrero 1561	Rosario, Santa Fe

Rusconi, Raúl	Calle 27-N° 630	25 de Mayo, Bs. As.
Rusconi, Raúl	Av. Ceballos 119	Chivilcoy, Bs. As.
Saba, Juan	Somellera 5488	Villa Lugano, Bs. As.
Saggese, Domingo	A. Mazza 1760	Rosario, Sta. Fe
Said, Jorge	Ecuador 888-7°	Buenos Aires
Said, Raúl	E. Mitre 75-7°	Buenos Aires
Salas Buzó, Guillermo	Bermúdez 1136	Buenos Aires
Salas Oliver, Pedro	Bvard. Oroño 836	Rosario, Santa Fe
Salazar, Juan C.	Pedernera 959	Barrio Maipú, Cba.
Salazar, Nancy M. de	Triunvirato 4013	Buenos Aires
Salazar Espinoza, Néstor	Triunvirato 4013 4° '19'	Buenos Aires
Salvarredy, Enrique	Colón 178	C. del Uruguay, E. Rios
Salvarredy, Ernesto	Colón 178	C. del Uruguay, E. Rios
Salti, Odette	Billinghurst 2495	Buenos Aires
Salvatori, Héctor	Alsina 1502	V. López, Bs. As.
Salz, Carlos	Alem 1417	Monte Grande, Bs. As.
Salleras, Alejandro	Alsina 174	Avellaneda, Bs. As.
Sampaolesi, Roberto	Corrientes 1296	Buenos Aires
Sanchez Peña, Carlos A.	Chile 944	Mendoza
Sanchez, Jorge D.	Ituzaingó 408	Zárate, Bs. As.
Sánchez, Rubén M.	9 de Julio 171-1°	Córdoba
Sanchik, Abraham	L. N. Alem 233	Córdoba
Sancholuz, Jorge	Chacabuco 344	Tandil, Bs. As.
Sancholuz, Jorge L.	Colón 3399	Mar del Plata, Bs. As.
San Martín, Fernando J.	Alvear 1320	Bánfield, Bs. As.
San Pedro, Arturo	Malabia 2274-11°	Buenos Aires
Sanso, Guillermo	Gral. Paz 32 E.	San Juan
Santacroce, José	J.L. de Cabrera Oeste 975	Córdoba
Santamarina de Fernández, B.	Rioja 642	Mendoza
Santos, Héctor	Olivieri 42-5°	Lanús, Bs. As.
Saragovi, Luis	Sarmiento 1434	Buenos Aires
Satler, Eduardo	Belgrano 232	Córdoba
Sausi, Alejandro	Av. Italia 1262	Rio Cuarto, Córdoba
Sauthier, Julio	Iriondo 441	San Justo, Santa Fe
Scaraffia, Helena Pedrani de	Aristides Villanueva 165	Mendoza
Scattini, Fernando	Alte. Brown 1239	Buenos Aires
Scattoni, Lía M. de	Saavedra 15	Buenos Aires
Scattoni, Omar	Casanova 249	Bahía Blanca, Bs. As.
Scavuzzo, Rodolfo	Roca 789	Esquel, Chubut
Scenna, Miguel A.	Gral. Roca 624	Bolívar, Bs. As.
Schlaen, Isaac	Colón 1260-15°	Rosario, Santa Fe
Schlaen, Julio	Olive 1159	Rosario, Santa Fe
Schulman, León	Gral. Paz 37	Bahía Blanca, Bs. As.
Schiaffino, Fernando	Cnel. D'Elia 1611 EP. Timbre 1°	Lanús O., Bs. As.
Scigolini, Horacio	Las Flores 628	Wilde, Bs. As.
Schijman, Rubén	J.B. Alberdi 6172	Buenos Aires
Schiratti, Alberto	Paraguay 1148	Buenos Aires
Schlesinger, Máximo	Panamá 573	Paraná, Entre Rios
Schujmajer, Isaac	Laprida 482	Lomas de Zamora, Bs. As.
Schvartzman, Samuel	Sarmiento 2195-8°	Buenos Aires
Schwender, Guillermo	San Martín 907	Reconquista, Sta. Fe
Scremin, Rodolfo	Mendoza 2984	Rosario, Sta. Fe
Segarra, José H.	San Lorenzo 160	Mendoza
Seggiaro, Myrian Berman de	Corrientes 643	Tucumán
Segovia, Alejandro	Urquiza 39	Villaguay, E. Rios

Segura, Abraham	Dean Funes 957	Córdoba
Seltzer, Isaac	Av. Mitre 2012-1°	Avellaneda, Bs. As.
Sená, José	Av. Quintana 326	Buenos Aires
Serena, Lucila	Calle 45–N° 985	La Plata, Bs. As.
Serres, Eduardo	Bulnes 2049–6°	Buenos Aires
Sidelnik. María H.	Independencia 1315	Mar del Plata, Bs. As.
Silva, Benito	Av. Maipu 1388	V. López, Bs. As.
Silverstein, Marcos	Larrea 1161	Buenos Aires
Sinópoli, Alberto	Acassuso 310	San Isidro, Bs. As.
Siotas, Jorge	Perú 79–5°P.	Buenos Aires
Siri, Alberto	Democracia 525	Bajo Palermo, Cba.
Sirito, César	Quintana 2059	Olivos, Bs. As.
Sitler, Rafael L.	Ecuador 1429	Buenos Aires
Sobolewsky, Bernardo	Homero 233	Buenos Aires
Soiza, Juan A.	R. Peña 1158–8°	Buenos Aires
Solivella Cuenca, Raúl	Blanco Encalada 5297–1° 'B'	Buenos Aires
Somma, Roberto	Sitio de Montevideo 66	Lanús, Bs. As.
Soraide, Eduardo R.	Libertador 257–1°	Córdoba
Sorana, Julio E.	Av. Córdoba 2965	Buenos Aires
Soriano, Julián	Rio Bamba 74–4°	Buenos Aires
Sosa Cazales, Julio	25 de mayo 3072	Mar del Plata, Bs. As
Sotelo, José A.	Belgrano 394	Gualeguay, E. Rios
Soto, Máximo	Entre Rios 480	Rosario, Santa Fe
Southall, Guillermo	O'Higgins 2352	Buenos Aires
Spatafore, Santiago	Castro 1643	Buenos Aires
Spector, Adolfo	Thames 2460	Buenos Aires
Spina, Ronald	Mitre 545	Morón, Bs. As.
Stefani, Carlos	Parera 164	Buenos Aires
Stella, Humberto	12 de octubre 1767	Buenos Aires
Stenbrun Bertoni, Miguel	Cabildo 714	Buenos Aires
Storero, Eduardo	Italia 1266	San Antonio de Padua, Bs. As.
Suaid, José A.	Av. Belgrano 189	Alta Gracia, Córdoba
Suárez, Alba	San Martín 164	Godoy Cruz, Mendoza
Sverdlick, José	B. Mitre 1221–4°	Buenos Aires
Swirynski, Natalio	Navarro 8	Beccar, Bs. As.
Taboada, Elvira	Sucre 558–8°	Córdoba
Tacite, Domingo	Jujuy 261–8°	Córdoba
Tagliero, Juan	Av. Lib. Gral. San Martín 1014	San Fernando, Bs. As.
Tapella, Luis (h)	Solís 1292-PB	Buenos Aires
Tapia, Josefina S. de	Spegazzini 530	Buenos Aires
Tarbine, Moisés	Entre Rios 1963	Córdoba
Tasada, Raúl	Bvard. Oroño 726	Rosario, Sta. Fe
Tealdi, Rubén	Santa Rosa 1366	Córdoba
Tello Delgado, José	Brown 158	Bahía Blanca, Bs. As.
Tenaglia, M. Escudero de	Belgrano 266–2°	San Martín, Bs. As.
Tenaglia, Roque	Belgrano 266–2°	San Martín, Bs. As.
Terre Vila, Luis R.	Santa Fe 2464	Rosario, Santa Fe
Texier, Alberto	Parera 121–5°	Buenos Aires
Therisod, Manuel	Sarmiento 877	Tandil, Bs. As.
Thierer, Bención	Olazábal 4735	Buenos Aires
Thwaites Lastra, Eduardo	Córdoba 1752–9°	Buenos Aires
Tiberti, Armando	Sarmiento y Ameghino	La Banda, Sgo. del Estero
Tiscornia, Atilio	Rivadavia 330	Comodoro Rivadavia, Chubut
Tiveron, Jorge	Calle 11 N° 514	La Plata, Bs. As.
Tomei, Eleonora	Avellaneda 4102	Buenos Aires

Torena, Roberto	Gral. Guemes 878	Salta
Torres, Juan R.	Avellaneda 313	Pte. R.S. Peña, Chaco
Torres Correa, Ricardo	9 de Julio 89	Tucumán
Tesello, Pedro	Belgrano 192	Córdoba
Tosi, Bruno	Calle 6 N° 690	La Plata, Bs. As.
Tosi, Enrique	Altolaguirre 2344	Villa Urquiza, Bs. As.
Tosi, Guillermo B.	Calle 6 N° 690	La Plata, Bs. As.
Tozzi, Jorge	Av. Galicia 672	Avellaneda, Bs. As.
Traverso, Ernesto	3 de febrero 721	Rosario, Sta. Fe
Traverso, Gabriel	Rivadavia 47	Villa Ramallo, Bs. As.
Travi, Orlando	Rivadavia 5483	Buenos Aires
Trivisonno, Jorge	Tucumán 1748	Buenos Aires
Tula Duca, Luis	Esquiú 801	Villa Cabrera, Cba.
Ugrin, María C.	Paraguay 2571-5°	Buenos Aires
Urrets Zavalía, Alberto	Arquitecto Thays 75	Córdoba
Vaccaro, Gerónimo	San Lorenzo 619	Corrientes
Valenzuela, Jorge	Parera 164	Buenos Aires
Valenzuela, María de los Angeles	Mitre 613	Venado Tuerto, Santa Fe
Vallejos, Benigno E.	Congreso 265/73	Tucumán
Varela, Olia R.	Acoyte 655-7°	Buenos Aires
Vassallo, Néstor	Bolivia 178-4°	Buenos Aires
Vaudagnotto, Osvaldo	San Martín 3362	Olavarría, Bs. As.
Vázquez de Parga, A.	Pueyrredón 2257	Buenos Aires
Vázquez, Santiago	9 de Julio 567	Nogoyá, Entre Rios
Vedoya, María E.	Azcuénaga 958-PB	Buenos Aires
Veja, Juan	Sarmiento 4288-2°	Buenos Aires
Véntola, Eduardo	Alberdi 1432	Buenos Aires
Véntola, Guillermo	Constitución 1058	San Fernando, Bs. As.
Véntola, Horacio	Av. San Martín 14331	Martínez, Bs. As.
Verisimo, Miguel	Fco. Bilbao 1721	Buenos Aires
Verna, Obdulio	Juan de Garay 3428	Olivos, Bs. As.
Vicario, Roberto	Soler 4557	Buenos Aires
Victorica, Luis	Sarmiento 1402	San Miguel, Bs. As.
Vidal Rioja, Dionisio	Calle 6 N° 1743	La Plata, Bs. As.
Videla, Julio C.	Carlos Calvo 2038	Buenos Aires
Vigo Ferreira, Nelson	Sarmiento 519	Concordia, Entre Rios
Vila Ortiz, Juan M.	Paraguay 40	Rosario, Santa Fe
Vilar, Carlos	Av. Sáenz 1060	Buenos Aires
Vilar, Oscar E.	Pampa 2654	Buenos Aires
Vilches, Pablo	Santa Fe 353	Cosquín, Córdoba
Vilela, Julio C.	Moreno 114-Of. 15	Tres Arroyos, Bs. As.
Villagra, Cornelio	Av. Patria 397	Córdoba
Villanueva, Amalia	Pueyrredón 2257	Buenos Aires
Villarrodona, Carlos	Urquiza 1285	Paraná, Entre Rios
Viña, Rosa	Nueva York 2783	Buenos Aires
Visiano, Osvaldo	Cucha Cucha 43	Sarandí, Bs. As.
Visintin, Marisa Coló de	Mariano Pelliza 4060	Olivos, Bs. As.
Vives, José R.	San Martín 520	Bernal, Bs. As.
Vittar, Antonio	San Nicolás 468	Rosario, Sta, Fe
Vodovosoff, Sergio	Fta. Sarmiento 1825-4°	Buenos Aires
Von Grolman, Gunther	Santa Fe 1460-5°	Buenos Aires
Vulicher, Norberto	Urquiza 69	San Nicolás, Bs. As.
Waisman, Gloria M. de	Mitre 192 Oeste	San Juan
Wasserman, Reynaldo	Rio de Janeiro 1063	Buenos Aires
Weigel Cortese, Humberto	Cnel. Diaz 1785	Buenos Aires

Weil, Bernardo	Urquiza 2736	Florida, Bs. As.
Weskamp, Federico	Laprida 1159	Rosario, Santa Fe
Weskamp, Rodolfo	Saavedra 20	Junín, Bs. As.
Weskamp Irigoyen, Rodolfo.	Saavedra 20	Junín, Bs. As.
Wignand, Heriberto	Perú 2515	San Justo, Bs. As.
Woelflin, Luis J.	Italia 837	Rosario, Santa Fe
Wouterlood, Pedro	Chutro 222	Córdoba
Yankelevich, Jaime	Loria 148	Buenos Aires
Yanovsky, Raúl	Juan B. Justo 3971	Buenos Aires
Zambelli, José A.	Cabildo 2938	Buenos Aires
Zambrano, Jorge C.	Cangallo 2082	Buenos Aires
Zambrano, Jorge (h)	Cangallo 2082	Buenos Aires
Zampini, Lilia	Calle 7 N° 1980	La Plata, Bs. As.
Zanelli, Arístides	Mansilla 3344−1°	Buenos Aires
Zanon, Carlos A.	Paraguay 1627−2°	Buenos Aires
Yashy, Carlos	Rosales 2880	Alto de San Vicente, Córdoba
Zaldívar, Roger	San Martín 1430	Mendoza
Zarate, Adolfo	Maza 3254	Rosario, Santa Fe
Závalo, Eduardo J.	Sobremonte 945	Rio Cuarto, Córdoba
Zeniquel, Justo	San Lorenzo 1356	Corrientes
Zeolite, Carlos I.	Mitre 1364	Mendoza
Zubelzu, Angeles B.	Pte. Roca 692−6°	Rosario, Santa Fe
Zubillaga, Juan B.	Ayacucho 291	Buenos Aires
Zunino, Alberto	Santa Fe 2590−2°	Buenos Aires
Zvik, Mauricio	Sen. Havegger 742	Reconquista, Santa Fe

NOSOCOMIA QUIBUS OCULIS AEGRI CURANTUR

Cátedras de Oftalmología

Universidad Nacional de Buenos Aires, Cátedra de Oftalmología. Profesor: Dr. José M. Roveda, Hospital Nacional de Clínicas, Córdoba 2149, Capital Federal.

Universidad Nacional de Córdoba, Cátedra de Oftalmología, Profesor: Dr. Alberto Urrets-Zavalia (h), Pabellón 'Rca. del Perú', Concepción Arenal 81, Córdoba.

Universidad Nacional de La Plata, Cátedra de Oftalmología. Profesor: Dr. Bruno Tosi, Calle 60, N° 120, La Plata (Bs. As.)

Universidad Nacional del Litoral Cátedra de Oftalmología. Profesor: Dr. Lorenzo Manavella, Hospital Centenario, Urquiza 3100, Rosario (Sta. Fe).

Universidad Nacional de Cuyo, Cátedra de Oftalmología. Profesor: Dr. Roger E. Zaldivar, Hospital Central, ler. piso, ala oeste, Mendoza.

Universidad Nacional del Nordeste, Cátedra de Oftalmología. Profesor: Dr. Manuel Chervin, Hospital 'J. F. Cabral', Rivadavia 1275, Corrientes.

Universidad Nacional de Tucumán, Cátedra de Oftalmología. Prof. Dr. Jorge Luis Castillo, Av. Benjamín Araoz 750, San Miguel de Tucumán.

Universidad Católica de Córdoba, Cátedra de Oftalmología. Profesor: Dr. Manuel Copello, Obispo Trejo 323, Córdoba.

Universidad Privada del Salvador, Cátedra de Oftalmología. Profesor: Dr. Roberto Sampaolesi, Callao 542, Capital Federal.

AUSTRALIA

SOCIETATES OPHTHALMOLOGICAE

Nationalis

The Australian College of Ophthalmologists

President: David O. Crompton
Vice-President: Lloyd Cahill
Immediate-Past President: Ronald F. Lowe
Honorary Treasurer: G. Burfitt-Williams
Honorary Secretary: Graeme Johnson, 27 Commonwealth Street, Sydney, New South Wales 2010
Censor-in-Chief: Peter A. Rogers

Councillors:

Queensland: L. J. Macintosh, J. V. T. Apel
New South Wales: C. H. Baker, E. J. Milverton, J. G. Henry, L. P. Robinson
Victoria: J. W. Bishop, B. A. Crawford, F. A. Billson
Tasmania: B. Taranto
South Australia: J. D. Lister, J. B. Murchland
West Australia: D. J. McAuliffe
ex officio members: G. W. Harley, T. Keldoulis

Regionales

Branches of the Australian College of Ophthalmologists in each State:

Queensland: Branch Secretary G. T. Porter, 131 Wickham Terrace, Brisbane, Queensland 4000. Number of members: 55
New South Wales: Branch Secretary E. J. Milverton, 16 Mary Street, Auburn, N.S.W. 2144. Number of members: 186
Victoria: Branch Secretary Lindsay Jones, 175 Bay Street, Brighton, Victoria 3186. Number of members: 108
Tasmania: Branch Secretary Gordon Wise, 174 Macquarie Street, Hobart, Tasmania 7000. Number of members: 11
South Australia: Branch Secretary D. R. Hall, 188 North Terrace, Adelaide, South Australia 5000. Number of members: 36
West Australia: Branch Secretary John. A. Rogers, 4 Ventnor Ave., West Perth, West Australia 6000. Number of members: 19

Total Membership of the College		
Ordinary members:	415	
Associate members:	26	
Honorary members:	42	
Grand total	483	

NOMINA ET DOMICILIA MEDICORUM AB OCULIS

Aboud, John	149 Wickham Terrace	Brisbane, Qld., 4000
Aitken, Adele L.	193 Macquarie Street	Sydney, N.S.W., 2000
Akkermans, Charles	267 Melbourne Street	North Adelaide, S.A., 5006
Ancell, Brian E. J.	178 North Terrace	Adelaide, S.A., 5000
Anderson, Archie S.	6 Gayner Court	Malvern, Vic., 3144
Anderson, Esme	20 Collins Street	Melbourne, Vic., 3000
Anderson, Peter F.	183 Macquarie Street	Sydney, N.S.W., 2000
Apel, John V. T.	137 Wickham Terrace	Brisbane, Qld., 4000
Appel, Godfrey	Suite 8, Wallace Way	Chatswood, N.S.W., 2067
Armstrong, Keith B.	231 Macquarie Street	Sydney, N.S.W., 2000
Armstrong, Thomas M.	175 Macquarie Street	Sydney, N.S.W., 2000
Baker, Cecil H.	33 Dowe Street	Tamworth, N.S.W., 2340
Banks, C. N.	324 Marrickville Road	Marrickville, N.S.W., 2204
Banks-Smith, G.	7 Mackenzie Street	Lindfield, N.S.W., 2070
Barnard, Young H.	'Alton', Wentworth Street	Manly, N.S.W., 2095
Barnett, Wm. J.	33 Dowe Street	Tamworth, N.S.W., 2340
Barty, G. M.	7 Ely Street	Wangaratta, Vic., 3677
Beaumont-Haynes, J.	184 Sydney Road	Fairlight, N.S.W., 2094
Beckett, H. C.	183 Macquarie Street	Sydney, N.S.W., 2000
Benjamin, David	66 High Street	Randwick, N.S.W., 2031
Bennett, Aubrey G.	76 Charters Towers Road	Townsville, Qld., 4810
Bennett, Donald C.	163 North Terrace	Adelaide, S.A., 5000
Benson, Colin J.	254 St. Georges Terrace	Perth, W.A., 6000
Bignell, John L.	2 Collins Street	Melbourne, Vic., 3000
Billson, Frank A.	428 St. Kilda Road	Melbourne, Vic., 3004
Bishop, Jas. W.	10 Wallace Street	Newtown, Geelong, Vic., 3220
Blair, J. Murray	123 Langtree Avenue	Mildura, Vic., 3500
Blakemore, C. G. A.	135 Macquarie Street	Sydney, N.S.W., 2000
Blaxland, F. J.	235 Macquarie Street	Sydney, N.S.W., 2000
Bond, Jennifer A.	153 Macquarie Street	Hobart, Tas., 7000
Bonner-Morgan, R. P.	4 Church Street	Morwell, Vic., 3840
Bonner-Morgan, Barbara	4 Church Street	Morwell, Vic., 3840
Borger, J. P.	20 Collins Street	Melbourne, Vic., 3000
Borowitz, Ariel	296 Glen Eira Road	Elsternwick, Vic., 3185
Bors, Frank H.	193 Macquarie Street	Sydney, N.S.W., 2000
Bougher, Gordon	4 Ventnor Avenue	West Perth, W.A., 6005
Boyd-Law, T.	P. O. Box 261	Ballina, N.S.W., 2478
Box, W. M.	89/113 Swanston Street	Melbourne, Vic., 3000
Bradley, Edgar	123 Rusden Street	Armidale, N.S.W., 2350
Branson, D. M.	231 North Terrace	Adelaide, S.A., 5000
Bremner, Mary H.	254 St. Georges Terrace	Perth, W.A., 6000
Brennan, Margaret	16 Errard Street North	Ballarat, Vic., 3350
Brett, P. R.	882 Whitehorse Road	Box Hill, Vic., 3128
Broadbent, John	P. O. Box 135	Goulburn, N.S.W., 2580
Bromley, J. H.	36 Ormonde Parade	Hurstville, N.S.W., 2229
Brown, Douglas	82 Market Street	Wollongong, N.S.W., 2500
Brummitt, D. A.	175 North Terrace	Adelaide, S.A., 5000
Brunckhorst, A. M.	114 Russell Street	Toowoomba, Qld., 4350
Bryan, Peter Kaye	20 Collins Street	Melbourne, Vic., 3000
Budge, A. C.		Devonport, Tas., 7310
Burfitt-Williams, G. C. T.	175 Macquarie Street	Sydney, N.S.W., 2000
Burkett, M. L.	15 Collins Street	Melbourne, Vic., 3000

Burnside, Colin C.	64 St. Johns Avenue	Gordon, N.S.W., 2072
Cahill, Lloyd	231 Macquarie Street	Sydney, N.S.W., 2000
Cairns, J. D.	12 Collins Street	Melbourne, Vic., 3000
Cameron, Malcolm E.	73 Wickham Terrace	Brisbane, Qld., 4000
Campbell, C. A. K.	160 Bolsover Street	Rockhampton, Qld., 4700
Campbell, Dame Kate	2 Collins Street	Melbourne, Vic., 3000
Carpenter, John B.	135 Macquarie Street	Sydney, N.S.W., 2000
Carroll, Anthony	Compass House, Featherstone Street	Bankstown, N.S.W., 2200
Carroll, H. B.	193 Macquarie Street	Sydney, N.S.W., 2000
Carroll, L. A.	105 Collins Street ..,.......	Melbourne, Vic., 3000
Carter, J. L. R.	41 Brisbane Street	Launceston, Tas., 7250
Chadha, Vidya B.	c/- Queen Elizabeth Hospital	Woodville, S.A., 5011
Chapman, M. J.	96 Shaftesbury Road	Burwood, N.S.W., 2134
Chatfield, R. K.	314 High Street	Penrith, N.S.W., 2750
Cheok, F. P. G.	193 Macquarie Street	Sydney, N.S.W., 2000
Cher, Ivan	52 Wallangra Road	Dover Heights, N.S.W., 2034
Chin, W. N.	55 Collins Street	Melbourne, Vic., 3000
Claffy, F. B.	235 Macquarie Street	Sydney, N.S.W., 2000
Clipsham, S. B.	North Shore Medical Centre, 66 Pacific Highway	St. Leonards, N.S.W., 2065
Colvin, Clifford S.	193 Anson Street	Orange, N.S.W., 2800
Colvin, John L.	251 Grattan Street	Carlton, Vic., 3053
Coop, D. H.	State Chambers, Civic Centre ...	Canberra, A.C.T., 2600
Cooper, Bryan	25 Homebush Road	Strathfield, N.S.W., 2135
Coote, B. D.	20 Collins Street	Melbourne, Vic., 3000
Counsell, W. D.	428 St. Kilda Road	Melbourne, Vic., 3004
Cowen, P. H.	2 Collins Street	Melbourne, Vic., 3000
Cowle, J. B.	110 Willoughby Road	Crows Nest, N.S.W., 2065
Crawford, B. A.	251 Grattan Street	Carlton, Vic., 3053
Crock, Prof. G. W.	Department of Ophthalmology, University of Melbourne, c/- Royal Victorian Eye & Ear Hospital	East Melbourne, Vic., 3002
Crompton, David O.	104 Brougham Place	North Adelaide, S.A., 5006
Cumming, Gordon	235 Macquarie Street	Sydney, N.S.W., 2000
Dart, J. L.	Box 361, P. O.	Surfers Paradise, Qld., 4217
Darvall, Roger	16 Tintern Avenue	Carlingford, N.S.W., 2118
Davies, George B.	48 Sale Street	Orange, N.S.W., 2800
Davies, Glynn Anthony ...	231 North Terrace	Adelaide, S.A., 5000
Davis, J.	51 Woodlands Rd.	East Lindfield, N.S.W., 2070
Deane-Butcher, W.	North Shore Medical Centre, 66 Pacific Highway	St. Leonards, N.S.W., 2065
Day, Ellen M.	2 Garden Street	Reservoir, Vic., 3073
Donaldson, E. J.	231 Macquarie Street	Sydney, N.S.W., 2000
Donovan, Brian J.	97 Scarborough Street	Southport, Qld., 4215
Douglas, R. L.	5 Masons Parade	Gosford, N.S.W., 2250
Duke, P. S.	135 Macquarie Street	Sydney, N.S.W., 2000
Dunlop, D. B.	17 Bolton Street	Newcastle, N.S.W., 2300
Du Temple, D. J.	152 Marsden Street	Parramatta, N.S.W., 2150
Elder, John R.	205 Auburn Street	Goulburn, N.S.W., 2580
English, Frank P.	113 Wickham Terrace	Brisbane, Qld., 4000
English, Peter B.	113 Wickham Terrace	Brisbane, Qld., 4000
Evanoff, E.	24 Mirool Street	Denistone, N.S.W., 2114
Favilla, Ian	4 Remy Court	Donvale, Vic., 3111
Fenton, F. G.	20 Collins Street	Melbourne, Vic., 3000

Findlater, J. H.	678 Military Road	Spit Junction, N.S.W., 2088
Finkelstein, E.	34 Paisley Street	Footscray, Vic., 3011
Flynn, Rev. Father F.	Box 82, P. O.	Port Moresby, T.P.N.G.
Flynn, Gregory	122 Gillies Street	Wollstonecraft, N.S.W., 2065
Fraser, Hugh	137 Wickham Terrace	Brisbane, Qld., 4000
Fogland, Wm. G.	17 Parker Avenue	Massena, New York, 13662
Foster, James B.	24 Queens Road	Melbourne, Vic., 3004
Foster, John L.	135 Wattle Valley Road	Camberwell, Vic., 3124
Freshney, E.	135 Macquarie Street	Sydney, N.S.W., 2000
Galbraith, J. E. K.	Cabrini Medical Centre, Coonil Crescent	Malvern, Vic., 3141
Gale, David	2 Collins Street	Melbourne, Vic., 3000
Gaston, W. Garfield	163 North Terrace	Adelaide, S.A., 5000
Gault, A. G.	2 Collins Street	Melbourne, Vic., 3000
Gibbons, N.	Johnstone Chambers, High Street	Maitland, N.S.W., 2320
Gibson, Brian Lockhart . . .	131 Wickham Terrace	Brisbane, Qld., 4000
Gibson, Walter Lockhart . . .	131 Wickham Terrace	Brisbane, Qld., 4000
Gill, C. J.	324 South Road	Moorabbin, Vic., 3189
Gillespie, R. E. R.	47 Berry Street	Nowra, N.S.W., 2540
Gillies, W. E.	110 Collins Street	Melbourne, Vic., 3000
Goddard, S. J.	541 Kiewa Street	Albury, N.S.W., 2640
Goldman, A.	64 Baden Powell Road	Frankston, Vic., 3199
Gorman, R. F.	1 Marsina Street	Darwin, N.T., 5790
Graham, Peter J.	14 Kingsway	Nedlands, W.A., 6009
Gray, W. C.	8 Main Street	Blacktown, N.S.W., 2148
Gregory, E. M.	22 Florence Street	Strathfield, N.S.W., 2135
Gregory-Roberts, F.	135 Macquarie Street	Sydney, N.S.W., 2000
Grice, Medody J.	16 Brisbane Street Annerley	Brisbane, Qld., 4103
Grover, V. K.	123 Langtree Avenue	Mildura, Vic., 3500
Hall, Donald R.	188 North Terrace	Adelaide, S.A., 5000
Halley, R. M.	1 Trail Street	Wagga Wagga, N.S.W., 2650
Halliday, F. B.	208 Rowe Street	Eastwood, N.S.W., 2122
Hanbury, Paul H.	Cnr. Pope & Smith Streets	Top Ryde, N.S.W., 2112
Handley, Harold A.	198 North Terrace	Adelaide, S.A., 5000
Hann, L. F.	187 Macquarie Street	Sydney, N.S.W., 2000
Hargrave, Michael	P. O. Box 599	Dubbo, N.S.W., 2830
Harkness, Margaret M.	175 North Terrace	Adelaide, S.A., 5000
Harley, G. W.	15 Collins Street	Melbourne, Vic., 3000
Harrington, N. N.	279 Hargreaves Street	Bendigo, Vic., 3550
Harrison, Andrew	131 Wickham Terrace	Brisbane, Qld., 4000
Harrison, Mark	137 Wickham Terrace	Brisbane, Qld., 4000
Hart, Daniel R. L.	137 Wickham Terrace	Brisbane, Qld., 4000
Hart, James L.	137 Wickham Terrace	Brisbane, Qld., 4000
Hart, John K.	North Shore Medical Centre, 66 Pacific Highway	St. Leonards, N.S.W., 2065
Hawkins, J. R.	22 Errard Street North	Ballarat, Vic., 3350
Hefferan, William Vincent	29 Brodie Street	Holland Park, Qld., 4121
Heinze, Julian	Cabrini Medical Centre, Coonil Crescent	Malvern, Vic., 3141
Hellein, Reginald	9 Richardson Street	West Perth, W.A., 6005
Henderson, P. N.	1 Fordham Road	Hawthorn, Vic., 3122
Henry, Allan V.	149 Wickham Terrace	Brisbane, Qld., 4000
Henry, J. Graham	152 Marsden Street	Parramatta, N.S.W., 2150
Herbstein, Amos	229 Macquarie Street	Sydney, N.S.W., 2000
Hercus, John	135 Macquarie Street	Sydney, N.S.W., 2000
Heron, R. J. A.	433 High Street	Maitland, N.S.W., 2320

Hertzberg, R.	42 Ormonde Parade	Hurstville, N.S.W., 2220
Higgins, Ralph A.	82 Market Street	Wollongong, N.S.W., 2500
Hill, B. G.	135 Macquarie Street	Sydney, N.S.W., 2000
Hilton, Alan Findley	131 Wickham Terrace	Brisbane, Qld., 4000.
Hinder, D. C. C.	Medical Centre, 100 Carillon Avenue	Newtown, N.S.W., 2042
Hipwell, G. C.	North Shore Medical Centre, 66 Pacific Highway	St. Leonards, N.S.W., 2065
Hobbs, Ian H.	79 Pennington Terrace	North Adelaide, S.A., 5006
Hodgkinson, B.	c/- 16 Roberts Street	North Balwyn, Vic., 3104
Hogg, J. E. P.	152 Marsden Street	Parramatta, N.S.W., 2150
Hollo, S. J.	229 Macquarie Street	Sydney, N.S.W., 2000
Hollows, F. C.	Department of Ophthalmology, c/- Prince of Wales Hospital, Avoca Street	Randwick, N.S.W., 2031
Hopkins, P. F.	152 Marsden Street	Parramatta, N.S.W., 2150
Hornbrook, John W.	235 Macquarie Street	Sydney, N.S.W., 2000
Horvat, M.	6/316 Wattletree Road	Malvern East, Vic., 3145
Houghton, P. B.	'Pine Lodge', Montana Parade	Croydon, Vic., 3136
Housego, C. J.	Park Avenue	Coffs Harbour, N.S.W., 2450
Howsam, Geoffrey	541 Kiewa Street	Albury, N.S.W., 2640
Howsam, K. G.	12 Morrison Place	East Melbourne, Vic., 3002
Hughes, H. L.	187 Macquarie Street	Sydney, N.S.W., 2000
Hunyor, A. B. L.	7 Help Street	Chatswood, N.S.W., 2067
Isaacs, A.	2 Collins Street	Melbourne, Vic., 3000
Isbell, G. P.	4 Waghorn Street	Ipswich, Qld., 4305
Jack, I. B.	357 Beamish Street	Campsie, N.S.W., 2194
James, A. A.	4 Brookvale House, Warringah Mall	Brookvale, N.S.W., 2100
James, H. M. R.	62 Auburn Road	Auburn, N.S.W., 2144
Johnson, Graeme W.	1 Wentworth Street	Manly, N.S.W., 2065
Johnson, Haddon H.	12a James Street	Mt. Gambier, S.A., 5290
Jones, Lindsay	175 Bay Street	Brighton, Vic., 3186
Joneshart, C. L.	16 Hillview Crescent	Newcastle, N.S.W., 2300
Jordan, A. S.	75 Winchester Street	Malvern, S.A., 5061
Kappagoda, M. B.	1/35 Milray Ave	Wollstonecraft, N.S.W., 2065
Karunaratne, D. M. S.	4 Robinson Ave	Beaumont, S.A., 5066
Keldoulis, T.	17 The Promenade	Cheltenham, N.S.W., 2119
Kelly, A. J.	244 Adelaide Street	Maryborough, Qld., 4650
Kennedy, Ian	60 Waters Road	Cremorne, N.S.W., 2090
Kennedy, John	67 Lake Street	Cairns, Qld., 4870
Kerkenezov, N.	96 Molesworth Street	Lismore, N.S.W., 2480
Kevin, J. B.	175 Macquarie Street	Sydney, N.S.W., 2000
Kilgour, K.	80 Woodland Street	Balgowlah, N.S.W., 2093
Killick, J. F.	56 Alexander Street	Manly, N.S.W., 2095
Kingsley, J.	187 Macquarie Street	Sydney, N.S.W., 2000
Kingston, R. A.	204 Byron Street	Inverell, N.S.W., 2360
Korach, E. V.	7 Bondi Road	Bondi Junction, N.S.W.,
Kurdian, b.	19/49 Osborne Road	Manly, N.S.W., 2095
Lamb, G. A. D.	18 Great Northern Highway	Midland, W.A., 6056
Landers, J. A. G.	104 Brougham PLace	North Adelaide, S.A., 5006
Lawrence, O.	5/780 Warrigal Road	Oakleigh, Vic., 3166
Leckie, T. D.	79 Bettinge Street	Bathurst, N.S.W., 2795
Lennox, A. A.	132 Kiora Road	Miranda, N.S.W., 2228
Lewis, N.	111 Collins Street	Melbourne, Vic., 3000
Lewis, P. J.	48 Sale Street	Orange, N.S.W., 2800

Libhaber, S.	61 Howitt Road	North Caulfield, Vic., 3161
Lidgett, K.	20 Collins Street	Melbourne, Vic., 3000
Lillicrap, G. R.	28 Stokes Street	Townsville, Qld., 4810
Linton, Robert G.	254 St. Georges Terrace	Perth, W.A., 6000
Lister, James D.	163 North Terrace	Adelaide, S.A., 5000
Lodge, John	Civic Centre	Canberra, A.C.T., 2600
Long, J.	81 Collins Street	Melbourne, Vic., 3000
Lorbeer, H.	145 Bell Street	Coburg, Vic., 3058
Loudon, R. D.	Compass House, Featherstone Street	Bankstown, N.S.W., 2200
Lowe, R. F.	82 Collins Street	Melbourne, Vic., 3000
Lowth, L. J.	The Arcade, Manuka	Canberra, A.C.T., 2603
Luke, C. J.	34 Woniora Road	Hurstville, N.S.W., 2220
Mangan, G.	Lister House, Baillie Street	Horsham, Vic., 3400
Mann, Prof. Ida	56 Hobbs Avenue	Nedlands, W.A., 6009
Mansfield, T. M.	9 Deanville Drive	Southport, Qld., 4215
Markwick, K. C.	20 Collins Street	Melbourne, Vic., 3000
Martin, Bruce B.	231 North Terrace	Adelaide, S. A., 5000
Martin, F. J.	14 Pearl Bay Avenue	Mosman, N.S.W., 2088
Martin, J. H. S.	2 Collins Street	Melbourne, Vic., 3000
Martin, Norman W.	149 Wickham Terrace	Brisbane, Qld., 4000
Maude, John D.	82 Market Street	Wollongong, N.S.W., 2500
Mellor, R. N.	105 Collins Street	Melbourne, Vic., 3000
Mercer, D. L.	69–71 Hay Street	Subiaco, W.A., 6008
Miller, T. J. B.	21 Braund Road	Fitzroy, S.A., 5082
Millar, R. B.	7 Homebush Road	Homebush, N.S.W., 2140
Milverton, E. John	16 Mary Street	Auburn, N.S.W., 2144
Mitchell, A.	116 Bradley Street	Goulburn, N.S.W., 2580
Mitchell, J. H.	21 Ringwood Street	Ringwood, Vic., 3134
Mitchell, L. J. C.	23 Grange Road	Toorak, Vic., 3142
Moore, Colin E.	104 Brougham Place	North Adelaide, S.A., 5006
Moore, Max C.	163 North Terrace	Adelaide, S.A., 5000
Morlet, G. C.	222 Barkers Road	Hawthorn, Vic., 3122
Morrissey, M. J.	152 Marsden Street	Parramatta, N.S.W., 2150
Morton, C. R.	114 Russell Street	Toowoomba, Qld., 4350
Morton, M. R.	68 Bellerini Street	Geelong, Vic., 3220
Moxham, R. M.	235 Macquarie Street	Sydney, N.S.W., 2000
Mulhearn, J. W.	22 Crown Road	St. Ives, N.S.W., 2075
Munro, R.	26 Clark Road	Ivanhoe, Vic., 3079
Munro, R. Bruce	102 Orton Street	Ocean Grove, Vic., 3226
Muntz, Wm. McL.	25 Ayres Road	West St. Ives, N.S.W., 2075
Murchland, John B.	163 North Terrace	Adelaide, S.A., 5000
Murphy, Justin	82 Collins Street	Melbourne, Vic., 3000
Murray, K. S.	125 Collins Street	Melbourne, Vic., 3000
MacArthur-Brown, J.	1114 Pacific Highway	Pymble, N.S.W., 2073
McAuliffe, David J.	30 Ord Street	West Perth, W.A., 6005
McCann, R. N.	82 Collins Street	Melbourne, Vic., 3000
McClelland, H. W. H.	P. O. Box 160	Cessnock, N.S.W., 2325
McGuinness, Edward F.	73 Wickham Terrace	Brisbane, Qld., 4000
McGuinness, Edward J.	73 Wickham Terrace	Brisbane, Qld., 4000
McGuinness, Roger	195 Macquarie Street	Sydney, N.S.W., 2000
Macindoe, N.	280 Burwood Road	Burwood, N.S.W., 2134
Macintosh, Laurel J.	201 Wickham Terrace	Brisbane, Qld., 4000
McKay, A. L.	30 Watt Street	Newcastle, N.S.W., 2300
MacLatchy, R. S.	254 St. Georges Terrace	Perth, W.A., 6000
McLarty, T. L.	188 North Terrace	Adelaide, S.A., 5000

MacMillan, K. C.	242 Cowper Street	Warrawong, N.S.W., 2502
McSweeney, D. C.	6 Glenrosa Road	Red Hill, Qld., 4059
McTeigue, C. J.	82 Collins Street	Melbourne, Vic., 3000
Nardi, W.	64 Woodlark Street	Lismore, N.S.W., 2480
Nicholls, B. W. G.	19 Milton Street	Canterbury, Vic., 3126
Nixon, G. K.	1 Trail Street	Wagga Wagga, N.S.W., 2650
Noble, John A.	135a Russell Street	Toowoomba, Qld., 4350
O'Connor, D. J.	82 Market Street	Wollongong, N.S.W., 2500
O'Connor, D. M.	P. O. Box 9	Dandenong, Vic., 3176
Ohlrich, John G.	149 Wickham Terrace	Brisbane, Qld., 4000
Owen, F. S.	16a Bolton Street	Newcastle, N.S.W., 2300
Parker, J. N.	81 Collins Street	Melbourne, Vic., 3000
Parker, R. W.	471 Lygon Street	Princes Hill, Vic.
Pavy, Ian Gordon	175 North Terrace	Adelaide, S.A., 5000
Pendergast, J.	193 Macquarie Street	Sydney, N.S.W., 2000
Perriam, D. J.	14 Gunther Parade	Pasadena, S.A., 5042
Peters, James	149 Wickham Terrace	Brisbane, Qld., 4000
Peters, S.	5 Helen Street	Geelong, Vic., 3220
Pettinger, D.	4 Vale Court	St. Ives, N.S.W., 2075
Phillips, Frank	148 Risdon Road	Moonah, Tas., 7009
Pickering, P. H.	16 Mary Street	Auburn, N.S.W., 2144
Pigott, Louis J.	137 Wickham Terrace	Brisbane, Qld., 4000
Pittar, G.	235 Macquarie Street	Sydney, N.S.W., 2000
Pittar, M. R.	P. O. Box 196	Tweed Heads, N.S.W., 2485
Pittar, Y.	P. O. Box 1039	Canberra City, A.C.T., 2601
Pockley E. V. Waddy	187 Macquarie Street	Sydney, N.S.W., 2000
Pockley, John A.	231 Macquarie Street	Sydney, N.S.W., 2000
Porter, G. T. J.	131 Wickham Terrace	Brisbane, Qld., 4000
Porter, W. T.	19 Union Street	Newcastle, N.S.W., 2300
Pountney, R. K.	17 Bolton Street	Newcastle, N.S.W., 2300
Powrie, R. M.	Taurana Hospital, Freemail Bag	Boroko, Papua, T.P.N.G.
Pradhan, J. S.	39 Field Street	Whyalla Playford, S.A., 5600
Price, Lennox	235 Macquarie Street	Sydney, N.S.W., 2000
Pyne, Remington J.	231 North Terrace	Adelaide, S.A., 5000
Quatermass, Mr. E.	52 Elphin Street	Launceston, Tas., 7250
Raad, G. R. A.	33 Colin Street	West Perth, W.A., 6005
Raiter, Isaac	4 Ventnor Avenue	West Perth, W.A., 6005
Readshaw, Grahame G.	137 Wickham Terrace	Brisbane, Qld., 4000
Redmond, K. B.	48 Sale Street	Orange, N.S.W., 2800
Renton, Robert	79 Pennington Terrace	North Adelaide, S.A., 5006
Rich, David	North Shore Medical Centre, 66 Pacific Highway	St. Leonards, N.S.W., 2065
Rigg, Robert Wm.	Box 713, P. O.	Southport, Qld., 4215
Roberts, John	32 Florence Street	Hornsby, N.S.W., 2077
Robertson, I. F.	2 Collins Street	Melbourne, Vic., 3000
Robinson, H. E.	Olympic Parade	Kangaroo Flat, Vic., 3555
Robinson, J. P.	95 Ryrie Street	Geelong, Vic., 3220
Robinson, L. P.	25 Blaxland Road	Bellevue Hill, N.S.W., 2023
Roche, M. F.	65 Nixon Street	Shepparton, Vic., 3220
Roche, J.	Colac District Hospital	Colac, N.S.W., 3250
Rodan, B. A.	5 Rasmissen Drive	Templestowe, Vic., 3106
Rodd, John	135 Macquarie Street	Sydney, N.S.W., 2000
Rogers, James S.	174 Macquarie Street	Hobart, Tas., 7000
Rogers, John A.	4 Ventnor Avenue	West Perth, W.A., 6005
Rogers, Peter A.	235 Macquarie Street	Sydney, N.S.W., 2000
Rose, Michael	950 Botany Road	Mascot, N.S.W., 2020

Rosen, E.	5 Rasmissen Drive	Templestowe, Vic., 3106
Rosen, P. A.	5 Rasmissen Drive	Templestowe, Vic., 3106
Rowlands, T. N.	195 Macquarie Street	Sydney, N.S.W., 2000
Rudd, Margaret E.	18 Garsia Street	Campbell, Canberra, A.C.T., 2601
Rutledge, Doreen	71 Wallumatta Road	Bayview, N.S.W., 2106
Ryan, E.	2 Collins Street	Melbourne, Vic., 3000
Ryan, H.	100 Collins Street	Melbourne, Vic., 3000
Saad, R. S.	7 Bapaume Road	Mosman, N.S.W., 2088
Saareste, A. G.	23 Railway Parade	Springwood, N.S.W., 2777
Salkeld, O. W.	200 Cothain Road	Kew, Vic., 3101
Sampson, Noel A.	97 Scarborough Street	Southport, Qld., 4215
Sarks, John	14 Norton Street	Leichhardt, N.S.W., 2040
Sarks, Shirley	14 Norton Street	Leichhardt, N.S.W., 2040
Scales, W. T. H.	71 Prince Street	Grafton, N.S.W., 2460
Scargill, S. W.	20 President Avenue	Caringbah, N.S.W., 2229
Scoles, F. Garrett	Box 70	Burleigh Heads, Qld., 4220
Scott, H.	68 Market Street	Wollongong, N.S.W., 2500
Serpell, G.	181 Victoria Parade	Fitzroy, Vic., 3065
Shanahan, Leo	P. O. Box 718	Canberra, A.C.T., 2601
Shortridge, D.	34 Church Street	Burwood, N.S.W., 2134
Shuter, D. J.	42 Beach Street	Frankston, Vic., 3199
Shuttleworth, T.	135 Bellevue Road	Bellevue Hill, N.S.W., 2023
Silva, Michael	308 Westfield Tower	Miranda Fair, N.S.W., 2228
Skeoch, Hugh	2 Milner Crescent	Wollstonecraft, N.S.W., 2065
Slade, John H.	79 Pennington Terrace	North Adelaide, S.A., 5006
Smith, P. Hardy	20 Collins Street	Melbourne, Vic., 3000
Spiro, Paul	137 Wickham Terrace	Brisbane, Qld., 3000
Spring, T. F.	20 Collins Street	Melbourne, Vic., 3000
Stark, Denis John	121 Wickham Terrace	Brisbane, Qld., 4000
Sterling-Levis, M.	324 Marrickville Road	Marrickville, N.S.W., 2224
Stern, Harry	12 Fairweather Street	Bellevue Hill, N.S.W., 2023
Stewart, J. M.	P. O. Box 9	Dandenong, Vic., 3175
Stobie, P. J.	182 Ward Street	North Adelaide, S.A., 5006
Strathdee, M. J. M.	41 Rawson Street	Epping, N.S.W., 2121
Stubbs, G. M.	110 Collins Street	Melbourne, Vic., 3000
Stuckey, G. C.	110 Hunter Street	Newcastle, N.S.W., 2300
Sullivan, Frank P.	131 Wickham Terrace	Brisbane, Qld., 4000
Sutherland, G.	81 Collins Street	Melbourne, Vic., 3000
Swan, David	19 King Street	Rockdale, N.S.W., 2216
Taranto, Barry	27 Harrington Street	Hobart, Tas., 7000
Taylor, J. N.	82 Collins Street	Melbourne, Vic., 3000
Taylor, R. F. L.	187 Macquarie Street	Sydney, N.S.W., 2000
Tester, M. P.	247 Ballina Street	Lismore, N.S.W., 2480
Thomas, Catherine S.	Box 512	Cairns, Qld., 4870
Thomson, G. G. B.	278 Burwood Road	Burwood, N.S.W., 2134
Thornton, D. J.	1 Trail Street	Wagga Wagga, N.S.W., 2650
Thyer, H. W.	2 Hackett Avenue	Millswood, S.A., 5034
Tidswell, T.	Park Street	Glenbrook, N.S.W., 2773
Tonkin, D. O.	267 Melbourne Street	North Adelaide, S.A., 5006
Topham, L. J.	Box 973	Townsville, Qld., 4810
Tostevin, A. L.	238 Melbourne Street	North Adelaide, S.A., 5006
Townshend, Francis L. A.	105 Davey Street	Hobart, Tas., 7000
Travers, Sir Thomas	251 Gratton Street	Carlton, Vic., 3053
Treloar, D.	135 Macquarie Street	Sydney, N.S.W., 2000
Trenerry, E. John	77 Ware Street	Fairfield, N.S.W., 2165

Troski, J.	82 Collins Street	Melbourne, Vic., 3000
Tye, A. A.	231 North Terrace	Adelaide, S.A., 5000
Vandeleur, K. W.	131 Wickham Terrace	Brisbane, Qld., 4000
Voloshin, Olga	20 Bulkara Road	Bellevue Hill, N.S.W., 2023
Waddy, P. M.	802/349 New South Head Road .	Double Bay, N.S.W., 2028
Waddy, R. G.	Mowll Village	Carlingford, N.S.W., 2118
Walker, T. D.	P. O. Box 580	Canberra City, A.C.T., 2601
Walsh, C. H.	183 Macquarie Street	Sydney, N.S.W., 2000
Walsh, Michael Anthony ...	65 Duke Street	Northam, W.A., 6401
Walter, C. J.	19 Union Street	Newcastle, N.S.W., 2300
Waterworth, David	59 Davey Street	Hobart, Tas., 7000
Waugh, M. L.	17 Bolton Street	Newcastle, N.S.W., 2300
Webster, Z.	15 Dee Why Square	Dee Why, N.S.W., 2099
West, R. H.	428 St. Kilda Road	Melbourne, Vic., 3000
Whaites, J. M.	17 East Street	Rockhampton, Qld., 4700
White, J. McB.	12 Collins Street	Melbourne, Vic., 3000
Whitford, R. S.	33 Colin Street	West Perth, W.A., 6005
Whitehouse, C. A.	12 Parr Parade	Narraweena, N.S.W., 2099
Whitington, R. E.	22 Macquarie Street	Taree, N.S.W., 2430
Wicks, Norman S. P.	267 Melbourne Street	North Adelaide, S.A., 5006
Williams, Darcy	82 Empire Circuit	Forrest, Canberra, A.C.T., 2603
Wilson, Brian G.	131 Wickham Terrace	Brisbane, Qld., 4000
Wilson, D. C.	24 Washington Street	Victoria Park, W.A., 6100
Wilson, E.	2a Bayswater Road	Kings Cross, N.S.W., 2011
Wilson, I. H.	33 Dowe Street	Tamworth, N.S.W., 2340
Wilson, R. G.	Shamrock Building, Williamson Street	Bendigo, Vic., 3550
Winn, R. W.	2 St. Johns Ave	Gordon, N.S.W., 2072
Wise, Gordon	174 Macquarie Street	Hobart, Tas., 7000
Wong, P. L.	272 Springvale Road	Glen Waverley, Vic., 3150
Wong-See, J.	City Mutual Building, Hobart Place	Canberra, A.C.T., 2600
Wood, Ronald F. J.	155 Wickham Terrace	Brisbane, Qld., 4000
Yates, Percy C.	4 Ventnor Avenue	West Perth, W.A., 6005
Yeates, S. Fergus M.	Ballow Chambers, Wickham Terrace	Brisbane, Qld., 4000

Associate members.

Austin, C. W.	17 High Street	Glen Iris, Vic., 3146
Billings, J. J.	141 Grey Street	East Melbourne, Vic., 3902
Bishop, M.	10 Wallace Street	Newtown, Geelong, Vic., 3220
Bryan, J. D.	153 Macquarie Street	Glen Iris, Vic., 3146
Cameron, L.	400 Swann Road	St. Lucia, Qld., 4067
Daley, E. A.	24 Nott Street	East Malvern, Vic., 3144
Dickenson, P.	4 The Grange Avenue	Canterbury, Vic., 3126
Doran, K. E.	176 Sandy Bay Road	Sandy Bay, Tas., 7005
Farrar, J. E.	9 Thyne Avenue	Launceston, Tas., 7250
Filipic, M.	Department of Pathology, Sydney Eye Hospital	Woolloomooloo, N.S.W., 2011
Firth-Smith, W.	15 Albion Street	Surrey Hills, Vic., 3127
Fisher, A.	1215 Hay street	West Perth, W.A., 6005
Gillis, S.	c/- Sydney Eye Hospital, Sir John Young Crescent	Woolloomooloo, N.S.W., 2011

Greer, C. H.	Department of Pathology, Royal Victoria Eye & Ear Hospital	East Melbourne, Vic., 3002
Hunter, I. J.	Department of Pathology, Bankstown Hospital	Bankstown, N.S.W., 2220
Jones, G.	200 Liebig Street	Warrnambool, Vic., 3280
Morson, S. M.	135 Macquarie Street	Sydney, N.S.W., 2000
Porter, C. J.	274 Toohey Road	Tarragindi, Qld., 4121
Rogers, Maureen	5 The Crest	Killara, N.S.W., 2071
Scott, E.	1 Alexander Drive	Mt. Lawley, W.A., 6050
Steen, A. S.	13 Warralong Crescent	Mt. Lawley, W.A., 6050
Taylor, H. J.	74 Sydney Street	Mackay, Qld., 4740
Vaughan, G. N.	5 Morrison Court	Box Hill North, Vic., 3129
Wilbur-Ham, B.	3 Balfour Street	Toorak, Vic., 3142
Williams, I. M.	10/393 Toorak Road	South Yarra, Vic., 3141

NOSOCOMIA QUIBUS OCULIS AEGRI CURANTUR

University Departments:

University of Melbourne,
Department of Òphthalmology: Professor G. W. Crock

University of Sydney,
Department of Ophthalmology: E. J. Donaldson, Director of Studies in Ophthalmology and Eye Health

University of New South Wales,
Department of Ophthalmology: Associate-Professor F. C. Hollows

Eye Departments in General Hospitals:

	No. of beds
Alfred Hospital, Melbourne, Victoria	10
Adelaide Childrens Hospital, Adelaide, South Australia	20
Mater Misericordiae, Brisbane, Queensland	16
Princess Alexandra's Hospital, Brisbane, Queensland	45
Prince of Wales Hospital, Randwick, New South Wales	20
Prince Henry's Hospital, Melbourne, Victoria	10
Queen Elizabeth Hospital, Adelaide, South Australia	12
Repatriation General Hospital, Adelaide, South Australia	20
Royal Perth Hospital, Perth, West Australia	20
Royal Adelaide Hospital, Adelaide, South Australia	32
Royal Children's Hospital, Brisbane, Queensland	12
Repatriation General Hospital, Brisbane, Queensland	15
Royal Victorian Eye & Ear Hospital	75
St. Vincents Hospital, Melbourne, Victoria	10
St. Vincents Hospital, Sydney, New South Wales	20
St. Andrew War Memorial Hospital, Brisbane, Queensland (Nancy & Maria Simpson Memorial Hospital for the Blind)	22

INSTITUTA SCHOLAEQUE CAECIS DESTINATAE

No specific data received.

AUSTRIA

SOCIETATES OPHTHALMOLOGICAE

Nationales

Österreichische Ophthalmologische Gesellschaft
President: Prof. Dr. K. Heinz
Secretary: Doz. Dr. W. Funder, 1. Augenklinik der Universität Wien, Spitalgasse 2, A – 1090 Wien
Number of members: 236

Verband der Augenärzte Österreichs
President: Dr. W. Friess
Secretary: Dr. H. Kemmetmüller, Johannesgasse 20, A – 1010 Wien
Number of members: 175

Regionalis

Ophthalmologische Gesellschaft in Wien
Secretary: Dr. K. Fanta, 1. Augenklinik der Universität Wien, Spitalgasse 2, A – 1090 Wien
Number of members: 165

NOMINA ET DOMICILIA MEDICORUM AB OCULIS

Aichmair, Hermann	Döblinger Hauptstraße 71	A-1190 Wien
Ambos, Ernst	Mozartstraße 71	A-4020 Linz
Antlanger, Helga	Gorianstraße 2	A-5020 Salzburg
Arnfelser, Hannelore	Gassergasse 2-8/3/5/24	A-1050 Wien
Asenbauer, Hans	Geyschlägergasse 2-12	A-1150 Wien
Astecker, Jörg	Herakhstraße 8	A-4810 Gmunden
Auerbach, Berthold	Anton Brucknerstraße 2	A-4820 Bad Ischl
Auffinger, Erwin	Bahnhofstraße 5	A-4400 Steyr
Autrata, Reinhold	Hermann Bahrstraße 6	A-1210 Wien
Avedikian, Hrant	Landesunfallkrankenh-Augenabt..	A-6800 Feldkirch
Bachna, Franz	Ybbsstraße 9	A-1020 Wien
Ballner, Heinz	Lagerhausstraße 2	A-2230 Gänserndorf
Bartl, Gustav	Auenbruggerplatz	A-8036 Graz
Bauer, Senta	Bahnhofstraße 53	A-3950 Gmünd
Beer, Franz	Mondscheingasse 1	A-8010 Graz
Benedikt, Olaf	Universitäts-Augenklinik	A-8020 Graz
Binder, Kurt	Währingerstraße 24/28	A-1090 Wien
Binder, Susanne	1. Univ. Augenklinik	A-1090 Wien
Bettelheim, Heinz	Josefstädterstraße 56	A-1080 Wien
Birkner, Waltraud	Grundlgasse 3	A-1090 Wien
Birnbacher, Theo	Neubaugürtel 23	A-1150 Wien

Blank, Adolf	Salzburgerstraße 8	A-4020 Ischl
Blecha, Walter	Neulinggasse 8	A-1030 Wien
Böck, Prof. Josef	Stadiongasse 2	A-1010 Wien
Braunsdorfer, Rita	Postgasse 1a	A-2620 Neunkirchen
Brausewetter, Gertrude	Spitalgasse 1	A-1090 Wien
Bruha, Helmut	Köhlergasse 18	A-1180 Wien
Caramanlis, Heidy	Rueppgasse 5/4	A-1020 Wien
Dechel, Karl	Klosterstraße 1	A-4840 Vöcklabruck
Derka, Heinz	Hauptstraße 26/V/4	A-1140 Wien
Doppel, Herta	Krausegasse 7a	A-1100 Wien
Eberhartinger, Wolfgang	Brüsselgasse 45-47/IV/1	A-1160 Wien
Eberhartinger, Maria	Schillerstraße 29	A-2340 Mödling
Eberle, Theodora	Währingerstraße 81	A-1180 Wien
Ebner, Rudolf	Wienerstraße 96	A-8605 Kapfenberg
Ebner, Sigrid	Elisabethstraße 59	A-8010 Graz
Ehrenecker, Franz	Preinsbacherstraße 5	A-3300 Amstetten
Erhalt, Heide	Universitäts-Augenklinik	A-8010 Graz
Ertl, Hans	Moritschstraße 5/II/1	A-9500 Villach
Exner, Dietrich	Stadtplatz 5	A-4400 Steyr
Eyb, Christian	Herrengasse 19	A-8750 Judenburg
Fanta, Prof. Helmut	Ferstelgasse 4/1	A-1090 Wien
Fanta, Klaus	1. Univ. Augenklinik	A-1090 Wien
Färber, Magdalena	Meranerstraße 8	A-6020 Innsbruck
Farkas, Andreas	Burgfried 38a	A-5400 Hallein
Fattinger, Wolfgang	Landstraße 32	A-4020 Linz
Fellner, Rudolf	Weißenkirchnerstraße 22	A-8020 Graz
Feßl, Rudolf	Untersteinerweg 7	A-5600 St. Johann/Pomgau
Friede, Friedrich	Pfarrgasse 15	A-4600 Wels
Fiala, Heinrich	Brünnerstraße 52	A-1210 Wien
Fischer, Franz	Opernring 17	A-1010 Wien
Fischer, Ingo	Freistädterstraße 96/19	A-4020 Linz
Fleischanderl, Arthur	Ringstraße 16	A-3500 Krems
Fleischanderl, Friedrich	1. Univ. Augenklinik	A-1090 Wien
Forte, Anton	Simmeringer Hauptstr. 60–64/1	A-1110 Wien
Frey, René Georg	Gersthoferstraße 142–146/20	A-1180 Wien
Freyler, Heinrich	Wiedner Hauptstraße 18	A-1040 Wien
Freyler, Heinrich	1. Univ. Augenklinik	A-1090 Wien
Friemel, Erika	Müllner Hauptstraße 48	A-5020 Salzburg
Friess, Walter	Kalchberggasse 10	A-8010 Graz
Fulmek, Rolf	Trautmannsdorfgasse 13/3/1	A-1130 Wien
Funder, Wolfgang	Mozartgasse 3/II/7	A-1040 Wien
Gatterbauer, Josef	Max Ott-Platz 6	A-5020 Salzburg
Geyer, Gertrud	Gersthoferstraße 22	A-1180 Wien
Gittler, Rudolf	Schlösselgasse 1	A-1080 Wien
Gogler, Eduard	Schubertstraße 9	A-4020 Linz
Göttinger, Wolfgang	Pensionsweg 12	A-8042 Graz
Graf, Friedrich	Wahlberggasse 3	A-1140 Wien
Graf, Margarete	Landstraßer Hauptstraße 46	A-1030 Wien
Graßberger, Hans	Kirchenplatz 1	A-4540 Bad Hall
Greil, Herbert	Maria Theresienstraße 7	A-6020 Innsbruck
Grossmann, Theodor	Heiliggeiststraße 8/p	A-6020 Innsbruck
Grün, Peter	Kupkagasse 6/4	A-1080 Wien
Grund, Johann	Landgutgasse 2	A-1100 Wien
Gsur, Lilli	Berlagasse 40/4/6	A-1210 Wien
Gürtler, Edmund	Friedmanngasse 17	A-1160 Wien
Habenberger, Rolf	Mandlgasse 23	A-1120 Wien

Habersack, Herbert	Stadlbauerstraße 6	A-4020 Linz-Urfahr
Hackl, Emmerich	Pillweinstraße 27	A-4020 Linz
Hainacher, Gregor	Stanislausgasse 2/14	A-1030 Wien
Hamburger, Prof. F. A.	Kollonitschstraße 10	A-2700 Wiener Neustadt
Handl, Otto	Dominikanerbastei 4/3	A-1010 Wien
Hanselmayer, Helmut	Bürgerringgasse 6	A-8010 Graz
Harmuth, Egon	Senefeldergasse 1/1	A-1100 Wien
Hart van Pelt, Lia	Augasse 1	A-7350 Oberpullendorf
Hatzl, Hertha	Favoritenstraße 4	A-1040 Wien
Haydn, Rudolf	Hietzinger Hauptstraße 5	A-1140 Wien
Haydn, Manfred	Dr. Franz Weissmannstraße 3 ...	A-3910 Zwettl
Hefel, Ferdinand	Angelika Kaufmannstraße 2a ...	A-6850 Dornbirn
Heftner, Franziska	Breitenfurterstr. 295–301/1	A-1230 Wien
Heider, Helmut	Wolf Dietrichstraße 4a	A-5020 Salzburg
Hein, Maria	Hauptplatz 118	A-8712 Niklasdorf
Heilig, Peter	Hackenberggasse 29/12	A-1190 Wien
Heinrich, Heribert	Porzellangasse 24	A-1090 Wien
Heinrich, Paul	Krankenh. der Barmherz. Schwes.	A-4020 Linz
Heinz, Prof. Karl.	Universitäts-Augenklinik	A-6020 Innsbruck
Heinz, Ottilie	Gärtnergasse 11	A-2100 Korneuburg
Heller, Harald	Alleestraße 22	A-9900 Lienz
Herbst, Martha	Kramergasse 1/2	A-9020 Klagenfurt
Herold, Inge	Daringergasse 18 b	A-1190 Wien
Hesse, Erich	Schlögelgasse 3	A-8010 Graz
Hlawacek, Irmgard	Hernsteinerstraße 15	A-2560 Berndorf
Hloch, Hedwig	Hauptstraße 2o	A-2340 Mödling
Hochmayr, Walpurga	Herrenstraße 43	A-4020 Linz
Hofmann, Prof. Hans	Merangasse 22	A-8010 Graz
Hommer, Gerald	Wienerstraße 4a	A-4020 Linz
Hommer, Kurt	Landstraße 49	A-4020 Linz
Holzer, Ernst	Hütteldorferstraße 81a/VII	A-1140 Wien
Hollegha, Christa	Hauptplatz 8	A-9100 Völkermarkt
Hrubesch, Maria	Bahnhofplatz 9	A-3500 Krems
Hruby, Prof. Karl	Pramergasse 5/13	A-1090 Wien
Hubmann, Armin	Klosterwiesgasse 24/1	A-8010 Graz
Hummer, Ekkehart	Matznergasse 20	A-1140 Wien
Hütter, Rudolf	Bambergerstraße (Sparkassenneubau)	A-9400 Wolfsberg
Jelinek, Gertrud	Venedigerau 4/3	A-1020 Wien
Jenewein, Gertrud	Dr. Pfeiffenbergerstr. 12	A-6460 Imst
Jochum, Wolfgang	Heschgasse 14	A-4840 Vöcklabruck
Kacetl, Erich	Neugasse 5	A-6900 Bregenz
Kadletz, Hermann	Bahngasse 46	A-2700 Wiener Neustadt
Karasek, Ernst	Am Kaisermühlendamm 1/15 ...	A-1223 Wien
Kask, Henrik	Stralehnergasse 15/4	A-1220 Wien
Kemmetmüller, Hermann ..	Johannesgasse 20	A-1010 Wien
Kenyeres, Peter	Hugo Riedlstraße 3	A-2130 Mistelbach
Keresztes, Anneliese	Nußdorferstraße 42	A-1090 Wien
Kessaris, Jean	Lazarettgasse 14	A-1090 Wien
Kiendler, Werner	Maria Theresienstraße 8	A-6020 Innsbruck
Kircher, Maria	Fleischmarkt 9/II	A-9020 Klagenfurt
Kiss, Walter	Josefsplatz 12	A-2500 Baden
Kleiner, Leo	Bahnhofstraße 3	A-6800 Feldkirch
Kleiner, Ilse	Bahnhofstraße 3	A-6800 Feldkirch
Kleinert, Heinrich	Schwarzpanierstraße 15/19	A-1090 Wien
Klemen, Ulrich	1. Univ. Augenklinik	A-1090 Wien

Klepetko, Blanka	Allgemeines Krankenhaus	A-2700 Wiener Neustadt
Klicpera, Walter	Karl Loystraße 13	A-4600 Wels
Klinger-Herber, Helene	Rilkestraße 20	A-4020 Linz
Knaipp, Herwig		A-8600 Bruck
Knittel, Kurt	Erlachgasse 106	A-1100 Wien
Kohlich, Gerhard	Kremser Landstraße 25	A-3100 St. Pölten
König, Walter	Bischofsplatz 1/I	A-8010 Graz
Kosmath, Betrix	Nußdorferstraße 61	A-1090 Wien
Kovalcik, Helga	Pfeilgasse 9	A-1080 Wien
Kraft, Hermann	R. Bieblstraße 36	A-5020 Salzburg
Kranewitter, Martin	Anichstraße 35	A-6020 Innsbruck
Krascenics, Otto	Heiligenstädterstraße 169	A-1190 Wien
Kuchner, Karl	Haeckelstraße 1	A-1235 Liesing
Kundigraber, Erich	Fleischmarkt 9	A-9020 Klagenfurt
Kunze, Reinhard	Bergmannstraße 4	A-6800 Dornbirn
Kurz, Leopold	Meißauerstraße 2/8/1	A-1222 Kagran
Kurz, Michael	Bahnhofstraße 6/1	A-5700 Zell/See
Kutos, Christine	Treustraße 52/2/18	A-1200 Wien
Kutos, Christine	Bockgasse 3	A-4020 Linz
Kutschera, Erich	Paffrathgasse 6	A-1020 Wien
Lechner, Peter	Margeretenstraße 25	A-1040 Wien
Leesemann, Peter	Klagenfurterstraße 24	A-9300 St. Veit/Glan
Leopold, Elisabeth	Billrothstraße 8-10/9/1	A-1190 Wien
Leopold, Rudolf	Stadtplatz 4	A-3400 Klosterneuburg
Leopold-Messer, Günther	Wiedner Hauptstraße 142	A-1050 Wien
Leopoldsberger, Wolfgang	Alter Markt 10/II	A-5020 Salzburg
Liebhart, Dorothea	Grieskirchnerstraße 14	A-4600 Wels
Liehn, Robert	Hauptplatz 9/11	A-8430 Leibnitz
Lisch, Karl	Christian Plattnerstraße 6	A-6300 Wörgl
Lisch, Walter	Salzburgerstraße 10	A-6300 Wörgl
Lob, Pauline	Schelleingasse 19	A-1040 Wien
Löffler, Karl	Per Albin Hanson-Ost, Zwölfpfen-niggasse 1	A-1100 Wien
Ludwig, Albert	Pfarrplatz 5	A-2500 Baden
Mallner, Josef	Bahnhofstraße 13	A-4600 Wels
Mallner, Erich	Bahnhofstraße 13	A-4600 Wels
Mansbart Wehinger, Antonie	Rudigierstraße 1	A-4020 Linz
Marx, Joachim	Josef Pirchlstraße 17	A-6370 Kitzbühel
Mejer, Fritz	Kirchengasse 25	A-1070 Wien
Messerklinger, Erika	Elisabethstraße 59	A-8010 Graz
Mettinger, Helmut	Karlsgasse 8	A-3430 Tulln
Michel, Julius	Dreifaltigkeitsstraße 3	A-5020 Salzburg
Michtner, Hertha	Neugasse 31	A-2020 Hollabrunn
Miller, Bruno	Meranerstraße 3	A-6020 Innsbruck
Misar, Rainer	Lainzerstraße 81	A-1130 Wien
Mittermair, Hildegard	Mozartstraße 38	A-4020 Linz
Molnar, Georg	8. Maistraße 18	A-9020 Klagenfurt
Mörl, Mathilde	Hormayerstraße 10	A-6020 Innsbruck
Much, Viktor	Weimarerstraße 8-10/II/3	A-1180 Wien
Mühlfellner, Josef	Kaiser Franz Josef-Kai 2/II	A-8010 Graz
Mulley, Lydia	Schillerstraße 2	A-9800 Spittal/Drau
Müller, Anton	Südtirolerplatz 7/1	A-8020 Graz
Müller, Josef	Joachimstraße 11	A-7000 Eisenstadt
Nagel, Rudolf	Kremsergasse 1	A-3100 St. Pölten
Nemec, Johann	Brunnengasse 50a	A-1160 Wien
Nemetz, Udo	Liechtensteinstraße 4	A-1090 Wien

Neubauer, Oskar	Westbahnstraße 1b	A-1070 Wien
Neuner, Hanspeter	Schalserstraße 2	A-6200 Jenbach
Neurauter, Hugo	Kaiserstraße 4/II	A-6900 Bregenz
Nitsch, Maximilian	Hernalser Hauptstraße 91	A-1170 Wien
Niulaszy, Ferdinand	Biberstraße 9	A-1010 Wien
Oberhummer, Marilies	Franz Josefstraße 5	A-8700 Leoben
Öhlknecht, Leopold	Josef Strommerstraße 22	A-3580 Horn
Orou, Franz	Unterer Stadtplatz 4	A-6060 Solbad Hall
Osinger, Kurt	Pötzleinsdorferstraße 10/3/1	A-1180 Wien
Ortner, Helmut	Laaerbergstraße 32/1/21	A-1100 Wien
Petri, Fritz	Hauptplatz 32	A-7100 Neusiedl/See
Petters, Kurt	Breitenfurterstraße 107-109	A-1120 Wien
Pfandl, Emil	Sterneckstraße 3/1	A-9020 Klagenfurt
Pfeffer, Bernadette	Roseggerstraße 6	A-8680 Mürzzuschlag
Philipp, Emmi	Defreggerstraße 19	A-6020 Innsbruck
Pilar, Otto	Parkstraße 30	A-4560 Kirchdorf/Krems
Pillat, Prof. Arnold	Himmelstraße 28a	A-1190 Wien
Pinkernell, Wilhelm	Freiliggrathstraße 13	A-2700 Wiener Neustadt
Possnigg, Irmgard	Jörgerstraße 9	A-1170 Wien
Preschitz, Helga	Altstadt 58	A-2460 Bruck
Pressina, Maria	Brauhausstraße 4	A-2320 Schwechat
Prokop, Olaf	Rathausplatz 5	A-3390 Melk
Proksch, Maria	Cobenzlgasse 26	A-1190 Wien
Prskavec, Friedrich	Jacquingasse 1/9	A-1030 Wien
Pulgram, Alois	Colloredogasse 35	A-1180 Wien
Purtscher, Ernst	Hadikgasse 50	A-1140 Wien
Rabensteiner, Adele	Opernring 4/I	A-8010 Graz
Raff, Maria	Nordwestbahnstr. 93-95	A-1200 Wien
Ramach, Friedrich	Mariahilferstraße 37	A-1060 Wien
Redl, Theodor	Gatterburggasse 10	A-1190 Wien
Reichel, Maria	Josefstädterstraße 7/12	A-1080 Wien
Reichelt, Günther	Heinrich Collinstraße 30	A-1140 Wien
Reinisch, Gerhard	Klammstraße 2	A-4020 Linz
Reinl, Hubert	Hauptplatz 9	A-9500 Villach
Renner, Alice	Rauscherstraße 10	A-1200 Wien
Renner, Anna-Maria	Mariahilferstraße 95/II/25	A-1060 Wien
Reunert, Petra	Vorgartenstraße 27/8/3	A-1200 Wien
Rhomberg, Andreas	Färberstraße 10/IV	A-6700 Bludenz
Riedl, Franz	Franz Josef-Straße 14/I	A-8700 Leoben
Rieger, Prof. Herwig	Museumstraße 15	A-4020 Linz
Rieger, Gebhard	Paracelsusinstitut	A-4540 Bad Hall
Riemer, Friedrich	Meidlinger Hauptstraße 49/1/4	A-1120 Wien
Ries, Agnes	Rugierstraße 26/15/2	A-1220 Wien
Rogenhofer, Alfred	Windspergerstraße 10	A-3340 Waidhofen/Ybbs
Römersdorfer, Erich	Ottakringerstraße 193	A-1160 Wien
Rotter, Hans	Praterstraße 193	A-1020 Wien
Rubey, Franz	Oswaldgasse 10/16	A-1120 Wien
Rummelhardt, Elfrida	Reichsratstraße 11/4	A-1010 Wien
Sackl, Hans Helmut	Stempfergasse 4	A-8010 Graz
Schäffl, Gottfried	Gentzgasse 104	A-1180 Wien
Schega, Egon	Gestettengasse 16/6/5	A-1030 Wien
Scheiber, Helmut	Griessstraße 20	A-4710 Grieskirchen
Schellberg, Hans	Lieberstraße 1	A-6020 Innsbruck
Schenk, Heinz	Spitalgasse 19	A-1090 Wien
Schindler, Rudolf	Bahnhofstraße 22/VI	A-9020 Klagenfurt
Schiel, Hildegard	Mozartstraße 38	A-4020 Linz

Schlagenhauf, Kurt	Annenstraße 55	A-8020 Graz
Schleifer, Gertrude	Hauptplatz 2/4	A-1238 Mauer
Schlusche, Paula	Hütteldorferstraße 171	A-1140 Wien
Schrott, Erika	Hans Gasserplatz 3/1	A-9500 Villach
Schreinzer, Werner	Wildagasse 10/16/10	A-1234 Wien
Schuler, Herbert	Ulrichstraße 12/I	A-6500 Landeck
Schuster, Herbert	Stammgasse 9/8	A-1030 Wien
Schwab, Franz	Brahmsplatz 7	A-1040 Wien
Schwaiger, H.	Müllner Hauptstr. Krankenh.	A-5020 Salzburg
Seböck, Irmgard	Börsegasse 14	A-1010 Wien
Seher, Kurt	Pilgramgasse 8	A-1050 Wien
Sehorst, Wilfried	1. Univ. Augenklinik	A-1090 Wien
Seidl, Wilfried	Hauptplatz 25	A-8570 Voitsberg
Sekyra, Heimo	Residenzplatz 5	A-5020 Salzburg
Skopek, Mathias	Landstraße 10	A-4020 Linz
Skorpik, Rudolf	Castellezgasse 2/9	A-1020 Wien
Slezak, Prof. Hans	Rathausstraße 15/8	A-1010 Wien
Sochor, Fritz	Bahnhofstraße 7	A-7400 Oberwart
Spiller, Heinrich	Braunspergengasse 27/V/1	A-1100 Wien
Spittermair, H.	Mozartstraße 38	A-4020 Linz
Stadler, Walter	Hauptplatz 29	A-4020 Linz
Stampfl, Berthold	Konrad-Voglstr. 6	A-4020 Linz
Stangler-Zuschrott, Elfriede	Landstr. Hauptstr. 141	A-1030 Wien
Steiner, Ludwig	O'Briengasse 43	A-1210 Wien
Stenzl, Alfred	Untersbergstr. 4/II	A-5020 Salzburg
Stellamor, Helga	Klimschgasse 14	A-1030 Wien
Stelzer, Adele	Schönbrunnerstraße 133	A-1050 Wien
Stelzer, Otto	Schönbrunnerstraße 133	A-1050 Wien
Stelzer, Rudolf	Beckgasse 15	A-1130 Wien
Stepanik, Prof. Jozef	Schlösselgasse 22	A-1080 Wien
Stidl, Adelinde	Skodagasse 19/11	A-1080 Wien
Stidl, Gerhard	Neubau 1-3	A-2000 Stockerau
Stieber, Rudolf	Anichstraße 32	A-6020 Innsbruck
Stierschneider, Heltraud	Lessinggasse 4/9	A-1020 Wien
Straka, Trude	Gutensteinerstr. 3	A-2753 Pisting
Subal, Elisabeth	Bösendorferstr. 5/9	A-1010 Wien
Suppantschitsch, Ernst	Werdertorgasse 5	A-1010 Wien
Synek, Herbert	Stadtplatz 6	A-5280 Braunau
Ternes, Titus	Krieglergasse 6/4	A-1030 Wien
Thaler, Arnulf	Penzingerstraße 29	A-1140 Wien
Thurnherr, Franz	Schulgasse 2	A-2700 Wiener Neustadt
Thöny, Ingeborg	Maria Theresienstr. 51	A-6020 Innsbruck
Till, Peter	2. Univ. Augenklinik	A-1090 Wien
Todter, Franz	Klostergasse 6-8	A-3100 St. Pölten
Trauschke, Friederike	Schwendergasse 24/5	A-1150 Wien
Trichtel, Fritz	Franz Josefstraße 4	A-3540 Bad Hall
Überreiter, Prof. Franz	Kärntnerring 10	A-1010 Wien
Unger, Heinz	Paris Lodronstraße 2	A-5020 Salzburg
Veitl, Hertha	Hernalser Hauptstr. 209	A-1170 Wien
Veitl, Walter	Hernalser Hauptstr. 209	A-1170 Wien
Vit, Heinrich	Wienerstraße 20	A-3100 St. Pölten
Volckmar, Hans	Hauptplatz 9/I	A-8010 Graz
Vukovich, Viktor	Rechte Wienzeile 85	A-1050 Wien
Wastl, Charlotte	Wallgasse 12	A-1060 Wien
Watzinger, Waltraud	Volksgartenstraße 7	A-8020 Graz
Watzl, Helmut	Hütteldorferstraße 355	A-1140 Wien

Widder, Wolfgang	Sparbesbachgasse 17	A-8010 Graz
Wiedner, Ekkehard	Marktgraben 12/I	A-6020 Innsbruck
Willomitzer, Herwig	Friedrichgasse 6/I	A-8010 Graz
Windhör, Richard	Europaplatz 7	A-3100 St. Pölten
Wimmer, Arnold	Krankenhaus Augenabt.	A-9010 Klagenfurt
Woitzuck, Maria	Parkstraße 10	A-2340 Mödling
Wolf, Margarete	Gumpendorferstraße 36	A-1060 Wien
Zechner, Elert	Landesunfallkrankenh. Augenabteilung	A-6800 Feldkirch
Zehetbauer, Georg	Max Emanuelstraße 7	A-1180 Wien
Ziegler, Arthur	Kolingasse 13	A-1090 Wien
Zimmermann, Stefan	Josefstädterstraße 21/1	A-1080 Wien
Zirm, Mathias	Auenbruggerplatz	A-8036 Graz
Zita, Karl	Traklgasse 4/33	A-1190 Wien
Zodl, Ute	Märzstraße 49/8	A-1150 Wien
Zotti, Anneliese	Uhlandgasse 3-5/I/43	A-1100 Wien
Zug, Franz	Brevilliergasse 18	A-2620 Neunkirchen
Zugschwerdt Bieber, Gertraud	Gentzgasse 6	A-1180 Wien
Zwiauer, Anton	Landeskrankenhaus	A-5020 Salzburg
Zymann, Eva	Würthgasse 11/14	A-1190 Wien

NOSOCOMIA QUIBUS OCULIS AEGRI CURANTUR

No. of beds

I. Augenklinik der Universität Wien, A-1090 Wien, Spitalgasse 2. Director: Prof. Dr.
K. Hruby 86

II. Augenklinik der Universität Wien, A-1090 Wien, Alserstraße 4, Director: Prof. Dr.
H. Slezak 80

Augenklinik der Universität Graz, A-8036 Graz, Auenbruggerplatz 4. Director: Prof. Dr.
H. Hofmann 150

Augenklinik der Universität Innsbruck, A-6020 Innsbruck, Anichstraße 35. Director: Prof.
Dr. K. Heinz 60

Augenabteilung des Krankenhauses der Stadt Wien Lainz, A-1130 Wien, Wolkersbergenstraße 1. Director: Prof. Dr. J. Stepanik 60

Augenabteilung der Krankenanstalt der Stadt Wien Rudolfstiftung, A-1030 Wien, Boerhaavegasse 8. Director: Prof. Dr. H. Fanta 58

Augenabteilung des Krankenhauses der Barmherzigen Brüder, A-1021 Wien, Große Mohrengasse 9. Director: Primarius Dr. H. Rotter 13

Augenabteilung des Hanusch Krankenhauses, A-1140 Wien, Heinrich Collinstraße 30. Director: Doz. Dr. U. Nemetz 62

Augenabteilung im Sanatorium Hera, A-1090 Wien, Löblichgasse 14. Director: Primarius Dr.
Niulaszy Ferdinand 20

Augenabteilung des Landeskrankenhauses Klagenfurt, A-9010 Klagenfurt, St. Veiterstraße
47. Director: Primarius Dr. R. Schindler 115

Augenabteilung des a.ö. Krankenhauses Horn, A-3580 Horn, Spitalgasse 10. Director:
Primarius Dr. L. Öhlknecht 36

Augenabteilung des a.ö. Krankenhauses der Stadt St. Pölten, A-3100 St. Pölten, Kremser
Landstraße 36. Director: Primarius Dr. H. Vit 64

Augenabteilung des a.ö. Krankenhauses der Stadtgemeinde Wiener Neustadt, A-2700 Wiener
Neustadt, Corviniusring 3-5. Director: Prof: Dr. F. Hamburger 36

Augenabteilung des a.ö. Krankenhauses der Stadt Linz, A-4020 Linz, Krankenhausstraße 9.
Director: Doz. Dr. K. Hommer 42

Augenabteilung des a.ö. Krankenhauses der Barmherzigen Brüder in Linz, A-4010 Linz,
Rudigierstraße 11-13. Director: Primarius Dr. E. Ambos 40

INSTITUTA SCHOLAEQUE CAECIS DESTINATAE

Blinden und Erzichungsanstalten
Bundes-Blinden-Erziehungsinstitut, Wittelsbachergasse 5, A-1020 Wien.
Odilien-Blindenanstalt Graz, Leonhardstraße 130, A-8010 Graz.
Kärntner Landes-Blindenanstalt Klagenfurt, Gutenbergstraße 9, A-9020 Klagenfurt.
Blinden-Lehr-und Erziehungsanstalt Innsbruck, Ing. Etzelstraße 71, A-6020 Innsbruck.

Sonderschulen für Sehgestörte Kinder
Zinkgasse 12-14, A-1150 Wien.

Blinden-Versorgungsheime
Osterreichische Blindenwohlfahrt, Blindenanstalten Josefstadt-Baumgarten, Josefstädterstraße 80,
A-1080 Wien.
Baumgartnerstraße 71-79, A-1140 Wien.
Odilien Blindenanstalt Graz, Leonhardstraße 130, A-8020 Graz.
Kärntner Landesblindenanstalt Klagenfurt, Gutenbergstraße 9, A-9020 Klagenfurt.
Tirolische Blindenanstalt Innsbruck, Ing. Etzelstraße 71, A-6020 Innsbruck.
Landes-Blindenheim Salzburg, Müllnerhauptstraße 56, A-5020 Salzburg.
Blindenheim St. Florian bei Linz, St. Florian A-4490.
Hilfsgemeinschaft der Blinden und Sehschwachen Österreichs, Treustraße 9, A-1200, Wien.
Blindenheim Harmonie Unterdambach.   Betten: 100
Blindenheim Waldpension Hochegg, A-2840 Grimmenstein.   Betten: 80

BELGICA ET LUXEMBURGIA

SOCIETATES OPHTHALMOLOGICAE

Société Belge d'Ophtalmologie
Board: Mme Brihaye Van Geertruyden, Mrs. P. Danis, M. Dehoux, J. François, H. Gildemyn, G. Massa, J. Michiels, J. Pigneur, R. Weekers, J. Zanen, P. Lebas
Secretary: P. Danis, avenue de la Folle Chanson 15, 1050 Bruxelles
Number of members: 456

NOMINA ET DOMICILIA MEDICORUM AB OCULIS

Abbeloos, E.	rue Joseph II, 37	Bruxelles
Absalone	rue du Pont Canal, 20	Jemappes (Hainaut)
Adam, Max	avenue Isidore Geyskens, 50	Bruxelles 16
Alaerts	boulevard Brand Whitlock, 36	1040 Bruxelles
Andre-van Leeuwen	avenue du Pesage, 129	Bruxelles
Apers, R. C. L.	Brederodestraat, 23	Anvers
Bacus-Luyckx, J.	boulevard Piercot, 48	4000 Liège
Baekeland, W.	rue Général Leman, 5	Bruges
Baekelandt, L.	Pantheonlaan, 46	1080 Brussel
Baes, Charles	drève du Duc, 18	Boitsfort
Bayet-Fourneau	place des Chasseurs, 6	Mons
Beeckman, G.	chaussée de Ninove, 698	1070 Bruxelles
Begaux-de Cock	Van Maerlandstraat, 52	2000 Antwerpen
Beheyt, J.	Eekhoutstraat, 37	Brugge
Beni Liliane	ch. de Jette 578	1090, Bruxelles
Benoit	avenue Rogier, 22	Liège
Bernolet, J.	Torenbrug, 2	Bruges
Berthelon, S.		Bruxelles
Bertrand, Paul	rue de la Croix-Rouge, 39	5100 Jambes
Bervoets, Serge	avenue Prudent Bols, 104	1020 Bruxelles
Biernaux, J.	rue de Montigny, 41	Charleroi
Bingen, F.	boulevard Général Jacques, 174	Bruxelles
Biver-Lejeune	rue de la Belle Maison, 25	4641 Olne (St.-Adelin)
Blanckaert, M.	Pasterstraat, 28	Ieper
Blaser, Hélène	Belgiëlei, 122	2000 Antwerpen
Blockeel	Consciencestraat, 42	Roeselaere
Blust	boulevard Emile Bockstael, 292	1020 Bruxelles
Bodson-Bozyk	avenue Guillaume Joachim, 19	Waremme
Bonhomme	rue Trappé, 24	Liège
Bonnet-de Rudder	avenue du Luxembourg, 34	Liège
Borremans, E.	rue François Gérard, 1	Wauthier-Braine
Bortels	avenue d'Italie, 169	Anvers
Bossaerts, H.	Frank Craeybeckxlaan, 29	Deurne
Bussu, André	boulevard Lambermont, 290	1030 Bruxelles
Botton	rue du Diamant, 70A	5306 Leignon Ciney
Bourgeois, R.	rue du Grand Veneur, 33	1170 Bruxelles
Boursin, P.	avenue d'Auderghem, 57a	Etterbeek
Bouton, J.	avenue Louise, 181	Bruxelles
Bragard, P.	rue du Palais, 130	4800 Verviers

Brandes, G.	rue Saint-Bernard, 58	Bruxelles
Breuseghem, R.	Schouwbroekstraat, 6	9921 Vinderhoute
Brihaye-Vangeertruyden	rue Vergote, 13	Bruxelles
Brouhon-Massillon	rue de la Station, 30	Barvaux s/Ourthe
Burvenich, P.	chaussée de Bruxelles, 65	Ledeberg (Gand)
Butaye-Teughels, Marie-Paule	Louisastraat 6	2800 Mechelen
Callier, J.	boulevard Tirou, 51	Charleroi
Cambie, E. J. A.	Gordunakaai, 76	9000 Gent
Candaele-Baeten, H.	Penitentenstraat, 20	Gand
Cardoen, T.	Wervikstraat, 69	Geluwe
Carlier, E.	rue Colonel Silvertop, 10	Boom
Carrier-Marechal	rue Forgeur, 13	Liège
Castel, Ch.	avenue Wuyts, 35	Merksem
Chanteux	Grand-Place, 17	Bertrix
Cheron, E.	boulevard Léopold III, 106	7600 Péruwelz
Claes	rue Joseph Cuylits, 25	Uccle-Bruxelles
Claes, Plovier	Broekstraat, 272	9160 Hamme
Claessen	avenue des Celtes, 50	Bruxelles
Closson-Maenhout	avenue de Janvier, 21	1200 Bruxelles
Coffyn	rue Haute, 39	Gand
Colette, P.	6, rue de la Loi	La Louvière
Collignon-Brach, J.	Hôpital de Bavière	Liège
Colmant	rue de la Jardinière, 220	Angleur
Colmant, J.	rue de Brantignies, 26	Ath
Cols, Ignace	Hemelakker, 6	Brasschaat
Comhaire, J.	avenue Rogier, 28	4000 Liège
Conreur, L.	rue Sans-Souci, 83	Bruxelles
Coppens, Albert A.	Lienaertstraat, 13	Alost
Coppens, André H.	Horriestraat 28	Roeselaere
Coppez, M.	place de Becquerelle, 1	Tournai
Coppez, P.	avenue de Tervueren, 73	Bruxelles
Coppieters, R.	Prinses Clementinelaan 145	9000 Gent
Corbeel-Alaerts	rue du Plagnia, 9	Rosière-Saint-André
Cornil	avenue des Français, 11	Tamines
Corswarem, F.	Ylerweglaan, 98	Ledeberg
Coucke, D.	Graaf Karel de Goedelaan, 10	8500 Kortrijk
Coulonvaux	rue J. Lion, 5	Dinant
Crunelle-Wyns, M.	rue de Namur, 73	Nivelles
Daels, H.	Beveilaai, 53	Courtrai
Danis, P.	avenue de la Folle-Chanson, 15	1050 Bruxelles
De Backer, P.	rue Saint-Georges, 15	Courtrai
De Backer, P.	Grand-Place, 14	Menin
De Becker, L.	Leopoldstraat, 31	Louvain
Debeir, O.	Albertlaan, 74	Knokke
De Blond, R.	Groendreef, 67	Lokeren
De Brabandere, J.	avenue Louise, 193	1050 Bruxelles
De Broeu	rue Jenneval, 33	Bruxelles
Declercq	avenue Fond'Roy, 21	1180 Bruxelles
Declercq-Denys	Maeger Scorrelaan, 39	Knokke
Decock, G.	Van Maerlantstraat, 52	Anvers
De Corte, H.	Nachtegalenlaan, 8	3078 Everberg
Defauw, N.	rue Docteur Vandurmen, 15	Saint-Nicolas (Waes)
Defossez, J.	Breidelstraat, 6	Torhout
De Graeve, A.	rue Royale, 55	Ostende
De Haese, W.	avenue Louis Jasmin, 109,	Bruxelles 15
De Hauwere, E.	Vrijheidstraat, 5	Alost

Dehaze	avenue d'Auderghem, 81	1040 Bruxelles
Dehoux	rue des Canonniers, 2	Nivelles
Dejardin-d'Horne, M.	ch. de Dave, 11	Wiere-Andoy (Namur)
De Laet, H.	avenue P. Stroobants, 46	Bruxelles
De Laey	Mechelsesteenweg, 184	Antwerpen
De Laey, J.-J.	Beukenlaan, 9	St-Denijs-Westrem
Delbauve	rue de la Station, 147	Mouscron
Delfosse	rue Jean Warocqué 12	La Louvière
Delhaie	rue de Wallonie, 14	Tournai
Delmarcelle	rue de Bruxelles, 132	Namur
Delmotte, J.	rue Roosevelt, 6	Gosselies
Delmotte, Michel	rue Konkel, 85	1150 Bruxelles
De Lombaert, C.	Versaierestraat 15	3790 Werugem
Delville-Hacourt	rue de l'Yser, 187	Ans-lez-Liège
Demolder, E.	avenue de Tervueren, 191	1160 Bruxelles
de Muelenaere, H.	avenue de Tervueren, 191	1160 Bruxelles
De Niel, J.	Nijverheidstraat	Sint-Niklaas
De Peuter, J. A.	Margravelei, 113	Anvers
Deprez-Binot, M. R.	rue du Bouxthay	Vottem (Liège)
De Proost. Fr.	Heydenberglaan, 99	1150 Brussel
Dereume-Decorte	avenue Prince Baudouin, 3	1410 Waterloo
Dernouchamps, J. P.	avenue Victor-Gilsoul, 46	1150 Bruxelles
De Roover, P.	Mont Saint-Martin, 28	4000 Liège
De Rouck, H. F.	Antwerpse steenweg, 52	Sint-Amandsberg
De Saedeleer	Vlamingstraat, 62	Bruges
De Smedt-Houtequiet	Capucijnenvoer, 42	3000 Leuven
D'espallier, J.	Mechelse steenweg, 265	Anvers
Destexhe, B.	rue de l'Eglise 124	4880 Creppe-Spa
De Sutter	rue Neuve, 15	Izegem
Detilleux, J. M.	avenue G. Versé, 4	1080 Bruxelles
Devaux	boulevard Audent, 17	Charleroi
Devis-Tuypens, L.	Moenebrachtstraat, 35	9582 Schendilbeke
De Vloo, N.	rue de Veeweyde, 115	1070 Bruxelles
De Vos, E.	rue du Sport, 260	Gand
Devos, H.	Brusselsesteenweg 322	Mechelen
De Vrieze, A.	Koning Albertstraat, 4	Courtrai
De Vuyst, Ch.	Groot-Brittanniëlaan, 56	Gent
De Walsche, L.	rue de la Victoire, 185	Bruxelles
De Weer, J. P.	rue des Chats, 27	Oudenaerde
Dewolf, J.	De Becker-Remy plein, 5	Kessel-Lo
De Zutter, R.	Koerselsesteenweg, 59	3950 Beringen
D'Haenens, J.	rue Euphr. Beernaert, 34	Ostende
Diepers, L.	Weg naar A, 37	Genk
Dierijck, Fr.	De Schuverlez 6	3500 Hemet
Dieudonne, G.	Résidence du Square, rue Théod. Prunieau, 6	Charleroi
Dindal-Monami	rue de Bruxelles, 17	Verviers
Doblowsky, E.	Graaf de Broquevillestraat, 1	Mol
Douchy	rue d'Elverdinghe, 11	Ypres
Donck, D.	Grand-Place, 18	Ypres
Dorzee, J.	avenue Paeppedelle, 42	Bruxelles
Doyen	place de l'Altitude 100, 10	1190 Bruxelles
Draps, Ed.	rue des Minimes, 22	Bruxelles
Dubois, J.	boulevard Louis Schmidt, 45	1040 Bruxelles
Dubois, J.	rue Grenot, 33	Belgrade (Namur)
Dubois, P.	rue de Behogne, 12	Rochefort

Dubuc, Michèle	rue Grande	5546 Doische
Duby, J.	avenue Herbofin, 3B	6600 Libramont
Duchateau-Boxus	boulevard d'Avroy, 75 E	4000 Liège
Dumont, Ch.	rue Dodonée, 5	1180 Bruxelles
Dumont	allée du Beau Chéniat, 1 bis	Loverval
Dumoulin, D.	Noordstraat 15	8480 Veurne
Dumoulin, Ph.	clos des Malouinières, 4	1150 Bruxelles
Dupoing-Jaucot	rue de la Station, 226	Châtelet
Dupont, W.	rue Albert Ier, 258	Genval
Eliaerts, H.	Turnhoutsebaan, 314	Borgerhout-Anvers
Evens, A.	avenue de Jette, 113	1090 Bruxelles
Evens, L.	Boseinde, 2	Neerpelt
Fanchamps	rue du Centre, 38	Verviers
Farnir, A.	Dieweg, 56a	1180 Bruxelles
Feron, A.	Stationstraat, 3	Temse
Feuillat, Fr.	Marnix laan, 39	1900 Overijse
Fievet, J.-P.	rue Klipveld, 76	1180 Bruxelles
Forez, J.	Résidence Europe, rue Peterinck, 10	Tournai
Fosse, G.	avenue Paul Hymans, 127	1200 Bruxelles
Fossion, L.	rue Louise, 3	Malines
François, J.	place de Smet de Naeyer, 15	Gand
François, P.	rue de Charleroi, 7	Nivelles
Françoisse	avenue F. Lambeau, 103	1150 Bruxelles
Freson, J.	rue Joseph, 20	Jemeppe-sur-Meuse
Fritz	avenue Louise, 202	1050 Bruxelles
Fumiere	rue de la Montagne, 34	1000 Bruxelles
Gabriel-Wille	Hoge Herviweg, 60	9830 St-Martens, Latem
Gailly-Preaux	rue Gatti de Gamond, 250	1180 Bruxelles
Galand, A.	Haultepenne	les Awirs-Engis
Garin	boulevard Audent, 23	6000 Charleroi
Garin, Philippe	boulevard Joseph II, 28	Charleroi
Gathy, Jean	chaussée de Mons, 52	Chimay
Geerts, L.	Torhoutse steenweg, 88	Sint-Andries
Gérard, Robert	avenue du Luxembourg, 9	Liège
Gerard-Novak	avenue Voltaire, 163	1030 Bruxelles
Gildemyn, H.	Tentoonstellinglaan, 54	9000 Gent
Gillis	avenue Montjoie, 22	Bruxelles
Gilson, M.	rue du Palais, 66	Verviers
Gilson, L.	rue du Palais, 66	Verviers
Gobin, M.	Gounodstraat, 1	Anvers
Goes, R.	Plantin en Moretus lei, 21	Anvers
Golard-Leblanc	avenue Bonaparte, 75	1180 Bruxelles
Gouders	rue Neuve, 97	Stavelot
Gougnard, Léon	avenue des Ormes, 25	4200 Cointe-Ougrée
Goux, J.-P.	avenue de l'Indépendance belge, 36	1080 Bruxelles
Grieten, J.	Bois de Marlomont, 61	Jalhay
Grillet, G.	Toekomstlaan, 1	Beerse (Antw.)
Gustin	Predikherenstraat, 17	Tongres
Guzik, A.	avenue du Domaine, 183	1190 Bruxelles
Habig	avenue d'Auderghem, 19	Bruxelles
Haegeman, G.	rue de la Gare, 51	Ninove
Halleux, F.	rue du Palais de Justice, 19	Huy
Hansenne, W.	avenue de Saturne, 15	1180 Bruxelles
Hansenne-Burguet, C.	Tiège, 72	4882 Sart-lez-Spa

Hanssens, M.	Gauweg 33	9150 Grembergen (Dendermonde)
Haustraete, Léon	avenue d'Italie, 98	Anvers
Haverals, G.	Bredabaan, 636	Merksem
Haverbeke, L.	Walenstraat, 5	Antwerpen
Heffinck, L.	rue Adam, 19	Grammont
Heintz, A.	rue de Neufchâteau	Bastogne
Heintz, P.	Koningin Elisabethlaan, 53	Brugge
Helin-Manderlier	rue Saint-Antoine, 3	Casteau
Henrard-Gourmet	place Coronmeuse, 10	Herstal
Henrotte-Houssa	Place du Congrès, 20	4000 Liège
Hermans	rue Potagère, 115	1030 Bruxelles
Hermans, G.	rue Potagère, 115	1030 Bruxelles
Hermia, J.-P.	rue Thierbise, 77	Montegnée
Herode, R.	boulevard L. Mettewie, 477	1080 Bruxelles
Hindrycks, G.	Korte Torhoutstraat, 11	Ypres
Hourlay, C.	boulevard Frère Orban, 8	4000 Liège
Hubert	boulevard Sainctelette, 126	Mons
Hubin	rue Grégoire Bodart, 8	Huy
Hugard, J.	Kortrijkstraat, 3	Pecq
Humbeek, Ed.	avenue Churchill, 138	Bruxelles
Humblet, M.	rue de Savary, 6	Courtrai
Huwart	rue Cayauderie, 38	Charleroi
Jacquemin, Pierre	rue Darchis, 25	Liège
Jacquemotte	square Gramme, 3	4000 Liège
Jadoul, P.	Prins Albertlaan, 50a	Saint-Trond
Jambe, H.	rue Jules Destrée, 282	Quaregnon
Jamotton, L.	avenue de Longwy, 128	6700 Arlon
Jansen, E.	Otterstraat, 18	Turnhout
Jansen-Tilmanne	Nouvelle Drève	Mariemont-Morlanwelz
Janssens, B.	avenue Désiré Yernaux, 23	Wavre
Jaumain, Cl.	rue Debast, 22	Quiévrain
Jeener, Fr.	avenue Goenmaere, 81 d	1160 Bruxelles
Joachim, M.	Clinique ophtalmologique, Hôpital de Bavière	Liège
Joiris	rue Jean Calas, 12	Seraing
Kallay, Oscar	boulevard de Smet de Nayer, 121	1090 Bruxelles
Kastelyn, Y.	chaussée de Ninove, 221	Dilbeek
Kelecom, J.	rue d'Amercœur, 49	4000 Liège
Kemp, Stephan	rue Cockerill, 10	6790 Athus
Kemp, Monique,	Rodenbachstraat 15	3500 Hasselt
Kempeneers, M.	Stationstraat, 58	9900 Eeklo
Kentgen-Troisfontaines	rue J. P. Carpay, 6	4000 Liège
Kerkhofs, G.	place des Bienfaiteurs, 9	1030 Bruxelles
Kestens	rue du Cièl, 10	Anvers
Kevers, G. H.	avenue des Martyrs, 200	Fléron
Kieffer, L.	avenue Nothomb, 20	Arlon
Kluyskens, J. M.	Krijgslaan, 1	Gand
Kozanecki, St.	rue du Printemps, 26	1328 Ohain
Kruijen, A.	Stationlaan, 35	Bilzen
Kuypers, C.	steenweg op Gent, 1108	Berchem-Sainte-Agathe
Lafaut, N. A.	Vlamingstraat, 62	8000 Brugge
Lambert, R.	boulevard Sainctelette, 25	7000 Mons
Lambrecht, J.	boulevard de la Sauvenière, 110	Liège
Lamotte, R.	rue Godefroid, 37	Namur
Laurys	rue Roi Albert, 83	Diest

Lauwers, R.	avenue des Azelées, 65	1030 Bruxelles
Lavergne, Gaston	boulevard de la Constitution, 99 .	Liège
Lebas	rue des Capucins, 57	Mons
Lebas, P.	rue des Capucins, 57	Mons
Lebas-Beernaerts	rue des Capucins, 57	Mons
Lebrun, G.	avenue du Polo, 64	1150 Bruxelles
Lecomte	avenue de Broqueville, 155	Bruxelles
Le jeune, J.	Veureweg, 11	Afsnee
Lekeux, M.	rue de Sclessin, 6	4000 Liège
Leman, Ph.	boulevard Léopold II, 94	Tournai
Lempereur-Cowez		6000 Charleroi
Lenaers	boulevard de la Sauvenière, 5	Liège
Lenaers, T.	rue Bailleux, 9	Embourg (Liège)
Leonard, Paul	Lange Leemstraat 128	2000 Antwerpen
Leplat, G.	rue des Anges, 19	Liège
Leuridan, O.,		8800 Borselen
Levecq, J. P.	Boulevard Sainctelette, 112	7000 Mons
Levecq-Fastrez	Boulevard Seinctelette, 112	7000 Mons
Liegeois, G.	rue Dartois, 8	Liège
Lievens	rue J. Plateau, 14	Gand
Lison, Fr.	rue de la Reinette, 73	Bruxelles
Lowyck, R.	1re Avenue, 27	Marcinelle
Luypaert, R.	R. avenue de Foestraats, 69	Uccle
Luyssaert, L.	Hoogstraat, 55	8580 Avelgem
Maertens, K.		8500 Kortrijk
Maes, O.	Leopoldlaan, 80	Lommel
Maes, E.	Nouvelle chaussée de Gand, 12	1720 Grand-Bigard
Maillart, N. M.	rue Alfred Giron, 15	1050 Bruxelles
Mairiaux, Edm.	rue Warocqué, 33	La Louvière
Maleux, M.	Grote Straat 10	3600 Genk
Marechal-Courtois	rue du Parc, 75	Liège
Mariaule, M.		
Martin, C.	avenue de l'Araucia, 5	1020 Bruxelles
Maryssael, R.	Beenhouwerstraat, 34	Bruges
Massa	rue Léopold, 71	Malines
Massa, J. M.	boulevard Campion, 22	Vilvorde
Massart	avenue Reine Astrid, 76	Namur
Massien, V.	rue du Lac, 30	1050 Bruxelles
Matton-Van Leuven, M.-Th.	de Smet de Naeyerplein, 5	Gand
Meunier, A.	rue Phillippe-le-Bon, 30	Bruxelles
Meur, G.	chaussée de Waterloo, 773	1180 Bruxelles
Michaux	rue Royale, 251	Bruxelles
Michiels, J.	rue de Tirlemont, 105	Louvain
Missiaen, Fr.	Tentoonstellingslaan, 64	Anvers
Missotten, R.	Kapelstraat, 40	Hasselt
Missotten, L.	Leo Dartelaan, 12	3030 Heverlee
Moens	Borluitstraat, 7	Gand
Monteiro-de Gandt	chemin des Mésanges, 85	5170 Profondville
Moons, Louis	Stationstraat, 87	2440 Geel
Mortelmans, L.	avenue Boekenberg, 164	Deurne-Anvers
Mousset-Walravens, Cl.	avenue Lebon, 51	1160 Bruxelles
Neetens, Adolphe	Lange Lozanastraat, 197	Anvers
Nelis, J.	rue Docteur Geens, 12	Tirlemont
Nenkin-Klaasen	Ferrerlaan, 117	Gand
Neuforge-Guiot, A.	rue Charles Périn, 4	7410 Ghlin
Nihard	quai Mativa, 13	Liège

Noel	avenue de Stassart, 3	Namur
Nonet-Reginster	rue Nijsten, 40	Liège
Novalet, P. G. S.	rue Hôtel des Monnaies, 118	1060 Bruxelles
Nuyens, N.	Hofkwartier, 26	Herenthals
Olemans, J. M.	rue Saint-Martin, 1	9600 Renaix
Ooms, P.	rue Deken Adams, 5	Turnhout
Page-Van Gompel	avenue René Gobert, 45	1180 Bruxelles
Parent, G.	rue de l'Abbaye, 56	1050 Bruxelles
Paris	boulevard Albert Ier, 62	Herstal
Parlier, M.-J.	Galgestraat, 29	Mechelen
Parmentier, N.	avenue de Woluwe-St.-Lambert, 29	1150 Bruxelles
Peigny, W.	rue de Bois-d'Haine, 64	7161 Haine-Saint-Paul
Peters	avenue des Alliés, 84	Louvain
Petitjean, M.	Afsneelaan, 109	9000 Gent
Pexters-Koch, M.	Hollandsveld laan, 34	3500 Leuven
Pigneur	rue Lelièvre, 4	Namur
Pirot, G.	rue de la Justice, 9	Liège
Pivont, A.	square J. Hiernaux, 3	Charleroi
Plasschaert	rue du Collège, 2	Saint-Nicolas-Waes
Poelman, A. H.	Voskenslaan, 71	Gand
Poncelet-Berleur	avenue Reine Astrid, 80	5000 Namur
Ponthot, J. M.	rue de Montigny, 31	Charleroi
Potvin	rue Neuman, 41	Braine-le-Comte
Prijot, E.	quai Churchill, 15	Liège
Rabaey, M.	Watervallestraat, 71	Bekegem
Raemaekers, G.	avenue Louise, 192	Bruxelles
Raoult, J.	boulevard Louis Schmidt, 31	1040 Bruxelles
Raskin	boulevard de Shirvel, 21	Hasselt
Raus, R.	Rondplein, 24	Mol
Rausin, G.	quai de Flandre, 7	Charleroi
Reiter, M. L.	rue Paul Bossu, 8	1150 Bruxelles
Renaut-Peeters	avenue Albert, 116	Bruxelles
Riga-Lespagnard	avenue Cardinal Mercier, 8	Bressoux-Liège
Robe-Vanwijck, A.	rue J. Merlot, 57	4900 Angleur
Roelens, M.	Kioskplaats, 14	Hoboken
Roger-Evrard	avenue Don Bosco, 25	Woluwe-Saint-Pierre
Roland	rue de l'Hôtellerie, 18	Lessines
Rommel, J.	Grote Markt, 28	8800 Roeselaere
Roquet, P.	route de Beaumont	Marchienne-au-Pont
Roussel	rue Forgeur, 29	Liège
Rysselaere, M.	Meersstraat, 88	Gand
Sallet, G.	Statiestraat, 20	9300 Aalst
Salome	rue de Lessines, 91	Grammont
Samain, H.	Rijsselse straat, 53	8500 Kortrijk
Santens, P.	Oostende straat, 1	Torhout
Scauflaire-Petit, Y.	rue du Nouveau-Monde, 28	Soignies
Schepens, Cl.	100 Charles River Plazza	Boston, Mass. 02114
Schmidt-Wibo	rue Saint-Bernard, 70	Bruxelles
Sels, J. F.	Antwerpsesteenweg, 381	2500 Lier
Sels, J. F.	Eikelstraat, 19	Lier
Sevrin, G.	rue du Nord, 42	1000 Bruxelles
Soil-Ketelbant	rue Marie-Henriette, 51	1050 Bruxelles
Soyer-Forêt	rue du Biseau, 15	Binche
Spiritus, M.	Tervuurse Vest, 21, Appt. 177	3030 Heverlee
Staudt, A.	rue du Prince Royal, 63	1050 Bruxelles

Stockmans, L.	Tolstraat, 56	Anvers
Sucs	rue de la Vallée, 14	1050 Bruxelles
Swinnen, F.	avenue Albert, 223	Bruxelles
Tenenbaum, J.	avenue de Neptune, 12	1190 Bruxelles
Theunis, Fr.	Thonissenlaan, 42	Hasselt
Thibert, H.	rue Raikem, 26	Liège
Thomas-Decortis, G.	rue Général Modard, 27	Loncin (Liège)
Thon-Neuprez	rue de la Belle-Voie, 17	Wavre
Toussaint, D.	avenue Belle-Vue, 118	Waterloo
Trau, R.	Rubenslei, 20-21	Anvers
VanBellegem-Dralands, G.	Groenstraat, 27b	3008 Veltem
Vandamme, J.	Politieke Gevangenenstraat, 23	Renaix
Van de Briel	rue de l'Harmonie, 10	Anvers
Van de Casteele, J.	Naamse Steenweg, 155	Heverlee
Van de Gaer, L.	Bergstraat, 23	Heist-op-den-Berg
Vandekerckhove, R.	Leopoldlaan, 36	De Pinte
Van den Abeele, L.	Oude Godstraat, 39	2520 Edegem
Van den Berghe, J.	Zuidstraat, 17	Roeselaere
Van den Dooren, E.	Stationstraat, 37	Oudenaerde
Van den Neste, C.	Twee Dreven, 51	9830 St-Martens, Latem
Vanderpoorten-Moens, E.	Clauslaan, 9	Gent
Van de Velde, J.	Wegvoeringstraat, 6	Wetteren
Van Ginneken, E.	Merksemheidelaan, 72	Merksem
Van Hess, F.	Noordstraat, 4	Gand
Van Hoonacker, E.	Stationstraat, 11	Kortrijk
Van Horenbeeck, A. G.	Jan Van Ryswycklaan, 16	Anvers
Van Houtte, L.	Van Arteveldeplein, 35	9000 Gent
Van Itterbeek-van Assche, E.	rue des Joyeuses Entrées, 2	Louvain
Van Langenhove, A.	square Riga, 12	1030 Bruxelles
Van Langenhove, E.	Karenveldstraat, 10	1890 Opwijck
Van Meensel-Fourneau	avenue Charles Woeste, 208	1090 Bruxelles
Van Mulders, L.	Markt, 17	Merchtem
Van Neste, L.	Wilgendreef, 34	Waregem
Van Oye	Rogierlaan, 26	8400 Oostende
Vanoye, R.	Kortrijkse steenweg, 251	9830 St-Martens, Latem
Van Steenberge, E.	Veldstraat, 10	Alost
Van Steerteghem, Ch.	avenue Molière, 234	1060 Bruxelles
Van Vlimmeren, H.	Herentalselaan, 259	2100 Deurne
Van Vooren, H.	Grote Markt, 118	Malines
Van Vooren, K.	Sint-Janstraat	Tielt
Van Wesemael	Hoogpoort, 57	Gand
Van Wezer, J. E. C. M.	Kapelstraat, 12	Hove Antwerpen
Van Wymeersch	Grand-Place, 34	Renaix
Vauthier-Balsacq	avenue Defré, 114	1180 Bruxelles
Verdonck, M.	Tolstraat, 64	Anvers
Vereecken, E.	Park Ryvissche, 66	9710 Zwynaarde
Verelst, J.	avenue Boileau, 10	1040 Bruxelles
Verbruggen, W.	Noeverselaan, 6	2650 Boom
Verheyden, Cl.	avenue Venizelos, 23	1070 Bruxelles
Verlaeken, L.	rue du Croissant, 81	Forest-Bruxelles
Verluyten, P.	Statiestraat, 51	Geel
Vermer, P.	rue En Rhée, 49	Dinant
Vernraeken, H.	Paleisstraat, 18	2000 Antwerpen
Verriest	Artoisstraat, 1	8000 Brugge
Verriest, G.	Coupure, 73	Gand
Verschure-Beka, A.-M.	rue de la Réunion, 1	7000 Mons

Verstrepen, S.	Dijkstraat, 17	Dendermonde
Vindevogel, S.	Statieplein, 6	Harelbeke
Vliegen, G.	Kerkstraat, 78	2000 Antwerpen
Warny-Hendrichs	rue Franz Merjay, 81	Ixelles
Wasteels, Monique	rue Sylvain Guyaux, 66	La Louvière
Watelet	boulevard Reine Astrid, 67	7100 La Louvière
Watillon	boulevard d'Avroy, 144	Liège
Wauters	rue de l'Association, 25	Bruxelles
Weckbecker, A.	avenue de Limburg Stirum, 11	Wemmel
Weekers, R.	Clinique ophtalmologique, Hôpital de Bavière	Liège
Weekers, J.-Fr.	Thier des Critchions, 169	Chênée (Liège)
Weetjens, B.	Opvoedingstraat, 79	9000 Gent
Wery, D.	avenue Montjoie, 63	1180 Bruxelles
Weyts, E.	avenue du Diamant, 168	1040 Bruxelles
Wibail, R.	avenue Brugmann, 425d	Bruxelles
Wibo-Durieu	rue Saint-Bernard, 70	Bruxelles
Willemssens, P.	rue Anselmo, 14	Anvers
Wirtel, A.	rue de Châtelet, 3	Loverval
Wisznia Kelman	avenue Winston Churchill, 174	Uccle, 1180 Bruxelles
Wouters, K.	Lantaarnpad, 16	Herentals
Wuilbaut, N.	rue Ortelius, 32	1040 Bruxelles
Wyndaele, C.	Koning Albertstraat, 25	3290 Diest
Zanen, A.	avenue Georges Bergmann, 65	1050 Bruxelles
Zanen, J.	rue Belliard, 74	1040 Bruxelles
Zwijsen, J.	Casinostraat, 7	Saint-Nicolas-Waas

NOSCOMIA QUIBUS OCULIS AEGRI CURANTUR

Clinique ophthalmologique de l'Université de Bruxelles, dir.: Prof. P. Danis.
Clinique ophthalmologique de l'Université de Gand, dir.: Prof. J. François.
Clinique ophthalmologique de l'Université de Liège, dir.: Prof. R. Weekers.
Clinique ophthalmologique de l'Université de Louvain, dir.: Prof. M. Appelmans.

INSTITUTA SCHOLAEQUE CAECIS DESTINATAE

Stedelijke lagere school voor slechtziende kinderen (garçons et filles entre 6 et 12 ans), Pierenbergstraat, 31, Antwerpen.

Koninklijk Instituut voor Blinde en Gezichtszwakke jongens, Snagaardstraat, 9, Brugge.

Koninklijk Instituut voor Blinde en Gezichtszwakke meisjes, Snagaardstraat, 9, Brugge.

Institut Provincial pour Sourds Muets, Aveugles et Amblyopes, 1, rue de Dilbeek, Berchem Sainte Agathe, Bruxelles.

Institut de Ganspoel. Enseignement spécial pour garçons et filles Aveugles et Amblyopes, Huldenberg, Bruxelles.

Institut Royal des Sourds et Aveugles, 1504, chaussée de Waterloo, Uccle (Bruxelles 18).

Institut Royal pour Sourds et Muets, Aveugles et Amblyopes, 278, Av. Georges Henri, Woluwé Saint-Lambert, Bruxelles.

Institut Provincial d'Etudes et de Traitements Psycho-Pédagogiques, Ghlin.

Institut Royal pour Sourds-Muets, Durs d'oreille, Troublés du language, Aveugles et Amblyopes, 80, rue Monulphe, Liège.

Readaptation, orientation professionnelle

Centres de rédaptation (pour hommes et femmes): St. Rafaëlshuis, Annunciatenstraat, 54, Brugge.
St. Godelieve Tehuis Markgravelei, 22, Antwerpen.

Services Psychotechniques

Psycho-Medisch Consultatiebureau. Sinte-Kathelijnestraat, 40 Brugge.
Centre d'Etudes et de Reclassement Professionnel des Handicapés Visuels, Départment de la Ligue.
     Braille, 57, rue d'Angleterre, Bruxelles 1060
Psycho-Medisch Consultatiebureau, Jan Mahieustraat 43, Roeselaere

Formation professionnelle

Licht & Liefde, Jerusalemstraat, 17, Brugge.
Ligue Braille, 57, rue d'Angleterre, Bruxelles 1060.
Koninklijke Maatschappij tot Onderstand der Blinden, Van Schoonbekestraat, 114, Antwerpen.

Cours menagers et de couture

Licht & Liefde, Brugge et Antwerpen.
Ligue Braille, Bruxelles, Charleroi, Gent, La Louvière, Namur, Tournai, Menin et à domicile.
Koninklijke Maatschappij tot Onderstand der Blinden, Antwerpen

Cours de Braille a domicile

Ligue Braille, 57, rue d'Angleterre, 1060 Bruxelles.

Cours par correspondance

Ligue Braille, 57, rue d'Angleterre, Bruxelles 1060.

BOLIVIA

SOCIETATES OPHTHALMOLOGICAE

Sociedad de Oftalmologica de Cochabamba

Secretary: Dr. Jaime Solares Zamora, Casilla Correo 1403, Cochabamba

No further data received.

BRASILIA

SOCIETATES OPHTHALMOLOGICAE

Nationales

Sociedade Brasileira de Oftalmologia
Rua Mexico, 111 grupos 1406/7/8-Centro,
20.000-Rio de Janeiro-Guanabara-ZC-00
Presidente: Prof. Paiva Gonçalves Filho
Vice-Presidente: Dr. Botelho Ferreira
Secretário Geral: Dr. Aroldo Lobo Mazza
1° Secretário: Dr. Marcelo Gonçalves
2° Secretário: Dr. Jorge Alberto Oliveira
Tesoureiro: Dr. Luiz Herculano Pinto Ernesto
Diretor de Cursos: Dr. Adalmir Morterá Dantas
Diretor de Publicações: Dr. Claudio Humberto Savastano Ramalho
Diretor de Biblioteca: Dr. Dario Dias Alves
Miembros: 1049

Conselho Brasileiro de Oftalmologia
Rue Jayme Benevolo, 23
Fortaleza – Ceará
Presidente: Prof. Leiria de Andrade Junior
Vice-Presidente:
Secretário: Prof. Renato de Toledo
Tesoureiro:

Regionales

Secção de Oftalmologia da Associação Bahiana de Oftalmologia
Hospital das Clinicas – Canela
Salvador – Bahia
Presidente: Dr. Roberto Lorens Marback

Sociedade de Oftalmologia do Ceará
Rua Pedro Primeiro, 997
Fortaleza – Ceará
Presidente: Dr. Antonio Mont'Alverne Lopes

Sociedade Campista de Oftalmologia
Av. Alberto Torres, 117
Campos – Estado do Rio de Janeiro
Presidente: Prof. Oswaldo C. Cardoso de Melo

Departamento de Oftalmologia de Associação Médica de Goiás

Caixa Postal 254
Goiânia – Goiás
Presidente: Dr. Durval Moraes de Carvalho

Associacão dos Ex-Residentes e Estagiários do Hospital São Geraldo

Hospital São Geraldo
Av. Prof. Alfredo Balena
Belo Horizonte – Minas Gerais
Presidente: Dr. Emyr Francisco Soares

Departamento de Oftalmologia da Associação Médica de Minas Gerais

Av. João Pinheiro, 161
Belo Horizonte – Minas Gerais
Presidente: Prof. Geraldo Queiroga

Departamento de Oftalmo-Otorrinol. da Sociedade de Medicina e Cirurgia de Juiz de Fora

Rua Braz Bernardino, 59
Juiz de Fora – Minas Gerais
Presidente: Dr. Marcos Saraiva

Associação Paranaense de Oftalmologia

Rua Ebano Pereira, 414 – 4° andar
Caixa Postal 550
Curitiba – Paraná
Presidente: Dr. Antonio Vantuil Samara

Departamento de Oftalmologia da Sociedade de Medicina de Pernambuco

Rua Osvaldo Cruz
Recife – Pernambuco
Presidente: Dr. Jayme Figueiredo

Centro de Estudos Ivo Correa Meyer

25ª Enfermaria da Santa Casa de Misericordia
Porto Alegre – Rio Grande do Sul
Presidente: Dr. Flávio Ferreira

Departamento de Oftalmo-Otorrinol. da Associação Médicas de Caxias do Sul

Av. Julio de Caxias, 2027
Caxias do Sul – Rio Grande do Sul

Sociedade de Oftalmologia do Rio Grande do Sul

Av. Senador Salgado Filho, 135 – 6° andar
Porto Alegre – Rio Grande do Sul
Presidente: Dr. Simão Brunstein

Academia de Oftalmologia de São Paulo
Av. Brigadeiro Luiz Antonio, 278
São Paulo – Estado de São Paulo
Presidente: Dr. Carlos Souza Dias

Associação Médica do Instituto Penido Burnier
Instituto Penido Burnier
Campinas – Estado de São Paulo
Presidente: Dr. Leoncio de Souza Queiroz Filho

Departamento de Oftalmologia de Associação Médica de Santos
Caixa Postal, 203
Santos – Estado de São Paulo

Sociedade Brasileira de Lentes de Contato
Rua México, 111 grupos 1406/7/8 – Centro
20.000 – Rio de Janeiro – GB.ZC-00
Presidente: Dr. Gilberto Lima de Arruda

Centro Brasileiro de Estrabismo
Rua Cincinato Braga, 59 apto. 582 – Bela Vista
01333 – São Paulo – Estado de São Paulo
Presidente: Dr. Carlos Souza Dias

NOMINA ET DOMICILIA MEDICORUM AB OCULIS

Alagoas

Araujo, Jeferson de lima ...	Trav. Franca Morel, 25	Maceió
Arruda, Aristeu	....	
Barbosa, Dario Ramos	Rua Dr. Paulo Netto, 255, Trapiche da Barra	Maceió
Breda, Arthur Guttemberg .	Av. Fernandes Lima, 315, Farol .	Maceió
Campos, Eunice de Lemos .	Rua do Comercio, 72	Maceió
Carleial, Oceano	Praça Floriano, 167	Penedo
Carleial, Papiniano	Av. Duque de Caxias, 1154	Maceió
Cortes, Durval	Rua 2 de Dezembro, 125	Maceió
Dias, Paul	....	
Lemos, Everaldo	Rua Antonio Cansanção, 1296 ..	Maceió
Lins, Ernande Roberto	....	
Lyra, Jorge	....	
Lyra, José Lins de Gusmão .	Av. Fernandes Lima, 416	Maceió
Monte, Hiran Pereira	Caixa Postal 16	Maceió
Mota, Valdomiro	Hospital Regional Santa Rita ...	Palmeira dos Indios
Omena, Olavo	Rua 2 de Dezembro, 119	Maceió
Pinto, Neves	Rua Duque de Caxias, 1016	Maceió
Ramos, Dalton de Oliveira .	Rua Bel. Milton Ramires, 67, Trapiche	Maceió

Rezende, Manoel Moura ...	Rua João Pessoa, 161, 1° andar .	Maceió
Rezende Neto, Manoel Moura	Rua João Pessoa, 161, 1° andar .	Maceió
Simões, Aristoteles	Praça Centenário, 951	Maceió

Amazonas

Delibo, Joel Clovis	Av. Tarumã, 952, 1° andar, Bairro Praça de Janeiro	Manaus
Monteiro, Roberto Cesar de Goes	Rua 10 de Julho, 93 apto. 102, Centro	Manaus
Nadaf, Calil de Moraes	Praça dos Remédios, 66	Manaus
Pereira, Avelino	Rua Leonardo Malcher, 742	Manaus
Russo, Paulo	Rua José Clemente, 216	Manaus
Sá, Franco de	Rua Barroso, 293	Manaus
Vasconcelos, Nilson	Rua Barroso, 62	Manaus

Bahia

Abdalla, Terezinha Maria Dutra	Rua Emidio dos Santos, 22 apto. 41, Barbalho	Salvador
Aguiar, Paulo Roberto Alcantara	Largo do Carneiro, 37 apto. 202, Nazaré	Salvador
Alakija, Cleonice de Assunção	Rua Siqueira Campos, 16	Salvador
Alencar, Procopio Pereira de	....	
Alves, Moacyr Galdino	Rua Claudio Manoel da Costa, 17 apto. 2	Salvador
Amaral, José Batista do ...	Rua Forte de São Pedro, 42 apto. 107	Salvador
Amorim Filho, Theonilo Uzeda	Av. 7 de Setembro, 341, apto. 801	Salvador
Andrade, Vavel José de		Itapetinga
Araujo, Aidil Brito	Av. Pres. Vargas, 108 apto. 603, Barra	Salvador
Araujo, Helio	Rua Eustaquio Bastos, 59, 1° andar	Ilheus
Assemany, Francisco Gomes	....	
Baleeiro, Astor	Rua Carlos Gomes, 2861, Edificio Castro Alves	Salvador
Barretto, Antonio Rafael Nery	Praça Adami, 44, 1° andar	Itabuna
Bastos, José Oliveira	....	
Bastos, Luiz Ferreira de Moura	Av. 7 de Setembro, 79, São Pedro	Salvador
Bezerra, America Lourdes ..	Rua Senador Costa Pinto, 23 apto. 303	Salvador
Branco, Eduardo Moreira ..	Rua C, 73, Pituba	Salvador
Branco, Ieda Cavalcante Rio .	Rua Teodoro Sampaio, 20, Barris.	Salvador
Branco, Pedro Teixeira Castelo	Av. 7 de Setembro, 245 apto. 11, Merces	Salvador

Branco Neto, Epaminondas Castelo .... Av. Euclides da Cunha, 47 apto. 701, Bairro Graça .... Salvador

Britto, Antonio Carlos Nogueira .... Av. Joana Angélica, 47 apto. 702. Salvador

Cabral, Ubirajara Chagas ... Rua Jardim Esperança, 13 apto. 22, Barbalho .... Salvador

Camera, José Albergarias de Carvalho .... Rua Inhuma, 10, Matatu .... Salvador

Campos, Aristeo .... Praça Dr. Antonio Muniz, 73 ... Ilheus

Carvalho, Guilherme Castro Lima de .... Rua Pedro Lessa, 2, Canela ..... Salvador

Carvalho, João Afonso de .. ..

Carvalho, Nelson Sena de .. Av. 7 de Setembro, 228 apto. 1101 .... Salvador

Chagas, Clorides Y.F. ..... Rua Greenfeld, 14 apto. 802 ... Salvador

Chaves, Geiza Maciel ...... Parque N.S. da Luz, Rua D N° 683, Pituba .... Salvador

Coelho, Anphilophio Francisco .... Rua Chile, 3, 2° andar .... Salvador

Cortes, Tania Lucia de Brito. Rua Brasilia, 5, Pituba .... Salvador

Costa, Emidia Maria Freitas . Av. 7 de Setembro, 555 apto 302, Condominio Quinta da Barra-Barra .... Salvador

Costa, Nelson dos Santos Vieira .... Rua 28 de Junho, 89 .... Ilheus

Coutinho, Edmilson Oliveira V. .... Av. Leovegildo Filgueiras, 107 apto. 803, Fazenda Carcia ... Salvador

Cruz, Luciene .... Cl. Oftalmologica do Hospital das Clinicas .... Salvador

Cunha, Maria Amelia Soares da .... Av. Princesa Leopoldina, 25, Graça .... Salvador

Cunha, Murilo Soares da ... Rua Rui Barbosa, 1, 1° andar ... Salvador

Dantas, Stenio .... Rua 7 de Setembro, 5 .... Itapetinga

Duarte, Pedro Amorim .... Praça Benjamin Constant, 16 ... Senhor do Bomfim

Esteves, Jorge Freitas ..... Rua Fernando Gomes, 38 apto. 32 .... Salvador

Falcão, Guilherme .... Rua Padre Vieira, 5, sala 30 .... Salvador

Falcão, Maria de Lourdes Lima .... Av. Leovegildo Filgueiras, 107 apto. 701, Garcia .... Salvador

Falcão, Newton Dias ...... Rua Renato Medrado, 14, apto. 804, Ed. Central Politeana ... Salvador

Fernandes, Luiz Maciel .... Av. Euclides da Cunha, 50 apto. 1102, Graça .... Salvador

Ferraz, M. Alves Pinto .... Horacio Urpia, 24 apto. 301, Graça .... Salvador

Ferreira, Ronaldo U. de Seixas .... IBOPC, Rua Pedro Lessa, 2, Canela .... Salvador

Ferreira, Zilda Lima ...... Rua Teixeira Leal, 15 apto. 502, Edificio Embaizador, Graça .. Salvador

Ferreira Neto, Ronaldo .... Av. Joana Angelica, 217 apto. 204, Nazaré .... Salvador

Figueiredo, Guilhardo de .. ..

Filardi, Altamiro Antonio .. Posto Federal do Tracoma Santana dos Brejos .... Via Lapa

Fonseca, Vera Lucia Seijo de Sá Sonseca .... Rua da Paz, 32 apto. 202, Graça . Salvador

Fontana, Rosa Maria de Noronha .... Av. Euclides da Cunha, 21/23 apto. 301, Graça .... Salvador

Franco, Paulo Cardoso de Menezes .... Rua Senador Costa Pinto, 49 apto. 1 .... Salvador

Freire, Maria Mesquita de Lima .... Rua Padre Feijo, 65, Canela .... Salvador

Freitas, Oswaldo Domiense de ....

Giudice, Rafael .... Rua Silva Jardim, 13 .... Jequie

Gomes, Nilson Ferreira .... Prof. Martagão Gesteira, 311 apto. 201 .... Salvador

Gomes, Wilson Ferreira .... Rua Pedro Leal, 3 apto. 31, Chame-Chame .... Salvador

Guerra Filho, José Martins Leitão .... Rua Francisco Ferraro, 25 A ... Salvador

Guimarães, Julio ....

Guimarães, Katia Nuno Marinho .... Rua Alm. Amintas Jorge, 1 apto. 101, Acupe, Brotas .... Salvador

Guimarães, Sergio Antonio Sena .... Rua José Paulino, 22, Brotas ... Salvador

Guimarães Filho, Julio ....

Ivo, Celia Leal .... Rua Marques de Caravelas, 47 ... Salvador

Lima, Darcy Martins ...... Rua Raul Drumond, 20 apto. 308, Barra .... Salvador

Lima, Djalma Martins ..... Rua Raul Drumond, 20 apto. 308, Barra .... Salvador

Lima, Hugo de Castro ..... Praça da República, 8 .... Vitória da Conquista

Lima, Humberto de Castro . Av. Euclides da Cunha, 9 apto. 1001, Graça .... Salvador

Lima, José Gonçalves de ... Praça Barão do Rio Branco, 26, Centro .... Juazeiro

Macedo Filho, Eurico Telles de .... Praça Rockfeller, 15 apto. 12, Barris .... Salvador

Machado, Thomas Dias .... Rua Padre Vieira, 11, 4° andar .. Salvador

Maia, Salviano ....

Maranhão, Lucio ....

Marback, Heitor .... Baixa de Bomfim, 236 .... Salvador

Marback, Roberto Lorens .. Baixa do Bomfim, 236, Itapagipe Salvador

Martins, Jayme Brown ....

Matos, Alfredo de Oliveira . Av. 7 de Setembro, 81 .... Salvador

Matos, Hugo Vieira .... Rua João Pessoa, 142 .... Vitória da Conquista

Meira, Antonio Tanajura Meira .... Rua Constancio Alves, 6 apto. 501, Saúde .... Salvador

Meira, Deolindo Vanderlei . Av. 7 de Setembro, 88 .... Salvador

Meira, Raimundo de Castro . Rua Constancio Alves, 6 apto. 501 B, Saúde .... Salvador

Meira, Romulo Luiz de C. . . . Rua Constancio Alves, 6 apto. 501, Saúde . . . . Salvador
Melo, Almiro Vieira de . . . . Av. 7 de Setembro, 283, A apto. 902 . . . . Salvador
Mendes, Marco Aurelio Oliveira . . . . Rua Bolivar América, 38, Nazaré . Salvador
Menezes, José Soares . . . . . Rua João Ribeiro Caldas, 9, Barris Salvador
Miranda Filho, Manoel Nobre de . . . . Rua Melquiades Moitinho, 3 . . . . 44900 – Irece
Monte, Manoel Ferreira . . . Rua Joel de Carvalho, 5 . . . . . . Alagoinhas
Muniz, Antonio Queiroz . . . Av. 7 de Setembro, 113, 6° andar Salvador
Nascimento, Anastacio . . . . Rua Alagoinhas, 75, Bairro Rio Vermelho . . . . Salvador
Nascimento, Antonio Costa . Rua Nilton Oliveira, 139 . . . . . . Salvador
Nobre, Ivan Novaes de Argolo . . . . Santa Casa de Misericordia, Hospital Santa Cruz . . . . Itabuna
Nobre, Mario de Argolo . . . Rua Cons. Paranhos, 32 . . . . Santo Amaro
Oliveira, Arlete Maria de . . . Areial de Baixo-31, Largo 2 de Julho . . . . Salvador
Oliveira, Balbino Antonio . . Praça da Bandeira, 34 . . . . Joazeiro
Oliveira, Eduardo Spinola P. de . . . . Ed. Com. A. Valerio de Carvalho, Praça Gampo Grande, 23 apto. 1101, Campo Grande . . . . . . Salvador
Oliveira, Fernando Principe de . . . . Ed. Com. A. Valerio de Carvalho, Praça Campo Grande, 23 apto. 1101, Campo Grande . . . . . . Salvador
Oliveira, Gileno Andrade . . Av. Presidente Vargas, 1700 apto. 101 . . . . Salvador
Oliveira, Osorio José de . . . Rua Mal. Floriano, 75, Canela . . Salvador
Oliveira, Sonia Noelia Silva . Rua Conçalves Dias, 20, Nazaré . Salvador
Oliveira Filho, Osorio José de . . . . Rua Mal. Floriano, 75, Canela . . Salvador
Papaleo, Felice . . . . Av. Sete de Setembro, 25, 1° andar . . . . Salvador
Passos, Armando Andrade de Almeida . . . . Rua Barros Falcão, 78, Matatu . . Salvador
Pastor, Daudete Gonçalves . Loteamento Jardim Atlântida Rua C N° 48, Barra . . . . Salvador
Paula, Adelia Maria Barros de . . . . Rua Itabuna, 7, Rio Vermelho . . Salvador
Pereira, Rita de Cassia Mota . Rua Manuel Barreto, 15 apto. 302, Graça . . . . Salvador
Pereira, Valdemir Uzel . . . . Av. 7 de Setembro, 57 apto. 202 . Salvador
Pinheiro, Carlos Aldir Ferraz Av. Euclides da Cunha, 50 apto. 1101, Craça . . . . Salvador
Ponde Filho, Joaquim . . . . . Rua Barão de Cotegipe, 927 sala 202 . . . . Feira de Santana
Pontes, Edilson Ribeiro . . . Av. Otavio Santos, 400 . . . . Vitória da Conquista
Portella, Dircelena M. Costa . Rua Visconde de Itaborai, 72, Amaralina . . . . Salvador
Queiroz, José Eutropio Souza Vaz de . . . . Rua Princeza Leopoldina, 52-A apto. 102, Barra Avenida . . . . Salvador

Ramalho, Humberto	Rua Padre Vieira, 5	Salvador
Ramos, Guilherme	Rua Padre Vieira, 11, 4° andar ..	Salvador
Ramos, Ruy Paschoal	Rua Visc. do Rio Branco, 35 s/110/11	Feirá de Santana
Reis, Auto	Rua Chile, 3, 2° andar	Salvador
Reis Filho, Manoel Alexandre dos	Av. Monteiro, 67, 2° andar	Salvador
Requião, Gladis Borges	Rua da Imperatriz, 83, Bomfim .	Salvador
Ribeiro, Maria Lucia	IBOPC, Rua Pedro Lessa, 2, Canela	Salvador
Rocha, Antonio Soares da	Av. Luiz Argolo, 102, Santo Antonio de Jesus	Salvador
Rolemberg Filho, Dacio Macedo	Rua Gabriel Soares, 40, São Pedro	Salvador
Sacramento, Maria Lucia do	Edificio Casa Grande da Barra, Rua Cristiano Ottoni, 1 apto. 901	Salvador
Sampaio, Aurivaldo Peixoto	Rua Santa Cruz, 6062	Itabuna
Santana, Antonio Luciano Soares de	Largo da Graça, 11 apto. 402, Graça	Salvador
Santana, João Marcelo Soares de	Av. 7 de Setembro, 325	Salvador
Santana, Maria C. G.	IBOPC, Rua Pedro Lessa, 2, Canela	Salvador
Santos, Aloyzio Borges dos .	Praça Tiradentes, 34	Amargoza
Santos, Dulce Barretos dos .	....	
Santos, Maria Laura Cardoso dos	Rua Padre Feijó, 72-A	Salvador
Santos, Osvaldete Durvalina .	Conjunto Stiep, Quadra 4, Travessa 5, Casa 10, Pituba	Salvador
Santos, Rita Lavina Pimenta.	Rua A, 261 apto. 203, Edificio Normalucia, Barra	Salvador
Santos, Vespasiano Gomes dos	Av. Euclides da Cunha, 74 apto. 401, Graça	Salvador
Santos, Walda Maria dos ...	IBOPC, Rua Pedro Lessa, 2, Canela	Salvador
Santos, Wilson Vianna Pacheco	Rua Bras do Amaral, 23	Salvador
Serravalle, Maria Celane F. .	Av. Salvador, 27, Bomfim	Salvador
Silva, Ailton Correia da	Rua Bruno Seabra, 17, Liberdade	Salvador
Silva, Eduardo Henrique Manso Cardoso e Silva ..	Rua Afonso Celso, 68, Barra	Salvador
Silva, Gelmires Almeida ...	Rua Pedro Americo, 10 apto. 603, Nazaré	Salvador
Silva, Margarida Pereira da .	Rua Prado Valadares, 3, 1° andar, Nazaré	Salvador
Silva, Marley Menezes	....	
Silva, Telma Maria Vargas Leal da	Lot. Antonio Carlos Magalhães Rua B. Casa 505, Pituba ...	Salvador
Silva, Vera Lucia dos Santos.	Rua Brigadeiro Pessoa da Silva, Vila São Paulo 1, Lapinha ...	Salvador
Simões, Elisio	Rua Chile, n° 27, 7° andar	Salvador
Sousa, Mariano José de	Rua Direita da Piedade, 6/8 apto. 09	Salvador

Sousa, Mario Borges de .... Av. Senhor dos Passos, 65 ...... Feira de Santana

Souza, Dinalva C. Guedes de Edificio Constantino apto. 604, Av. Antonio Carlos Magalhães, Pituba, Parque Julio Cesar ... Salvador

Souza, Serafim Santana de . Rua Forte de São Pedro, 42 apto. 107 .... Salvador

Spinola, Edmundo .... Rua da Graça, 17 .... Salvador

Spinola, Harlley .... Rua Constancio Alves, 6 ap. 501, Saúde .... Salvador

Tavares, Marilena Lopes ... IBOPC, Rua Pedro Lessa, 2, Canela .... Salvador

Teixeira, Edna Rita de Lima. IBOPC, Rua Pedro Lessa, 2, Canela .... Salvador

Terraça, Sonia Maria Fernandes .... Rua Renato Medrado, 25 apto. 302. Politeama .... Salvador

Tito, Ramilson Pereira .... IBOPC, Rua Pedro Lessa, 2, Canela .... Salvador

Tolomei, Domingos Raphael Micheli .... Rua da Italia, 9 .... Jequié

Veloso, Sonia .... Ladeira de São Bento, 4, 36° andar .... Salvador

Vieira, Luiz Barreto ...... Edificio Santa Rita Av. 7 de Setembro, 31, sala 608 .... Salvador

Viena, Carlos Antonio Goes Av. Joana Angélica, 59 apto. 101, Nazaré .... Salvador

Ceará

Almeida, Francisco Waldo Pessoa de ....

Andrade, José Maria de .... Rua Torres Camara, 135 .... Fortaleza

Andrade Junior, Leiria de .. Rua Padre Valdevino, 2255, Aldeota .... Fortaleza

Araujo, Marcia Maria ae ... Rua Jaime Benevolo, 23 . ..... 60.000. Fortaleza

Araujo Filho, Francisco ... Rua 24 de Maio, 1400 .... Fortaleza

Brito, Maria José de ....

Callou, Antonio Lyrio .... Rua Major Sampio, S/N .... Barbalha

Carneiro, José Hyder Dantas Av. Ruy Barbosa, 2665, Aldeota . Fortaleza

Cartaxo, Décio Teles ...... Rua Silva Pauleti, 160 .... Fortaleza

Cartaxo, Maurilio O. de Souza .... Rua Eduardo Bezerra, 895, São João do Tanapé .... Fortaleza

Castro, Leda Maria Smith Rodrigues .... Rua Pereira Filgueiras, 1961 .... Fortaleza

Castro, Valzenir Rodrigues de .... Rua Pereira Filgueiras, 1961 .... Fortaleza

Chaves, Guaracy Maia ..... Rua Tomas Acioli, 466, Estancia . Fortaleza

Chaves, José Carlos .... Av. João Pessoa, 4149 .... 60.000, Fortaleza

Ferreira, Helio Goes ...... Av. Tristão Gonçalves, 358 ..... Fortaleza

Figueiredo, Hugo Santana de Rua da Conceiçao, 393 .... Juazeiro do Norte ......

Freitas, Francisco Valter da Justa .... Rua São Francisco, 966, Bairro Aldeota .... Fortaleza

Gomes, José Nilson Ferreira. Praça General Tiburcio, 132 .... Sobral

Guerra, Carlos Alfredo Cisne	Rua João Brigido, 1840, Caixa Postal 887 Dionisio Torres ..	Fortaleza
Juaçaba, Roberto Caminha .	Av. Dez. Moreira da Rocha, 1313, Aldeota	Fortaleza
Leal, Cyro Carneiro	Rua Floriano Peixoto, 915	Fortaleza
Leal, Sylvio Ideburque	Rua 24 de Maio, 1289	Fortaleza
Leite, Fernando	Rua Gal. Guilherme Rocha, 1201.	Fortaleza
Lopes, Antonio Mon'Alverne ne	Rua Pocinhos, 33	Fortaleza
Macedo, Francisco Sales de .	Rua José Sombra, 490, Parque Araxá	Fortaleza
Magalhães, José	Av. Duque de Caxias, 1529	Fortaleza
Maranhão, Lucio Leite	Av. Duque de Caxias, 991, Centro	Fortaleza
Mello Filho, João Costa ...	Av. Visconde de Caiuipe, 2346 ..	Fortaleza
Mendes Filho, João	Rua Barão do Rio Branco, 1006, 1° andar	Fortaleza
Menezes, José Afranio Memoria de	Rua Antonio Augusto, 1079, Aldeota	Fortaleza
Monte, Fernando Queiroz ..	Rua Princeza Izabel, 1956	Fortaleza
Moura, Leopoldo Farias ...	Av. Tristão Gonçalves, 950	Fortaleza
Nogueira, João Maia	....	Orós
Nunes, Francisca Angela de Oliveira	Rua J. da Penha, 617	Fortaleza
Oliveira, Edmilson Barros de	Av. Santos Dumont, 830	Forteleza
Oliveira, J.E. Motta Barros de	Rua Afonso Celso, 180, Aldeota .	Fortaleza
Oliveira, Zairton Gaspar ...	Rua Guilherme Rocha, 263, 5° andar	Fortaleza
Pinheiro, Ocelo	....	
Ponte, Walter Machado da .	Rua Gonçalves Ledo, 660, Aldeota	Fortaleza
Praça, Antonio Sequeira ...	Av. Almirante Barroso, 727 apto. 303, Praia de Iracema	Fortaleza
Rangel, Antonio Mont'Alverne	Rua Osvaldo Cruz, 2095	Fortaleza
Ribeiro, José Luciano Xavier	Rua Campos Sales, 168, Benfica .	Fortaleza
Silva, José Arimathea Monte	Rua Joaquim Ribeiro, 161	Sobral
Silva, Luiz Carlos Sales de Castro e	Rua Guilherme Rocha, 10702, Jacarecanga	Fortaleza
Soares, Ricardo de Gouveia .	Praça José de Alencar	Fortaleza
Teixeira, Helenita Magalhães	Rua Mons. Bruno, 2215, Aldeota .	Fortaleza
Teles, Ebert	Rua Dr. João, Pessoa, 103	Crato
Ximenes, Odimar Napoleão .	Av. 13 de Maio, 319	Fortaleza

Distrito Federal

Almeida, Marco Aurelio B. de	SQS 306 BL G apto. 201	Brasilia
Almeida, Marilene G.	Edificio São Paulo apto. 219/220.	Brasilia
Alves, Jurandir Augusto de A.	Clinica Oftalmológica, Hospital Distrital	Brasilia
Andrade, Paulo Gomes de ..	Hospital do Estado Maior das Forças Armadas, Setor Residencial Interno, Casa 11	Brasilia

Barreto, Jaison Tupy . . . . . Deputado Federal, Camara dos
Deputados . . . . Brasilia
Borges, Donato Rispoli . . . . SQS 212 BL. D apto. 524 . . . . . . Brasilia
Costa, Claudio . . . . Edificio JK, Sala 33 . . . . Brasilia
Costa, José Domingos . . . . . Hospital dos Servidores da União,
Ipase, L 2 Norte . . . . Brasilia
Costa, Roberto Bassit Lamei-
ro da . . . . SQS 308 Bloco I apto. 410 . . . . . Brasilia
Crispim, Arlindo Dafico . . . Hospital Santa Luzia, Av. W 3 Q.
716 E Lote 05 Brasilia
Faria Junior, José Rodrigues
de . . . . Quadra N A, 5, Lote 24, Tagua-
tinga . . . . Brasilia
Ferreira, Milton Celestino . . SQS 307, BL. H. apto. 304 . . . . . Brasilia
Ferreira, Valter Vianna . . . . Instituto de Olhos de Brasilia,
SGS, Edificio Embaixador,
S-312-314 . . . . Brasilia
Gonçalves, Elizabeto Ribeiro Instituto de Olhos de Brasilia,
SCS, Edificio Embaixador,
S-312-314 . . . . Brasilia
Gracindo Neto, Ignacio
Brandão . . . . SQS 413 BL. T. apto. 107, Asa
Sul. . . . . Brasilia
Guimarães, Ana Maria Lira . SQS 303 BL. G apto, 201 . . . . . . Brasilia
Leal, Ediwaldo Martins . . . . SQS 404, BL. A apto. 304 . . . . . 70.000, Brasilia
Lemos, José de Bouza . . . .
Lima, Augusto Juvenal
Marques . . . . SQS 307 BL. I apto. 402 . . . . . . Brasilia
Lindoso, Iara Barbosa . . . . . SQS 206 BL. C apto. 202 . . . . . . Brasilia
Maldi, Vanildo . . . . Hospital das Forças Armadas, SR I
BL. I apto. 205 Estrada Con-
torno do Bosque . . . . Brasilia
Medeiros, João Eugenio
Gonçalves de . . . . Edificio Gilberto Salomão,
3-105-105, Setor Comercial
Sul . . . . Brasilia
Menezes, Eduardo Almeida
de . . . . Edificio São Paulo, s/219-220
Setor Comercial Sul . . . . Brasilia
Motta, Dirceu Guido . . . .
Mousinho, Evalde de Al-
meida . . . . SQN 406 BL. 63 apto. 303 . . . . . Brasilia
Nolli, Osmar James . . . . SHCGN Quadra 711 BL. E apto.
402 . . . . Brasilia
Palmieri, João Cristovão . . . SQS 307 BL. 6 apto. 101 . . . . . . Brasilia
Paschoal, Marco Antonie
Vieira . . . . SQS 308 BL. I apto. 411 . . . . . . Brasilia
Paula, Celio Heitor de . . . . . SQS 206 K 304 . . . . Brasilia
Pereira, Celso Generoso . . . Super Quadra 305 BL. K apto.
602, ASA SUL . . . . Brasilia
Pereira Neto, Laurentino . . Clinica Oftalmologica, Hospital
Distrital . . . . Brasilia
Reis, Hamilton Tavares . . . . SQS 106 Bloco F apto. 204 . . . . Brasilia
Rodrigues, Maria Clara . . . .
Santos, José Felipe dos . . . . Edificio Ceará, 9° andar, Sector
Comercial Sul . . . . Brasilia

Santos, Mario	SQS 407 BL. 'O' apto. 205	Brasilia
Santos, Oliveiros Castro dos .	SQS 199 BL. B. apto. 306	Brasilia
Sawaki, Emilia Kazue	SQS 404 BL. 'L' apto. 207	Brasilia
Senna, Roberto Antonio Soares de	SQS 302 BL. H. apto 506	Brasilia
Serralvo, Ariovaldo	SQS 305 BL. apto. 305, Plano Piloto	Brasilia
Silva, Maria Elizabeth Arrais de Castro Rodrigues da .	SQS 307 BL. E apto. 605	70.000, Brasilia
Sousa, Carlos Alberto Acioly de	SQS 106 BL. F apto. 204	Brasilia
Souza, Glower Leonidas Coelho de	Super Quadra 305, BL. D apto. 605, Asa Sul	Brasilia
Teles, Antonio Carlos Machado	HI Sul Ch 1 Lote 42	Brasilia

Espirito Santo

Anacleto, Ercilia	Rua Gama Rosa, 20, Centro	Vitória
Arantes, Iran Malfitano	Av. Republica, 224 apto. 603 ...	Vitória
Arantes, Suely de Assis	Av. Cesar Hilal, 808, Praia do Sua	Vitória
Barbieri Filho, Argeo	Rua 7 de Setembro, 200, Centro .	Vitória
Barcellos, Wilmington Ayrola	Av. Cesar Hilal, Ed. Adelia apto. 1, Praia do Suá	Vitória
Barreto, Gentil	Praça Geronimo Monteiro, 45, Sobrado	Cachoeiro de Itapemirim
Buaiz, Benjamin	Av. Pres. Florentino Avidos, 502	Vitória
Casotti, Paulo José	Rua Barão do Itapemirim, 31 ...	Cachoeiro do Itapemirim
Castro, Izaumi Dias de	Av. João Felipe Calmon, 768 ...	Linhares
Favarato, Hernandez	Rua Vasco Coutinho, 111	Vitória
Freitas, Elviro Athayde de Freitas	Rua Barão de Itapemirim, 14 ...	Cachoeiro do Itapemirim
Gomes, Adir	Rua Graciano Neves, 266 apto. 402	Vitória
Gozman, Ricardo C.	Rua 7 de Setembro, 215	Vitória
Guio, Almir	Rua de Vintem, 189 apto. 2	Vitória
Heringer, Carlos Gomes ...	Rua Senador Salgado Filho, 12, Jucutuquara	Vitória
Imperial Neto, Mario Corte .	Rua Dom Pedro II, 160	Colatina
Lessa, Glades	....	
Lima, Mario Correa	Av. João Blei, 11	Castelo
Lopes, José, Roberto Negri .	Rua do Rosário, 121 apto. 5	Vitória
Magalhães, Caetano	....	
Mario, Célia Figueiredo Souza	Rua Pedro Carlos de Souza, 217, Ilha de Santa Maria	Vitória
Meira, Anamaria de Figueiredo	Av. Beira Mar, 2755, Caixa Postal 577	Vitória
Meira, Manoel Gomes	Av. Beira Mar, 2755	Vitória
Moises, Kamel Camech	Rua Erotides Rezende, 43	Vitória
Moraes, Milton Nunes de ..	Av. Getulio Vargas, 314, 1° andar	Colatina
Neves, Raul de Oliveira	Rua Colatina, 333	Vitória
Passos Junior, Carlyle	Rua Antonio Aguirre, 69	Vitória

Pavan, Dermeval Castiglioni .	Av. Marcos Azevedo, 299	Vitória
Pereira, Ismael Gonçalves ..	Rua Pinto Homem de Azevedo, 101, Jucutuquara	Vitória
Re, Antonio Cezar	Rua Santo André, 68, Vila Rubim	Vitória
Rebouças, José de Almeida .	Caixa Postal 85	Vitória
Ribeiro, Paulo Eduardo Magalhães	Rua Barão de Monjardim, 182 apto. 103	Vitória
Schilgen, Carlos Lindenberg von	Av. Saturnino de Brito, 595	Vitória
Schwab, Rutelea Firme	Rua Valerio Coser, S/N, Bairro Cobilandia	Vila Velha
Silva, José Maria S.	Caixa Postal 337	Colatina
Silva, Rosa Maria da	Rua Maria Amalia, 786	Vila Velha
Souza, L. Poltronieri de ...	....	Aracruz
Tironi, Walace	Av. Saturnino de Brito, 1175 apto. 703, Praia de Canto ...	Vitória
Vianna, Paulo Ney	Casa de Saúde e Maternidade São Pedro, Bairro Gilberto Machado	Cachoeiro do Itapemirim

Estado do Rio de Janeiro

Abido, Jamil	Rua Tenente Gel. Cardozo, 768 .	Campos
Affonso, Adyr	Rua José Alvarenga, 499 sala 4 ..	Caxias
Almeida, Luiz Geraldo de Queiroz e	Rua Carlos Lacerda, 45	Campos
Amorelle, Alexandre	....	
Anderaos, Jorgina	Rua Eduardo Junqueira, 20 ...	Volta Redonda
Araujo, Rosalmir Baptista de	Rua Cel. Moreira Cesar, 180 apto. 802, Icaraí	Niterói
Assad, Carlos Augusto	Rua Voluntários da Pátria, 530 ..	Campos
Azeredo, Icnael Gomes de .	Rua Assis Ribeiro, 47	Itaperuna
Azeredo, Regina Celi Silveira F.	Rua Marques do Paraná, 253 apto. 305, Centro	Niterói
Azevedo, Amin de	Rua Cristovão Leal, 39	Barra Mansa
Azevedo, Democrito Jonathas	Basé Aérea Nalval de	São Pedro da Aldeia
Azevedo, Rosali Sampaio ..	Rua Visc. do Rio Branco, 765 apto. 1003	Niterói
Badini, Adilson Faria	Rua Miguel de Frias, 211 apto. 701, Icaraí	Niterói
Badini, Maria Helena Gonçalves	Rua Miguel de Frias, 211, apto. 701, Icaraí	Niterói
Baracuhy, Helena Vieira ...	Rua Teodorico Fonseca, 282 ...	Marques de Valença
Barbosa, Carlos Waldyr	Rua 10, 37, Engenhoca	Niterói
Barreto, Waldemar, Paes ...	Rua Azevedo Sodré, 92, Paraizo .	São Gonçalo
Bastos, Hayrton Moreira ...	Av. Cardose Moreira, 191	Itaperuna
Batista, Carlos Roberto S. ..	Av. Amaral Peixoto, 455 apto. 611, Centro	Niterói
Bianco, André	Hospital C.N.S.	Volta Redonda
Blum, Ronaldo Celso Leon .	Rua Romeu, 41	Nova Iguaçú
Bonini, Marco Antonio	Praia do Icaraí, 137, Icaraí	Niterói
Branco, Accacio de Souza ..	Praça Ruy Barbosa, 205, apto. 601	Petropolis

Camargo, Sandra Mar	Rua São Paulo, 28, Centro	Niterói
Campos, Edgar	Av. 15 de Novembro, 970, 3° andar	Petropolis
Campos, Sheila Mara Gomes.	Rua Joaquim Tavora, 270, Icaraí	Niterói
Carmo, Wanderley José Carvalho do	Rua Yago Valerio, 1109, Of. Velha	Barra do Piraí
Carraro, José Luis de Barros.	Rua D. Guilhermina, 109	Barra do Piraí
Carvelho, Othon Barros de .	Rua Dr. Pereira Nunes, 90 apto. 302, Bairro Ingá	Niterói
Ceia, Mario Lopes de	Rua Santos Dumont, 83 apto. 1002	Nova Iguaçú
Cesario, Manoel	Rua Frei Angelo, 652	São Fidelis
Chaves, Carles Alberto Azevedo	Rua dos Leites, 69 sala 5	Santo Antonio de Padua
Ciabatari, Reinaldo Tadeu Aylla	Av. Oliveira Botelho, 1075 casa 31	Teresopolis
Cnop Junior, Lemant de ...	Praia de Icaraí, 119 apto. 304, Icaraí	Niterói
Combat, Nivaldo	Rua Boqueirão Pequeno, 456, Bairro Estrela do Norte	São Gonçalo
Costa, Amaro Moreira da ..	Rua Conceição, 137 apto. 707 ..	Niterói
Costa, Jorge Daure	Rua Gal. Silvestre Rocha, 134, Jardim Icaraí	Niterói
Cruz, Arlete Velasco	Estrada Froes, 701	Niterói
Cunha, Itubias de Azevedo .	Rua Barão do Amazonas, 514 apto. 410, Centro	Niterói
Cunha, Luiz Carlos	Av. Amaral Peixoto, 593	Barra do Piraí
Curi, Renato Luiz Nahoum .	Rua Miguelote Viana, 17, Jardim Icaraí	Niterói
Cury, Wenry W.	Av. Ari Parreiras, 438, Canto do Rio	Niterói
Dantas, Adalmir Morterá ..	Rua Miguel de Frias, 37 apto. 103, Icaraí	Niterói
Duarte, Augusto de Queiroz	Rua Herotides de Oliveira, 29, Terreo- Campo de São Bento .	Niterói
Erthal, Celso	Edificio Erthal s-101-2	Bom Jardim
Fernandes, Rubenm Salles .	Av. Amaral Peixoto, 55, 4° andar.	Niterói
Ferraz, Denir	Rua 33, 146	Volta Redonda
Franceshi, José de Nzare Valmont	Av. Vicente Federici, 40 apto. 101, Icaraí	Niterói
Gomes, Gastão Pinto	Rua Presidente Pedreira, 189 apto. 901, Ingá	Niterói
Goulart, José Bastos	Rua Frutuoso Rangel, 137	Nova Iguaçu
Gripp, Antonio Carlos Werner	Rua Antero Perlingeiro, 39, Centro	Macaé
Gripp, Luiz Alberto Emerick	Rua Pres. Domiciano, 227 apto. 403	Niterói
Guerra, Manuel Alberto Barbosa	Rua Barão de Miracema, 225 ...	Campos
Haack, Alfred W.	Av. 15 de Novembro, 970 apto. 405	Petropolis

Innocente, Enio Leite ..... Alameda São Boaventura, 584,
Bairro Fonseca .... Niterói
Inocente, Raul .... Rua Casimiro de Abreu, 23 apto.
101, Ingá .... Niterói
Jogaib, Maria Estephane ... Rua Andrade Pinto, 275 apto.
201 .... Niterói
Knust Sobrinho, José Carlos. Rua Joaquim Tavora, 221 apto.
604, Icaraí .... Niterói
Kunsel, Herbert Georg .... Rua Suissa, 189 .... Nova Friburgo
Laaf, Siegfried .... Rua Miguel de Frias, 245 apto.
602, Icaraí .... Niterói
Lemos, Virgilie Tito de .... Rua Alice Pinheiro, 55, Quar-
teirão Ingelheim .... Petropolis
Lessa, Magda Vianna ...... Rua Gal. Pereira da Silva, 246
apto. 201, Icaraí .... Niterói
Levy, Ivan de Uzeda Maciel Rua Mariz e Barros, 272 ...... Niterói
Lima, F. Silva .... Rua Alberto Braune. 127 ...... Nova Friburgo
Lima, Sandro Castilho .... Rua Abelardo Matta, 261 ...... São Gonçalo
Lima, Telemaco Boldrim de
Freitas .... Rua Joaquim Maximo Soares,
178, Sobrado .... Nilopolis
Liporaci, Francisco Anto-
nino .... Rua Eduardo Junqueira, 846 ... Barra Mansa
Lohmann, Julio Constant .. Rua Gal. Kondon, 175 apto. 102,
São Francisco .... Niterói
Machado, Humberto Braga
Siqueira .... Rua Gel. Moreira Cezar, 259 apto.
402 .... Niterói
Machado, Renato Pereira .. Av. Amaral Peixoto, 370, sala
1202, Centro .... Niterói
Magalhães, Samuel T. ....
Maia, Jeão ....
Manhães, Francisco S. Alle-
mand .... Rua Benta Pereira, 62 .... Campos
Mannarelli, Roberto Augusto Av. Brig. Lima Silva, 1269, sala
113 .... Duque de Caxias
Mansur, Cleber Mucio
Damasco .... Rua Francisco de Souza, 67 .... Rio Bonito
Mariath, José Meirelles ....
Martins, Dirceu Badini .... Rua Alberto Braune, 86, sala 208. Nova Friburgo
Mary, Fernando .... Rua Aurelino Leal, 105 apto.
201, Centro .... Niterói
Medeiros, Carlos .... Av. 15 de Novembro, 179 ...... Petropolis
Melara, Carlos Henrique ... Rua Belizario Augusto, 90 apto.
204, Icaraí .... Niterói
Mello, Osvaldo C. Cardoso
de .... Rua Barão de Cotegipe, 86, 1°
andar .... Campos
Mendes, Ubiratan Faria .... Trav. Augusto Fragoso, 29 ..... Petropolis
Menezes, Astrogildo T .... Rua Lopes Trovão, 199 .... Niterói
Menezes Neto, Antonio
Inacio de .... Praia de Icaraí, 341, BL. B apto.
1201, Icaraí .... Niterói
Miguel, Fuad Antonio ..... Rua João Sobral Bitencourt, 103 . Campos
Moyses, Marcos Fernandes . Colégio Naval, casa 4 .... Angra dos Reis
Monteiro, Maria de Gama .. Rua Tiradentes, 22 .... Niterói

Moraes, Flavio Abi-Ramia de	Rua Dr. Geraldo Martines, 201, Santa Rosa	Niterói
Moraes, Maria Lucia Mendes de	Rua Eduardo Junqueira, 20	Volta Redonda
Paes, Edalvo Henriques	Rua Cons°. José Fernandes, 250 .	Campos
Passerino, Francisco José ..	Hotel Iberia, Rua Visc. do Rio Branco, 389	Niterói
Peçanha, Cyro Almeida	Caixa Postal 69	Três Rios
Pena, Ari de Souza	Rua Maestro Felicio Toledo, 551 sala 207/8 Edificio Palácio dos Jornalistas	Niterói
Pepeira, José	Rua Maestro Djalma do Carmo, 322	Nilópolis
Perisse, Artevelle	Rua Cel. Pimenta, 239	Itaperuna
Pimentel, Antonio Pedro ..	Rua Lopes Trovão, 32 apto. 1302, Icaraí	Niterói
Pimentel, Paulo	Rua 15 de Novembro, 134	Niterói
Rezende, João Andrade ...	Rua Cristovão Leal, 39	Barra Mansa
Ribeiro, Antonio Carlos Hallays Ribeiro	Rua Goitacazes, 338, São Francisco	Niterói
Ribeiro Filho, Armando M. Ferreira	Rua Sebastiãe Herculano de Matos, 127, Centre	Nova Iguaçú
Rodrigues, Mario Affonso Vasconcelos	Av. 15 de Novembro, 888, sala 806	Petropolis
Schott, Antonie Carlos	Rua João Pessoa, 168, Icaraí ...	Niteró
Silva, Carlos Edson e Silva .	Rua Antonio Silva, 42, Fonseca .	Niterói
Silva, Levy Lopes da	Rua Noronha Torrezão, 165	Niterói
Silva, Roberto Lucio Caetano da	Alameda Barcelos, 44, Icaraí ...	Niterói
Siqueira, Inimá de Almeida .	Rua Itaperuna, 114, Santa Rosa .	Niterói
Souza, Luiz Gastão Costa ..	Rua General Osorio, 89 apto. 104	Petropolis
Telles, Miguel Plinio Rivello Telles	Rua Maestro Felicio Toledo, 551 salas 207/8, Edificio Palacio dos Jornalistas	Niterói
Valentim, Marcos Adilson ..	Rua Ana Maria, 43	Belfort Roxo
Varginha, Jonas da Silva ...	Rua Mal. Trompowski, BL. B-2 apto. 301, Aman	Rezende
Vasconcelos, Renato Araujo de	Rua Dr. Celestino, 42 apto. 406 .	Niterói
Wangler, Arthur Adolpho Pessolani	Rua Voluntários da Pátria, 396 ..	Campos
Zaidan, Rosuel	Rua 25-A, 81 sala 308/09, Edificio Justina Mollica	Volta Redonda
Zanerotti, Delfio Brandão ..	....	
Zangalli, Antonio Luiz	Rua Belizario Augusto, 90 apto. 204, Icaraí	Niterói
Zukeran, Tioei	Rua Telio Barreto, 595	Macaé

Goiás

Almeida, Cristiano Teixeira de	....	

Alto, Florisvaldo Pereira Pouso	Praça da Bandeira, 3	Piracanjuba
Amaral, Matilde F. de	Av. B, 770, Setor Oeste	Goiania
Araujo, João Severino de ..	Rua Goiás, 245	Inhumas
Assemany, Francisco Gomes	Hospital São Patricio. Rua 3. 78	Ceres
Ayres, Francisco	Caixa Postal 440	Goiania
Ayres, Marilia	Caixa Postal 440	Goiania
Camara, Danilo Leopoldo da	Rua 1° de Maio, 185	Anapolis
Camargos, Marcos Lacel ...	Hospital N.S. de Fátima	76360 – Mineiros
Carvalho, Adylson Nery ...	Avenida Goiás, 439	Jataí
Carvalho, Durval Moraes de .	Av. Goiás, 606 sala 802	Goiania
Castro, Antonio Domingos de	Edificio Princeza Izabel, Av. Goiás, 971, apto. 404	Goiania
Castro, Lincoln Caiado de ..	....	
Costa, Jeronimo Manoel da .	Av. Tocantins, 858, Ed. Jarina ..	Goiania
Coutinho, Wilson Santana ..	....	
Cristino Sobrinho, Leonardo	. Rua Getulino Artiaga, 103	Ipameri
Cruvinel, Ricardo Campos .	Rua Cel. Vaiano, 425	Rio Verde
Faria, Edson Linch de	....	
Ferreira, Aderbal G. Souza .	Rua Castro Alves, 686	76300 – Jataí
Ferreira, Odilon Vasconcelos	Av. Goiás, 60 apto. 205	Goiania
Filgueiras Junior, Francisco .	Rua Severino Teodoro	Mineiros
Jucenwicz, Leszek Marian Karclewicz	....	
Lima, Elizeu de	Av. Goiás, 760	Anapolis
Mota, Josue José da	Rua 3, 628, 1° andar, sala 111 ..	Goiania
Paranhos. Augusto	Rua 4, 38 apto. 4	Goiania
Pereira, Olinto Manso	....	
Pereira, Ozanno Leite	Rua 19 n° 71 BL. B apto. 1305 .	Goiania
Rassi, Fued Raul	....	
Rego, Braulio Brandão	Hospital São Pio X, Praça São Pio X, 84	Ceres
Ribeiro, Ruberpaulo de Mendonça	Rua 83 D, 101, Setor Sul	Goiania
Rocha, Gilberto Resende ..	....	Gurupi
Rocha, José Maria Garcez ..	Hospital N.S. do Carmo	Ourinhos
Roriz, Idan	Rua 7 de Setembro, 293	Anapolis
Seba Neto, João	Rua 9, 30, Setor Oeste	Goiania
Seboni, Sedda	Casa de Saude Santa Izabel	Itumbiara
Silveira, José Peixoto	....	
Vaz, Sebastião Aureliano ..	Rua Santa Rita, 78, 1° andar ...	Itumbiara
Veloso, Luiz Onofre	Hospital São Geraldo, Rua 9 B, Setor Oeste	Goiania

Guanabara

Abramovic, Pedro Mathias .	Rua Pedro Américo, 348 apto. 302, Glória	Rio de Janeiro, GB. ZC-01
Abrantes, Alfredo José	Rua Barão do Flamengo, 17 apto. 1102, Flamengo	Rió de Janeiro, GB. ZC-01
Abud, Jorge Felipe	Clinica Oftalmológica do Hospital da Lagon, INPS Rua Jardim Botanico, 501, Jardim Botanico	Rio de Janeiro, GB. ZC-20

Aguiar, Pedro Moacyr de ..	Rua Aurea, 96, Santa Tereza ...	Rio de Janeiro, GB. ZC-45
Alanati, Alberto	Rua Constante Ramos, 64 apto. 202, Copacabana	Rio de Janeiro, GB. ZC-07
Albuquerque, Sergio Neves Cavalcanti de	Rua Antonio Basilio, 505, casa 1, Tijuca	Rio de Janeiro, GB. ZC-09
Alencar, Adroaldo de	Rua Anita Garibaldi, 43 apto. 801, Copacabana	Rio de Janeiro, GB. ZC-07
Almeida, Eduardo Lopes de	Rua Conde de Bomfim, 370 apto. 414, Tijuca	Rio de Janeiro, GB. ZC-09
Almeida, Guilherme de	Rua Cambauba, 1698, Jardim Guanabara, Ilha do Governador	Rio de Janeiro, GB. ZC-32
Alves, Aderbal de Albuquerque	Rua General Urquiza, 136 apto. 202, Leblon	Rio de Janeiro, GB. ZC-95
Alves, Dario Dias	Praia do Flamengo, 254 apto. 601, Flamengo	Rio de Janeiro, GB. ZC-01
Alves, Jader da Silva	Rua Viuva Dantas, 451 apto. 109, Campo Grande	Rio de Janeiro, GB. ZC-26
Alves, Moises Severiano ...	Rua do Caja, 316, Penha	Rio de Janeiro, GB. ZC-22
Amaya, Paulo Shigueru	Rua Dois de Dezembro, 22 apto. 808, Flamengo	Rio de Janeiro, GB. ZC-01
Amaral, Nelson Moura Brasil do	Praia do Flamengo, 274 apto. 601, Flamengo	Rio de Janeiro, GB. ZC-01
Amaral, Otavio Moura Brasil do	Rua Uruguaiana, 25, 1° andar, Centro	Rio de Janeiro, GB. ZC-21
Amahal, Ozanan	Rua Otavio Correia, 53, Urca ...	Rio de Janeiro, GB. ZC-82
Amaral Filho, Oswaldo Moura Brasil do	Av. Atlantica, 2856 apto. 202, Copacabana	Rio de Janeiro, GB. ZC-07
Ambrosio, Renato	Rua Voluntários da Pátria, 114 apto. 808 Botafogo	Rio de Janeiro, GB. ZC-02
Ambrosio, Vera Martins ...	Rua Voluntários da Pátria, 114 apto. 808, Botafogo	Rio de Janeiro, GB. ZC-02
Amorim, Carlos Alberto ...	Rua Vitório da Costa, 88 apto. 301, Botafogo	Rio de Janeiro, GB. ZC-02
Amorim Filho, Theonilo ...	Rua Joaquim Nabuco, 197 apto. 601 Copacabana	Rio de Janeiro, GB. ZC-37
Amorim Neto, Olinto José Gonçalves de	Hotel Barão de Tefé, Av. Barão de Tefé, 99, Saúde	Rio de Janeiro, GB. ZC-05
Andó, Joãe	Rua Condessa Belmonte, 211 apto. C-05, Engenho Novo ..	Rio de Janeiro, GB. ZC-16
Andrade, Aloisio Moreira ..	Rua Constante Ramos, 73 apto. 703, Copacabana	Rio de Janeiro, GB. ZC-07
Andrade, Carlucio	Rua General Artigas, 72 apto. 101, Leblon	Rio de Janeiro, GB. ZC-95
Andrade, Fernando Gabriel de	Av. Copacabana, 162, 11° andar, Copacabana	Rio de Janeiro, GB. ZC-07
Andrade, Genesio Jeronimo de	Rua Djalma Ulrich, 110 apto. 304, Copacabana	Rio de Janeiro, GB. ZC-07
Andrade, Gilberto Fornaciari de	Av. Engenheiro Richard, 200, Grajaú	Rio de Janeiro, GB. ZC-11

Andrade, Gilson Fornaciari
de ....   Rua Itabaiana, 271, Grajaú .....   Rio de Janeiro, GB. ZC-11
Andrade, João Crisostomo
de ....   Rua Barão de Itambi, 7 apto. 603,
                             Botafogo ....   Rio de Janeiro, GB. ZC-01
Andrade, José Guilherme
Ottoni de ....   Rua Aarão Reis, 37 apto. 102,
                             Santa Tereza ....   Rio de Janeiro, GB. ZC-45
Andrade, Luiz Evandro
Brandão de ....   Rua Oliveira da Silva, 48 apto. 8,
                             Tijuca ....   Rio de Janeiro, GB. ZC-09
Andrade, Luiz Moreira de .. Rua Barão de Flamengo, 35 apto.
                             821, Flamengo ....   Rio de Janeiro, GB. ZC-01
Andrade Junior, Fernando
Gabriel de ....   Av. Copacabana, 162, 11° andar,
                             Copacabana ....   Rio de Janeiro, GB. ZC-07
Anesio, Alfredo Ary ....
Antunes, Leda Maria Pinto . Rua Dr. Bulhoes, 278, Engenho
                             Novo ....   Rio de Janeiro, GB. ZC-13
Aquino Filho, Leonardo
Tonas de ....   Rua Manuela Barbosa, 33 apto.
                             402, Meier ....   Rio de Janeiro, GB. ZC-16
Arabe, Dorival ....   Av. Copacabana, 1032, apto. 906,
                             Copacabana ....   Rio de Janeiro, GB. ZC-07
Aragão, Jesuino Lins de ... Rua Honorio de Barros, 38 apto.
                             304, Flamengo ....   Rio de Janeiro, GB. ZC-01
Aragão, Raimundo Ozildo
Rocha de ....   Escola de Saúde do Exercito, Rua
                             Moncorvo Filho, 20, Centro .   Rio de Janeiro, GB. ZC-14
Arakaki, Celso Masao .....   Rua 2 de Dezembro, 35 apto.
                             704, Flamengo ....   Rio de Janeiro, GB. ZC-01
Arakaki, Kanziro ....   Rua Rodrigo de Brito, 14 apto.
                             403, Botafogo ....   Rio de Janeiro, GB. ZC-82
Arantes, Marcelo Guimarães.   Rua Itaipava, 17 apto. 307, Gávea   Rio de Janeiro, GB. ZC-20
Araujo, Evelyn James .....   Rua Voluntários da Pátria, 139
                             apto. 802, Botafogo ....   Rio de Janeiro, GB. ZC-02
Araujo, Francisco A. Bar-
reira de ....   Rua Dona Delfina, 162 apto. 201,
                             Tijuca ....   Rio de Janeiro, GB. ZC-09
Araujo, Jarbas Galvão de .. Rua Carlos Sampaio, 106, apto.
                             30, Esolanada do Senado ....   Rio de Janeiro, GB. ZC-86
Araujo, Rubeval ....   Hospital Pedro Ernesto (Residen-
                             te) Av. 28 de Setembro, 87,
                             Vila Izabel ....   Rio de Janeiro, GB. ZC-11
Areal, Marco Antonio Este-
ves ....   Rua Bueno de Paiva, 28, Meier ..   Rio de Janeiro, GB. ZC-16
Armando, Deborah do A.
Marcondes ....   Travessa Soledade, 29, Praça da
                             Bandeira ....   Rio de Janeiro, GB. ZC-29
Arroyo, Antonio Del .....   Cl. Ottalmologica do Hospital
                             Pedro Ernesto, Av. 28 de
                             Setembro, 87, 4° andar, Vila
                             Izabel ....   Rio de Janeiro, GB. ZC-11
Arruda, Gilberto Lima de .. Rua Sorocaba, 464 sala 409,
                             Botafogo ....   Rio de Janeiro, GB. ZC-02

Arruda, Jonas de	Av. Lineu de Paula Machado, 788, Jardim Botanico	Rio de Janeiro, GB. ZC-20
Arruda, Marcelo Lima de ..	Av. Lineu de Paula Machado, 788, Jardim Botanico	Rio de Janeiro, GB. ZC-20
Athayde, Helio Pacheco ...	Rua Tavares Bastos, 19, Catete ..	Rio de Janeiro, GB. ZC-01
Azevedo, Ennio	Rua Siqueira Campos, 180 apto. 303, Copacabana	Rio de Janeiro, GB. ZC-07
Azevedo, Luiz Fernando da Mota	Av. Heitor Beltrão, 81, Tijuca ...	Rio de Janeiro, GB. ZC-10
Azevedo, Marcio da Rocha .	Rua Visc. de Santa Izabel, 460 apto. 103, Grajaú	Rio de Janeiro, GB. ZC-11
Baltz, Willy Nicolino	Av. 17 Casa 316, Vila dos Oficiais Galeäo, Ilha do Governador ..	Rio de Janeiro, GB. ZC-32
Barboza, Luiz Roberto Colombo	Hospital Pedro Ernesto, Oftalmologia, Av. 28 de Setembro, 87, 4° andar, Vila Izabel	Rio de Janeiro, GB. ZC-11
Barbuto, Claudio Roberto .	....	
Barcaui, Pedro Paulo	Rua Visc. de Pirajá, 12 apto. 801, Ipanema	Rio de Janeiro, GB. ZC-37
Baron, Clarice	Rua Santa Clara, 340 apto. 902, Copacabana	Rio de Janeiro, GB. ZC-07
Barros, Arnoldo Gomes de .	Hospital Pedro Ernesto, Oftalmologia, Av. 28 de Setembro, 87, 4° andar, Vila Izabel ...	Rio de Janeiro, GB. ZC-11
Barros, Joaquim de Azevedo	Rua Alvaro Ramos, 245 apto. 301, Botafogo	Rio de Janeiro, GB. ZC-82
Bastos, Reynaldo Araujo ..	Rua Marques de Abrantes, 118 apto. 1004, Botafogo	Rio de Janeiro, GB. ZC-01
Batti, Maria Irene Bez	Rua Sa Ferreira, 178 apto. 406, Copacabana	Rio de Janeiro, GB. ZC-07
Bellizzi, Ataliba Macieira ..	Rua Barão da Torre, 521 apto. C. 01, Ipanema	Rio de Janeiro, GB. ZC-95
Benchimol, Eliezer	Rua República do Perú, 124 apto. 201, Copacabana	Rio de Janeiro, GB. ZC-07
Benchimol, Raphael	Av. Atlântica, 2016 apto. 701, Copacabana	Rio de Janeiro, GB. ZC-07
Berbary, Carlos Antonio Andrade	Rua Carlos Sampaio, 351 apto. 703, Esplanada do Senado ...	Rio de Janeiro, GB. ZC-86
Berner, Max Herbert	Rua Ribeiro de Almeida, 2 apto. 2, Laranjeiras	Rio de Janeiro, GB. ZC-01
Bessa, Carlos Henrique	Rua Prudente de Morais, 1179 apto. 302, Ipanema	Rio de Janeiro, GB. ZC-95
Bezerra, Francisca das Chagas	Residente do Hospital Estadual Getulio Vargas, Rua Lobo Junior, 2293, Penha Circular .	Rio de Janeiro, GB. ZC-22
Bezerra, Maria Gonçalves ..	Clinica Oftalmológica do Hospital dos Servidores do Estado, Rua Sacadura Cabral, 178, 5° andar, saúde	Rio de Janeiro, GB. ZC-05
Bichara, José	Hospital da Policia Militar, Rua Estácio de Sá, 20, 4° andar, Estácio de Sá	Rio de Janeiro, GB. ZC-10

Binda, Vivaldo .... Rua Pedro Américo, 110 apto.
806, Catete .... Rio de Janeiro, GB. ZC-01

Birenbaum, Salomão ...... Rua Barão de Ubá, 346, Praça da
Bandeira .... Rio de Janeiro, GB. ZC-29

Bittar, Nazir .... Rua Belfort Roxo, 296 apto. 103,
Copacabana .... Rio de Janeiro, GB. ZC-07

Blois, Alahir .... Rua Prof. Arthur Ramos, 132
apto. 202, Leblon .... Rio de Janeiro, GB. ZC-95

Bobadilla, Carlos E. Eslava . Rua Uruguai, 279 apto. 405,
Tijuca .... Rio de Janeiro, GB. ZC-05

Borges, Antonio Fernando
Allemand .... Praça Gal. Portinho, 6 apto. 602,
Maracanã .... Rio de Janeiro, GB. ZC-29

Botelho, Luiz Carlos
Almeida .... Rua Cardeal D. Sebastião Leme.
236 apto. 302, Bairro de
Fátima .... Rio de Janeiro, GB. ZC-45

Botelho, Ya-Ery Guimarães . Rua Filinto Almeida, 45 apto.
301, Cosme Velho .... Rio de Janeiro, GB. ZC-01

Braga, José Garcia .... Hospital Pedro Ernesto-Residente,
Av. 28 de Setembro, 87, Vila
Izabel .... Rio de Janeiro, GB. ZC-11

Branco, Eduardo Moreira .. Rua Senador Vergueiro, 135 apto.
308, Flamengo .... Rio de Janeiro, GB. ZC-01

Brandão, Oto Gil Pires .... Rue José Higino, 37, casa 6, apto,
202, Tijuca .... Rio de Janeiro, GB. ZC-09

Bressan Filho, Antonio .... Rua Bento Lisboa, 184 apto.
1109, Catete .... Rio de Janeiro, GB. ZC-01

Bressan Filho, Augusto .... Rua 2 de Dezembro, 77 apto,
903, Flamengo .... Rio de Janeiro, GB. ZC-01

Brito, Carlos Alberto de
Sousa .... Rua Amaral, 27 apto. 205,
Andaraí .... Rio de Janeiro, GB. ZC-11

Brito, Eduardo Augusto de
Caldas .... Rua Domingos Ferreira, 221 apto.
401, Copacabana .... Rio de Janeiro, GB. ZC-07

Brunstein, Guilherme ..... Rua Barata Ribeiro, 13 apto. 201,
Copacabana .... Rio de Janeiro, GB. ZC-07

Bteshe, Saul ....
Bufolin, Dival .... Rua Visc. da Pirajá, 525 apto.
606, Ipanema .... Rio de Janeiro, GB. ZC-95

Bunges, Bernardo Frederico . Praça Saens Pena, 55 apto. 707,
Tijuca .... Rio de Janeiro, GB. ZC-09

Cabral, Luiz Liberato ..... Rua Mariz e Barros, 39 apto. 909,
Praça da Bandeira .... Rio de Janeiro, GB. ZC-29

Caire, Lincoln .... Rua Dias da Cruz, 59, 4° andar,
Meier .... Rio de Janeiro, GB. ZC-16

Camarota, Virginia Isabel
Soutello .... Rua Constant Ramos, 43 apto.
701, Copacabana .... Rio de Janeiro, GB. ZC-07

Camera, Silvio .... Rua Conselheiro Zenha, 19 apto.
406, Tijuca .... Rio de Janeiro, GB. ZC-09

Campos, Evaldo de Men-
donça .... Rua Maris e Barros, 470 apto.
606, Tijuca .... Rio de Janeiro, GB. ZC-29

Campos, Silvio de	Rua São Clemente, 514 apto. 404, Botafogo	Rio de Janeiro, GB. ZC-02
Campos, Sylvio Leal Costa de	Rua Timoteeo da Costa, 215 apto. 204, Leblon	Rio de Janeiro, GB. ZC-95
Campos, Vera Correia	Rua Uruguai, 57 apto. 602, Tijuca	Rio de Janeiro, GB. ZC-09
Canedo, Pedro Chaves	Rua 5 de Julho, 336 apto. 502, Copacabana	Rio de Janeiro, GB. ZC-07
Cantergiani, Ivo	Rua Barão da Torre, 404 apto. 102, Ipanema	Rio de Janeiro, GB. ZC-95
Capella, Antonio Pires	Av. Braz de Pina, 804 apto. 202, Penha	Rio de Janeiro, GB. ZC-22
Cardoso, Gilza Rosa e Silva .	Rua Visc. de Pirajá, 596 apto. 503, Ipanema	Rio de Janeiro, GB. ZC-95
Cardoso, Mary Margareth Viana	Av. N.S. de Copacabana, 968 apto. 602, Copacabana	Rio de Janeiro, GB. ZC-07
Carmo, Wanderley José Carvaho do	Av. Prado Junior, 281 apto. 1014, Copacabana	Rio de Janeiro, GB. ZC-07
Carpes, Luiz Carlos Fontoura	Clinica Professor José Kos, Rua Moncorvo Filho, 104, Centro	Rio de Janeiro, GB. ZC-14
Carrijo, José Moreira	....	
Carvalho, Aloisio de	Travessa Nestor Victor, 63 apto. 101, Tijuca	Rio de Janeiro, GB. ZC-10
Carvalho, Antonio Batista de	Rua Conde de Bomfim, 500 apto. 702, Tijuca	Rio de Janeiro, GB. ZC-09
Carvalho, Audir Marinho de .	Rua Senador Vergueiro, 45 apto. C-04, Flamengo	Rio de Janeiro, GB. ZC-01
Carvalho, Carlos Fernando de	Rua Paissandú, 191 apto. 505, Flamengo	Rio de Janeiro, GB. ZC-01
Carvalho, José Siqueira de .	Av. N.S. de Copacabana, 1236, 4° andar, Copacabana	Rio de Janeiro, GB. ZC-37
Carvalho, Lery Teixeira de .	Rua Nacional, 131, Jacarepaguá .	Rio de Janeiro, GB. ZC-89
Carvalho, Maria Heloisa Paulo Filho	Rua Mal. Mascarenhas de Moraes, 143 apto. 304, Copacabana ..	Rio de Janeiro, GB. ZC-07
Carvalho, Murilo Fontoura .	Rua Mal. Mascarenhas de Moraes, 143 apto. 304, Copacabana ..	Rio de Janeiro, GB. ZC-07
Carvalho, Nelson Monteiro de	Rua Souza Lima, 366 apto. 10001, Copacabana	Rio de Janeiro, GB.
Carvalho, Nerma Lindgren de	Rua Pereira Nunes, 152 apto. A, Tijuca	Rio de Janeiro, GB. ZC-11
Carvalho, Olavo Souza	....	
Carvalho, Olga Manhães ...	Av. Copacabana, 40 apto. 1101, Copacabana	Rio de Janeiro, GB. ZC-07
Carvalho, Paulo Mauricio Mendes de	Rua dos Artistas, 235 apto. 201, Aldeia Campista	Rio de Janeiro, GB. ZC-11
Carvalho, Vicente Muniz de	Rua Nascimento Silva, 213 apto. 303, Ipanema	Rio de Janeiro, GB. ZC-95

Castro, Milton de .... Av. Copacabana, 95 apto. 401,
Copacabana .... Rio de Janeiro, GB. ZC-07

Castro, Nilo de .... Policlinica Geral, Av. Nilo
Peçanha, 38, 4° andar, Centro Rio de Janeiro, GB. ZC-00

Castro, Werther Leite de ... Rua Barão da Torre, 231, Fundos
apto. 401, Ipanema .... Rio de Janeiro, GB. ZC-37

Catelan, José Hubert ...... Rua Senador Vergueiro, 138 apto.
210, Flamengo .... Rio de Janeiro, GB. ZC-01

Cavalcanti, Dilma Nunes de
Sá .... Rua Lauro Muller, 36 apto.
1101-Botafogo .... Rio de Janeiro, GB. ZC-01

Cavalcanti, Edson Guedes .. Rua Correa Dutra, 119 apto. 808,
Flamengo .... Rio de Janeiro, GB ZC-82

Cavalcante, Gilvanda Maria
Morais .... Rua Vicosa, 32, Penha .... Rio de Janeiro, GB. ZC-01

Cavalcanti, João Celso
Uchoa .... Rua Basileia, 64 apto. 101, Tijuca Rio de Janeiro, GB. ZC-22

Chacur, Salvador .... Av. Epitacio Pessoa, 4000 apto.
602, Lagoa .... Rio de Janeiro, GB. ZC-09

Cyrino, Orlando .... Rua Major Rubens Vaz, 596,
Gávea .... Rio de Janeiro, GB. ZC-20

Coelho, Carlos Alberto .... Rua Projetada 2, 239, Jardim Rio
de 'A'-Campo Grande ...... Rio de Janeiro, GB. ZC-20

Coimbra, Oseas .... Rua M, 3, Campo des Afonsos .. Rio de Janeiro, GB. ZC-26

Cola, Nevio Edenir .... Av. 28 de Setembro, 167 apto.
302, Vila Izabel .... Rio de Janeiro, GB. ZC-27

Colombo, Sergio Cezar .... Rua Pedro Americo, 204 apto. 6,
Catete .... Rio de Janeiro, GB. ZC-11

Contino, Miguel Mattoso .. Rua Domingos Ferreira, 63 apto.
506, Copacabana .... Rio de Janeiro, GB. ZC-01

Corlett, José .... Rua Jundiá, 49, Bento Ribeiro .. Rio de Janeiro, GB. ZC-07

Correia, Carlosalberto ..... Rua Julio de Castilhos, 23 apto.
801, Copacabana .... Rio de Janeiro, GB. ZC-83

Costa, Alvaro .... Rua Debret, 23, 11° andar,
Centro .... Rio de Janeiro, GB. ZC-37

Costa, Cicero Gonçalves ... Rua Teles, 254 apto. 301, Jacarepaguá .... Rio de Janeiro, GB. ZC-00

Costa, Edson Stravalli da .. Rua Candido Benicio, 2151 apto.
404, Jacarepaguá .... Rio de Janeiro, GB. ZC-89

Costa, Fernando Otavio da . Rua Dez. Isidro, 126 BL. B. apto.
302, Tijuca .... Rio de Janeiro, GB. ZC-89

Costa, José Augusto Medei-
ros Ferro .... Rua das Laranjeiras, 40 apto. 501,
Laranjeiras .... Rio de Janeiro, GB. ZC-09

Costa, José Herculano ..... Rua Miguel Lemos, 51 apto. 603,
Copacabana ....

Costa, Theophilo Machado
de Araujo .... Rua Figueiredo Magalhães, 263
apto. 904, Copacabana ..... Rio de Janeiro, GB. ZC-07

Costa, Wilton .... Rua Senador Vergueiro, 146 apto.
403, Botafogo .... Rio de Janeiro, GB. ZC-07

Costa Filho, Adroaldo de
Alencar .... Rua Anita Garibaldi, 43 apto.
801, Copacabana .... Rio de Janeiro, GB. ZC-01

Costa Filho, Maximiliano .. Rua do Matoso, 182 apto. 305,
Praça da Bandeira .... Rio de Janeiro, GB. ZC-07

Rio de Janeiro, GB. ZC-10

Coutinho, Fernando Dantas .	Rua Felisberto de Menezes, 31 apto. 803, Tijuca	Rio de Janeiro, GB. ZC-29
Couto, Sueli	Rua Afonso Pena, 66 apto. 1209, Tijuca	Rio de Janeiro, GB. ZC-10
Cruz, Isaac Gonzalez	Rua São Roberto, 64 apto. 301, Estácio de Sá	Rio de Janeiro, GB. ZC-10
Cukierman, Jaques	Rua Barão de Mesquita, 186 apto. 402, Andaraí	Rio de Janeiro, GB. ZC-11
Cukierman, Samuel	Rua Barão de Itambi, 14 apto. 601, Botafogo	Rio de Janeiro, GB. ZC-01
Cunha, Deodal da Conceição Diniz	Rua Lauro Muller, 46 apto. 608, Botafogo	Rio de Janeiro, GB. ZC-82
Cunha, Elvira Thompson da .	Rua Joaquim Nabuco, 98 apto. 102, Copacabana	Rio de Janeiro, GB. ZC-37
Cunha, Henrique de Brito e .	Rua Figueiredo Magalhães, 421 apto. 902, Copacabana	Rio de Janeiro, GB. ZC-07
Cunha, Mario Bomfim Pereira da	Rua Teixeira de Melo, 43 apto. 302, Ipanema	Rio de Janeiro, GB. ZC-95
Cunha, Nelson José	Santa Casa de Misericordia, 1ª enfermaria, Rua Santa Luzia, 206, Centro	Rio de Janeiro, GB. ZC-39
Cunha, Sergio Franklin de Souza	Rua Cruz e Souza, 112 apto. 301, Frente, Encantado	Rio de Janeiro, GB. ZC-38
Cunha, Tania Mara	Rua Toneleros, 366 apto. 902, Copacabana	Rio de Janeiro, GB. ZC-07
Dalfre, José Luiz	Rua Carius, 431 apto. 201, Campo Grande	Rio de Janeiro, GB. ZC-26
Dantas, Francisco Apocalypse	Rua Lucilia, 126, Campo Grande .	Rio de Janeiro, GB. ZC-26
Deboni, José Apparecido . .	Rua Inhanga, 30 apto. 301, Copacabana	Rio de Janeiro, GB. ZC-07
Delgado, Eliane Gomes	Rua Siqueira Campos, 16 apto. 604, Copacabana	Rio de Janeiro, GB. ZC-07
Di Ciero, Constantino	Rua das Laranjeiras, 243 apto. 602, Laranjeiras	Rio de Janeiro, GB. ZC-01
Di Piero, Maria Lucia Paulo Filho	Av. N.S. de Fátima, 63, Bairro de Fátima	Rio de Janeiro. GB. ZC-86
Dias Filho, Alexandre	Rua Conselheiro Lampreia, 374, Cosme Velho	Rio de Janeiro, GB. ZC-01
Dias, Arthur Borges	Rua Dias da Rocha, 39 apto. 102, Copacabana	Rio de Janeiro. GB. ZC-07
Dias, Flavio Rezende	Praça Cruz Vermelha, 12, Terreo, Cruz Vermelha	Rio de Janeiro. GB. ZC-86
Dias, Moacyr Fernandes . . .	Rua Francisco Eugenio, 176, B.C. 8, São Cristovão	Rio de Janeiro, GB. ZC-08
Diniz, Aluizio Antonio Balieiro	Rua Gilberto Cardoso, 300 apto. 803, Leblon	Rio de Janeiro, GB. ZC-95
Donato, Salvatore	Rua Senador Nabuco, 354, Vila Izabel	Rio de Janeiro, GB. ZC-11
Dresch, Milton	Oculistas Associados Praça Cruz Vermelha, 12, Terreo, Centro .	Rio de Janeiro, GB. ZC-86

Duarte, José Bento ....   Rua Min. Alfredo Valadão, 77 apto. 1004, Copacabana ....   Rio de Janeiro, GB. ZC-07

Duarte, Waldemiro Gonçalves ....   Rua Sen. Vergueiro, 107 apto. 701, Flamengo ....   Rio de Janeiro, GB. ZC-01

Duran, Jaime Pericas ......   Rua Buenos Aires, 220, Sobr., Centro ....   Rio de Janeiro, GB. ZC-00

Encina, Roque Antonio Meilicke ....   Hospital do IASEG, Oftalmologia, Av. Henrique Valadares, 141, Esplanada do Senado .... · Rio de Janeiro, GB. ZC-86

Ernesto, Luiz Herculano Pinto ....   Rua Silva Rabello, 40, 2° andar, Meier ....   Rio de Janeiro, GB. ZC-16

Estrada, Werther Duque ...   Praça Cardeal Arcoverde, 25, 2° andar, Copacabana ....   Rio de Janeiro, GB. ZC-07

Fabiano, Paulo Cesar Franco   Av. Prado Junior, 281, apto. 1014, Copacabana ....   Rio de Janeiro, GB. ZC-07

Falcão, Angélica Maria Pitta .   Clinica Oftalmológica do Hospital São Francisco de Assis, Av. Presidente Vargas, 2863, Centro ....   Rio de Janeiro, GB. ZC-14

Faria, Emanuel de ....   Rua Ferreira Vianna, 56 apto. 702, Flamengo ....   Rio de Janeiro, GB. ZC-01

Faria, Jeãe Luiz Bassan ....

Farias, Antonio Afonso Reis ....   Rua Senador Vergueiro, 114 apto. 701, Flamengo ....   Rio de Janeiro, GB. ZC-01

Farias, Sergio Lopes de ....   Rua Barão do Flamengo, 28 apto. 902, Flamengo ....   Rio de Janeiro, GB, ZC-01

Fatorelli, Afonso ....   Rua Abelardo de Barros, 21 apto. 201, Tijuca ....   Rio de Janeiro, GB. ZC-01

Favarato, Hernandez ......   Rua Sá Ferreira, 138 apto. 1003, Copacabana ....   Rio de Janeiro, GB. ZC-37

Favaron, José ....   Rua dos Araujos, 11-A BL. 3 apto. 401, Tijuca ....   Rio de Janeiro, GB. ZC-09

Feijó, Ney ....   Rua Ramon Franco, 108 apto. 201, Urca ....   Rio de Janeiro, GB. ZC-82

Fernandes, Ignez Zita Q. de A. ....   Rua Alm. Guilhem, 234 apto. 302, Leblon ....   Rio de Janeiro, GB. ZC-95

Fernandes, João Alberto da Silva ....   Rua Almirante Guinle, 234 apto. 302, Leblon ....   Rio de Janeiro, GB. ZC-95

Fernandes, Ruy Costa .....   Rua Carlos de Goes, 469 apto. 301, Leblon ....   Rio de Janeiro, GB. ZC-95

Fernandes, Sergio Pinho Costa ....   Rua Carlos de Goes, 469 apto. 301, Leblon ....   Rio de Janeiro, GB. ZC-95

Ferrari, Geraldo Magela Gomes ....   Rua Voluntários da Pátria, 187 apto. 306, Botafogo ....

Ferrari, Guido ....   Rua Humberto de Campos, 635 apto. 402, Leblon ....   Rio de Janeiro, GB. ZC-95

Ferraro, Humberto Ramos .   Rua José Higino, 332 apto. 201, Tijuca ....   Rio de Janeiro, GB. ZC-09

Ferreira, Botelho ....   Rua Hilário de Gouveia, 88 apto. 402, Copacabana ....   Rio de Janeiro, GB. ZC-07

Ferreira, Carlos Alberto ...	Rua Conrado Niemeyer, 28 apto. 302, Copacabana	Rio de Janeiro, GB. ZC-07
Ferreira, Gerson de Paiva ..	Rua São Paulo, 37, Sampaic	Rio de Janeiro, GB. ZC-15
Ferreira, Gregorio P. Gimenez	Av. Henrique Valadares, 141, Esplanada do Senado	Rio de Janeiro, GB. ZC-86
Ferreira, José Alves	Av. Rio Branco, 185, 14° andar, Centro	Rio de Janeiro, GB. ZC-21
Ferreira, Luiz Eurico	Av. N.S. Copacabana, 1052, 4° andar, Copacabana	Rio de Janeiro, GB. ZC-07
Ferreira, Marcello Martins ..	Av. Copacabana, 3700 apto. 301, Copacabana	Rio de Janeiro, GB. ZC-37
Ferreira, Oziel Marques	Av. Prado Junior, 335 apto. 1011, Copacabana	Rio de Janeiro, GB. ZC-07
Ferreira, Ronald	Rua Zizi, 4, Lins de Vasconcelos .	Rio de Janeiro, GB. ZC-16
Ferreira, Tulio Hostilio Correia	Rua Ministro Alfredo Valadão, 35 apto. C-06, Copacabana	Rio de Janeiro, GB. ZC-07
Ferreira Filho, Oswaldo Odilon	Rua Paula Freitas, 62 C-5 apto. 1, Copacabana	Rio de Janeiro, GB. ZC-07
Fialho, Luiz Alfredo Abreu	Rua Fernando Ferrari, 61 apto. 611, Botafogo	Rio de Janeiro, GB. ZC-01
Fialho, Sylvio de Abreu ...	Av. Atlântica, 3892, 1° andar, Copacabana	Rio de Janeiro, GB. ZC-37
Fialho, Tito de Abreu	Rua Izidro de Figueiredo, 30 apto. 201, Maracanã	Rio de Janeiro, GB. ZC-11
Fidelman, Salomãe	Rua Gago Coutinho, 62 apto. 701, Laranjeiras	Rio de Janeiro, GB. ZC-01
Figueira, Alvaro	Rua Sãe José, 90, 10° andar, Centro	Rio de Janeiro, GB. ZC-00
Figueiredo, Juarez Correia de	Rua Santa Luzia, 173 apto. 101, Maracanã	Rio de Janeiro, GB. ZC-11
Figueiredo, Nicanor Prezidio de	Rua Uruguaiana, 55 sala 721, Centro	Rio de Janeiro, GB. ZC-21
Filippo, Nicola de	Rua Carlos Sampaio, 351 apto. 703, Esplanada do Senado ...	Rio de Janeiro, GB. ZC-86
Finkel, Edith	Rua Toneleros, 203 apto. 1001, Copacabana	Rio de Janeiro, GB. ZC-07
Fonseca Neto, Mancel Bernardes da	Praia de Botafogo, 340 apto. 1021, Botafogo	Rio de Janeiro, GB. ZC-02
Fontes, Paulo Cesar Silva ..	Rua Visc. de Santa Izabel, 162 apto. C = 02, Vila Izabel	Rio de Janeiro, GB. ZC-11
Freire, João Baptista de ... Macedo	Rua Muniz Barreto, 93, Botafogo	Rio de Janeiro, GB. ZC-02
Freire, José de Mello Carvalho Moniz	Rua Prof. Quintino Vale, 78 apto. 102, Estácio de Sá	Rio de Janeiro, GB. ZC-10
Freire, José Sergio Cunha ..	Rua Santa Cristina, 29 apto. 204, Santa Tereza	Rio de Janeiro, GB. ZC-45
Freire, Mario Aparecido ...	Rua Gustavo Augusto de Rezende, 250 Quadra 'E' BL. 28 apto 101, Ilha de Governador	Rio de Janeiro, GB. ZC-32
Freitas, Francisco	Rua Carlos de Vasconcelos, 142 apto. 706, Tijuca	Rio de Janeiro, GB. ZC-09

Freitas, Paulo Vasques de ..	Rua Teixeira de Melo, 10 apto. 201, Ipanema	Rio de Janeiro, GB. ZC-95
Frota, Lauro	Rua Senador Vergueiro, 207 apto. 1109, Flamengo	Rio de Janeiro, GB. ZC-01
Furtado, Heitor Baptista ...	Rua Firmino da Silva, 41, Jacare-paguá	Rio de Janeiro, GB. ZC-89
Gagno, Fortunato	Clinica Oftalmologica do Hospital N.S. das Dores, Santa Casa, Av. Ernani Cardoso, 21, Casca-dura	Rio de Janeiro, GB. ZC-12
Gallo, Teresinha do Nasci-mento	Rua Buarque de Macedo, 37 apto. 604, Catete	Rio de Janeiro, GB. ZC-01
Galvão, Neurisvan Pereira ..	Av. Franklin Roosevelt, 84 apto. 604, Centro	Rio de Janeiro, GB. ZC-39
Garrido, Alina Fernandez ..	Rue Souza Franco, 245 casa 2, Vila Izabel	Rio de Janeiro, GB. ZC-11
Gazaneo, Francisco	Rua Aquidaban, 805 c-61 apto. 301, Lins	Rio de Janeiro, GB. ZC-16
Giardulli, Antonio	Praça Almirante Jaceguai, 61 apto. 201, Bairro de Fátima	Rio de Janeiro, GB. ZC-86
Gloria Filho, Elmo	Rua Barão da Torre, 42 apto. 901, Ipanema	Rio de Janeiro, GB. ZC-95
Godoy, Renato Coelho de .	Rua Grajaú, 206 apto. 105, Grajaú	Rio de Janeiro, GB. ZC-11
Gomes, Cesar Ronaldo Vieira	Av. Prado Junior, 308 apto. 404, Copacabana	Rio de Janeiro, GB. ZC-07
Gomes, José Candido Fiuza .	Rua Voluntários da Pátria, 330 apto. 201, Botafogo	Rio de Janeiro, GB. ZC-02
Gomes, Maristela Lobão ...	Rua Maestro Vila Lobos, 1 apto. 606, Tijuca	Rio de Janeiro. GB. ZC-10
Gomes, Samuel Bolshaw ...	Rua Sá Ferreira, 166 apto. 101, Copacabana	Rio de Janeiro, GB. ZC-07
Gonçalves, Carlos Américo de Paiva	Rua Oton Bezerra de Melo, 109, Gávea	Rio de Janeiro, GB. ZC-20
Gonçalves, Carlos de Paiva .	Rua Mário de Andrade, 44, Bota-fogo	Rio de Janeiro, GB. ZC-02
Gonçalves, José Edmar	Rua Senador Correia, 44 apto. 204, Laranjeiras	Rio de Janeiro, GB. ZC-01
Gonçalves, Luciano	Rua Paissandú, 385 apto. 301, Flamengo	Rio de Janeiro, GB. ZC-01
Gonçalves, Marcelo	Rua São José, 90 sala 1201, Cen-tro	Rio de Janeiro, GB. ZC-00
Gonçalves, Orlando	Rua Fernando Mendes, 28 apto. 708, Copacabana	Rio de Janeiro, GB. ZC-07
Gonzaga, Renato	Rua Figueiredo Magalhães, 219 apto. 603, Copacabana	Rio de Janeiro, GB. ZC-07
Gonzales, Justo Adolfo	Clinica Oftalmológica do Hospital Miguel Couto, Rua Mario Ribeiro, Gávea	Rio de Janeiro, GB. ZC-20
Gosling, Fernando José Bas-baum	Rua Garcia D'Avila, 34 apto. 201, Ipanema	Rio de Janeiro, GB. ZC-95

Gottsmann, Ricardo Wolfgang	Rua Santo Amaro, 33 apto. 605, Glória	Rio de Janeiro, GB. ZC-01
Goulart, Claudio	Oculistas Associados, Praça Cruz Vermelha, 12, Terreo, Centro	Rio de Janeiro, GB. ZC-86
Goulart, José Ronald Andrade	Rua Maestro Francisco Braga, 502 apto. 204, Copacabana	Rio de Janeiro, GB. ZC-07
Gouveia, Anibal	Rua Buenos Aites, 104, 6 andar, Centro	Rio de Janeiro, GB. ZC-00
Gracindo Neto, Ignacio Brandão	Rua Meira de Vasconcelos, 149, Andaraí	Rio de Janeiro, GB. ZC-11
Graziano, Socio	Rua Sacadura Cabral, 117 apto. 1208, Saúde	Rio de Janeiro, GB. ZC-05
Gryner, David	Av. N.S. de Copacabana, 912 apto. 901, Copacabana	Rio de Janeiro, GB. ZC-07
Guaranha, Claudio Odone		
Guimarães, Ildefonso	Rua Ribeiro Guimarães, 150 apto. 1002, Aldeia Campista	Rio de Janeiro, GB. ZC-11
Guimarães, Juvenil	Rua da Conceição, 31, 5° andar, Centro	Rio de Janeiro, GB. ZC-21
Guimarães, Roberto Franklin Lemos	Av. Atlântica, 752 apto. 1202, Copacabana	Rio de Janeiro, GB. ZC-07
Guimarães, Remeu Francisco Junqueira	Rua Moncorvo Filho, 95 apto. 501, Centro	Rio de Janeiro, GB. ZC-14
Guaraná, Fernando	Rua Jardim Botanico, 211, Jardim Botanico	Rio de Janeiro, GB. ZC-20
Guedes, Armando Augusto	Rua Farani, 60 apto. 108, Botafogo	Rio de Janeiro, GB. ZC-02
Guilliod, Carlos Renee	Rua Joaquim Palhares, 608 apto. 1003, Estácio de Sá	Rio de Janeiro, GB. ZC-29
Haberlehner, Carmen Maciel	Rua Prof. Luiz Catanhede, 62 ap. s. 103, Laranjeiras	Rio de Janeiro, GB. ZC-01
Higa, Vilian Hiroyuki	Trav. Protogenes Guimarães, 60 apto. 302, Catete	Rio de Janeiro, GB. ZC-01
Kac, Sansãe Isaac	Rua Marques de Abrantes, 158 apto. 302, Botafogo	Rio de Janeiro, GB. ZC-01
Kassab, Carlos Mauricio	Rua dos Oitis, 65, Gávea	Rio de Janeiro, GB. ZC-20
Kassuga, Rubens Hasegawa	Av. N.S. Copacabana, 1052, 4° andar, Copacabana	Rio de Janeiro, GB. ZC-07
Kiralyhegy, Jorge	Rua Gustavo Sampaio, 460 apto. 902, Leme	Rio de Janeiro, GB. ZC-07
Kirjner, Moacyr	Rua Duvivier, 86 apto. 502, Copacabana	Rio de Janeiro, GB. ZC-07
Kischinevsky, Adolfo	Rua General San Martin, 900 apto. 701, Leblon	Rio de Janeiro, GB. ZC-95
Kleinberg, Celso	Av. Pasteur, 196 apto. 1002, Botafogo	Rio de Janeiro, GB. ZC-82
Lacerda, Savas	Rua dos Romeiros, 211, Penha	Rio de Janeiro, GB. ZC-22
Langone, Antonio Carlos	Rua Carolina Santos, 33, Lins	Rio de Janeiro, GB. ZC-16
Lanna, Nilton		
Lanna, Oscarina de Oliveira		
Laurini, Valny Antonio	Rua Turf Club, 12 apto. 705, Maracanã	Rio de Janeiro, GB. ZC-11

Lavos, Raul Rodrigues .... Rua Pinheiro Machado, 181 apto.
705, Laranjeiras .... Rio de Janeiro, GB. ZC-01
Leal, Ana Carmen de Rosa . Rua Hilário de Gouvea, 88 apto.
502, Copacabana .... Rio de Janeiro, GB. ZC-07
Leal, Ede .... Rua Buarque de Macedo, 31 apto.
201, Flamengo .... Rio de Janeiro, GB. ZC-01
Leal, Margareth Emilia Leal . Rua Djalma Ulrich, 183 apto.
605, Copacabana .... Rio de Janeiro, GB. ZC-07
Leão, João Baptista Furtado Rua Antonio Basili, 483 apto.
701, Tijuca .... Rio de Janeiro, GB. ZC-09
Leite Filho, Luiz Augusto
Morizot .... Rua Prudente de Moraes, 564
apto. 103, Ipanema .... Rio de Janeiro, GB. ZC-37
Leite Filho, Solidonio ..... Rua Lobo Junior, 2293, Penha .. Rio de Janeiro, GB. ZC-22
Lemos, Alfredo Heliton de . Rua Uruguai, 57 apto. 104, Tijuca Rio de Janeiro, GB. ZC-09
Lemos Filho, Jair .... Av. Copacabana, 249 apto. 503,
Copacabana .... Rio de Janeiro, GB. ZC-07
Lessa, Maria de Lourdes Mar-
tins .... Rua Uruguai, 380 apto. 803,
Bloco A, Tijuca .... Rio de Janeiro, GB. ZC-09
Lima, Adelaide de Lucena
Lima .... Rua Alvaro Chaves, 28 apto. 603,
Laranjeiras .... Rio de Janeiro, GB. ZC-01
Lima, Arlindo Marques .... Rua São Francisco Xavier, 392
apto. 602, Tijuca .... Rio de Janeiro, GB. ZC-11
Lima, Fontes .... Av. Osvaldo Cruz, 108 apto. 301,
Flamengo .... Rio de Janeiro, GB. ZC-01
Lima, Gelson de Souza .... Rua Gustavo Sampaio, 520 apto.
204, Leme .... Rio de Janeiro, GB. ZC-07
Lima, Gerson de Abreu e .. Rua Amoroso Costa, 273, Tijuca . Rio de Janeiro, GB. ZC-09
Lima, José Victorino de
Araujo .... Av. Copacabana, 1018 apto. 504,
Copacabana .... Rio de Janeiro, GB. ZC-07
Lima, Murilo Valeriano de . Rua Mal. Mascarenhas de Moraes,
129 apto. 501, Copacabana .. Rio de Janeiro, GB. ZC-07
Lima, Raul dos Santos .... Praça Serzedelo Correia, 15, sala
806, Copacabana .... Rio de Janeiro, GB. ZC-07
Lins, Camilo Moraes de A. . Rua Decio Vilares, 169 apto. 201,
Copacabana .... Rio de Janeiro, GB. ZC-07
Lobato, Luiz Carlos Doura-
do .... Rua Francisco Manoel, 61, Ben-
fica .... Rio de Janeiro, GB. ZC-08
Lobo, Roberto de Castro ..
Lopes, Érico Augusto ..... Rua Sá Viana, 20-A C. 3, Grajaú . Rio de Janeiro, GB. ZC-11
Lopes, José Roberto Negri . Rua Barata Ribeiro, 628 apto.
901, Copacabana .... Rio de Janeiro, GB. ZC-07
Lourenço, Vera Lucia ..... Rua Dr. Padilha, 520 apto. 204,
Engenho de Dentro .... Rio de Janeiro, GB. ZC-13
Louzada, Joaquim .... Rua Soares Cabral, 71 apto. 202,
Laranjeiras .... Rio de Janeiro, GB. ZC-01
Louzada, Nelson Terra .... Rua Prof. Ortiz Monteiro, 36
apto. 104, Laranjeiras ...... Rio de Janeiro, GB. ZC-01
Luiz, João Carlos ....
Luna Neto, Alfredo Mauricio
de .... Av. Paulo de Frontim, 751 apto.
501, Rio Comprido .... Rio de Janeiro, GB. ZC-10

Lustosa, Tales Cardoso	Av. Osvaldo Cruz, 96 apto. 905, Flamengo	Rio de Janeiro, GB. ZC-01
Luz, Gualton Garcez da ...	Rua Bolivar, 125 apto. 301, Copacabana	Rio de Janeiro, GB. ZC-07
Lyra, João Carlos Fernandes de Gusmão	Av. Epitacio Pessoa, 2566 apto. 401, Leblon	Rio de Janeiro, GB. ZC-95
Macedo, Francisco Willys ..	Praia de Botafogo, 360 apto. 806, Botafogo	Rio de Janeiro, GB. ZC-02
Machado, Estevão Pedro Pessanha	Rua Ferdinando Laboriau, 175, Tijuca	Rio de Janeiro, GB. ZC-09
Machado, Lais Delduque Vieira	Travessa José Higino, 150, Tijuca.	Rio de Janeiro, GB. ZC-09
Maciel, Tania Maria Guitton.	Rua Souza Franco, 245 casa 2, Vila Izabel	Rio de Janeiro, GB. ZC-11
Magalhães, Aloisio de Almeida	Rua Laranjeiras, 430 apto. 406, Laranjeiras	Rio de Janeiro, GB. ZC-01
Magalhães, Antonio Ediberto	Policlinica de Botafogo, Av. Pasteur, 72, Botafogo	Rio de Janeiro, GB. ZC-82
Magalhães, Jorcenio de Alencar	Rua Andrade Neves, 256-F-apto. 301, Tijuca	Rio de Janeiro, GB. ZC-09
Magalhães, Pedro de Almeida	Rua Visconde de Silva, 43, Botafogo	Rio de Janeiro, GB. ZC-02
Maia, Hugo Ribeiro Soares .	Av. Julio Furtado, 236 apto. 203, Grajaú	Rio de Janeiro, GB. ZC-11
Maior, Luiz Alberto Souto .	Rua Padre Francisco Lana, 136 apto. 104, Vila Izabel	Rio de Janeiro, GB. ZC-11
Malta, Luiz Fernando Pimentel	Av. Epitacio Pessoa, 2180 apto. 101, Ipanema	Rio de Janeiro, GB. ZC-37
Maranhão Neto, Manoel A. de Albuquerque	Rua Prof. Gastão Bahiana, 111 apto. 201, Copacabana	Rio de Janeiro, GB. ZC-07
Marcon, Gladis Marchiori ..	Rua Constant Ramos, 162 apto. 702, Copacabana	Rio de Janeiro, GB. ZC-07
Marcovecchio, José	Rua General Severiano, 40 apto. 722, Botafogo	Rio de Janeiro, GB. ZC-82
Marques, Zuleika Dias	Rua Mal. Bitencourt, 215, Riachuelo	Rio de Janeiro, GB. ZC-15
Martinez, Oilides Conte ...	Rua Senador Vergueiro, 219 apto. 1106, Flamengo	Rio de Janeiro, GB. ZC-01
Martins, Oswaldo	Rua Dr. Miguel Vieira Ferreira, 141, apto. C. 02, Ramos	Rio de Janeiro, GB. ZC-24
Mattos, Maria Amelia Costa Mello	Hospital Pedro Ernesto, Oftalmologia Av. 28 de Setembro, 87, 4° andar, Vila Izabel	Rio de Janeiro, GB. ZC-11
Mauro, Antonio	Rua Dona Cecilia, 27, Rio Comprido	Rio de Janeiro, GB. ZC-10
Mazza, Aroldo Lobo	Rua Figueiredo Magalhães, 808 apto. 101, Copacabana	Rio de Janeiro, GB. ZC-07
Medeiros, Aracilda	Rua Gal. Ribeiro da Costa, 56 apto. 403, Leme	Rio de Janeiro, GB. ZC-07

Medeiros, Luiz Augusto de . Av. Rio Branco, 135 sala 1004, Centro .... Rio de Janeiro, GB. ZC-21

Medeiros, Maria Edilce Teixeira .... Rua Carolina Santos, 95 apto. 208, Meier .... Rio de Janeiro, GB. ZC-16

Medeiros, Roberto Barbosa de .... Rua Timoteo da Costa, 297 apto. 1601, Leblon .... Rio de Janeiro, GB. ZC-95

Medina, Darcy de Souza ... Rua Bom Pastor, 541, Tijuca ... Rio de Janeiro, GB. ZC-09

Meireles, Renato Dantas ... Rua Humaitá, 261 apto. 403, Humaitá .... Rio de Janeiro, GB. ZC-02

Mello, Ajhax Medeiros de .. Rua Saravatá, 35 apto. 403, Mal. Hermes .... Rio de Janeiro, GB. ZC-27

Mello, Paulo Augusto de A. . Rua José Linhares, 111 apto. 301, Leblon .... Rio de Janeiro, GB. ZC-95

Mello Junior, José Maria de . Rua Santa Clara, 161 apto. 804, Copacabana .... Rio de Janeiro, GB. ZC-07

Melman, José .... Rua Aristides Spinola, 49 apto. 304, Leblon .... Rio de Janeiro, GB. ZC-95

Melo, Guilherme Tavares da Cunha .... Estrada do Capão, 71, Jacarepaguá .... Rio de Janeiro, GB. ZC-89

Melo, José Luiz Bandeira de . Rua São Salvador, 59 apto. 206, Laranjeiras .... Rio de Janeiro, GB. ZC-01

Melo Filho, Agenor .... Hotel Barão de Tefe, Av. Barão de Tefé, 99, Saúde .... Rio de Janeiro, GB. ZC-05

Mendes, Murilo de Souza .. Av. João Ribeiro, 5, Sobrado, Pilares .... Rio de Janeiro, GB. ZV-13

Mendes, Roberto Bastos ... .

Mendes, Wilton Medeiros .. Rua Lisboa, 62, Circular da Penha Rio de Janeiro, GB. ZC-22

Mercante, Alberto S. ...... Rua Haddock Lobo, 191 apto. 801, Tijuca .... Rio de Janeiro, GB. ZC-10

Mernes, Ruben Ramon Balbuena .... Rua Conde de Bomfin, 369 apto. 811, Tijuca .... Rio de Janeiro, GB. ZC-09

Milsztajn, Jaime .... Rua Domingos Ferreira, 149 apto. 403, Copacabana .... Rio de Janeiro, GB. ZC-07

Miranda, Lincoln Gutemberg de .... Rua Montenegro, 64 apto. 203, Ipanema .... Rio de Janeiro, GB. ZC-95

Miranda, Mauro dos Santos . Av. Copacabana, 1032 apto. 906, Copacabana .... Rio de Janeiro, GB. ZC-07

Monteiro, Adelino Joaquim Coelho .... Rua Mambarés, 247, Mal. Hermes Rio de Janeiro, GB. ZC-27

Monteiro, Antonio Rezende de Castro .... Rua Santa Clara, 289 apto. 504, Copacabana .... Rio de Janeiro, GB. ZC-07

Monteiro, Carlos Alberto de Almeida .... Rua Prof. Estelita Lins, 148 apto. 305, Laranjeiras .... Rio de Janeiro, GB. ZC-01

Monteiro, Fernando ...... Rua Souza Lima, 366 apto. 1001, Copacabana .... Rio de Janeiro, GB. ZC-37

Monteiro, Paulo .... Rua Anita Garibaldi, 60 apto. 213, Copacabana .... Rio de Janeiro, GB. ZC-07

Montenegro, Janete Machado Alves .... Rua Voluntários da Pátria, 88 apto. 303, Botafogo .... Rio de Janeiro, GB. ZC-02

Moraes, Alcides Viana de ..	Av. Prado Junior, 308 apto. 404, Copacabana	Rio de Janeiro, GB. ZC-07
Moraes, Cezano Rosa	Rua Buarque de Macedo, 25 apto. 701, Catete	Rio de Janeiro, GB. ZC-01
Moreira, Fernando de Almeida	Praça Cruz Vermelha, 12, Terreo, Centro	Rio de Janeiro. GB. ZC-86
Mororo, Sonia Regina	Rua da Patria, 510 apto. 202, Agua Santa	Rio de Janeiro, GB. ZC-13
Motta, Geraldo	Av. Afranio de Melo Franco, 265 apto. 603, Leblon	Rio de Janeiro, GB. ZC-95
Muniz, Eldo	Rua Soares Meireles, 367 apto. 201, Pilares	Rio de Janeiro, GB. ZC-13
Murillo, Wilde Arze	Rua Dias da Rocha, 39 apto. 301, Copacabana	Rio de Janeiro, GB. ZC-07
Nadaf, Salim Moises	Rua 2 de Dezembro, 62 apto. 503, Flamengo	Rio de Janeiro, GB. ZC-01
Nadalini, Walter Roberto ..	Praça Serzedelo Correia, 15 sala 806, Copacabana	Rio de Janeiro, GB. ZC-07
Nakamura, Paulo Fukuji ...	Rua Eng. Gama Lobo, 114, Vila Izabel	Rio de Janeiro, GB. ZC-01
Nakase, Yoshikazu	Rua Carlos Sampaio, 351 apto. 703, Espl. do Senado	Rio de Janeiro, GB. ZC-86
Nascimento, Liane	Praça Cruz Vermelha, 12, Terreo, Centro	Rio de Janeiro, GB. ZC-86
Neurauter, Romano	Rua Buarque de Macedo, 32 apto. 603, Flamengo	Rio de Janeiro, GB. ZC-01
Neves Junior, José de Souza.	Av. Bartolomeu Mitre, 340 apto. 301, Leblon	Rio de Janeiro, GB. ZC-95
Noronha, Mario Jorge Rosa de	Praia do Flamengo, 82 apto. 502, Flamengo	Rio de Janeiro, GB. ZC-01
Nougue, Luiz	Rua Evaristo da Veiga, 49 apto. 401, Centro	Rio de Janeiro, GB. ZC-06
Novais, José Luiz	Rue Debret, 23, 2° andar, Centro	Rio de Janeiro, GB. ZC-00
Nunes, Carlos Lopes	Rua Itabaiana, 263 apto. 201, Grajaú	Rio de Janeiro, GB. ZC-11
Obrzut, Krystina Helena Hillekes	Rua Barão da Torre, 259 apto. C-01, Ipanema	Rio de Janeiro, GB. ZC-95
Oliveira, Donato de	Rua Teodur Herzl, 56 apto. 104, Botafogo	Rio de Janeiro, GB. ZC-02
Oliveira, Elisabeth Araujo Jorge Marques de	Rua Domingos Ferreira, 236 apto. 703, Copacabana	Rio de Janeiro, GB. ZC-07
Oliveira, Fernando de	Rua Buenos Aires, 180 S/10ja, Centro	Rio de Janeiro, GB. ZC-00
Oliveira, Jorge Alberto Soares de	Rua Visc. de Santa Cruz, 243 casa 1, Engenho Novo	Rio de Janeiro, GB. ZC-15
Oliveira, Oswaldo Barbosa de	Rua Prof. Gabizo, 281 apto. 301, Tijuca	Rio de Janeiro, GB, ZC-29
Oliveira, Paulo Antonio de .	Av. Suburbana, 10.136 apto. 202, Cascadura	Rio de Janeiro, GB. ZC-12
Pacheco, J. Regis	Av. Rainha Elizabeth, 234 apto. 402, Copacabana	Rio de Janeiro, GB. ZC-37

Paes, Dirceu .... Rua Candido Mendes, 263 apto.
203, Glória .... Rio de Janeiro, GB. ZC-06
Pais, Columbino de Moraes
Teixeira .... Rua Otavio Correia, 53, Urca ... Rio de Janeiro, GB. ZC-83
Paiva, Marcos dos Santos .. Rua Arthur Menezes, 16 apto.
102, Maracanã .... Rio de Janeiro, GB. ZC-11
Paixão, Marcus Antonio No-
gueira .... Rua Bento Lisboa, 24 apto. 903,
Catete .... Rio de Janeiro, GB. ZC-01
Pantaleão, Eduardo Pinto .. Rua Barata Ribeiro, 208 apto.
801, Copacabana .... Rio de Janeiro, GB. ZC-07
Paula, Roberto Dias de .... Rua Aiaca, 184, Vila Mariopolis,
Anchieta .... Rio de Janeiro, GB. ZC-27
Paulo Filho, Antonio ..... Av. N.S. de Fátima, 63, Bairro de
Fátima .... Rio de Janeiro, GB. ZC-86
Paulo Filho, Rubem Dolanda Av. N.S. de Fátima, 63, Bairro de
Fátima .... Rio de Janeiro, GB. ZC-86
Paz Filho, Antonio Fernan-
des da .... Rua Hadock Lobo, 401 apto.
601, Tijuca .... Rio de Janeiro, GB. ZC-10
Pecego, José Guilherme de
Carvalho .... Rua Barão da Torre, 277 apto.
401, Ipanema ....
Pecora, Nicola .... Rua Santa Clara, 161 apto. 201,
Copacabana .... Rio de Janeiro, GB. ZC-07
Pegado, Luiz Carlos da Silva . Av. N.S. de Copacabana, 862
apto. 501, Copacabana ..... Rio de Janeiro, GB. ZC-07
Pegado, Paulo Cesar de Bar-
ros .... Rua Dr. Nicanor, 165, Inhauma . Rio de Janeiro, GB. ZC-13
Peixoto, Maria Margarida .. Rua General Severiano, 70,
Botafogo .... Rio de Janeiro, GB. ZC-82
Peliks, Simon .... Av. Vis. de Albuquerque, 15 apto.
C-01, Leblon .... Rio de Janeiro, GB. ZC-95
Pereira, Celio de Castro .... Rua São Luiz Gonzaga, 730 sobr.,
São Cristovão .... Rio de Janeiro, GB. ZC-08
Pereira, Celso Marra ...... Av. Paulo e Sousa, 194 apto. 202,
Maracanã .... Rio de Janeiro, GB. ZC-11
Pereira, Isidorio Romão ... Caixa Postal 8015, Bonsucesso .. Rio de Janeiro, GB. ZC-24
Pereira, Ismar de Castro
Alves .... Rua Prof. Ortiz Monteiro, 15
apto. 402, Laranjeiras ...... Rio de Janeiro, GB. ZC-01
Pereira, José Ribamar ..... Av. Suburbane, 2600, Higien-
ópolis .... Rio de Janeiro, GB. ZC-24
Pereira, Luiz Fernando San-
tos Pacheco .... Av. Rainha Elizabeth, 234 apto. Rio de Janeiro, GB. ZC-37
402, Copacabana ....
Pereira, Maria Tereza Mon-
teiro .... Rua Andrade Pertence, 32 apto.
102, Catete .... Rio de Janeiro, GB. ZC-01
Pereira, Miriam Celeste .... Clinica Oftal. do Hospital São
Francisco de Assis, Av. Presi-
dente Vargas, 2863, Centro .. Rio de Janeiro, GB. ZC-14
Pereira, Sandra da Silva .... Rua Ferreira Leite, 133 casa 1,
Abolição .... Rio de Janeiro, GB. ZC-13
Pereira, Silvio Sergio de
Canto .... Rua Conde de Bomfim, 239 apto.
204, Tijuca .... Rio de Janeiro, GB. ZC-09

Pereira Filho, Narciso de Almeida	Rua Conselheiro Zenha, 51 apto. 304, Tijuca	Rio de Janeiro, GB. ZC-09
Perez, Aurelio M. Cazal	Rua Marques de Abrantes, 152 apto. 905, Flamengo	Rio de Janeiro, GB. ZC-01
Pimentel, Hugo	Rua Pernambuco, 1019 apto. 302, Engenho de Dentro	Rio de Janeiro, GB. ZC-13
Pina, Armando Carlos de ..	Trav. Francisco Ramos, 78, Olaria	Rio de Janeiro, GB. ZC-22
Pinguelli, Antonio Benedicto	Av. do Exercito, 13 apto. 606, São Cristovão	Rio de Janeiro, GB. ZC-08
Pinto, Expedito Geraldo S. .	Rua Mariz e Barros, 933 apto. 702, Tijuca	Rio de Janeiro, GB. ZC-29
Pinto, Geraldo Celio Gomes.	Rua Padre Andre Moreira, 331, Meier	Rio de Janeiro, GB. ZC-16
Pinto, John Murray de Miranda	Rua Barão de Ipanema, 102, apto. 604, Copacabana	Rio de Janeiro, GB. ZC-07
Pinto, José Mariano	Rua Jorge Rudge, 86 apto. 203, Vila Izabel	Rio de Janeiro, GB. ZC-11
Pinto, Paulo Rodrigues	Rua Carlos Sampaio, 351 apto. 703. Centro	Rio de Janeiro, GB. ZC-86
Pinto, Sergio Augusto	Rua Alberto Leite, 85, Meier ...	Rio de Janeiro, GB. ZC-16
Pinto Junior, Gabriel de Assumpção	Hospital de Clínicas Brasil-Portugal, Rua Carolina Machado, 38, Cascadura	Rio de Janeiro, GB. ZC-12
Pio, Helio Santos	Av. Bartolomeu Mitre, 553 apto. 305, Leblon	Rio de Janeiro, GB. ZC-95
Pires, Marco Antonio Estevão	Clinica Oftalmológica do Hospital São Francisco de Assis	Rio de Janeiro, GB. ZC-14
Porcaro, Ferdinand	Rua Teodoro da Silva, 320 apto. 201, Vila Izabel	Rio de Janeiro, GB. ZC-11
Portes, Luiz Carlos Pereira .	Trav. Tamoios, 40 apto. 1001, Botafogo	Rio de Janeiro, GB. ZC-01
Porto, Luiz Fernando Guimarães da Silva	Rua Arthur Araripe, 77 apto. 202, Gávea	Rio de Janeiro, GB. ZC-20
Prado Junior, João	Hotel Barão de Teffé, 99, Saúde .	Rio de Janeiro, GB. ZC-05
Pretti, Dalva Marilia	Rua São Salvador, 65 apto. 302, Flamengo	Rio de Janeiro, GB. ZC-01
Procopiak, Egeu	Rua Marques São Vicente, 431 apto. 805, Gávea	Rio de Janeiro, GB. ZC-20
Proença, Lino Gaspar	Rua Sacadura Cabral, 117 apto. 1112, Saúde	Rio de Janeiro, GB. ZC-05
Provenzano, Sylvio	Rua Pirassununga, 59 apto. 202, Tijuca	Rio de Janeiro, GB. ZC-09
Queiroz, Antonio Carlos Fonseca de	Rua Barão da Torre, 270, Fundos apto. 202, Ipanema	Rio de Janeiro, GB. ZC-95
Queiroz, Francisco de Assis .	Rua Belfort Roxo, 231 apto. 407, Copacabana	Rio de Janeiro, GB. ZC-07
Queiroz, Nivaldo Batista Queiroz	Rua Correa Dutra, 99 apto. 1008, Flamengo	Rio de Janeiro, GB. ZC-01

Queiroz, Olga de Azevedo .. Rua Leonidia, 145 apto. 107,
                           Olaria .... Rio de Janeiro, GB. ZC-22
Rached, Fuad Jacob Abi ... Rua Senador Vergueiro, 123 apto.
                           401, Flamengo .... Rio de Janeiro, GB. ZC-01
Ramalho, Claudio Humberto '
  Savastano .... Rua Senador Furtado, 39 apto.
                           210, Tijuca .... Rio de Janeiro, GB. ZC-29
Ramalho, Melo .... Av. N.S. de Copacabana, 664
                           apto. 303, Copacabana ..... Rio de Janeiro, GB. ZC-07
Ramos, Dorival Ventura ... Av. Copacabana, 1085 apto. 204,
                           Copacabana .... Rio de Janeiro, GB. ZC-07
Ramos, Osmany .... Rua Siqueira Campos, 121 apto.
                           204, Copacabana .... Rio de Janeiro, GB. ZC-07
Ramos, Sebastião Coutinho . Rua Pereira Nunes, 192-C-V apto.
                           202, Aldeia Campista ...... Rio de Janeiro, GB. ZC-11
Ramos, Tulio .... Praça Eugenio Jarim, 22 apto.
                           301, Copacabana .... Rio de Janeiro, GB. ZC-07
Rancel Filho, Helio de Mi-
  randa .... Rua Barão de Pirassinunga, 7
                           apto. 204, Tijuca .... Rio de Janeiro, GB. ZC-09
Rebello, Orlando da Silva .. Rua Mal. Mascarenhas de Moraes,
                           103, apto. 1001, Copacabana . Rio de Janeiro, GB. ZC-07
Rebouças, Julio Cesar ..... Av. Braz de Pina, 122, Terreo,
                           Penha .... Rio de Janeiro, GB. ZC-22
Regis, Edson Paulo Rondon . Rua São Januário, 375 apto. 405,
                           São Cristovão .... Rio de Janeiro, GB. ZC-08
Rezende, Geraldo Augusto
  de .... Rua Gal. Glicerio, 364 apto. 201,
                           Laranjeiras .... Rio de Janeiro, GB. ZC-01
Rezende, Sebastião .... Praia de Botafogo, 340 apto. 241,
                           Botafogo .... Rio de Janeiro, GB. ZC-02
Rezende Filho, Joviano de . Praça Cruz Vermelha, 12, Ierreo,
                           Centro .... Rio de Janeiro, GB. ZC-07
Ribeiro, Bernardo Elifas ... Cl. Oftalmológica do Instituto
                           Benjamin Constant, Av. Pas-
                           teur, 350, Praia Vermelha ... Rio de Janeiro, GB. ZC-82
Ribeiro, Marcio Cottini .... Rua Prof. Alfredo Gomes, 3, Bo-
                           tafogo .... Rio de Janeiro, GB. ZC-02
Ribeiro, Joaquim Vidal Leite Rua Turf Clube, 12 apto. 303,
                           Maracnã .... Rio de Janeiro, GB. ZC-11
Ribeiro, Theodoro .... Av. Rio Branco, 108, 18° andar,
                           Centro .... Rio de Janeiro, GB. ZC-21
Rigo, Paulo Henrique da
  Silva .... Rua Utrillo, 20 apto. 402, Del
                           Castilho .... Rio de Janeiro, GB. ZC-16
Rizzo, Umberto Antonio .. Rua Martins Ribeiro, 12 apto.
                           704, Laranjeiras .... Rio de Janeiro, GB. ZC-01
Rocha, Henrique Celso de
  Rezende .... Rua Dr. Marques de Canário, 24
                           apto. 509, Gávea .... Rio de Janeiro, GB. ZC-20
Rocha, Jairo Borges da .... Rua Silverio, 15 apto. 303, Casca-
                           dura .... Rio de Janeiro, GB. ZC-12
Rocha, Maria Emilia Vital da Av. Mem de Sá. 247 apto. 405,
                           Centro .... Rio de Janeiro. GB. ZC-86
Rocha, Luiz Carlos .... Rua F-60 apto. 301, Padre Miguel Rio de Janeiro, GB. ZC-00
Rocha, Neulisses Gama .... Hospital Pedro Ernesto, Oftal-
                           mologia, Av. 28 de Setembro,
                           87, 4° andar, Vila Izabel .... Rio de Janeiro, GB. ZC-11

Rodrigues, Eunice	....	
Rodrigues, José Balles ter ..	....	
Rodrigues, Miriam Leal	Rua das Laranjeiras, 143 apto. 805, Laranjeiras	Rio de Janeiro, GB. ZC-01
Ronai, Hermann Lorant ...	Rua Uruguai, 468 apto. 606, Tijuca	Rio de Janeiro, GB. ZC-09
Ropa, Alain Laurent Daniel .	Rua Francisco Sá, 5 apto. 304, Copacabana	Rio de Janeiro, GB. ZC-37
Rosan, Atair	Av. Copacabana, 371 apto. 1109, Copacabana	Rio de Janeiro, GB. ZC-07
Rossi Filho, Libero	Rue Gal. Cristovão Barcelos, 251 apto. C.01, Laranjeiras	Rio de Janeiro, GB. ZC-01
Ruiz, Romualdo de Freitas .	Rua Mario Barreto, 28-A, Tijuca .	Rio de Janeiro, GB. ZC-09
Sá, Geraldo Matos de	Rua das Laranjeiras, 210 apto. 1204, Laranjeiras	Rio de Janeiro, GB. ZC-01
Sacchetin, Waldeluir Dublin .	Hospital Pedro Ernesto-Residente, Av. 28 de Setembro, 87, Vila Izabel	Rio de Janeiro, GB. ZC-11
Saliba, Wilson Florantino dos Santos	Rua Belfort Roxo, 20 apto. 1103, Copacabana	Rio de Janeiro, GB. ZC-07
Salomão Filho, Nami	Rua Correia Dutra, 52 apto. 102, Flamengo	Rio de Janeiro, GB. ZC-01
Samara, Miriam Abi	Rua Domingos Ferreira, 188 apto. 902, Copacabana	Rio de Janeiro, GB. ZC-07
Sampaio, Aristides de Barros	Rua Viuva Dantas, 80 sala 311, Campo Grande	Rio de Janeiro, GB. ZC-26
Sampaio, Humberto Alves .	Rua Xavier da Silveira, 90 apto. 704, Copacabana	Rio de Janeiro, GB. ZC-07
Sampaio, José Lourenço Brasil	Praça da República, 93 apto. 504, Centro	Rio de Janeiro, GB. ZC-14
Santos, Ary Barbosa	Cl. Oftal. do Hospital de Bonsucesso-INPS, Av. Londre, Bonsucesso	Rio de Janeiro, GB. ZC-24
Santos, Carlos Alberto dos .	Rua Maxwel, 211 casa 2, Andaraí	Rio de Janeiro, GB. ZC-11
Santos, Evaldo Machado dos	Rua Aires Saldanha, 136 apto. 604, Copacabana	Rio de Janeiro, GB. ZC-07
Santos, Maria da Graça Silveira dos	Rua Barão, 2, Jacarepaguá	Rio de Janeiro, GB. ZC-89
Santos, Paulo Cesar dos ...	Rua Domingos Ferreira, 63 apto. 1207, Copacabana	Rio de Janeiro, GB. ZC-07
Sbragio, Antonio Carlos ...	Rua São Francisco Xavier, 342 apto. 820, Maracanã	Rio de Janeiro, GB. ZC-11
Sbrissa, Renato Acosta	Av. Copacabana, 759 apto. 705, Copacabana	Rio de Janeiro, GB. ZC-07
Serpa, Josée	Rua Buenos Aires, 204, 2° andar, Centro	Rio de Janeiro, GB. ZC-00
Silva, Arildo da	Rua Antonio Basilio, 269 apto. 404, Tijuca	Rio de Janeiro, GB. ZC-09
Silva, Carlos Afonso	Hotel Barão de Tefé, Av. Barão de Tefé, 99 Saúde	Rio de Janeiro, GB. ZC-05
Silva, Carlos Fernando Ferreira da	Rua Santa Clara, 33 apto. 722, Copacabana	

Silva, Dilson Marques da ...	Rua Barão de Itaipú, 148, Andaraí	Rio de Janeiro, GB. ZC-11
Silva, Ivan José da	Rua Eng. Gastão Lobão, 169, Meyer	Rio de Janeiro, GB. ZC-16
Silva, Jacer Ferreira da	Rua Tadeu Kosciusco, 19 apto. 1003, Centro	Rio de Janeiro, GB. ZC-86
Silva, Jorge Pereira Dias da .	Rua Santa Clara, 50 sala 304, Copacabana	Rio de Janeiro, GB. ZC-07
Silva, Julio Ramos da	Rua Gal. Ribeiro 'a Costa, 230 apto. 1205, Leme	Rio de Janeiro, GB. ZC-07
Silva, Leifson Holder da ...	Rua Paula Freitas, 19 apto. 911, Copacabana	Rio de Janeiro, GB. ZC-07
Silva, Lucia Krauss	Av. Maracanã, 566 apto. 803, Maracanã	Rio de Janeiro, GB. ZC-11
Silva, Milton Marques e	Rua Dr. Satamini, 91 apto. 201, Tijuca	Rio de Janeiro, GB. ZC-10
Silva, Roberval Tavares da .	Rua Pedro Americo, 151 apto. 906, Catete	Rio de Janeiro, GB. ZC-01
Silva, Zanizor Rodrigues da .	Av. N.S. de Fátima, 86 apto. 701, Bairro de Fátima	Rio de Janeiro, GB. ZC-86
Silva Filho, Amaro Pereira da	Rua Manuel Miranda, 199 apto. 201, Engenho Novo	Rio de Janeiro, GB. ZC-15
Silva Filho, João Ferreira da.	Av. Atlântica, 3700 apto. 702, Copacabana	Rio de Janeiro, GB. ZC-37
Silveira, Luiz Antonio Lopes	Rua Tenente Possolo, 24 apto. 31, Centro	Rio de Janeiro, GB. ZC-86
Silveira, Luiz Carlos Ribeiro da	Clinica Oftalmologica do Hospital dos Servidores do Estado, Rua Sacadura Cabral, 178, 5° andar, Saúde	Rio de Janeiro, GB. ZC-05
Simões, José Ribeiro	Rua 9, 57 apto. 102, IAPI, Penha	Rio de Janeiro, GB. ZC-22
Sirimarco, Luiz Fernando ..	Cl. Oftal. do Hospital São Francisco de Assis, Av. Pres. Vargas, 2863, Centro	Rio de Janeiro, GB. ZC-14
Shor, Leon	Rua Conde de Bomfim, 116 apto. 302, Tijuca	Rio de Janeiro, GB. ZC-09
Souto, Rodovalho Rego ...	Rua Graça de Melo, 640 R-G, C. 26 ap. 202, Cavalcanti	Rio de Janeiro, GB. ZC-12
Souza, Antonio Ildefonso de	....	
Souza, Caleb Ribeiro de ...	Rua Uruguai, 339 apto. 609, Tijuca	Rio de Janeiro, GB. ZC-09
Souza, Eduardo Moreira de .	Rua Amaral, 61, Andaraí	Rio de Janeiro, GB. ZC-11
Souza, Ernesto Albino de ..	Av. Radial Sul, 25 apto. 306, Botafogo	Rio de Janeiro, GB. ZC-02
Souza, Gerson Lopes de ...	Rua Miraluz, 202, Bonsucesso ..	Rio de Janeiro, GB. ZC-24
Souza, José Julio de	Praça Tiradentes, 31 apto. 402, Centro	Rio de Janeiro, GB. ZC-58
Sousa, Julio da Costa	Rua Souza Valente, 20 apto. 2, São Cristovão	Rio de Janeiro, GB. ZC-08
Souza, Paulo Borges de	Rua Barão de Mesquita, 463 apto. 105, Andaraí	Rio de Janeiro, GB. ZC-11
Souza, Ricardo Lucio de ...	Rua Conde de Bomfim, 113 apto. 202, Tijuca	Rio de Janeiro, GB. ZC-09

Spindola, Atilio de A. Ferreira	Rua Montenegro, 71 apto. 802, Ipanema	Rio de Janeiro, GB. ZC-95
Studart, Armando Barroso .	Rua das Plameiras, 93 apto. 203, Botafogo	Rio de Janeiro, GB. ZC-02
Tannus, José Baruich Schuwartz	Rua dos Araujos, 52 apto. 401, Tijuca	Rio de Janeiro, GB. ZC-09
Tauhata, Ataliba	Clinica Oftalmológica do Hospital de Bonsucesso-INPS, Av. Londres-Bonsucesso	Rio de Janeiro, GB. ZC-24
Tavares, Amélio	Rua Senador Dantas, 117 apto. 1215, Centro	Rio de Janeiro, GB. ZC-06
Tavares, João Elviro	Rua 7 de Setembro, 88, 2° andar, Centro	Rio de Janeiro, GB. ZC-21
Tavares, Wilton Campos ...	Rua Ferreira Viana, 53 apto. 203, Flamengo	Rio de Janeiro, GB. ZC-01
Tavares Filho, Amélio	Rua Senador Dantas, 117 sala 1215, Centro	Rio de Janeiro, GB. ZC-06
Teixeira, Edmar Machado ..	Praia do Flamengo, 374 apto. 302, Flamengo	Rio de Janeiro, GB. ZC-01
Teixeira, Herculano Reis de A.	Rua Senador Vergueiro, 56 apto. 701, Flamengo	Rio de Janeiro, GB. ZC-01
Teixeira, João Baptista Braga	Rua 5 de Julho, 63 apto. 101, Copacabana	Rio de Janeiro, GB. ZC-07
Teixeira, Josué Moreira	Rua Conde de Porto Alegre, 431, Rocha	Rio de Janeiro, GB. ZC-15
Teixeira, Wiliam Alves	....	
Telles, Luiz Fernando	Rua Joaquim Nabuco, 149 apto. 301, Copacabana	Rio de Janeiro, GB. ZC-37
Terto, José Nelson Pereira .	Rua Candido Mendes, 236 BL. B. apto. 811, Glória	Rio de Janeiro, GB. ZC-06
Tokunaga, Seizi	Rua da Glória, 268 apto. 204, Glória	Rio de Janeiro, GB. ZC-06
Tosi, José Raphael	Praça Saens Pena, 55 Fundos apto. 106, Tijuca	Rio de Janeiro, GB. ZC-09
Tozzatto, Lelia	Rua da Selva, 120, Tijuca	Rio de Janeiro, GB. ZC-09
Tupinambá, Luiz Fernando .	Rua Visc. de Pirajá, 28 apto. 503, Ipanema	Rio de Janeiro, GB. ZC-95
Uchoa, Ivaldo de Mendonça	Rua Dr. Satamini, 84 apto. 405, Tijuca	Rio de Janeiro, GB. ZC-10
Valdetaro, João	Rua Pàulo Cesar de Andrade, 232 apto. 102, Laranjeiras	Rio de Janeiro, GB. ZC-01
Vaz, Luiz Bernardino Aguiar	Rua Senador Vergueiro, 93 apto. 408, Flamengo	Rio de Janeiro, GB. ZC-01
Veiga Filho, Silvio Luiz ...	Rua Souza Lima, 432 apto. C-01, loja, Copacabana	Rio de Janeiro, GB. ZC-37
Velasco, Miguel Angelo Padilha	Rua Aarão Reis, 37 apto. 102, Santa Tereza	Rio de Janeiro, GB. ZC-45
Veloso, Paulo Cruz Monteiro	Rua Senador Nabuco, 100, Vila Izabel	Rio de Janeiro, GB. ZC-11
Vianna, Ronald Galvarro ..	Rua Dr. Niemeyer, 37 apto. 102, Engenho de Dentro	Rio de Janeiro, GB. ZC-13

Vidaurreta, Alberto Rodrigues	Rua Dias da Cruz, 155 sala 506-107, Meier	Rio de Janeiro, GB. ZC-16
Vieira, Gilberto Doin	Rua Alzira Bramdão, 11 apto. 504, Tijuca	Rio de Janeiro, GB. ZC-09
Vieira, Heitor Manoel Farani	Rua Conde de Bomfim, 1156 apto. 103, Tijuca	Rio de Janeiro, GB. ZC-09
Vieira, José Maria Alves	Rua Barão do Flamengo, 28 apto. 703, Flamengo	Rio de Janeiro, GB. ZC-01
Vieira, Marcio Barbosa	Rua Guaju, 57, Meier	Rio de Janeiro, GB. ZC-16
Vieira, Raimundo Braga Fernandes	Clinica Oftalmológica do Hospital dos Servidores do Estado, Rua Scadura Cabral, 178, 5° andar, Sáude	Rio de Janeiro, GB. ZC-05
Vilela, Marlene Santiago	Rua Dr. Satamini, 39 apto. 302, Tijuca	Rio de Janeiro, GB. ZC-10
Vilhena, Hiran Mattos de	Rua Sanáta Alexandrina, 1151, Rio Comprido	Rio de Janeiro, GB. ZC-10
Wajnberg, Marcos Isaac	Rua Toneleros, 106 apto. 502, Copacabana	Rio de Janeiro, GB. ZC-07
Winter, Jorge	Rua Visc. de Caravelas, 57, Botafogo	Rio de Janeiro, GB. ZC-02
Wolosker, Marcos	Av. Oswaldo Cruz, 115 apto. 102, Botafogo	Rio de Janeiro, GB. ZC-01
Yamane, Riuitiro	Rua Prof. Gastão Bahiana, 496 apto. 1802, Copacabana	Rio de Janeiro, GB. ZC-07
Yamane, Yoshifumi	Av. Osvaldo Cruz, 115 apto. 907, Flamengo	Rio de Janeiro, GB. ZC-01
Zago, Luiz Alberto	Av. Ataulfo de Paiva, 386 apto. 306, Leblon	Rio de Janeiro, GB. ZC-95
Zarur, Almiro	Rua Pernambuco, 360, Engenho de Dentro	Rio de Janeiro, GB. ZC-13
Zenicola, Ruth Nascimento	Rua Dois de Dezembro, 131 apto. 803, Catete	Rio de Janeiro, GB. ZC-01
Zukeram, Emilio Soitsi	Rua Santo Amaro, 196 apto. 106, Catete	Rio de Janeiro, GB. ZC-01

Maranhão

Andrade, Conceição Macau		
Azevedo, Crisanto Carneiro de	Av. Getulio Vargas, 87	São Luiz
Chagas, Maria Magnolia de Jesus	Rua Senador João Pedro, 9J	São Luiz
Dias, Walter Ferreira	Rua Jose Bonifácio, 321	São Luiz
Diniz, Jose Venancio Braga	Rua Joaquim Tavora, 356, 4° andar, Edificio Sulacap	São Luiz
Lima, William Moreira	Rua Osvaldo Cruz, 1282	São Luiz
Monte, Asterio Pinto do	Av. Santos Dumont, 100 Bairro, Tirirical	São Luiz
Oliveira, Francisco Gomes de	Av. Getulio Vargas, 137, Apeadouro	São Luiz
Queiroga, Augusto	Casa de saude Santa Luzia	Imperatriz
Ramos, Antonio Jose	Clinica Oftal. Hospital Tarquino Lopes F°, Praça Neto Guterrez S/N	São Luiz

Rego, Dirsa Nogueira de Moraes	Rua Astolfo Marques, 237	São Luiz
Reis, Abreu	Rua Nina Rodrigues, 168	São Luiz
Santana, Pedro Neiva de ...	Avenida Beira Mar, 448	São Luiz
Silva, Antonio Ribeiro da ..	Rua Godofredo Viana, 240	65000, Sao Luiz
Teixeira, Luiz Sergio Carvalho	Av. Getulio Vargas, 1973	São Luiz
Vale, Jose Jeronimo Facure .	....	

Mato Grosso

Azevedo, Muller Peixoto de .	Rua da Constituição, 1051	Campo Grande
Basmage, Jose	Clinica de Campo Grande, Rua Gal. Rondon, 735	Campo Grande
Chiconelli, Rubens	Rua Antonio João, 35	Cuiaba
David, Hermindo de	Hospital Nazareno	79700, Fatima do Sul
Foster, Arnaldo	Av. Marechal Dutra, 1033	Rondonopolis
Guimarães, Manuel	Caixa Postal 126	Campo Grande
Kalix, Nicola Miguel	Rua General Mello, 291	Cuiaba
Lani, Luiz Eleutherio	Hospital Geral	Campo Grande
Medeiros, Pedro Ozório Barbosa de	Rua Mal. Mallet, 725	Aquidauana
Miranda Filho, Arlindo Bastos de	Serviço de saude da 2A Brigada Mixta	Corumba
Monteiro, Paulo Antonio Costa	Rua 14 de Julho, 570, s- 301 ...	Campo Grande
Moraes, Abel	Av. Cuiaba S/N	78500 Rondonopolis
Moutinho, Jose Fernando ..	....	Corumba
Pereira, S. Eloy	Rua 14 de julho, 570, s. 302	Campo Grande
Ribeiro, Aureo Garcia	Rua Marcelino, Pires, 1495	Dourados
Vilela, Rafael Mendonça ...	Praça Barão do Rio Branco, 116 .	Caceres
Vinagre, Pedro Mauro de Barros	Rua Dom Aquino, 1175	Corumba
Yamaki, Kojum	Rua Antonio Maria Coelho, 249 .	Campo Grande

Minas Gerais

Abreu, Jose Procopio de ...	Av. Independência, 882	Divinopolis
Abreu, Luiz Carlos Pascoutto	Hospital São Geraldo, Av. Alfredo Balena, S/N Santa Efigenia ..	Belo Horizonte
Abreu, Mauro Schqueri de .	Clinica Oftal. do Hospital Marcio Canha	Ipatinga
Adami, Marcos Eduardo ...	Rua Minas Gerais, 435	Poços de Caldas
Agostini Neto, João	Rua Thome de Souza, 679 Funcionários	Belo Horizonte
Almeida, Darcy de	Praça Tiradentes, 86	Teofilo Otoni
Almeida, Hernderson Celestino de	Rua Antilhas, 49	Belo Horizonte
Almeida, Homero Gusmão de	Rua Rio de Janeiro, 909 apto. 304	Belo Horizonte
Almeida, Jose Vilela Henderson	Cl. Oftal. do Hospital S. Geraldo, Av. Prof. Alfredo Balena	Belo Horizonte

Almeida, Lucio de	Hospital Felicio Rocho, Av. Contorno, 9530	Belo Horizonte
Almeida, Luiz Martins de ..	Caixa postal 242	Governador Valadares
Amaral, Ozanan Gazolia do .	Rua N.S. da Saúde, 43	Uberaba
Andrade, Rubens Carvalho de	Rua Zacarias Rolemberg, 43, Mangabeiras	Belo Horizonte
Andrade Junior, Rubens de .	Rua Gal. Const. Valadares, 501 .	Juiz de fora
Antunes, Paulo de Souza ..	Rua Cal. Antonio Sobreira, 111, Bom Pastor	Juiz de Fora
Anuea, Wilde Lima de	Rua 15 de novembro, 190	Porto Novo do Cunha
Araujo, Fernando de Deus .	Rua Espírito Santo, 495, apto. 1203	Belo Horizonte
Araujo, Gelmires Machado de	Hospital São Geraldo, Av. Alfredo Balena, Santa Efigenia	Belo Horizonte
Araujo, Vanio Pontes de ...	Hospital São Geraldo, Av. Alfredo Balena, Santa Efigenia	Belo Horizonte
Avila, Murila Ribeiro de ...	Rua Barão da Ponte Alta, 10 ...	Uberaba
Azevedo, João Garcia de ...	....	
Bachur, Sebastião Roberto .	Av. Francisco Sales, 1585 apto. 32, Funcionários	Belo Horizonte
Bandeira, Fernando	Edif. Banco Agro Pastoril, s. 103-104	Governador Valadares
Barbosa, Jose Araujo	Rua Carneiro Junior, 175	Itajuba
Barbosa, Pedro	Rua João Gomes Eusebio, 20 ...	Carlos Chagas
Bastos, Dalmo	Farmacio Santa Maria	Leopoldina
Bonfioli, Alfredo Bernardo Loureiro	Av. do Contorno, 5009, Serra ...	Belo Horizonte
Bonfioli, Amélio	....	
Bracho, Alberto Enrique Atencio	Hospital São Geraldo, Av. Alfredo Balena, Santa Efigenia	Belo Horizonte
Brito, Wagner Lucena	Hosp. S. Geraldo, Av. Alfredo Balena, Santa Efigenia	Belo Horizonte
Cabral, Edi Stilver Cardozo .	Hosp. S. Geraldo, Av. Alfredo Balena. Santa Efigenia	Belo Horizonte
Caixeta, Antonio Vieira ...	Praça Antonio Dias, 620	38700, Patos de Minas
Caldo, Benito Onofre	Rua Cel. Antonio da Silva, 168 ..	Caratinga
Calixto, Nazzim da Silveira .	Rua Grão Mogol, 1177	Belo Horizonte
Campos, Adelmo	Av. João Pinheiro, 557	Uberlandia
Campos, Emilio Castelar ...	....	
Cançado, Darcio Martins ...	Rua Dep. Lourenço de Andrade, 97	Passos
Capelo, Gloria Maria Wanderley	Hospital S. Geraldo, Av. Alfredo Balena, Santa Efigenia	Belo Horizonte
Cardoso, Renato Dias	Hospital São Geraldo, Av. Alfredo Balena, Santa Efigenia	Belo Horizonte
Carneiro, Helio Cavalcante .	Rua Cel Carlos Brandão, 99	Uberaba
Carneiro, João Honorio ...	Rua Cel. Carlos Brandão, 99	Uberaba
Carrijo, Eleovir Peixoto ...	Hospital Santo Antonio, Rua Rio Branco, 636	Araguari
Carvalho, Vicente Muniz ...	Hospital São Geraldo, Av. Alfredo Balena, Santa Efigenia	Belo Horizonte
Castelanos, Jose	....	

Castro, Jose Tarcisio de ...	Rua Amercio Macedo, 491	Belo Horizonte
Castro, Leopoldo C. de	Rua Itajuba, 733, Floresta	Belo Horizonte
Cavalcante, Bandeira	Av. Olegário Maciel, 507	Caratinga
Cecilia, Helio Lima Santa ..	Av. Afonso Pena, 297, 7° andar .	Uberlandia
Cecilia, Ruy Lima Santa ...	Rua Samuel Santos, 313	Araguari
Chamone, Dirceu	Hospital São Geraldo, Av. Alfredo Balena, Santa Efigenia	Belo Horizonte
Chaves, Antonio Carlos Lopes	Hospital São Geraldo, Av. Alfredo Balena, Santa Efigenia	Belo Horizonte
Claret, Antonio	Vila dos Oficiais, 21	Sao João Del Rey
Conte, Orvile Colombo de .	Rua Pernambuco, 619	Belo Horizonte
Correa, Gildrades da Costa .	Hospital São Geraldo, Av. Alfredo Balena S/N, Santa Efigenia ..	Belo Horizonte
Correa, Wiliam Bonaparte ..	Rua 7, 1007	Ituiutaba
Coscarelli, Ennio	Rua São Paulo, 638, 4° andar ...	Belo Horizonte
Coscarelli, Leticia Antonini .	Rua São Paulo, 638, 3° andar ...	Belo Horizonte
Costa, Jose Daphnis Mil-Homens	Rua Delfim Moreira, 619	Varginha
Coutinho, Lima	Rua Artur Bernardes, 178	Itauna
Covolo, Alcir Berreta	Hospital São Geraldo, Av. Alfredo Balena, Santa Efigenia	Belo Horizonte
Cruz, Jose Custodio da Costa	Rua Halfeld, 651, s. 501	Juiz de Fora
Cunha, Carlos Rodrigues ...	Rua dos Andradas, 88	Uberaba
Cunha, Marcio Antonio Rodrigues da	Av. João Pinheiro, 292	Uberlandia
Cunha, Tania Mara	Rua Santos Dumont, 289	Juiz de Fora
Dahbar, Nadim	Rua Floriano Peixoto, 847	Juiz de Fora
Delvaux, Euclides	....	
Dias, Gerson	Caixa postal 282	Itajuba
Dias, João	....	
Donato Neto, Elias	Hospital São Geraldo, Av. Alfredo Balena, Santa Efigenia	Belo Horizonte
Duarte, Elcio Faria	Av. Rio Branco, 1804, apto. 320	Juiz de Fora
Dutra, Galba Volpini	Rua Albita, 334 apto 3	Belo Horizonte
Elias, Nelson	Rua D-Aparecida, 227	Guaxupé
Faria, Helio Souto Maior de	Av. Contorno, 7337	Belo Horizonte
Fernandes, Maria Cristina Guerra	Rua Espírito Santo, 1095 apto 1 .	Juiz de Fora
Fernandes, Paulo Mandel-stam	Hospital São Geraldo, Av. Alfredo Balena, Santa Efigenia	Belo Horizonte
Ferreira, David Rodrigues ..	Rua Abaete, 254 Bomfim	Belo Horizonte
Ferreira Neto, Nicomendes .	Rua Conde Linhares, 55 apto 104, Bairro, Cidade Jardim ..	Bela Horizonte
Figueiredo, Joaquim Barbosa de	Rua 13 de maio, 485	37570, Ouro Fino
Filippo, Geraldo de	Caixa postal 61	Barbacena
Fonseca, Guilherme de Assis	....	
Fonseca, Leonidia Freire ..	Rua Poços de Caldas, 165	39860, Nanuque
Fraga Filho, Tomaz Jacinto de	Rua Ceara, 42	Juiz de Fora
Frange, Frederico Alonso ..	Rua Pires de Campos, 81	Uberaba
Freitas, Nairo Alves de	Clinica Oftal. da Santa casa de misericordia, Santa Efigenia .	Belo Horizonte
Freitas, Natan	Rua dos Santos, 290	Montes Claros

Freitas Filho, Justino de ...	Caixa postal 197	Varginha
Galvão, Paulo Gustavo	Rua São João do Paraízo, 247 Bairro, Sion	Belo Horizonte
Garzedin, Gilson Motta	Rua Espírito Santo, 841, apto 902	Belo Horizonte
Giudice, Mário Del	Praça do Rosário, 1	Viçosa
Godinho, Cleber Jose	Rua Bahia, 1192 apto 710	Belo Horizonte
Gomes, Breno Furtado	Rua São Paulo, 89315–810	Belo Horizonte
Gomes, Geraldo Magalhẽs ..	Rua Cal. Prates, 200	Montes Claros
Gomes, Julio Maria	Clinica Oftal. do Hospital Marcio Cunha	Ipatinga
Gomes, Roberto Magalhães .	Rua Cel Joaquim Costa, 160	Guaxupé
Gonçalves, Edahir	Av. João Pinheiro, 761 apto. 12 .	Uberlandia
Contijo, Paulo Pinto	Santa casa de misericordia – oftal., Santa Efigenia	Belo Horizonte
Contijo, Roberto Assumpção	Rua Santa Catarina, 941	Belo Horizonte
Gorenstein, Saulo	Hospital São Geraldo, Av. Alfredo Balena, Santa Efigenia	Belo Horizonte
Gouveia, Amilcar Xavier de .	Caixa postal 524	Juiz de Fora
Gouveia, Antonio	Rua Halfeld, 603, salas 201/2 ...	Juiz de Fora
Gualberto, Osvaldo de Andrade	Rua Caetano Dias, 95, Serra	Belo Horizonte
Guaracy, Jair S.	Rua D. Vigoso, 223	Juiz de Fora
Guimarães, Marcio	Rua Tupi, 265 apto. 403, Centro	Belo Horizonte
Guimarães, Odair	Hospital São Geraldo, Av. Alfredo Balena, Santa Efigenia	Belo Horizonte
Hercos Filho, João	Hospital Santa Luzia, Av. Santos Dumont	Uberaba
Holanda, Jose Everton de Almeida	Hospital São Geraldo, Av. Alfredo Balena, Santa Efigenia	Belo Horizonte
Hueb, Aziz Miguel	Rua Aigismundo Mendes, 104 ..	Uberaba
Izecksohn, David	Rua Afonso Pena, 255	Araguari
Kascher, Jose Martins Nominato	Rua Campos Sales, 472	30000, Belo Horizonte
Ladeira, Nivaldo Barbosa Dias	Av. Minas Gerais, 1225	Governador Valadares
Laender, Renato Cruz	Rua Rio Verde, 529, Sion	Belo Horizonte
Laguardia, Paulo Eustachio .	Av. Getulio Vargas, 632 apto. 501	Juiz de Fora
Lanna, Antonio Elisio	Rua Cantidio Drumond, 37	Ponte Nova
Leal Filho, Sylvio Ideburque	Hospital São Geraldo, Av. Alfredo Balena, Santa Efigenia	Belo Horizonte
Leite, Eduardo Henrique ..	Rua Salinas, 719 apto. 4	Belo Horizonte
Leite, Juarez Ferreira	Rua Dr. Marcolino, 37	Patos de Minas
Lessa, Elio Rocha	Hospital de olhos Santa Luzia ...	Montes Claros
Lima, Fernando Soares de Souza	Hospital São Geraldo, Av. Alfredo Balena, Santa Efigenia	Belo Horizonte
Lima, Manoel Gonçalves de .	Av. Conrorno, 9797 apto. 220, Prado	Belo Horizonte
Lima, Winnie Maria S. de Souza	Av. Olegario Maciel, 274 apto. 814, Centro	Belo Horizonte
Macedo, Zita de Brito Freite	Rua Epamínondas Otoni, 360 ..	Teofilo Otonio
Monnaka, Lygia H. de Magalhães	Rua Dante, 249 apto 301	Belo Horizonte

Moreira, Marlene de Melo Bomdim	Rua Artur Joviano, 111 apto. 301 Anchieta	Belo Horizonte
Muzzi, Carmelo Antonio ...	Hospital S. Geraldo, Av. Alfredo Balena, Santa Efigenia	Belo Horizonte
Lignani Neto, Luiz	Av. Alberto Laender, 111	Teofilo Otoni
Lima, J. de Oliveira	....	
Lima, Manoel Gonçalves de .	Hospital S. Geraldo, Av. Alfredo Balena, Santa Efigenia	Belo Horizonte
Lima, Raul Soares de Souza .	Rua São Paulo, 2210	Belo Horizonte
Magalhães, Gilberto de	Clinica Santa Paula	37550, Pouso Alegre
Maia, João Andre da Costa .	Av. Contorno, 9711, 150 apto. Barro Preto	Belo Horizonte
Maia, Marco Aurelio de Morais	Rua Batista de Oliveira, 1000 ...	Juiz de Fora
Maior, Marcio Ribeiro Sotto.	Rua Batista de Oliveira, 1298 ...	Juiz de Fora
Maior, Ruben Sotto	Rua Halfeld, 744, 3° andar	Juiz de Fora
Martins, Herminio Rocha ..	Rua Halfeld, 640	Juiz de Fora
Mascarenhas, Bolivar D. ...	Rua Gal. Osorio, 25	Curvello
Masini, Jose Henrique	Rua Oscar Vidal, 55	Juiz de Fora
Medeiros, Osvaldo Travassos de	Hospital São Geraldo, Av. Alfredo Balena, Santa Efigenia	Belo Horizonte
Medeiros, Oswaldo	Hospital São Geraldo, Av. Alfredo Balena, Santa Efigenia	Belo Horizonte
Meireles, Guilherme	Rua Aguapei, 87	Belo Horizonte
Mendonça, Cesar	Hospital São Geraldo, Av. Alfredo Balena, Santa Efigenia	Belo Horizonte
Menicucci, Ene	Rua do Ouro, 20 Bairro, Serra ..	Belo Horizonte
Merch, Adyr Haddad	Rua Coronel Novais, 36	Carangola
Miraglia Junior, Orestes ...	Rua Ludgero Dolabela, 224 apto. 202, Gutterres	Belo Horizonte
Moraes, Helio	Hospital S. Geraldo, Av. Alfredo Balena, Santa Efigenia	Belo Horizonte
Moreira, Jose Caputo	Rua Olegário Maciel, 22	Uberaba
Moura, Roberto Abdala ...	Rua Goitacazes, 103 s. 905	Belo Horizonte
Nascimento, Heider Augusto do	Rua Mauricio de Menezes, 38 Bairro, Olga Burnier	Juiz de Fora
Neto, Leopoldo Pacini	....	
Neves, Julio Teixeira	Rua São Paulo, 409, 8° andar ...	Belo Horizonte
Neves, Sylvio Lucio de Paula	Rua Dr. Olavo Tostes, 110 apto. 105	Muriaé
Odilon F. Filho, Oswaldo ..	Av. Francisco Sales, 427	Belo Horizonte
Oliveira, Décio Brito de ...	Rua Grão Para, 1010	Belo Horizonte
Oliveira, Ildefonso Jose de .	Rua Angelo de Quadros, 649 ...	Montes Claros
Oliveira, Luiz Roberto Melo de	Hospital São Geraldo, Av. Alfredo Balena, Santa Efigenia	Belo Horizonte
Orefice, Fernando	Hospital Felicio Rocho, Av. Contorno, 9530	Belo Horizonte
Paletta, Geraldo	Rua Oscar Vidal, 79	Juiz de Fora
Palis, Samir	Av. 21, 1513	Ituiutaba
Panico, Paulo Henrique Frasseschi	Rua Tome de Souza, 679 apto. Cobertura	Belo Horizonte
Paschoalino, Helcio Costa ..	Rua Oswaldo Cruz, 145	Juiz de Fora
Passos Filho, Antonio Azevedo	Rua Rio de Janeiro, 462 s. 2310 .	Belo Horizonte

Patrão, Renato Lansac	Rua 20, 960	Ituiutaba
Patrus, Agostinho	Rua da Capelinha, 550 Bairro, Serra	Belo Horizonte
Paulo, Cesar Marques Netto .	Rua Espírito Santo, 994	Juiz de Fora
Penna, Abner de Souza	Rua Moacyr Birro, 637, Caixa Postal 5	Cel. Fabriciano
Penna, Gesse de Oliveira ...	Clinica oftal. da Santa casa de misericórdia, Santa Efigenia .	Belo Horizonte
Pereira, Isidorio Romão ...	....	
Pereira, Jose Queiroz	Praça Santa Rita, 192	Cataguazes
Peret, Paulo	Rua São Paulo, 893, 8° andar ...	Belo Horizonte
Pinto, Olavo Alberto Gomes.	Rua Junqueira, 444	São Lourenço
Pires, Ari Alvares	Rua Viçosa, 250, Carmo	Belo Horizonte
Pires Filho, Luiz	Praça. Cel. Prates, 52	Montes Claros
Prata, Nilton	Cl. Oftal. da Faculdade de medicina do Triangulo Mineiro ...	Uberaba
Queiroga, Geraldo	Rua Felipe dos Santos, 382	Belo Horizonte
Queiros, Luiz Cesar Galvão de	Hospital São Geraldo, Av. Alfredo Balena	Belo Horizonte
Queiroz, Eduardo Carlos ...	Rua Aimores, 1056 apto. 6	Belo Horizonte
Ramos, Jose Custodio Pires .	Rua Olegario Macie, 184	Aimore
Rassi, Alan Ricardo	Hospital São Geraldo, Av. Alfredo Balena	Belo Horizonte
Rassi, Darlan	Hospital São Geraldo, Av. Alfredo Balena	Belo Horizonte
Reis, Francisco Nogueira ..	Rua Dep. Ribeiro Rezende, 161 .	Varginha
Reis, Romeu	Av. Minas Gerais, 275	Governador Valadares
Rezende, Oswaldo Henrique V. de	Rua Delfim Moreira, 375	Varginha
Rezende, Oswaldo Valadão .	Rua Delfim Moreira, 375	Varginha
Ribeiro, Ivan Pena	Rua Carangola, 145 apto. 301 ..	Belo Horizonte
Ricciardi, Braz Antonio Ribeiro	Rua Estevao Pires, 822 apto. 13, Serra	Belo Horizonte
Ricciardi, Leia Maria Mundim	Rua Prof. Estevão Pires, 822 apto. 13, Serra	Belo Horizonte
Rocha, Hilton	Rua Rio de Janeiro, 2251	Belo Horizonte
Rodarte, Osmar	Rua Bernardo Guimarães, 1477 .	Belo Horizonte
Rodrigues, Maria de Lourdes	Hospital São Geraldo, Av. Alfredo Balena	Belo Horizonte
Sã, Sandoval Henrique	Praça Alcides de Paula Gomes ...	Frutal
Sa Filho, Lourival Franco de	Hospital São Geraldo, Av. Alfredo Balena	Belo Horizonte
Salerno, Newton Rodrigues .	Rua Araguari, 65 apto 1406	Belo Horizonte
Salgado, Fabio de Augusto .	Cl. Oftal. da Santa casa de misericórdia, Santa Efigenia	Belo Horizonte
Sanabio, Clairmin Geraldo Horta	Rua João Domingos da Fonseca, 101	Formiga
Sanna, Jaime Balmes Pires .	Rua Paulo Afonso, 526, Santo Antonio	Belo Horizonte
Santana, Mauricio Ananias de	Rua da Gloria, 153 apto 201 ...	Juiz de Fora
Santo, Antonio Octavio E. .	Av. Afonso XIII, 435 apto. 202, Gutierrez	Belo Horizonte

Santos, Christiano F. Barsante	Rua Guajajaras, 65 apto 301, Centro	Belo Horizonte
Santos, Clecius	Hospital São Geraldo, Av. Alfredo Balena	Belo Horizonte
Santos, Lindorifico Esteves dos	Rua Esp. Santo, 341, 6° andar ..	Belo Horizonte
Sepulveda, Otavio Marcos ..	Rua Campo Alegre, 29, Floresta .	Belo Horizonte
Signorelli, Carlos Roberto ..	Hospital São Geraldo, Av. Alredo Balena S/N, Santa Efigenia ..	Belo Horizonte
Silva, Antonio Carlos Ferreira da	Rua Padre Jose Maria Xavier, 40 .	São João Del Rey
Silva, Antonio Izidoro	Rua do Ouro, 167	Belo Horizonte
Silva, Felicio Aristoteles da .	Hospital São Geraldo, Av. Alfredo Balena, Santa Efigenia	Belo Horizonte
Silva, Helcio de Faria	Trav. Leonelo Fortini, 17 A	36100 Juiz de Fora
Silva, Ismael Ribeiro da ...	Rua Carlos Rodrigues, 54	Uberaba
Silva, Jair Ribeiro da	Rua Prof. Chagas, 204	Poços de Caldas
Silva, Jeronimo Dias da	Rua PE-Augusto, 397 apto. 101 .	Montes Claros
Silva, Lycio Cortizo da	Rua Timbiras, 673 Bairro, Funcionarios	Belo Horizonte
Silva, Marcelo	Rua João de Matos, 130, Renascença	Belo Horizonte
Silva, Maria Jose Soares da .	Av. do Contorno, 9530	30000, Belo Horizonte
Silva, Nicanor Simeão da ..	Av. 1° de Junho, 427	Divinopolis
Silva, Paulo Patricio de M. E.	Rua Gal. Afonso Moniciro, 130 .	Barbacena
Silva Neto, Teofilo Pereira da	Hospital São Geraldo, Av. Alfredo Balena, Santa Efigenia	Belo Horizonte
Silveira, Oswaldo Gomes da .	Rua Carijos, 136 apto 701	Belo Horizonte
Silveira, Zultenio da da Silva	Rua Alvaro Santos, 23, Vila Paris	Belo Horizonte
Soares, Eduardo Jorge Carneiro	Rua Levindo Lopes, 61 apto. 203	Belo Horizonte
Soares, Emir Francisco	Av. Almirante Alexandrino, 570 apto. 104	Belo Horizonte
Soares, Gilson Tadeu	Hospital São Geraldo, Av. Alfredo Balena, Santa Efigenia	Belo Horizonte
Soares, Pedro Vieira	Rua Senador Pompeu, 212 apto. 32, Serra	Belo Horizonte
Spessatto, Nolvar Selvino ..	Hospital São Geraldo, Av. Alfredo Balena	Belo Horizonte
Stephan, Otto Emilio	Trav. Sen. Joaquim Bernardes, 41 41	Pouso Alegre
Tannus, Amilson Guimarães.	Av. Afonso Pena, 245, A	Uberlandia
Tasca, Marco Aurelio	Av. Braz Bernardino, 241 apto. 201, Centro	Juiz de Fora
Tavares, Angalo Laborne ..	Rua São Paulo, 638, 4° andar ...	Belo Horizonte
Tavares, Cazimiro Laborne .	Rua Conde Linhares, 240, Cidade Jardim	Belo Horizonte
Teixeira, Maria Celia Ciarlini	Hospital São Geraldo, Av. Alfredo Balena, S/N, Santa Efigenia ..	Belo Horizonte
Trindade, Maria de Nazare Filgueiras	Hospital São Geraldo, Av. Alfredo Ralena, Santa Efigenia	Belo Horizonte
Urbano, Lucia Carvalho de Ventura	Hospital São Geraldo, Av. Alfredo Balena, Santa Efigenia	Belo Horizonte

Valle Filho, Jose Antonio do	Praça Malo Viana, 45	Januaria
Vasconcellos, Ignacio	Praça da Matrix, 56	Ponte Nova
Ventura, Fernando A de Oliveira	Hospital São Geraldo, Av. Alfredo Balena, S/N Santa Efigenia . .	Belo Horizonte
Viana, Eduardo Veloso	Rua Cel. Jose Ferreira, 246	Uberaba
Vianna, Paulo C. Carvalho de Velloso	Trav. Cel. Jose Ferreira, 246, São Sebastião	Uberaba
Vianna, Walmo Soares	Hospital São Geraldo, Av. Alfredo Balena	Belo Horizonte
Vieira, Antonio Carlos	Hospital Felício Rocho	Belo Horizonte
Vieira, Marcelo Infante	Av. Rio Branco, 2406, 3° andar .	Juiz de Fora
Vieira Filho, Humberto Martins	Av. Amazonas, 135	Belo Horizonte
Villela, Geraldo	Rua Firmino Sales, 340	Lavras
Villela, Jose Mauro	. . . .	
Weber, Marcio Tadeu Vaz de Mello	Rua Santos Dumont, 401	Juiz de Fora
Zingoni, Gersio	Caixa Postal 416	Poços de Caldas

Pará

Abreu, Lobato de	Av. Nazare, 325	Belem
Amaro, Jorge Hage	Av. Generalìssimo Deodoro, 883 Bairro Umarizal	Belem
Amorim, Luiz Marcelo Bayma de	Trav. Soares Carneiro, 795, Telegrafo	Belem
Arêde Filho, Armando Ribeiro	Av. Pres. Vargas, 197 apto 605 . .	Belem
Barreto, Aracy	Av. Governador Malcher, 223 . . .	Belem
Dias, Paulo	Rua Braz de Aguiar, 774, Nazaré .	Belem
Fernandes, Paulo Mandelstam	Av. Roberto Camelier, Vila Mata 3, Jurunas	Belem
Ferreira, Eliane Santos	Conj. do I.A.P.I. BL. 8 Casa H, São Braz	Belem
Ferreira, Naeli Diros	Trav. Dom Romulo de Seixas, 586	Belem
Fortes, Adevaldo de Oliveira	Av. São Jeronimo, 749, Nazare . .	Belem
Jateni, Maria de Nazareth Franco	Av. Pdre Eutiquio, 1867, Bairro B. Campos	Belem
Lemos, Sarah R. Ferreira de .	Edificio Importadora, Av. Pres. Vargas, 197, s- 204-206	Belem
Lopes, Pedro Gomes de Oliveira	Trav. Quintino Bocaiuva, 680 . . .	Belem
Martins, Mario Antonio . . .	Casa de saude Santa Lucia, Rua Dr. Moraes, 24 . . . . . :. . . .	Belem
Moraes, Manoel Brito de	Rua Jeronimo Pimentel, 696, Umarizal	Belem
Neves, Raymundo Nonnato Aranha	Av. Independencia, 1032, apto. 602	Belem
Nogueira, Luiz Gonzaga Cardoso	Trav. Estrela, Edif. Estrela apto. 405 A	Belem

Pimentel, Carlos A. de O. .. Rua Marechal Deodoro, 1122 ... Belem
Queiros, Joaquim Marinho
de .... Edif. Comendador Pinho, Trav.
Campos Sales, 63 S-1001 .... Belem
Silva, Hugo Laercio Azevedo
da .... Rua Cons° Furtado, 1246 ...... Belem
Tobias, Dilermando ...... Av. 15 de Agosto, 91, s. 113 .... Belem
Vasconcelos, Oriente ..... Rua 28 de Setembro, 269 ...... Belem
Vieira, Ofir Dias .... Rua Manuel Barata, 1555, Bairro,
Reduto .... Belem

Paraíba

Almeida, Agripino Caval-
cante de .... Rua Maciel Pinheiro, 320 ...... Campina Grande
Araujo, Willian Xavier de .. Rua Venancio Neiva, 82, 1° andar Campina Grande
Arruda, Ramonilson ...... Av. N.S. de Fatima, 1916 ...... João Pessoa
Barreto, Luiz Gonzaga .... Casa de saude Dom Paiva, Rua 13
de maio, 331 .... João Pessoa
Branco, Carlos Agripino ... Av. João Machado, 477 .... João Pessoa
Camarão, Cesar Gadelha ... Rua Major Lindolfo Pires, 12,
Centro .... Souza
Dantas, Jose Anchieta de
Galvão .... Rua Francisca Moura, 586,
Centro .... João Pessoa
Granville, Roberto .... Praça Dom Ulrico, 63 .... João Pessoa
Guimarães, Sabino Rolin .. Rua João Pessoa, 380 .... Cajazeiras
Holanda, Crysostomo Luce-
na de .... Av. Getulio Vargas, 299 .... Campina Grande
Maciel, Edgley .... Edificio Arius s-11 E 13, Rua
Maciel Pinheiro .... Campina Grande
Oliveira, Roberto A. Pinto
de .... Rua Maciel Pinheiro, 320 ...... Campina Grande
Pereira, Tito Livio de Sa ... Av. Professora Maria Sales, 431,
Tambau .... João Pessoa
Santos, João Caetano dos .. ..
Sarafin, Pericles Vitorio ... .
Silva, Amaury Vicente .... Clinica de olhos Santa Iuzia, Praça
Getulio Vargas, 22 .... Patos
Souza, João Lucio de ..... Rua Epitácio Pessoa, 26 .... Pianco
Souza, Newton Jorge de ... Hospital Santa Izabel .... João Pessoa
Ventura, Antonio Aurelio de
Oliveira .... Rua Maciel Pinheiro, 320 ...... Campina Grande
Wanderley, Alberto Urouiza Clinica São Camilo, Rua Prof.
Jose Coelho, 25 .... João Pessoa

Paraná

Adam, Rubens de Quadros . Rua Dr. Alfredo Bufren, 86, 15°
andar .... Curitiba
Alcantara, Lauro João Lobo. Av. Visconde de Guarapuava,
4747 .... Curitiba
Amaral, Jose Eduardo Lou-
reiro do .... Hospital e Maternidade São Paulo Cianorte
Angelucci, Celso Francisco . Rua Mariano Torres, 110 apto. 5 . Curitiba

Araujo, João Carlos Ferraz de	....	
Athayde Neto, Aristides de .	Rua Saldanha Marinho, 334	Curitiba
Bacelar, Décio da Silva	Hospital Santo Antonio, Caixa Postai 44	Mandaguari
Barros, Luiz A. Rego	Rua Professora E. Rego Barros, 50	Curitiba
Bazanella, Adherbal	Av. Brasil, 4130	Maringa
Berg, Artur Van Den	Av. São Paulo, 132	Londrina
Bittencourt, Luiz A. Machado	Rua 15 de novembro, 556, S/405/7	Curitiba
Bockman, Nelson	....	
Braga, Carlos	Hotal Diplomata	Foz do Iguaçu
Braga, Renato de Quinta-nilha	Rua Cel. Alcantara, 208	Jacarezinho
Brik, Maurício	Rua Voluntários da Pátria, 475 apto. 402	Curitiba
Brofman, Ronaldo	Rua Visc. do Rio Branco, 1799 .	Curitiba
Campos, Artur Jose	Rua Voluntário da Pátria, 475 ..	Curitiba
Campos, Carneiro de	Instituto Santa Luzia, Av. São Paulo, 732	Londrina
Gascardo Filho, Francisco .	Hospital São Jose	Cianorte
Checchia, Antonio	Av. Vicente Machado, Edif. Ita-poã, 1° andar	Ponta Grossa
Checcia, Deonea P.	Rua Santana, 507	Ponta Grossa
Correa, Fausto Melo	Ed. Banrisul, conj. 1003, 4, Rua Marechal Floriano	Curitiba
Costa, Ariovaldo Roque da .	Av. Paraná, 14, 4	Umuarama
Coutinho, Valdir de O.	Av. Duque de Caxias, 151	Maringa
Daher, Fahed	Rua Rio Branco, 460	Apucarana
Daher, Fahiz Jorgo	Hosp. e Mat. São Paulo, Rua Monteiro Lobato, 289	Rolândia
Daher, Nagib	Rua Rio Branco, 460	Apucarana
Daieldo, Mario Moreira	....	Toledo
Daniel, Segundo	Edificio Asa, S. 1.311, Praça General Osório	Curitiba
Doveinis, Sérgio	Av. Brasil, 4340	Maringá
Duarte, Antonio Lucio	Policlinica São Vicente de Paula .	Francisco Beltrão
Durant, Bernardo Pericas ..	Rua Mal. Deodoro, 167, 1° andar.	Curitiba
Faria, Samir Carlos Teixeira .	Rua Barão do Serro Azul, 110, Centro	Curitiba
Ferraz, Osman	Av. Bandeirantes, 645	Londrina
Ferreira, Carlos Cesar	Rua Voluntários da Pátria, 475, S/402	Curitiba
Ferreira, Celso do Amaral ..	Rua São Leopoldo, 28, Bairro — Jardim Centenário ....:...	Curitiba
Ferreira, Felizardo Leite ...	Rua Alberico Figueira, 50 ,.....	Curitiba
Ferreira Filho, Leonidas do Amaral	Av. 15 de novembro, 556, sala 405	Curitiba
Figueiredo, Luiz Armando .	Rua Prof. João Candido, 344 S/101	Londrina
França, Rubem Nogueira de .	Rua Angelo Sampaio, 2566	Curitiba
Freitas Filho, João Baptista de	Rua Ibiporã, 344	Pato Branco

Fujji, Yoshihiro	Rua Piaui, 588, Centro	Londrina
Furquim Neto, Benedito	Posto Federal do Tracoma	Maringa
Galperin, Aron	Av. 15 de novembro, 1041	Maringa
Garmatter Junior, Julio	Rua Ubaldino do Amaral, 124	Curitiba
Granier, Jean Dominique	Caixa postal 409	Guarapuava
Grupenmacher, Paulo Zelter.	Rua Barão do Bio Branco, 63 S/911	Curitiba
Hatanaka, Michideru	Av. Minas Gerais, 40	Carnelio Procópio
Hilgert, Celso Petter	Policlinica Pato Branco	Pato Branco
Homaiser, Jose Augusto	Rua Paulo Pedrosa de Alencar, 4468	Umuarama
Hoyama, Pakeo	Edifício Senzala, Rua Goias, 1126 apto 35 B	Londrina
Jojima, Marabu	Rua Barão do Rio Branco, 63 S. 507	Curitiba
Kondo, George	Av. Brasil, 3.253	Maringa
Krueger, Egon Armando	Rua Ebano Pereira, 335	Curitiba
Largura, Walmor	Av. São Paulo, 132	Londrina
Lerner, Moises	Rua Emiliano Pernetta, 736	Curitiba
Lima, Concessa Maria Mendes	Rua Carlos Cavalcanti, 273 apto. 132, Centro	Curitiba
Luz, Gualton Garcez da	Travessa Agostinho Macedo, 156, Bairro Taboão	Curitiba
Maimone, Nelson	Av. Brasil, 3765	Maringa
Meweghel, Marlia de Oliveira		Pendeirantes
Miranda, Carlos G.	Av. Brasil. S/N	Cascavel
Monteiho, Rubens Costa	Rua Amapa, 744	Paranavai
Moreira, Carlos Augusto	Rua Marechal Deodoro, 211, conj. 605	Curitiba
Moreira, Saly Maria Bugman.	Rua Marechal Deodoro, 211, apto 605	Curitiba
Moreira Filho, Carlos Augusto	Rua Visconde de Nacar, 860	Curitiba
Mota Filho, Eduardo Froes da	Av. Brasil, 3325	Maringa
Mutti, Vicente D.	Rua 15 de novembro, 595, Caixa postal 286	Irati
Naito, Tadashi	Rua Santos Dumont. 2467	Maringa
Nassif, Antonio Celso Nunes	Praça Zacarias, 36, 8° andar	Curitiba
Nitta, Kunihiro	Caixa postal 318	Maringa
Nogueira, Clarisvaldo	Rua Manoel Ribas, 450	Paranavai
Novais, Dantom	Av. Minas Gerais, 34	Cornelio Procopio
Peixoto, Walmyer Almeida	Praça. Zacarias, Ed. Santa Maria, 3° andar	Curitiba
Penteado, Renato Rocha	Rua Visc. de Nacar, 431 apto. 208.	Ponta Grossa
Piechnik, Mathias	Rua Cel. Dulcidio, 1080	Curitiba
Pimpão, Nelson Biasone Ferreira	Rua Piaui, 580	Londrina
Pinto, Anor Dittert	Rua Bom Jesus, 134	Rio Negro
Rebello, Raquel	Rua Lamenha Lins, 261	Curitiba
Ribas, Roberto Hiram	Rua Lamenha Lins, 261	Curitiba
Rosa, Jose		
Sakata, Kenji	Rua Barão do Rio Branco, 63 s. 507	Curitiba
Saliba, Antonio	Rua Augusto Ribas, 486	Ponta Grossa

Samara, Antonio Vantuil .. Rua Carmelo Rangel, 600 ...... Curitiba

Santos, Paulo Cesar dos ... Rua Cons. Araujo, 271 apto. 2, Centro .... Curitiba

Schaedler, Hilario ....

Schwartz Filho, Humberto . Rua Barão do Cerro Azul, 252, apto. 104 .... Curitiba

Sessak, Romão .... Praça Willie Davids, 795 .... Londrina

Silveira, Ody Traback ..... Av. Rio de Janeiro, 765 .... Londrina

Simas Fernando .... Av. Vicente Machado, 972 ..... Curitiba

Siqueira Neto, Otavio ..... Rua Balduino Taques, 480 ..... Ponta Grossa

Soares Filho, Francisco de Paula .... Edificio, ASA, Praça Gal. Osório Curitiba

Stabile, Jose Justino ...... Rua Erastos Gaetner, 1637 apto. 202, Bacacheri .... Curitiba

Stramare, Tito Lívio ...... Rua Dom Fernando Taddei, 861 Jacaresinho

Sue, Takashi .... Caixa postal 1632 .... Curitiba

Szymanski, Constantino Leszek .... Av. Brasil, 2784 .... Cascavel

Thá, Rosaldo .... Rua Comendador Araujo, 279 apto. 701 .... Curitiba

Ulzefer, Edimar .... Rua São Paulo, 640 .... Cascavel

Uscocovich, Carlos Orejuela . Inst. de oftal. e otorrino e endosc., Rua Souza Naves, S/N . Cascavel

Vida, Alcione Bonancin ... Hospital e maternidade de Palotina .... Palotina

Vieira, Jose ....

Vieira, Lino Pineda .... Rua Manoel Ribas, 850 .... Paranavai

Vieira, Sidney Iglestas ..... Rua Emiliano Perneta, 837 apto. 1401, Centro .... Curitiba

Wambier, Ary Riesemberg . Rua Engenheiro Schamber, 928, 2° andar .... Ponta Grossa

Werner, Ciro Nael .... Rua Maringa, 752 Caixa postal 1447 .... Londrina

Zorning, Luiz Fernando ... Rua Candido Lopes, 205, conj. 13, 1° andar .... Curitiba

Pernambuco

Albuqerque, Inácio Cavalcante de .... Rua do Progresso, 71 .... Recife

Almeida, Eduardo Eustaquio de ....

Almeida Filho, Odilon Oliveira de ....

Alves, Sergio Guilherme ... Rua Minas Gerais, 80 .... Recife

Andrade, Francisco Lessa de Av. Beira Mar, Rio Doce .... Olinda

Antunes, Zinio da Silva .... Edificio Santo Albino, Av. Guararapes, 86 s. 703 .... Recife

Araujo, Edinaldo Coelho de . Rua Professora Lourdes Dutra, 42, Agua Fria .... Recife

Arruda, Adolfo Pereira de .. Rua Dom Sebastião Leme, 127, Graças .... Recife

Barbosa Filho, Jose Diomedes .... Rua Arlindo Gouveia, 39 apto. 319, Madalena .... Recife

Barreto, Silvio Paes .... Av. Roda e Silva, 1687 .... Recife

Batista Filho, Jose .... Praça Jardim, 16 .... Garanhuns

Beltrão, Jose de Vasconcelos	Rua da Imperatriz, 187, 1° andar.	Recife
Cavalcanti, Eduardo	Ed. Ouro Branco s-605	Recife
Cavalcanti Neto, Severiano de S.	Rua Jader de Andrade, 148, Casa Forte	Recife
Costa, Aylton Ferreira da ..	Rua Dr. Jose Mariano, 406	Garanhus
Costa, Alcides Fernandes da.	Rua Jader de Andrade, 321, Casa Forte	Recife
Cunha, Diomedes Leonardo da	....	
Dias, Aurimenes	Hospital São Sebastião	Caruaru
Figueiredo, Henrique Cesar .	Ed. Armando Bastos, 6° andar, Av. Guararapes, 210	Recife
Figueiredo, Jayme	Praça do Entroncamento, 104 ..	Recife
Florencio, Heriberto Monteiro	Rua Coronel Limeira, 28	Caruaru
Fonseca, Propercio Gomes da	Hospital Militar de Recife	Recife
Freitas, Manoel Cavalcanti Gomes de	Rua da Amizade, 94 apto. 601 Bloco B, Graças	Recife
Galvão, Roberto	Av. Visconde de Suassuna, 505 ..	Recife
Gomes, Alvaro	....	
Humberto, Vasconcelos Beltrão	Rua Dr. Jose Maria, 171, Bairro, Encruzilhada	Recife
Lins, Mem Sampaio Barreto .	Rua Nova, 356, 1° andar	Recife
Lins, Nilo Emanoel Barreto .	Rua Nova, 356	Recife
Lira, Pedro Cavalcanti	Rua Cardeal Arcoverde, 197, Graças	Recife
Lopes, Afranio Roberto Ferreira	....	
Lopes, Newton Guimarães Cardoso	....	
Mayer, Mozar Barros	Rua Barão de Itamaraca, 455, Espinheiro	Recife
Medeiros, Afonso Ligorio de	Av. Visconde de Suassuna, 505 ..	Recife
Menezes, Paulo Jose de	Av. Gal. San Martin, 2144, San Martin	Recife
Paiva, Clovis	Rua dos Navegantes, 2465, Boa Viagem	Recife
Pessoa, Roberto Salazar da Veiga	Rua Alfredo Ozorio, 363, Tamarineira	Recife
Ramalho, Dario de Paiva ...	Av. João Pessoa, 768	Arcoverde
Ramos Junior, Luiz	....	
Rego, Luiz Gonzaga	....	
Saldanha, Ernani Nogueira .	Rua São Félix, 187, Bairro, Campo Grande	Recife
Sampaio, Jose Livonio	Rua do Progresso, 368 apto. 43, Boa Vista	Recife
Santos, Ely Almeida	Rua Santa Leonor, 56	Recife
Silva, Ermano Flavio Alves da	Rua Samuel Campelo, 192 Espinheiro	Recife
Souza, Jorge de	....	
Suassuna, Anacleto	Rua Bruno Maia, 181 apto. 503 .	Recife

Valença, Durval Selva ..... Av. Visconde de Suassuna, 505 .. Recife
Valença, Tubal .... Av. Beira Rio, 651, Bairro, Mada-
lena .... Recife
Valente, Adolpho .... Rua da Hora, 519, apto. 606, Es-
pinheiro .... Recife
Vaz, Levi Tenorio .... Rua Leonardo Pacheco Duque, 36 Arcoverde
Ventura, Altino .... Rua do Progresso, 71 .... Recife
Vieira, Ruth Maria G. ..... Rua João de Barros, 255 .... Recife
Vilaça, Jose Araujo .... Rua Nova, Ed. Santana S- 306 .. Recife
Zaverucha, Abrahão ...... Rua Eng. Paulo Bittencourt, 65 . Recife

Piauí

Carvalho, Evaldo .... Rua Anfrisio Lobão, 1235 ..... Terezina
Carvalho, Jose Epifanio de . Rua Machado de Assis, 1490 ... Teresina
Cerqueira, Jose Mendes de . Praça Getulio Vargas, 594 ...... Piracuruca
Costa, Abilio de Lima ..... Rua 7 de setembro, 118 .... S. Raimundo Nonato
Costa, Gilberto Martins de
Araujo .... Rua São João, 512 .... Floriano
Costa, Sebastião Martins de
Araujo .... Rua Euripedes de Aguiar, S.N. .. Floriano
Gonçalves, João Orlando
Ribeiro .... Rua Areolino de Abreu, 1476 ... Terezina
Gonçalves, Paulo Tarso Ri-
beiro .... Rua Nogueira Tapeti, S.N. ..... Oeiras
Magalhães, Mansueto Martins Rua General Osório, 2061 ..... Terezina
Sampaio, Angelo Gil Ferreira
de .... Clinica Oseas Sampaio, Rua David
Caldas, 173-N .... Terezina
Silveira, Durwagner Barros
da .... Rua Félix Pacheco, 1101 ...... Terezina

Rio Grande do Norte

Araujo, Manoel Teixeira de . Rua João Pessoa, 219, 2° andar,
Edifício Sisal .... Natal
Couto, Fernando A. Martins
do .... Praça 30 de setembro, 129 ..... Messoro
Dantas Filho, Inamar ..... Rua Joaquim Fabricio, 245, Pe-
tropolis .... Natal
Evangelista, Luiz .... Praça da Conceição .... Macau
Fernandes, Raul Pessoa .... Rua Vigario Bartolomeu, 592 ... Natal
Flor, Tania Gomes .... Rua Marechal Deodoro .... Natal
França Filho, Luiz .... Av. Salvado Filho, 1653, Tirol .. Natal
Fulco, Marcos Francisco de
Assis .... Av. Rodrigues Alves, 738, Triol . Natal
Garcia, Carlos Alexandre de
A. ....
Medeiros, Ivo .... Rua Monsenhor Jose Paulino,
1063, Centro .... Natal
Melo, Manoel Villar de ....
Monte, João Maria de Miran-
da .... Rua Maxaranguape, 619, Tirol .. Natal
Monte, Luiz Gonzaga de
Miranda .... Rua Afonso Pena, 1034, Bairro,
Tirol .... Natal

Oliveira, João Carrilho de ..	Av. Maranhão, 1244	Mossoro
Sa, Maria S.C. de	Av. Deodoro, 670 apto. 903	Natal
Silva, Jose de Anchieta Ferreira da	Rua Manoel Machado, 370	Natal
Silveira, João Luiz Borba da.	....	

Rio Grande do Sul

Abreu, Jose Darly	Rua Andre Marques, 643	97100 Santa Maria
Aires, Jose Alberto	Rua Marques de Caxias, 288	Rio Grande
Alegre, Irai Albuquerque Porto	Faculdade Catolica de Medicina, Rua Sarmento Leite, 245 ...	Porto Alegre
Altmayer, João Hugo	Rua General Portinho, 446	Rio Grande
Altmayer, Jose Antonio ...	Rua Dr. Nascimento, 763	Rio Grande
Almeida, Jorge	Rua Marechal Floriano, 744	96800 Santa Cruz do Sul
Alvares, Helio	Enf. 25, Santa Casa	Porto Alegre
Alvarez, Marlene	Rua Floriano Peixoto, 1.548 ...	Santa Maria
Alves, Fernando Voges	Rua Republica, 87, 1° andar	Porto Alegre
Alves, Jose Moreira	Rua Octavio Rocha, 40, 2° andar.	Porto Alegre
Andreazza, Ely Jose	Av. Julio de Castilhos, 1989	Caxias do Sul
Antunes, Marilene Freitas ..	Av. A, 8, Vila Icaro	Canoas
Araujo, Belo João	Enf. 25, Santa Casa	Porto Alegre
Argemi Filho, Jose Maria ..	Rua 15 de Novembro, 2.207	Uruguaiana
Arroyo, Angel Del	Enf. 25, Santa Casa	Porto Alegre
Athayde, Orlando Dias	Villa Dr. Pestana	Ijui
Ayres, Alberto Jose	Av. Silva Paes, 443	Rio Grande
Azambuja, Mario Araujo ...	Rua Carlos de Carvalho, 63	Porto Alegre
Baglioni, Getulio	Rua Gal. Marques, 807	São Borja
Barbosa, Gil Horta	Caixa Postal 364	95.100 Caxias do Sul
Barbosa, Luiz Antonio Horta	Rua 13 de Maio, 489	Caxias do Sul
Barbosa, Paulo Horta	Rua Sarmento Leite, 187	Porto Alegre
Basile, Breno	Rua Tamandare, 303	Livramento
Bastos, Helio	Hospital Militar	Cachoeira do Sul
Bastos, Sau da Silva	Rua General Neto, 109 apto. 72 .	Novo Hamburgo
Becker, Marco Antonio	Av. João Pessoa, 41 apto. 520 ..	Porto Alegre
Behrendt, Rodolf	Av. Getulio Vargas, 1331	Porto Alegre
Beltrão, Aecio Cesar	Rua Riachuelo, 1583 apto. 21 ..	Porto Alegre
Beltrão, Romeu	Rua Mal. Floriano, 1100	Santa Maria
Bem, Victor Hugo Cardone de	Rua Duque de Caxias, 541 apto. 1003, Centro	Porto Alegre
Bocaccio, Francisco Jose de Lima	Rua Toblas Barreto, 71	Porto Alegre
Bof, Arnaldo	Rua General Vitorino, 254 apto. 704	Porto Alegre
Bolli, Paulo Afonso S.	Hospital São Francisco	Porto Alegre
Bona, Celso de	Enf. 25, Santa Casa	Porto Alegre
Brasil, Eduardo Assis	Galeria Chaves, 2° andar	Porto Alegre
Brasil, Oscar	....	
Bruck, Regis Correa	Av. Guaiba, 4060	Porto Alegre
Brunstein, Simão	Av. Salgado Filho, 28	Porto Alegre
Buede, Carlos	Av. Senador Salvado Filho, 233 S/54	Porto Alegre
Camilotti, Teodorico W. ...	Rua do Acampamento, 326	Santa Maria
Capuano, Atilio Jose	....	

Cardon, Efraim	Rua Prof. Annes Dias, 154-S/601, Centro	Porto Alegre
Cardon, Joni	Rua Jose Bonifacio, 719, Bonfim.	Porto Alegre
Carrion, Carlos Augusto Machado	Rua Luciana de Abreu, 450	Porto Alegre
Castagno, Roger Lahorgue .	Rua Anchieta, 2112	Pelotas
Castagno, Sidney	Rua Anchieta, 256	Pelos
Castro, Arthur Viliamil de .	Av. Barão de Upacaray, 1101 ...	Dom Pedrito
Castro, Djalma Fiuza de ...	Rua Bernardino Angelo, 1103 ..	Dom Pedrito
Cattoi, Nestor Sergio	Rua Julio de Castilhos, 621 apto. 405	Lajeado
Cavalheiro, Jacir Bonat	Rua Andrade Neves, 821	Pelotas
Cezar, Reinaldo Fernando .	Rua do Acampamento, 326	Santa Maria
Chassavoimaister, Geraldo .	Rua Dr. Fernando Vieira, 501 apto. 34	Porto Alegre
Cini, Carlos	Rua Duque de Caxias, 613	Cruz Alta
Cini, Mario	Rua Quintino Bocaiuva, 1035 ...	Porto Alegre
Coelho, Renan	Rua 7 de Setembro, 961	Cachoeira do Sul
Correa, Gildrades da Costa .	Rua dos Andradas, 1273	97100 Santa Maria
Correa, Nelson Ritencourt .	Rua Dr. Flores, 245, apto 31 ...	Porto Alegre
Costa, Nadyr Pereira da ...	Rua Mal. Floriano, 427 S- 202 ..	Santa Cruz do Sul
Coulon, Carlos Arthur	Rua do Guia Lopes, 587	Caxias do Sul
Couto, Hilton Santos	Rua João Brasil, 942	Rosário do Sul
Covolo, Alcir Beretta	Rua Dr. Bozano, 1661 apto. 302 .	Santa Maria
Crosseti, Francisco	Rua do Acampamento, 434	Santa Maria
Crosseti, José Erasmo	Rua do Acampamento, 334	Santa Maria
Cunha, Luiz Phelipe da	Rua Bento Gonçalves, 221	Passo Fundo
Degrazia, Carlos Oswaldo ..	....	
Degrazia, Newton Carlos ...	Rua Bento Marins	Uruguaiana
Donato, Donato Di	Rua Gomes Jardim, 1188	Porto Alegre
Duarte, Manoel C.	Galeria Chaves S-23	Porto Alegre
Duarte Neto, Plotino Amaro	Rua 24 de Octubro, 847, Bairro Independência	Porto Alegre
Durval, Paulo	Rua Dr. Cassiano, 105	Pelotas
Esteves, Aldehyr Luiz	Rua Uruguai, 240	Porto Alegre
Esteves, Elizabeth H.	Rua Fernando Gomes, 38 apto. 32.	Porto Alegre
Esteves, Paulo Fernando ...	Av. Bagé, 1400, Bairro. Petropolis	Porto Alegre
Ferraz Filho, Diogo	Av. João Pessoa, 735	Porto Alegre
Ferreira, Flávio	Av. Protasio Alves, 865 apto. 703	Porto Alegre
Foernges, Aldo Bruno	Rua dos Andradas, 1727, 8° andar	Porto Alegre
Fontoura, Saul	Rua Independencia, 98	Porto Alegre
Fortes, João Borges	Rua dos Andradas, 1664 apto. 26, 5° andar	Porto Alegre
Fortes, Manuel Inacio Mansur	Rua Bento Gonçalves, 123 D ...	Bagé
Frasseto, Gilmore	Rua Mal. Floriano, 1031, 1° andar	Santa Maria
Freitas, Jovino da Silva	Av. Brasil. 234 apto. 3	Passo Fundo
Galbinski, David	Rua Dr. Flores, 262, Conj. 84, 8° andar	Porto Alegre
Gama, Jose Carlos Costa ...	Praça Dom Feliciano, 126 apto 152	Porto Alegre
Geiger, Delton Ney	Edificio Dr. Honorato, 1° andar, Rua 7 de setembro, S/N	Cachoeira do Sul
Giugno, Olimpio	Rua Osvaldo Aranha S.N.	Veranopolis

Goldhardt, Bruno B.	....	Panambi
Gomes, Antonio Alverne Ferreira	Rua Santo Antonio, 299, apto. 102	Porto Alegre
Goncalves, Danilo	Av. Tupi Silveira, 1649	Bagé
Gonçalves, Paulo Miranda ..	Rua Venancio Aires, 2003	São Luiz Gonzaga
Gontan, Antonio Carlos Crossetti	Rua Mal. Floriano, 433 apto. 102	Santa Cruz do Sul
Gorrese, Pascoal Pery	....	
Goulart, Joaquim Paulo de O.	....	Jaguarão
Grimaldi, João Caetano ...	Rua Irmão Weibert, 364, Partenon	Porto Alegre
Hansen, Jardeci Machado ..	....	
Hoefel, Jorny C.	Av. Independencia, 701	São Leopoldo
Horst, Udo	Enf. 25, Santa Casa	Porto Alegre
Jorge, Nivea Burgos	Av. Independencia, 270	Porto Alegre
Juchem, Claudio Alberto da Fontoura	Rua Barão de Santo Angelo, 11 apto. 302	Porto Alegre
Knijnik, Leon	Rua General João Tales, 424 apto. 5	Porto Alegre
Kopper, Alipio	....	
Kruel, Antonio Loureiro ...	Av. Brasil, 1089	Passo Fundo
Kruel, Ivo	Rua dos Andradas, 1727, 6° andar	Porto Alegre
Kwitko, Idel Luiz	Rua Venancio Aires, 928 apto. 401	Porto Alegre
Lara, Armando de	Rua Coronel Bordini, 803	Porto Alegre
Leite, Wilson de Oliveira ...	Rua Intendente Alfredo Azevedo, 580, Bairro, Gloria	Porto Alegre
Lenzi, Raphael Jose Antonio	Rua Dr. Flores, S.N.	Nova Prata
Leo, Renato Carlos de	Rua dos Andradas, 1737	Porto Alegre
Leutchuk, Antonio	Hospital São Jose	Tres Passos
Lubisco, Humberto	Rua dos Andradas, 1137 apto. 1110, 12° andar	Porto Alegre
Maltchik, Jaime	Rua Ramiro Barcelos, 1591	Porto Alegre
Marcon, Italo Mundialino ..	Rua Vicente da Fontoura, 2342 apto. 102, Bairro, Petropolis .	Porto Alegre
Marcon, Natalino	Rua 13 de Maio, 336	Veranopolis
Mariath, Alfredo	....	
Marranguello, Italo	Rua Ramiro Barcelos, 1868 apto. 21	Porto Alegre
Marroni, Belmonte	Rua Mal. Floriano S.N	Soledade
Martini, Artemio	Rua Bento Gonçalves	97650, Itaqui
Martins, Alberto Eduardo ..	Hospital de caridade	Taquara
Martins, Dinarte Silveira ...	Rua Fernando Gomes, 174	Porto Alegre
Martins, Luthero Dutra	Rua Cel. Chicuta, 175	Passo Fundo
Mascarenhas, Arthur	Rua dos Andradas, 1727	Porto Alegre
Mazzei, Dirceu	Rua dos Andradas, 1727, 4° andar	Porto Alegre
Medeiros, Dirceu Camargo de	Clinica N.S. da aparecida, Rua do Comércio. S/N	Frederico Westphalen
Medici, Mario Garrastasu ..	Posto de higiene de Jaguarão ...	Jaguarão
Meyer, Paulo Mendes Correa	Rua Quintino Bocaiuva, 325 apto. 5, Bairro Moinhos de vento ..	Porto Alegre

Meyer, Rivadavia Mendes Correa	Rua Sarmento Leite, 187	Porto Alegre
Mendes, Alexandre Argollo .	....	
Mentz, Ernani	Rua dos Andradas, 1727 apto 21 .	Porto Alegre
Mesko, Iremar Couto	Rua Francisco Ferrer, 385 apto. 22	Porto Alegre
Metsavaht, Renato	Hospital N.S. Pompéia	Caxias do Sul
Morais, Gabriel Ferreira de .	Rua 24 de Maio, 38	Cachoeira do Sul
Morais, Jorge	....	
Morais, Salucio Breno de ..	Av. Andrade Neves, 417	Cachoeira do Sul
Muller, Egon Roeber	Hospital Tuparendi	Tuparendi (via Santa Rosa)
Muller, Lauro L.	Edifício Cruzeiro do Sul, 2° andar	Porto Alegre
Nesi, Vicente Carmine	....	
Nevedoski, Victor	Rua Ramiro Barcelos, 2171 apto. 42	Porto Alegre
Nicolini, Jair J.	Rua Cel. Chicuta, 175	Passo Fundi
Noal, Antoninho	Rua Venancio Aires, 893	Santa Maria
Obara, José	Rua do Cômércio, 69	Ijui
Oliveira, Luiz Renato Garcez	....	
Oliveira, Wanderley Kneipp de	Rua Com. Batista, 26	Porto Alegre
Olszewski, Edmundo	Praça D. Feliciano, 56 apto. 82 ..	Porto Alegre
Olszewski, Sergio	Praça Dom Feliciano, 56 apto 82 .	Porto Alegre
Osorio, Luiz Assunção	Rua Gal. Vitorino, 161, 2° andar .	Porto Alegre
Palludo, Marny	Rua Osvaldo Aranha, 232 apto. 5.	Porto Alegre
Passos, Paulo	Caixa Postal 66	Bagé
Pellegrini, Renato Danilo W..	Rua Andrade Neves, 35	Rio Pardo
Pellin, Roberto	Av. Wenceslau Escobar, 3239, Tristeza	Porto Alegre
Pereira, Paulo H. Leggerini .	Rua Luciana de Abreu, 461	Porto Alegre
Piltcher, Isaac Levin	Rua 15 de Novembro, 703 apto. 11	Pelotas
Pinto, Ary Antonio	Galeria Chaves, 1° andar	Porto Alegre
Pinto, Policarpo Marlei	Rua Venancio Aires, 479	Alegrete
Pires, Alberto	Rua Marques de Caxias, 288	Rio Grande
Pithan, Lincoln Abrett	Rua Vasco Alves, 294	Alegrete
Primio, Raul Franco de	Rua Venancio Aires, 946	Porto Alegre
Raase, Hugo	Hospital Tuparendi	Santa Rosa
Ramos, Rubens S.	Rua do Guia Lopes, 1041	Caxias do Sul
Ramos, Segic Manoel	Av. Julio de Castilhos, 1983	Caxias do Sul
Raskim, David	Rua Fernandes Vieira, 204 apto. 302, Independencia	Porto Alegre
Raskim, Simão	Av. Rio Branco, 731	Santa Maria
Reller, Nelson	Rua Duque de Caxias, 798 apto. 33	Porto Alegre
Rizzato, Roberto Rossi	Rua do Acampamento, 326	Santa Maria
Rocha, Ailton Lovato da ..	Rua Capivari, 240	Porto Alegre
Rocha, Nelson	Rua Major Ouriques, 760	Cachoeira do Sul
Roeber, Guilherme Roberto	Rua Cel. Martins, 1195	Cruz Alta
Romani, Flavio Antonio ...	Rua do Acampamento, 434	Santa Maria
Rossi Filho, Armindo	Rua do Acampamento, 326	Santa Maria
Rotman, Hugo	....	
Sabani, Moyses	Rua General João Telles, 399 ...	Porto Alegre
Salengue, Gervasio Belchior .	Rua 15 de Novembro, 253	Pelotas
Salim, Carlos	Hospital Santa Terezinha	Erechim
Sander, Pedro	Av. João Pessoa, S.N.	Canela

Sanmartin, Zeniro Jose	Av. Farrapos, 1432 apto. 11, Floresta	Porto Alegre
Santiago, Jose de Oliveira ..	Rua dos Andradas, 1711 sala-501.	Porto Alegre
Santos, Paulo Roberto dos .	Rua Duque de Caxias, 1594 apto. 901 Centro	Porto Alegre
Santos, Valdir G. dos	....	
Schafer, João Carlos Bauer .	Rua Miguel Teixeira, 83 apto. 63, Cidade Baixa	Porto Alegre
Schaffer, Paulo Roberto ...	Rua dos Andradas, 918 apto. 904	Porto Alegre
Schermann, Alfredo	Rua dos Andradas, 1664, 3° andar	Porto Alegre
Schermann, Israel	Rua dos Andradas, 1664, 3° andar	Porto Alegre
Schirmer, Marion Bastola ..	Rua 7 de Setembro, 848	Cachoeira do Sul
Schirmer, Mirton Bastola ..	Rua Marechal Floriano, 666	Palmeira das Missões
Schmidt, Victor	Rua Quintino Bocaiuva, 1010 ...	Porto Alegre
Schmitz, Jones Jose Araujo .	Travessa Republica, 74	Santa Rosa
Sebastiany, Gilson	Av. João Antonio, 747	Sobradinho
Seibel, Valter A. Ayres	Rua Silva Paes, 443	96200, Rio Grande
Seligman, Mauricio	Rua Venancio Aires, 964	Porto Alegre
Seligman, Rafael	Av. Dr. Bozano, 1120, 1° andar .	Santa Maria
Silva, Roberto Silveira da ..	....	
Silva Filho, Francisco das Chagas	Rocca Salles	Estrela
Silveiro, Antonio Augusto .	Av. Encantado, 148 apto. 302 ..	Porto Alegre
Silveira, Fernando Gomes da	Caixa Postal 247	Erechim
Silveira, Luiz Fernando da .	....	
Silveira, Ruy Barbosa da ...	Rua Euclides da Cunha, 14	Alegrete
Silveira Neto, João Alfredo .	Av. João Pessoa, 651	90000, Porto Alegre
Snel, Ito	Hospital Policlinica Arroio da Seca	Estrela
Soares, João Paulo Correa ..	....	
Soria, Freddy Flaviano Torrico	Rua Julio de Castilhos, 640	Osório
Souza, Carlos Gomes da Silva e	Rua Floriano Peixoto, 888 – altos, Centro	Santa Maria
Souza, João Edson Scherer de	Rua Pedro Vargas, 578	Carazinho
Spessatto, Nolvar	Rua Floriano Peixoto, 130	Santa Maria
Spolidoro, Angelo Raphael .	....	
Sprinz, Simão	Rua Fernandes Viera, 238 apto. 701	Porto Alegre
Stanziola, Roberto Oreste ..	Rua Ramiro Barcelos, 1709 apto.. 6	Porto Alegre
Steffem, Alcidio Paulo	Rua Santo Angelo, 414	Santa Rosa
Taicher, José C.	Rua Joaquim Nabuco, 957	93300, Novo Hamburgo
Tavares, Raimundo Nonato da Silva	Rua Cel. Sezefredo, 371	São Gabriel
Teixeira Neto, Corçom	Rua Cel. Cipriano Ferreira, 481 .	Porto Alegre
Telicheveski, Isaac	....	
Telles, Nelton Guimarães ..	Rua Felipe de Oliveira, 1193, Bairro, Petropolis	Porto Alegre
Terrosso, Fernando	Rua Luiz Lorea, 381	96200, Rio Grande
Tombesi, Regis Lambert ...	Praça Saturnino de Brito, 16	Santa Maria
Trois, Sylvio Martins	Rua Candido Falcão, 1869	São Borja

Veronese, Pedro .... Rua Marques do Herval, 1331 ... Santo Angelo
Viecelli, Sergio Vito ...... Rua Uruguai, 610 .... Santana do Livramento
Vissirini, Caetano .... Rua Borges de Medeiros, 809 ... Caxias do Sul
Wagner, Alvino .... Av. Farrapos, 2302 .... Porto Alegre
Wallenhauit, Siegfried Paulo
  Germano .... Rua Mariz e Barros, 193 .... Cruz Alta
Wallwitz, York Arminio E.
  Von .... Rua General Sampaio, 126 ..... Bagé
Walmarath, Jose Antonio .. ..
Withz, Germano Von Wal .. Av. 7 de Setembro, 1168 ...... Bagé
Zanette, Waldomiro João .. Enf. 25, Santa casa .... Porto Alegre
Zanol, Ademar Levi ...... Rua Professor Braga, 79 apto. 55 . Santa Maria
Zeillmann, Fausto Feres ... Hospital São Vicente de Paulo,
  Rua Venancio Aires. 163 .... Cruz Alta

Santa Catarina

Agumi, Seiko .... Rua Benjamin Constant, S/N ... Caçador
Almeida, Joubert Barros de . Rua Pres. Nereu Ramos, 73, 2º
  andar .... Lages
Araujo, João .... Rua Hercilio Luz S/N .... Lages
Barbosa, Aylton Alves .... Rua Ferreira Lima, 13 apto. 404 . Florianópolis
Barreto, Julibyo Jupy ..... Rua Silva Jardim, 222 .... Florianópolis
Beltrão, Luiz Calderan .... Caixa Postal 289 .... Joaçaba
Canter, Moacir .... Rua do Principe, 330 apto. 812 . Joinville
Carbonell, Washington F. .. Caixa Postal 234 .... Brusque
Chanem, Emir Amin ...... Rua Abdon Baptista, 172 ...... Joinville
Chanem, Sadala Amin ..... Rua Abdom Batista, 172 ...... Joinville
Coral, Cleusa .... Rua Abdon Baptista, 172 ...... Joinville
Dumsch, Arnaldo .... Hospital N/S, do Sagrado Cora-
  ção, Descanso .... São Miguel do Oeste
Ferro, Antonio Roberto de
  Moura .... Av. 7 de Setembro, 353 .... Rio do Sul
Fonseca, Gilberto Guerreiro
  da .... Rua Felipe Schmidt, 99 .... Florianópolis
Fontes, Henrique Jose Filo-
  meno .... Rua Alves de Brito, 15, Centro .. Florianópolis
Freusberg, Otto .... Largo de São Sebastião, 9 ...... Florianópolis
Heuzi, Fernando Luiz ..... Rua 15 de Novembro, 1135 .... Blumenau
Kechelei, Hans Egon ...... Hospital Sagrada Família ..... São Bento do Sul
Lawinski, Jacob .... Rua Dorval Malquiades de Souza,
  29, 4º andar .... Florianópolis
Liberato, Afonso Celso .... Rua 15 de Julho, 32 .... Itajai
Lunardi, Valmor Ernesto .. Hospital Santo Antonio .... Chapeco
Mendes, Aramis Ritzmann . Rua Ruy Barbosa, 20 .... Florianópolis
Miranda, Manoel .... Hospital de Tubarão .... Tubarão
Neves, Decio R. Madeira ... Largo Benjamin Constant, 21 ... Florianópolis
Niemeyer, Erico Rocco .... Rua Paraguay, 71, Caixa Postal
  381 .... Blumenau
Packeter, Henrique .... Caixa Postal 199 .... Criciuma
Peters, Carl Heinz .... Rua 7 de Setembro, 1560 ...... Blumenau
Rahal, Jose Carlos .... Caixa Postal 405 .... Joaçaba
Ramos,   Airton   Rogério
  Ribeiro .... Rua Nereu Ramos, 100 .... Lajes
Santhiago, Wilson Gomes .. Hospital Santa Izabel .... Blumenau
Santhiago, Wilson Holtrup . Rua Almirante Tamandaré, 737,
  Vila Nova .... Blumenau

Serrão, Eneas	Orleães, Lauro Muller	Estado de Santa Catarina
Silva, Getulio Alvino	Praça Hercilio Luz, 67	Porto União
Urban, Aldo Floriano	Rua Mario Lobo, 45	Joinville
Vieira, Julio Doin	Rua Bocaiuva, 6	Florianópolis
Zaguini, Hélio Luiz	Rua Hercílio Luz, 16	Itajai

São Paulo

Abramowicz, Doris Blay ...	Rua Oscar Freire, 836 apto. 134, Gerqueira Cesar	01426 São Paulo
Abreu, Jose Maria P. Queiroz	Rua Coronel Quirino, 1131, Cambui	Campinas
Abreu, Manoel Penteado Queiroz	Rua Viscondessa de Campinas, 400	Campinas
Abucham, Julio	Rua Sampaio Viana, 125 apto. 22, Paraiso	04004, São Paulo
Abucham, Roberto	Rua Conselheiro Brotero, 1417 apto 12	São Paulo
Abud, Emilio	Rua 7 de Abril, 118, 4° andar ...	São Paulo
Abujamra, Suel	Rua Sampaio Viana, 125 apto. 83, Paraiso	04004, São Paulo
Aguiar, Alexandre	Rua Deputado Emilio Carlos, 130 Bairro de Limão	2721 São Paulo
Aguiar, Luiz Amador	Cl. Oftal. da S. Casa de Misericordia, Rua Dr. Cezario Mota Junior, 112, Vila Buarque ...	01221 São Paulo
Agujar, Jose Pessoa	Rua 15 de Novembro, 930	Piracicaba
Aguiar Filho, João de Campos	Rua Paula Souza, 277	Sorocaba
Aidar, Mauricio Marinho ...	Viaduto 9 de Julho, 181, 9° andar	São Paulo
Aihara, Teruo	Rua Benjamin Constant, 54	Suzano
Albertão, Claudomiro	Rua Dr. Gurgel, 102	Presidente Prudente
Albuquerque, Zid	Rua D. Jose de Barros, 168, 3° andar	São Paulo
Alencar, Pedro de	Rua 15 de Novembro, 58, Itararé.	São Paulo
Alencar Neto, Rufino Antunes	Rua Coropes, 281 A, Pinheiros ..	São Paulo
Alexandre, Luiz Gonzaga ..	Av. Brig. Luiz Antonio, 4166, Jardim Paulista	São Paulo
Almada, Alexandre Terra ..	Rua Loefgren, 1690 apto. 4, Vila Clementino	04040 São Paulo
Almanza, Dario W. Waldivia.	Caixa Postal 84	São Paulo
Almeida, Aluysio Machado de	Rua Riachuelo, 66, Conj. 61	Santos
Almeida, Antonio Augusto de	Instituto Penido Burnier	Campinas
Almeida, Cardoso de	Rua Cel. Oliveira Lima, 173	Santo André
Almeida, Celio de	Av. Rodrigues Alves, 6-52	Bauru
Almeida, Domingos Savio de Aquino	Rua Dr. Rodrigues Azevedo, 188	Lorena
Almeida, Geraldo Vicente de	Rua Duarte Da Costa, 60, Lapa .	05080 São Paulo
Almeida, Gilberto Leal de ..	Instituto Penido Burnier	Campinas
Almeida, Osvaldo	Av. Andrade Neves, 223........	Campinas
Almeida, Salvador S.	Av. Rodrigues Alves, 652	17100 Bauru
Almeida, Ulisses de Barros .	Rua Dr. Hermas Braga, 702, Bairro Nova Campinas	13100 Campinas

Almeida, Jr., Custodio de .. ..

Almeida Filho, Joscary de   Rua Quintino Bocaiuva, 629,
                             Brooklin Paulista ....   04623 São Paulo
Almeida Filho, Jose Ary de . Rua Quintino Bocaiuva, 629 ....   Itapetininga
Alves, Carlos Alberto Rodri-
gues ....
Alves, João ....   Av. Andrade Neves, 223 ....   Campinas
Alves, João Batista Camargo. Rua Major Quedinho, 99, 9°
                             andar ....   São Paulo
Alves, Luis ....   Av. Angelica, 1311 apto. 502 ...   São Paulo
Alves, Manoel Luiz ....   Rua Marechal Deodoro, 1191 ...   São Bernardo Do Campo
Alves, Osorio Augusto ....   Rua Cel. Quirino, 982 ....   Campinas
Alves Filho, Osorio ....   Rua Andrade Neves, 223 ......   Campinas
Alvite, Alderico ....
Amaral, Juares Cerqueira do   Rua Rio Grande Do Sul, 181 ...   São Caetano do Sul
Amaral, Roberto Franco do .   ...
Amaral Filho, Arthur Vicen-
te ....   Rua Cel. Xavier de Toledo, 266,
                             11° andar ....   São Paulo
Amarante, Olavo Pires do ..   ..
Amaro, Walter A. D. ......   Rua Silva Bueno, 1902, Bela Vista   04208 São Paulo
Amendola, Arnaldo Carda-
monte ....   Rua Cons. Brotero, 1379, apto.
                             22, Santa Cecilia ....   01232 São Paulo
Andrade, Ataliba Camargo
de ....   Rua 13 de Maio, 69 ....   Campinas
Andrade, Demetrio ....   Rua 26, N. 764 ....   14780 Barretos
Andrade, Geraldo de Castro   Rua 13 de Maio, 147 ....   Campinas
Andrade, João Batista de
Camargo ....   Rua 13 de Maio, 1418, apto. 81
                             Bela Vista ....   01327 São Paulo
Andrade, Lauro Camargo ..   Rua 13 de Maio, 69 ....   Campinas
Angelucci, Celso Francisco .   Cl. Oftal. do Hosp. São Paulo,
                             Rua Botucatu, 720, Vila Cle-
                             mentino ....   04023 São Paulo
Antunes, Valcir Coronado .   Rua Maua, 91 ....   Assis
Anunciação, Adriano Pinto
da ....   Rua Francisco Haro Caparroz,
                             351 ....   São Paulo
Appendino, Walter ....   Rua Ceara, 336 ....   Catanduva
Aprigliano, Orlando ......   Al. Joaquim Eugenio de Lima,
                             268 apto. 21 A, Jardim
                             Paulista ....   01403 São Paulo
Araujo, Antonio Euripedes
Gomes ....   Ed. Vital Brasil, Rua Goias, 255,
                             Conj. 42, 4° andar, Gonzaga .   Santos
Araujo, Hildebrando Macedo
de ....   Rua Lucas Obes, 52 apto. 4 ....   São Paulo
Araujo, Jose Cezar Machado
de ....   Rua da Penha, 1286 ....   Sorocaba
Arian i, Paulo ....   Rua Gal. Osorio, 183 ....   Campinas
Arruda, Egidio Correa da
Costa ....   Rua 14 de Julho, 14 ....   Campinas
Attadia, Egle Renata ......   Av. São Luis, 192 apto. 1309 ...   São Paulo
Attanes, Maury ....   Rua Nebraska, 325 ....   São Paulo
Augusto, Moema Rocha ...   Av. independencia, 1351 ......   Ribeirão Preto

Avelino Sobrinho, Jose Gomes	Av. Francisco Glicerio, 980, apto. 91	Campinas
Avila, Rubens Giraldo	Cl. Oftal. da S. Casa de Misericordia, Rua Dr. Cezario Mota Junior, 112, Vila Buarque ...	01221 São Paulo
Azeredo, Almiro	Faculdade de Medicina	Ribeirão Preto
Azevedo, Marcelo Laurentino de	Cl. Oftal. do Hosp. das Clinicas ..	São Paulo
Bachi, Herculano	Av. Dois, 160	Rio Claro
Bacchi Junior, Herculano ..	Rua 6 N. 1009, apto. 102	Rio Claro
Bacchi, Irineu Pacheco	Rua Saldanha Marinho, 995, Cidade Jardim	Piracicaba
Balbo, Roque Jose	Hosp. Vera Cruz	Campinas
Baptistela, Roberto	Alameda Vital Brasil, 190, Jardim Aurea	Mogi Mirim
Barbaro, David Jose Souza .	Rua Duque de Caxias, 763	Bededouro
Barbieri Neto, Jose	Av. Espanha, 558	Araraquara
Barbosa, Jacy	Rua Francisca Miquelina, 191 ...	São Paulo
Barbosa, Roberto Angelo ..	Rua Duque de Caxias, 954	13100 Campinas
Barbosa Filho, Luiz	Rua Riachuelo, 42, 2° andar	11100 Santos
Barreto, Carlos A. Maia Menna	Av. Guanabara, 64	Andradina
Barreto, Fernando de Mattos	Av. Ipiranga, 313, 8° andar, Centro	01046 São Paulo
Barros, Antenor de Toledo .	Rua 21 de Abril, 268	Lins
Barros, Antonio Jordão de .	Rua Gal. Osorio, 753	Ribeirão Preto
Barros, Cecilia Marina Paes de	Rua Leoncio de Carvalho, 166, Paraiso	04003 São Paulo
Barros, Maria Estela Mendonça de	Rua Napoleão de Barros, 276, Vila Mariana	04024 São Paulo
Barros, Oswaldo Monteiro de	Rua Itapeva, 300	São Paulo
Barros, Paulo M. de	Av. 17 N. 757	14780 Barretos
Bartolomeu, Aldo	Av. Dr. Arnaldo, 1372, Sumaré .	São Paulo
Bastos, Luiz Ferreira M. ...	Rua Dez. Elizeu Guilherme, 32, Paraiso	04004 São Paulo
Bei, Paulo	Av. Angelica, 2355	São Paulo
Belletato, Arnald o	Rua das Paineiras, 16	Santo André
Bellhaus, Morad Saman	Rua Antonio Bicudo, 355, apto. 3 Pinheiros	São Paulo
Bellini, Angelo Rogers	Av. Angelica, 2121 apto. 43, Santa Cecilia	01227 São Paulo
Belluzzo, Marcelo	Casa de Saude, São João Batista .	Andradina
Belmonte, Edard	Rua São Beno, 32, 1° andar	Sorocaba
Benito, Nelson	Rua Cel. Xavier de Toledo, 98, 4° andar	São Paulo
Berenguer, Sylvio de Menezes	Av. Borges Correia, 1483	Araraquara
Bergamaschi, Mario Italo ..	Av. 7 de Setembro, 2875	São Carlos
Berretini, Gino Luiz	Praça Maua, 29, 4° andar	Santos
Berti, Alberto	....	
Berti, Armando	Alameda Santos, 734, 14° andar Cerqueira-Cesar	01418 São Paulo
Berton, João Fernando	Cl. Oft. da F.C.M. Santa Casa de Misericordia, Rua Benjamin Constant, 1657	Campinas

Bertotti, Ruy Celeste	Rua Cons° Antonio Prado, 9 – 66	Bauru
Betinfane, Alberto Jorge ...	Hospital das Clinicas, Oftal.	São Paulo
Bicas, Harley Edison Amaral	Rua João Penteado, 310	Ribeirão Preto
Blois, Alcides Saverio	....	
Bonancmi, Adriano	Av. Bosque da Saude, 681	São Paulo
Bonfim, Paulo C.	Rua Vol. Delmiro Sampaio, 35 Santo Amaro	04754 São Paulo
Bonini, Ivo Sidnei	Viaduto 9 de Julho, 181, 9° andar	São Paulo
Bonomo, Pedro Paulo de Oliveira	Rua Barão de Itapetininga, 297, 3° Andar. Centro	01402 São Paulo
Borba, Luiz de Assis Pacheco	Rua Frei Caneca, 433, Bela Vista	São Paulo
Botelho, Jose Arruda	Rua Lourenço Castanho, 83	São Paulo
Boteon, Joel Edmur	Largo do Arouche, 418 apto. 225, Vila Buarque	São Paulo
Braga Neto, Antonio B. Silva	....	
Branco, Benicio de Castello .	Rua Tiradentes	Araçatuba
Branco, João B. Castelo ...	Rua Tiradentes, 6	16100 Araçatuba
Brandas, Paulo	Hospital São Judas	Jau
Brandão, Francisco Paulo ..	Rua Edgard Ferraz, 215	Jau
Brandão, Sergio Carlos	....	
Brochado, Mario Ferraz ...	Av. Mal. Deodoro, 38 apto. 64 Gonzaga	Santos
Broto, Wilson	Rua Duarte de Carvalho, 123 ...	São Paulo
Brusadin, Orlando	....	
Bueno, Adalberto Siqueira .	Av. Guanabara, 161	Andradina
Buffoni, Carlos Milton	Rua Benjamin Constant, 548 ...	São Jose. Rio Pardo
Burnier, Feliciano Penido ..	Instituto Penido Burnier	Campinas
Caldeira, Jorge Alberto Fonseca	Rua Amalia Noronha, 289, Jardim America	São Paulo
Camargo, Jaime de	Cl. Oft. da Faculdade de Medicina	Mogi das Cruzes
Camargo, Joaquim Arruda .	Av. Duque de Caxias, 728	Araraquara
Gamargo, Mario Luiz de ...	Rua Jesuino Arruda, 254 apto. 96, Itaim	04532 São Paulo
Camargo, Ruy	Av. Rangel Pestana, 2.236	São Paulo
Cambrascelli, Jose Luiz	Rua Marques do Herval, 654	Taubaté
Campanari, Oswaldo Doretto	Av. Sampaio Vidal, 535, Ed. Ouro Verde	Marilia
Campos, Carlos de Souza ..	Rua Saldanha Marinho, 321	Campinas
Campos, Hamilcar Cesar Pecego de	Praça Osvaldo Cruz, 138, Conj. 111, Santo Amaro	São Paulo
Campos, Luiz Machado	Rua Cons. Prade, 134	Birigui
Campos, Pery Alves	Rua Cel. Xavier de Toledo, 234, Centro	São Paulo
Canettieri, Francisco	Rua Dom Bosco, 533	Lorena
Carneiro, João	Rua Marconi, 131, S. 309	São Paulo
Carnio, Gilberto	Cl. Oft. da Santa Casa de Misericordia	11100 Santos
Carvalho, Celso Antonio de .	Rua Grecia, 233, Jardim Europa .	01450 São Paulo
Carvalho, Militão Villela de .	Rua Cel. Lucio Leonel, 161	Casa Branca
Carvalho, Oswaldo	Rua Presidente Vargas, 33	Marilia
Carvalho Neto, Vicente	Rua Bartira, 347, Perdizes	São Paulo
Castanheira, Eddio Calixto .	Rua Prudente de Morais, 97	Araçatuba
Castanheira, Jose Calixto ..	Rua Prudente de Morais, 87	Araçatuba

Castelani, Jose	Rua Cel. Xavier de Toledo, 210 9° andar, Centro	01048 São Paulo
Castro, Jairo Amancio de ..	....	
Castro, Luiz Alfredo Lopes de	Rua Teodoro Sampaio, 399, Pinheiros	05405 São Paulo
Castro, Manoel Domingos de	Av. Rebouças, 2267	São Paulo
Castro Filho, Sylvio Magalhães	....	
Catapano, Vicente	Rua Alvaro Ramos, 1979	São Paulo
Celeste, João	Rua 7 de Abril, 118 apto. 302 ..	São Paulo
Centurion, Virgilio A.N. ...	Av. Paulista, 352, 4° andar, Bela Vista	01310 São Paulo
Chama, Raul	Rua 24 de Maio, 35, Conj. 1007, 10° andar	São Paulo
Checchinato, Clovis Deziderio	Rua do Rosario, 78	Jundiai
Chechinato, Danilo Deziderio	Rua do Rosario, 88	13200 Jundiai
Chimelo, Diomar	Rua Alagoas, 152	158 00 Catanduva
Chuljc, Sung	Rua Santa Tereza, 21, 4° andar, Centro	01016 São Paulo
Cianciarullo, Jerry Vicente .	Av. Gal. Olimpio da Silveira, 528 apto. 202	São Paulo
Cielo, Alcides del	C.E.O. Moacir Alvaro, Rua Condessa de São Joaquim, 288, Bela Vista	01320 São Paulo
Ciero, Martinho di	....	
Cintra, Dino de Aguiar	Rua Dr. Gurgel, 548	Presidente Prudente
Cintra, Jonas Ricardo Martins	Rua Santo André, 228	Jaboticabal
Cintra, Luiz Gonzaga	Rua Andrade Neves, 558	Campinas
Cisoto, Pedro	Rua Cuiaba, 236	Catanduva
Cobra, Castor João	....	
Coelho, Elien Bussmeyer ..	Cl. Oftal. de E.P.M, Hosp. São Paulo, Rua Botucatu, 720 ...	04023 São Paulo
Coletes, Adauto Gonçalves .	Rua Barão Do Rio Branco, 541 .	Garça
Colmenero, Armindo Terra .	Rua Dom Gaspar Affonseca, 2, Bairro, Gonzaga	Santos
Conceição, Alcindo Duarte .	Av. Andrade Neves, 223	Campinas
Concilio, Luiz	Av. Aclimação, 268	São Paulo
Consolmagno, Lagardeth ..	Rua Alfredo Jose Caetano, 1240 ·	Piracicaba
Consoni Filho, Ernesto	Rua Muniz de Souza, 985 apto. 34, Cambuci	01534 São Paulo
Correa, Gilberto Delfino ...	Cl. Oftal. da S. Casa de Misericordia, Rua Dr. Cezario Mota Junior, 112, Vila Buarque ...	01221 São Paulo
Cossermelli, Wilson	Av. Paulista, 66 apto. 51	São Paulo
Costa, Ademar	Rua Inglaterra, 600	São Paulo
Costa, Alberto da Silva	Rua Voluntarios da Franca, 1583	Franca
Costa, Gomes da	Av. Rangel Pstana, 2354	São Paulo
Costa, Hermes Pereira	....	1460 Sertãozinho
Costa, Laudo Silva	....	
Costa, Marilisa Nano	Cl. Oftal da F.C.M.S. Casa de Misericordia, Rua Benjamin Constant, 1657	Campinas

Costa, Milton Menezes	Av. Pompéia, 141	São Paulo
Costa, Orlando F.	Cl. Oftalmologica Da S. Casa de Misericordia	11100 Santos
Costa Filho, Jose Gomes da.	Av. Rangel Pestana, 2308	São Paulo
Cotrim, Sergio	Rua Herval, 715, Belem	São Paulo
Cremonesi, Antonio	Rua Alvaro Ferreira dem Moraes, 159	Ourinhos
Criado, Luiz Carlos	Rua Juatindiba, 502 apto. 82 ... Parque da Mooca	São Paulo
Crochim, Salomão	Av. Celso Garcia, 3384 apto. 11 .	São Paulo
Crosio, Henrique Barbosa ..	Rua Visconde de Inhauma, 1444 .	Ribeirão Preto
Crosta, Fernando Antonio Russo	Rua Arthur Prado, 434 A apto. 83. Liberdade	01322 São Paulo
Cruz, Geovah Paulo da	E. Italia, Av. Ipiranga, 344, S/52 B Centro	01046 São Paulo
Cruz, Maria Luiza Funes Navarro da	Av. da Saudade, 3752, Santa Cruz	São Jose do Rio Preto
Cruz, Victor Bastos Navarro da	Av. da Saudade, 3752	São Jose do Rio Preto
Cugurra, Luiz	Rua Capitão João Cesario, 78, Penha	03603 São Paulo
Cunha, Moacyr Silveira	Rua Bahia, 563	São Paulo
Cunha, Rubens Lustosa ...	Rua Bahia, 563	São Paulo
Cunha, Sergio Lustosa da ..	Rua Bahia, 563, Higienopolis ...	01244 São Paulo
Curiati, Antonio Salim	Rua Rio Grande do Sul, 1750 ...	Avare
Cursino, Jose Wilson	Rua Visc. do Rio Branco, 330 apto. 11	Taubate
Cvintal, Tadeu	Rua Carlos Sampaio, 304, 2° andar, Bela Vista	01333 São Paulo
Dalmonte, Luiz Vicente Oliveto	Av. Vicente Carvalho, 38 apto. 72 Boqueirão	Santos
Damasceno Jr, João Bastista.	Rua São Pedro, 966	Mirassol
Delgado, Adhemar	....	
Delmanto, Aleixo Rubens ..	Rua Pensilvania, 553, Cidade Monções	04564 São Paulo
Delmanto, Olavo	Rua Silva Bueno, 519, 4° andar .	São Paulo
Delmanto, Orlando	....	
Delsin, Benedito Alves	Rua Marechal Deodoro, 3096, 2° andar	São Jose do Rio Preto
Dias, Carlos Ramos de Souza	Rua Cincinato Braga, 59 apto. 582, Bela Vista	01333 São Paulo
Dias, João Souza	....	
Dias, Marcio Peres	Cl. Oftal. Da S. Casa de Misericordia, Rua Dr. Cezario Mota Junior, 112, Vila Buarque ...	01221 São Paulo
Dores, Candido Augusto Bresser	Av. Higienopolis, 195 .apto. 113, Higienopolis	01238 São Paulo
Doria, Osvaldo C.	Av. Rangel Pestana, 2251, S/110	São Paulo
Dreyer, Luiz Armando	Rua Siqueira Campos, 466	Presidente Prudente
Duailibi, Walter	....	
Eduardo, Jose de Paula	Rua Itacolomi, 44 apto. 502, Higienopolis	São Paulo
Eduardo, Nelson de Paulo ..	Hotel Municipal	Jaboticabal

Eiger, Moises Luiz	Rua Vol. da Patria, 2403	02010 São Paulo
Eliezer, Coliolano Pompeu	Av. Jabarquara, 774 apto, 12, Vila Paulista	04360 São Paulo
Endo, Roberto Mitiaki	Rua Barra Funda, 794, Barra Funda	01152 São Paulo
Endo, Yoshio	Rua Carlos Tiago Pereira, 72, Jardim da Saude	04150 São Paulo
Estevez, Elcio Sanchez	Rua Santa Catarina, 30 Caixa Postal 40	Votuporanga
Esteves, Jose	Rua Barão de Itapetininga, 255, S/903	São Paulo
Ewbank Junior, David	Rua Marechal Deodoro, 399	Franca
Falcão, Edgar Cerqueira	Rua Martins Afonso, 34	Santos
Falcão, J. Marinho		
Falcão, Pedro	Av. Paulista, 266, Bela Vista	01310 São Paulo
Falcão, Teofilo de Cerqueira	Rua São Francisco, 61, 2° andar	Santos
Faluh, Paulo	Av. Santo Amaro, 791. Conj. 18, Vila Nova Conceição	04505 São Paulo
Faraldo, Carlos	Cl. Oftal. Faculdade de Ciencias Medicas	Botucatu
Faria, Francisco Carlos Pessoa	Rua Barão de Itapetininga, 207, 12° andar, Centro	01042 São Paulo
Faria, Jovino de	Av. Angelica, 765 apto. 603	São Paulo
Fausto, Ebe Rosseti	Rua Prof. Francisco Castro, 70	São Paulo
Fattore, Roberto Alonso	Rua Barão de Amazonas, 1199 apto. 4	Ribeirão Preto
Felberg, Romeu	Praça João Mendes, 42, 3° andar, Centro	01501 São Paulo
Felix, Salim	Rua Jose Bonifacio, 61	Guaratingueta
Fenley Junior, Eduardo	Rua Vieira Bueno, 374	Americana
Ferderman, Isaac	Instituto Penido Burnier	Campinas
Fernandes, Fernando Corpa	Hosp. São Paulo, Dep. de Oftal., Rua Botucatu, 720, Vila Clementino	São Paulo
Ferrara, Francisco	Av. Republica do Libano, 1204	São Paulo
Ferraz, Aloisio Carlos	Rua Barata Ribeiro, 50 apto. 72	Campinas
Ferraz, Eloy Lopes	Clinica Lopes Ferraz	15400 Olímpia
Ferreira, Aloysio Affonso	Instituto Penido Burnier	Campinas
Ferreira, Claudio Roque Buono	Rua Dante Carraro, 110, Pinheiros	05422 São Paulo
Ferreira, Domingos Carvalho		
Ferreira, Edilberto Capps	Rua Martin Francisco, 159 apto. 123, Vila Buarque	01226 São Paulo
Ferreira, Milton	Rua Joaquim Floriano, 164, Itaim	04534 São Paulo
Ferreira, Newton	Rua Cel. Xavier de Toledo, 234	São Paulo
Ferreira, Webber Martins	Av. Rodrigues Alves, 6, 52	Bauru
Figueiredo, Fernando C.		
Figueiredo, Helio de Azevedo	Rua Rita Candido Nogueira, 233	Cravinhos
Figueiredo, Oscar		
Figueiredo, Pedro dos Santos		
Figueiredo, Sebastião Carlos de	Rua Padre Anchieta, 1653	Franca
Fleider, Chaya Bela	Rua Bandeirantes, 135 apto. 53, Bom Retiro	01124 São Paulo

Foloni, João Batista	Rua 4 de Abril, 263	Marilia
Fonseca, Hermes Pereira da .	....	
Fonseca, Manoel Correa da .	Rua Benjamim Constant, 61, 9° andar	São Paulo
Fonseca, Yara Giaccone da .	Rua São Zeferino, 119, Agua Fria	São Paulo
Fontanini, Sergio	Rua Azevedo Costa, 374	Lorena
Fortes, Helio Martins	....	
Foschine, Roberto	....	
Franco, Gilberto Junqueira .	Av. Paulista, 1745 apto. 1718 ...	São Paulo
Franco, João Ribeiro	Rua Arruda Alvim, 161 apto. 101, Pinheiros	05410 São Paulo
Franco, Renato Melo	....	
Freitas, João Alberto Holan- landa de	Instituto Penido Burnier, Rua Dr. Mascarenhas, 249, Caixa Postal 284	Campinas
Freitas, Marta M. Lavor Ho- landade	Instituto Penido Burnier, Caixa Postal 284	Campinas
Freitas, Walter F.	Al. Joaquim Eugenio de Lima, 268, Jardim Paulista	01403 São Paulo
Freitas, Walter Gonçalves de.	Av. Tucuruvi, 259, Tucuruvi	02305 São Paulo
Furman, Jose	Av. Angelica, 2635, 7° andar San- ta Cecilia	São Paulo
Furnaro, Jose Roberto	Av. São Luiz, 258, S/605, Centro	01046 São Paulo
Furquim, Paulo	Rua Bernardino de Campos, 1256	Olimpia
Furquim, Rubens	Rua Eurico Sodre, 192	Lins
Galasso, Moacir G.	Rua Amaro Cavalheiro, 508, Pin- heiros	São Paulo
Gallo, Armando	Viaduto 9 de Julho, 181, 9° Andar, Centro	01050 São Paulo
Gallo, Hugo Jose Pagano ...	Instituto Penido Burnier, Caixa Postal 284	Campinas
Gallo Filho, Alberto	Rua Capitão Jose de Souza, 24 ..	Campinas
Galotti, Oswaldo	Rua Dr. Jose Queiros Aranha, 65 apto, 423, Vila Mariana	04106 São Paulo
Gama, Antonio Anacleto Espinola da	....	
Gama Filho, Durval da	Rua Domingos de Moraes, 770, Vila Mariana	04009 São Paulo
Gamba, Leonel Henrique La.	Cl. Oft. Faculdade de Ciencias Medicas	Botucatu
Ganeu, Ismael Abdo	Cl. Oftal. da E.P.M., Hosp. São Paulo, Rua Botucatu, 720, Vila Clementino	04023 São Paulo
Garbin, Helio	Instituto Penido Burnier, Caixa Postal 284	Campinas
Garcia, Jair	Rua Vol. da Patria, 2128, San- tana...................	02010 São Paulo
Garcia, Luiz Fernando Este- ves	Rua Maranhão, 1510	Avare
Garletti, Enio	Rua Jaguaribe, 252 apto. 903, Santa Cecilia	São Paulo
Gasparini, João Basilio	Rua Fernandes Sampaio, 2 D, Jar- dim Sampaio	02041 São Paulo
Gasparini Jr, Orlando	Rua Tiradentes, 29, 6° andar ...	Araçatuba

Gasparini, Mario	....	
Gasparini Sobrinho, João ..	Cl. Oftal. do HSPE, Rua Pedro de Toledo, 1800, Vila Clementino	04039 São Paulo
Gattas, Anderson	Rua Americo Brasiliense, 620 apto. 2	Ribeirão Preto
Gatti, Roberto Ferrari	Rua Oratorio, 77, Mooca	03117 São Paulo
Geraldo, Antonio Carlos ...	Rua 15 de Novembro, 337	Dracena
Gesuele, Arnaldo N.	Rua Martins Fontes, 164, 1° andar, Centro	01050 São Paulo
Ciachetti, Dirceu	Rua Barão de Arary, 609, 5° andar	Araras
Gigante, Edmilson	Rua Dr. Gurgel, 497	Presidente Prudente
Gil, Jose Bernardes Almeida.	Rua Joinville, 524, Vila Mariana .	04008 São Paulo
Goldchmit, Marcos	Rua Gregorio Pais de Almeida, 754, Pinheiros	05450 São Paulo
Gomes, Julio Pereira	Rua Marconi, 94, 4° andar, Centro	01047 São Paulo
Gomes Sobrinho, Jose Pereira	Al. Gabriel Monteiro da Silva, 496	São Paulo
Gonçalves, Arnaldo	Rua Itapeva, 490, Conj. 88	São Paulo
Gonçalves, Maria Jacinta Vieira	Rua Monte Cassino, 265, Jardim São Bento	02526 São Paulo
Gonçalves, Waldemar Guedes	Av. Rui Barbosa, 135, S/4.5.6. ..	Assis
Gondin, J. Alencar	Praça da Republica, 15	11100 Santos
Gorga, Adolfo Francisco H.	Cl. Oftal. da Faculdade Medicina	Marilia
Grippa, Armando	....	
Grizzo, Braulio	Rua Leonardo Cavalcante, 28 ...	Jundiai
Grotta, Adolpho Souzza ...	Rua Jose Bonifacio, 250	São Paulo
Guarnieri, Luiz Carlos	Rua Marechal Deodoro, 1191 ...	09700 São Bernardo do Campo
Guarnieri, Naor	Rua São Paulo, 1179	Votuporanga
Guerreiro, Nelson de Carvalho	Praça Luis Gama, 38	Pirajui
Guimarães, Dionisio	Rua Saldanha Gama, 158	São Paulo
Guimarães, Jair Xavier	Rua Batista Capelos, 207, Aclimação	São Paulo
Guimarães, Laerte	Alameda Casa Branca, 355	São Paulo
Guimarães, Osmar	Rua Arthur Martins, 36	Sorocaba
Guimarães, Ricardo Vaz ...	Rua Ricardo Pinto, 8	Santos
Guimarães, Rubens X.	Rua Batista Capelos, 226, Aclimação	São Paulo
Guimaraẽs, Wilson	....	
Gusmão, Cadmo Accioly de	Cl. Oftal. da S. Casa de Misericordia, Rua Dr. Cezario Mota Junior, 112, Vila Buarque ...	01221 São Paulo
Habib, Jose Tanuri	Rua Julio Prestes, 757	Ribeirão Preto
Hashimoto, Mauro Fideo ..	Rua Fiação da Saude, 128, Bl. C1 apto. 41, Vila Mariana	São Paulo
Hasimoto, Yasuo	Rua Herval, 608, Belenzinho ...	03062 São Paulo
Havas, Luiz Carlos	Rua Dona Ana Neri, 232 A 238, Mooca	03106 São Paulo
Haddad, Emilio	Av. 7 de Setembro, 22	Itapolis
Helal Junior, John	Rua Dr. Bianchi Bertoldi, 100 apto. 111, Pinheiros	São Paulo

Heimbeck, Felipe Jorge ...	Cl. Oftal. Faculdade de Ciencias Medicas	Botucatu
Hayashi, Samuel	Rua Caquito, 63, Penha	São Paulo
Hayashida, Akira	Rua Pedro de Toledo, 1260	Araçatuba
Hercos, Jorge Miziara	Rua Antonio de Rodoy, 3330 ..	15100 São Jose do Rio Preto
Hida, Milton Massato	Rua General Telles, 403	Botucatu
Higashitani, Iassuo	Rua Cosns° Brotero, 1208 apto. 44, Santa Cecilia	01232 São Paulo
Higuchi, Toshihiko	Av. Agami, 217, Indianopolis ...	São Paulo
Hirai, Alcides	Cl. Oftal. da E.P.M., Hosp. São Paulo, Rua Botucatu, 720, Vila Clementino	04023 São Paulo
Hirch, Abrahão C.	Rua Jose Bonifacio, 250, 8° andar, Centro	01003 São Paulo
Hoyama, Pakao	....	
Holzchuh, Nilo	Cl. Oftal. da S. Casa de Misericordia, Rua Dr. Cezario Mota Junior, 112, Vila Buarque ...	01221 São Paulo
Horovitz, Josef	Rua Hadock Lobo, 1663/71, Cerqueira Cesar	01414 São Paulo
Horta, Jose	Rua Felicio Marcondes, 197	Guarulhos
Iacovini, Atilio Smilari	Rua 11 de Agosto, 34	São Paulo
Iamashita, Takeo	Praça da SE, 323 apto. 51/52, Centro	01001 São Paulo
Imamura, Paulo Mitsuro ...	Rua Barão de Itapetininga, 297, 3° andar, Centro	01042 São Paulo
Inada, Americo Noriaki ...	Cl. Oftal. da Faculdade Reg. de Medicina, Av. Brig. Faria Lima, 5416	São Jose do Rio Preto
Insfran, Nestor Sanchez ...	Rua Capote Valente, 452, Pinheiros	05409 São Paulo
Ishimoto, Kaneo	....	
Ismar, Antonio	Cl. Oftal, da S. Casa de Misericordia	11100 Santos
Izecksohn, Leonardo	Rua Ministro Ferreira Alves, 181, Pompeia	São Paulo
Jardim, Gualter Silva	....	
Jervasio, Luiz Francisco ...	Av. Celso Garcia, 2294, S/20, Bairto Braz	São Paulo
Jorge, Tuffi	Rua Carlos Gomes, 1625	Araraquara
Jose, Newton Kara	Av. Brig. Luiz Antonio, 3775 Jardim Paulista	01401 São Paulo
Kage, Kazuto	Rua Tamandare, 693 apto 44, Liberdade	01525 São Paulo
Kamei, Kanto	Rua Dr. Sampaio Viana, 26, Paraiso	04004 São Paulo
Katayama, Getulio	Rua Dr. Julio Prestes, 821	Itapetininga
Kawano, Agnaldo Jose	Rua Jose Ferreira da Rocha, 19, Jardim Mont Kemel	05633 São Paulo
Kennerley, Rodger Gordon .	Rua Raimundo de Brito, 47, Aclimação	São Paulo
Kley, Ruben Reis	Rua Oscar Freire, 1447, Pinheiros	05409 São Paulo
Koba, Nilda	Av. Francisco Salles Damasco, 488	Cacapava
Kogan, Pleise	Rua da Graça, 215, 1° andar, Conj. 14, B. Retiro	São Paulo

Komatsu	Rua 15 de Novembro, 925	Piracicaba
Konno, Motomo	Cl. Oftal. da S. Casa de Misericordia, Rua Dr. Cezario Mota Junior, 112, Vila Buarque	01221 São Paulo
Kuwahara, Yasuharu	Av. da Liberdade, 91, 4° andar, Liberdade	01502 São Paulo
Lacerda, Rogerio	Rua Dez. Vicente Penteado, 120, Jardim America	01440 São Paulo
Lambert, Hayrton	Rua Condessa de São Joaquim, 288, Bela Vista	01320 São Paulo
Lambert, Luiz Roque	Rua Dr. Cezario Mota, 393, S/3 e 4	Santo André
Lambrimidis, Constantino D.	Cl. Oftal. s. Casa da Rua Dr. Cezario Mota Jr., 112	01221 São Paulo
Lamy Filho, Candido	Rua Dona Ana Pimentel, 282	São Paulo
Lanceloti, Luiz Carlos	Unidade de Saude	15378 Ilha Solteira
Lancia, Antonio Maury	Rua Carneiro de Souza, 18	12100 Taubate
Laranjeira, Luzita Maria Xambre	Cl. Oftalmologica da F.CM.S. Casa de Misericordia, Rua Benjamin Constant, 1657	Campinas
Lauretti Filho, Argemiro	Cl. Oftal. da Faculdade de Medicina, Caixa Postal. 301	Ribeirão Preto
Leal, Jairo Pires	Cl. Oftal. da Faculdade de Medicina	Mogi das Cruzes
Leão, Adelmo de Souza	Rua Barão de Jundiai, 418	Jundiai
Leite, Antonio Olive		
Leite, Geraldo Nogueira	Rua Angelo Bertoncini, 141	Assis
Lepper, Fernando Max	Rua Loureiro Baptista, 45, Vila Maiana	04019 São Paulo
Lepper, Geraldo	Rua Loureiro Baptista, 45	04019 São Paulo
Lerro, Clovis Fernandes	Rua Marechal Deodoro, 1759	São Bernardo do Campo
Liborio, Jose Roberto	Rua Capitão Thiago Luz, 81, 1° andar, Santo Amaro	São Paulo
Lima, Antonio Jose Lopes	Rua Dr. Carlos Chagas, 405, Jardim Esplanada	São Jose dos Campos
Lima, Jose Carlos de Souza	Rua Bahia, 563	São Paulo
Lima, Luiz Carvalho	Rua Teodoro Sampaio, 2763, Pinheiros	05405 São Paulo
Lima, Luiz G. Carvalho	Rua Laerte Assunção, 437, Jardim America	São Paulo
Lima, Sergio de Souza Pereira	Expedicionario Castro Garcia, 288	14400 Franca
Lira, Wilson Rolemberg	Rua Siqueira Campos, 452	Monte Aprazivel
Livramento, J. M. Bueno do	Rua Pedro II, 76, 2° andar	Santos
Lobo, Fabio Guimarães	Av. Santo Amaro, 204, Conj. 12	São Paulo
Luca, Jayme Vicente de	Rua 7 de Setembro, 2263	São Carlos
Luca, Sergio Paulo de	Rua Major Diogo, 666 apto. 92, Bela Vista	01324 São Paulo
Lui Netto, Adamo	Rua Duque de Caxias, 565	Taquaritinga
Luongo, João	Pca. Clovis Bevilacqua, 351, 1° andar	São Paulo
Luz, Benedito Maw Batista da	Rua Santa Filomena, 145	São Bernardo do Campo

Macchiaverni Filho, Nelson .   Cl. Oftal. da F.C.M.S. Casa de Misericordia, Rua Benjamin Constant, 1657 . . . .   Campinas

Macedo, Carlos Rodrigues ..   . .

Machado, Domingos . . . . . .   Av. da Liberdade, 47, 1° andar, Liberdade . . . .   01502 São Paulo

Machado, Geraldo de Castro.   Rua Dom Pedro II, 54 . . . .   Santos

Machado, Jose Geraldo de Castro . . . .   Av. Washigton Luiz, 542 apto. 131 . . . .   Santos

Machado, Nicolino Rebello .   Rua Pedro Segundo, 54 . . . .   Santos

Madeira, Ibrahim Carlos . . .   Rua Antonio Neri, 519 . . . .   Tieté

Magaldi, Maria Celeste Carvalho de . . . .   Rua Imaculada Conceição, 92, Santa Cecilia . . . .   São Paulo

Magalhães, Hilton Natal . . .   Casa de Saude Corregos . . . .   Dois Corregos

Magalhães, Paulo Braga de .   Rua Sampaio Vidal, 975, Jardim Paulistano . . . .   01443 São Paulo

Magalhães, Thomas Figueiredo . . . .   Av. Gabriel Monteiro da Silva, 1480 . . . .   São Paulo

Magalhães, Wilton . . . .   Av. Ipiranga, 1147, 1° andar . . . .   São Paulo

Maglioca Junior, Gilberto ..   Rua Ximbo, 201, Aclimação . . . .   04108 São Paulo

Magnani Filho, Rodolpho ..   Rua General Galvão, 256 . . . . . .   Jau

Maia, Sergio Alcantara . . . .   Rua Jaciporã, 119, Sumaré . . . . .   01256 São Paulo

Maiello, Luiz Antonio . . . . .   Cl. Oftal. do HSPE, Rua Pedro de Toledo, 1800, Vila Clementino . . . .   04039 São Paulo

Maiolino, Mario . . . .   Rua Herval, 608, 6° andar . . . . .   São Paulo

Mais, Francisco Arthur . . . .   Av. João Mendes Jr., 247, Bairro, Cambui . . . .   Campinas

Malavazzi, Edmar Haddad ..   Rua Amador Florence, 85 . . . . .   Campinas

Malavazzi, Mario Jose . . . . .   Rua Barreto Leme, 1112 . . . . . .   13100 Campinas

Malini, Luiz Gonzaga . . . . .   Rua Guaricanga, 138, Lapa . . . . .   05075 São Paulo

Malta, A. . . . .   Av. Angelica, 1045, Santa Cecilia   São Paulo

Manaia, Oswaldo Nunes . . .   Rua Amador Bueno, 275 . . . . . .   Ribeirão Preto

Mandelli Jr, Jose . . . .   Rua Delfino de Melo, 42 . . . .   Laranjal Paulista

Manetta, Lino . . . .   Rua Cel. Oliveira Lima, 492 . . . .   09000 Santo André

Maniscalco, Jose Francisco .   Av. Sampaio Vidal, 457 . . . .   Marilia

Mantovani, Luiz Carlos . . . .   Rua Inglaterra, 261 . . . .   Jundiai

Manzano, Marco Antonio ..   Rua Fernão Dias, 54, Pinheiros ..   05427 São Paulo

Marão, Sebastião . . . .

Marco, Erlan de . . . .   Rua Dr. Diogo de Faria, 900, Vila Clementino . . . .   04037 São Paulo

Marinho, Clovis . . . .

Marino Neto, Cesario . . . . .   Rua Oratorio, 48, Mooca . . . . . .   03116 São Paulo

Marino Neto, Rosario . . . . .   Rua Vergueiro, 3476 . . . .   São Paulo

Marinus, Cyrus de J. F. . . . .   Rua Cel. Xavier de Toledo, 234, Centro . . . .   01048 São Paulo

Marques, João Souza . . . . .   Praça Conego Joaquim Alves, 93 .   Batatais

Marques, Jose Carlos . . . . . .   Instituto Penido Burnier, Caixa Postal 284 . . . .   Campinas

Marques Netto, Paulo Cesar .   Cl. Oftal. da S. Casa de Misericordia, Rua Dr. Cezario Mota Junior, 112, Vila Buarque . . .   01221 São Paulo

Marquesi, Jose Paulo de Figueiredo .... Rua Oscar Freire, 1360 apto. 41, Jardim America .... São Paulo

Martins, Ary Moacir ...... Rua Quintino Bocaiuva, 191 .... Jau

Martins, Jose Maria Aiello .. Rua Jundianopolis, 304 .... Jundiai

Martins, Jose Maria Q. .... Rua Dr. Frederico Steidel, 219 apto 62, Santa Cecilia ...... São Paulo

Martins, Moacir .... Rua Edgar Ferraz, 353 .... 17200 Jau

Martins, Rubens Jose Macedo .... Rua Prudente de Moraes, 1242 .. Ribeirão Preto

Marum, Daniel .... Praça João Mendes, 42, 5° andar, Centro .... 01501 São Paulo

Marum, Sergio Pelegrini ... Rua Abilio Soares, 989, Paraiso . 04005 São Paulo

Mattiussi, Gloria Maria Celli . Rua Mario Amaral, 329 Paraiso . 04002 São Paulo

Mattos, Jose Belfort ...... Rua Barão de Itapetininga, 297, 3° andar .... São Paulo

Mattos, Manoel Barros .... Rua Voluntarios da Patria, 2128, Santana .... 02010 São Paulo

Mattos, Rubens Belfort .... Caixa Postal 4086 .... São Paulo

Mattos Junior, Rubens Belfort .... Rua Barão de Itapetininga, 297, 3° andar, Centro .... 01402 São Paulo

Mello, Paulo Augusto de Arruda .... Alameda Itu, 1209 apto. 61 Cerqueira Cesar .... 01421 São Paulo

Mello, Wilson de .... Praça N.S. da Conceição, 740 ... Franca

Mendes, Clemente J. ...... Rua Dr. Veiga Filho, 422 apto. .. 111, Santa Cecilia .... 01229 São Paulo

Menezes, Antonio Ismar Marçal .... Av. Pinheiro Machado, 1033, 1035, Jose Menino .... Santos

Menezes, Virgilio L. de .... Praça do Patriarca, 96, S. 43 .... São Paulo

Messetti, João Alberto .... Rua 4, Cj, 127 .... Rio Claro

Meyer, Milton Correa ..... Rua Cap. Prudente, 50 .... São Paulo

Miyata, Alice F. .... Departamento de Oftal., Hosp. das Clinicas, Rua Bernardino de Campos, 1000 .... Ribeirão Preto

Midoricava, Ruy .... Hosp. das Clinicas, Oftal., Rua Bernardino de Campos, 1000 . Ribeirão Preto

Miki, Tomitaro .... Rua Teodoro Sampaio, 2537, Pinheiros .... 05405 São Paulo

Miraglia, Orestes .... Rua Dodrigues Alves, 585 ...... Bauru

Miranda, Francisco de Assis Torres .... Rua Saint Martin, 24, 68 ...... Bauru

Moassab, Marcio Barbosa .. Rua Visconde do Rio Branco, 176. .... Taubaté

Moekel, Ernesto Rubens ... Praça do Matriz, 79 .... 18270 Tatui

Molez, Antonio Braz ...... Cl. Oftal. de S. Casa da Misericordia, Rua Dr. Cezario Mota Jr., 112 Vila Buarque ...... 01221 São Paulo

Monteiro, Alberto .... Rua Amador Bueno, 489 ...... Ribeirão Preto

Monteiro, Cassio Galvão ... Rua Mercedes Lopes, 41, Vila Santana .... 03614 São Paulo

Morabito, Arnaldo .... Av. Duque de Caxias, 283 ...... Araraquara

Moraes, Jose Benedito de .. ..

Moreira, Jose Belmiro de
Castro .... Av Angelica, 2355, 6° andar,
Conj. 61, Santa Cecilia ..... 01227 São Paulo

Moreira, Jose Nelson An-
drade .... Hosp. das Clinicas .... Botucatu

Mori, Hisato .... Rua Flaviano de Mello, 822 .... Mogi das Cruzes

Mori, Yoitiro .... Cl. Oftal. da Fac. de Ciencias
Medicas e Biologicas .... Botucatu

Morinishi, Yaeko .... Praça Benedito Calixto, 186 apto.
97, Pinheiros .... 05406 São Paulo

Moro, Jomar Wladimir dal . Rua Maranhão, 26 apto. 62,
Higienopolis .... São Paulo

Moura, Sergio Pompeia
Ramos de .... Rua Gonçalves Ledo, 488, Ipiranga .... 04216 São Paulo

Muller, Mario .... Rua Altino Arantes, 933 .... Casa Branca

Multehinik, Elias .... Rua Vol. da Patria, 1413, Santana 02011 São Paulo

Munhcs, Rubens .... Rua Caetes, 687 .... Tupã

Nakano, Kozo .... Rua Correia Dias, 34, 8° andar,
Paraizo .... São Paulo

Nammur, Emilio .... Rua Tutoia, 78 .... São Paulo

Nascimento, Heitor .... Instituto Penido Burnier, Rua Dr.
Mascarenhas, 249 .... Campinas

Nassif, Jorge .... Rua Cel. Francisco Martins, 363 . Igarapava

Nazareth, Sellmann .... Praça São Jose, 2835 .... São Jose do Rio Preto

Nedstein, Isaac .... Rua Barão de Itapetininga, 297,
3° andar .... São Paulo

Neves, Emerson F. Pereira
das .... Rua Itapeva, 486 a 490, Conj. 66,
Bela Vista .... 01332 São Paulo

Neves, Herbert Luiz A. .... Cl. Oftal. da S. Casa da Misericordia .... 13100 Campinas

Nicolella, Januario Neto ... Rua Barão Mota Paes, 53 ...... Pinhal

Niemeyer, Waldemar ...... Rua Barão de Itapetininga, 120,
S/217, 8 .... São Paulo

Nigro, Nelson .... Praça Cunha Bueno, 1250 ...... Guararapes

Nobrega, João Francisco
Centola .... Rua São Sebastião, 817 ...... Ribeirão Preto

Nocera, Jose Hamilton .... Cl. Oftal. da F.C.M.S. Casa de
Misericordia, Rua Benjamin
Constant, 1657 .... Campinas

Noda, Aquira .... Rua Brig. Luis Antonio, 878,
Conj. 32 .... São Paulo

Nomura, Hissashi .... Rua Flaviano de Mello, 822 .... Mogi das Cruzes

Novais, Armando de Arruda. Rua Barão de Itapetininga, 46, 7°
andar, Centro .... 01042 São Paulo

Novo, Carlos da Silva ..... Rua Barão de Itapetininga, 46, 7°
andar .... São Paulo

Nunes, Nelia .... Viaduto 9 de Julho, 181, 9°
andar .... São Paulo

Nunes, Saulo Pinto .... Rua Sud Menucci, 197, Vila
Mariana .... São Paulo

Olivalves, Edilberto .... Rua Silvia, 276, 4° andar, Bela
Vista .... 01331 São Paulo

Oliveira, Helion de Mellee .. Instituto Penido Burnier, Rua Dr.
Mascarenhas, 249 .... Campinas

Oliveira, Ivan de	Rua Rodrigues Alves, 636	Lins
Oliveira, J. Garcia de	Rua Voluntarios da Patria, 1413, 1° andar	São Paulo
Oliveira, Luiz Valentie de ..	Rua 9 de Julho, 1625	São Carlos
Oliveira, Orlando Naves de .	Rua Luiz Coelho, 308, Conj. 66, Consolação	01309 São Paulo
Oliveira, Saulo Jose Prata de.	Rua Visc. do Rio Branco, 893 ..	Taquaritinga
Oliveira Junior, Assis Pinto de	Rua Guaripocaba, 8, Bom Retiro .	01134 São Paulo
Orsolini, Oswaldo	Rua Pereira Bueno, 118	Pirassununga
Ortolan Junior, Guilherme .	Rua Epitacio Pessoa, 858	Sertãozinho
Paccola, Virgilio	Rua 11 de Agosto, 100	Ribeirão Preto
Pacheco, Jose Carlos Gouvea	Rua Marques de Itu, 266, Conj. 81/82, Vila Buarque	01223 São Paulo
Padovan, Alfredo Helio Ribeiro	Rua Djalma Dutra, 480	Botucatu
Padua, Waldomiro	Rua Prof. Batista Andrade, 148, Bras	São Paulo
Pagnocca, Diogenes	Rua Dr. Erico Sodre, 192	Lins
Palamone, Luiz Bento	Rua Italia, 1657	Araraquara
Palazzo, Nicola Conrado Italo	Largo de Pinheiros, 47, Pinheiros .	05424 São Paulo
Pardo, Jose	Praça 9 de Julho, 41	Catanduva
Passerotti, Sergio	Cl. Oftal. de HSPE, Rua Pedro de Toledo, 1800, Vila Clemen- tino	04039 São Paulo
Pastore, Celio	Rua Visc. do Rio Branco, 504 ..	Taquaritinga
Pedro, Fuad Jose	Rua Antonio Carlos Mori, 46 ...	Ourinhos
Pelicioni, Americo	Av. Rio Branco, 211 S/17-18, Campos Eliseos	01205 São Paulo
Pellicano, Aristides	Rua Barão de Jundiai, 901	Jundiai
Pentagna, Oreste	Al. Ribeiro da Silva, 26 apto. 104, Campos Eliseos	01217 São Paulo
Pentagna, Pasquale	Av. do Estado, 716	16300 Penapolis
Pereira, Francisco Santiago .	Rua Campos Sales, 606	Santo André
Pereira, Jamir Laudares	Instituto Penido Burnier, Rua Dr. Mascarenhas, 249	Campinas
Pereira, Jose Roberto Alves .	Cl. Oftal. da S. Casa de Misericor- dia, Rua Dr. Cezario Mota Jr., 112, Vila Buarque	01221 São Paulo
Pereira, Lineu Rubens Car- valho	Caixa Postal 283	Dracema
Pereira, Lucio Arthur	Rua Amador Bueno, 181, 2° andar	Santos
Pereira, Luiz Carlos	Rua Cel. Joaquim do Prado, 59 .	Cruzeiro
Pereira, Milton	....	
Pereira, Sebastião	Rua Humberto 1, 371, Vila Mariana	São Paulo
Peret Filho, Francisco Amedée	....	
Perrella, Jose Cesar	Rua Flaminio Lessa, 197	Guaratingueta
Pierre, Renato Alberto	Av. Adolfo Pinheiro, 610, Santo Amaro	São Paulo
Pimentel, Myrthes	....	
Pina Neto, Luiz	Rua Bahia, 684	São Paulo
Pinho, Edson	Av. 21, 300	Barretos

Pinto, Arlindo . . . . Rua Augusta, 838 . . . .

Pinto, Augusto Nilson Ro-
mariz . . . . Instituto Penido Burnier, Rua Dr.   São Paulo
                                    Mascarenhas,   249,   Caixa
                                    Postal 284 . . . .   013100 Campinas

Pinto, Fabio Gilson Cavalca . Praça dom Pedro II, 46 . . . .   Guaratingueta

Pinto, Leila Maria Marciano . Alameda Uapes, 515, Planalto
                                    Paulista . . . .   São Paulo

Pinto, Luiz Cesar Cavalca . . Instituto Penido Burnier, Caixa
                                    Postal 284 . . . .   Campinas

Pires, Antonio Fernando . . . Rua São Samuel, 129, Vila Maria   04120, São Paulo

Pires, Fernando . . . . Rua Indiana, 385, Brook Paulista   04562 São Paulo

Piza, Plinio de Toledo . . . . . Rua 7 de Abril, 118, 8° andar,
                                    Centro . . . .   01044 São Paulo

Pola, Romeu . . . . Rua Americo Samarone, 303, Vila
                                    Moinho Velho . . . .   04284 São Paulo

Polati, Mariza . . . . Al. Franca, 1041, apto. 21, Jar-
                                    dim Paulista . . . .   01422 São Paulo

Poletto, Ivo Luiz . . . . Praça Oswaldo Cruz, 47, Conj. 33,
                                    Paraiso . . . .   04004 São Paulo

Posada, Manoel . . . . Av. da Liberdade, 47, 1° andar,
                                    Liberdade . . . .   01502 São Paulo

Praca Filho, Alencar Leite . Departamento de Oftalmologia
                                    Faculdade de Ciencias Medicas   Campinas

Pradella, Geraldo . . . . Rua Quintino Bocaiuva, 435 . . . .   São João da Boa Vista

Prado, Durval Livramento . . Av. Ipiranga, 313, 8° andar . . . . .   São Paulo

Prado Junior, João . . . . Praça Teodoro de Carvalho, 24
                                    apto. 11, Vila Mariana . . . . . .   São Paulo

Prata, João Antonio . . . . . . Rua Vieira de Moraes, 1746,
                                    Campo Belo . . . .   São Paulo

Previdelli, Alderico . . . . Rua Gal. Glicerio, 456 . . . .   Taquaritinga

Primiano, Benito Ricardo . . Rua Carlos Gomes, 2149 . . . . . .   Araraquara

Prospero, Nicanor Tadeu . . Rua Raul Pompeia, 547, Pompeia   São Paulo

Puzzi, Domingos Luciano . . Praça Toledo Barros, 155, 8°
                                    andar . . . .   Limeira

Puzzi, Jose . . . . Rua Conselheiro Saraiva, 492 . . .   Limeira

Quafa, Ahmad Samir . . . . . Rua Francisco Cruz, 255, Vila
                                    Mariana . . . .   04117 São Paulo

Queiroz, Antonio Cavalcante
de . . . . Av. Brig. Luiz Antonio, 2191, 1°
                                    andar . . . .   São Paulo

Queiroz, Leoncio de Souza . Instituto Penido Burnier . . . .   Campinas

Querido Filho, Licurgo . . . . Rua Dr. Souza Alves, 778 . . . . . .   Taubaté

Ramalho, Murillo Oliveira . . Rua Matias Cardoso, 49, Pinheiros   05425 São Paulo

Raskin, David Grois Amm . Rua Marechal Deodoro, 865,
                                    apto. 64 . . . .   Campinas

Reale, Jose . . . . Av. Rangel Pestana, 1292 apto.
                                    14 . . . .   São Paulo

Rebocho, Paulo R. C. . . . . . R. Agrario Souza, 186 . . . .   São Paulo

Regatieri, Ademir de O. . . . Cl. Oftal. da E.P.M., Hosp. São
                                    Paulo, Rua Botucatu, 720,
                                    Vila Clementino . . . .   04023 São Paulo

Rego, Eduardo de Almeida . Av. Sampaio Vidal, 457, 1° andar.   Marilia

Reichl, Geza . . . . Rua Igarapava, 49, Itaim . . . .   São Paulo

Reis, Jessy Vilela . . . . Rua Tiradentes, 82 . . . .   Araçatuba

Reis, Jose Carlos . . . . Rua Colonia da Gloria, 225, Jar-
                                    dim Gloria . . . .   São Paulo

Reis, Jose Vilela	Caixa Postal 198	A raçatuba
Reno, Julio	Rua Amador Bueno, 60	Santos
Ribeiro, Arthur Jupiacaba Tiburcio	Av. Jorge Tibiriça, 508	Cruzeiro
Ribeiro, Diogenes Conella	Rua Dr. Altino Arantes, 203	Ourinhos
Ribeiro, Jose Francisco Gomes	Largo do Cambuci, 66, 2° Andar	São Paulo
Ribeiro, Ovidio	Rua Gabriel dos Santos, 253 S/121, Santa Cecilia	01231 São Paulo
Ribeiro, Silvio	Av. Altino Arantes, 165	Ourinhos
Rizzi, Alexandre Belfort	Rua Barão de Itapetininga, 297, 3° andar	São Paulo
Rocco, Alfredo	Rua Barão de Itapetininga, 297, 3° andar, Centro	01042 São Paulo
Rocha, Jose Martins	Instituto Penido Burnier, Caixa Postal 284	Campinas
Rodriguez, João Ramão	Instituto Penido Burnier, Caixa Postal 284	Campinas
Rodrigues, M. de Lourdes Veronese	Rua Cerqueira Cesar, 1189	014100 Ribeirão Preto
Rollemberg, Ivan Valle	Rua Rubião Junior, 3042	São Jose do Rio Preto
Romão, Erasmo	Departamento de Oftalmologia Faculdade de Medicana	Ribeirão Preto
Romeiro Filho, Manoel Inacio	Rua Sergipe, 478	Catanduva
Rosa, Celio Lobo		
Rosa, Francisco Almeida	Rua Barão de Itapetininga, 207, 12° andar	São Paulo
Rosa, Luis Azevedo	Rua Cel. Souza Franco, 205	Mogi das Cruzes
Rosario, Elcio Ramos	Rua Vol. de São Paulo, 3117	São Jose do Rio Preto
Rosas, Wilson Jehovah	Rua 11, N 305 Caixa Postal 265	15.700 Jales
Rosemberg, Moacir Horacio	Rua Itacolomi, 523, Higienopolis	01239 São Paulo
Ross, James	Praça da Republica, 386, 2° andar, Centro	01045 São Paulo
Rossi, Pedro	Rua Jaguaribe, 25 apto. 13	São Paulo
Rymer, Samuel	Rua Antonio Carlos, 196, apto. 68, Bela Vista	São Paulo
Saad, Sami		
Sabbag, Michael	Rua Dr. Deodate Wertheimer, 267, S/15	Mogi das Cruzes
Sacchetin, Woyne Figner	Departamento de Oftalmologia, Hosp. das Clinicas	Ribeirão Preto
Sadala, Jose	Av. La Salle, 363	Araraquara
Safadi, Nadir Jorge	Rua Itapeva, 486 a 490, Conj. 66, Bela Vista	01332 São Paulo
Saihg, Wilson Hayek	Av. 19, N 574	Barretos
Salaroli, Jose B.		
Sales, Paulo Ramos	Rua Gregorio Serrão, 49 apto. 2b, Vila Mariana	04106 São Paulo
Salgado, Luiz Queiroz	Hosp. das Clinicas, Av. Dr. Eneas de Aguiar	São Paulo
Saliba, Jorge	Rua Alfredo Jose Caetano, 111	Piracicaba
Salles, Libanio de Padua	Rua Humaita, 191, Bela Vista	01321 São Paulo
Salles, Luiz Braz	Rua Mooca, 2420, Conj. 11	São Paulo
Sallun Filho, Raul Cassad	Av. Barão de Itapura, 1182	Campinas
Sampaio, Jose Maria Rollemberg	Rua Rubião Junior, 3042	São Jose do Rio Preto

Sanchez, Celia .... Cl. Oftal. da. F.C.M., Rua Benja-
                          min Constant, 1657 .... Campinas
Sanda, Luiz Ossamu ...... Rua Sinimbu, 148, apto 71,
                          Liberdade .... São Paulo
Sano, Valter Isuneiti ..... Rua Pero Neto, 228, Saude ..... 04053 São Paulo
Santanda, Tooku .... Cl. Oftal. Faculdade de Ciencias
                          Medicas e Biologicas .... 18600 Botucatu
Santos, Carlos Alberto M.
  Mira .... Rua Pamplona, 68, Bela Vista ... São Paulo
Santos, Clecius A. Cirilo Dos Rua Dr. Julio Prestes, 249 ..... Americana
Santos, Jose Benedito dos .. Rua Maranhão, 1219 .... 18740, Avare
Santos, Osório Musa dos ... Largo 13 de Maio, 490, 5° andar . Santo Amaro
Santos, Raul Saraiva ...... Rua Martim de Sá, 65, Vila Maria-
                          na .... 04128 São Paulo
Santos, Salmo dos .... Av. Alvaro Ramos, 2379, 4. Para-
                          da .... 03331 São Paulo
Santos Filho, Benedito de
  Paula .... Rua Marques de Itu, 58, 9° andar,
                          Vila Buarque .... São Paulo
Sborgia, João .... Rua Marcondes Salvado, 149 ... Ribeirão Preto
Scavoni, Felício .... Rua Benjamin Constant, 77, 7°
                          andar .... São Paulo
Schelb, Clinton .... Dep. de Oftal. Hospital das Clini-
                          cas, Rue Bernardino de Cam-
                          pos, 1000 .... Ribeirão Preto
Schiavo, Savio .... Rua Cel. Xavier de Toledo, 234,
                          1° andar, Centro .... 01048 São Paulo
Shuindt, Sergio .... Rua Vol. de São Paulo, 2953 fun-
                          dos, Centro .... São Jose do Rio Preto
Schwartz, Tommy .... Rua Dr. Veiga Filho, 375 apto 5
                          B, Higienopolis .... São Paulo
Sebrão, Paulo Renato .....
Semeghini, Theodosio Derio.. Av. 8, 490 .... Fernandopolis
Shalabi, Zelia .... Rua Itarare, 255 apto 1, Bela
                          Vista .... 01308 São Paulo
Shiguimatsu, Soiti .... Rua dos Chanes, 164, Vila Helena São Paulo
Shimanoe, Wagner K. ..... Rua Cond. de São Joaquim, 160
                          apto 31, Bela Vista .... 01320 São Paulo
Shinzato, Jose .... Instituto São Lucas, Rua Cel.
                          Monteiro, 317 .... São Jose dos Campos
Shinzato, Syogi .... Rua Cel. Monteiro, 317 .... São Jose dos Campos
Silva, Alberto A. de Cunhae . Rua Pará, 319 .... Catanduva
Silva, Aparecida Suely Messa
  P. da .... Cl. Oftal. da Faculdade de Medi-
                          cina de Campinas, Rua Benja-
                          min Constant, 1657 .... Campinas
Silva, Avelino Gomes da ... . São Paulo
Silva, Carlos Alberto Peixoto
  da .... Rua Inhambu, 600, Vila Ubera-
                          binha .... 04520 São Paulo
Silva, Cid Marques da ..... Rua 7 de Abril, 118, 12° andar .. São Paulo
Silva, Eduardo Costa e .... Rua Oratório, 67, Alto Mooca .. São Paulo
Silva, João Amaro F. ..... Rua Vergueiro, 263 apto. 122,
                          Liberdade .... 01504 São Paulo
Silva, Jose Carlos da ...... Rua Coronel Simões, 649 ...... São Manoel
Silva, Jose Luiz Lemos da .. Rua Pernambuco, 147, 4° andar,
                          Higienopolis .... 01240 São Paulo

Silva, Landoaldo Brandão da	....	
Silva, Luiz Carlos Sales de C. e	Rua Garibaldi, 1148	Ribeirão Preto
Silva, Napoleão João da ...	Rua Augusta, 2676 apto. 53, Cerqueira Cesar	01412 São Paulo
Silva, Nelson Cavalheiro ...	Av. Europa, 587, Jardim Europa .	São Paulo
Silva, Paulo Lemos Gomes da	Rua Martins Fontes, 164 Conj. 109–111, Centro	01050 São Paulo
Silva, Rogério Marcos da ...	Rua Quintino Bocaiuva, 307, 2° andar	São Paulo
Silva, Valdir Balarin	Rua 5°, 423	Rio Claro
Silva, Wander Agmont	Av. Santo Amaro, 1919 apto. 401, Vila Olimpia	São Paulo
Silveira, Jose Bresser da ...	Praça da Sé, 411, s. 3	São Paulo
Silvino, Wilmar Roberto ...	....	
Simões, João Castro	Cl. Oftal. da Santa Casa da Misericordia	11100, Santos
Simone, Luiz	Rua Jose Bonifácio, 132	Mogi das Cruzes
Siqueira, Alvaro Ferraz de .	Praça Ademar de Barros, 67	Mococa
Siqueira, Felipe	Rua Ceara, 157	Higienopolis
Siqueira, Helvecio Botelho .	Rua 9, 1101	Santa Fé do Sul
Sirio, Nilmo Jose	Praça da Matriz, 15	Santo Anastácio
Smanski, C. L.	Caixa Postal 2447	São Paulo
Soares, Abilio Nogueira ...	Rua Antonio Alves, 13-26	Bauru
Soares, Jose Jaime Tavares .	Rua Manoel Coelho, 298	09500, São Caetano do Sul
Soares, Reginaldo Parreira .	Instituto Penido Burnier, Caixa Postal 284	Campinas
Saccol, Ovidio	Rua Cotoxo, 970, Vila Pompéia .	05021 São Paulo
Soussumi, Yusaku	Rua Gal. Carneiro, 1557	Franca
Souza, Jose Araujo Rolim de	....	
Souza, Jose Lucas de	Rua Braulio Gomes, 25 S/609, Centro	01047 São Paulo
Souza, Jose Maria Ramos de	Rua Itapeva, 300, Bela Vista	01332 São Paulo
Souza, Nivaldo Vieira de ...	Rua Quintino Bocaiuva, 484, Bairro, Higienopolis	Ribeirão Preto
Souza, Olavo A. C. de	Rua Paula Souza, 622	Itu
Souza, Olavo Silva	Rua Paula Souza, 622	Itu
Souza, Ovidio Portugal de ..	Rua Expedicionários, 473	Ourinhos
Spadaro Junior, Francisco .	Rua Caetes, 819	Tupã
Suenaga, Jorge Katue	Vila Irene, 32	Mogi das Cruzes
Suenaga, Mário Katue	Caixa Postal 307	Mogi das Cruzes
Susana Junior, Remo	Rua Camilo, 222, Vila Romana .	05045 São Paulo
Suzuki, Hisashi	Rua Arthur Azevedo, 129 apto. 2, Cerqueira Cesar	05404 São Paulo
Szlnory, Soltan	Rua Peixoto Gomide, 77, Jardim Paulista	01409, São Paulo
Szymanski, Lech Michael ..	Cl. Oftal. do Hosp. das Clinicas, Av. Dr. Eneas C. Agniar, Cerqueira Cesar	05403, São Paulo
Taddei, Mauricio Onesti ...	Av. São Francisco, 61, conj. 21, 2° andar	Santos
Taka, Tomoji	Rua Barão de Jaceguai, 99, Campo Belo	04606 São Paulo
Takahaschi, Walter Yukiniko	Cl. Oftal. do Hospital das Clinicas, Cerqueira Cesar	05409 São Paulo

Tanganelli, Santos Pedro ...	Rua Sampaio Vidal, 1109, Jardim Paulista	São Paulo
Tasso, Carlos	Rua Figueira, 837, S. 215	São Paulo
Tavares, Dalmo	Rua Padre Luiz, 17, 3° andar ...	Sorocaba
Tavares, Milton	Rua Monsenhor João Soares, 294.	Sorocaba
Tavares, Walter	Rua Mons. João Soares, 294	18100, Sorocaba
Teixeira, Dagoberto	Alameda Navarro de Andrade, 376, Caixa Postal 332	Adamantina
Teixeira, Valdete Maia	Rua Dr. Martinico Prado, 241, Santa Cecilia	São Paulo
Tierno, Domingos Colombo .	Rua Renato Paes de Barros, 142 apto. 63	São Paulo
Tirabosqui, Pedro Roberto .	Cl. Oftal, da Fac. da Ciencias Med. e Biologicas	Botucatu
Tock, Josef	Av. Republica do Libano, 1873, Ibirapuera	04501, São Paulo
Toledo, Celso	Rua Gaspar Libero, 383, S. 10, D.	São Paulo
Toledo, Milton	Instituto Penido Burnier	Campinas
Toledo, Renato de	Rua Sena Madureira, 744, Vila Clementino	04021 São Paulo
Toledo, Sylvio de Almeida .	Rua Braulio Gomes, 25, 6° andar, Centro	01047 São Paulo
Toledo Filho, Milton Baptista de	Instituto Penido Burnier, Rua Dr. Mascarenhas, 249	13100, Campinas
Toller, Getulio Freitas	Rua 28, 1230	Barretos
Tomonami, Emi	Cl. Oftal. da Fac. de Ciencias Med. c. Biologicas	Botucatu
Tosi, Jose Carlos	Rua Prof. Jose Ranieri, 3-44	Bauru
Treiger, Raphael	Rua Prates, 39 apto 65, Bom Retiro	São Paulo
Tupinamba, Alexandre da Silveira	Rua Antonio Carlos, 582, 2° andar, B. Vista	São Paulo
Tupinamba, Jacques	Rua Antonio Carlos, 582, 2° andar B. Vista	São Paulo
Ubaiz, Mamede Ali	Rua 28, 1230	14780, Barretos
Uchoa, Plinio	Rua Cerqueira Cesar, 623	Ribeirão Preto
Ueno, Hideo	Rua Benjamin Constant, 54	Suzano
Uesugui, Carlos Fumiaki ...	Rua Marques de Itu, 382 apto. 131, Vila Buarque	01223 São Paulo
Ungaretti, Drina Coelho ...	Rua D. Balduina, 234, Sumaré ..	São Paulo
Uras, Ricardo	Rua Senador Paulo Egidio, 15 apto. 507-08	São Paulo
Valle, Sebastião Ribeiro de .	Rua Quintino Bocaiuva, 254	Caconde
Valle, Sergio do	Viaduto 9 de Julho, 181, 9° andar	São Paulo
Vasconcelos, Carlos Eduardo	Rua Cel. Souza Reis, 94	São Paulo
Velasquez Filho, Jose	Rua Capitão Tiago Luz, 81, 1° andar, Santo Amaro	São Paulo
Veloso, Eraldo de Albuquerque	Rua Dr. Costa Valente, 144 S-25 .	São Paulo
Vergueiro, Nestor Almeida .	Rua 15 de Novembro, 12	Pinhal
Vianna, Geraldo Ferreira ..	Rua Bernadino de Campos, 1427 .	Ribeirão Preto
Vianna, Raul de Camargo ..	Av. Dr. Nelson D'Avila, 164	São Jose dos Campos
Vicente, Jose Julio Boldrini .	Cl. Oftal. da E.P.M. Hosp. São Paulo, Rua Botucatu, 720, Vila Clementino	04023 São Paulo

Vidigal, Diaulas	Rua Augusta, 2895, C. 52, Consolação	São Paulo
Vieira, Antonio Penha	Rua Dr. Julio Cardoso, 1600 ...	Franca
Vieira, Benedito Borges ...	Rua Domicio da Gama, 108, Perdizes	São Paulo
Vieira, Jose Ignacio	Rua Monteiro Mello, 209, 1° andar, Lapa	05050 São Paulo
Vieira, Sidney Iglesias	Instituto Penido Burnier, Rua Dr. Mascarenhas, 249	13100, Campinas
Vilela, Francisco	Rua Tiradentes, 82	Arapatuba
Vilela, Rubens M.	Av. Jabaquara, 983, Mirandopolis	04045 São Paulo
Villi, Fabio	Rua Jaragua, 817, Bom Retiro ..	01129 São Paulo
Violante, Antonio Carlos ..	Rua Teixeira da Silva, 393 apto. 91, Paraizo	04002 São Paulo
Violante, Mario	....	
Wehbe Junior, Jamil	Rua Cel. Oliveira Lima, 158	Santa Andre
Wenceslau, Antonio	Rua Clemente Alvares, 87, Lapa .	05047 São Paulo
Willmersdorf, Jorge Cavalheiro	Rua Monsenhorndrade, 36 apto. 56, Braz	03000 São Paulo
Vilella, Antonio	Rua Tiradentes, 87	16100, Araçatuba
Yamashiro, Sussumo	Rua Cel. Jose Monteiro, 317	12200 São Jose dos Campos
Yamo, Kazumi	Rua Prof. Tranquilli, 288, Vila Mariana	04126 São Paulo
Yasuda, Naoto	Av. Fagundes Filho, 1021, Vila Monte Alegre	04304 São Paulo
Yokomizo, Nelson	Rua Cons. Furtado, 151 conj. 73, Liberdade	São Paulo
Yoshikava, Takasho	Cl. Oftal. do HSPE, Rua Pedro de Toledo, 1800, Vila Clementino	04039 São Paulo
Younan, Ibrahim	Rua Ondina, 427	São Jose do Rio Preto
Zacharias, Ferjalla	....	Alto de Santana
Zapata, Rene Sanchez	Instituto Penido Burnier, Caixa Postal 284	Campinas
Zenha, Jose Carlos	Rua Padre Chico, 180, Vila Pompéia	São Paulo
Zezzi, Gilberto	Rua Dom Pedro, 209	Marilia
Zinsly, Bolivar	Rua Cel. Monteiro, 317	São Jose dos Campos

Sergipe

Brizuela, Abraham Eduardo Mejia	Porto Velho Hotel, Porto Velho .	Território de Rondonia
Fontes, Roberto José Bahia .	Rua Raimundo Costa Carvalho, 162	Estância
Goes, Max Rollemberg	Rua Maroim, 624	Aracajú
Gomes, Joseval Silva	Rua de Araua, 291	Aracajú
Maciel, Raimundo Emanuel Menezes	Cl. Oftal. da Faculdade de Ciencias Medicas da UFS, Av. Dezembarcador Naynard, 174	Aracajú
Marques, Ademilde	Rua Amazonas, 785, Bairro, Siqueira Campos	Aracajú
Moraes, Antonio Carlos Vieira de	Cl. Oftal. da Faculdade de Ciencias Médicas da UFS, Av. Dezembargador Maynard, 174	Aracajú
Oliveira, Naira Maynart de .	Rua Riachuelo, 106	Aracajú

Porto, Lauro de Brito	Rua Boquim, 67	Aracajú
Santana, Alvaro Azevedo ..	Rua de Campos, 82	Aracajú
Simões, Juliano Calasans ...	Rua Dom Jose Thomaz, 62	Aracajú
Tavares, Marilena Lopes ...	Av. Pedro Calasans, 797	Aracajú
Pereira, Calos Umberto	Rua Silvio Romero, 95, Santo Antonio	Aracajú

NOSOCOMIA QUIBUS OCULIS AEGRI CURANTUR

Faculdade de Medicina da Universidade Federal de Alagoas
Prof. Jefferson de Lima Arauje, Trav. Franca Morei, 25, Mació, Alagoas

Escola de Ciências Médicas de Alagoas
Prof. Everaldo Lemos, Rua Antonio Cansanção, 1296 Macció, Alagoas

Faculdade de Medicina da Fundação Universidade do Amazonas
Prof. Roberto de Goes Monteiro, Rua 10 de Julho, 93 apto 102, Centro, Manaus, Amazonas

Faculdade de Medicina da Universidade Federal da Babia
Prof. Heitor Marback, Baixa do Bomfim, 236, Salvador, Bahia

Escola de Medicina e Sáude Pública da Universidade Católica de Salvador
Prof. Humberto de Castro Lima, Av. Euclides da Cunha, 9 apto. 1001, Salvador, Bahia

Faculdade de Medicina da Universidade Federal do Ceará
Prof. José Maria de Monteiro e Andrade, Rua Torres Camara, 135, Fortaleza, Ceará

Faculdade de Ciências da Saúde
Campus Universitário, Asa Norte, Brasilia, Distrito Federal

Faculdade de Medicina da Universidade Federal do Espirito Santo
Prof. José de Almeida Rebouças, Caixa Postal 85, Vitória, Espirito Santo

Escola de Medicina da Santa Casa de Misericordia de Vitória
Prof. Argeo Barbieri Filho, Rua 7 de Setembro, 200, Vitória, Espirito Santo

Faculdade de Medicina da Universidade Federal Fluminense
Prof. Henry Curi, Av. Ari Parreiras, 438, Canto do Rio, Niterói, Estado do Rio de Janeiro

Faculdade de Medicina de Petrópolis
Prof. Accacio de Souza Branco, Praça Ruy Barbosa, 205 apto. 601, Petropolis, Estado do Rio de Janeiro

Faculdade de Medicina de Campos
Prof. Oswaldo C. Cardoso de Melo, Rua Barão de Cotegipe, 86, 1° andar, Campos, Estado do Rio de Janeiro

Escola de Ciências Médicas de Volta Redonda
Prof. Joviano de Rezende Filho, Praça Cruz Velmelha, 12, Terreo, Centro, 20.000, Rio de Janeiro, GB. ZC-86

Faculdade de Medicina de Valença da Fundação Educacional Dom André Arcoverde
Prof. Morizot Leite Filho, Av. N.S. Copacabana, 583 apto. 814, Copacabana, 20.000, Rio de Janeiro, GB. ZC-07

Faculdade de Medicina da Fundação Universitaria Sul-Fluminense
Prof. Jonas de Arruda, Av. Lineu de Paula Machado, 788, Jardim Botanico, 20.000, Rio de Janeiro, GB. ZC-20

Faculdade de Medicina de Teresópolis
Prof. Fernando Dantas Coutinho, Praça Cruz Vermelha, 12, Terreo, Centro, 20.000, Rio de Janeiro, GB. ZC-86

Faculdade de Medicina da Universidade Federal do Rio de Janeiro
Prof. Sylvio Abreu Fialho, Rua 7 de Setembro, 88, 6° andar, Centro, 20.000, Rio de Janeiro, GB. ZC-21

Escola de Medicina e Cirurgia do Rio de Janeiro
Prof. Antonio Paulo Filho, Av. N.S. de Fátima, 63, Bairro de Fátima, 20.000, Rio de Janeiro, GB. ZC-86

Faculdade de Ciências Médicas da Universidade do Estado da Guanabara
Prof. Werther Duque Estrada, Rua Barata Ribeiro, 48, apto. 402, Copacabana, 20.000, Rio de Janeiro, GB. ZC-07

Escola Médica do Rio de Janeiro da Universidade Gama Filho
Prof. Luiz Eurico Ferreira, Av. N.S. Copacabana, 1052, 4° andar, Copacabana, 20.000, Rio de Janeiro, GB. ZC-07

Escola de Medicina, Fundação Técnico Educacional Souza Marques
Prof. Paiva Gonçalves Filho, Praça Serzedelo Correia, 15, 3° andar, Copacabana, 20.000, Rio de Janeiro, GB. ZC-07

Centro de Ciências Biológicas
Prof. Eloy Pereira, Rua 14 de Julho, 570 apto. 303, Campo Grande, Mato Grosso

Faculdade de Medicina, Fundação Universidade do Maranhão
Prof. Astério Pinto do Monte, Av. Santos Dumont, 100, Bairro Tirirical, São Luiz, Maranhão

Faculdade de Medicina da Universidade Federal de Minas Gerais
Prof. Hilton Rocha, Rua Rio de Janeiro, 2251, Belo Horizonte, Minas Gerais

Faculdade de Ciências Médicas de Minas Gerais
Prof. Geraldo Queiroga, Rua Felipe dos Santos, 382, Belo Horizonte, Minas Gerais

Faculdade de Medicina da Universidade Federal de Juiz de Fora
Prof. Ruben Sotto Maior, Rua Halfeld, 744, 3° andar, Juiz de Fora, Minas Gerais

Faculdade Federal de Medicina do Triângulo Mineiro
Prof. Eduardo Velloso Vianna, Rua Cel. José Ferreira, 246, Uberaba, Minas Gerais

Faculdade de Medicina de Itajubá da Asoc. de Integração Social de Itajubá
Prof. Domingos Sávio de Aquino Almeida, Rua Dr. Rodrigues Azevedo, 188, Lorena, Estado de São Paulo

Escola de Medicina e Cirurgia de Uberlândia
Prof. Edahir Gonçalves, Av. João Pinheiro, 761 apto. 12, Uberlândia, Minas Gerais

Faculdade de Ciências Médicas 'Dr. José Antonio Garcia Coutinho'
Prof. Gilberto de Magalhães, 37550, Pouso Alegre, Minas Gerais

Faculdade de Medicina de Barbacena da Fundação Presidente Antonio Carlos
Prof. Geraldo De Felippo, Caixa Postal 61, Barbacena, Minas Gerais
Prof. Paulo Patricio de Moura e Silva, Rua Gal. Afonso Monteiro, 130, Barbacena, Minas Gerais

Faculdade de Medicina do Norte de Minas Gerais
Prof. Elio Rocha Lessa, Hospital de Olhos Santa Luzia, Montes Claros, Minas Gerais

Faculdade de Medicina da Universidade do Pará
Prof. Aracy Barreto, Av. Governador Malcher, 223, Belém, Para

Faculdade de Medicina do Pará
Rua Braz de Aguiar, 774, Nazaré, Belém, Pará

Faculdade de Medicina da Universidade Federal da Paraiba
Prof. Roberto Granvile, Praça Dom Ulrico, 63, João Pessoa, Paraiba

Faculdade de Medicina de Campina Grande
Prof. Roberto Albrantes Pinto de Oliveira, Rua Maciel Pinheiro, 320, Campina Grande, Paraiba

Faculdade de Medicina da Universidade Federal do Paraná
Prof. Egon Armando Kruger, Rua Ebano Pereira, 335, Curitiba, Paraná

Faculdade de Ciências Médicas da Universidade Católica do Paraná
Prof. Francisco de Paula Soares Filho, Edifício Asa, Praça Gal. Osório, Curitiba, Paraná

Faculdade Evangélica de Medicina do Paraná
Prof. Carlos Augusto Moreira, Rua Mal. Deodoro, 211, conj. 605, Curitiba, Paraná

Curso de Medicina do Centro de Ciências da Universidade Estadual de Londrina
Prof. Osman Simei Baema Ferraz, Av. Bandeirantes, 645, Londrina, Paraná

Faculdade de Medicina da Universidade Federal de Pernambuco
Prof. Clovis de Azevedo Paiva, Rua dos Navegantes, 2465, Boa Viagem, Recife, Pernambuco

Faculdade de Ciências Médicas de Pernambuco
Prof. Clovis de Azevedo Paiva, Rua dos Navegantes, 2465, Boa Viagem, Recife, Pernambuco

Faculdade de Medicina da Fundação Universidade Federal do Piauí
Prof. João Orlando Ribeiro Gonçalves, Rua Areolino de Abreu, 1476, Terezina, Piauí

Faculdade de Medicina da Universidade Federal do Rio Grande do Sul
Prof. Luis Assumpção Osório, Rua Gal. Vitorino, 161, 2° andar, Porto Alegre, Rio Grande do Sul

Fundação Daculdade Católica de Medicina de Porto Alegre
Prof. Rivadavia Corrêa Meyer, Rua Sarmento Leite, 187, Porto Alegre, Rio Grande do Sul

Faculdade de Medicina da Universidade Católica de Pelotas
Prof. Ivano Marques da Rocha, Pelotas, Rio Grande do Sul

Faculdade de Medicina de Pelotas
Prof. Isaac Piltcher, Rua 15 de Novembro, 11, Pelotas, Rio Grande do Sul

Centro de Ciências Biomédicas da Universidade Federal de Santa Maria
Prof. Armindo Rossi Filho, Rua do Acampamento, 326, Santa Maria, Rio Grande do Sul

Faculdade de Medicina do Rio Grande
Prof. João Hugo Altmayer, Rua General Portinho, 446, Rio Grande, Rio Grande do Sul

Faculdade de Medicina da Universidade de Caxias do Sul
Prof. Rubens Ramos, Rua do Guia Lopes, 1041, Caxias do Sul, Rio Grande do Sul

Faculdade de Medicina de Passo Fundo da Universidade de Passo Fundo
Prof. Luthero Dutra Martins, Rua Cel. Chicuta, 175, Passo Fundo, Rio Grande do Sul

Faculdade de Medicina da Universidade Federal de Santa Catarina
Prof. Otto Freusberg, Largo de São Sebastião, 9, Florianópolis, Santa Catarina

Faculdade de Medicina da Universidade de São Paulo
Prof. Paulo Braga de Magalhães, Rua Sampaio, Vidal, 975, São Paulo, Estado de São Paulo

Escola Paulista de Medicina
Prof. Renato de Toledo, Rua Sena Madureira, 744, São Paulo, Estado de São Paulo

Faculdade de Ciências Médicas da Santa Casa de São Paulo
Prof. Athur Vicente do Amaral Filho, Rua Cel, Xavier de Toledo, 266, 11° andar, São Paulo, Estado de São Paulo

Faculdade de Medicina de Ribeirão Preto da Universidade de São Paulo
Prof. Almiro Pinto de Azeredo, Depto. de Oftalmologia, Hospital das Clínicas, Ribeirão Preto, Estado de São Paulo

Faculdade de Medicina de Sorocaba da Pontificia Universidade Católica de São Paulo
Prof. Benedito de Paulo Santos Filho, Rua Marques de Itú, 58, 9° andar, Vila Buarque, São Paulo, Estado de São Paulo

Faculdade de Ciências Médicas da Universidade Estadual de Campinas
 Prof. Antonio Augusto de Almeida, Instituto Penido Burnier, Campinas, Estado de São Paulo

Faculdade de Ciências Médicas e Biológicas de Botucatú
 Prof. Milton Massato Hida, Rua General Telles, 403, Botucatú, Estado de São Paulo

Faculdade de Ciências Médicas de Santos
 Prof. Plinio de Toledo Piza, Rua 7 de Abril, 118, 8° andar, 01044 São Paulo, Estado de São Paulo

Faculdade de Medicina de Marilia
 Prof. José Francisco Maniscalco, Av. Sampaio Vidal, 457, Marilia, Estado de São Paulo

Faculdade de Medicina de Taubaté
 Prof. José Carlos Gouvêa Pacheco, Rua Marques do Itú, 266, 8° andar, Vila Buarque, 01223 São Paulo, Estado de São Paulo

Faculdade de Medicina de São José de Rio Preto
 Prof. Ibrahim Younan, Rua Ondina, 427, São José do Rio Preto, Estado de São Paulo
 Prof. Benedito Alves Delsin, Rua Mal. Deodoro, 3096, 2° andar, São José do Rio Petro, Estado de São Paulo

Faculdade de Medicina de Mogi das Cruzes
 Prof. Hisato Mori, Rua Flaviano de Mello, 822, Mogi das Cruzes, Estado de São Paulo
 Prof. Hissashi Nomura, Rua Flaviano de Mello, 822, Mogi das Cruzes, Estado de São Paulo

Faculdade de Medicina da Fundação Universitaria do ABC
 Prof. Jorge Cavaleiro Wilmersdorf, Rua Monsenhor Andrade, 36 apto. 56, Braz, 03008 São Paulo, Estado de São Paulo

Faculdade de Medicina de Jundiaí
 Prof. Newton Kara José, Av. Brigadeiro Luiz Antonio, 3775, Jardin Paulista, 01401 São Paulo, Estado de São Paulo

Faculdade de Medicina de Catanduva da Fundação 'Padre Albino'
 Catanduva, Estado de São Paulo

Faculdade de Medicina de Santo Amaro
 Santo Amaro, São Paulo, Estado de São Paulo

Faculdade de Medicina de Braganca Paulista
 Bragança Paulista, Estado de São Paulo

Faculdade de Medicina da Universidade Federal de Sergipe
 Prof. Lauro de Brito Porto, Rua Boquim, 67, Aracajú, Estado de São Paulo

INSTITUTA SCHOLAEQUE CAECIS DESTINATAE

cegos

Instituto de Cegos do Brasil Central, Rua Marquez do Paraná, 79, Bairro EE.UU. Uberaba, MG 65

Instituto São Rafael, Av. Augusto de Lima, 2109, Belo Horizonte, MG. 157

Instituto de Cegos, Propriedade da Santa Casa de Misericordia do Recife, Rua Guilherme Pinto, 146, Capunga, Recife, Pernambuco 35

União Auxiliadora dos Cegos do Recife, Rua Sete, 240, Alto José do Pinho, Casa Amarela, Recife Pernambuco 18

Instituto de Proteçao Aos Cegos e Sardos Mudos, Rua São Pedro, 93, Rocas, Natal, Rio Grande do Norte 75

Lar das Moças Cegos, Escola Residencial, Av. Ana Costa, 198, Vila Matias, Santos, SP 31
Instituto para Cegos Santa Luzia, Rua Rio Grande do Sul, 23, Aracatuba, São Paulo 13
Instituto Santa Luzia, Ginásio e Escola Profissional p/ Cegos, Av. Cavalhada, 3.999, Porto
  Alegre, RGS 141
Associação Linense para Cegos, Av. Nilo Noronha, 656, Lins SP ...:.................... 31
Escola Luis Braille, Rua Andrade Neves, 3084, Pelotas, RGS 10
Instituto Paranaense de Cegos, Av. Visc. de Guarapuava, 4186, Curitiba, Paraná 214
Abrigo de Cegos, Rua Redenção, 72/82, Belém, São Paulo, SP ....
Abrigo de Cegos Santa Luzia, Rua Silva Jardim, 69, Santos, SP ....
Abrigo dos Cegos Joana D'Arc, Rua Visconde de Cairú, 228, Santos, SP ....
Ação Social de Educação e Assistencia aos Cegos, Av. 13 de Maio, 47, 16° andar, Grupo
  1809, Rio de Janeiro, GB ....
Aliança dos Cegos de São Paulo, Rua Jaguarani, 310, Jabaquara, SP ....
Assistência Linense de Instrução para Cegos, Caixa Postal 118, Lins, SP ....
Associação Aliança dos Cegos, Rua 24 de Maio, 47, São Francisco Xavier, Rio de Janeiro,
  GB ....
Associação Brasileira de Cegos, Rua Herval de Gouvea, 24, Madureira, Rio de Janeiro, GB ..
Associação de Cegos de Juiz de Flora, Av. dos Andradas, 455, Juiz de Fora, MG ....
Associação de Cegos de Ribeirão Preto, Rua Duque de Caxias, 625, Ribeirão Preto, SP ....
Associação de Cegos Luiz Braille, Edificio Feira de Amostras, 6ᵛ andar, Belo Horizonte, MG
Associação de Cegos Piauí, Rua Barroso, 450, Teresina, Piaui ....
Associação de Cegos São Judas Tadeu, Rua das Rosas, 127, Bosque da Saúde, São Paulo, SP.
Associação Dorina Nowill Para Estudantes Deficientes Visuais, Av. Independência, 1941,
  Ribeirão Preto, SP ....
Associação Filantrópica do Amparo aos Cegos, Rua Antonio Rodrigues, 998, Caixa Postal
  88, Presidente Prudente, SP ....
Associação Fluminense de Amparo aos Cegos, Rua Santa Rosa, 82, Santa Rosa, Niteroi,
  Estado do Rio ....
Associação Linense de Assistência aos Cegos, Rua São Benedito, 181, Lins, SP ....
Associação para Cegos 'Hellen Keller', Rua Floriano Peixoto, 669, Ribeirão Preto, SP .....
Associação Paulista de Redenção aos Cegos, Rua Vera, 2.A, Vila Matilde, SP ....
Associação Pró-Biblioteca e Alfabetização para Cegos, Alameda Surutai, 350, Jardim Paulis-
  ta, São Paulo, SP ....
Associação Promotora de Instrução e Trabalho para Cegos, Rua Conselheiro Nebias, 649,
  Santos, SP ....
Associação União Geral dos Cegos, Travessa Teixeira, 21, Engenho Novo, Rio de Janeiro,
  GB ....
Comissão De Prevenção à Cegueira, Instituto Benito Burnier, Campinas, São Paulo ....
Cruzada de Recuperação e Assistência aos Cegos, Rua Tiradentes, 148, Niteroi, Estado do
  Rio ....
Departamento de Trabalho pata Cegos, Rua Juca Quito, 618, Jaboticabal, SP ....
Escola de Enfermagem da Cruz Vermelha Brasileira, Seção Braille, Rua Libero Badaró, 595,
  4° andar, São Paulo, SP ....
Escola de Recuperação de Cegos, Serviço de Assistência à Mendicância, Rua Simões Dias,
  794, Aracaju, Sergipe ....
Escola Luiz Braille, Rua Dr. José Brusque, 240, Pelotas, RGS ....
Escola para Cegos Godofredo Viana, Praça São João, 22, CP 244, São Luiz, Maranhão ....
Escola para Cegos Monsenhor Tobias, Rua Fernandes Barros, 161, Maceió ....
  Couto, Largo de Nazaré, Salvador, Bahia ....
Federação dos Cegos Laboriosos, Rua Cardoso de Almeida, 844, Perdizes, SP ....
Fundação Contra a Cegueira Santa Luzia, Hospital Santa Luzia, Praça Conselheiro Almeida
Fundação para o Livro do Cego no Brasil, Rua Dr. Diogo de Faria, 358, Vila Clemente, São
  Paulo, SP ....
Institutição das Cegas Helen Keller, Rua Perseverança, 24, Rocha, Rio de Janeiro, GB .....
Instituto Araraquarense de Assistência do Cego Trabalhador, Rua Itália, 1223, Araçatuba,
  SP ....

Instituto Campineiro dos Cegos Trabalhadores, Av. Washington Luiz, 570, Campinas, SP ..
Instituto de Cegos da Bahia, Rua Militão Lisboa, 55, Salvador, Bahia ....
Instituto de Cegos da Paraiba Adalgisa Cunha, Av. Santa Catarina s/n, Mandacarú, João
  Pessoa, Paraíba ....
Instituto de Cegos de Pernambuco, Av. Guilherme Pinto, 141, Capunga, Recife, Pernambuco
Instituto de Cegos do Ceará, Av. Bezerra de Menezes, 892, São Geraldo, Fortaleza ....
Instituto de Cegos São Geraldo, Rua G, 57, Parque Peruche, Casa Verde, São Paulo, SP ....
Instituto de Proteção aos Cegos, Caixa Postal 38, Campina Grande, Paraiba ....
Instituto dos Cegos da Bahia, Rua Augusto Guimarães, 44, Salvador, Bahia ....
Instituto dos Cegos da Paraíba, Av. Epitácio Pessoa, 568, João Pessoa, Paraiba ....
Instituto Evangélico dos Cegos, Rua Ana Leonídia, 166, Rio de Janeiro, GB ....
Instituto Evangelico para Cegos, Rua Germano Dantas, 485, Engenho de Dentro, Rio de
  Janeiro, GB ....
Instituto Jundiaiense Profissional para Cegos Luiz Braille, Av. Sebastião Mendes Silva, 539,
  Jundiaí, SP ....
Instituto Luiz Braille, Rua Cazuru, 789, Botucatu, SP ....
Instituto Luiz Braille de Marilia, Av. Republica, 935, Marilia, SP ....
Instituto Luiz Braille de Santos, Av. Marechal Deodoro, 136, Santos, SP ....
Instituto Luiz Braille do Estado do E. Santo, Av. Vitória, Vitória, Espirito Santo ....
Instituto Matogrossense para Cegos, Rua 7 de Setembro, 456/458, Campo Grande, Mato
  Grosso ....
Instituto Montessoriano Alvaro Maia, Rua Paraiba, Adrianópolis, Manaus, Amazonas .....
Instituto Paranaense para Cegos, Av. Guarapuava, 4186, Curitiba, Paraná ....
Instituto Profissional de Cegos Santa Terezinha, Rua Galiléia, 14, Casa Verde, São Paulo, SP
Instituto Profissional dos Cegos de Catanduva, Rua Espirito Santo, Vila São Jorge, Catan-
  duva, SP ....
Instituto Profissional para Cegos Padre Chico, Rua Dr. Moreira de Godoi, 456, Ipiranga, São
  Paulo, SP ....
Instituto Profissional Paulista para Moças Cegas, Rua Mooca, 3931, São Paulo, SP ....
Instituto Tiradentes para Cegos, Rua D. Pedro I, 1106, Fortaleza, Ceará ....
Lar Campineiro das Moças, Rua Dr. Quirino, 1856, Campinas, SP ....
Lar Padre Luiz Orione, Bairro de São Francisco, Niteroi, Estado do Rio ....
Liga de Proteção aos Cegos do Brasil, Rua Dias da Cruz, 371, Meier, Rio de Janeiro, GB ...
Liga Nacional de Prevenção da Cegueira, Rua Uruguaiana, 25, 1° andar, Rio de Janeiro, GB .
Linense de Assistência, Instrução e Trabalho para Cegos, Av. Paulo Geraldi, 166, Lins, SP ..
Núcleo Profissional de Cegos, Rua do Vergueiro, 576, Piracicaba, São Paulo ....
Núcleo Profissional de Cegos, Av. Conselheiro Bebias, 649, Santos, SP ....
Núcleo Profissional de Cegos, Rua 7 de Setembro, 344, Sorocaba, SP ....
Sociedade Beneficente dos Cegos de Recife, Estrada dos Remédios, 1558, Recife, Pernam-
  buco ....
Sociedade Franca de Instrução e Trabalhos para Cegos, Rua Água Santa, 103, Vila Nova,
  Franca, São Paulo ....
Sociedade Organizadora de Trabalho para Cegos, Rua 17, 44, Barretos, SP ....
União dos Cegos do Brasil, Rua Clarimundo de Melo, 216, Piedade, Rio de Janeiro, GB ....
União Profissional dos Cegos, Av. Rio Branco, 621, Natal ....

BRITANNIA

SOCIETATES OPHTHALMOLOGICAE

Nationales

Faculty of Ophthalmology

At the Royal College of Surgeons, Lincoln's Inn Fields, London, WC2H 3PN
President: Mr. E. C. Zorab
Vice-Presidents: Mr. J. R. Hudson, Mr. M. J. Roper-Hall
Honorary Treasurer: Mr. J. E. Coates
Honorary Secretary: Mr. Lorimer Fison
Number of members: 588

Ophthalmological Society of the United Kingdom

At The Royal College of Surgeons, Lincoln's Inn Fields, London, WC2H 3PN
President: Mr. L. E. Werner
Vice-Presidents: Mr. S. J. H. Miller, Mr. J. H. Dobree, Mr. A. G. Palin, Mr. K. C. Wybar
Honorary Treasurer: Mr. Frank W. Law
Honorary Secretaries: Mr. P. A. MacFaul, Mr. J. L. Kennerley Bankes
Editor: Mr. P. D. Trevor-Roper
Ex Officio: Representatives of Affiliated Societies
Number of members: 1395

Oxford Ophthalmological Congress

Master: Dr. D. Christison
Deputy Master: Mr. A. C. L. Houlton
Editorial Secretary: Mr. S. I. Davidson
Honorary Secretary-Treasurer: Mr. W. Martin Walker, 690 Warwick Road, Solihull, Warwickshire
Number of members: 1000

Section of Ophthalmology, Royal Society of Medicine

1 Wimpole Street, London, W1M 8AE
President: Mr. E. C. Zorab
Honorary Secretaries: Mr. Brian Harcourt, Mr. Peter Fells
Number of members: 355

Regionales

Midland Ophthalmological Society
President: Mr. K. Rubinstein
Vice-President: Mr. G. Siggins

President-Elect: Mr. H. F. T. MacFetridge

Honorary Treasurer: Mr. I. A. R. Brown

Honorary Secretaries: Mr. Vernon H. Smith, Birmingham & Midland Eye Hospital, Church Street, Birmingham, B3 2NS. Mr. D. S. Thomson, Lansdown Lodge, Lansdown Road, Cheltenham, Glos.

Number of members: 159

North of England Ophthalmological Society

President: Mr. J. Lindley Smith

Vice-President: Mr. T. Stafford Maw

Honorary Treasurer: Mr. Peter Wilson

Honorary Secretary: Mr. R. Ivor T. Lloyd, Northfield, Park Road, Menston, Ilkley, Yorks.

Number of members: 180

Scottish Ophthalmological Club

President: Mr. Charles Cockburn

Vice-President: Mr. R. J. S. Smith

Honorary Secretaries: Dr. James Hughes, 6 Wester Coates Avenue, Edinburgh, EH12 5LS. Mr. W. Wilson, 34 Calderwood Road, Newlands, Glasgow, S.3

Southern Ophthalmological Society

President: Mr. J. N. Ormrod

Vice-President: Mr. J. Whitwell

Immediate Past President: Mr. M. J. Gilkes

Honorary Clinical Secretary: Mr. H. N. O'Donaghue

Honorary Secretary & Treasurer: Mr. E. Milwyn Evans, 'Leybourne', Old Roar Road, St. Leonards-on-Sea, Sussex

Number of members: 116

South Western Ophthalmological Society

President: Mr. T. Stuart-Black Kelly

Vice-Presidents: Mr. G. Hibbert, Mr. C. A. Brown

Honorary Secretaries: Mr. V. J. Marmion, Mr. N. L. Dallas, Bristol Eye Hospital, Bristol, BS1 2LX

Number of members: 89

NOMINA ET DOMICILIA MEDICORUM AB OCULIS

Abrams, J. D.	99 Harley Street	Londen, W.1
Absolon, M. J.	Southampton Eye Hospital, Wilton Avenue	Southampton, SOQ WWW
Acheson, R. R.	40 Jeffreys Way	Stonegallows, Taunton
Adam, Alastair	11 Blantyre Terrace	Edinburgh, EH10 5AD

Adams, John Boyd	The Beeches, 14 Mansion House Road	Paisley, Renfrews
Adams, M. H.	Canberra, Rock, Nr. Wadebridge .	Cornwall
Adlakha, D.	15 Walmley Road	Sutton Coldfield. Warwicks.
Ahmad, K.	15 Holmston Road	Ayr
Ahmad, N.	Sussex Eye Hospital, Eastern Road	Brighton
Ainslie, Derek	36 Weymouth Street	London, WIN 3LR
Aitchison, Henry H.	5 Brandling Park	Newcastle-on-Tyne, 2
Ali, M.	51 Ambleside, Bartley Green ...	Birmingham, B32 3HR
Allen, Percival L.	142 Alexandra Road	Farnborough, Hants.
Almosulli, H. H.	48 Elm Walk	Raynes Park, London, S.W.20
Alvi, A. R.	58 Parsonage Road	Manchester, 20
Amies, D. R.	Ophthalmic Department, Royal Air Force Hospital	Ely, Cambs.
Anderson, John	54 Hornton Street	London, W.8
Anderson, L.	Janefield, 43 Hillview Road, Cults	Aberdeen
Anderson, P.	12 St. John's Hill	Shrewsbury, Salop.
Anwar, Mohammed	24 Colwyn Avenue	Perivale, Middx.
Applin, H. W.	Sandilands, Cooks Cross	South Molton, N. Devon
Arnott, E. J.	82 Harley Street	Londen, W.1
Arundell, P. W.	13 Liverpool Terrace	Worthing, Sussex
Ashraf, Ali M.	Stobhill Hospital	Glasgow, N1
Ashton, Prof. Norman H. ..	2 The Cloisters, Westminister Abbey	London S.W.1
Ashworth, A. N.	Cranford, 3 St. Helens Close	Southsea, Hants
Ashworth, Bryan	36 Barnton Court	Edinburgh, EH4 6EH
Assinder, E. W.	The New House	Snittersfield, Nr. Stratford on Avon
Auplish, R. N.	Moorfields Eye Hospital City Road	London, E.C.1
Austin, J. H.	15 Chadbrook Crest, Brook Road	Birmingham, 15
Averill, T. L. F.	c/o Bank of New South Wales, 14 Kingsway	London, W.C.2
Awdry, Philip N.	23 Banbury Road	Oxford, OX2 6NX
Aynsley, T. Rutherford ...	23 Rothesay Road	Bournemouth
Ayoub, J. E. M.	11 Wimpole Street	London, W.1
Bacon, Edward	Bridle Way, South-down Road, Shawford	Winchester, Hants
Badr, Ihsan, A. Z.	St. Paul's Eye Hospital, Old Hall Street	Liverpool
Bain, W. E. S.	4 Roehampton Wick, 401 Upper Richmond Road	London, S.W.15
Banik, J. L.	Royal Infirmary	Preston, Lancs.
Bankes, J. L. K.	27 Harley Street	London, W1N IDA
Barber, Norman K.	32 Fields Park Road	Newport, Mon
Barclay, Alexander P.	10 St. David's Drive	Broxbourne, Herts
Barling, G. M.	51 Thorpe Road	Peterborough
Barnes, Dagmar	c/o Bank of New South Wales, Sackville Street	London, W.1
Barras, T. C.	Kinfauns, Fort Road	Gosport, Hants., PO12 2DT
Barron, Agnes M. K.	10 Golf Place, Greenock	Renfrews
Barry D. R.	Birmingham & Midland Eye Hospital, Church Street	Birmingham, B3 2NS
Bartholomew, R. S.	Eye Department, Royal Infirmary, P. O. Box 72	Dundee, DDI 9ND

Barton, J. R. S.	9 Haines Park	Taunton
Barton, Maurice H.	Rushall Field Farm	Woodhouse, Nr. Loughborough, Leics.
Basu, D. K.	William Goodenough House (Flat 302), Mecklenburgh Square ..	London, W.C.1
Batheja, N. S.	110 Spencefield Lane	Leicester
Batten, K. L.	c/o Williams & Glyns Bank Ltd., 22 Whitehall	London, S.W.1
Beattie, P. H.	28 Newmarket Road	Norwich, NOR 26D
Bedford, G. T.	25 Croslands Park	Barrow-in-Furness, Lancs.
Behrman, S.	33 Harley Street	London, W.1
Belsey, R. L.	Brookfield, Oxenhope	Keighley, Yorks.
Bennett, A. E.	7 Court Drive, Shillingford	Oxford, OX9 8ER
Bennett, Fiona M.	4 Earls Court Gardens	Aberdeen
Bevan, G. H.	21 Moor Crescent	Gosforth, Newcastle-on-Tyne, 3
Beveridge, Brian F.	c/o Lloyds Bank Ltd., 708 High Road	London, E.11
Bhalerao, V. R.	78 Newgate Avenue	Appley Bridge, Nr. Wigan, Lancs., WN6 9JJ
Bhargava, Satish K.	4 Freshfield Road	Heaton Mersey, Stockport, SK4 3HN
Billinghurst, Margaret	8 Haverfield Gardens	Kew, Surrey
Binnie, Bertram	5 Rysland Crescent, Newton Mearns	Glasgow
Birch, H. E. W.	Bungalow 8, Royal Victoria Hospital, Gloucester Road	Boscombe, Bournemouth
Birchall, C. H.	42 Craiglea Drive	Edingburgh, EH10 5PF
Bird, Alan	155 Turney Road	London, S.E.21
Birks, Doreen A.	19 St. Leonard's Terrace	London, S.W.3
Bishop, Patricia J.	7 Glade Gardens, Shirley	Croydon, Surrey
Blach, R. K.	88 Harley Street	London, W.1
Black, George	43 Park Square	Leeds, LS1 2NP
Blacklidge, T. S.	173 Newton Drive	Blackpool
Blair, C. J. L.	28 Hillbrow	Richmond, Surrey TW10 6BH
Blaxter, P. L.	The Uplands, Fulshaw Park	Wilmslow, Cheshire
Boase, A. J.	Kilworth, Meresfield	Uckfield, Sussex
Boomla, Darius F.	58 Rennets Wood Road	London, S.E.9
Booth, A. H.	32 Castle Gate	Nottingham
Boucherat, Robert	16 Laneham Close	Bessacarr, Doncaster
Bowen, D. I.	19 Granton Close	Formby, Lancs., L37 3PH
Brammar, D. K.	14 Storth Avenue	Sheffield, S10 3HL
Brewerton, R.	11 Rickmansworth Road	Watford
Bridgeman, The Hon. G. J. O.	Watley House	Sparsholt, Winchester
Briggs, Allan H.	Lincoln House, 56/58 Clasketgate	Lincoln
Britten, M. J. A.	Eshton, Withinlee Road	Prestbury, Cheshire
Brodrick, J. D.	22 Bents Drive	Ecclesall, Sheffield, S11 9RP
Brogan, Agnes M.	9 Romney Avenue	Glasgow, S.4
Bron, A. J.	18 Woodside Avenue	London, N.6
Brooks, R. Philip	20 Western Road	Southall, Middlesex
Brown, C. A.	16 Grove Road	Coombe Dingle, Bristol, BS9 2RQ
Brown, H. J.	538 Wellingborough Road	Weston Favell, Northampton

Clarke, Derek H.	18 Starrock Road	Coulsdon, Surrey
Clements, D. B.	3 Thornhill Close, Granville Park	Aughton, Nr. Ormskirk, Lancs.
Clemett, R. S.	7 Wellington Avenue	Worcester Park, Surrey
Clifton, Frank	3 Sussex Gardens	Petersfield, Hants.
Clover, Peter T.	11 Kingsdown Road	Surbiton, Surrey
Coates, J. E.	27 Friargate	Derby, DE1 1BY
Cobb, Benjamin	3 Grange Grove	London, N.1
Cockburn, Charles	12 Rubislaw Terrace	Aberdeen
Coddington, W. G.	Springwood, Writmore Heath	Newcastle, Staffs., ST5 5JA
Cogan, J. E. H.	8 Lonsdale Gardens	Tunbridge Wells
Cogan, J. F.	Brookside, Knowsley	Prescot, Lancs.
Cohen, S. G.	58 Ripplevale Grove	London, N.1
Compton, Stanley	28 Epsom Road	Guildford, Surrey
Condon, Patrick	Eye Department, Bromley General Hospital, Cromwell Avenue	Bromley, Kent
Conway, J. S.	30 Middleway	London, N.W.11
Cook, C. A.	13 Clarence Terrace, Regent's Park	London N.W.1
Cook, John H.	112 Sutton Common Road	Sutton, Surrey
Cormack, J. G.	6 Marlee Road, Broughty Ferry	Dundee
Corrigan, M. J.	Greenacres, Cassett Avenue	Southampton
Cory, C. C.	Lench, Blawford Road	Reigate, RH2 7DC
Cory, J. W. E.	45 Hardwick Lane	Bury St. Edmunds
Cowley, R.	27 The Crescent	Linthorpe, Middlesbrough
Cracknell, D. G.	154 Swithland Lane	Rothley, Leics.
Craig, A. W.	3 Stepney Drive	Scarborough
Crawford, R. A. D.	80 Gladstone Road	Broadstairs, Kent
Crews, S. J.	77 Wellington Road	Edgbaston, Birmingham, 15
Crick, R. P.	Private Patients Wing, King's College Hospital, Denmark Hill	London, S.E.5
Crombie, A. L.	19 Graham Park Road	Gosforth, Newcastle upon Tyne, 3
Cross, Alexander G.	27 Harley Street	London, W1N 1DA
Cullen, J. F.	244 Colinton Road	Edinburgh, EH14 1DL
Currie, J. G. D.	4 Imperial Square	Cheltenham
Curtis, F. J.	Reeves Cottage	Leigh, Nr. Reigate, Surrey
Curwood, B. C.	56 Russell Road, Clifton	Bristol, 13
Curzon-Miller, A. G.	Penhayes, Meneage Road	Helston, Cornwall
Dalgleish, Roy	18 Darley Avenue	West Didsbury, Manchester, 20
Dallas, Neil L.	Chantry House	Abbot's Leigh, Nr. Bristol
Darby, D. J.	73 Harley Street	London, W1
Darbyshire, F. J.	c/o Barclays Bank Ltd., 95 Victoria Street	London, S.W.1
Dark, A. J.	Eye Department, Hallamshire Hospital	Sheffield
Darvell, R. H. J.	49 Chesham Road	Amersham, Bucks.
Das, S. N.	11 Eton Grove	London, N.W.9
Davidson, Sidney I.	1 Dowhills Drive	Blundellsands, Liverpool, L23 8SU
Davies, E. W. G.	27 Harley Street	London, W1N IDA
Davies, L. W.	22 Woodlands	Gosforth, Northumberland, NE3 4YL
Davies, Margaret	22 Arundel Court, Duppas Road	Croydon, CRO 4BP
Davies, M. S.	The Forest, Benenden	Cranbrook, Kent
Davies, T. Gwilym G.	2 Scarsdale Avenue	Littleover, Derby, DE3 6ER

Dawson, D.	464 Duffield Road	Allestree, Derby
De, Santimoy	6a Augustus Road	Edgbaston, Birmingham, B15 3NR
Debnath, S. C.	62 Parkfield Avenue	Hillingdon, Middx.
De Courcy, Thomas L.	The Cronk	Port Lewaigue, Nr. Ramsay, I.O.M.
De Saram, R. B.	29 The Avenue, Branksome Park	Poole, Dorset
Dhillon, G. S.	23 Barnton Court	Barnton Grove, Edinburgh, 4
Dobree, J. H.	113 Harley Street	London, W.1
Dodd, C. L.	Manchester Royal Eye Hospital Oxford Road	Manchester, 13
Doggart, James H.	Albury Park, Albury	Guildford, Surrey
Doig, W. M.	12 Thorn Drive, High Burnside	Rutherglen, Glasgow
Dollar, Jean M.	6 Devonshire Place	London, W.1
Donoghue, Cecilie	97 Courthill Avenue	Glasgow, S.4
Dorrell, E. D.	8 Butts Hill Road	Woodley, Berks.
Dorrell, E. W.	1a Erleigh Road	Reading
Douglas, A. A.	White House	Newtyle, Angus
Douglas, Elma P.	47 Dowanhill Street	Glasgow, G11 5HB
Doyle, D.	35 Thorn Road	Bearsden, G61 4BS
Doyle, Janet	35 Thorn Road	Bearsden, G61 4BS
Dudgeon, John	71. Lochmaben Road	Crookston, Glasgow, G52
Duguid, I. M.	73 Harley Street	London, W.1
Duke - Elder, Sir Edward	28 Elm Tree Rd. St. John's Wood	London N.W.1
Durran. John	West Winnocks, Mount Tabor Road	Kinnoull, Perth
Duthie, O. M.	22 St. John Street	Manchester, 3
Eadie, S. P.	79 Downs Court Road	Purley, Surrey
Earl, C. J.	Private Consulting Room, National Hospital, Queen Square	London, W.C.1
Easty, David	Bristol Eye Hospital	Bristol, BS1 2LX
Efimba, V. A.	Eye Department, St. James' Hospital	London, S.W.12
Elkington, A. R.	61 Doneraile Street	London, SW6 6EW
Ellis, Jean R.	62 Kilmardinny Crescent, Bearsden	Glasgow, G61 3NR
Ellis, R. P.	Royal Eye Infirmary	Plymouth, Devon, PL4 6PL
Elsby, James M.	Storeton, Westwood Road	Ryde, Isle of Wight
Emery, D. G.	'Breckland' Griffins Hill, Bristol Road	Birmingham 29
Ensor, G. F.	56 Warwick Road	Bishop's Stortford, Herts.
Eustace, Peter	8 Leigham Drive	Harborne, Birmingham
Evans, A. T. G.	Ivy House, Ghyll Road	Scotby, Carlisle, Cumberland
Evans, E. Milwyn	Leybourne, Old Roar Road	St. Leonards-on-Sea, Sussex
Evans, H. M.	59 Hamilton Avenue, Harborne	Birmingham 17
Fagan, J. H. W.	51 Mount Harry Road	Sevenoaks, Kent
Fawssett, Kenneth	4 St. John's Road	Newbury, Berks.
Fells, Peter	133 Hendon Lane	Finchley, London, N3 3PR
Fenton, P. J.	Bere Farm House	North Boarhunt, Fareham, Hants.
Fergus, A. N.	Buffbeards, Hindhead Road	Haslemere, Surrey
Ffooks, Oliver O. F.	Lammas House, Ling Lane	Scarscroft, Nr. Leeds
Ffytche, T. J.	1 Wellington Square	Chelsea, London, S.W.3
Finch, Judith	121 Oakham Road, Rividale	Warley, Worcs.
Fisher, R. F.	4 Blacksmith's Hill	Sanderstead, Surrey
Fison, L. G.	62 Wimpole Street	London, W1M 7DE
Fitzmaurice, D. J.	23 Woodlands Way	Barton, Nr. Preston, Lancs.

Folca, P. J.	Brookhill Cottage, Castle Road ..	Kingswear, Devon
Forsyth, K. B.	Astley Towne	Stockport-on-Severne, Worcs.
Foster, John	17 North Hill Road	Leeds, 6
Foulds, Prof. W. S.	Department of Ophthalmology, University of Glasgow	Glasgow, G11 6NT
Frankenthal, J.	Sunderland Eye Infirmary, Alexandra Road	Sunderland
Franks, Ursula	7 Reres Road	Broughty Ferry, Dundee
Fraser, H.	36 The Ropewalk	Nottingham
Fraser, Ian C.	Old School House, School Gardens, Castle Street	Shrewsbury
Freedman, Arnold	The Eye Hospital, Walton Street .	Oxford
Freedman, S. Sydney	5 Chiswick Place	Eastbourne
Freeman, John D. J.	277 Glouchester Road	Cheltenham, GL51 7AA
Friedmann, Allan I.	Frognal Gardens	London, N.W.3
Galbraith, A. L.	50 Bromyard Road, St. Johns ...	Worcester
Galbraith, Samuel	57 Blairbeth Road	Burnside, Rutherglen, Glasgow
Galloway, N. P. R.	Robinscroft, Rempstone	Loughborough
Galloway, N. R.	Langham House, Elm Bank	Nottingham, NG3 5AJ
Galton, E. M. G.	5 West Heath Lodge, Branch Hill	London, N.W.3
Gann, John H.	5 Gaul Road	March, Cambs.
Gardiner, P. A.	30 Weymouth Street	London, W.1
Gardner, Catherine A.	29 Ness Bank	Inverness
Garner, Alec	Department of Pathology, Institute of Ophthalmology, Judd Street	London, WC1H 9QS
Garrow, William G.	Charlesville, Stotfield	Lossiemouth, Morayshire
Garston, J. B.	20 Gorsey Lane	Bowdon, Cheshire
Gartside, Edward	6 Bodenham Road	Folkestone, Kent
Gavey, C. J.	Westminster Hospital	London, S.W.1
Gebertt, Stanislaw	8 Stuart Avenue	Perth, Scotland
Gentles, A. W.	51 Kent Road	Harrogate, HG1 2EU
George, J. B.	c/o Messrs. Glyn Mills & Co., Krikland House, Whitehall ...	London, S.W.1
Ghosh, S.	c/o Royal Eye Hospital, St. George's Circus	London, S.E.1
Ghosh, T. N.	61 C Queen's Road	Aberdeen
Ghoshal, T. K.	115 Northgate	Wakefield
Gibbs, D.	'Waterfrets' Burnt House Lane, Speldhurst	Tunbridge Wells, Kent
Gilkes, M. J.	30 The Drive	Hove, Sussex, BN3 3JD
Gillan, R. U.	55 Harley Street	London, W.1
Gillespie, Ian	Southampton Eye Hospital, Wilton Avenue	Southampton, SO9 4XW
Glasspool, M. G.	15 Bushy Park Gardens	Teddington, Middx.
Gloster, J.	Institute of Ophthalmology, Judd Street	London, WC1H 9QS
Glover, E. C.	62 Wimpole Street	London, WIM 7DE
Goddard, Una K.	193 Woodhall Way	Molescroft, Beverley, Yorks.
Goldsmith, Sir Allen	63 Harley Street	London, W.1
Goldsmith, H.	538 Derby Road, Wollaton Park .	Nottingham, NG7 2GY
Gordon, W. Lindsay	182 Wake Green Road, Moseley .	Birmingham, 13
Goulstine, D. B.	3 St. George's Terrace	East Bolden, Co. Durham
Gow, Alastair C.	17 Monument Road	Ayr

Graham, Charles W. . . . . . .   54 Learmonth Court . . . .   Edinburgh, EH14 IPB
Graham, Malcolm V. . . . . . .   Montrose, Ty Gwyn Avenue . . . .   Cardiff
Graham, P. . . . .   73a Cathedral Road . . . .   Cardiff, CF1 9HE
Gray, T. D. H. . . . .   41 Rodney Street . . . .   Liverpool
Grayson, M. C. . . . .   4 Bishops Close . . . .   Whitchurch, Cardiff
Greaves, Desmond P. . . . . .   56 Wimpole Street . . . .   London, WIM 1DF
Green, Lionel M. . . . .   55 Harley Street . . . .   London, W.1
Greeves, P. R. . . . .   Summer Leas . . . .   Yelverton, S. Devon
Gregory, Irene D. R. . . . . . .   2a Southlands Grove, Bickley . . .   Bromley, Kent, BR1 2DQ
Gregory, T. S. S. . . . .   Bignell House . . . .   Nr. Bicester, Oxon.
Griffith, T. P. . . . .   78 Leathwaite, Loop Road South   Whitehaven, Cumberland
Griffiths, J. D. . . . .   Belvoir Lodge, Upper Old Field
                                        Park . . . .   Bath, Somerset
Griffiths, Peter . . . .   Eye Department, The General
                                        Hospital . . . .   Burton-on-Trent
Groves, J. S. . . . .   5 Davenport Road . . . .   Coventry
Gundry, M. F. . . . .   Maltmans, Headcorn . . . .   Ashford, Kent
Gurd, Dudley P. . . . .   Shanklin Lodge, Eastern Villas
                                        Road . . . .   Southsea, Hants.
Hadley, D. A. . . . .   66 Kingfisher Drive, Ham . . . . . .   Richmond, Surrey
Hahn, H. J. . . . .   c/o Medical Dept. Ministry of
                                        Defence (Naval), Lillie Road .   London, SW6
Haining, W. M. . . . .   Department of Ophthalmology,
                                        University of Dundee, 10 Dud-
                                        hope Terrace . . . .   Dundee
Haley, A. H. . . . .   Llaindelyn . . . .   St. Clears, Carms.
Hall, Roger D. . . . .   Worcester Eye Hospital, Barbour-
                                        ne Road . . . .   Worcester, WR1 1RY
Hall-Parker, Beresford . . . . .   North Riding Infirmary . . . .   Middlesbrough, Teesside
Hall, I. B. . . . .   396 Albert Drive . . . .   Pollokshields, Glasgow, G41
                                                                                    4JP
Halliwell, T. J. . . . .   29 Central Hill . . . .   London, SE19 1BW
Hamilton, Elizabeth F. . . . .   3 East Donnington Street . . . . . .   Darvel, Ayrshire
Hamilton, W. D. E. . . . .   3 Dorset Road . . . .:. .   Windsor, Berks.
Hamilton, W. H. C. M. . . . .   14 Mansion Row, Old Brompton   Gillingham, Kent
Handscombe, Marion C. . . .   8 Spencer Road . . . .   Coventry, CV5 6PA
Harcourt, R. B. . . . .   43 Park Square . . . .   Leeds, 1
Harden, A. F. . . . .   17 Carver Road . . . .   Herne Hill, London, S.E.24
Hardman, L. B. . . . .   21 Oldham Road . . . .   Grasscroft, Nr. Oldham
Harper, G. L. . . . .   Brondanw, Allanson Road . . . . .   Rhos-on-Sea, Denbighshire
Harrington, R. W. . . . .   5 Great Western Terrace . . . .   Glasgow, W2
Harris, W. . . . .   131 The Ridings, Rothley . . . . . .   Leicestershire, LE7 7SL
Harry, John . . . .   31 Woodhatch Spinney . . . .   Coulsdon, Surrey, CR3 2SU
Hart, C. T. . . . .   4 Imperial Square . . . .   Cheltenham
Hart, J. C. Dean . . . .   Bristol Eye Hospital, Lower
                                        Maudlin Street . . . .   Bristol
Hartley, Leslie B. . . . .   Orkney, Golf Drive . . . .   Camberley, Surrey
Hartley, R. C. . . . .   Royal Eye Infirmary . . . .   Plymouth, Devon
Hasan, Mahmud-Ul . . . .   c/o 3up left, Gourock Street . . . .   Glasgow, C5
Hashimi, M. . . . .   28 Drax Avenue . . . .   London, S.W. 20
Haslam, G. C. . . . .   6 Alicia Avenue, Kenton . . . .   Harrow, Middx.
Hassan, Mumtaz . . . .   Eye Department, King's Mill Hos-
                                        pital . . . .   Sutton-in-Ashfield, Notts.
Haworth, S. M. . . . .   7 Berkeley Avenue . . . .   Nottingham, NG3 5BU
Hayes, Lydia M. . . . .   5 Canynge Square . . . .   Clifton, Bristol, 8
Healy, J. J. . . . .   Invercauld, New Road . . . .   Llanellli, Carms.

Heath, Christopher	Nanslone Mill	Penwortha Coombe, Nr. Perranporth, Cornwall
Heath, W. E.	Furners	Wittersham Kent, TN30 7EA
Heaton, J. M.	58A Wimpole Street	London, W.1
Heckford, Frank	Berwick Cottage, Pelham Fields .	Ryde, Isle of Wight
Hempel, Andrew	42 Bramham Gardens, Nr. Earl's Court	London, S.W.5
Henson, Audrey	8 Stafford Street	London, W.1
Hibbert, F. G.	96 Eaton Crescent	Swansea, Glam., SA1 4QP
Higginbottom, Walter M. ..	8 Agbrigg Road, Sandal	Wakefield, Yorks.
Higgitt, A. C.	7 Perceval Avenue	Hampstead, London, N.W.3
Hill, Prof. D. W.	Royal College of Surgeons, Lincoln's Inn Fields	London, WC2A 3PN
Hill, K. Reed	48 Harley Street	London, W.1
Hillman, J. S.	6 Hampshire Drive, Augustus Road	Birmingham, B15 3NZ
Hirtenstein, Arnost	52 Bradford Street	Walsall, Staffs., WS1 3QD
Hitchings, R. A.	33 Chase Side	Enfield, Middx.
Ho, Hilton	33 Glanleam Road	Stanmore, Middlesex
Hoare, H. G. W.	Longfield, 196 Stow Hill	Newport, Mon, NPT 4HB
Hobbs, H. E.	46 Wimpole Street	London, W1M 7DG
Holding-Parsons, G. G. K. ..	Asperra, Haven Road	Canford Cliffs, Bournemouth, Hants.
Hollingsworth, A.	Highview, Watts Palace Lane	Northiam, Sussex
Holroyd, J. B. M.	16 Hall Park Rise, Horsforth	Leeds, LS18 5LW
Hopkins, David	6 Mornington Villas, Manningham Lane	Bradford
Hossain, A. T. M. Moazzam	75 Cowley Road	Ilford, Essex
Houlton, A. C. L.	23 Banbury Road	Oxford
Howat, J. M. L.	28 Claremont Place	Newcastle-on-Tyne, NE2 3AH
Howat, Thomas K.	22 Sandyford Place	Glasgow, G3 7NG
Hudson, J. M.	4 Wirral Road	Northfield, Birmingham, B31 1NZ
Hudson, J. R.	36 Wimpole Street	London, WIM 7EE
Hughes, James	6 Wester Coates Avenue	Edinburgh, EH12 5LS
Humfrey, S. H. G.	The Granary	Dallington, Northampton
Hunter, Peter J. L.	423 Unthank Road	Norwich, NOR 27E
Hunter, R. D.	395 Albert Drive	Glasgow, S.1
Husain, S. A.	35 Beechwood Gardens, Clayhall	Ilford, Essex, IGS OAL
Hypher, T. J.	26 Chalmers Road	Cambridge
Ingram, D. Vernon	4 Tongdean Road	Hove, Sussex, BN3 6QR
Ingram, H. Vernon	Uplands, Dudsbury Crescent ...	Ferndown, Dorset
Ingram, R. M.	118 Northampton Road	Kettering, Northants.
Jack, R. C.	29 Billing Road	Northampton
Jackson, C. R. S.	30 Blacket Place	Edinburgh, EH9 1RL
Jackson, H. S.	17 Harley Street	London, W1N 1DA
Jackson, L. S.	12 Clarendon Place	Stirling, Scotland
Jacobs, H. B.	49 Queen Anne Street	London, W.1
Jaffe, Roy	128 Harley Street	London, W.1
Jagger, Derek B.	South Lodge, Highlands Close ..	Farnham, Surrey
Jaiswal, Ramesh C.	30 Angus Gardens	London, N.W.9 SLE
James, D. Geraint	149 Harley Street	London, WIN IHG
Jamie, Elizabeth D.	50 Harley Street	London, W.1
Janus, Fred	26 St. John Street	Manchester, 3
Jardine, P.	2 Clifton Park	Bristol

Jay, Barrie S.	10 Beltane Drive, Seymour Road	London, SW19 5JR
Jenner, Paul W.	6 Somerhill Avenue	Hove, 2, Sussex
Johnston, I. G.	Military Hospital	Catterick Camp, Yorks.
Johnstone, I. Lloyd	15 Grange Court, Grange Court Road	Bristol, BS9 4DW
Jones, A. S.	Wildcroft, Bourneside, Wentworth	Virginia Water, Surrey
Jones, Prof. B. R.	Department of Clinical Ophthalmology, Institute of Ophthalmology, Judd Street	London, WC1H 9QS
Jones, D. E. P.	29 Hantone Hill, Bathampton . . .	Bath, Somerset
Jones, Eleanor	168 Milton Road	Cambridge
Jones, Kenyon	Whitecross, Llandre	Bow Street, Cards.
Jones, M. A.	9 Gladstone Road	Sheffield, S10 3GT
Jones, Ralph F.	Langdale House, Buccleuch Road, Branksome Park	Poole, Dorset
Joyce, Martin	162 Old Bath Road	Cheltenham, GL53 7DR
Kadri, S. W. M.	Department of Ophthalmology, St. James's Hospital	Leeds, LS9 7TF
Kanagasundaram, C. R.	54 Moorside South, Fenham	Newcastle-upon-Tyne, Staffs.
Kane, Iris	10 York Road	Woking, Surrey
Kanski, J. J.	4 Hardwick Green, Clevelands . .	London, W13 8DN
Kapur, S. B.	23 Farnham Close	London, N.20
Karim, M. A.	c/o 91 Cleave Road	Gillingham, Kent
Kaushal, Krishan	47 Warmington Road	Liverpool, 14
Keast-Butler, John	39 de Freville Avenue	Cambridge, CB4 1HW
Keith, C. G.	127 Harley Street	London, W.1
Kelly, T. Stuart-Black	Linden, Weston Road	Bath
Kelsey, J. H.	28 Weymouth Street	London, W1N 3FA
Kemp, M. H.	Worcester Eye Hospital, Barbourne Road	Worcester
Kempster, R. C.	86 Homewood Road, Northenden	Manchester, 22
Kennedy, Hugh B.	34 Leven Street	Glasgow, G43 2DA
Kent, P. J. M.	North Staffs Royal Infirmary . . .	Stoke-on-Trent, Staffs.
Kerr, J. N.	27 Inglemere Road, Forest Hill . .	London, S.E.23
Kerr-Taylor, Helen	Hill House	Shotley, Nr. Ipswich, Suffolk
Kersley, H. Jonathan	32 Warrington Crescent	London, W9 1EL
Kesby, B. R.	210 Compton Road	Wolverhampton, Staffs.
Kesson, Anna J.	16 Kew Terrace	Glasgow, G12 OTE
Khan, M. A. A.	100 Compton Place, Carpenders Road	Watford, Herts.
Khwaja, I. A.	Flat 29, Gilmore House, 113 Clapham Common, North Side	London, S.W.4
Killen, B. U.	32 Mount Road, Penn	Wolverhampton, WV4 5SW
King, E. F.	29 Clarendon Gardens	London, W.9
King, J. A.	11 Hillview	Edinburgh, EH4 2AB
Kinnear, W. F.	Twigmoor House, Messingham Lane	Scawby, Brigg, Lincs., DN20 9AZ
Kirkham, Trevor H.	Department of Ophthalmology, St. Thomas's Hospital	London, S.E.1
Klein, Miklos	96 Harley Street	London, W.1
Kletz, Teviot G.	24 Guessens Road	Welwyn Garden City
Knight-Jones, David	White Gates, Wood Lane	Gedling, Notts.
Kodicek, J. H.	11 Bulstrode Gardens	Cambridge

Kohistani, M. Wali	Royal Victoria Hospital	Westbourne, Bournemouth
Lakhanpal, G. K.	Manchester Royal Eye Hospital, Oxford Road	Manchester
Lalla, M. M.	St. Woolos Hospital	Newport, Mon.
Lambah, Paul	Chase Batch, Coniston Way	Cannock, Staffs.
Lang, Ronald	Sevington, Epsom Road	Guildford, Surrey
Langley, D. A.	30a Wimpole Street	London, W.1
Law, Frank W.	Flat 14, 59 Weymouth Street ...	London W1N 3LH
Laxminarasimhaiah, T. H. ..	7 Denison Road, Hazelgrove	Stockport, Cheshire
Learmont, David	17 Lexden Road	Colchester
Leaver, P. K.	17 Meynell Gardens	London, E9
Lee, W. R.	Tennent Institute of Ophthalmology, Western Infirmary ..	Glasgow
Leigh, M. Eileen	2 Park View Road, Ealing	London, W.5
Leighton, D. A.	Royal Eye Hospital, Oxford Road	Manchester, M13 9WH
Leishman, R.	11 Sandyford Place	Glasgow, C.3
Levy, A. H.	19 Campden Hill Court, Campden Hill Road	London, W.8
Levy, Jack	18 Nethermains Road	Milngavie, Glasgow
Lewis, D. R. H.	2 Osgood Avenue	Green Street Green, Nr. Orpington, Kent
Littledale, E. J.	Felton House, High Street	Old Portsmouth, Hants.
Lloyd, J. P. Francis	Diamond Horse, Sennen Cove ...	Penzance, Cornwall
Lobascher, D. J.	77 South End Road	London, N.W.3
Lobb, Dorothy M.	217 Broad Walk	London, S.E.3
Locket, N. Adam	Appleton, Royston Groce, Hatch End	Pinner, Middx.
Long, Kathleen M.	13 The Avenue, Spinney Hill ...	Northampton
Longmore, C.	Ivy House	Shenstone, Nr. Lichfield, Staffs.
Loudon, Isobel	Dykescroft	Galston, Ayrshire
Lubran, J.	Heatherbank, 342 Brook Lane	Sarisbury, Nr. Southampton
Luke, Irving	9 Princess Court, 74 Compayne Gardens	London, N.W.6
Lumley, W. C.	89 Hallows Lane	Dronfield, Nr. Sheffield
Lurie, Leonard	75 Harley Street	London, W.1
Lyall, M. G.	Neuk, Bieldside	Aberdeen
Lyle, Eric H.	The Woodlands, Ricketts Hill, Tatsfield	Westerham, Kent
Lyle, T. Keith	23 Harley House, Marylebone Road	London, N.W.1
Lyne, A. J.	149 Oundle Road	Orton Longueville, Peterborough
Lyons, D. E.	18 Ruabon Road	Manchester, 20
Lyons, Edward	Bron-y-Graig	Llanddulas, Nr. Abergele, Denbighshire
Lytton, Alfred	Fairleigh Cottage	Highleigh, Nr. Chichester, Sussex
McAdam, A. H.	117 Gayton Road	King's Lynn, Norfolk
McCabe, E. J.	'Inverall' 44 Rosemary Hill Road, Streetly	Sutton Coldfield, Warwicks.
McCall, J. Keith	Balnacraig, Langbank	Port Glasgow, Renfrews.
McCann, J. A.	31 Rodney Street	Liverpool, 1
McClemont, J.	9 The Green	Hurworth-on-Tees, Co. Durham
McCurry, A. L.	Robinsmead, 148 Main Street, Snittland	Leicester

McEwan, Charles G.	73 Blairbeth Road, Burnside	Rutherglen, Lanarks.
MacFaul, P. A.	63 Harley Street	London, W1N 1DD
MacFetridge, H. F. T.	Hinton, Elm Road	Hereford
MacFetridge, M. E.	Hinton. Elm Road	Hereford
McGavin, D. D. Murray	6 Carse View Drive, Bearsden ...	Glasgow
McGill, J. I.	Lyne Lodge	Virginia Water, Surrey
MacGillivray, Allister M. ...	23 Farington Street	Duudee
McGrand, James C.	Pemberley, Sleepers Hill	Winchester, Hants.
McKelvey, A. J. W.	Rosemead, Crellow Hill, Stithians	Truro, Cornwall, TR3 7AQ
McKelvie, A. R.	c/o Lloyds Bank, 160 High Street	London, W3
Mackie, E. Gordon	357 Fulwood Road	Sheffield, S10 3 BQ
Mackie, Ian A.	99 Harley Street,	London, W1
Maclean, Charles M.	Rhyber Lodge, Cleghorn Road ..	Lanark
Maclean, Pamela	9 Church Street, Monifieth	Dundee, DD5 4JP
McLenachan, John	939 Walmersley Road	Bury, Lancs.
Maclure, Gordon M.	36 The Avenue, Linthorpe	Middlesbrough, Teesside, TS5 6PD
McMillan, James	Wellesley Cottage	Upper Basildon, Berks
McNaught, Ella	3 Ossian Road	Glasgow, G43 2JJ
McOwan, B. M.	36 The Avenue, Linthorpe	Middlesborough
Macpherson, D. G. S.	113 The Drive	Hove, 3, Sussex
McPherson, H. J.	25 Dreghorn Loan, Colinton ...	Edinburgh, 13
McWilliam, R. J.	20 Westminster Terrace, Sauchie-hall Street	Glasgow, C.3
Mahto, R. S.	6 Cranwells Park, Weston	Bath, BA1 2YD
Malik, M. H. K.	30 Crockerton Road	London, S.W.17
Mallett, John M.	Derwent House, 15a Montpelier Road, Ealing	London, W.5
Manson, Neil	2 Westfield Drive, Gosforth	Newcastle-on-Tyne, NE3 4XT
Mantinband, M.	7 Treborough House, Nottingham Place	London, W.1
Mapstone, Roy	Winder, Oaksway, Gayton	Wirral, Cheshire
Marmion, V. J.	Bristol Eye Hospital, Lower Maudlin Street	Bristol, BS1 2LX
Marsh, R. J.	36 Reigate Road	Ewell, Surrey
Marshall, B. A.	47 Warnington Drive	Bessacarr, Doncaster
Martin, Brian	Southbank	Collingham, Nr. Wetherby, Yorks.
Martin, J. P.	2 Radway Crescent	Southampton
Martin-Doyle, C.	The Swiss Cottage, Old Church Road, Colwell	Malvern, Worcs
Martyn, Margaret H. E.	Cawthorne House, Nottingham Road	Ravenshead, Nottingham
Mathalone, M. B. R.	2 Woodlands, Road	Surbiton, Surrey
Mathers, R. M.	322 Blackness Road	Dundee
Matthews, P. H. N.	The Leicester Clinic, Scraptoft Lane	Leicester, LE5 1HY
Maw, T. Stafford	1 Shepherd's Avenue	Worksop, Notts.
May, William	11 Beach Avenue	Barton-on-Sea, Hants.
Meadows, S. P.	142 Harley Street	London, W1
Mehta, H. K.	Moneifion, Treborth Road	Bangor
Memon, M. A.	1a Grove Park	London, E.11
Merriman, W. G.	4 Great Stuart Street	Edinburgh, EH3 6AW
Millar, Geoffrey T.	91 Morningside Drive	Edinburgh, EH10 5NN
Miller, Dorothy	109 Harley Street	London, W.1

Miller, Stephen J. H.	149 Harley Street	London, W1N 2DE
Millington, D.	278 Rocky Lane, Great Barr	Birmingham, 22A
Mills, Paul V.	Harwin, Ty Gwyn Road	Cyncoed, Cardiff
Milne, J. D.	65 The Grove	Gosforth, Newcastle-on-Tyne, 3
Milne, K. P.	c/o Glyn Mills & Co., Kirkland House, Whitehall	London, S.W.1
Milne, W. S.	19 King's Gate	Aberdeen
Milner, J. G.	30 a Wimpole Street	London W.1
Moore, J. Gibson	132 Harley Street	London W.1
Moore, I. H. G.	Baptist Church House, Priory Road	Dudley, Worcs.
Moores, N. S.	137 Harley Street	London, W.1
More, B.	538 Lanark Road West, Balerno .	Midlothian
Morgan, Gwyn	Institute of Ophthalmology, Judd Street	London, WC1H 9QS
Morgan, O. G.	Primrose Cottage	Walberswick, Suffolk
Moss, D.	45 Pangfield Park, Allesley Park	Coventry, CV5 9NN
Moss, John	130 Wendover Road	Stoke Mandeville, Bucks.
Munro, S. S. F.	Gwynant, St. Margaret's Road ..	Hereford
Munton, C. G. F.	86 Amsbury Road	Hunton, Nr. Maidstone, Kent
Murray, Nina ·..........	6 The Square, Buxton	Buxton
Murray, T. G.	197 London Road	Portsmouth, Hants.
Murray, W. N.	Glenburn, Burnside Road	Fochabers, Morayshire, N32 7EV
Mushin, Alan S.	935 Finchley Road	London, N.W.11
Mustardé, John C.	3 Longbank Road	Ayr
Nafie, M. W.	25 Prince Avenue	Southend-on-Sea, Essex
Nagasubramanian, S.	Institute of Ophthalmology, Judd Street	London, WC1H 9QS
Nairac, M. I.	Masters Keep, Standish Court ...	Stonehouse, Glos.
Nanjiani, M. R.	24 Dunrobin Avenue	Elderslie, Renfrews.
Naunton, W. J.	35 Surrey Street	Norwich
Neubert, F. R.	Roseneath, The Grange	St. Peter Port, Guernsey, C.1
Nixon, J. M. G.	Willis House	West Orchard, Nr. Shaftesbury, Dorset
Nixseaman, D. H.	38 Burness Avenue, Alloway ...	Ayr, KA7 4QB
Nolan, John	6 Avenue Victoria, Roundhay ..	Leeds, LS8 H2
Nutt, A. B.	344 Glossop Road	Sheffield, S10 2HW
O'Connell, Margaret M.	Merthyr General Hospital, Merthyr	Tydfil, South Wales, CF47
O'Connor, Ivan M.	34 Halton Lane, Wendover	Aylesbury, Bucks.
O'Donoghue, Hugh N.	13 Kingsmere Road	London, SW19 6PY
O'Driscoll, T. G.	c/o Oldchurch Hospital	Romford, Essex
Ogg, A. J.	14 The Close	Salisbury, Wilts.
O'Neill, T. M.	14 New Dover Road	Canterbury
O'Riordan, M. D.	15 Cedar Court, Somerset Road .	London, S.W.19
Ormrod, J. N.	Barry Cottage, Pheasant Lane ...	Loose, Nr. Maidstone, Kent
O'Rourke, Patrick	Sunderland Eye Infirmary, Alexandra Road	Sunderland
Orr, H. Campbell	8 Summerfield Road, Chapel Ash.	Wolverhampton
Orr-Ewing, Catherine	69 Upper Park Road	London, N.W.3
Osmond, A. H.	116 Heene Road	Worthing
Oughton, Nora M.	Southlands, Walgrave	Northampton
Owen, R. A.	Twitten End, Bickley Park Road	Bromley, Kent, BRI 2AY

Packer, R. E.	The Pines, The Links	Pembrey, Carms.
Palin, Anthony G.	Litfield House, Clifton Down ...	Bristol, BS8 3LS
Palmer, C. A. L.	79 Upper Hanover Street	Sheffield. 3
Pancham, P. K.	16 Castledykes Road	Dumfries
Parkinson, M. J.	High Trees, Waldringfield	Woodbridge, Suffolk
Parsons-Smith, B. Gerald ..	Charing Cross Hospital, Fulham Road	London, W6 8RF
Parton, John B.	Brown Roofs, Copsem Lane	Esher, Surrey
Parvis, A. H.	62 Endlesham Road	London, SW12 8JL
Paterson, Gillian	150 Thurlow Park Road, W. Dulwich	London, S.E.21
Paterson, M. W.	12 Kirklee Road	Glasgow, G12 0ST
Paterson, Robert W. W.	116 Mearns Road, Clarkston	Glasgow
Patterson, Alan	36 Victoria Road	Freshfield, Nr. Liverpool, L37 7DD
Paul, M.	89 Redhouse Road, Tettenhall ..	Wolverhampton, WV6 8XQ
Pearce, J. L.	Windrush House, Half Shire Lane	Blakedown, Nr. Kidderminster
Peiris, C. S. L.	14 Lulworth Road	Birkdale, Southport
Penman, Gerard G.	Silversmith's	Sherborne, Dorset
Percival, S. P. B.	Cannonfield, Muston Road	Hunmanby, E. Yorks.
Pereira, J. F.	The Manor House, Fornham-All-Saints	Bury St. Edmunds, Suffolk
Perkins, Prof. E. S.	Institute of Ophthalmology, Judd Street	London, WC1H 9QS
Perriam, D. J.	53 Rosebery Gardens	London, N8 8SH
Petrie, W.	6 Corrennie Drive	Edinburgh, 10
Philipp, Arthur	Fairwood	Llangunnor, Carmarthen
Philips, Prof. C. I.	Eye Pavilion, Chalmers Street ...	Edinburgh, EH3 9HA
Phillips, J. L. J.	33 Vardean Gardens	Brighton, BN1 6WJ
Phillpotts, J. S.	11 Little Warren Close	Guildford, Surrey
Pierse, Dermot, M. Ch.	45 Coombe Road	Croydon
Pilcher, R. K.	c/o Midland Bank 59 Old Christchurch Road	Bournemouth, Hants.
Pillai, S.	7 Rhyd-yr-helig, Sketty	Swansea, Glam.
Pirie, C.	35 Spottiswoode Gardens, St. Andrews	Fife
Pitts, S. M.	4 Siskin Road, Pedmore	Stourbridge, Worcs.
Porter, Richard	33 Mitford Close, Oxclose	Washington, Co. Durham
Prasad, Shyam S.	c/o Corneo-Plastic Unit, Queen Victoria Hospital	East Grinstead, Sussex
Price, D. M. Clewett	19 Oaklands Park	Bishop's Stortford, Herts.
Price, T. J. Grahame	Central Medical Establishment, P. O. Box 22, Royal Air Force, Kelvin House, Cleveland Street	London, W.1
Priestley, T. B.	3 Mornington Villas	Bradford, 8
Primrose, John A. E.	42 Harley Street	London, W.1
Pritchard, G. C.	83 Alleyn Park	London, SE21 8AA
Rahman, M.	146 Cheviot Gardens	London, N.W.2
Raichand, Motilal	Victoria Hospital	Burnley, Lancs.
Rampling, A. E.	'Lisbamandra' Fort Road, Alverstoke	Gosport, Hants.
Ramsell, T. G.	38 Forest Road, Meols, Hoylake .	Wirral, Cheshire, L47 6AX
Ranner, N. E. A.	44 Cadigan Court, Mulgrave Road	Sutton, Surrey
Ray, P. K.	65 Morningfield Road	Aberdeen, AB2 4AP

Redmond, S. P.	Lincoln House, 56/58	Clasketgate, Lincoln.
Reich-d'Almeida, F. B.	Department of Pathology, Institute of Ophthalmology, Judd Street	London, WC1H 9QS
Reis, J. L.	1 Albert Drive	London, S.W.19
Rennie, A. G. R.	58 Castlehill Drive, Newton Mearns	Glasgow
Rerrie, J. D.	Kent County Ophthalmic Hospital	Maidstone, Kent
Rice, N. S. C.	Grey Cottage, Heronsgate	Rickmansworth, Hets.
Rich, W. J. C.	15 Southernhay East	Exeter
Richards, Andrew B.	54 Popes Grove	Twickenham, Middx.
Richards, R. L.	29 Ness Bank	Inverness
Richer, R. G.	28 Newbridge Crescent	Wolverhampton
Riddell, Prof. W. J. B.	24 Gladstone Place	Aberdeen, AB1 6XA
Ridgway, A. E. A.	12 Pereira Road	Birmingham, 17
Ridley, Frederick	Pitts Walk, Bowling Green Close, Roehampton	London, SW15 3TE
Ridley, Harold	53 Harley Street	London W.1
Rintoul, Andrew J.	Royal Naval Hospital	Haslar, Hants.
Rizk, S. N. M.	18 The Avenue	Mansfield, Notts.
Roberts, D. St. Clair	Sussex Eye Hospital, Eastern Road	Brighton
Robertson, I. R.	47, Sea View Road	Sunderland, Co. Durham, SR2 9HA
Robinson, G. E.	101 Bramcote Drive West	Beeston, Nottingham
Robson, S. R.	105 Princes Road	Leicester
Roddie, Alastair	The Knoll, 81 Harpers Lane	Bolton, BL1 6HU
Rodger, F. C.	Stratton Firs	Cirencester, Glos.
Roffey, B. W.	Fir Lodge, Hopesay	Craven Arms, Shropshire
Rolfe, Muriel E.	The Limes	East Malling, Kent
Romanes, G. J.	32 Prince of Wales Road	Dorchester, Dorset
Romano, J. H.	96 Harley Street	London, W1
Roper-Hall, M. J.	38 Harborne Road, Edgbaston	Birmingham, B15 3HE
Rose, F. C.	35 Harley Street	London, WIN IHA
Rosen, E. S.	53 Firswood Mount	Gatley, Cheshire
Rostron, K. W. B.	Penquite	Lelant, near St. Ives
Rowsell, Philip G.	1 Dorchester Court, Wray Common Road	Reigate, Surrey
Roy, A. M.	16 Pearl Court	Eastbourne
Ruben, C. M.	12 Harley House, Upper Harley Street	London, NW1. 4PR
Rubinstein, K.	10 Pritchatt's Road	Edgbaston Birmingham, 15
Rudd, Charles	5 Pritchatt's Road	Edgbaston, Birmingham, B15 2QU
Rumble, J. A.	2 Punchbowl Cottages, Church End, Paglesham	Rochford, Essex, SS4 2DH
Rushton, R. H.	20 Holwood Road	Bromley, Kent, BR1 3EB
Rusk, Maeve	51 Old Edinburgh Road	Inverness
Russell, A. A.	2 Mortonhall Road	Edinburgh, 9
Russell, R. W. Ross	5 Roedean Crescent	London, S.W.15
Sabherwal, S.	Birmingham & Midland Eye Hospital, Church Street	Birmingham, 3
Salmon, J. D.	Woodbridge	Woldingham, Surrey
Sampson, Robert	Grey Gables, Broadhempston	Totnes, Devon
Sanders, M. D.	9 Alma Terrace, Allenstreet	London W.8

Sandhu, B. S.	132 Harley Street	London, W.1
Sarwar, M.	Edgehill	Wheatley, Oxon.
Savin, Lewis H.	20 Wimpole Street	London, W.1
Savory, Mary	6 Devonshire Place	London, W.1
Schloss, Anne	46 Strathearn Road	Edinburgh, 9
Schwerdt, F. C. C.	Grindle House, Clyst St. Mary	Exeter
Scott, A. Stewart	13 St. John Street	Manchester, 3
Scott, Prof. George I.	20 Heriot Row	Edinburgh, EH3 6EN
Scott, J. D.	Eye Department, Addenbrooke's Hospital, Hills Road	Cambridge
Searle, C. W. A.	17 Lower Common South, Putney	London, S.W.15
Sellers, J. I.	Abbeys House	Claxton, York, YO6 7SD
Sellors, P. J. H.	High Burrows, The Drive	Belmont, Surrey
Sethi, B. P.	15 Yetlands, Dalston	Carlisle, CA5 7PB
Setna, P. H.	27 Clifton Drive South, Ansdell	Lytham St. Annes, Lancs.
Shah, M.	62 Tyneham Road, Merton Park	London, SW19
Shah, Piyush	Heathfield Hospital	Ayr
Shannon, Thomas	Oakroyd, Foxholes Road	Horwich, Lancs.
Shapland, C. Dee	Cornerways, Orley Farm Road	Harrow-on-the-Hill
Sharma, B. D.	32 Kenmore Way	Carluke, Lenarks
Sharma, S. K.	42 Parkstone Road	Poole, Dorset
Sheldon, J. V.	Victoria Hospital	Burnley, Lancs.
Sheriff, S. M. M.	22 The Avenue, Southlands	Mansfield, Notts.
Shrivastava, B. D.	Boston General Hospital	Boston, Lincs.
Shuttleworth, F. N.	Chiswick House, 3 Chiswick Place	Eastbourne
Sibthorpe, J. O.	Ansteys, New Road	Hemingford Abbots, Hunts.
Siddique, S. M.	20 Pledwick Lane, Sandal	Wakefield, Yorks.
Siggins, G. F. G.	27 Westbourne Road	Edgbaston, Birmingham B15 3TX
Sikka, O. P.	5 Scartho Road	Grimsby, Lincs.
Simmons, G. L.	Ely Court	Staplehurst, Kent
Simpson, Elizabeth D. L.	9 Boyne Terrace Mews, Holland Park	London. W.11
Sinclair, C. Gordon	Hatfield Mount	Norton, Worcester
Smail, J. M.	Yew Tree Lodge, 49a The Mount	Shrewsbury
Smiley, W. K.	Ilex House, Orchehill Rise	Gerrads Cross
Smith, Arthur	Badgers Holt, Sawley	Ripon, Yorks, HG4 3EP
Smith, H. Benedict	56 Rodney Street	Liverpool, 1
Smith, H. Chalmers	1 Fairview	Cardross, Dumbartonshire
Smith, J. L. S.	19 Oxford Road, Birkdale	Southport
Smith, Mark E.	Hatch House	Ingrave, Nr. Brentwood, Essex
Smith, M. W.	7 Chad Road, Edgbaston	Birmingham, B15 3EN
Smith, Redmond	2 Harley Street	London, W.1
Smith, R. J. S.	43 Belmont Road, Kilmacolm	Renfrews, PA13 4LN
Smith, Sydney B.	20 St. John Street	Manchester, M3 4FA
Smith, Vernon H.	8 Moorcroft Road, Moseley	Birmingham, B13 8LX
Smith, W. A. M.	2 Arnwood Drive	Glasgow, W.2
Snodgrass, Marjory B.	Greenways, Kirkintilloch	Glasgow
Snow, J. T.	20 Ethelbert Road	Canterbury, Kent
Sollom, A. W.	Maryland, Perton Road, Wightwick	Wolverhampton
Somerset, Edward J.	5 Fulwith Road	Harrogate, Yorks.
Somerville, F.	31 Wilmington Square	London, W.C.1
Soni, K. G.	8 Peel Walk, Harborne	Birmingham, 17

Souper, Dorothy K.	75 Thorpe Road	Norwich
Sparks, I.	Guilsford, Ounsdale Road	Wombourn, Nr. Wolverhampton
Speight, I. B.	42 Welholme Avenue	Grimsby
Spero, L. P.	23 Bury Lodge Gardens, Alverstoke	Gosport, Hants.
Spiro, Isidore	42 Harley Street	London, W.1
Stallard, H. B.	112 Harley Street	London, W1N 1AF
Stanworth, A.	87 Devonshire Road, Dore	Sheffield, S17 3NU
Starbuck, Mary J.	48 St. Lawrence Forstal	Canterbury, Kent
Starr, P. A. J.	100 Harley Street	London, W.1
Stead, Stanley	4 Paulton Drive, Bishopston	Bristol, BS7 8JJ
Steele, Arthur D. McG.	18 Holland Road	London, W.14
Stephenson, Robert W.	Morningside, Prestbury	Cheltenham, Glos., GL52 3AY
Stevens, A. Vivian	52a Sloane Square	London, S.W.1
Stevens, Philip R.	493 Preston New Road, Yew Tree Brow	Blackburn, BB2 7AN
Stokoe, N. L.	3 Merchiston Park	Edinburgh, 10
Strachan, I. M.	41 Stumperlowe Park Road	Sheffield, 10
Strong, J. D. E.	Holly Lodge, West Overton	Marborough, Wilts.
Strong, J. R.	Flat 6, 53 Drayton Gardens	London, SW10
Tachiaos, P.	St. Paul's Eye Hospital, Old Hall Street	Liverpool, 3
Tandon, H. P.	27 Rhona Drive	Great Sankey, Nr. Warrington, WA5 3PB
Tattersfield, J. F.	30 Sauncey Avenue	Harpenden, Herts.
Taylor, Enid	60 Woodvale	London, N10 3DN
Taylor, Peter	17 Moor Park Avenue	Preston, PR1 6AN
Taylor, W. O. Gibson	16 Ronaldshaw Park	Ayr
Thomas, E. K. Roy	Ty-r-nant, St. James' Gardens	Swansea
Thomas, J. B. Trevelyan	2 Clarendon Road	Bournemouth
Thomas, P. A.	33 Marlbrook Lane	Marlbrook, Nr. Bromsgrove, Worcs.
Thomas, Sir Tudor	Oakhurst, Tygwyn Road, Penylan	Cardiff, CF2 5JG
Thomson, A. M. Wright	16 Kirklee Road	Glasgow, G12 OST
Thomson, D. S.	4 Imperial Square	Cheltenham
Thomson, J. Masterton	Hill-Top, Whidborne Close, Kilmorie	Torquay, Devon
Thorne Thorne, B.	4 Tongdean Road	Hove, Sussex, BN3 6QB
Todd, R. M.	35 Bushfield Road,	Albrighton, Nr. Wolverhampton
Traill, R.	Bellevue, Sunnylaw	Vridge of Allan, Stirlings.
Tree, Mark	148 Lordswood Road, Harborne	Birmingham, 17
Trevor-Roper, Patrick D.	3 Park Square West	London, N.W.1.
Tripathi, R. C.	105 Sunnyfield, Mill Hill	London, N.W.7
Tsolakis, Stelios	85 Linden Gardens	London, W.2
Tulloch, Alexander K.	20 Jedburgh Road	Dundee
Tulloh, C. G.	33 Old Sneed Park	Bristol, BS9 1RG
Tulloh, Ernest P.	21 Boscombe Spa Road	Bournemouth
Turner, D.	25 Denholm Terrace	Greenock, Renfrews.
Vacalopoulos, C. P.	Royal Eye Infirmary, Greenhill	Weymouth, Dorset
Vale, Eileen M.	3 Clock Tower Court, West Parade	Bexhill-on-Sea, Sussex
Vasey, Jean M.	104 Hayes Road	Bromley, Kent
Vaughan-Jones, R.	133 Carisbrooke Way	Cyncoed, Cardiff

Viswanathan, Bharathi	39 Oakfield Road	Newport, Mon.
Vodden, V. M.	20 Beverley Road	Leamington Spa, Warwicks.
Walker, Colin B.	Southampton Eye Hospital, Wilton Avenue	Southampton
Walker, W. Martin	609 Warwick Road	Solihull, Warwicks.
Waller, W. D.	Huxley, Lock Road	Marlow, Bucks.
Walsh, E. P.	4 Pomeroy Road, Uplowman Road	Tiverton, Devon
Walsh, P.	The Woodlands, Oaken Lanes ...	Coadsall, Staffs.
Walter, Margaret V.	Church Farm House	Ripple, Nr. Deal, Kent
Walters, C.	89 Regents Road	Leicester
Walton, W. F.	Cranmere	Bishopsteignton, S. Devon
Ward, D. M.	The Hermitage, Ringmore	Shaldon, S. Devon
Ward, R. D.	17 Westmead, Roehampton	London, S.W.15
Waters, Brian	P.M.O.'s Residence, 2 Hill Crest, Britannia Royal Naval College.	Dartmouth, Devon
Watson, David M.	Flat 3, Regis House, 49 Beaumont Street	London, W.1
Watson, P. G.	22 Parkside	Cambridge, CB1 1JE
Wear, A. R.	New Croft, Wetheral	Cumberland
Weatherill, J. R.	16 Cecil Avenue, Baildon	Shipley, Yorks.
Weir, Rosemary	The Moorings, Gareloch Road ..	Rhu, Dumbartonshire
Welham, R. A. N.	Royal Berkshire Hospital	Reading, RG1 5AN
Werb, A.	130 Bridge Lane	London, N.W.11
Westlake, D. J.	The Sloop, Beech Waye	Gerrard's Cross, Bucks.
Whitting, Maurice H.	109 Harley Street	London, W.1
Whittington, Theodore H. ..	23 Chiltern Road	Sutton, Surrey
Whitty, H. P. B.	47 Oatlands Drive	Weybridge, Surrey
Whitwell, John	Bagatelle, Burton Road, Branksome Park	Bournemouth, Hants.
Whyte, D. K.	84 Balnakyle Road, Lochardie ..	Inverness
Wilkie, J. L.	47 Knoll Avenue	Darlington, DL3 8PT
Willetts, G. S.	41 Wenlock Drive, Villa Park ...	Escrick, York.
Williams, B. Innes	Fairlie House, The Grove	Epsom, Surrey
Williams, H. P.	102 Swan Court, Chelsea Manor Street	London, SW3 5RU
Williams, R. C.	53 Park Avenue North	Harpenden, Herts.
Williamson, John	Eye Department, Southern General Hospital	Glasgow, S.W.1
Wilson, A. Eric	17 Mount Street	Taunton, Somerset
Wilson, M. S.	78 Harley Street	London, W1N 1AF
Wilson, Peter	7 Halifax Road, Edgerton	Huddersfield, HD3 3AN
Wilson, T.	22 Rennie Street	Falkirk, Stirlingshire
Wilson, William	34 Calderwood Road, Newlands .	Glasgow, S.3
Winning, James	26 Kirkhill Road	Strathaven, Lanarkshire
Winstanley, J.	10 Pembroke Villas, The Green .	Richmond, Surrey
Woodhouse, Derrick F.	161 Compton Road	Wolverhampton
Wright, J. E.	Hillside, Quickley Lane	Chorleywood, Herts.
Wright, Peter	23 Harley House, Marylebone Road	London, N.W.1 5HE
Wright, Robert E.	Beech Cottage, Church Road ...	Fleet, Hants.
Wybar, Kenneth C.	8 Welbeck House, Welbeck Street	London, W1M 7HB
Wyllie, Anne M.	Queen Alexandra Hospital, Cosham	Portsmouth, PO6 3LY
Young, J. D. H.	3 Farm End	Woodstock, Oxon.
Young, John H.	75 Gregory Boulevard	Nottingham, NG7 5JA

Youngson, R. M.	c/o Royal Army Medical College,	
	Millbank	London, SW1
Yow, Charles W. N.	Chalgrove, Peterborough Hill ...	Harrow-on-the-Hill
Zorab, E. C.	20 Brunswick Place	Southampton, SO1 2AQ
Zwink, F. B.	Woodthorpe, St. Mary's Avenue,	
	Wanstead	London, E.11

NOSOCOMIA QUIBUS OCULIS AEGRI CURANTUR

No. of beds

Birmingham & Midland Eye Hospital, Church Street, Birmingham, B3 2NS	97
Bristol Eye Hospital, Lower Maudlin Street, Bristol, BS1 6SY	104
Caenarvon Eye & Cottage Hospital, Caernarvon	30
Dundee Eye Institution, Dundee, Angus	
Eye, Ear & Throat Hospital (for Shropshire & Wales), Shrewsbury, Shropshire, SY1 IJS	67
Glasgow Eye Infirmary, 2 Sandyford Place, Glasgow, C3	72
Glasgow Ophthalmic Institution, Glasgow	
Greenock Eye Infirmary, Greenock, Renfrewshire	15
Kent Coutry Ophthalmic & Aural Hospital, Church Street, Maidstone, Kent	100
Manchester Royal Eye Hospital, Oxford Road, Manchester, M13 9WL.................	192
Moorfields Eye Hospital, City Road, London, EC1	210
Moorfields Eye Hospital, High Holborn, London, WC1	100
North Riding Infirmary, Eye, Ear & Throat Centre, Middlesborough, Teesside	114
Nottingham Eye Hospital, The Ropewalk, Nottingham	63
The Oxford Eye Hospital, Walton Street, Oxford	52
Royal Eye Hospital, St. George's Circus, Southwark, London, SE1 OBA...............	124
Royal Eye Infirmary, Plymouth, Devon	50
Royal Victoria Eye Infirmary, Paisley, Renfrewshire, PA1 3RQ	25
St. Paul's Eye Hospital, Old Hall Street, Liverpool 3	112
Southampton Eye Hospital, 2 Wilton Street, Southampton, Hampshire, SO9 4XW	46
Sunderland Eye Infirmary, Alexandra Road, Sunderland, Co. Durham	60
Sussex Eye Hospital, Eastern Road, Brighton, Sussex, BN2 5BF	56
Victoria Eye Hospital, Eign Street, Hereford	25
West of England Eye Infirmary, Magdalen Street, Exeter, EX2 4HT	62
Western Ophthalmic Hospital, 155 Marylebone Road, London, NE1	58
Weymouth & Dorset County Royal Eye Infirmary, 9 Greenhill, Weymouth, Dorset	25
Wolverhampton & Midland Counties Eye Infirmary, Compton Road, Wolverhampton, Staffs.	103
Worcester Eye Hospital, Barbourne Road, Worcester	18

Ophthalmic Departments in the Teaching Hospitals

Aberdeen Royal Infirmary, Foresthill, Aberdeen, AB9 2ZB
Charing Cross Hospital, Fulham Palace Road, London, W6 8RF
Dundee Royal Infirmary, Barrack Road, Dundee
Glasgow Royal Infirmary, Glasgow
Guy's Hospital, London Bridge, SE1 9RT
King's College Hospital, Denmark Hill, London, SE5
The London Hospital, Turner Street, London, E1 2AD
The Middlesex Hospital, Mortimer Street, London, W1P 7PN
Royal Free Hospital, Gray's Inn Road, London, WC1X 8LF
Royal Infirmary, Lauriston Place, Edinburgh, 3
Royal Victoria Hospital, Grosvenor Place, Belfast
Southampton General Hospital, Southampton
St. Bartholomew's Hospital, West Smithfield, London, EC1A 7BE

St. George's Hospital, Hyde Park Corner, London, SW1
St. Mary's Hospital, Praed Street, Paddington, W2 1NY
St. Thomas's Hospital, Lambeth Palace Road, London, SE1 7EH
United Birmingham Hospitals, Birmingham
United Bristol Hospitals, Bristol
United Cambridge Hospitals, Cambridge
United Leeds Hospitals, Leeds
United Liverpool Hospitals, Liverpool
United Manchester Hospitals, Manchester
United Newcastle-upon-Tyne Hospitals, Newcastle-upon-Tyne
United Nottingham Hospitals, Nottingham
United Oxford Hospital, Oxford
United Sheffield Hospitals, Sheffield
University College Hospital, Gower Street, London, WC1E 6AU
University Hospital of Wales, Cardiff
Western Infirmary, Glasgow, G11 6NT
Westminster Hospital, Horseferry Road, London, SW1

INSTITUTA SCHOLAEQUE CAECIS DESTINATAE

England and Wales:
Director of Social Services, Anglesey County Council, Shire Hall, Llangefni, North Wales.
Ashton-under-Lyme District Society for the Blind, 17 Mottram Road, Stalybridge, Cheshire.
Barrow, Furness and South Cumberland Society for the Blind, 4 Slater Street, Barrow-in-Furness, Lancashire.
Director of Social Services, Bedfordshire County Council, County Hall, Bedford.
Berkshire County Blind Society, 5 Erleigh Road, Reading, Berkshire.
Director of Social Services, Birmingham City Council, PO Box 15, 102 Edmund Street, Birmingham, B3 3DT
Birmingham Royal Institution for the Blind, Queen Alexandra Technical College, 49 Court Oak Road, Harborne, Birmingham, 17.
Boston and Holland Blind Society, 14 Tower Road, Boston, Lincolnshire.
Brighton Society for the Welfare of the Blind, 142 Preston Road, Brighton, BN1 6Af
Director of Social Services, Captain's Walk, Brecon, Wales.
Bucks Association for the Blind, Pebble Lane, Aylesbury, Bucks.
Director of Social Services, Caernarvonshire County Council, County Offices, Caernarvon.
Cambridgeshire and Isle of Ely County Council, Social Services Department, Castle Court, Shire Hill, Cambridge, CB3 QAP
Director of Social Services, Cardiganshire County Council, 5 Llanbadarn Road, Aberystwyth, Cardigans.
Director of Social Services, Carmarthenshire County Council, 3 Red Square, Carmarthen.
Catholic Blind Institute, 26 North Street, Liverpool, L2 9RX
Chester Blind Welfare Society, 67 Liverpool Road, Chester, CH2 1AP
Colne and District Society for the Blind, Acornlea House, Foulridge, Nr Colne, Lancs.
Director of Social Services, County Hall, Station Road, Truro, Cornwall.
Cumberland and Westmoreland Welfare Trust for the Blind, 15 Fisher Street, Carlisle, CA3 8RW
Director of Social Services, Social Services Department, Denbighshire County Council, Llanrhydd Street, Ruthin, Denbighshire, LL15 1PR
Social Services Department, County Offices, Matlock, Derbyshire.
Director of Social Services, County Hall, Exeter, Devon, EX2 4QR
Institution for the Blind of Dewsbury, Batley and District, 64 Daisy Hill, Dewsbury, Yorks.
Director of Social Services, Dorset County Council, County Hall, Dorchester.
Director of Social Services, Durham County Council, County Hall, Durham.

Director of Social Services, County Council of Essex, Kensal House, 77 Springfield Road, Chelmsford, Essex.
Director of Social Services, Glamorgan County Council, County Council Offices, Greyfriars Road, Cardiff, CF1 3LL
Director of Social Services, Gloucestershire County Council, Bearland Wing, Shire Hall, Gloucester, GL1 2TW
Director of Social Services, 36 Brighowgate, Grimsby, Lincolns.
Guernsey Association for the Blind, Constable Office, St. Peter Port, Guernsey, Channel Islands.
Director of Social Services, Hampshire County Council, The Castle, Winchester, Hants.
Director of Social Services, Herefordshire County Council, 17 St Owen Street, Hereford.
Social Services Department, Hertfordshire County Council, County Hall, Hertford.
Heywood and Whitefield Blind Welfare Society, Social Centre for the Blind, 1 Starkey Street, Heywood, Lancs.
Director of Social Services, County Offices, Bridge Street, Huntingdon.
Isle of Wight Society for the Blind, 107 Staplers Road, Newport, Isle of Wight.
Jersey Society for the Education and Welfare of the Necessitous Blind, Hillway, Rue de la Blanche Pierre, St Lawrence, Jersey, Channel Islands.
Jewish Blind Society, 1 Craven Hill, Lancester Gate, London, W2 3EN
Director of Social Services, Kent County Council, Social Services Department, Springfield, Maidston, Kent.
Director of Social Services, Kesteven County Offices, Sleaford, Lincs.
Medical Officer of Health, Health Department, East Cliff County Offices, Preston, PR1 3JN, Lancs.
Royal Leicestershire, Rutland and Wycliffe Incorporated Society for the Blind, Margaret Road, Leicester, LE5 5FU
Lindsey Blind Society, 45 Newland, Lincoln.

London:

Chief Officer of the Social Services Department, Greater London Council, County Hall, London, S.E.1.
and Director of Social Services of the London Boroughs of: – Barking, Barnet, Bexley, Brent, Bromley, Camden, City of London Westminster, Croydon, Ealing, Enfield, Greenwich, Hackney, Hammersmith, Harringey, Harrow, Havering, Hillingdon, Hounslow, Islington, Kensington and Chelsea, Kingston upon Thames, Lambeth, Lewisham, Merton, Newham, Redbridge, Richmond upon Thames, Southward, Sutton, Tower Hamlets, Waltham Forest, and Wandsworth.
London, Association for the Blind, Pelican House, 88–92 Peckham Road, London, SE15 5LH
Macclesfield Society for the Blind, 15 Queen Victoria Street, Macclesfield, SK116LP, Cheshire.
Social Services Department, Slaway House, Aytoun Street, Manchester, M1 3ET
Merioneth County Council, County Offices, Dolgellou, Merioneth.
Merthyr Tydfil Institution for the Blind, 88 Portmorlais, Merthyr Tydfil, Glamorgan.
Social Services Department, Monmouth County Council, Victoria Street, Cwmbran, Monmouthshire, NP4 3XY
Montgomeryshire County Council, County Offices, Welshpool, Montgomeryshire.
National Blind Helpers League, 18 Rainbow Court, Paston Ridings, Peterborough, PE4 6UP
Director of Social Services, County Hall, Martineau Lane, Norwich, NOR 47A, Norfolk.
North Regional Association for the Blind, Headingley Castle, Headingley, Leeds, LS6 2DQ
Director of Social Services, Northamptonshire County Council, Social Services Department, Wooton Hall, Market Square, Northampton.
Director of Social Services, Eldon House, Regent Centre, Gosforth, Newcastle upon Tyne, NE3 3NF
Royal Midland Institution for the Blind, Chaucer Street, Nottingham, NG1 5LR
Director of Social Services, Oxfordhsire County Council, The Moors, Kidlington, Oxford.
Social Services Department, Pembrokeshire County Council, Perrott's Road, Haverfordwest, Pembrokeshire.
Social Services Department, County Hall Llandrindod Wells, Radnorshire.

Royal National Institute for the Blind, 224–6–8 Great Portland Street, London, W1N 6AA
St. Dunstan's Orginasation for Men and Women Blinded on War Service, St. Dunstan's, PO Box 58, 191 Old Marylebone Road, London, NW1 5QN
St John's Guild for the Blind, 44 Abindgon Road, Luton, Beds.
Social Services Department, Shropshire Voluntary Association for the Blind, Shire Hall, Abbey Foregate, Shrewsbury, SY2 6NL, Salop.
Director of Social Services, Bath City Council, 12 Charlotte Street, Bath, Somerset.
Southern Regional Association for the Blind, 32 Old Queen Street, London, SW1H 9HP
Director of Social Services, Staffordshire County Council, Council Social Services Department, 69–70a Foregate Street, Stafford.
Director of Social Services, East Suffolk County Council, Milner House, County Hall, Ipswich, Suffolk.
Director of Social Services, East Sussex County Council, PO Box 5, County Hall, St Annes Crescent, Lewes, Sussex.
Director of Social Services, West Sussex County Council, Social Services Department, Wren House, Country Hall Chichester, Sussex, PO19 1RN
Wales and Monmouthshire Council for the Blind, Cardiff Institute for the Blind, 20 Newport Road, Cardiff.
Walsall CBC Institution and Workshops for the Blind, Hatherton Road, Walsall, WS1 1XX
Director of Social Services, Warwickshire County Council, The Shire Hall, Warwick.
Westmoreland County Council, County Hall, Kendal, Westmoreland.
Western Regional Association for the Blind, 39 East Street, Newton Abbot, Devon, TQ12 2JP
Director of Social Services, Wiltshire County Council, County Hall, Trowbridge, Wilts.
Wolverhampton, Dudley and Districts Institute for the Blind, Wolverhampton Road East, Wolverhampton, Staffs, WV4 6AZ
Director of Social Services, Worcestershire County Council, Infirmary Walk, Worcester.
Director of Social Services, York Corporation, Ryedale Building, 60 Piccadilly, York, YO1 1PP
Director of Social Services, County Hall, Beverley, Yorks. (East Riding).
Director of Social Services, County Hall Northalerton, Yorks. (North Riding).
Director of Social Services, Social Services Department, 87 Northgate, Wakefield, Yorks. (West Riding).

Scotland:

Aberdeen Town and County Association for Teaching the Blind at their Homes, 20 Bon Accord Square, Aberdeen, AB1 2DJ
Senior Assistant, Social Work Department, Clackmannanshire County Council, Ochil House, Manshill, Alloa, Clacks.
Society for the Blind in Dumfries and Galloway, 24 Catherine Street, Dumfries, DG1 1HZ
Dundee Society for the Welfare of the Blind, 39 St. Andrew's Street, Dundee, DD1 2EU
The Royal Asylum and School, Craigmillar Park, Edinburgh, EH16 5NA
Fife Society for the Blind, 1 Townsend Place, Kirkcaldy, Fife.
Forfarshire Mission to the Blind, Ravenswood, New Road, Forfar, Angus, DD8 2AF
Northern Counties Institute for the Blind, 38 Ardconnel Street, Inverness.
Corporation of Glasgow, Social Work Department, 73 John Street, Glasgow, C.1.
Perthshire and Kinross-shire Society for the Blind, 8 St. Leonard's Bank, Perth, PH2 8EB
County Director of Social Work, Stirling County Council, County Offices, Langgarth, Stirling.
Director of Social Work, Social Work Department, Zetland County Council, 64 St Olaf Street, Lerwick, Zetland, AB3 OEN

BULGARIA

SOCIETATES OPHTHALMOLOGICAE

Société d'Ophtalmologie Bulgare

Secrétaire: Prof. Dr. Nicola Konstantinov, I Rue Dante, Sofia 42

NOMINA ET DOMICILIA MEDICORUM AB OCULIS*

Anastasoff, A.	Augenarzt	Russe
Antonoff, G.	Augenabteilung	Michailowgrad
Argiroff, D.	Gurko, 39	Sofia
Atzeff, G.	Augenabteilung	Swistoff
Baitscheff, T.	Augenklinik	Plovdiv
Banaliewa, S.	Wolgograd, 16	Sofia
Bankoff, P.	Georgi Sofiski, 30	Sofia
Batschwarowa	Augenarzt	Plovdiv
Benewa, D.	Positano, 11-A	Sofia
Boikikeff, N.	Wolgograd, 16	Sofia
Bojtschewa, E.	Sliwniza, 309	Sofia
Christoff, Ch.	Bezirkskrankenhaus	Pernik
Daboff, S.	Tr. Kitantscheff, 55	Sofia
Deneff, W.	Gogol, 3	Sofia
Dimitroff, K.	Augenabteilung	Blagoewgrad
Dimitroff, P.	Augenklinik	Plovdiv
Dimitrowa, W.	Georgi Sofiski, 1	Sofia
Dimowa, L.	Augenabteilung	Stara-Sagora
Djakoff, D.	Boteff, 120	Sofia
Dotschefr, D.	Augenabteilung	Plewen
Dotzeff, G.	Augenabteilung	Pernik
Dudulowa, R.	93-B, Sofia	Rakowski
Ewtimoff, K.	Augenabteilung	Haskowo
Gaberoff, T.	Augenabteilung	Pasardschik
Ganeff, P.	Augenabteilung	Tirnowo
Gantscheff, N.	Ruski, 17	Sofia
Gasibarowa, L.	Augenabteilung	Sliwen
Georgiewa, L.	Miko-Papo, 65	Sofia
Georgiewa, L.	Augenabteilung	Plewen
Goleminowa, Rosa	Georgi Sofiski, 1	Sofia
Golomeewa, V.	Miko-Papo, 65	Sofia
Guschguloff, I.	Augenabteilung	Sliwen
Hadschiiwanoff, I.	Augenabteilung	Russe
Handschieff, D.	Augenabteilung	Tolbuhin
Hantowa, N.	Georgi Sofiski, 1	Sofia
Hasan, W.	Militärkrankenhaus-Augenabteilung	Sofia
Hristoskowa, E.	Transportkrankenhaus-Augenabteilung	Sofia
Iwanoff, I.	Augenabteilung	Burgas
Iwanoff, I.	G. Dimitroff, 43	Sofia

*) Empruntés de l'Edition VI

Jankoff, L.	Augenabteilung	Tscherwen-Breg
Kantschewa, T.	Augenabteilung	Warna
Karalamboff, B.	Augenabteilung	Warna
Kirowa, K.	Augenabteilung	Lom
Koen, E.	Augenklinik	Plovdiv
Konstantinoff, L.	Petöfi, 34	Sofia
Konstantinoff, N.	Dante-str., 1	Sofia
Koschuhsroff, S.	Wolgograd, 16	Sofia
Kowatschewa, Wera	Georgi Sofiski, 1	Sofia
Kuloff, W.	Augenabteilung	Kolarowgrad
Lasaroff, G.	Augenabteilung	Lowetsch
Lasaroff, L.	Augenabteilung	Gabrowo
Lenkoff, S.	Georgi Sofiski, 30	Sofia
Lukoff, L.	Wolgograd, 16	Sofia
Notowa-Usunowa, M.	G. G. Deschd, 34	Sofia
Pantschewa, B.	Boteff, 120	Sofia
Paskaleff, N.	Augenabteilung	Warna
Pawlowa, T.	Augenabteilung	Stara-Sagora
Pentschewa, L.	Augenabteilung	Russe
Petroff, P.	Augenabteilung	Wratza
Platikanowa, I.	Augenabteilung	Tirnowo
Popelenkoff, T.	Krankenhaus des Innenministeriums	Sofia
Radeff, R.	Augenabteilung	Russe
Radonowa, M.	Bezirkskrankenhaus	Küstendil
Rangeloff, B.	Augenabteilung	Wratza
Rankoff, B.	Positano, 48	Sofia
Ratscheff, R.	Augenabteilung	Widin
Rjaskoff, S.	Sliwniza, 309	Sofia
Sagorscheff, E.	Kolaroff, 60	Sofia
Sarbjanowa, A.	Augenabteilung	Burgas
Schumkowa, N.	Wolgograd, 16	Sofia
Sdrawkoff, Ch.	Axakoff, 20	Sofia
Siljanovski, N.	Augenabteilung	Smoljan
Simeonoff, T.		Plewen
Sinigerski, A.	Augenabteilung	Wratza
Slateff, P.	Augenabteilung	Tolbuhin
Stankoff, S.	Augenabteilung	Kolarowgrad
Stilianoff, N.	Augenabteilung	Rasgrad
Stlianoff, S.	Augenabteilung	Botewgrad
Stoentschewa, P.	Augenabteilung	Plewen
Sutschlowa, G.	Augenabteilung	Russe
Swetogorski, P.	Augenabteilung	Widin
Taneff, B.	Gradska-Bolnitza	Plovdiv
Taskoff, G.	Augenabteilung	Targowiste
Tersieff, R.	Bezirkskrankenhaus	Plovdiv
Todorowa, E.	Augenabteilung	Plewen
Toleff, P.	Augenabteilung	Russe
Tomoff, Ch.	Augenabteilung	Plewen
Tschakoff, G.	Sliwniza, 309	Sofia
Valkanoff, Valkan	Augenklinik	Plovdiv
Vassileff, I.	Dobar Junak, 19	Sofia
Wassileff, B.	Augenabteilung	Silistra
Wassileff, W.	Augenklinik	Plovdiv
Wassileff, W.	Adalbert-Antonow, 23	Sofia
Wassilewa, W.	Wolgograd, 16	Sofia

Wladimiroff, W.	Augenabteilung	Haskowo
Wladimiroff, W.	Augenabteilung	Dimitrowgrad
Wladimiroff, W.	Augenabteilung	Orjahowo
Zenewa, M.	Augenabteilung	Tirnowo
Zivkoff, E.	Bürusoff, 42	Sofia

CANADA

SOCIETATES OPHTHALMOLOGICAE

Nationalis

The Canadian Ophthalmological Society
President: Dr. J. P. Harshman
President-Elect: Dr. S. M. Drance
Secretary: Dr. G. A. Thompson, Suite 401, 1849 Younge Street, Toronto, Ontario M4S 1Y2
Treasurer: Dr. S. Y. Shirley
Executive Director: Dr. G. Nason
Number of members: 586

Regionales

Newfoundland Medical Association
Sectretary: Dr. R. D. Lawton, 135 Military Rd., St. John's, Newfoundland

Nova Scotia Society of Ophthalmology & Otolaryngology
Secretary: Dr. E. v. Rafuse, 1531 Oxford St., Halifax, Nova Scotia

Quebec Association of Ophthalmologists
Secretary: Dr. A. R. Labelle, 350 Hall St., St. Lambert, Quebec

Section of Ophthalmology – Ontario Medical Association
Secretary: Dr. J. C. Ball, 131 Ontario St., St. Catharines, Ontario

In Manitoba (Name of group not known)
Secretary: Dr. Norman A. Wine, 513 Boyd Bldg., 388 Portage Ave, Winnipeg 1, Manitoba

Alberta Ophthalmology & Otolaryngology Society
Secretary: Dr. D. T. R. Hassard, 410 Physician's & Surgeons Bldg, 8409-112th St., Edmonton, Alberta

British Columbia Oto-Ophthalmological Society
Secretary: Dr. H. N. Fitterman, 2025 West 42nd Ave, Suite 320, Vancouver 13, British Columbia

NOMINA ET DOMICILIA MEDICORUM AB OCULIS

Adams, S. T.	Room 269, Montreal General Hospital	Montreal, Que.
Addison, D. J.	Suite 302, 267 O'Connor St. . . .	Ottawa, Ont.
Aikenhead, J. F.	214-6th Ave, S.W.	Calgary, Alta. T2P OR1
Alaton, I.	1050 Avenue Rd.	Toronto, Ont. M5N 2C7
Alberga, V. H.	Suite 109, 2789 Jane St.	Downsview, Ont. M3N 2J2
Albertson, M. E.	Suite 903, 170 St. George St. . . .	Toronto, Ont. M5R 2N8
Alexander, J. C. C.	213 Church St.	Oakville, Ont.
Alexander, R. L.	Suite 204, 59 Yonge St. N.	Richmond Hill, Ont.
Ali, S. H.	43 Victoria St.	Amherst, N.S.
Allen, J. D.	278 O'Connor St.	Ottawa, Ont. K2P 1V4
Allin, W. D.	Suite 204, 178 John St.	Brampton, Ont.
Amyot, M.	Suite 220, 30 St. Joseph Blvd. E. .	Montreal, Que.
Anderson, D. L.	205, Medical Arts Bldg.	Edmonton, Alta. T5K OK9
Anderson, D. M.	56 Grand Ave. N.	Galt, Ont.
Anderson, J. D.	Medical Arts Clinic	Regina, Sask.
Andrews, C. H.	Suite 302, Medical Bldg.	Prince Albert, Sask. S6V 3K
Anhalt, E. F.	425 St. Mary Ave.	Winnipeg, Man R3C ON2
Armstrong, W. L.	Bank of Commerce Bldg, Suite 700, 1175 Douglas St.	Victoria, B.C.
Armstrong, W. S. S.	Suite 408, McLeod Bldg, 100th St.	Edmonton, Alta. T5J OP1
Arstikaitis, M.	123 Edward St.	Toronto, Ont.
Ash, D. G. G.	Medical Arts Clinic	Regina, Sask.
Audet, J.	655 est, Grand Allee	Quebec, Que.
Bailey, N. L.	Suite 403, 1120 Yates St.	Victoria, B.C.
Baird, C. D.	43 Victoria Ave	Chatham, Ont. N7L 2Z9
Baird, J. T.	McConnel Medical Centre	Cornwall, Ont.
Baird, R. P.	230 Frederick St.	Kitchener, Ont.
Ball, J. C.	131 Ontario St.	St. Catharines, Ont. L2R 5J9
Ballantyne, J. F.	326 Queen's Ave.	London, Ont. N6B 1X4
Bateman, C. R.	606 Waterloo Sq.	Waterloo, Ont. N2J 1P2
Bee, R. W.	800 Corbin Ave	New Britain, Conn. 06051
Begg, I. S.	2550 Willow St.	Vancouver, B.C.
Belanger, G.	475 Talbot, Blvd.	Chicoutimi, Que.
Bellefeuille, F.	875 Boul. des Récollets	Trois Rivières, Que.
Bending, G. C.	1515 N. W. Harrison Blvd.	Corvallis, Oreg.
Bennett, G.	Suite 6, 220-4th Ave	Kamloops, B.C.
Benoit, C. F.	Suite 203, 419 Graham Ave.	Winnipeg, Man.
Berger, B.	1541 West Broadway Ave.	Vancouver, B.C.
Bernier, R. G.	Suite 220, 30 est Boul. St. Joseph	Montreal, Que.
Bernstein, M.	220 Tecumseh Rd. W.	Windsor, Ont. N8X 1G1
Best, R. G.	Suite 405, Canada Bldg.	Windsor, Ont. N9A 1A8
Beswick, J. A.	Suite 12, 2860 Ellesmere Rd. . . .	West Hill, Ont.
Beuglet, E.	Suite 605, Medical Arts Bldg. . . .	Windsor, Ont. N9A 4J9
Bhadresa, G. M.	202 Royal Bank Bldg.	Red Deer, Alta. T4N 1Y1
Biehn, J. T.	282 Wellington St.	Sarnia, Ont. N7T 1H2
Bigúe, P.	449-3rd Ave	Quebec, Que.
Bissada, M.	2157 est Fleury	Montreal, Que.
Black, D.	Suite 226, 170 St. George St. . . .	Toronto, Ont. M5R 2N8
Blanchette, R.	1384 est rue Jean-Talon	Montreal, Que.
Boley, J. P.	1279 Ouellette Ave.	Windsor, Ont.
Boulanger, J.	45 Ste. Ursule St.	Quebec, Que.
Bowen R. A.	Suite 406, 235 Bastion St.	Nanaimo, B.C.

Boxer, L.	Suite 440, 3550 Côte des Neiger Rd.	Montreal, Que.
Boyd, T. A. S.	Room 129 Clinical Sciences Bldg. University of Alberta	Edmonton, Alta. T6G 2G3
Bradley, B. M.	139 Wellington St.	Sarnia, Ont. N7T 1G4
Bradley, J.	Suite 3, 1092-101 St.	North Battleford, Sask. S9A 2X6
Brault, J.	418 Sherbrooke St. E.	Montreal, Que.
Brent, H. P.	Suite 212, 20 Wynford Dr.	Don Mills, Ont.
Britton, M. H.	272 St. George St.	Moncton, N.B.
Britton, W. A.	Suite 704, 1081 Carling Ave. ...	Ottawa, Ont. K1Y 4G2
Brosnan, J. D.	Suite 1230, 750 West Georgia St.	Vancouver, B.C.
Brouillette, G.	Hopital Hotel Dieu de Montreal, Service L'ophthalmologie, 3840 rue St. Urban	Montreal, Que
Brownstein, S.	Royal Victoria Hospital, Department of Ophthalmology, Room 7, 687 Pine Avenue W. .	Montreal, Que.
Bruce, S. B.	289 Dufferin Ave.	London, Ont. N6B 1Z1
Brunet, M.	Suite 220, 30 St. Joseph Blvd. E. .	Montreal, Que.
Brunette, J. R.	30 St. Joseph. Blvd. E.	Montreal, Que.
Buncic, J. R.	Eye Clinic Hospital for Sick Children, 555 University Ave	Toronto, Ont.
Burran, E. L.	545 Lawrence Ave.	Kelowna, B.C.
Bustillo, J. L.	Suite 630, 10830 Jasper Ave. ...	Edmonton, Alta. T5N 3W6
Cairns, J. A.	Suite 601, 145 E. 13th St.	N. Vancouver, B.C.
Callahan, W. P.	183 St. Clair Ave. W.	Toronto, Ont.
Cambon, E. N.	1701 West Broadway Ave.	Vancouver, B.C.
Campbell, J. S.	207, Cuthbertson Block	Thunder Bay, Ont.
Capombassis, P. A.	Suite 250, 5025 Sherbrooke St. W.	Montreal, Que.
Cardarelli, G. ....·	2452 A. Dufferin St.	Toronto, Ont. M6E 3T1
Caux, J. N.	65 est Grand-Allee	Quebec, Que.
Chen, R. Y.-S.	Suite 504, 370 Steeles Ave. E. ..	Brampton, Ont.
Cheskes, A.	Suite 210, 170 Bloor St. W.	Toronto, Ont.
Chevrette, L.	Suite 311, 3875 rue St-Urbain ..	Montreal, 131, Que.
Chisholm, L. D. J.	Suite 503, 1849 Yonge St.	Toronto, Ont. M4S 1Y2
Chornell, J. G.	Suite 502, 10240-124 St.	Edmonton, Alta T5N 3W6
Chubb, P. D.	Suite 96, 520-17th Ave.	W. Vancouver, B.C.
Clinckett, F. R.	267 O'Connor St.	Ottawa, Ont. K2P 1V3
Cloutier, R.	Suite 1503, 625 President Kennedy	Montreal, Que.
Cobb, G. M. ·...........	1707 Weston Rd.	Weston, Ont.
Cody, P. C.	809-41st Ave.	Vancouver, B.C.
Cohen, A.	720 West Broadway Ave.	Vancouver, B.C.
Collyer, R. T.	326 Queen's Ave.	London, Ont. N6B 1X4
Cooper, M.	Suite 1, 1500 Royal York Rd. ..	Weston, Ont. M9P 3B6
Cormier, J. G.	Box 537, Dorchester St.	Sydney, N.S.
Corriveau, A. R.	150 Metcalfe St.	Ottawa, Ont. K2P 1P5
Cote, G.	Hopital St. Sacrement	Quebec, Que.
Coulas, L. G.	3535 Lakeshore Blvd. W.	Tornonto, Ont.
Couldwell, W. J.	Suite 706, 625-5th Ave.	New Westminster, B.C.
Crabb, A. M.	88 Wentworth St. S.	Hamilton, Ont.
Cragg, C. E. A.	327 Charlotte St.	Peterborough, Ont. K9J 7C3
Crawford, J. S.	Room M 165, 555 University Ave.	Toronto, Ont. M5G 1X8

Crewson, A. L.	132 Second St. W.	Cornwall, Ont. K6H 5V1
Criswick, V. G.	Suite 210, 1900 Richmond Ave. .	Victoria, B.C.
Croisetiere, F.	176 est boul, St. Joseph	Montreal, 151 Que.
Cruickshanks, B.	160 Essex St.	Sarnia, Ont. N7T 4R7
Cruise, J. T.	Suite A, 818 Douglas St.	Victoria, B.C.
Csordas, J. E.	Suite 605, Medical Arts Bldg. ...	Hamilton, Ont.
Cullen, G. C. R.	22575 Lougheed Hwy.	Maple Ridge, B.C.
Culvur, R. L.	397 Palliser Sq. E.	Calgary, Alta T2G OP5
Culver, R. W.	397 Palliser Sq. E. 115-9th Ave. S.E.	Calgary, Alta. T2G OP5
Dagenais, R.	780 Ste-Foy	Longueil, Que.
Dale, J. P. B.	Suite 706, 625-5th Ave.	New Westminister, B.C.
Davidson, H. J.	224 Charlotte St.	Sydney, N.S.
Davis, P. L.	Suite 1114, 1414 Drummond St. .	Montreal, Que.
Dawson, P. S.	Suite 420, 2550 Côté des Neiges .	Montreal, Que.
de Groot, J-A.	Suite 220, 30 est Blvd St. Joseph .	Montreal, Que.
Dekany, E. C.	Suite 203, 15 Roncesvalles Ave. .	Toronto, Ont. M6R 2K2
Delisle, P. H.	1401, 18e rue	Quebec, Que.
de Margerie, J. M.	Faculty of Medicine, University of Sherbrooke	Sherbrooke, Que.
Demers, J-P.	Suite 1503, 625 President Kennedy	Montreal, Que.
Demers, P. E.	985 Royal	Trois Rivières, Que.
Deschenes A.	627 est Jacques-Cartier	Chicoutimi, Que.
Dickson, D. H.	Suite 201, 164 Queen St. E.	Brampton, Ont.
Dillane, J. G.	Suite 708, Medical Arts Bldg. ...	Hamilton, Ont. L8N 1T8
Dixon, W. S.	Suite 503, 1849 Yonge St.	Toronto, Ont. M4S 1Y2
Dobbin, M. C.	Suite 100, 688 Coxwell Ave. ...	Toronto, Ont. M4C 3B7
Donegan, E. A.	Suite 256, 75 Spadina Cr. E.	Saskatoon, Sask. S7K 3H3
Dorsey, D. M.	154 James St. S.	Hamilton, Ont. L8P 3A2
Dorsey, M.	154 James St. S.	Hamilton, Ont. L8P 3A2
Drance, S. M.	2550 Willow St.	Vancouver, B.C.
Drysdale, I. O.	707 Charlotte St.	Peterborough, Ont.
du Toit, M. M. S.	8th Ave. & 8th St. S. W.	Calgary, Alta. T2P 1H9
Dubé, I.	2705 Blvd. Laurier Ste-Foy	Quebec, Que.
Dugre, J.	1000 Ste-Foy Rd.	Quebec, Que.
Dumas, J.	30 St. Joseph Blvd. E.	Montreal, Que.
Duncan, H. A. G.	Suite 508, 1538 Sherbrooke St. W.	Montreal, Que.
Duquette, C.	Suite 126, 794 5e rue	Shawinigan, Que.
Dyson, C.	Dept. of Ophthalmology, 3 North, Victoria Hospital	London, Ont. N6A 4G5
Eager, R. F.	Suite C, 5827 Main St.	Niagara Falls, Ont.
Easterbrook, W. M.	Suite 303, 1849 Yonge St.	Toronto, Ont. M4S 1Y2
Edelstein, E.	6000 Côté des Neiges	Montreal, Que.
Edwards, G. K.	340 McLeod St.	Ottawa, Ont. K2P 1A3
Elder, J. R.	Suite 206, 1333 Sheppard Ave. E.	Willowdale, Ont. M2J 1V1
Elliot, A. J.	2550 Willow St.	Vancouver, B.C.
Elliot, W. J.	Box 519	Parksville, B.C.
Elvin, N. L.	Suite 309, Medical Arts Bldg. ...	Winnipeg, Man. R3C OL6
Engen, E. S.	345 Victoria St.	Kamloops, B.C.
Ewing, C. C.	University Hospital, Dept. of Ophthalmology	Sasktoon, Sask.
Fainstein, S. B.	385 The West Mall	Etobicoke, Ont. M9C 1E7
Fejer, T. P.	2nd Floor, 1365 Yonge St.	Toronto, Ont. M4T 2P7
Feldman, F.	Suite 206, 99 Avenue Rd.	Toronto, Ont.

Fichman, S. H.	Suite 460, 6000 Côté des Neiges Rd.	Montreal, Que.
Flegg, K. R.	1081 Carling Ave.	Ottawa, Ont. K1Y 4G2
Fleming, K. O.	Suite 721, 925 West Georgia St.	Vancouver, B.C.
Flindall, R. J.	Suite 111, 2197 Riverside Dr.	Ottawa, Ont. K1H 7X3
Forman, J. A.	Suite 209, 1538 Sherbrooke St. W.	Montreal, Que.
Fouron, P.	599 Ave. Pere Michaud	Joliette, Que.
Foy, E. F.	Suite 405, 10830 Jasper Ave.	Edmonton, Alta.
Frankelson, E. N.	Dept. of Ophthalmology, College of Medicine, University of Saskatchewan	Saskatoon, Sask. S7N 0W8
Frenkling, S. R.	Suite 106, 77 The Queensway W..	Mississauga, Ont.
Fraser, W. F.	Suite 207, 340 McLeod, St.	Ottawa, Ont. K2P 1A4
Gagné, C. A.	15 Ave Begin	Lévis, Que.
Gagnon, A.	258 Iberville Blvd.	Repentigny, Que.
Gagnon, R.	Suite 1503, 625 President Kennedy	Montreal, Que.
Gaukrodger, W. T.	Suite 301, 180 Metcalfe St.	Ottawa, Ont. K2P 1P5
Gauthier, P.	250 est rue King	Sherbrooke, Que
Gauvin, P.	Suite 1503, 625 President Kennedy	Montreal, Que.
Gelinas, C.	15 Ave. Begin	Lévis, Que.
Genereux, A. G.	Suite 408, Canada Bldg.	Saskatoon, Sask. S7K 0B3
George, O. D.	253 Main St.	Yarmouth, N.S.
Ghosh, M.	Department of Ophthalmology, 1 Spadina Cres.	Toronto, Ont. M5S 2J5
Gibson, S. W. N.	Suite 309, 4900 Kingsway	South Burnaby, B.C.
Gillan, J. G.	206 Sheppard Ave. W.	Willowdale, Ont.
Gimbel, H. V.	1711-4th St. S.W.	Calgary, Alta T2S 1V8
Glenister, E. I.	1592 Oxford St.	Halifax, N.S.
Goel, J. N.	11 George St. S.	Galt, Ont.
Golesic, S.	955 Queen St. E.	Sault Ste. Marie, Ont.
Gordon, E.	Suite 3337, 1 Place Ville Marie	Montreal, Que.
Goedon, R.	Suite 100, Medical Centre Bldg. 8th Ave. 8th St.	Calgary, S.W. Alta.
Grader, J.	Suite 207, 1415 Lawrence Ave. W.	Toronto, Ont. M6L 1A9
Graham, J. E.	Suite 305, 20 Wynford Dr.	Don Mills, Ont. M3C 1J4
Graham, J. S.	3006-32nd Ave.	Vernon, B.C.
Gransden, G. M.	299 Main St.	Chilliwack, B.C.
Gravel, H.	55 Church St.	Verdun, Que.
Gravel, J. P.	1601 Boul. Laurier	Quebec, Que.
Green, D. H.	790 Sherbrook St.	Winnipeg, Man.
Grégoire, B.	Suite 306, 261 Montreal Rd.	Ottawa, Ont. K1L 6C4
Grégoire, J.	Suite 706, 555 Murray	Sherbrooke, Que.
Grieve, H. G.	Suite 701, 1430 Beach Dr.	Victoria, B.C.
Greves, J. K. G.	Medical Centre Maple Ave.	New Glasgow, N.S.
Griffith, W. R.	Suite 440, 11th Ave & Rose, Medical Dental Bldg.	Regina, Sask.
Groshaw, R. E.	1730 Weston Rd.	Weston, Ont.
Guest, W. C.	Suite 309, Medical Arts Bldg.	Winnipeg, Man. R3C 0L6
Halliday, J. A.	315 Brant Ave.	Brantford, Ont. N3T 3J8
Halliwell, D.	Suite 204, 1175 Cook St.	Victoria, B.C.
Hamilton, H. S.	15240 Thrift Ave.	White Rock, B.C.
Hammerling, J. S.	6777 Quinpool Rd.	Halifax, N.S.

Hand, R. F.	Suite 404, 5880 Spring Garden Rd.	Halifax, N.S.
Harper, D. W. H.	2451 A Bloor St. W.	Toronto, Ont. M6S 1P7
Harris, G. S.	Suite 507, 750 West Broadway Ave.	Vancouver, B.C.
Harrison, E. Q.	366 Central Ave.	London, Ont. N6B 2E2
Harshman, J. P.	2401 Bloor St. W.	Toronto, Ont. M6S 1P1
Hassard, D. T. R.	Suite 410, 8409-112th St.	Edmonton, Alta. T6G 1K6
Hausler, H. R.	477 Parkside Dr.	Toronto, Ont.
Hayes, B. G.	Suite 204, 300 King St. W.	Oshawa, Ont.
Hayes, R. T.	42 Coburg St.	St. John, N.B.
Hill, C. E.	158 St. George St.	Toronto, Ont. M5S 2G2
Hill, J. C.	Suite 333, 170 St. George St.	Toronto, Ont.
Hiltz, J. W.	120 Eglinton Ave. E.	Toronto, Ont. M4P 1E2
Hindle, N. W.	Suite 111, Medical Arts Bldg. 6th Ave. 3rd St.	Calgary, Alta. T2P 0R8
Hollands, R. H.	Suite 201, 1750 E. 10th Ave.	Vancouver, B.C.
Hook, J. H.	51-6th St. E.	Medicine Hat, Alta. T1A 7H
Horton, J. G.	Suite 102, 6 Glen Wood Pl.	Brockville, Ont. K6V 2T3
Howden, G. D.	Suite 500, 1175 Douglas St.	Vancouver, B.C.
Hunter, W. S.	176 St. George St.	Toronto, Ont. M5R 2M7
Hutchison, W. G.	85 Westmount Rd.	Guelph, Ont.
Hyslop, W. A.	Suite 608, Maritime Bldg.	New Glasgow, N.S.
Inch, F. A. B.	Suite 700, Medical Arts Bldg.	Hamilton, Ont.
Innes, R. M. R.	Suite 626, 718 Granville St.	Vancouver, B.C.
Irving, J. A.	3195 Granville St.	Vancouver, B.C.
Jamieson, D.,M.	100 Queen St. S.	Kitchener, Ont. N2G 1V8
Jamieson, J. S.	Suite 11, 347 Sherbrooke St.	North Bay, Ont.
Jans, R. G.	700-8th St. S.W.	Calgary, Alta. T2P 2A7
Jarvis, G. J.	2917 Bloor St. W.	Toronto, Ont. M8X 1B4
Johnson, D. G.	Suite 706, 625-5th Ave.	New Westminster, B.C.
Johnson, E. A.	1028 Bel-Aire Dr. S.W.	Calgary, Alta. T2V 8B9
Johnston, A. C. W.	Suite 270, 5780 Cambie St.	Vancouver, B.C.
Julien, P. E.	794-5th St.	Shawinigan Falls, Que.
Julien, P. G.	1695 Rue Girouard	St. Hyacinthe, Que.
Karsgaard, A. T.	425 St. Mary Ave.	Winnipeg, Man. R3C 0N2
Katz, A. H.	5845 Côté des Neiges Rd.	Montreal, Que.
Kaufman, M. I. H.	4773 Sherbrooke St. W.	Montreal, Que.
Kazdan, J. J.	Suite 9,4 Finch Ave. W.	Willowdale, Ont.
Kazdan, M. S.	Suite 304, 99 Avenue Rd.	Toronto, Ont.
Keays, C. F.	5880 Spring Garden Rd.	Halifax, N.S.
Kellett, J. R.	1251 West King Edward Ave.	Vancouver, B.C.
Kelly, R. G. C.	Suite 902, 1849 Yonge St.	Toronto, Ont. M4S 1Y2
Kelly, R. G. M.	Suite 301, 3025 Hurontario St.	Mississauga, Ont.
Khalil, M. K.	Suite 250, 5025 Sherbrooke St. W.	Montreal, Que.
Kiff, R. D.	17 Dunedin St.	Orillia, Ont.
Kirker, G. E. M.	72 Bayview Dr. S. W.	Calgary, Alta.
Kirkham, T. H.	The Montreal Children's Hospital, 2300 Tupper St.	Montreal, Que.
Kirschberg, L. S. S.	Suite 25, 1390 Sherbrooke St. W.	Montreal, Que.
Knowles, V. R.	Suite 312, Medical Arts Bldg.	Saskatoon, Sask. S7S 3H3
Koziak, P. H.	Suite 709, Tegler Bldg.	Edmonton, Alta. T5J 0T8
Kral, K.	Apt. 615, University Towers, 1201 Richmond St.	London, Ont. N6A 3L6
Krolman, G. M.	Suite 201, 414 Graham Ave.	Winnipeg, Man R3E 0W3

Kuder, G. G.	85 Westmount Rd.	Guelph, Ont. N1N 5J2
Kwitko, M. I.	Suite 440, 6000 Côté des Neiges Rd.	Montreal, Que.
Kyle, J. L.	6150 Valley Way	Niagara Falls, Ont.
Labelle, A. R.	964 Cherrier St.	Montreal, Que.
Labelle, P.	Suite 220, 30 est Boul. St. Joseph	Montreal, Que.
Laflamme, M.	Suite 40, 55 rue de l'Eglise	Verdun, Que.
Lamer, L.	Suite 250, 450 Sherbrooke St. E.	Montreal, Que.
Lapointe, G. A.	627 est Jacques-Cartier	Chicoutimi, Que.
LaRochelle, P. R.	219 Notre Dame Nord	Thetford Megantic, Que.
Lavoie, R. G.	Suite 201, 915 St. Cyrille Blvd. W.	Quebec, Que.
Laws, H. W.	81 Brinkerhoff St.	Plattsburgh, N.Y. 12901
Lawton, R. D.	135 Military Rd.	St. John's, Nfld.
Leitch, T. J. G.	Suite 350, 8702 Meadowlark Rd.	Edmonton, Alta. T5R 5W5
Lemire, J.	Suite 250, 450 Sherbrooke St. E.	Montreal, Que.
Lennox, B. M.	143 Ontario St.	St. Catharines, Ont.
Leong, S. T.	Suite 505, Canada Trust Bldg.	Lethbridge, Alta.
Lerman, S.	Room 1211, McIntyre Bldg. McGill University	Montreal, Que.
Lerner, M.	Suite 512, 388 Portage Ave.	Winnipeg, Man. R3C 0C8
Letarte, F.	84 St. Louis St.	Quebec, Que.
Levine, M. H.	452 Main St. E.	Hamilton, Ont.
Lewis, J. E.	24 Pine St. S.	Timmins, Ont.
Liddy, B. St. L.	National Defence Medical Centre, Alta Vista Dr.	Ottawa, Ont.
Lindsay, A.	458 Main St.	Kentville, N.S.
Little, J. G.	268 Dundas St. E.	Belleville, Ont. K8N 1E6
Little, John M.	1 Cedar Ave.	Pointe Claire, Que.
Lloyd, L. A.	Suite 507, 170 St. George St.	Toronto, Ont. M5R 2M8
Locke, J. C.	Suite 1012, 1414 Drummond St.	Montreal, Que.
Longinotto, M. B.	Suite 210, 1711-4th St. S.W.	Calgary, Alta.
Lorenzetti, D. W. C.	Suite 1322, 1650 Cedar Ave.	Montreal, Que.
Luke, S. K.	Suite 510, 75 Donway West	Don Mills, Ont. M3C 2E9
Lussier, M.	30 St. Joseph Blvd. E.	Montreal, Que.
MacAulay, M. G.	330 Mt. Tolmie Ridge Apts., 1900 Mayfair Dr.	Victoria, B.C.
Macdonald, D. K.	Suite 911, 1849 Yonge St.	Toronto, Ont. M4S 1Y2
MacDonald, R. K.	Suite 421, 170 St. George St.	Toronto, Ont. M5R 2M8
MacFarlane, E. B.	Suite 610, Medical Arts Bldg.	Hamilton, Ont.
MacIvor, J.	986-3rd Ave. E.	Owen Sound, Ont. M4K 2K9
MacKay, J. A.	51-6th St. E.	Medicine Hat, Alta. T1A 7H4
MacMillan, C. C.	42 Wellington Row	St. John, N.B.
MacRae, D. M.	5880 Spring Garden Rd.	Halifax, N.S.
MacRae, D. R.	27 Leinster St.	St. John, N.B.
Macrae, H. M.	Suite 226, 170 St. George St.	Toronto, Ont. M5R 2M8
Macrae, W. G.	6 Jack Frost Lane	Ruxton, Md. 21204
Macrodimitris, A. G.	Suite 203, 419 Graham Ave.	Winnipeg, Man. R3C 0M3
Marcrosson, K. I.	21 Clinic Block	Yorkton, Sask. S3N 1E5
McCartney, H. J.	707 Charlotte St.	Peterborough, Ont. K9J 7B3
McCreery, R. G.	Suite 130, 5780 Cambie St.	Vancouver, B.C.
McCulloch, J. C.	Room 115, 1 Spadina Cres.	Toronto, Ont. M5S 2J5
McCunn, P. D.	Suite 206, 340 McLeod St.	Ottawa, Ont. K2P 1A4
McDiarmid, R. O.	Suite 35, Clement Block, Rosser Ave.	Brandon, Man. R7A 0L3

McDonald, D. J.	2917 Bloor St. W.	Toronto, Ont.
McFarlane, D. C.	382 Queen's Ave.	London, Ont. N6B 1X6
McGillivray, D. M.	88 Wentworth St. S.	Hamilton, Ont.
McGrath, J. P.	20 Cornwallis St.	Kentville, N.S.
McGrath, W. P.	1310 Ouellette Ave.	Windsor, Ont. N8X 1J8
McKerricher, D. E.	Suite 405, 235 Bastion St.	Nanaimo, B.C.
McKinlay, W. D.	Suite 730 Birks Bldg.	Vancouver, B.C.
McKinna, A. J.	Director Dept. of Ophthalmology, Univ. Hospital, 339 Windermere Rd.	London, Ont.
McLean, J. A.	Suite 1211, 750 West Broadway Ave.	Vancouver, B.C.
McLean, M. J.	Suite 1211, 750 West Broadway Ave.	Vancouver, B.C.
McLellan, J. R.	Box 712, 164 Charlotte St.	Sydney, N.S.
McMillan, D. W.	Suite 305 Northgate Bldg.	Edmonton, Alta.
McNicholas, P. D.	1 A Church Hill	St. John's, Nfld.
Madronich, J. S.	Suite 311, Medical Arts Bldg. ...	Hamilton, Ont.
Magder, H.	Suite 460, 6000 Côté des Neiges Rd.	Montreal, Que.
Magee, D. R.	Suite 309, Medical Arts Bldg. ...	Winnipeg, Man. R3C 0L6
Mahood, A. W.	Elmira Medical Centre	Elmira, N.Y. 14901
Mailer, C. M.	Suite 8, 225 Queen's Ave.	London, Ont. N6A 1J8
Mailloux, L.	525 Cherrier St.	Montreal, Que.
Maisonville, P. St. L.	Suite 109, 3195 Granville St. ...	Vancouver, B.C.
Malenfant, M.	Hotel Dieu de Sherbrooke	Sherbrooke, Que.
Mallek, H.	736 Granville St.	Vancouver, B.C.
Mann, W. H.	10 Hincks St.	St. Thomas, Ont. N5R 394
Maranda, E.	216 St. Vallier St. W.	Quebec, Que.
Marchildon, A.	3045 LaPromenade	Ste-Foy, Que.
Marshall, M. R.	Apt. 1704, 355 St. Clair Ave. W. .	Toronto, Ont.
Martin, A. J.	1629 Baker St.	Cranbrook, B.C.
Martin, W. R. J.	Suite 309, 4900 Kingsway Ave. .	South Burnaby, B.C.
Matheson, D. C.	4900 Kingsway Ave.	South Burnaby, B.C.
Mathieu, M.	Suite 220, 30 St. Joseph Blvd. E.	Montreal, Que.
Matvenko, J.	1175 Douglas St.	Victoria, B.C.
Mendelson, J.	Suite 203, Boyd Bldg.	Winnipeg, Man.
Mercier, M.	15 Ave. Begin	Lévis, Que.
Miller, M. S.	Suite 404, 906-8th Ave. S.W. ...	Calgary, Alta.
Mills, D. W.	Suite 505, 200 Queen's Ave. ...	London, Ont. N6A 1J3
Milot, J.	Suite 312, 30 St. Joseph Blvd. E.	Montreal, Que.
Minnes, J. F.	3195 Granville St.	Vancouver, B.C.
Mitchell, D. C.	The Medical Arts Bldg, 145 Queenston St., Suite 402	St. Catharines, Ont.
Molloy, J. H.	5880 Spring Garden Rd.	Halifax, N.S.
Monfette, C.	364 Sherbrooke St. E.	Montreal, Que.
Moore, C. H.	Suite 403, 1120 Yates St.	Victoria, B.C.
Moreside, J. W.	170 Fitzroy St.	Charlottetown, P.E.I.
Morgan, A. L.	Suite 1116, 123 Edward St.	Toronto, Ont.
Morgan, J. F.	Hotel Dieu Hospital	Kingston, Ont.
Morgan, R. A.	Suite 1152, 10830 Jasper Ave. ..	Edmonton, Alta.
Morin, J. D.	1050 Avenue Rd.	Toronto, Ont.
Mortimer, C. B.	Suite 1001, 170 St. George St. ..	Toronto, Ont. M5J 1A2
Morton, P. L.	Suite 8, 825 Coxwell Ave.	Toronto, Ont. M4C 3E7
Mount, H.,T. J.	340 McLeod St.	Ottawa, Ont. K2P 1A4

Murphy, S. B.	Royal Victoria Hospital, Department of Ophthalmology, 687 Pine Ave. W.	Montreal, Que.
Murray, D. K.	5974 Spring Garden Rd.	Halifax, N.S.
Murray, R. G.	University of Saskatchewan	Saskatoon, Sask. S7N 0W8
Must, C. J.	327 Charlotte St.	Peterborough, Ont. K9J 7C3
Myers, L.	Suite 303, 25 Brunswick Ave.	Toronto, Ont. M5S 2L9
Nadeau, N.	4 Prince William St.	Cambellton, N.B.
Neveu, M.	875 Rue des Recollets.	Trois Rivières, Que.
Newbigin, B.	325 A Lakeshore Rd. E.	Port Credit, Ont.
Nicholls, J. V. V.	Suite 203, 111 Waterloo St.	London, Ont. N6B 2M4
Nicol, W. G.	Suite 307, 1199 Cedar Ave.	Trail, B.C.
Noble, R. I.	790 Sherbrook St.	Winnipeg, Man.
Noiseaux, J. J. J.	Suite 404, 12245 rue Grenet.	Montreal, Que.
Norton, H. J. Jr.	797 Elmwood Ave.	Rochester 20, N.Y.
O'Brien, D. B.	6389 Coburg Rd.	Halifax, N.S.
Oliver, G. L.	450 Central Ave.	London, Ont. N6B 2E8
Orquin, J.	Suite 18, 5582 Gatineau	Montreal, Que.
Pager, R.	Suite 220, 30 St. Joseph Blvd. E. .	Montreal, Que.
Paine, D. L. E.	Suite 404, 1120 Yates St.	Victoria, B.C.
Panisset, A.	Suite 1503, 625 President Kennedy	Montreal, Que.
Panneton, A.	985 Royale	Trois Rivières, Que.
Parker, D.	Suite 441, Palliser Sq, W, 131-9th Ave. S.W.	Calgary, Alta. T2P 1K1
Parker, J. A.	Room 105, University Wing, Toronto General Hospital	Toronto, Ont.
Pashby, T. J.	Suite 1, 20 Wynford Dr.	Don Mills, Ont. M3C 1J4
Patrick, A.	Suite 201, 9950-107th St.	Edmonton, Alta. T5K 1G5
Pearce, W. G.	2-131, Clinical Sciences Bldg, University of Alberta.	Edmonton, Alta. T6G 2G3
Pearman, R. W.	Suite 250, 5025 Sherbrooke St. W.	Montreal, Que.
Peramaki, R. T.	Suite 406, 96 Larch St.	Sudbury, Ont.
Perron, L.	964 Cherrier St.	Montreal, Que.
Perry, R. J.	Etherington Hall, Stuart St.	Kingston, Ont.
Pinkerton, R. M. H.	Etherington Hall, Stuart St.	Kingston, Ont.
Plamondon, J. L. M.	30 Cote du Palais	Quebec, Que.
Plante, A.	Hotel Dieu de Roberval	Roberval, Que.
Podedworny, W. M.	Suite 1, 225 James St. S.	Hamilton, Ont. L8P 3B2
Poirier, G.	1401, 18e rue	Quebec, Que.
Powell, E.	Suite 104, Medical Arts Bldg.	Thunder Bay, Ont.
Prasloski, P. F.	Suite 204, 625-5th Ave.	New Westminster, B.C.
Pratt-Johnson, J. A.	Suite 714, 750 West Broadway Ave.	Vancouver, B.C.
Probert, L. A.	Suite 510, Scott Bldg.	Moose Jaw, Sask.
Pyper, J. E.	386 Cambria St.	Stratford, Ont. N5A 1J4
Querengesser, E. I.	473 Queen St. S.	Kitchener, Ont. N2G 1N8
Quigley, J. H.	1674 Oxford St.	Halifax, N.S.
Rafuse, E. V.	1531 Oxford St.	Halifax, N.S.
Ramsay, R. M.	Suite 125, Medical Arts Bldg.	Winnipeg, Man. R3C 0L6
Ramsey, M. S.	Suite 21, Box 16, R.R. #1	Tantallon, Halifax, N.S.
Ramsey, R. B.	Suite 222, 1414 Drummond St. .	Montreal, Que.
Read, R. M.	Suite 12, 5880 Spring Garden Rd.	Halifax, N.S.
Reed, H. N.	425 St. Mary Avenue	Winnipeg, Man. R3C 0N2
Rees, D. L.	Suite 303, Medical Arts Bldg.	Edmonton, Alta. T5K 0K9

Regan, G. T.	66 Waterloo St.	St. John, N.B.
Renpenning, H. J.	112 Palisades	Saskatoon, Sask. S7K 0J8
Rentiers, P. K.	Suite 306, 2151 McCallum Rd.	Abbotsford, B.C.
Revie, I. H. S.	Suite 407, 428 Portage Ave.	Winnipeg, Man
Richards, J. S. F.	2550 Willow St., Dept. of Ophthalmology	Vancouver, B.C.
Richardson, O. B.	1314 Clonsilla Ave.	Peterborough, Ont. K9J 2Z2
Ridgway, C. R.	9950-107 St.	Edmonton, Alta.
Rodrigue, D.	Suite 1401, 18 Rue	Quebec, Que.
Rombough, W. G.	301 Frederick St.	Kitchener, Ont. N2H 2N6
Rooney, J. T.	Suite 35, 907 Rosser Ave.	Brandon, Man.
Rose, H. A.	P.O. Box, 520	Yellowknife, N.W.T.
Rose, J. A.	Suite 306, Medical Arts Bldg.	Winnipeg, Man. R3C 0L6
Roseborough, G. F.	851 Pandora Ave.	Victoria, B.C.
Rosen, D. A.	Etherington Hall, Stuart St.	Kingston, Ont. K7L 2B6
Rosenbaum, P.	1414 Drummond St.	Montreal, Que.
Ross, H. W.	Suite 301, 9656 King George V1 Highway	Surrey, B.C.
Ross, R. A.	Suite 123, 725 Carmi Ave.	Penticton, B.C.
Rousseau, A. P. J.	2790 Mont-Royal St.	Quebec, Que.
Rowe, W. J.	Suite 123, 725 Carmi Ave.	Penticton, B.C.
Roy, P. E.	Suite 160, 1500-18e Rue	Quebec, Que.
Saheb, N. E.	Suite 502, 3665 Rodgewood	Montreal, Que.
Samis, W. D.	Suite 904, 1849 Yonge St.	Toronto, Ont. M4S 1Y2
Sapp, G. A.	Suite 404, 5880 Spring Garden Rd.	Halifax, N.S.
Schirmer, K. E.	5300 Côté des Neiges Rd.	Montreal, Que.
Schneider, R. J.	University Hospital	Saskatoon, Sask. S7N 0W8
Scott, J. H.	Room 300, 740 Rosser Ave	Brandon, Man. R7A 0K9
Shafto, C. M.	438 Palliser Sq. W.	Calgary, Alta. T2P 1K1
Shamess, S. A.	Box 849	Sault Ste. Marie, Ont.
Shea, M.	Suite 828, 170 St. George St.	Toronto, Ont. M5R 2M8
Sheldon, G. M.	16 B Yonge St. N.	Richmond Hill, Ont.
Shenken, E.	Suite 603, 2 St. Clair Ave. W.	Toronto, Ont. M4V 1L5
Sheridan, B. B. M.	4 Taschereau St.	Hull, Que.
Shirley, S. Y.	Suite 301, 180 Metcalfe St.	Ottawa, Ont. K2P 1P5
Sholdra, E. P.	Suite 404, 120 Holland Ave	Ottawa, Ont.
Shusterman, M.	72 St. Clair Ave. W.	Toronto, Ont.
Shutt, H. K. R.	6004-144 St.	Edmonton, Alta.
Siddall, J. R.	Suite 309, 4900 Kingsway	South Burnaby, B.C.
Sillers, D. E.	1707 Weston Rd.	Weston, Ont.
Silver, S.	38 Coburg St.	St. John, N.B.
Simard, M.	475 Bldg., Talbot	Chicoutimi, Que.
Simon, F.	Suite 385, The West Mall	Etobicoke, Ont. M9C 1E7
Simpson, D. G.	Suite 1402, 750 West Broadway Ave.	Vancouver, B.C.
Sinton, E. J.	Suite 608, 4808 Ross St.	Red Deer, Alta. T4N 1X5
Sipos, J. K.	Suite 118, 612 St. Johns Rd.	Pointe Claire, Que.
Slatt, B.	Suite 918, 1849 Yonge St.	Toronto, Ont. M4S 1Y2
Smart, R. E.	Prescott Rd, R.R. # 1	Brockville, Ont. K6V 5T1
Smith, D. R.	Suite 107, 250 Lawrence Ave W.	Toronto, Ont. M5M 1B2
Smith, E. L.	Suite 914, 750 West Broadway Ave.	Vancouver, B.C.
Smith, E. W.	Suite 408, Canada Bldg.	Saskatoon, Sask.
Smith, R. S.	Park Medical Bldg, 1635 Abbott St.	Kelowna, B.C.

Smith, S. S.	Suite 101, 1711-4th St. S.W.	Calgary, Alta. T2S 1V8
Sneed, R. J.	Suite 1001, Second St. W.	Ashland, Wis. 54806
Sniderman, B. P. P.	Suite 406, 99 Avenue Rd.	Toronto, Ont. M5R 2G5
Sniderman, H. R.	Suite 406, 99 Avenue Rd.	Toronto, Ont. M5R 2G5
Somerville, G. M.	206 Sheppard Ave. W.	Willowdale, Ont.
Speakman, J. S.	170 St. George St.	Toronto, Ont. M5R 2M8
Spearman, W. F.	267 O'Connor St.	Ottawa, Ont. K2P 1V3
Spencer, J. R.	Suite 22, 347 Sherbrooke St.	North Bay, Ont.
Spitzer, M. L.	215 King St. W.	Dundas, Ont.
Spooner, E. G.	Medical Arts Bldg.	Regina, Sask.
Standret, D. T.	672 Brant St.	Burlington, Ont.
Stasior, O. G.	668 Madison Ave.	Albany, N.Y. 12208
Steidl, P. E. M.	418 Sherbrooke St. E.	Montreal, Que.
Stein, H. A.	3000 Lawrence Ave. E.	Scarborough, Ont.
Stewart, A. J.	750 West Broadway Ave.	Vancouver, B.C.
Stewart, D. G.	The Polyclinic – 170-172 Fitzroy St.	Charlottetown, P.E.I.
Sutherland, R. L.	Suite 806, 8th Ave. & 8th St. S.W.	Calgary, Alta. T2P 1H9
Swaine, F. M.	Suite 104, 208 Dundas St. E.	Belleville, Ont.
Sweeney, D. B.	Suite 105, 3000 Lawrence Ave. E.	Scarborough, Ont.
Szasz, J.	550 Ingersoll Ave.	Woodstock, Ont. N4S 4Y2
Szeps, J.	P.O. Box 1196, 194 Wellington St.W.	Chatham, Ont. N7M 5L7
Taj, A. H.	Western Memorial Hospital	Corner Brook, Nfld.
Tanenbaum, H. L.	Suite 828 W, Jewish General Hospital, 3755 Cote Ste. Catherine Rd.	Montreal, Que.
Tanner, W. H. R.	Suite 45, Academy Medical Bldg.	Calgary, Alta. T2S 1W1
Tanzer, H.	17 Elfindale Cr.	Willowdale, Ont. M2J 1B6
Taube, J. I.	Suite 1007, Hume-Nansur Bldg.	Indianapolis, Ind. 46204
Teichman, B.	Suite 206 A. 99 Avenue Rd.	Toronto, Ont. M5R 2G5
Ten Cate, A. G.	135 Ormond St.	Brockville, Ont. K6V 5Y2
Terry, E.	1509 Sherbrooke St. W.	Montreal, Que.
Tessier, L. J.	1249 St. Joseph Blvd. E.	Montreal, Que.
Thibaudeau, J.	250 King St. E.	Sherbrooke, Que.
Thompson, C. A.	232 Queen's Ave.	London, Ont.
Thompson, C. O.	265 Brant Ave.	Brantford, Ont. N3T 3J6
Thompson, G. A.	Suite 401, 1849 Younge St.	Toronto, Ont. M4S 1Y2
Thompson, G. H.	1175 Douglas St.	Victoria, B.C.
Tipler, H. A. B.	199 Ontario St.	St. Catharines, Ont.
Toews, R. R.	Suite 602, 5400 Portage Rd.	Niagara Falls, Ont.
Tremblay, R. P.	Suite 220, 235 E. Dorchester St.	Montreal, Que.
Trottier, M.	Suite 404, 12245 rue Grenet	Montreal, Que.
Turnbull, J. B.	3514 Lakeview Ave.	Regina, Sask.
Turnbull, W.	Suite 322, 1414 Drummond St.	Montreal, Que.
Tweedy, R. A. J.	14 Willow Court	Welland, Ont.
Vachon, A.	C.P. # 215	LaSalle, Que.
Vaile, S. J.	Suite 918, 1849 Yonge St.	Toronto, Ont. M4S 1Y2
Valberg, J. D.	Suite 307, 267 O'Connor St.	Ottawa, Ont. K2P 1V3
Vanderburg, D. L.	16 O'Brien St.	Orillia, Ont.
Veronneau, S.	755 Park Ave.	New York, N.Y. 10021
Viger, R. J.	1230-11th St. Huntingdon W.	Virginia, 25701
Walsh, P. J. P.	121 Wellington St. W.	Barrie, Ont.
Warner, D. M.	Suite 1402, 750 West Broadway Ave.	Vancouver, B.C.

Warnica, J. K.	Suite 112, 121 Wellington St. ...	Barrie, Ont.
Watson, A. G.	Suite 406, 267 O'Connor St. ...	Ottawa, Ont. K2P 1V3
Weaver, M. A.	88 Wentworth St. S.	Hamilton, Ont.
Werner, N. H.	Suite 404, 309 Hargrave St.	Winnipeg, Man. R3B 2J8
Whiston, G. J.	15 Cranston Ave.	Dartmouth, N.S.
White, P. D.	481 Park St.	Kitchener, Ont. N2G 1N7
Wiebe, H. L. R.	Suite 2, 13665-96th Ave.	Surrey, B.C.
Wiggins, R. L.	Suite 402, 1120 Yates St.	Victoria, B.C.
Wilczek, Z. M. J.	Suite 212, 2489 Bloor St. W. ...	Toronto, Ont.
Wilkie, J. S.	201-1750 East 10th Ave.	Vancouver, B.C.
Willis, N. R.	Suite 505, 200 Queens Ave.	London, Ont. N6A 1J3
Willis, W. E.	Hotel Dieu Hospital, Dept. of Ophthalmology	Kingston, Ont.
Wilson, W. M. G.	Suite 30, 3195 Granville St.	Vancouver, B.C.
Wior, G. A.	1538 Sherbrooke St. W.	Montreal, Que.
Wiss, F. R.	224 Elm St. W.	Sudbury, Ont. P3C 1V3
Witelson, H. C.	Medical Arts Bldg.	Hamilton, Ont.
Witzel, S. H.	Suite 203, 713 Davis Dr.	Newmarket, Ont.
Wolstein, E.	Suite 307, 267 O'Connor St. ...	Ottawa, Ont. K2P 1V3
Woodall, G. P.	109 Gardenia Court	Oshawa, Ont.
Woywitka, N. W.	Suite 309, 10049 Jasper Ave. ...	Edmonton, Alta. T5J 1T7
Wright, E. N.	Suite 106, Medical Arts Bldg. ...	Thunder Bat, Ont.
Wright, W. R.	206 Rookwood Ave.	Fredericton, N.B.
Wyatt, H.,T.	Charles Camsell Hospital, 12815-115 Ave.	Edmonton, Alta. T5M 3A4
Young, R. W.	Suite 203, 603 Davis Dr.	Newmarket, Ont.
Young, W.	Suite 301, 9656 King George Highway	Surrey, B.C.
Zahoruk, R. M.	McMaster University Medical Centre, Department of Opthalmology, Room 4 U 4	Hamilton, Ont.
Zucker, B. B.	2 St. Clair Ave. W.	Toronto, Ont.
Zuege, P.	453 Palliser Sq., 115-9th Ave. S.E.	Calgary, Alta.

Senior Members

Bendor-Samuel, J. E. L. ...	425 St. Mary Avenue	Winnipeg, Man. R3C 0N2
Briant, T. E.	36 Highland Gardens	Welland, Ont.
Conroy, J. B.	1000 Moss St.	Victoria, B.C.
Coupal, J. L.	221 River Rd.	Eastview, Ont.
Crewson, W. L.	147 Kent St.	Hamilton, Ont. L8P 3Z2
Cunningham, E. R.	1215 W. 13th Ave.	Vancouver, B.C.
Elkington, E. H. W.	572 Island Rd.	Victoria, B.C.
Gilhooly, J. P.	80 McLaren St.	Ottawa, Ont. K1V 8L9
Godin, P. E. A.	3445 Drummond St., Apt. 307 ..	Montreal, Que.
Gordon, R. I.	140 Aberdeen Rd.	Kitchener, Ont.
Gorrell, D. S.	3516 Henderson Rd.	Victoria, B.C.
Graham, H. M.	5807 Wallace St.	Vancouver, B.C.
Grove, J. H.	2649 Flannery Dr.	Ottawa, ont. KIV 8L9
Henderson, R. H.	76 Norwood Cr.	Waterloo, Ont.
Holland, L. G.	6905 Tupper Cr.	Halifax, N.S.
Ingham, G. H.	113 William St.	Stratford, Ont.
Johnston, J. F. A.	176 St. George St.	Toronto, Ont. M5R 2M7
Johnston, K. B.	Box 40	Como, Que.
Kirkpatrick, H. W.	440 Park St.	Kentville, N.S.
Lacerte, J.	34 Fabrique	Quebec, Que.
Langille, J. A.	107 Church St.	Amherst, N.S.

Ling, C. H.	20 Glengarry Dr.	Winnipeg, Man.
Luke, W. R. F.	7 Pineforest St.	Toronto, Ont.
MacDonald, A. E.	Suite 511, 170 St. George St.	Toronto, Ont. M5R 2M8
MacDonald, D. C.	97 Carlton Towers, 325-5th Ave. N.	Saskatoon, Sask. S7K 2P7
Rook, L. A.	Box 998	Vernon, B.C.
Savisky, M. F.	7432 Leary Cres.	Sardis, B.C.
Stoddard, R. H.	967 Ivanhoe St.	Halifax, N.S.
White, G. B.	239 Sugarloaf St.	Pt. Colborne, Ont.

NOSOCOMIA QUIBUS OCULIS AEGRI CURANTUR

There are no special Eye Hospitals in Canada.
They are all departments of a General Hospital.

INSTITUTA SCHOLAEQUE CAECIS DESTINATAE

Schools for the Blind at:
Vancouver, B.C. .... 125 pupils
Brantford, Ont. .... 200 pupils
Montreal, Que. (2 schools) .... —
Quebec, Que. .... —
Halifax, N. Scotia .... 162 pupils

CHILI

SOCIETATES OPHTHALMOLOGICAE

Sociedad Chilena de Oftalmología
Secretary: Dr. Miguel Kottow, Evaristo Lillo 393, Las Condes
No data received.

COLOMBIA

SOCIETATES OPHTHALMOLOGICAE

Sociedad Colombiana de Oftalmología
Secretary: Dr. Rafael Bahamon, Bogotá

No data received.

CUBA

SOCIETATES OPHTHALMOLOGICAE

Sociedad Cubana de Oftalmologia

Presidente: Dr. Rolando Hernández Leal
Vice-Presidente: Dr. Elio Marrero Faz
Secretario: Dr. Rolando López Cardet, 3ra N⁰ 371, e/ San Leonardo y Kessell, Rpto. Apolo, La Habana
Vice Secretario: Dr. Jesús Rigueiro Vázquez
Tesorero: Dr. Othón Gómez Ruíz
Vocales: Dra. Elizabeth Chávez Quiñones, Dr. Fausto Tablada
Miembros: 387

NOMINA ET DOMICILIA MEDICORUM AB OCULIS

Alemany Martorell Jaime ..	15 No. 705, e/ A. y Paseo	Vedado, La Habana
Almonte Aras, Placido	Calle F # 64, e/ 3ra. y 5ta.	Vedado, La Habana
Armas Leon, Mirtha de	15 # 334, Apto. 303	Vedado, La Habana
Arrue Arguelles, Justino ...	Depto. Oftalmologia, Hospital Provincial 'M. Ascunce'	Camaguey
Benacet Buruaga, Hugo	Calle 30 # 758, e/ Kohly y 41 ..	Alto-Vedado, La Habana
Boffil Delgado, Francisco ..	Cisnero Betancourt No. 569	Los Pinos, Habana
Camacho Caballero, Olga ..	Hospital de Moron	Camaguey
Cantera, Irma de la	Hospital Pando Ferrer 76 y 31 ..	Marianao
Cardenas Torriente, Violeta	Vista Alegre No. 306 e/ Cortina y J. B. Zayas Vibora	La Habana (5)
Castellanos Dumois, Arquimides	Hospital 'Cmdte. Fajardo' Zapata y C	Vedado, La Habana
Castro Mestre, Angel	Dpto. de Oftalmologia, Hosp. Calixto Carcia	La Habana (4)
Cavero Encuentra, Julia ...	41 # 810	Cienfuegos, Las Villas
Chavez Quiñones, Elizabeth	Palatino # 115 e/ Salvador y Esperanza	Cerro, La Habana
Cisneros Lavadi, Alberto ...	Dpto. Oftalmologia, Hospital Militar	Santiago de Cuba, Oriente
Coello Trimiño, Natalia ...	Gloria # 72	Santa Clara, Las Villas
Colom, Gladys	Paseo No. 455 bajos	Vedado, La Habana
Colon Sanchez, Emilio	Paseo No. 455, bajos, e/ 19 y 21 .	Vedado, La Habana
Diaz Guerra, Hilda	Avenida Novena # 4221 e/ 42 y 44	Marianao, La Habana
Dominguez Llarena, Hector	Gral. Peraza # 17	Moron, Camaguey
Fernandez Bergados, Felipe	Parque # 4413 e/ Garrido y Carolina	Guanabacoa, La Habana
Fernandez Colas, Caridad ..	Animas # 612, bajos e/ Lealtad y Perseverancia	La Habana
Ferrer, Elsa	Ronda # 15, Apto. 2 e/ Neptuno y San Miguel	La Habana
Ferrer, Lourdes	Dpto. Oftalmologia, Hospital Militar	Marianao (13)

Ferrerons, Florencio ......   San Carlos # 957 e/ Sto. Tomas y
                                Benjumeda ....   La Habana
Garcia, Carlos ....   Hospital de Manzanillo ....   Oriente
Gelado Espinosa, Jose .....   Dpto. Oftalmologia, Hospital
                                Lenin ....   Holguin, Oriente
Gil Lopez Himely, Jose ....   Teneria # 54 ....   Cardenas, Matanzas
Gómez Ruíz, Othón ......   Calle D 321 Apto 12 e/ 13 y 15 .   Vedado, La Habana
Gonzales Bez, Jose ....   Calle E # 67 ....   Lawton, La Habana
Gonzalez Gonzalez, Raul ..   Calle Medio # 100 ....   Prov Matanzas
Gonzalez Morffa, Carlos ...   Luis Estevez # 169 ....   Santa Clara, Las Villas
Guerra Gomez, Luisa .....   Ave. 17 # 6421, Apto. 3 ....   Marianao (13)
Gutierrez Paris, Pablo .....   Animas No. 1008 Apto. A (altos)   La Habana
Guzman Montalvo, Nelson .   Dpto. Oftalmologia, Hospital de
                                Guantanamo ....   Oriente
Hechevarria Duque, Yolanda   Hospital de Remedios ....   Las Villas
Hernandez Gonzalez, Rodol-
fo ....   54 # 3513 e/ 37 y 35 ....   Cienfuegos, Las Villas
Hernandez Leal, Rolando ..   26C # 8 e/ 47 y Fondo de Alde-
                                coa ....   Nuevo Vedado, La Habana
Herrera Hdez, Norma .....   Dpto. Oftalmologia, Hospital Pro-
                                vincial ....   Matanzas
Horta Hdez, Ivo O. ....   24 # 303 e/ 5ta. y 3ra ....   Miramar, Marianao
Jara Casco, Eugenio ......   Paseo No. 455 e/ 19 y 21 ....   Vedado, La Habana
Joa, Elena ....   Linea # 1212, Apto. 4 ....   Vedado, La Habana
Lima Capote, Sara ....   Centro Medico, Sol esq. Colon ..   Pinar del Rio
Lopez Cascale, Alberto ....   Ave. 13 No. 6203 altos ....   Almendares, Marianao
Lopez Cardet, Rolando ....   3ra No. 371, e/ San Leonardo y
                                kessell. Rpto Apolo ....   La Habana
Mark Labrado, Gladys ....   San Lazaro No. 701 ent. S. Maria-
                                no y Sta. Catalina ....   Vibora, La Habana (5)
Marrero Faz, Elio ....   Dpto. Oftalmologia, Hospital Pro-
                                vincial ....   Santiago de Cuba, Oriente
Marrero de la Rosa, Antonio   Calle 21 # 452, altos ....   Vedado, La Habana
Martinez Glez, Jose ....   Dpto. Oftalmologia, Hospital Mili-
                                tar ....   Santiago de Cuba, Oriente
Martinez Rivalta, Jorge ....   Dpto. Oftalmologia, Hospital Mili-
                                tar ....   Marianao (13)
Matilla Segui, Jose ....   Cisneros # 15 ....   Camaguey
Mayor Cancio, Rosa Esther .   Calle 12 No. 512. Apto. 2 e/ 21 y
                                23 ....   Vedado, La Habana
Mendoza Cruz, Rolando ...   Hospital Provincial ....   Santiago de Cuba, Oriente
Mendoza Rojo, Evelio .....   Gral. Lee # 58, Apto. 6 e/ Rabi y
                                Flores ....   Santos Suarez, La Habana
Menendez Gonzalez, Fernan-
do ....   E 407, Apto. 210 ....   Vedado, La Habana
Morejon Sanz, Antionio ...   Dpto. Oftalmologia Hospital
                                Lenin ....   Holguin, Oriente
Odelin Lopez, Pablo ......   Hospital de Guantanamo .....   Oriente
Olivares, Maria J. ....   Dpto. Oftalmologia, Hospital
                                Lenin ....   Holguin, Prov. Oriente
Oliver Carreras, Jose ......   Hospital Provincial ....   Matanzas
Olmeda, Ernesto ....   Ave. 401 # 18015, altos ....   Santiago de Las Vegas, La
                                                                   Habana
Ordaz Cabrera, Maria Luisa .   36 # 351 esq. Ave. del Bosque ..   Nuevo Vedado, La Habana
Pelaez Molina, Orfilio .....   Estrada Palma # 412 ....   Vibora, Habana

Pereyras Costa, Rolando ...	Calle 10 # 65 e/ A y C, Altahabana	La Habana
Perez Tamayo, Bertila	Hogar de Digtroficos Antiguo Hosp. Infantil, Plaza de Sn. Juan de Dios	Camaguey
Pinelo Alcaide, Dolores	Calle H No. 116 ent. Calzada y 5ta	Vedado, La Habana (4)
Puente Coroneaux, Jorge V.	Avenida 86 # 18703, Rpto. Fontanar	Prov. La Habana
Puig Mora, Martha	Depto. Oftalmologia Hospital Cmdte. Fajardo Zapata y C ..	Vedado, La Habana (4)
Ramil Peña, Irene	Hospital de Florida	Camaguey
Ramos Medina, Carmen ...	Albergue de Medicos # 6	Nueva Gerona, Isla de Pinos
Ricardo Lorenzo, Rosa Amalia	Linea # 309 e/ H e I	Vedado, La Habana
Rigual, Jose	Depto. Oftalmologia, Hospital Militar	Marianao (13)
Rigueiro Vazquez, Jesus	Ave. 9a. # 4411, Apto. 6	Almendares, Marianao
Rios Torres, Marcelino	Hospital de Placetas	Las Villas
Rivero Perez, Ramon	Calle 84 # 901 e/ 9 y 11	Marianao, La Habana
Rodriguez, Josefa	Servicio Oftalmologia, Hospital Clin. Quirurgico, Ave 26 y R. Boyeros	La Habana
Rodriguez, Noelio	Calle G No. 604	Vedado, La Habana
Rodriguez Cuellar, Jose ...	San Cristobal # 15	Santa Clara, Las Villas
Rodriguez Perez, Mario	Calle 6 # 503 e/ 21 y 23	Vedado, La Habana
Rubio Figueredo, Flora ...	Centro Medico, Sol esq. a Colon .	Pinar del Rio
Rubio Garces, Emilio	Maximo Gomez No. 516, Esq. Tacon	Guines, Prov. Habana
Rubio Merejo, Lourdes	Dpto. Oftalmologia, Hospital de Sagua la Grande	Las Villas
Sanchez Borroto, Peiro	Bartolome Maso # 75	Colon, Prov. Matanzas
Sanchez Rivera, Orlando ...	B No. 609 entre 25 y 27	Vedado, La Habana (4)
Santiesteban, F. Rosaralis ..	Dpto. Oftalmologia, Hospital Prov. 'M. Ascunce'	Camaguey
Tablada Fauto	Ave. 1ra. y Calle 0 Apto. 321, Edificio Rio Mar	Marianao, La Habana
Torre de la Ordetx, Guillermo	15 # 955 e/ 8 y 10	Vedado, La Habana
Valdes Rodriguez, Carmen .	Ave. 13 No. 6013, Apto. 3 ent. 60 y 62	Marianao (13)
Varela Ramos, Georgina ...	Calle 7 # 185 Rpto. Vista Hermosa	Camaguey
Vazquez Olazabal, Oneida .	San Nicolas No. 404, Apto. 3 esq. a San Rafael	La Habana (2)
Vera Gamisan, Rosa S.	Pezuela No. 309, Ent. Prensa y Colon	Cerro, La Habana (6)
Vidal Sainz, Tulia	30 # 758 e/ Ave. Kohly y 41, altos	Vedado, La Habana
Villar, Rosendo	Nazareno # 61 e/ Colon y Maceo	Santa Clara, Las Villas
Vizcaino Londian, Jorge ...	Gloria # 72	Santa Clara, Las Villas

NOSOCOMIA QUIBUS OCULIS AEGRI CURANTUR

Hospital 'Ramón Pando Ferrer', Dir.: Dr. Othón Gómez Ruíz

INSTITUTA SCHOLAEQUE CAECIS DESTINATAE

Escuela 'Abel Santamaria' (para ciegos y ambliopes no recuperables).
Centro Especial de Oftalmología, 45 alumnos de visión recuperable.

CYPRUS

SOCIETATES OPHTHALMOLOGICAE

Cyprus Ophthalmological Society

Bureau: Pancyprian Medical Association, Princess Zena de Tysa Bldg., Nicosia 118
Chairman: Dr. V. Karatzas
Secretary: Dr. A. G. Lapithis, 40 Evagoras Ave., Pantheon Bldg., Nicosia 118
Members: Dr. Ion Economides, Dr. A. Kaniklides, Dr. V. Christodouloy
Number of members: 20

NOMINA ET DOMICILIA MEDICORUM AB OCULIS

Alp, Ozday A.	c/o Turkish Hospital	Nicosia
Anastasiades, Takis	1, Kalvou str.	47067 Nicosia
Charalambous, Phobus	Hospital Limassol	3111 Limassol
Christodouloy, Vassos	25, Ethnikis Antistaseos	3076 Limassol
Christopoulos, Polys	1b, Salamis Ave	76213 Nicosia
Constantinides, Costas	10 Jules Vern str.	73664 Limassol
Economides, Ion	Skyros str. Lordos Bldg	77321 Nicosia
Francos, John	44, Stassinos Ave	62541 Nicosia
Hilimintris, Angelos	1, Hippocrates str.	63421 Famagusta
Ihan, Hurmuz E.	c/o Turkish Hospital	Nicosia
Kaniklides, George	12, Apost. Varnavas str.	62465 Famagusta
Kaniklis, Andreas	52, Gr. Afxentiou str.	65333 Famagusta
Karatzas, Vassilis	18 Them. Dervi str.	42338 Nicosia
Lapithis, Aristides	40, Evagoras Ave	43169 Nicosia
Loizou, Gregory	17, X. Xenierou str.	75337 Nicosia
Pierides, Lyriacos	2, Argyrocastrou str.	77471 Nicosia
Pouppis, Vassos	16, Loukis Akritis str.	71191 Limassol
Said, Hassan Mihad	c/o Turkish Hospital	Nicosia
Salik, Hassan Tahsin G.	c/o Turkish Hospital	Nicosia
Sarris, Solon	23, Katsonis str.	65740 Nicosia
Siganos, Socratis	c/o Medical Association	45640 Nicosia
Tziros, Christos	3, Simos Mendardos str.	62353 Larnaca
Tsolakis, Panayiotis	Famagusta Hospital	62011 Famagusta
Vorgas, Andreas	1, Socratous str.	67533 Famagusta

NOSOCOMIA QUIBUS OCULIS AEGRI CURANTUR

	No. of beds
General Hospital, Nicosia (Directors: Dr. K. Pierides, Dr. I. Economides)	18
General Hospital, Famagusta (Director: Dr. P. Tsolakis)	4
General Hospital, Larnaca (Director: Dr. C. Tziros)	3
Dr. A. G. Lapithis' Clinic, Nicosia	5
Dr. Gegory Loizou's Clinic, Nicosia	6
Dr. S. Sarris's Clinic, Nicosia	5
Dr. P. Christopoulos's Clinic, Nicosia	5

Dr. A. Hilimintris's Clinic, Famagusta 5
Dr. A. Vorkas's Clinic, Famagusta 5
Dr. A. Kaniklis's Clinic, Famagusta 6
Dr. V. Pouppis's Clinic, Limassol 15
Dr. V. Christodouloy's Clinic, Limassol 9
Dr. C. Constantinides's Clinic, Limassol 6
Turkish Hospital, Nicosia 4

INSTITUTA SCHOLAEQUE CAECIS DESTINATAE

'St. Barnabas' School for the Blind, Nicosia: 60 pupils. Director: Mr. N. Ierides.
   School for the Blind in Turkish Quarter (estimated pupils 15).
   'Hosted for Blind Adults, boys en girls, Nicosia: 16 adults

DANIA

SOCIETATES OPHTHALMOLOGICAE

Nationalis

The Danish Ophthalmological Society

President: Jens Edmund
Vice-President: Niels Ehlers
Secretary: N. T. Rosenberg
Bureau: Øjenafdelingen, Rigshospitalet Blegdamsvej, 2100 København Ø
Number of members: 182

Regionales

The Copenhagen Ophthalmologists Organization

Secretary address: Flyvemedicinsk Øjenklinik, Rigshospitalet, Tagensvej 18, 2200 København N
Number of members: 48

Provincial Ophthalmologists Organization

Secretary address: Øjenafdelingen, Centralsygehuset, 9800 Hjørring
Number of members: 62

NOMINA ET DOMICILIA MEDICORUM AB OCULIS

Anthonisen, H.	Toftebæksvej 2	2820 Lyngby
Backhaus, B.	V. Voldgade 7-9	1552 København V
Bardram, Tiegen M.	Dybendalsvej 57	2000 København F
Barfoed, P.	Tidseltoft 13	7100 Vejle
Bech, K.	Kristianiagade 6,	2100 København Ø
Boberg-Ans, J.	Ole Bruunsvej 12	2920 Charlottenlund
Brinkbo, B.	Bredgade 5	7400 Herning
Bruntse, Else	Øjenafdelingen, Centralsygehuset.	7400 Herning
Bruun-Jensen, J.	Smedegade 6	4200 Slagelse
Brændstrup, Johanne	Sortedam Dossering 95 B	2100 København Ø
Braendstrup, P.	Sortedam Dossering 95 B	2100 København Ø
Bülow, N.	Henningsens Alle 25	2900 Hellerup
Byrn, W.	Øregårdsalle 15	2900 Hellerup
Bøjer, J.	Adelgade 42	9500 Hobro
Christensen, J. Spangsberg	Øjenafdelingen, Kolding Sygehus	6000 Kolding
Christensen, Sigbrit	Trørødvej 30	2950 Vedbæk
Clemmesen, V.	Ramsherred 19 A	4700 Næstved
Dalsgaard-Nielsen, E.	Vagtelvej 52 A	2000 København F
Damgård-Jensen, E.	Ryesgade 8	8000 Århus
Diemar, S.	Kystvej 1	8500 Grenø

Dreisler, K. K.	Jernbaneplads 2	4300 Holbæk
Dreyer, V.	Frederiksgade 10	1265 København K
Edmund, J.	Frederiksberg Alle 60	1820 København V
Ehlers, H.	Dag Hammarskjöldsalle 1	2100 København Ø
Ehlers, N.	Øjenafdelingen, Århus Kommune-hospital	8000 Århus C
Eisum, F.	Fortevej 6	8240 Risskov
Eldrup-Jørgensen, P.	Søvang 8	2970 Hørsholm
Esbjerg, H. O.	Torvegade 1	5000 Odense
Esbjerg Jørgensen, O.	Hovedvejen 158	2600 Glostrup
Fabricius, Agnethe	Østergade 27	1100 København K
Fabricius-Jensen, H.	Toldbodvej, Snoghøj	7000 Fredericia
Falbe-Hansen, I.	Evaldsvej 11	2960 Rungsted Kyst
Fastrup, H.	Kirkegade 11	8900 Randers
Faurschou Jensen, S.	Hækkehusvej 42	5681 Bellinge
Fledelius, M.	Æblevangen 6	9800 Hjørring
Fock, Vagn	Næsset 27	8700 Horsens
Fogt, J.	Albanitorv 5	5000 Odense
Frandsen, Anna	Brudevænget 31	Stavnholt, 3520 Farum
Frandsen, E.	Fredericiegade 17	6000 Kolding
Frandsen, Helga	Esperancealle 16	2920 Charlottenlund
From, Johan	Svejagervej 7	2900 Hellerup
Galskov, Aa.	'Skovgården' Asminderød Mark	3480 Fredensborg
Glissov, B.	Øjenafdelingen, Centralsygehuset	4700 Næstved
Godtfredsen, E.	Aurehøjvej 23	2900 Hellerup
Goldschmidt, E.	Øjenafdelingen, Odense Sygehus	5000 Odense
Gregersen, E.	Langs Hegnet 22	2800 Lyngby
Halske, Jens Vagn	Amagerbrogade 7, mezz	2300 København S
Hanum, S.	Fisketorvet 2	4200 Slagelse
Hartkopp, O.	Øjenafdelingen, Centralsygehuset	4800 Nykøbing F
Heegaard, S.	Brogårdsgade 14	7800 Skive
Heidensleben, E.	Roskildevej 264	2610 Rødovre
Hein, S.	Bispegade 17	6100 Haderslev
Holm, K.	Ericastien 18	2820 Gentofte
Holm-Pedersen, E.	Søndergade 7	8000 Århus
Hvidberg-Hansen, J.	Konkylievej 3	8250 Egå
Jensen, H. J.	Lille Torv 6	8000 Århus C
Jensen, J.	Kongesvej 63	6400 Sønderborg
Jensen, O. A.	Annasvej 9	2900 Hellerup
Jensen, P.	Møllestien 8	2800 Lyngby
Jensen, Søren	Tornekrogen 48	3500 Værløse
Jensen, Vagn J.	Flinteløkken, Hostrupskov	6200 Abenrå
Jensen, V. A.	Øjenafdelingen, Århus Kommune-hospital	8000 Århus C
Johansen, E. V.	Østergade 4	6700 Esbjerg
Kall, E.	Mylius Erichsensalle 35	2900 Hellerup
Kessing, S. Vedel	Jernbanegade 4, I	1608 København V
Kjeldsen, M. H.	Højderyggen 11	Bredballe, 7100 Vejle
Kjer, P.	Strandvej 84	2900 Hellerup
Knerrumgård, E.	Kongevej 100	5000 Helsingør
Kjærgård, G.	Falkoneralle 80	2000 København F
Knudtzon, K.	Sundvænget 29	2900 Hellerup
Kindt, P.	Algade 28	9000 Ålborg
Konnerup, F.	Fælledvej 40	7000 Fredericia
Krarup Jensen, I.	Svejbækhus, Kalsholtvej, Svejbæk	8600 Silkeborg

Kristensen, P.	Grandalsvej 34	7700 Thisted
Kruse, F.	Øjenafdelingen, Kommunehospitalet	1399 København K
Ladekarl, P.	Lille Odinshøj	3140 Alsgårde
Ladekarl, S.	Nrd. Strandvej 56	3000 Helsingør
Larsen, Godfred	Øjenafdelingen, Centralsygehuset	8900 Randers
Larsen, Hans-Walther	Brasehøj 16	2900 Hellerup
Larsen, Victor	Østerbrogade 60	2100 København Ø
Lawætz, B.	Østbanegade 5	2100 København Ø
Lorentzen, S. E.	Sønderbakken 20	2820 Gentofte
Lund, Steffen	Højbro Plads 19	1200 København K
Madsen, P. H.	Øjenafdelingen, Roskilde Amts-og Bys sygehus	4000 Roskilde
Mahneke, A.	V. Voldgade 7-9	1552 København V
Malling, H.	Nørremøllevej 80	8800 Viborg
Marner, Else	V. Voldgade 7-9	1552 København V
Mellemgaard, Lis	Slotsvænget 19	3400 Hillerød
Moestrup, B.	Skudsvej 7	9800 Hjørring
Mortensen, Kjeld	Avænget 14	4600 Køge
Møllenbach, C. J.	Oslo Plads 14	2100 København Ø
Møller, P. M.	Hunderupvej 204 B	5000 Odense
Møller Nielsen, N. O.	Hvedevænget 30	7500 Holstebro
Nordentoft, Birthe	Hasserisvej 242	9000 Ålborg
Nordentoft, V.	Hasserisvej 242	9000 Ålborg
Nordsted, A.	Østeraa 9	9000 Ålborg
Norn, M. S.	Vanløse Byvej 16	2720 Vanløse
Nørgaard, B.	Ermelundsvej 71	2820 Gentofte
Nørholm, Inger	Hegnsvej 91	2850 Nærum
Nørskov, K.	Anemonevej 60	2820 Gentofte
Ohrt, V.	Sct. Georgsvej 18	9000 Ålborg
Olsen, Jess	Helsingørgade 52	3400 Hillerød
Porsaa, K.	Skovvangen 32	2920 Charlottenlund
Pouplier, G.	Munkegården	5700 Svendborg
Preisler, E.	Banegårds Plads 6	8000 Århus C
Qvist, A.	St. Nicolajgade 1	5700 Svendborg
Rask, J. A.	Sct. Anne Plads 2	5000 Odense
Rasmussen, K.	Algade 28 A	4000 Roskilde
Rasmussen, Knud Erik	Skriverengen 5	2791 Dragør
Ravn-Sørensen, C. H.	Vestergade 14	5000 Odense
Reeh Pedersen, L.	Christoffers alle 133	2800 Lyngby
Ring, J. O.	Lindevej 1	4760 Vordingborg
Rosenberg, N. T.	Kløvervænget 26	5000 Odense
Rud, E.	AErøvej 38	9900 Frederikshavn
Ry Andersen, S.	Øjenpatologisk Institut ved Københavns Universitet Rigshospitalet, Tagensvej 18	2200 København N
Sebber, E.	Valby Langgade 86 A	2500 Valby
Seedorff, H. H.	Odensgade 5	2100 København Ø
Seedorff, Tove	Duevej 101	2000 København F
Simonsen, S. E.	Gartnervænget 35	3520 Farum
Sjøntoft, F.	Østergade 18	1100 København K
Sjærbæk Olesen, O.	Skovvejen 47	8600 Silkeborg
Skeller, E.	Lyngby Hovedgade 27	2800 Lyngby
Skydsgaard, H.	Sølvgade 36	1307 København K
Sparrested, A.	Fredericiagade 35	7500 Holstebro
Spiers, F.	Østergade 4	8600 Silkeborg

Svane-Knudsen, P.	Fredericiagade 17	6000 Kolding
Thorkildgaard, O.	Råshusvej 2	4300 Holbæk
Thykier-Nielsen, E.	Frederikssundsvej 119	2700 Brønshøj
Vedel Jensen, N.	Øjenafdelingen, Centralsygehuset	9800 Hjørring
Vesterdal, E.	Bülowsvej 18 B	1870 København V
Vilstrup, Grethe	Amager Landvej 30	2770 Kastrup
Vogelius, H.	Toftegårds Alle 43	2500 Valby
Vorting, S. J.	Asavænget 6	2800 Lyngby
Warburg, Mette	Sortedam Dossering 95 A	2100 København Ø
Wegener, J.	Kløvervænget 26 D	5000 Odense
Westerlund, E.	Kongensgade 25	4800 Nykøbing F
Vibek, Inge Lis	Søndergade 23	4900 Nakskov
Wille-Jørgensen, A.	Store Torv 2	7700 Thisted
Willumsen, N.	Grønnevej 9	5992 Troense
Winther, E.	Christiansmindevej 13	4300 Holbæk
Work, Kresten	Paradisvænget 12	2840 Holte
Østerberg, G.	St. Jacobs Plads 6	2100 København Ø
Østerby, E.	Solklintvej 16	8250 Egå
Øtheer, A.	Øjenafdelingen, Sygehuset	Thorshavn, Færøerne

NOSOCOMIA QUIBUS OCULIS AEGRI CURANTUR

No. of beds

Rigshospitalets øjenafdeling (The University Eyeclinic, Copenhagen) Director: E. Gregersen, J. Edmund ... 35

Rigshospitalets øjenafdeling Tagensvej 18, 2200 København N. Director: B. Lawaetz, H. H. Seedorff ... 22

Århus Kommunehospitals øjenafdeling (The University Eyeclinic, Århus) 8000 Århus C. Director: Viggo A. Jensen, Niels Ehlers ... 38

Kommunehospitalets øjenafdeling Ø. Farimagsgade 3, 1399 København K. Director: Poul Braendstrup, M. Norn, K. Nørskov, S. E. Lorentzen ... 43

Frederiksberg Hospitals øjenafdeling, Ndr. Fasanvej 59, 2000 København F. Director: Knud Bech ... 16

Øjenafdelingen, Københavns Amstssygehus i Gentofte, Niels Andersensvej 65, 2900 Hellerup. Director: P. Kjer, Hans-Walther Larsen ... 28

Sct. Josephs Hospital, øjenafdelingen, 6700 Esbjerg. Director: E. V. Johansen ... 15

Sct. Josephs Hospital, Sjaellandsgade 46, 7000 Fredericia øre-, naese-, hals- og øjenafdeling. Director: F. Konnerup ... 16

Frederikshavn Sygehus, øjenafdelingen, 9900 Frederikshavn. Director: E. Rud ... x)

Faerøerne, Landssjúkrahúsid, øjenklinik, 3800 Torshavn. Director: Anders Øther ... x)

Herning Centralsygehus, 7400 Herning. Director: Else Bruntse ... x)

Hjørring Sygehus, øjenafdelingen, 9800, Hjørring. Director: N. Vedel-Jensen, B. Moestrup. 12

Sct. Hedvigs Hospital, øjenafdelingen, 6000 Kolding. Director: Emil Frandsen, P. Svane-Knudsen ... 20

Nykøbing Fl. Centralsygehus, Øjenafdelingen, Fjordvej 15, 4800 Nykøbing Fl. Director: E. Westerlund ... 12

Naestvéd Centralsygehus, øjenafdelingen, 4700 Naestved. Director: V. Clemmesen, B. Glissov ... 18

Odense Sygehus, øjenafdelingen (The University Eyeclinic, Odense), Sdr. Boulevard 29, 5000 Odense. Director: P. M. Møller, E. Goldschmidt, S. Faurschou Jensen ... 28

Randers Centralsygehus, Øjenklinik Ø. Østervangsvej 26, 8900 Randers. Director: Godfred Larsen ... x)

Amtssygehuset, Roskilde, øjenafdelingen, 4000 Roskilde. Director: K. Rasmussen, P. H. Madsen ... 20

Thisted Sygehus, Øjenafdelingen, 700 Thisted. Director: A. Wille-Jørgensen, Preben Kristen-
sen .... x)
Sct. Maria Hospital, 7100 Vejle, Director: P. Barfoed 15
St. Ansgar Hospital, Fiskergade 7-9, 6200 Åbenrå. Director: Vagn Jensen .... x)
Ålborg Sygehus, Øjenafdelingen, 9000 Ålborg. Director: V. Ohrt 20
Øjenafdelingen, Det kgl. Blindeinstitut, Kastelsvej 60, 2100 København Ø. Director:
H. Skydsgaard .... x)

INSTITUTA SCHOLAEQUE CAECIS DESTINATAE

No. of pupils

Statens Institut for blinde og svagsynde i København, Rymarksvej 1, 2900 Hellerup 240
Refnæsskolen, Kystvjen, 4400 Kalundborg 150
Bredegaard – (Institution for weakminded blinds), 3480 Fredensborg 20
Hestehavehus (Department of Refnæsskolen), Kalundborg 10
Klintegården (Department of Refnaesskolen), Kalundborg 20
Hjem for arbejdsføre blinde kvinder (Home) for blind women able to work), Mariendalsvej
20, 2000 København F 12
Raklevgården (Home for blind young men), Raklev, 4400 Kalundborg 25
Plejehjemmet Solgaven, Amerikavej, 9500 Hobro 56

FINLANDIA

SOCIETATES OPHTHALMOLOGICAE

Suomen Silmälääkäriyhdistys – Finlands Ögonläkarförening, r.y.
(The Ophthalmological Society of Finland)
President: Prof. Henrik Forsius
Secretary: Pentti Pakarinen, Haartmanink, 4 C, 00290 Helsinki 29

Suomen Silmälääkärit-Finlands Ögonläkare
(Finnish Ophthalmologists)
President: Ilkka Raivio
Secretary: Anja Mustakallio, Solnantie 9 A 6, 00330 Helsinki 33

NOMINA ET DOMICILIA MEDICORUM AB OCULIS

Aantaa, Yrjö	Katajanokank. 3 A 5	00160 Helsinki 16
Adel, Aune	Satamakatu 5 B 22	00160 Helsinki 16
Ahlas, Antti	Linnank. 13 b as. 9	20100 Turku 10
Ahlas, Leena	Linnank. 13 b as. 9	20100 Turku 10
Ahonen, Aino	Uramontie 44	11120 Riihimäki 12
Airas, Kaija	Jaanintie 34 E 81	20540 Turku 54
Ant-Wuorinen, Alli-Sisko	Rintamamiehentie 30	06100 Porvoo 10
Appelqvist, Auli	Kankolankatu 11 A	15900 Lahti 90
Arentz-Grastvedt, Björn		81100 Kontiolahti
Aulamo, Rauno	Puutarhakatu 23 D	33210 Tampere 21
Aulavuo, Elsa	Haarniskatie 6 A 6	00910 Helsinki 91
Aurekoski, Heikki	Mariankatu 18 Y 3	67200 Kokkola 20
Björkenheim, Barbro	Kirkkokatu 9	48100 Kotka 10
Castrén, Jorma	Merikatu 5 A	00140 Helsinki 14
Dickhoff, Kai von	Aurorankatu 9 B 7	00100 Helsinki 10
Elenius, Prof. Valter	Vähä-Hämeenkatu 7 C	20500 Turku 50
Ennevaara, Kai	Keskussairaala	87140 Kajaani 14
Erkkilä, Heikki	Koskelant. 30 D 31	00610 Helsinki 61
Esilä, Raili	Päivärinnankatu 3 B	00250 Helsinki 25
Eskelin, Lars-Erik	Meritullinkatu 7 A	00170 Helsinki 17
Fieandt, Olof von	Kasarminkatu 10 A	00140 Helsinki 14
Forsius, Prof. Henrik	OYKS Silmätautien os. Kajaanintie 50	90230 Oulu 23
Grop, Kurt	Hietalahdenkatu 1 L	65130 Vaasa 13
Hakosalo, Heljä	Kastellintie 64	90220 Oulu 22
Haramo, Raili	Louhentie 5 D	02130 Tapiola 3
Harjula, Reijo	Maunukselank. 6-8 A 6	50100 Mikkeli 10
Heikkilä, Heikki	Likolammenkatu 4 C	33300 Tampere 30

Helminen, Tauno	Munkkiniemen puistotie 21 A	00330 Helsinki 33
Helve, Jyrki	Helatie 4 A 2	90250 Oulu 25
Honkonen, Esko	Puistokatu 7 b A	00140 Helsinki 14
Horsmanheimo, Aulis	Helenankuja 5	02700 Kauniainen
Hyry, Antti	Maakuntakatu 14	96100 Rovaniemi 10
Hyvärinen, Lea	Satukallio B 12	02200 Niittykumpu
Häkkinen, Leena	Yliopistonk. 11 a D 48	20110 Turku 11
Ihalainen, Anja	Itäkangastie 8 B 11	90500 Oulu 50
Ilvessalo-Setälä, Maija	Pyhän Laurintie 5 A	00340 Helsinki 34
Junnola, Kalevi	Tuomiokirkonkatu 17 A	33100 Tampere 10
Juurikkala, Anita	Hiihtäjäntie 4 B 23	00810 Helsinki 81
Juusela, Arto	Ulvilantie 11 b F 133	00350 Helsinki 35
Jägerroos, Paavo	Keskussairaala	70210 Kuopio 21
Jäntti, Keijo	Tuureporinkatu 14 C	20100 Turku 10
Jönsas, Carl-Håkan	Hedelmäkatu 2 D	33270 Tampere 27
Kaarakka, Olavi	Sahalankatu 11	60100 Seinäjoki 10
Kaivonen, Matti	Keskuskatu 23 A 22	48100 Kotka 10
Kankaanpää, Heikki		53130 Lappeenranta 13
Karjalainen, Kari	Heikinmäki A 9	02170 Haukilahti
Karli, Hillevi	Gräsantie 15 E 43	02700 Kauniainen
Karma, Anni	Koskitie 32 B	90500 Oulu 50
Karo, Terttu	Kauppiaskatu 2	20100 Turku 10
Katavisto, Martti	Nepenmäenkatu 1 C 10	80200 Joensuu 20
Kaunisto, Nanny	Fredrikinkatu 32	00120 Helsinki 12
Kause, Eeva-Raija	Haukitie 6	02170 Haukilahti
Klemetti, Anneli	Keskussairaala	40620 Jyväskylä 62
Knape, Birgitta	Fredrikinkatu 66 B 30	00100 Helsinki 10
Koivusalo, Pirkko	Kuoretie 4 B	02170 Haukilahti
Kontturi, Kyösti	Tiirasaarentie 32	00200 Helsinki 20
Koponen, Jarkko	Leipäläntie 17	20300 Turku 30
Korhonen, P. Kalevi	Kalevankatu 54	45200 Kouvola 20
Koskenoja, Matti	Keskussairaala	40620 Jyväskylä 62
Koskiahde, Veli	Vitanova	20960 Turku 96
Koskinen, Kaarina	Armas Lindgrenint. 11 D	00570 Helsinki 57
Krause, Ulf	Kajaanintie 50	90220 Oulu 22
Kyrki, Liimi	Haulitie 2	90250 Oulu 25
Kytilä, Juha	Hakalankatu 2	60100 Seinäjoki 10
Laaka, Ville	Laivastokatu 12 B 54	00160 Helsinki 16
Laatikainen, Leila	Lohenpyrstö 2 C	00650 Helsinki 65
Lahti, Alpo	Ulvilantie 19 L 4	00350 Helsinki 35
Lampisjärvi, Antti	Hollantilaisentie 1	00330 Helsinki 33
Larmi, Tauno	Haukiverkko 15 A	02170 Haukilahti
Lavikainen, Pertti	Keskussairaala E 5	48210 Kotka 21
Lehtinen, Yrjö	Pohjolank. 43 A 4	00610 Helsinki 61
Lehtonen, Jarmo	Aleksi 12	15110 Lahti 11
Lehvä, Lauri	Leivonkuja 16	36220 Suorama
Leikola, Johannes	Tyyppäläntie 8 F 48	40250 Jyväskylä 25
Leivo, Pirkko	Pihlajatie 28 B	00270 Helsinki 27
Liesmaa, Martti	Väinämöisenk. 9 B 19	00100 Helsinki 10
Lindberg, Prof. John	Vuorikatu 16	00100 Helsinki 10
Linkova, Matti	Kivitorpantie 5 A 18	00330 Helsinki 33
Listola, Jouni	Keskussairaala	50100 Mikkeli 10
Lähde, Yrjö	Haukkamäenkatu 4 A 8	33560 Tampere 56
Majaniemi, Taina	Honkatie 30 as. 7	20540 Turku 54
Mali, Anssi	Yrjönk. 6-8 B 21	53600 Lappeenranta 60
Marjanen, Sinikka	Yliopistokatu 11 a	20110 Turku 11

Merenmies, Esteri	Kangaspellontie 5 A	00300 Helsinki 30
Merenmies, Lauri	Kangaspellontie 5 A	00300 Helsinki 30
Meretoja, Jouko	P. Rautatiekatu 60	11120 Riihimäki 12
Miettinen, Pentti	Likolammenkatu 6 D	33300 Tampere 30
Miettinen, Rauno	Ampuhaukantie 5 A 6	90250 Oulu 25
Molnár, Maja-Liisa	Linnankatu 47 A 18	20300 Turku 30
Mustakallio, Anja	Solnantie 9 A 6	00330 Helsinki 33
Mustonen, Eila	Syrjäkatu 6 as. 4	90140 Oulu 14
Mäntyjärvi, Maija	Huuhankatu 8 B 11	70600 Kuopio 60
Mäntylä, Pekka	Poutuntie 7 A 5	00400 Helsinki 40
Nieminen, Kauko	Hämeenkatu 15 B 10	33100 Tampere 10
Niiranen, Matti	Vaahteratie 5 D	02130 Tapiola 3
Niittyviita, Aimo	Etelärantakatu 16 A 3	94100 Kemi 10
Nikoskelainen, Eeva	Jyrätie 3 P	20540 Turku 54
Nordman, Erik	Kupittaankatu 154	20810 Turku 81
Ojala, Liisa	Relanderinaukio 2 F	00570 Helsinki 57
Oksala, Prof. Arvo	Honkatie 28 as. 2 ꝟ.	20540 Turku 54
Olin-Lamberg, Carin	P. Suotie 17	02700 Kauniainen
Olsbo, Anja	Carpelanint. 8 B	10600 Tammisaari, TMS
Oravisto, Terttu	Sjöströmintie 1	00570 Helsinki 57
Orma, Heta	Kulosaaren Puistot. 38	00570 Helsinki 57
Outinen, Lasse	Näsilinnank. 42 A 13	33200 Tampere 20
Paakkala, Anna-Maija	Vanha pappila	36200 Kangasala
Pajari, Antti	Keskussairaala	57120 Savonlinna 12
Pakarinen, Pentti	Ylänkötie 3 N	00650 Helsinki 65
Palkama, Prof. Arto	Sandelsink. 2 B 34	00260 Helsinki 26
Pelkonen, Ulla	Runeberginkatu 56 B	00260 Helsinki 26
Pihkala, Irja	P. Hesperiank. 13 B	00260 Helsinki 26
Pohjanpelto, Pekka	Honkapirtintie	15900 Lahti 90
Pohjola, Seppo	K.-S. rak. 7 a	53130 Lappeenranta 13
Pursiainen, Lea	Maaherrankatu 18 A 8	50100 Mikkeli 10
Raitta, Christina	Koivuniementie 16	00930 Helsinki 93
Raivio, Ilkka	Kauppalantie 22	02700 Kauniainen
Raivio, Terhi	Kauppalantie 22	02700 Kauniainen
Ralli, Reijo	Kiskontie 10 B 31	00280 Helsinki 28
Raski, Kauko	Runeberginkatu 39 A	00100 Helsinki 10
Rokkanen, Aila	Marjaniemenranta 29	00930 Helsinki 93
Routti, Reijo	Lemminkäisenkatu 19	20720 Turku 72
Rysä, Pekka	Rentukkatie 17 A 2	90800 Oulu 80
Rytkölä, Tapani	Magnus Hagelstamink. 2	02700 Kauniainen
Saari, Matti	Toppelundintie 7 D 42	02170 Haukilahti
Saikku, Liisa	Mannerheimintie 132 B	00270 Helsinki 27
Salmi, Pekka	Friittala, Suurpää	28400 Ulvila
Salminen, Lotta	Vähä-Hämeenkatu 7 C 51	20500 Turku 50
Salonen, Antti	Kuusitie 9 A 27	00270 Helsinki 27
Sammalkivi, Jarmo	Keskussairaala	13200 Hämeenlinna 20
Sarmela, Timo	Vanhatie 26 A 4	15240 Lahti 24
Simojoki, Wellamo	Träskända, Metsäläntie	02940 Aurora
Sopanen, Veli	Multiniemeranta 20	78300 Varkaus 30
Stenius, Sten	Kymenlaaksonkatu 20	48100 Kotka 10
Sulamaa, Simo	Kirkkotie 19 D	02700 Kauniainen
Suo, Kaarlo	Palokunnantie 22	158 Lahti 80
Suvanto, Erkki	Pohjoispuisto 4 B 29	28100 Pori 10
Suvanto, Jaakko	Hallinraitti 2 A 3	60200 Seinäjoki 20
Takki, Kirsti	Ersintie 1 B	02700 Kauniainen

Takki-Luukkainen, Inka-Taina	Solnantie 12	00330 Helsinki 33
Takkunen, Eivor	Alkutie 32 J	00660 Helsinki 66
Tammisto, Prof. Tapani	Oikotie 10	02260 Finnå
Tarkkanen, Prof. Ahti	Maamonlahdentie 3 as. 5	00200 Helsinki 20
Teir, Prof. Harald	Rakuunantie 5 A	00330 Helsinki 33
Tenhunen, Tuija	Väinämöisenkatu 1	00100 Helsinki 10
Terho, Erkki	Albertinkatu 11 C	90100 Oulu 10
Tevajärvi, Maj-Britt	Kerankuja 5	02700 Kauniainen
Tiainen, Kaisa	Kihokkitie 14	90160 Oulu 16
Tiainen, Martti	Kaskikatu 4 B 8	00320 Jyväskylä 32
Tieva, Osmo	Huhtiniemenk. 26 as	53600 Lappeenranta 60
Tommila, Veikko	Kauppalantie 24	02700 Kauniainen
Tuomaala, Paavo	Vitkantie 2 as. 3	96100 Rovaniemi 10
Tuomioja, Maunu	Bulevardi 17 A 10	00120 Helsinki 12
Tuovinen, Erkki	Kulosaaren Puistot. 42	00570 Helsinki 57
Unto, Eira	Vanha Hämeent. 109 B 5	20540 Turku 54
Ursin, Kai af	Hämeenkatu 9 A 4	33100 Tampere 10
Vainio-Matilla, Birgitta		28400 Ulvila
Valle, Olavi	Asunto E 11	48210 Kotka 21
Vannas, Antti	Pohj. Ranta 10 A	00170 Helsinki 17
Vannas, Prof. Salme	Pohj. Ranta 10 A	00170 Helsinki 17
Varonen, Toini	Vallitunsaari 13 A	94100 Kemi 10
Vasama, Ritva	Koukkutie 4	33530 Tampere 53
Venäläinen, Unto	Sibeliuksenk. 5 A 15	13100 Hämeenlinna 10
Wessman-Viertola, Leila	Urheilukatu 28 A 11	00250 Helsinki 25
Viherluoto, Kaarina	Mannerheimintie 114 D	00250 Helsinki 25
Viikari, Kaisu	Rykmentintie 43 as. 20	20880 Turku 88
Wittfooth, Kirsti	Keskussairaala Vaasanpuistikko 3 A	65100 Vaasa 10
Voipio, Hannu	Urheilukatu 52	00250 Helsinki 25
Vuopala, Veikko	Sirppitie 13 as. 2	90530 Oulu 53
Vänttinen, Sinikka	Snellmaninkatu 1 B 21	70100 Kuopio 10
Ylösjoki, Kirsti	Sepänkatu 15 B 30	00150 Helsinki 15
Zewi, Moses	Maariankatu 3 A	20100 Turku 10
Zitting, Erna	Erottajankatu 9	00130 Helsinki 13
Äikäs, Tapani	Ratakatu 7 A	00120 Helsinki 12

NOSOCOMIA QUIBUS OCULIS AEGRI CURANTUR

	No. of Beds Sairaalapaikkoja
University Centralhospital, Dept. of Ophthalmology, Helsinki (Head: Prof. Salme Vannas)	126
University Centralhospital, Dept. of Ophthalmology, Turku (Head: Prof. Arvo Oksala)	45
University Centralhospital, Dept. of Ophthalmology, Oulu (Head: Prof. Henrik Forsius)	52
University Centralhospital, Dept. of Ophthalmology, Kuopio (Head: −)	24
Eye Department of the Centralhospital, Hämeenlinna (Head: Jarmo Sammalkivi)	9
Eye Department of the Centralhospital, Joensuu (Head: Martti Katavisto)	20
Eye Department of the Centralhospital, Jyväskylä (Head: Matti Koskenoja)	18
Eye Department of the Centralhospital, Kajaani (Head: Kai Ennevaara)	13
Eye Department of the Centralhospital, Kemi (Head: Aimo Niittyviita)	15
Eye Department of the Centralhospital, Kokkola (Head: Heikki Aurekoski)	12
Eye Department of the Centralhospital, Kotha (Head: Matti Kaivonen)	23
Eye Department of the Centralhospital, Lappeenranta (Head: Seppo Pohjola)	15
Eye Department of the Centralhospital Mikkeli (Head: Reijo Harjula)	11

INSTITUTA SCHOLAEQUE CAECIS DESTINATAE

GALLIA (la France)

SOCIETATES OPHTHALMOLOGICAE

Nationalis

Société Française d'Ophtalmologie

Président: Prof. René Hugonnier
Vice-Président: Dr. Henri Miller
Secrétaire-Général: Prof. Christian Haye
Trésorier: Dr. Jean-Paul Boissin
Siège: 9 Rue Mathurin-Régnier, 75015 Paris 15
Membres: ca. 2500

Regionales

Société d'Ophtalmologie de Paris
Secrétaire Général: Dr. J. P. Bailliart, 47, rue de Bellechasse, 75007 Paris

Société d'Ophtalmologie de l'Est
Secrétaire Général: Prof. C. Thomas, 133, rue Saint-Dizier, 54000 Nancy

Société d'Ophtalmologie de Lyon
Secrétaire: Dr. J. Audibert, 54, rue Jacquart, 69004 Lyon

Société d'Ophtalmologie du Midi
Secrétaire Général: Prof. Agr. P. V. Berard, 48, rue de Breteuil, 13006 Marseille

Société d'Ophtalmologie de Bordeaux et du Sud-Ouest
Secrétaire Général: Prof. E. Bessiere, 9, rue Hustin, 33000 Bordeaux

Société d'Ophtalmologie de l'Ouest
Secrétaire Général: Dr. A. Baron, 5, rue Bonne-Louise, 44 Nantes

Société d'Ophtalmologie du Nord
Secrétaire Général: Prof. Pierre Francois, 41, rue d'Artois, 59000 Lille

NOMINA ET DOMICILIA MEDICORUM AB OCULIS

Abecassis, André	Centre d'Exp. Médicales du Personnel navigant, Hôpital des Armées 'Lyautey'	67-Strasbourg-Neudorf
Abitbol, Yvan	54, avenue Paul-Valéry	95-Sarcelles

Abravanel, Annette	30, rue Bobillot	75013 Paris
Achard, Marcel	53, Grande-Rue	25-Besançon
Adenis, Jean-Paul	16, rue Victor-Chabot	87100 Limoges
Afchard, Charles	12, rue Gambetta	58000 Nevers
Aflalo, Guy	48, avenue Anatole-France	54000 Nancy
Agenos, Bernard	Résidence du Parc St-Hilaire, 45, boulevard Pont-Achard	86-Poitiers
Albarea-Levy, Eliane	7, rue Georges-Berger	75017 Paris
Albault, André	32, avenue Billières	31-Toulouse
Albinet, Jacques	48, rue de Galinié	81-Mazamet
Alcayde, Michel	Le Saint-Denis, rue Caizergues-de-Pradines	34000 Montpellier
Alexandrescu, Mariana	13, rue du Lieuvin	75015 Paris
Algan, Bernard	25, rue du Grand-Verger	54-Nancy
Almalric, Pierre M.	Centre Medical Ophtal. 6, rue Saint-Clair	81000 Albi
Amar, Léo	Palais Armenonville, Rond-Point-Duboys-d'Angers	06-Cannes
André, Jacques	28, rue des Ardennes	50-Cherbourg
Andrieu, Gabriel	9, boulevard de Strasbourg	83-Toulon
Antoine, Françoise	101, rue Saint-Dizier	54-Nancy
Antoine, Renée	Parc Beauregard B1.C. n° 2	13-Aix-en-Provence
Apprill-Lamp, Marie-Thérèse	2, rue de l'Industrie	68-Mulhouse
Aran, Philippe	13, rue du Castillet	66000 Perpignan
Archaix, Roger P.	94, rue de la République	85-Fontenay-le-Comte
Ardichen, J.	3, place du Capitole	31-Toulouse
Ardouin, Maurice	Beau Soleil au Pont-Réan	35170 Bruz
Arnaud, Bernard	832, rue des Sorbes, 'Le Lavandou'	34000 Montpellier
Arncodo, Jacques	12, Prado Parc, 411, avenue du Prado	13008 Marseille
Arnoux, Louis	3, rue du Capitaine-de-Bresson	05-Gap
Arnoux, Marcel	66 d, rue Sainte	13001 Marseille
Aron, Jean-Jacques	28, avenue Raphaël	75016 Paris
Artières, Pierre	20, boulevard Victor-Hugo	30-Alès
Artigues, Jean-Marie	3, place du Réduit	64-Bayonne
Asseman, Roger	13, place Sébastopol	59-Lille
Aubert, Lucien	397, rue Paradis	13008 Marseille
Aubry, Jean-Pierre	26, rue Maries	81000 Albi
Aubry, Michel	20, rue F. Sarloveze	60-Compiègne
Aubry, Pierre	Passage Barbafust	80-Abbeville
Audibert, Jacques	54, rue Jacquard	69004 Lyon
Audibert, Pierre	16, rue Jean-Jacques-Rousseau	44-Nantes
Audoueineix, Emile	32, rue Auvray	72-Le Mans
Aurientis, Jean	9, avenue Victor-Hugo	13-Aix-en-Provence
Auvert, Bertranne	78, avenue de Suffren	75015 Paris
Averbuch, Michel	258 bis, rue des Pyrénées	75020 Paris
Avrillon, Jean	31, boulevard Exelmans	75016 Paris
Bach, Claude	1, place de l'Homme-de-Fer	67-Strasbourg
Baculard-Bodenes, Madeleine	1, place Alphonse-Deville	75006 Paris
Baikoff, Georges	2, rue Racine	44000 Nantes
Bailbe, Noël	19, place de la Banque	66-Perpignan
Bailliart, Jean-Pierre	47, rue de Bellechasse	75007 Paris
Ballereau, Luc	7, rue Jules-Polo	44000 Nantes
Balon, Michel	21, rue Auber	75009 Paris
Barbançon, Sege René	18, avenue de Verdun	79-Niort

Bard, Jean	202, boulevard Jean-Jaurès	92-Boulogne
Barisain-Monrose, Pierre ...	70, rue Henri-Vadon	83-Saint-Raphaël
Baron, André	5, rue Bonne-Louise	44-Nantes
Baronet, Philippe	32, rue Alsace-Lorraine	31-Toulouse
Barret, Philippe	32, avenue Mozart	75016 Paris
Barrioulet, Yves	22, boulevard Henri-Sizaire	81-Castres
Barrut, Marc	27, place Grandclément	69-Villeurbanne
Bartoli, Dominique	16, rue Neuve-de-la-République .	10-Sainte-Savine
Barut, Charles Pierre	15, boulevard Gambetta	38-Grenoble
Barut, Charles	31, rue Ferrandière	69002 Lyon
Baudrillart, Pierre	10, rue de Vouillé	75015 Paris
Baumgartner-Keppi, Marguerite	114, route de Mittelhausbergen	67-Strasbourg-Cronenbourg
Beal, Francis	45, rue de Chanzy	59-Tourcoing
Beauchamp, Pierre	15, rue Sadi-Carnot	14000 Caen
Beauchef, Michel	22, rue des Tanneurs	61-L'Aigle
Bec, Pierré	34, rue de Rémusat	31-Toulouse
Bechac, Gérard	21, rue de Languedoc	31-Toulouse
Béchetoille, Alain	140, Faubourg-Saint-Martin	75010 Paris
Bégué, Jean-Jacques	60, avenue Marcel-Cachin	92-Châtillon-sous-Bagneux
Bélicard, Pierre	6, place des Jacobins	69002 Lyon
Bellier, Frank B.	14, rue Jean-Perreal	69008 Lyon
Benand, Robert	26, rue Anatole-France	93-Aulnay-sous-Bois
Benichou, David	33, rue de Berri	75008 Paris
Bénit-Gerdessus, Marie – Thérèse	29, allée Jean-Jaurès	31-Toulouse
Benmansour, Hadi	276, boulevard Saint-Germain ..	75007 Paris
Benner, Rolf	2, rue de Zurich	68-Mulhouse
Benoit, Alain	4, place Vaillant-Couturier	91-Corbeil
Bentami, Abdennour	10, rue de Pologne	78-Saint-Germain-en-Laye
Berard, Pierre-Vital	48, rue de Breteuil	13006 Marseille
Berche, Jacques	43, Grande-Rue	94-Nogent-sur-Marne
Berche, Léon	32, rue Victor-Hugo	62-Lens
Berdugo, Jacques	5, place Foch	95880 Enghien-les-Bains
Berkman, Nicole	19, boulevard de Courcelles	75008 Paris
Bermond, Charles	19 bis, cours Maréchal-Foch	40-Dax
Bernard, Jean-Antoine	21, rue de Civry	75016 Paris
Bernard-Mettil, Pierre	3, rue de Médicis	75006 Paris
Berrondo, Paul	7, rue Vauban	64-Bayonne
Bertezene, Pierre	13, rue du Castillet	66-Perpignan
Berthemy, Claude	9, rue Moncey	25-Besançon
Bertin, François	7, rue Trémoille	35-Vitré
Bertrand, Jean-Jacques	43, boulevard Malesherbes	75008 Paris
Bertrand, Léon	2, place Marcel-Naudot	21300 Chenove
Besnainou, Lucien	11, place de la Nation	75011 Paris
Besnainou, Roger	1, rue Saint-Paul	60-Beauvais
Bessière, Edouard	9, rue Hustin	33-Bordeaux
Bessin, André	5, place des Vieilles-Halles	61-Argentan
Bessou, Paul	27, rue des Potiers	31-Toulouse
Biais, Bertrand	70, rue J.-J.-Rousseau	18-Bourges
Biard, Louis	2, rue René-Barthélémy	92260 Fontenay-aux-Roses
Bideau, René	94, rue Félix-Faure	92-Colombes
Bigonnet, Jean	6, rue Arnaud-de-Fabre	84-Avignon
Bigorgne, Josette	15, avenue Emile-Savigner	49240 Avrillé
Bineau, Jean-Marc	28, rue Béranger	76600 Le Havre
Binet, Jacques	8, rue de la Grosse-Armée	18-Bourges

Boureau, Martine	7, rue Portalis	75008 Paris
Bourely, Jacques	51, avenue de l'Aigue	21200 Beaune
Bourgeois, Hubert	7, chemin de Charrière-Blanche	69130 Ecully
Bourget, Jacques M. R.	10, rue Alsace-Lorraine	86-Poitiers
Bourret, Léon	2, rue Félix-Faure	06-Cannes
Bousseau, Maurice	Polyclinique du Parc, 10, rue du Clos	91-Ris-Orangis
Boutron, Robert	14, rue de Bruxelles	75009 Paris
Bouzaid, Raymond	15 *ter*, rue des Tournelles	94-L'Hay-les-Roses
Boyer, Raoul	La Sarrasine	84470 Châteauneuf-de-Gadagne
Brachet, Alain	5, rue Berteaux-Dumas	92-Neuilly-sur-Seine
Brasseur, Gérard	3, Parc de la Scie	76130 Mont-Saint-Aignan
Braun-Vallon, Suzanne	19, rue de Miromesnil	75008 Paris
Brégeat, Paul	9, rue Théodule-Ribot	75017 Paris
Bremmé-Helm, Claude	72 boulevard de Port-Royal	75005 Paris
Brémond, Jean	59, boulevard de la Libération	13001 Marseille
Bretagne, Alain	9, rue des Carmes	54-Nancy
Bretagne, Paul	79, rue de Badonviller	54-Nancy
Brini, Alfred	8, rue des Arquebusiers	67-Strasbourg
Bronner, Albert	2 *A*, rue Schwilgué	67-Strasbourg
Bronstein, Jacques	133, avenue Gambetta	93-Bagnolet
Bronstein, Lydie	3, rue des Acacias	75017 Paris
Brugère, Christian	3, rue de Verdun	69500 Bron
Brun, Patrice P.	'Le Petit Brotteaux', 25, rue Jean-Broquin	69006 Lyon
Brun, Francis	3, rue Liogier	42100 Saint-Etienne
Bruneau, J.	12, rue Margueritte	75017 Paris
Bruneau de La Salle, Jacq.	15, rue Sadi-Carnot	14-Caen
Brunelle, Jean-Claude	85 *ter*, rue Jeanne-d'Arc	76-Rouen
Brus, Charles	15, boulevard De-Lattre-de-Tassigny	40-Mont-de-Marsan
Bruyas, Guy	14, rue Latapie	64-Pau
Buisson, Suzanne	2, rue Saint-Jacques	38-Grenoble
Buovolo, Jacques	5, place du Théâtre	17-Saintes
Burette, André	25, boulevard du Maréchal-Leclerc	51-Reims
Burger, André	7, rue du Dôme	67-Strasbourg
Burnet, Yves	203, avenue du Maréchal-Foch	92-Bagneux
Bursaux, Michel	23, rue Lochet	51-Châlons-sur-Marne
Cabantous, Michel	12, rue d'Italie	13-Aix-en-Provence
Cahn, Roger	3, rue Rolland	22-Dinan
Cailleux, Jean-Claude	12, rue du Petit-Salut	76000 Rouen
Cailleux, Michel	28, boulevard du Général-de-Gaulle	76-Dieppe
Calabre, Camille	23, rue Gubernatis	06-Nice
Calix, Marc	1, rue Victor-Hugo	31-Toulouse
Calmettes, Louis	27, rue de Metz	31000 Toulouse
Calvet, Henri	3, avenue Pierre-1er-de-Serbie	75016 Paris
Cambrillat, Georges	80, avenue Victor-Hugo	26-Valence
Camezind, Michel	8, rue Ozenne	31000 Toulouse
Campinchi, René P.	61, rue La Boétie	75008 Paris
Canonne, Charles	9, rue Théophile-Boyer	59-Le Cateau
Canque, Marthe	10, boulevard Vaquez	63-Royat
Canque, Michel	2, avenue Julien	63-Clermont-Ferrand
Cantat, Marie-Antoinette	14, place Pierre-de-Coubertin	63-Clermont-Ferrand

Cantonnet, Pierre	9, Villa Poirier	75015 Paris
Caquet-Schmid, Nicole	12, rue de Bourgogne	75007 Paris
Carli, Jacques	55, rue des Poilus	13-La Ciotat
Carlotti, Pierre-François	4, Jardin Alsace-Lorraine	06-Nice
Carnus, Charles	11, boulevard d'Estourmel	12-Rodez
Carton, Michel	8 bis, rue du Maréchal-Foch	59-Dunkerque
Castel, Jean	18, Grande-Rue	29-Morlaix
Cattoir, Renée	84, rue Pelleport	75020 Paris
Catros, André	4, rue d'Isly	35-Rennes
Cau, Jean	54, rue de Montebello	50-Cherbourg
Cauny, Michèle	53, boulevard Victor-Hugo	92-Neuilly-sur-Seine
Cavicchi, Licio	32, rue Thomas-Couture	60-Senlis
Cayrou, Maurice	1 bis, rue de la Porte-du-Moustier	82000 Montauban
Cazaban, René	Clinique du Parc	34-Castelnau-le-Lez
Ceddaha, Marcel	136, boulevard Voltaire	75011 Paris
Cellier, Claude	14, rue des Recollets	19-Brive
Chabat, Henriette	26, boulevard Bonne-Nouvelle	75010 Paris
Chabot, Jacqueline	190, rue de Saint-Genès	33-Bordeaux
Chalono, Jeannine	35 B, avenue Aristide-Briand	93-Stains
Chalvignac, André	30, rue des Clers	57-Metz
Chambon, Pierre	3, place d'Armes	12-Rodez
Champetier-Chave, Henriette	30, avenue Victor-Hugo	26-Valence
Champion, Jacques	2, rue Félix-Gras	84-Avignon
Chanteau, Yves	23, place des Otages	29 N-Morlaix
Chappé, Roger	23, rue Gargoulleau	17-La Rochelle
Chapuis-Maurette, Michèle	15, boulevard Raspail	84-Avignon
Charasse, René	31, rue du Progrès	13005 Marseille
Charier, Christiane	16, avenue du Midi	94100 Saint-Maur-des-Fossés
Charles, Jean	3, rue Marcellin-Berthelot	89000 Auxerre
Charleux, Jacques	29, place Bellecour	69002 Lyon
Charnay, Claude	11, avenue de Paris	24-Périgueux
Charpentier, Pierre-Louis	37, rue Adolphe-Besson	77-Chelles
Chassaing, Jean	23, avenue de la Gare	19-Brive
Chatellier, Philippe	8, rue des Saussaies	75008 Paris
Chauviré, Etienne	44, place de la République	69002 Lyon
Chavanné, Henri	2, rue Sala	69002 Lyon
Chermezon, Jean-Paul	89, avenue Mozart	75016 Paris
Chesnais, Augustin	1, rue de Verdun	35-Fougères
Chevaleraud, Jacques	8, avenue Bertie-Albrecht	75008 Paris
Chevannes, Hervé	20, rue Copernic	44-Nantes
Chevassus, Jean	7, place Michelet	43-Le Puy-en-Velay
Chiche, Roland	45, boulevard Barbès	75018 Paris
Chilkowsky, Catherine	10, rue d'Auvilliers	91290 Arpajon
Chiozza, Emile	7, boulevard de Strasbourg	83-Toulon
Chovet, Marcel	Tour 5, allée Albeniz, parc du roi d'Espagne	13008 Marseille
Chrisment, Jacques	15, quai Maréchal-Leclerc	88-Saint-Dié
Claux, Jean-Michel	46, avenue Roger-Salengro	94-Champigny-sur-Marne
Clavel, André	86, rue Judaïque	33-Bordeaux
Clay-Frayssinet, Claude	25, avenue Mac-Mahon	75017 Paris
Clop, Henri	7, rue Henri-Gréville	49-Angers
Cochet, Paul	16, rue de Magdebourg	75016 Paris
Cochois, Jean-P.-E.	55, rue Albert-de-Mun	44-Saint-Nazaire
Coeytaux, Michel	2, boulevard Henri-Paul-Schneider	71-Le Creusot
Colinot, Paul	17, rue de l'Horloge	27-Vernon
Collet-Vichot, Odile	116, rue de Rennes	75006 Paris

Collier, Michel	26, rue Serviez	64-Pau
Collin, Olivier	4, place de l'Hôtel-de-Ville	74-Thonon-les-Bains
Collin, Pierre	68, rue d'Antibes	06-Cannes
Colombier, George William	11, square Mérimée	06-Cannes
Comiti-Sarrola, Georgette	29, boulevard Dubouchage	06-Nice
Common, Pierre	152, boulevard de Strasbourg	76-Le Havre
Constantinides, Georges	9, rue Henri-Dunant	59-Lille
Corbel, Michel	88, rue Jean-Sans-Peur	59-Lille
Corcelle, Louis	16, rue d'Aviau	33-Bordeaux
Cordier, Jacques	34, rue Gambetta	54-Nancy
Cornand, Georges	43, boulevard Grignan	83100 Toulon
Cornibert, Jean	10, rue du Colonel-de-Grancey	21-Dijon
Corréard, René	22, rue Gambetta	77-Meaux
Coscas, Gabriel	192 bis, rue de Vaugirard	75015 Paris
Coste, Maurice	22, rue Robert-de-Luzarches	80-Amiens
Costeau, Jacques	9, rue de la Loge	34000 Montpellier
Costil, Maurice	11, rue Perronet	92-Neuilly-sur-Seine
Cotten, Mari-Thérèse	8, rue Edouard-Detaille	92100 Boulogne
Couadau, Etienne	56, rue de Boussières	59-Hautmont
Couadau, Henri	3, rue Albert-Lautman	31-Toulouse
Couderc, Jean-Louis	3, rue du Bourg-l'Abbé	75003 Paris
Coulier, Jean-Pierre	9, avenue du 8 Mai	13400 Aubagne
Courtin, Joseph	31, rue Amiral-Courbet	80-Amiens
Courvoisier, Fabienne-Noëlle	2, rue Charles-de-Vergennes	21-Dijon
Couter, Pierre	13, rue Soupirants	62-Calais
Couzi, Jacques	57, avenue P.-V.-Couturier	94-Vitry-sur-Seine
Crehange, Jacques	50, avenue Mathurin-Moreau	75019 Paris
Crouzet, Jean	3, avenue Valvein	93-Montreuil-sous-Bois
Cueto-Alvarez, Pablo	11, rue Crozatier	75012 Paris
Cugnier-Bellière, Monique	3, quai Barlier	70-Vesoul
Cuq, Gérard-Jean	4, place Saint-Sernin	31-Toulouse
Curioni, Marguerite	8, rue de Buzenval	75020 Paris
Curmi, Augustin	231, rue J. et R.-Kennedy	13-Salon-de-Provence
Cuvillier, Annie	6 bis, rue Jean-Moulin	94300 Vincennes
Daban, Paul	30, boulevard Chasles	28-Chartres
Dagorne, Jean	5, rue Maréchal-Joffre	76-Le Havre
Dahan, Jacques	7, rue Roger-de-Nezot	78100 Saint-Germain-en-Laye
Dalger, Georges	2, avenue de la Mitre	83-Toulon
Damois, François	9, rue Emile-Duployé	76000 Rouen
Daraux, Henri	5, place Wilson	31-Toulouse
Darcy, Janine	204, boulevard Raspail	75014 Paris
Darleguy, Paul	35, rue de Suffren, Le Mourillon	83-Toulon
Dauban, Françoise	1, place Cabrol	12-Decazeville
Daumail, Jean	41, boulevard Pasteur	63-Clermont-Ferrand
Dauthuile, Pierre	Santa Lucia, 1, avenue Thiers	06-Menton
Debbasch, Silvio	47, avenue d'Alembert, Parc de Sceaux	92160 Antony
Debrousse, Jean	12, rue Gambetta	58-Nevers
Decaudin, André	44, rue de Lille	75007 Paris
Decorps, Paul	15, rue du Huit-Mai 1945	75010 Paris
Decour, Humbert	OPH, 'Les Tournelles'	63-Vertaizon
Déduit, Yolande	1, rue Goethe	67000 Strasbourg
Defives, Michel	2, rue du Pont-à-Seille	57-Metz
Defoug, Denise	7, rue Servandoni	75006 Paris
Degabriel, Jacques	Dompierre-sur-Charente	17-Chérac

Dehorter-Duez, Claude	110, rue Royale	59-Lille
Dejean, Charles	1, Carré du Roi	31100 Montpellier
Delarra, Pierre	46, rue Delsaulx	59-Valenciennes
Delaveuve, Jacques	7, rue de la Gare	88100 Saint-Dié
Delbos, Roger	20, place du Monument	15-Riom-ès-Montagne
Delbosc, Georges	122, cours Jean-Jaurès	38-Grenoble
Delcroix, André	24, rue L.-de-Bettignies	59-Saint-Amand
Deleuil, André	14, rue Esparriat	13-Aix-en-Provence
Delfour, Georges	3, rue Alexandre-Fourtanier	31-Toulouse
Delord, Robert	3, rue Sainte-Ursule, (boulevard des Arènes)	30-Nîmes
Delorme, Rose-Marie	49, rue Pasteur	44-Bouguenais
Deloron, Gilbert	56, rue du Maréchal-Joffre	92-Colombes
Delpech, Jacques	33, rue des Châlets	31-Toulouse
Delplace-Combe, Marie-Paule	18, Résidence 'La Mauberdière' .	37-Saint-Avertin
Delpuget, Jacques-Henri ...	Clinique des Charmilles, 12, boulevard Brossolette	91-Arpajon
Delpy, Jacques	74, avenue de Grammont	37-Tours
Delthil, Simone	46, rue de Naples	75008 Paris
Delyfer, Gilbert	Parc du Château, Résidence Les Chênes-Verts	33-Mérignac
Demailly, Philippe	41, avenue Kléber	75016 Paris
Demichel, Patrick	Centre Médical, place de l'Europe, Cité du Grand Parc	33-Bordeaux
Demillière, Bernard	322, avenue Berthelot	69-Lyon
Demonte, Henri	9, rue Lazare Escarguel	66-Perpignan
Deneuville, Jean	33, rue des Tennerolles	92-Saint-Cloud
Denis, Alain	10, rue Delayant	17-La Rochelle
Denis, Anne	immeuble Provence, 73, rue de Suresnes	92380 Garches
Denys, Albert	rue du Champ-de-la-Croix	86100 Chatellerault
Déodati, Félix	4, place Matabiau	31-Toulouse
Deplaix, Claude	4, rue de la Basilique	58-Nevers
Depouilly, Louis	17, place Bossuet	21-Dijon
Dernoncour, Yvon	69, rue Ordener	75018 Paris
Dervieux, Antoine	26, boulevard Magenta	75010 Paris
Desbordes, Pierre	118, avenue de Paris	94-Vincennes
Descamps, Jean	13, rue Victor-Hugo	60-Creil
Deschatres, Alain	65, avenue Paul-Doumer	92-Rueil-Malmaison
Després, Albert	49, avenue Ledru-Rollin	94-Le Perreux
Desprez, Pierre	5, rue de Saint-Exupéry	39-Champagnole
Desvignes, Pierre	27, rue du Cherche-Midi	75006 Paris
Deswarte, Jean	22, avenue de Ferrière	59-Maubeuge
Devoize, Jacques	8, boulevard du 14-Juillet	89-Sens
Dhermy, Pierre	70, rue Maurice-Thorez	92000 Nanterre
Didierlaurent, Andrée	31, rue Rebatel	69003 Lyon
Dietz, Pierre René	2, rue de Gonzague	08100 Charleville-Mézières
Dillemann, Annick	29, rue Labrouste	75015 Paris
Diss, Paul-Gérard	rue Eugène-Piron	13-Salon-de-Provence
Dittersdorf, Anita	2 ter, avenue d'Aléry	74-Annecy
Doise, Pierre	82, avenue Anatole-France	59-Anzin
Dollfus, Marc-Adrien	Fleurheim	27480 Lyons-la-Forêt
Dollard, Henri	2 bis, rue du Général-de-Gaulle ..	34-Sète
Domercq, Maurice	2, rue des Cordeliers	64-Pau
Dor, Edouard	3, rue Dormoy	42-Saint-Etienne
Dorlencourt, Michel	208, avenue Aristide-Briand	92-Bagneux

Dorne, Pierre Alain Jr.	21, rue Colbert	30-Nîmes
Doucet, Pierre	9, rue Montpensier	64-Pau
Douillet, Albert	9, rue Henri-IV	80-Amiens
Dran, Régine	18, rue Léon-Giraud	75019 Paris
Drouin, Pierre	26, rue de l'Etoile	72-Le Mans
Druault-Toufesco, Nicolas .	13, rue du Petit-Pré	37-Tours
Dubar, Jean	2, boulevard Jean-Jaurès	92-Boulogne-sur-Seine
Dublineau, Philippe	26, boulevard du Maréchal-Foch .	49000 Angers
Dubois, Jean-Claude	7, rue Coursarlon	18000 Bourges
Dubois-Poulsen, André	8, avenue Daniel-Lesueur	75007 Paris
Ducam, Michèle	56, rue de Fécamp	75012 Paris
Ducarre, Claude	12, rue Jean-Jaurès	74-Annecy
Ducret, Jacques	10, place Jules-Méline	88-Remiremont
Ducros, Jean	6, boulevard Joseph-Vallier	38-Grenoble
Dufour, Daniel	34, rue Caumartin	59-Lille
Dugelay-Magnaud, Juliette .	62, rue Martre	92-Clichy
Dulière, Luc	Résidence Jeanne-d'Arc, avenue de Pierrevert	04-Manosque
Dumas, Jacques	2, avenue Julien	63-Clermont-Ferrand
Dumont, Louis	12, rue de l'Université	59-Douai
Dumont, Pierre	2, rue Danton	75006 Paris
Dupont-Delcourt, Michel ..	86, rue de Famars	59-Valenciennes
Dupuy, Monique	3, rue Albert-de-Mun	33000 Bordeaux
Durand, Luc	2, quai Saint-Antoine	69002 Lyon
Durand, Rémi	10, rue Saint-Antoine	60-Compiègne
Durbet, Gérard	Résidence Jeanne-d'Arc, avenue de Pierrevert	04100 Manosque
Duriez, Jean-Claude	59, rue Lafaurie de Monbadon ..	33-Bordeaux
Duval, Raoul	463, rue de l'Eglise	76-Bois-Guillaume
Eberhardt, Jean	61, avenue Francis-Tonner	06-Cannes-la-Bocca
Einholtz, Edgard	6, avenue de la Gare	36-Châteauroux
Elgolli, Mohamed	93 boulevard Magenta	75010 Paris
Elie, Emile	12, rue de la Tour	85-Les Sables-d'Olonne
Elie, Gabriel	1, place Général-Leclerc	29 N-Brest
Eliet, Jacques	2, rue Victor-Hunger	14-Vire
Epifanie, Richard	3, rue des Jacobins	09-Pamiers
Escoute, Régine	95, Cours Lieutaud	13006 Marseille
Espesson, Yves	22, cours Fauriel	42-Saint-Etienne
Etchats, André	17, Lices du Nord	81-Albi
Etienne, Jean-Paul	23, rue de Luynes	28200 Châteaudun
Etienne, Raymond	31, rue Ferrandière	69002 Lyon
Fabre, Philippe	45, rue Paul-Pons, B.P. 55	26400 Crest
Falies, Jean-F.	Cannes Marina	06210 Mandelieu
Farbos, Jean-Pierre	209, rue Eau-de-Robec	76000 Rouen
Fargette, Lucien	2, rue Anatole-Bailly	45-Orléans
Farnarier, Georges	225, avenue des Caillols	13012 Marseille
Fau, Alain	62, avenue Foch	54-Nancy
Fau, Robert	10, place Bellegarde	24-Bergerac
Faure, Jean-Pierre	53, rue d'Ablon	91-Athis-Mons
Favory, Albert	43, rue de Bellechasse	75007 Paris
Felgines, Jean-Pierre	41, rue Réaumur	17-La Rochelle
Ferrand, Jean	40, boulevard Voltaire	13006 Marseille
Ferraris-Richard, Odile	4, rue du Général-Leclerc	95210 Saint-Gratien
Ferrero, Nicole	5, rue de Conti	95-L'Isle-Adam
Ferrez, Beranrd L.	8, rue des Loges	95-Montmorency
Feuvrier, Yves-Michel	2, rue de Rohan	35-Rennes

Fiel, Jeannine-Renée	17, avenue de Lattre	88-Epinal
Filhastre, Henri	26, boulevard Michelet	13008 Marseille
Filippi, René	4, rue Saint-Antoine	30-Nîmes
Filloux, Pierre Marie	17, rue de la Petite-Cité	27-Evreux
Fimbel, Jean	11, avenue M.-Faure	26-Valence
Fischer, Michel	Clinique Saint-Joseph, 2, rue A. M. Javouhey	77300 Fontainebleau
Flandin, Jean	1, rue Roger-Payol	26-Montélimar
Florquin, Annick	8, rue de la Ronce	92410 Ville-d'Avray
Foissin, Jean	4, rue Royale	74-Annecy
Foltz, André	44, rue Lesage	51-Reims
Fontaine, Marine	17, rue Rousselet	75007 Paris
Fontan, Pierre	3, rue Alexandre-Fourtanier	31-Toulouse
Fontenaille, Nicole	19, rue Racine	44000 Nantes
Forest, André	89, avenue de Villiers	75017 Paris
Forest, Charles	2, avenue Bugeaud	75016 Paris
Forgeron, Pierre	133, avenue Carnot	91-Savigny-sur-Orge
Fortier, Jacqueline	150, rue de Tolbiac	75013 Paris
Fortin, Janine	9, rue du Lieutenant	53-Laval
Fouanon, Christian E.	2, rue Guépin	44000 Nantes
Foucault, Claude	44, rue Desmoueux	14-Caen
Fougeres, Rozen Erwane	132, boul. Montparnasse	75014 Paris
Fouin, Georges	Le Fontainebleau, 26, boulevard Dubouchage	06000 Nice
Fourcade, Jean	4, place A.-Fallières	47-Agen
Fourcade, Maurice	17, boulevard Foch	83-Draguignan
Francfort, Gérard	36 bis, rue du Briolet	55100 Verdun
Franck, Jean-Paul	61, rue des Aqueducs	69005 Lyon
François, Pierre	41, rue d'Artois	59-Lille
Frankel, Hélène	14, rue Massenet	75016 Paris
Fraysse, Rolland	clinique Pasteur; 138, rue de Funay	72-Le Mans
Freyche, Claude	3, place Alexandre-Moret	74-Annemasse
Frileux, René	18 bis, boulevard de la Bastille	75012 Paris
Fritsch, René	2, place Victor-Hugo	38-Grenoble
Fritz, Bernard	128, route de Bischwiller	67-Strasbourg-Shiltigheim
Fruchtenreich, Michel D.	43, rue Raymond-Poincaré	54000 Nancy
Gabersek, Victor	Pavillon de la Grille, Salpêtrière, 47, boulevard de l'Hôpital	75013 Paris
Gaboriau, Jacques	56, rue de la Gare	79-Niort
Gacon-Lamendour, Rose	Hôpital des Armées Sainte-Anne, Service d'Ophtalmologie	83-Toulon
Gaillard, Gilberte	3 bis, rue de l'Alboni	75016 Paris
Galdin, Pierre	2, place Du Guesclin	30-Nîmes
Gally, Jean	62, rue Antoine-Marty	11-Carcassonne
Ganem, Jean	10, rue Danton	75006 Paris
Garipuy, Jean	38, rue du Taur	31-Toulouse
Garnier, Jean-Paul	22, rue du Champ-Jacquet	35-Rennes
Garnier, Robert	4, place Maurice-Marchais	56-Vannes
Garric, René	17, place Winston-Churchill	87-Limoges
Garrigue, Henri	3, boulevard Henri-IV	75004 Paris
Gassenc, Robert	20, rue de Bretagne	27-Bernay
Gaud, François	8, rue de Copenhague	75008 Paris
Gauffre, Raymond	46, boulevard de la République	34-Béziers
Gauthier, André	Résidence de la Mer, boulevard de la Mer	64-Hendaye-Plage

Gay, Jean	16, avenue de Romans	38-Voiron
Gelassin, Jacques	6, rue Félix-Faure	17500 Jonzac
Gemin, Yves	60, rue Saint-André-des-Arts	75006 Paris
Gerbert, Ernest	66, avenue Gabriel-Péri	93-Saint-Ouen
Gerhard, Jean-Pierre	16, place d'Austerlitz	67-Strasbourg
Gérin, Georges	68, boulevard de la Libération	13004 Marseille
Gharbi, Albert	30, boulevard Gambetta	06-Nice
Gherardi-Bakalova, Marguerite	25, rue du Sergent-Bauchat	75012 Paris
Chiloni, Hélène	33, rue de la Brèche-aux-Loups	75012 Paris
Ghnassia, Jean-Paul	95, boulevard Carnot	06-Cannes
Giafferi, Dominique	66, boulevard Péreire	75017 Paris
Gille, Claude	15, rue Saint-Denis	76-Rouen
Gillet, Jean-Michel	Hôpital Francis-Picaud S.P. 69-253	
Ginguené, Alain	2 bis, rue Harouys	
Girard, Charles	17, boulevard Foch	44-Nantes
Girard, Georges	43, rue des Lilas	83-Draguignan
Girard, Pierre	17, boulevard Foch	75019 Paris
Giraud, Gustave	2, avenue Julien	83-Draguignan
Giudici, Pierre	2, rue de Friedland	63-Clermont-Ferrand
Goddé, Denise	20, rue de Longchamp	13006 Marseille
Goetz, Gérard	64, avenue de la République	75016 Paris
Goffart, Ivan	Clinique Pasteur, 138, rue de Funan	68000 Colmar / 72100 Le Mans
Gognes, Micheline	7, rue Paul-Doumer	02-Saint-Quentin
Golfier, Lise	274, rue de Vaugirard	75015 Paris
Golovine, Serge	7, Rond-Point Mirabeau	75015 Paris
Goni, Louis	1 rue Sadi-Carnot	07-Annonay
Gonnet, Claude	2, place Saint-Louis	03-Vichy
Gotlib, Olivier	15, rue Théodule-Ribot	75017 Paris
Goumet, Georges	18, boulevard Voltaire	75011 Paris
Goupil, Henry	7, rue Arthur-Leduc	14-Caen
Gouray, Alain	6, place Ed.-Normand	44-Nantes
Goure, Pierre	12, rue Raymond-IV	31-Toulouse
Gourinat, Pierre	59, avenue de la Révolution	87-Limoges
Gouriou, Jean	32, quai du Léon	29N-Landerneau
Grall, Yvon	9, rue Berteaux-Dumas	92200 Neuilly-sur-Seine
Grange, Henri	14, avenue de Saxe	69006 Lyon
Grange, Jean D.	63, avenue du Maréchal-de-Saxe	69003 Lyon
Granveaud, Bernard	5, rue du Grand-Puits	13-Martigues
Gras-Boujol, Marie-José	16, avenue d'Estienne-d'Orves	91-Juvisy
Graziani, Antoinette	77, Cours Napoléon	20-Ajaccio
Grelier, Jean	Clinique Francheville	24000 Périgueux
Grenier, Jacques	238, rue Garibaldi	69003 Lyon
Grilleau, Joël	7, Cité Champagne	75020 Paris
Grollenund, Marc	Gouville	21160 Marsannay-la-Côte
Gross, Bernard	44, rue Victor-Hugo	62-Boulogne-sur-Mer
Gros, Philippe	87, Grande-Rue	62200 Boulogne-sur-Mer
Gubert, Nicole	1, rue de Staël	75015 Paris
Gudys, Joseph	17, rue Monsigny	75002 Paris
Guidoni, Georges	6, rue Voltaire	11-Narbonne
Guignot, Robert	23, rue des Trois-Faucons	84-Avignon
Guillaumat, Louis	22, place des Vosges	75004 Paris
Guillemin-Delsarte, Micheline	1, place de la Commanderie	54000 Nancy

Guillerez, François-Régis ..	5, rue des Lombards	51-Châlons-sur-Marne
Guillermin, Robert	33, rue Camille-Arnaud	07-Tournon
Gulin, Francis	19, boulevard de Magenta	75010 Paris
Gur, Alain	27, rue de la Paix	10-Troyes
Guyader, Charles	83, rue Jean-Jaurès	29 N-Brest
Guyard, Maurice	42, avenue Foch	06-Nice
Guyot, Dominique	17, boulevard Raspail	75007 Paris
Guyot-Sionnest, Monique ..	15, rue Joseph-Bara	75006 Paris
Hache, Jean-Claude	221, boulevard de la Liberté	59-Lille
Haineaux, Jean	28, rue de la Gare	79-Niort
Halbron, Pierre	6, boulevard Flandrin	75016 Paris
Halimi, Raoul	71, rue Saint-Antoine	75004 Paris
Hallay, Jacques	19, place Jean-Payra	66-Perpignan
Hallot-Boyer, Pierre	18, place du Pélican	49-Angers
Hamada, Reijiro	Hôtel-Dieu, Service d'Ophtalmologie, place du Parvis-Notre-Dame	75004 Paris
Harmard, Henry	14, rue Chauveau-Lagarde	75008 Paris
Haudiquet, Georges	19, rue de l'Olivier	13005 Marseille
Hausseray, Claude	20, rue Victor-Hugo	59-Douai
Haussy, Roger d'	20, rue Macquart	59-Lille
Haut, Jean	229, boulevard Raspail	75014 Paris
Haye, Christian	23 bis, avenue Niel	75017 Paris
Hebert, Claude	51, boulevard de Richelieu	02100 Saint-Quentin
Heinrich, René	17, rue Eugénie	67-Strasbourg-Neudorf
Heitz, Robert	64, Grande-Rue	67-Haguenau
Helmstetter, Mathilde	12, rue des Frères	67-Saverne
Henry, Christian	Les Baudras, 7, rue Jean-Zay ...	71-Sanvignes-les-Mines
Henry, Christian	291, rue Jeanne-d'Arc	54000 Nancy
Henry, Jacques	30, rue des Missionnaires	78-Versailles
Hermann, Pierre	3, rue Saint-Léonard	49-Angers
Herr, François	4, rue des Clefs	68-Colmar
Hervouët, François	16, boulevard Guist'hau	44-Nantes
Heumann, Marcel	1, rue des 4-Cheminées	92-Boulogne-s/Seine
Hillemand-Philbert, Monique	42, rue du Général-Leclerc	76-Rouen
Hissler, Roger	116, route du Polygone	67100 Strasbourg-Neudorf
Hoel, Jean-Henri	36, rue Ambroise-Paré	53-Laval
Hofmann, Henri	32, rue d'Aiguillon	29 N-Brest
Holl, Charles	49, avenue Roger-Salengro	68-Mulhouse
Hollier-Larousse, Hélène ...	10, rue H.-Maze	78-Viroflay
Hong-Tuan, Tanh	20, rue Charles-Baudelaire	75012 Paris
Horowitz, Georgette	11, rue de Sontay	75016 Paris
Hubert, Régine	62, rue Saint-Lazare	75009 Paris
Hubert, Alain	8, rue Hoche	35-Rennes
Hudelo, André	3, rue de Cérisoles	75008 Paris
Hudelo, Jean	10, rue Galilée	75016 Paris
Hugonnier, René	Hôpital Edouard-Herriot, Pavillon C	69003 Lyon
Humeau, Marie-Françoise ..	Le Pavillon	14860 Ranville
Hurstel, Raoul	74, rue Rodier	75009 Paris
Hurstin, Albert	93, avenu Gambetta	75020 Paris
Ingignoli, Bernard A.	5, faubourg Saint-Jacques	26000 Valence
Iris, Françoise	7, boulevard Montparnasse	750006 Paris
Istre, Michel	26, rue Dr-Mazet	38-Grenoble
Jacquemaire, André	17, rue Gambetta	59-Douai
Jacquemart, Michel	24, rue Carnot	93-Noisy-le-Sec

Jacques, Roland	rue du Pont-de-Boulogne	80-Abbeville
Jambon-Genet, Madeleine ..	8, place Bellecour	69002 Lyon
James, Paul	2, avenue du Six-Juin	14-Caen
Janus, Yves	14, rue Dagobert-Fischer	67700 Saverne
Jarlot, Roger	3, place Gambetta	75020 Paris
Jarny, Jean	13, cours Cambetta	65-Tarbes
Jarry, Claude A.	58, boulevard d'Inkermann	92200 Neuilly-sur-Seine
Jarry, Claude	73, avenue Paul-Doumer	75016 Paris
Jayle, Gaëtan-Edouard	79, rue du Dr-Escat	13006 Marseille
Jeanrot, François	12, boulevard Carnot	81-Castres
Jeglot, André	2, rue Michel-Brodon	50-Saint-Lô
Jehanin, Herve	15, quai Lamartine	35-Rennes
Jezegabel, Claude	8, rue de Bordeaux	37-Tours
Jonquères, Jacques	67, boulevard Saint-Germain ...	75005 Paris
Joseph, Etienne	20, rue Alphonse-de-Neuville ...	75017 Paris
Joseph, Jean-Claude	27, rue Pasteur	85-La Roche-sur-Yon
Joullie, Robert	11 bis, rue de Lorraine	32-Auch
Jourdes, Jean-Claude	17, rue Borelly	12200 Villefranche-de-Rouergue
Jourdy, Pierre	6, rue Marcel-Renault	75017 Paris
Jousset, Michel .	9, boulevard Dubois	28-Dreux
Julien, Raymond-Georges ..	33, rue Condillac	33-Bordeaux
Jullich, Lucien	2, rue Général-Dagobert	50-Saint-Lô
Julou, Jean	5, rue Catulienne	93-Saint-Denis
Junod, Suzanne	111, rue Saint-Jacques	13006 Marseille
Kaminzer, Fernand	25, rue Edouard-Verpraet	59-Fourmies
Kastler, Mireille	1, rue du Val-de-Grâce	75005 Paris
Keraudy, Monique	3, rue du Pont	78510 Triel-sur-Seine
Kessis, Eugène		24-Cazoules
Klein, Marcel	161, rue de Tolbiac	75013 Paris
Koutseff, André	5, place de la Liberte	83-Toulon
Kraft, David	85, avenue du Général-Leclerc ..	75014 Paris
Krajevitch, Elianora	125, boulevard Saint-Germain ..	75006 Paris
Krebs, Alain	6, rue de Champagne	78200 Mantes-la-Jolie
Kreis, Françoise	7, rue Georges-Berger	75017 Paris
Laage de Meux, Patrice de .	6, boulevard Wilson	06-Antibes
Labatut, Robert	5, rue Drapès	89-Sens
Lachèze, Georges	avenue Victor-Hugo	19-Brive
Lacourt, Jean	9, avenue Reille	75014 Paris
Lacroix, André	Villa Gure Egoitya, Avenue des Fleurs	64100 Bayonne
Lafon, Anselme	6, place de l'Hôtel-de-Ville	30-Nîmes
Lafosse, Jean	88, avenue Parmentier	75011 Paris
Lagrange, Anne-Marie	28, rue Lauriston	75016 Paris
Laignier, Marcel	75 bis, avenue Marceau	75016 Paris
Lajoux, Jean	2, rue Parc	25300-Pontarlier
Laliam, Mohamed	22, rue d'Avejan	30-Alès
Lamouric, Jean Joseph	90, rue Nationale	56-Pontivy
Lançon, Michel	111, route Nationale de Saint-Louis	13015 Marseille
Lanfranchi, Jacques	35, boulevard Victor-Hugo	06-Nice
Langlois, Jean	15, rue Saint-Denis	76-Rouen
Lanthony, Philippe	37, rue des Archives	75004 Paris
Laporte, Bernard	52, rue de Paris	78-Maisons-Laffitte
Laporte, Pierre	7, rue de Silhol	07-Aubenas
Laporte, Pierre-M.	14, rue de l'Arquebuse	51-Reims

Lapras, Pierre	12, rue Picot	83-Toulon
Larmande, Aimé	Allée Brûlée	37-Chambray-lès-Tours
Laroche, Georges	2, avenue Victor-Hugo	92-Meudon
Laroche, Marie-Angèle	Hôpital de Montfermiel	93-Montfermeil
Laubies, André	93, avenue des Minimes	31-Toulouse
Laude, René	82, boulevard Général-Leclerc	59-Roubaix
Laulan, Jean	128, rue Croix-de-Séguey	33-Bordeaux
Laval, Marc	39, boulevard des Capucines	75002 Paris
Lebigre, Bernard	11, passage Lelong	95320 Saint-Leu-la-Forêt
Lebouc, Lucienne	8, rue Anatole-de-la-Forge	75017 Paris
Le Bourhis, Guy	17, avenue Colbert	83-Toulon
Le Bourhis-Martel, Jacqueline	5, rue du Calvaire	44-Nantes
Le Bozec, Ernest	8, rue Colbert	29-Brest
Le Breton Oliveau, Guy	32, rue Auvray	72-Le Mans
Lecaillon-Thibon, Bernard	4, rue des Jotglars	66000 Perpignan
Lecoq, Pierre, Joël	104, boulevard Arago	75014 Paris
Le Digabel, Patrick	10, place Mercadieu	31-Muret
Le Douaran, Louis	15, rue de Clisson	56-Lorient
Ledoux, Claude	146, boulevard Henri-Sellier	92-Suresnes
Lefouin, Martine	16, rue Auguste-Blanqui	94250 Gentilly
Lefranc, Daniel	17, rue Saint-Côme	17000 La Rochelle
Lefranc, Jacques	22, rue du Champ-Jacquet	35000 Rennes
Lefrère, André	12, rue de la Tour	85-Les Sables-d'Olonne
Legeard, Jean	Chemin La Marque	30-Bagnols-sur-Cèze
Legland, Jacques	41, rue Saint-Albin	59-Douai
Le Goff, Jean	17, rue Alfred-de-Musset	40-Dax
Legrand, Jules	11, rue Copernic	44-Nantes
Legras, Michel	16, rue Berteaux-Dumas	92200 Neuilly-sur-Seine
Legros, Jacques	109,cours National	17100 Saintes
Le Hunsec, Jean	5, rue Gustave-Flaubert, Résidence Parc-Château	33-Mérignac
Lelouch-Benichou, Jacqueline	39, avenue de Clichy	75017 Paris
Lemaire, Madeleine	115-119, rue Lecourbe	75015 Paris
Lemaitre, Jean	17, rue Belvalette	62-Boulogne-sur-Mer
Lemasson, Christian	2 bis, rue Carnot	16000 Angoulême
Léopold, Philippe	24, cours Louis-Berriat	38-Grenoble
Le Pape, Françoise	36, quai de Brest	29-Châteaulin
Le Petit, Jean	12, rue A.-M.-Javouhey	61-Alençon
Lepètre, Caroline	27, rue Saint-André-des-Arts	75006 Paris
Lépine, Bernard	8, rue Emile-Allez	75017 Paris
Lequin, Michèle	4, rue Sigorgne	71-Mâcon
Lerat, Marcel	7, rue Cassini	44-Nantes
Le Rebeller, Marie-José	108, avenue du Président-Robert-Schumann	33-Le Bouscat
Lesage, Daniel	11, rue A.-Huet	76-Le Havre
Lesage, Jean-Paul	23, rue Neuve-du-Patis	45-Montargis
Lescure, Francis	Ecole Vétérinaire	31-Toulouse
Lesenne, Edouard	30, rue Saint-Vincent-de-Paul	59-Roubaix
Lesoutivier-Lévy, Danièle	9, rue Dareau	75014 Paris
Leurent, Philippe	153, rue de la Bassée	59-Lille
Le Van, Nham	115, rue de Flandre	75019 Paris
Levasseur, Jean-Claude	21, rue Diderot	92-Asnières
Lévy, Jean-Paul	1 bis, rue Mozart	57-Metz
Lévy, Robert-Lucien	18, rue du Général-de-Castelnau	67000 Strasbourg

Levy-Carlotti, Janine	9, rue Albert-de-Lapparent	75007 Paris
Lhuillier, Pierre	43, rue des Tourneurs	31-Toulouse
Limon, Sylvie	4, rue Lagarde	75005 Paris
Liscoet, Hubert	25, rue de la Gare	22000 Saint-Brieuc
Lobstein, André	1, rue Saint-Thomas	67-Strasbourg
Lods, Francoise	24, rue Verdi	06-Nice
Lombard, Gabriel	175, rue de la Pompe	75016 Paris
Longo, Anne-Marie	3, avenue Maréchal-Lyautey	83-Hyères
Lorin, Pierre	1, avenue Leclerc	08200 Sedan
Lorrain, Alfred	47, boulevard Riquet	31-Toulouse
Loubère, Jean	15, rue Louis-Barthou	64-Pau
Louly, Raymond	6, rue Saint-Pol	59-Cambrai
Loyer, Jules	Clinique Sainte-Thérèse	22-Lannion
Lozivit, Pierre	11 bis, rue Massenet	06000 Nice
Luca, Francisca	22, rue Legendre	75017 Paris
Luce, Rémi	12, rue Paul-Souday	76-Le Havre
Lucot, Jean	9, rue Aimé Clément	05-Gap
Lumbroso, Pierre	25, boulevard Gergovia	63-Clermont-Ferrand
Lustig, Jacques	199, avenue Daumesnil	75012 Paris
Lustman, Marcel	99, rue de Longchamp	75016 Paris
Lyèvre, Jean-Jacques	12, Grande-Rue	25-Audincourt
Mage, Robert	4, rue du Grand-Mouton	36-Châteauroux
Magnard, Georges	40, rue Malesherbes	69006 Lyon
Magnard, Pierre	6, rue Sébastien-Gryphe	69007 Lyon
Malabre, Jean	8, avenue de la Libération	87-Limoges
Malbrel, Pierre	48, avenue Linné	59-Roubaix
Maleki, Medhi	29, avenue de la Motte-Picquet	75007 Paris
Malméjac, Nicole	54, rue Marcel-Sembat	78140 Velizy
Malnou, François	51, quai Aristide-Briand	19-Tulle
Malo, Camille	Polyclinique, avenue Florian-de-Kergorlay	14800 Deauville
Malterre, Michel	43, avenue Rockfeller	69003 Lyon
Maman, Maurice	136, boulevard National	13003 Marseille
Man, Hoang-Xuan	21, boulevard Saint-Germain	75005 Paris
Mandelkern, Jean-Claude	79, cours Fauriel	42100 Saint-Etienne
Mandonnet, Maurice	5, avenue de Grande-Bretagne	63-Clermont-Ferrand
Manent, Pierre	13, avenue de l'Esplanade	67-Strasbourg
Marchal, Eric	63, Promenade des Anglais	06-Nice
Marchal, Hélène	19, rue Félix-Faure	54-Nancy
Margaillan, Alain	14, rue J.-Labat	64-Bayonne
Margerin, R.	12, Avenue Montdigne	75008 Paris
Margo, Henry	45, rue de Poterie	50-Valognes
Maria, Yves	59, rue Spontini	75016 Paris
Marie, Albert	13 bis, avenue de Brazza	93-Noisy-le-Sec
Marigny, Gabriel de	Centre Hospitalier Régional	38000 Grenoble
Marion, Pierre	1 bis, rue Porte-du-Moustier	82-Montauban
Marmier, Robert	43, rue La Bruyère	75009 Paris
Marteret, Henri	10, Cité Malesherbes	75009 Paris
Marteville, Jean	26, rue des Minimes	41-Blois
Martin, André	91, avenue Hoche	92-Colombes
Martin, Georges	Les Chrysanthèmes, avenue Joseph-Reinach	04-Digne
Martin-Sibille, Yves	Ecole du Service de Santé Militaire, 14, avenue Berthelot	69007 Lyon
Martinez, André	22 ter, rue des Essarts	69500 Bron
Martinot, Pierre Philippe	18, rue des Otages	80-Amiens

Marx, Paul	2, rue Edouard-Gamelin	76-Mont-Saint-Aignan
Masclef, Pierre	186, boulevard de Créteil	94100 Saint-Maur-des-Fossés
Masingue, Pierre	7, avenue Saint-Roch	59300 Valenciennes
Massin, Marcel	5, Villa Jocelyn, square Lamartine	75016 Paris
Masson, Philippe	28, rue Jaillant-Deschainets	10-Troyes
Masson, Roger	8, place du Commerce	75015 Paris
Massonnet-Naux, Michelle	6, rue Nouvelle	49-Saumur
Massot, Jean	73 bis, rue Gilbert	86-Châtellerault
Mastagli, Louis-A.	2, rue Rameau	78-Versailles
Matavulj, Nada	Hôpital Civil, Clinique Neurologique	67-Strasbourg
Mathieu, Claude	34, rue de la Verrerie	75004 Paris
Maugery, Gilbert	158, rue Nationale	69-Villefranche-sur-Saône
Maugery, Jean-Philippe	24, chemin de Montriblond	69160 Tassin-la-Demi-Lune
Mauler, Jean-Jacques	Sainte-Fontaine	57-Freyming
Maussion, Lucien	29 bis, rue Pierre-Demours	75017 Paris
Mawas, Edouard	38, rue de Courcelles	75009 Paris
Mawas, Huguette	2, boulevard Suchet	75016 Paris
Mawas, Jacques	2, Boulevard Suchet	75016 Paris
Mawas-Pack, Lucie	32, avenue de Brimont	78400 Chatou
Mazel, René	107, rue des Bourguignons	92-Bois-Colombes
Mazuel, Rémy	220, avenue du Maine	75014 Paris
Medeiros, Francois de	14, rue Pigalle	75009 Paris
Meiffret, Alain	128, avenue de la République	83-Toulon
Meignan, Eugénie	58, avenue Diderot	94-Saint-Maur
Menager-Sangy, Paule	24, rue de Charenton	75012 Paris
Mercadier, Jacques	7, avenue du 22-Août-1944	34-Béziers
Mercier, Jacques	17, quai du Foix	41-Blois
Mercier, Jacques	56, avenue Julien	63-Clermont-Ferrand
Mergier, Jean	12, avenue Franklin-Roosevelt	92-Suresnes
Merigot de Treigny, Pierre	1, Square de Latour-Maubourg	75007 Paris
Merle, Claude	23, rue Paul-Bert	03-Moulins
Merle, Marie-Claude	41, rue de Reuilly	75012 Paris
Mesmay-Sillat, Blanche de	10, place du Collège	71-Chalon-sur-Saône
Métaireau, Jean-Pierre	6, place Edouard-Normand	44-Nantes
Metge, Paul	22, rue Bel-Air	13006 Marseille
Métral, Jean-Marie	9, rue Sala	69002 Lyon
Mettais, Pierre	23, avenue du Bel-Air	75012 Paris
Meunier, André	10, boulevard Chasles	28-Chartres
Meyer, Alain	71, rue Gambetta	52-Saint-Dizier
Meyer, Marie-Claude	29, boulevard Edgar-Quinet	75014 Paris
Meyniel, Joseph	20, place du Palais-de-Justice	15000 Aurillac
Michat, Georges	7, allée Paul-Riquet	34-Béziers
Michel, Augustin	39, boulevard de Montmorency	75016 Paris
Michel, Jean-Bernard	29, rue Manin	75019 Paris
Michel, Jean-Guy	Villa Arcadie, rue Auguste-Rencir, 140, rue de France	06-Nice
Miller, Henri	19, boulevard Beauséjour	75016 Paris
Minier, Yves	place de la République	65-Lourdes
Miroux-Orsatelli, Catherine	5, place de l'Abbaye	94000 Créteil
Modrin, Daniel	75, avenue Frédéric-Mistral	84100 Orange
Molkhou, Aline	2, avenue Henri-Dunant	93270 Sevran
Moncade, Jacqueline-Laure	56, rue Tiquetonne	75002 Paris
Mondon, Henri	77, boulevard Saint-Michel	75005 Paris
Monier, Raymond	9, avenue du 8-Mai	13-Aubagne
Monod, Francis-André	4, rue Saint-Vivien	17-Saintes

Monroux, Paul	5, rue Charles-Chautard	41100 Vendôme
Montauffier, René	7, rue Vauban	83-Toulon
Montibert, Jean	6, place des Jacobins	69002 Lyon
Montouroy, Roger	2, rue de Lesson	17-Rochefort-sur-Mer
Montoux, Pierre	3, rue Blanc-Dutrouilh	33-Bordeaux
Montvigner-Monnet, Régine	33, rue Félix-Chautemps	73200 Albertville
Morand-Baril, Danielle	38, avenue Foch	94-Fontenay-sous-Bois
Morault, Yves	16, rue d'Elbeuf	76-Rouen
Morax, Pierre V.	14, avenue Pierre-Ier-de-Serbie	75016 Paris
Moreau, Pierre	10, boulevard de la Trémouille	21-Dijon
Morel, Jules	56, rue Jean-Bart	59-Lille
Morel-Charron, Jacqueline	106, boulevard Jourdan	75014 Paris
Morin, Guy	23, rue Chartraine	27-Evreux
Moser, Michel	34, rue Denis-Papin	41-Blois
Mouillon, Michel	Centre Hospitalier de Grenoble, Service d'Ophtalmologie	38700 La Tronche
Moulinard, Louis	69, rue Saint-Blaise	61-Alençon
Mouls, Pierre	56, rue du Pavé-Blanc	92140 Clamart
Mourier, Jean-François	41, avenue de Saxe	69000 Lyon
Mouton, Jean	3, rue de l'Ecu	41-Romorantin
Mouzet-Bories, Madeleine	82, boulevard de la Marne	94-La Varenne Saint-Hilaire
Mugneret, Georges	12, rue Pelletier-de-Chambure	21000 Dijon
Mulsant, Jean	La Dépendaire	71840 Chevagny-les-Chevrières
Muratet, Jacques	1, rue du Général-Faidherbe	09100 Pamiers
Musset, Pierre	2, rue Saint-François	29 S-Quimper
Musso, Jean-Pierre	92, avenue de Grammont	37-Tours
Musso-Artigues, Eveline	23, rue Moncade	64-Orthez
Naneix, Georges	11, rue d'Alsace	49-Angers
Narodetzky, Boris	41, rue de Passy	75016 Paris
Nataf, Robert	1, avenue Auguste-Plat	91130-Ris-Orangis
Nataf, Roger	138, rue de Courcelles	75017 Paris
Nattaf, Simon	48, rue Monsieur-le-Prince	75006 Paris
Naudin, Pierre	4, avenue Thiers	77-Melun
Nayral, Georges	17, avenue Pétrarque	84200 Carpentras
Nextoux, René	127, rue du Faubourg-Poissonnière	75009 Paris
Nègre, Louis	85, rue de Rivoli	75001 Paris
Nguyen Van Ba	131, rue de Paris	93-Montreuil
Nicolas, Jean-Georges	91, rue Croix-de-Seguey	33-Bordeaux
Nordmann, Jean	28, rue Erwin	67 Strasbourg
Normand, Henri	37, avenue du Général-Leclerc	72-Le Mans
Offret, Guy	16, rue Logelbach	75017 Paris
Offret, Hervé Antoine	16, rue Logelbach	75017 Paris
Omar Askaryar, Mohammad	68, rue du Château-des-Rentiers	75013 Paris
Onfray, Michel	6, avenue de la Motte-Picquet	75007 Paris
Oppert, Georges	5, rue Mallet-Stevens	75016 Paris
Orliac, Pierre	38, boulevard Gambetta	46-Cahors
Ourgaud, Albert	5, boulevard Notre-Dame	13006 Marseille
Pagès, Robert	Résidence Le Richelieu, 50, avenue Albert-Camus	86-Châtellerault
Pallas, Max	21, rue Paul-Mamert	33-Bordeaux
Parizot, Hubert	12, rue Carnot	92-Bois-Colombes
Partiot, Guy	43, avenue de la République	94-Saint-Maur
Pataa, Claude	5, rue du Président-Roosevelt	03-Vichy
Patault, Marc	60, rue A.-Brunet	18-Vierzon

Prevost Boure, François	60, rue de la Bretonnerie	45-Orléans
Prévot, Georgés	23, rue de la République	45-Orléans
Prieur, M.	22, rue de Madrid	75008 Paris
Profizi, Jean Charles	7, rue Racine	83-Toulon
Prost, Jacques	29, rue Saint-Désiré	39-Lons-le-Saunier
Protais, Hélène	116, rue du Général-Leclerc	76000 Rouen
Prudhomme, Jacques	1, rue du Château-du-Roi	46-Cahors
Prudhommeaux, Pierre	6, rue Segrais	14-Caen
Pruvost, Francis	47, rue de Châteaudun	28-Chartres
Puistienne, Jacques	80, boulevard Général-Leclerc	59-Roubaix
Quentin, Jean	5, place Godinot	51-Reims
Quere, Maurice	247, avenue de Grammont	37-Tours
Queroix, Michel	39 bis, boulevard Husson	91-Viry-Châtillon
Quivy, Etienne	188, rue de Saint-Genès	33000 Bordeaux
Raffray, Jean	107, rue Jean-Jaurès	92-Puteaux
Ramain, Paul	26, rue Eugène-Mercier	51-Epernay
Ramanantsoa, Raymond	6, rue du Maréchal-Fayolle	13004 Marseille
Rampin, Serge	23, rue Thiers	13100 Aix-en-Provence
Ranoux, Arsène	10, boulevard Victor-Hugo	24100 Bergerac
Rapilly, Claude	6, avenue du 6-Juin	14-Caen
Raspiller, Antoine	Résidence Parc Olry, Entrée F, 91, avenue de Strasbourg	54000 Nancy
Ravault, Maurice	44, rue Montgolfier	69006 Lyon
Ravon, Paul	5, place de l'Hôtel-de-Ville	42-Saint-Etienne
Raynaud, Guy	62, rue Baudricourt	75013 Paris
Raynaud, Jean-Marie	8, Grande-Rue Jean-Moulin	34-Montpellier
Razemon, Philippe	54, rue de la Madeleine	59000 Lille
Reboul, Henri	5, place de l'ancienne Poste	26-Montélimar
Rechter, Odette	37, rue Julien-Lacroix	75020 Paris
Reeb-Schilovitz, Joëlle	2, rue Arthur-Papon	77-Gretz-Armainvilliers
Regnault, François, René	21, rue Croulebarbe	75013 Paris
Reich, Stéphane	85, avenue du Général-Leclerc	75014 Paris
Renard, Gabriel	16, Boulevard Raspail	75007 Paris
Renard, Georges	26, rue de Denver	29 N-Brest
Renaudin, Paul	47, B. rue Poincaré	67-Sélestat
Reny, André	Résidence Montet-Octroi, 8, Square de Liège	54500 Vandoeuvre-les-Nancy
Reny, Pierre	11, rue des Clercs	57-Metz
Reversé, Bernard	10, rue du Bailliage	76-Rouen
Reydy, Roger	Traverse les Rosiers, Bât. JN	13014 Marseille
Rey-Goetz, Marie-Louisie	87, avenue d'Altkirch	68-Mulhouse
Reynon, Marcel	7, place Gustave-Rivet	38-Grenoble
Richard, Yves	65, avenue du Dr-Arnold-Netter	75012 Paris
Rico, Marcel	6 bis, rue de Russie	06-Nice
Ricois, Daniel	19, rue Danielle-Casanova	77-Montereau
Rietzler, François-Xavier	9, quai d'Alsace-Lorraine	77000 Melun
Rigal, Jean-Marie	7, avenue Georges Clémenceau	34500 Béziers
Rigaud, Lucien	immeuble Olympe, 2, rue Franklin	66-Perpignan
Rigault, Claude	6, rue Flourens	34-Béziers
Rigord, Yves	6, avenue Clotis	83-Hyères
Riu, Robert	11, place général-de-Gaulle	20200 Bastia
Rivain, Annie	3, square Mont-Cassin	49000 Angers
Rivière, Roger	9, rue Goethe	75016 Paris
Rizzi, Claude	26, place du Peuple	42-Saint-Etienne

Robin, André	19, cours Bugeaud	87-Limoges
Robinet, Gérard	34, boulevard Carpeaux	59-Valenciennes
Roblot, Jean	13, boulevard Victor	75015 Paris
Roche, Charles	36, boulevard Gambetta	30-Nimes
Rocher, Jean	33, rue Saint-Patrice	76-Rouen
Roger, Jacques	21, rue Jean-Macé	29 N-Brest
Roger, Jean	105, avenue du Roule	92-Neuilly-sur-Seine
Rogez, Jean-Pierre	43, avenue de Paris	79000 Niort
Rognant, Jean-Yves	6, avenue des Thermes, Les Ambassadeurs	73-Aix-les-Bains
Rollat, Jean de	23 *bis*, boulevard Gambetta	52-Chaumont
Rollet, Jacques	3, place Bellecour	69002 Lyon
Rollin, Jean-Pierre	56, faubourg-de-Montbéliard	90000 Belfort
Romanet, René	37, rue Sommeiller	74-Annecy
Roques, Alain	5, rue du Lycée	06-Nice
Roques, Michel	11, rue Louis-Barthou	64000 Pau
Roquigny, Jean-Pierre	40, rue Benjamin-Constant	18200 Saint-Amand-Montrond
Rosan, Henri	5, rue Granvelle	25-Besançon
Roset, Georges	Clinique Sainte-Odile, avenue Foch	54-Longwy
Rossano, Roger	113, rue de la Tour	75016 Paris
Rossazza, Christian	39, rue Laponneraye	37000 Tours
Roth, André	Centre Hospitalier Universitaire .	25000 Besançon
Rouche, Robert	70, rue du Palais-de-Justice	77-Melun
Rouchy, Jean-Pierre	11, avenue Elisée-Reclus	75007 Paris
Rougerie, Michel	22, rue Salberie	49-Cholet
Rougier, Jacques	4, rue de la Charité	69002 Lyon
Routher, François	59, boulevard Pasteur	63-Clermont-Ferrand
Roumagnou, Jacques	boulevard Jean-Jacques-Rousseau.	13500 Martigues
Roussel, Paul	rue des Coquières, Bât. 1	13-Aubagne
Rousselie, Françoise	3, avenue Daumesnil	94160 Saint-Mandé
Rousselin, Claude	17, boulevard Victor-Hugo	78-Poissy
Roux, André	86, cours Lieutaud	13006 Marseille
Roux, Charles	9, rue de Faucigny	74-Sallanches
Roux, Henri	17, boulevard Laromiguière	12-Rodez
Roux, Madeleine	4, avenue de la Gare	71-Autun
Roux, René	24, rue Vaugelas	74-Annecy
Rouzaud, Paul	4, rue Marcel-de-Serres	34-Montpellier
Royer, Jean		Chatillon-le-Duc, par 25-Besançon
Royer, Michel	11, boulevard Anatole-France	93-Aubervilliers
Rüe, Christian de la	5, rue Tardif	14-Bayeux
Ruellan, Yves-Marie	10 *bis*, rue de Madame	78000 Versailles
Ruelle, Jeanne	197, rue Championnet	75018 Paris
Ruolt, Jean	29, faubourg National	67-Strasbourg
Ryzman, Paul	4, rue des Anglais	75005 Paris
Sacrez, Pierre	1, rue Pont-à-Seille, Tour Coislin.	57-Metz
Sageot, Marie-Claude	16, rue Claude-Groulard	76200 Dieppe
Saint-Martin, Olivier de	46, cours Victor-Hugo	33-Arcachon
Saïto, Tamotsu	1, rue A.-Gervais	92-Issy-les-Moulineaux
Sala, Robert	62-64, avenue de la République .	93-La Courneuve
Salmon, André	44, avenue Merlin	57-Thionville
Salvanet, Annie	40, boulevard de Charonne	75020 Paris
Samaran, Max	3, place du Réduit	64100 Bayonne
Sandère, Edmond	196, avenue de Versailles	75016 Paris

Santiard, Bernard	11, Grande-Rue	70-Gray
Santini, Gérard	11, rue Antheaulme	77-Nemours
Saracco, Jacques	21, avenue du Prado	13006 Marseille
Saraux, Henri	2, square Alboni	75016 Paris
Sarniguet-Badoche, Jeanne	123, rue de Reuilly	75012 Paris
Sauvan, Jean	7, place Félix-Baret	13006 Marseille
Schemmel, Alain	9, rue V.C. Artige	07-Aubenas
Schillaci-Ferrand, Geneviève	'Le Ribera', 523, rue Paradis	13008 Marseille
Schilovitz, Guy	2, rue Arthur-Papon	77-Gretz-Armainvilliers
Schmidt, Louis	35, rue Néricault-Destouches	37-Tours
Sedan, Robert	18, quai de Rive-Neuve	13007 Marseille
Ségur, Monique	20, rue des Platrières	94-Créteil
Seigneur, Benjamin	34, avenue de la Marne	92-Asnières
Semonin, Pierre	1, place F.-Rude	21-Dijon
Sénéchal, André	3, square Moncey	75009 Paris
Serpin, Gilbert	11 bis, rue Montlosier	63-Clermont-Ferrand
Seznec, Paul	26, rue Henri-Heine	75016 Paris
Siboni, Désiré	238, rue de Belleville	75020 Paris
Slaouti, Paul	Résidence Le Gambetta, 38, avenue Gambetta	23-Guéret
Smati, Abdel Hamed	7 bis, rue du Général-de-Gaulle	89-Sens
Sobrepère, Georges	17, rue des Abeilles	13001 Marseille
Sole, Pierre	Le Bassinet	53-Cunlhat
Solignac, Jean Alphonse	38, avenue du Château	94-Vincennes
Sorato, Mario	17, rue de la Bretonnerie	45-Orléans
Soulie, Claude	74, boulevard Beaumarchais	75011 Paris
Sourdille, Jacques	194 bis, rue de Rivoli	75001 Paris
Sourdille, Philippe	16, boulevard Guist'hau	44-Nantes
Sourdille, Pierre	23, rue du Quinconce	49-Angers
Spielmann, Claude	11, rue de la Ravinelle	54-Nancy
Spira, Claude	3, boulevard des Brotteaux	69006 Lyon
Stam, Colette	23, avenue des Chartreux	13004 Marseille
Stefanini, Jean-Paul	2, place Foch	20-Ajaccio
Steiner, Charles	24, rue de la Moder	67-Haguenau
Stintzy, François	2, Petite rue du Vieux-Marché-aux-Vins	67-Strasbourg
Storch, Bernard	31, rue Brisson	42-Roanne
Storch, Jean	6, place de Verdun	42300 Roanne
Subileau, Jean	60, rue de Londres	75008 Paris
Surugue, Paul	90, rue de Belleville	75020 Paris
Svilarich, Jean-Claude	76, rue Emile-Martin	18000 Bourges
Tabarly, Franck	65, rue d'Alsace-Lorraine	31-Toulouse
Tapie, Robert	79, cours Desbrey	33-Arcachon
Tardieux, Charles	57, boulevard Victor-Hugo	06-Nice
Tarlé, Emile	5, rue de la Monnaie	18000 Bourges
Tarris, Joé	2, rue Chartran	92-Neuilly-sur-Seine
Tassy, Alain	29, boulevard Georges-Clemenceau	13004 Marseille
Tatry, Christiane	24, rue Albert-Thuret	94-Chevilly-Larue
Teisseire, Josette	30, avenue Junot	75018 Paris
Temple, Jacques	23, rue de l'Aiguillerie	34-Montpellier
Terrassier, Jean-Jacques	16, rue du Moulin-de-Pierre	92130 Issy-les-Moulineaux
Tessier, Paul	26, avenue Kléber	75016 Paris
Teulières, Jean	19, cours de Verdun	33-Bordeaux

Thalabard, Joseph	Sous-Directeur du Service de Santé de la Première Région militaire, Q.G. du Camp des Loges	75998 Paris
Théron, Henri-Paul	22, rue du Dr-Lamare	78100 Saint-Germain-en-Laye
Thimen, Nathalie	50, rue Michel-Ange	75016 Paris
Thomas, Charles	133, rue Saint-Dizier	54-Nancy
Thomas, Robert	11, avenue Clemenceau	44-La Baule
Tibi, Armand	3, rue Victor-Duruy	75015 Paris
Timsit, Elie	71, avenue d'Arches	08-Charleville-Mézières
Tissot, Roger	14 *bis*, rue Jean-Jaurès	08-Sedan
Tognet, Jacques	23, rue Gambetta	42-Saint-Etienne
Torre, François	5, rue des Meuniers	94-Vincennes
Toubin, Josette	138, avenue Berthelot	69007 Lyon
Toufic, D. Nicolas	69, rue Haxo	75020 Paris
Touraille, Simone	64 *bis*, rue de Monceau	75008 Paris
Tranier, Guy	72, avenue des Pyrénées	33-Villenave-d'Ornon
Trémoulet, Odette	33, rue Félicien-David	75016 Paris
Trepsat, Christiane	5, avenue Foch	69006 Lyon
Troche, Maurice	10, rue Rémilly	78-Versailles
Tromeur, Yves	3, place Saint-Mathieu	29-Quimper
Tronche, Pierre	25, rue Marivaux	63-Clermont-Ferrand
Urgancioglu, Méri	Fondation ophtalmologique A.-de-Rothschild, 29, rue Manin	75019 Paris
Urvoy, Martine	Castel Saint-Martin, 4 *bis*, rue Saint-Martin	35-Rennes
Valdman, Jean-R.	35, avenue Foch	75016 Paris
Valery, Jean	18, rue Nungesser-et-Coli	75016 Paris
Vallès, André	119, rue Paradis	13006 Marseille
Valtot, Françoise	72, boulevard de Bercy	75012 Paris
Valty, Sylviane	65, boulevard des Invalides	75007 Paris
Vanhoutte, André	boulevard Louise-Michel	59-Somain
Velter, François	Chalet Marie-Thérèse	88-Saint-Dié
Verdickt, Pierre	103, rue de Beaumont	59-Roubaix
Vergez, André	4, rue Mignard	75016 Paris
Vergez, Marc	14, boulevard Carnot	31000 Toulouse
Vergne, Jean	172, avenue Jean-Jaurès	92-Clamart
Vergne, Pierre	6, rue Chambellan	21-Dijon
Vergnes, Roger	46, rue de Metz	31-Toulouse
Verin, Phillippe	54, rue de Verdun	33130 Bègles
Vermorel, Bernard	228, boulevard Raspail	75014 Paris
Veyrier, Bernard	17, Chemin de l'Ouest	30400 Les Angles
Viallefont, Henri	27, rue de Maguelone	34-Montpellier
Viateau, Alyse	7, Allée des Chênes	93-Clichy-sous-Bois
Viaud, Léonce	43, rue Gimelli	83-Toulon
Viaud-Hudlet, Catherine	45, rue Huguerie	33-Bordeaux
Vidal, Colette	14, place de la Corderie	16-Cognac
Vidal, Raoul	133 *bis*, avenue de Versailles	75016 Paris
Viel, Pierre	18, rue Alexandre-Legros	76-Fécamp
Viellard, Robert	12, place du Général-de Gaulle	71100 Chalon-sur-Saône
Vignat, Jean-Pierre	4, rue Léon-Lagrange	93160 Noisy-le-Grand
Vigo, Maurice	10, rue des Augustins	66-Perpignan
Vincent, Jean	7, avenue du Midi	87-Limoges
Vincent, Jean-Marie	31, rue Boulay-de-la-Meurthe	88-Epinal

Vitte, Gérard	57, rue de la Ravinelle	54-Nancy
Vittrant, Jacques	6, rue Racine	02200 Soissons
Vivié, Edouard	9, place de l'Hôtel-de-Ville	06-Cannes
Voegtle, Yves	place Louis-LaCombe	46100 Figeac
Voinot, Jacques	89, Grande-Rue	25-Besançon
Voisin, Jean	6, rue de Babylone	75007 Paris
Vola, Jean-Louis	La Pélissière, boulevard de Gabès, 455, avenue du Prado	13008 Marseille
Vouters, Jules	56, rue de Bourgogne	59-Lille
Wagner, Christian	70, avenue Gustave-Flaubert	76000 Rouen
Waksmann, Jacques	Centre médical, rue Sery	76-Le Havre
Wannebroucq-Leroyer Colette	132, route Nationale	59-Lille
Warter, Gérard	22, rue Monsieur-Le-Prince	75006 Paris
Wertheimer, Jean	82, boulevard des Belges	69006 Lyon
Wiart, Jean-Louis	6, avenue du 6-Juin	14-Caen
Wintzenrieth, Bayard	26, place de la République	87000 Limoges
Woillez, Marcel	118, rue Jacquemars-Gielée	59-Lille
Zapp-Decker, Renée	14, rue de la Vallée	57350 Stiring-Wendel
Zaretzki, Martine	78, rue Brillat-Savarin	75013 Paris
Zarrabi, Khosrow	28, rue Troyon	92310 Sèvres
Zenatti, Claude	54, Cours de Vincennes	75020 Paris
Zenatti-Lafargue, Josette ..	41, rue Pierre-Sémard	94370 Sucy-en-Brie

NOSOCOMIA QUIBUS OCULIS AEGRI CURANTUR

Chefs de Service et Consultations d'Ophtalmologie dans les Hopitaux de Paris et de Villes de Facultés

Paris

I. Etablissements de l'Assistance Publique

Ambroise Paré: Dr. Vergez
Beaujon: Dr. Sénéchal
Bicêtre: Prof. Agr. Aron
Bichat: Dr. Blancard
Broussais: Prof. Haye Christian
Cochin: Prof. Brégeat
Cretail: Prof. Coscas
Franco-Musulman (Bobigny): Dr. Voisin
Hérold (enfants): Dr. Voisin
Hôtel-Dieu: Prof. G. Offret
Laënnec: Prof. Agr. Auvert
Lariboisière: Prof. Agr. Saraux
Necker-Enf.-Mal: D. Polliot
Paul-Brousse: Prof. Agr. Aron
Pitié: Dr. Joseph, Prof. Agr. F. Rousselie
Saint-Antoine: Dr. Morax
Saint-Lazare:
Saint-Louis: Prof. Agr. M. Fontaine
Tenon: Dr. Forest
Trousseau (enfants): Dr. Campinchi

II. Etablissements indépendants de l'A.P.

Centre National d'Ophtalmologie des Quinze-Vingts (13, rue Moreau, Paris 12°)
Prof. Agr André Dubois-Poulsen, Dr. Denise Goddé-Jolly, Dr. Louis Guillaumat, Dr. Marcel Massin

Fondation Ad. de Rothschild (rue Manin, Paris 19°)
Dr. Edouard Mawas, Dr. Jean Garnem, Dr. Pierre Halbron, Dr. Paul Payrau

Hôpital Saint-Joseph, (1, rue Pierre-Larousse, Paris 14°)
Centre Médico-Chirurgical Foch (Suresnes: Dr. Vergez)

Angers
Clin. Opht. de la Faculté, Prof. Hermann

Besançon
C.H.U., Prof. Agr. Jean Royer

Bordeaux
Clin. Opht. de l'Un.: Hôp. Saint-André: Prof. Bessiere et Prof. Agr. Verin. Prof. Agr. Le Rebeller Marie-José
Hôpital des Enfants, Prof. Agr. Corcelle

Caen
Ecole Nation. de Médecine, C.H.R.: Dr. Prud'Hommeaux

Clermont-Ferrand
Clinique Annexe d'Ophtalmologie de la Faculté: Prof. F. Rouher; Dr. Sole

Dijon
Prof. Agr. Pierre Moreau

Grenoble
C.H.R. (La Tronche): Prof. J.-L. Bonnet

Lille
Clin. Opht. de l'Un.: Cité Hospitalière: Prof. Pierre François et Prof. Agr. Marcel Woillez
Clin. Opht. Fac. Libre: Disp. Saint-Philibert: Dr. Baude
Hôpital Militaire Scrive: Dr. Cl. Dehorter-Duez

Limoges
Clin. Opht. de la Faculté: Prof. Agr. André Robin

Lyon
Cliniques Ophtalmologiques de l'Université;
Hôpital de la Croix-Rousse: Prof. Georges Bonamour
    Maître de Conférence-Agrégée: Mme Mireille Bonnet
    Assistants-Chefs de Clinique: Dr. Malterre, Dr. M.-L. Pommier
Hôpital Edouard-Herriot: Prof. René Hugonnier
    Maîtres de Conférences-Agrégés: Dr. Maurice Ravault, Dr. Luc Durand
    Ophtalmologiste Chef de Service: Dr. R. Etienne
Hôpital Saint-Luc: Dr. Chavanne
Hôpital Saint-Joseph: Dr. Chauvire, Dr. Sermet
Hôpital Saint-Charles: Dr. Ilinca Bonnet
Hôpital Les Charmettes: Dr. Grange

Infirmerie Protestante: Dr. Arnal, Dr. Jean Wertheimer
Hôpital dispensaire Ecole Croix-Rouge à Bron: Dr. Spira, Dr. Charleux, Dr. M.-L. Pommier.

Marseille
Clin. Opht. de l'Université: Hôtel-Dieu: Prof. Jayle, Prof. Agr. P.-V. Berard, Prof. Agr. Saracco
Hôpital de la Conception: Prof. Agr. Ourgaud
Hôpital Saint-Joseph: Dr. Marcel Arnoux
Hôpital Nord: Prof. Farnarier, Prof. Agr. Saracco

Montpellier
Clinique Opht. Univ., Centre Gui-de-Chauliac (Clinique St-Eloi): Prof. Charles Boudet

Nancy
Clin. Opht. de l'Univ.: Hôpital Central: Prof. Ch. Thomas, Prof. Agr. Jacques Cordier, Prof. Agr.
    Bernard Algan, Prof. Agr. A. Reny

Nantes
Clin. Opht.: Prof. Legrand, Dr. Baron
Hôpital Saint-Jacques: Prof. Agr. Hervouet
Hôpital de l'Hôtel Dieu: Prof. Agr. Maurice Quéré

Reims
C.H.U., Docteur A. Burette

Rennes
Clin. Opht. Pontchaillou: Prof. Ardouin, Prof. Agr. Martine Urvoy

Rouen
Ecole Nationale de Médecine: Dr. Reverse

Strasbourg
Clin. Opht. de l'Université: Hôp. Civ.: Prof. Bronner
    Maîtres de Conférences Agrégés: Prof. Brini, Prof. Gerhard

Toulouse
Clin. Opht. de l'Université: Hôpital de la Grave: Prof. Calmettes, Prof. F. Deodati, Prof. Agr. P. Bec

Tours
Clin. Opht. du C.H.U.: Prof. Larmande

INSTITUTA SCHOLAEQUE CAECIS DESTINATAE

Quelques établissements spécialisés pour amblyopes

Nous n'avons pu, faute de place, fournir une liste complète. Les ophtalmologistes intéressés pourront se la procurer à la Fédération Nationale des Associations de Parents d'Enfants Déficients Visuels (F.N.A.P.E.D.V.), 28, place Saint-Georges, 75442 Paris, Cedex 09.

Allier, Yzeure, 'Les Charmettes', Institut Médico Pédagogique et Professionnel.

Bouches-du-Rhone, Marseille 6ème, Ecole de Déficients sensoriels, 77, Rue Grignan (G. et F.). Etablissement public, géré par le Ministère de l'Education Nationale.

Marseille 7ème, Institut Régional de Jeunes Sourds et Jeunes Aveugles, 3, Rue Abbé Dassy (G.). Géré par l'Association de Patronage de l'Institut Régional, 8, Montée de l'Oratoire, Marseille 7ème.

Marseille 7ème, Institut Régional de Jeunes filles aveugles, 8, Montée de l'Oratoire (G. et F.). Géré par l'Association de patronage de l'Institut (même adresse).

Cote d'Or, Dijon, 'Clos Chauveau' Centre de Rééducations spécialisées (G. et F.). Géré par l'Oeuvre des Pupilles de l'Ecole Publique de la Côte d'Or, 1, Place de la Banque.

Cotes du Nord, Plenee Jugon, Centre Educatif Rural d'aveugles (G). Géré par 'La Croisade des Aveugles', 15, Rue Mayet, Paris 6ème.

Haute Garonne, Ramonville Saint-Agne, Centre de Lestrade, Institut d'Education Sensorielle (G. & F.). Géré par l'Association pour la sauvegarde des Enfants Invalides, 22, Rue Croix Baragnon.

Ramonville Saint-Agne, Centre spécialisé d'Enseignement secondaire 'Le Parc Saint-Agne' (G. & F.). Dépend de l'Association pour la Sauvegarde des Enfants Invalides (22, Rue Croix Baragnon, Toulouse

Ramonville Saint-Agne, Centre Medico Professionnel (G. & F.). Géré par l'Association pour la Sauvegarde des Enfants Invalides (même adresse que ci-dessus).

Gironde, Bordeaux, Institution Régionale des Sourds Muets et Jeunes Aveugles, 61, Rue de Marseille (G).

Merignac, Centre pour faibles de vue: Avenue Aristide Briand (G. et F.). Géré par l'Association de Patronage, 61, Rue de Marseille, Bordeaux.

Talence, Institution des Jeunes Aveugles, Place de l'Eglise (G. et F.).

Ille-et-Vilaine, Rennes, Lycée de Bréquigny, 4 classes dispensant l'enseignement du ler cycle du second degré.

Indre-et-Loire, Tours, Institut Médico-Pédagogique 'Beau Site' (G. et F.). Déficients visuels de 6 à 16 ans.

Loire Atlantique, Chauve, Centre Educatif Ménager Rural d'Aveugles (F.). Dépend de la Croisade des Aveugles, 15, Rue Mayet, 75 Paris 6ème.

Nantes, Institut Départemental 'La Persagotière,' 30, Rue du Frère Louis (G. et F.).

Nantes, C.E.S. de la Géraudière, Annexe du Chemin des Landes.

Maine-et-Loire, Angers, Institut Montéclair Centre Hospitalier, (G. & F.). Géré par le Centre Hospitalier Régional d'Angers.

Marne, Reims, Institut Régional de Rééducation Sensorielle et Motrice, 4, Avenue du Général Eisenhower (Code postal: 51.100 Reims).

Meurthe-&-Moselle, Nancy, Institution des Jeunes Aveugles, 8, Rue de Santifontaine (Code postal: 54.000 Nancy).

Nancy, Beauregard (G. & F.). Lycee Georges de la Tour Avenugles et amblyopes-internat. Enseignement du second degré. Les élèves sont admis à partir de la classe de seconde.

Morbihan, Auray, Institution La Chartreuse (F). Géré par la Congrégation des Filles de la Sagesse.

Nord, Lille, Institution de Jeunes Sourdes et Jeunes Aveugles, 131, Rue Royale (F). Géré par la Congrégation des Filles de la Sagesse.

Ronchin, Institut Départmental des Sourds-Muets et Aveugles à Lille (G. & F.).

Puy-de-Dome, Clermont-Ferrand, Centre de Rééducation pour Déficients visuales, 30, Rue Sainte-Rose (G. & F.).

Clermont-Ferrand, Ecole Victor Duruy, Rue de Châteaudun.

Hautes-Pyrenees, Arrens, Centre Médico Professionnel Jean, Thébaud (Code postal Arrens 65.400 Argeles Gazost).

Bas-Rhin, Strasbourg, Centre Louis Braille pour déficients visuels, 80, Route de Neuhof (Code postal 67.100 Strasbourg). Géré par la Congrégation des Soeurs de la Croix.

Still, Institut des Aveugles (G. & F.). Géré par la Congrégation des soeurs de la Croix à Strasbourg.

Haut-Rhin, Illzach, Institut Médico-Pédagogique 'Le Phare' 16, Rue de Kingersheim (G. & F.).

Rhone, Lyon-Vaise (9ème), Institut des Jeunes Aveugles, 12, Rue Saint-Simon (G. & F.).

Villeurbanne, Ecole de Rééducation pour Déficients visuels, 20, Rue Louis Braille (G. & F.). Géré par l'Association Départmentale d'l'Oeuvre des Pupilles de l'Ecole Publique du Rhône. 52, Avenue du Maréchal Foch, Lyon 6ème.

Saone-&-Loire, Lugny, Institut Médico-Pédagogique de Cruzille.

Paris, Paris, 7ème, Institut National des Jeunes Aveugles, 58, Boulevard des Invalides (G. & F.). Organisme de tutelle: Ministère des Affaires sociales.

Paris, 7ème, Centre de Rééducation de l'Association Valentin-Haüy, 5, Rue Duroc (G. & F.).

Paris, 7ème, Centre Général des Aveugles en Rééducation, 11 ter, Rue Amélie (G. & F.).

Paris, 1 lème, Centre de formation professionnelle pour aveugles et grands infirmers, 59, Boulevard de Belleville (G. & F.).

Paris, 14ème, Institut d'Education Sensorielle pour Jeunes Filles Aveugles, 88, Avenue Denfert Rochereau (G. & F.).

Paris, 18ème, C.E.G. Rue Gustave Rouanet.

Seine Maritime, Meufmesnil- Offranville, Section spécialisée de C.E.T. (Collège d'Enseignment technique) (G. & F.).

Mesnil-Esnard, Centre pour amblyopes 'Normandie Lorraine' (G. & F.).

Yvelines, Marly-le-Roi, Centre de Réadaptation pour Aveugles récents, 3, Rue de Louvois (G. & F.).

Rambouillet, Lycée. A partir de la classe de seconde.

Tarn-et-Garonne, Montauban, Institut-Medico-Educatif pour Handicapés moteurs. Géré par la Sauvegarde des Enfants Invalides (Toulouse)

Var, Toulon, Ecole Publique de Plein air 'La valbourdine,' 10, Boulevard Bianchi.

Vienne, Larnay, près de Poitiers, Institution de Jeunes Sourds et de Sourds Aveugles (G. et F.). Géré par la Congrégation des Filles de la Sagesse à St. Laurent S/Sevre 85, Vendée.

Poitiers, Institution de Jeunes Sourds et Sourds Aveugles, 116, Avenue de la Libération (G.). Géré par l'Association de Patronage de l'Institution des Jeunes Sounds du Centre Ouest de la France.

Essonne, Chilly-Mazarin, Centre Educatif, 30, Avenue Mazarin (F.). Dépend de l'Association Valentin-Haüy, 5, Rue Duroc, 75 Paris 7ème.

Montgeron, Ecole Nationale pour déficients visuels, Code Postal 91230 Montgeron. Etablissement d'enseignment public. Garçons et filles déficients visuels (1/20° à 3 ou 4/10°) agés de 8 à 18 ans à l'admission.

Hauts-de-Seine, Saint-Cloud, Classes spécialisées annexées au C.E.T., 41, Rue Pasteur.

Val-de-Marne, Saint-Mande, Institut Départemental des Aveugles de la Seine, 7, Rue Mongenot (G. & F.).

Vitry, Ecole de Plein Air, 10, Rue de France. Classes de 6è, 5è, 4è.

GERMANIA (D.B.R.)

SOCIETATES OPHTHALMOLOGICAE

Nationalis

Deutsche Ophthalmologische Gesellschaft
Ständiger Sitz in Heidelberg
Vorsitzender: Prof. Dr. G. Meyer-Schwickenrath
Schriftführer: Prof. Dr. W. Jaeger, Univ. Augenklinik, Bergheimerstrasse 20, Heidelberg
Mitgliederzahl: 1528

Regionales

Rheinische-Westfälische Gesellschaft für Augenheilkunde
Vorsitzender: Prof. Dr. H. J. Küchle
Schriftführer: Dr. G. Berneaud-Kötz, Cronenfelderstr. 56, 56 Wuppertal-Cronenberg
Mitgliederzahl: 400

Württembergische Augenärztliche Vereinigung
Vorsitzender: Prof. Dr. H. Harms
Schriftführer: Dr. L. Schöninger, Charlottenstr. 21a, 7 Stuttgart-S
Mitgliederzahl: 200

Bayerische Augenärztliche Vereinigung
Vorsitzender: Prof. Dr. H. J. Merté
Schriftführer: Dr. C. Zenker, Augenklinik Herzog Carl Theodor, 8 München 19
Mitgliederzahl: 150

Vereinigung Rhein-Mainischer Augenärzte
Vorsitzender: Prof. Dr. H. J. Schlegel
Schriftführer: Dr. O. Remler, Hugenottenallee 116, 6078 Neu-Isenburg
Mitgliederzahl: 180

Berliner Augenärztliche Gesellschaft
Vorsitzender: Prof. Dr. Hugo Hager
Schriftführer: Prof. Dr. H. F. Tiburtius, Augenklinik des Klinikums, Hindenburgdamm 30, 1 Berlin-Steglitz
Mitgliederzahl: 80

Vereinigung Nordwestdeutscher Augenärzte

Vorsitzender und Schriftführer: Prof. Dr. W. Papst, Augenklinik des Allgemeinen
Krankenhauses, 2 Hamburg-Barmbeck
Mitgliederzahl: 300

NOMINA ET DOMICILIA MEDICORUM AB OCULIS

Abarbanell, Hermann	Vor der Burg 8	3300 Braunschweich
Abarbanell	Delinsweg 3a	2000 Hamburg 64
Abdullah, A.	Bahnhofstraße 15	8480 Weiden
Abele, H. J.	Lindenstraße 3	4000 Düsseldorf
Abels, Hans	M.-Luther-Straße 9	5110 Alsdorf
Adelstein, Prof. F.	Univ.-Augenklinik	6300 Gießen
Adelung, I. Ch.	Lange Straße 4	7941 Riedlingen
Adleff, Ernst	Bahnhofstr. 46e	4618 Kamen
Aengenheyster, G.	Bahnhofstr. 3	4430 Burgsteinfurt
Agricola, H.	Schwenckstr. 35	2000 Hamburg 19
Aigster, Hans	Weißenburger Straße	8480 Weiden
Albers, D.	Marienstraße 19	7000 Stuttgart 1
Albers, Werner	Imbuschweg 46	1000 Berlin 47
Albrecht, L.	Mainzer Straße 1a	5427 Bad Ems
Albrecht, Manfred	W.-Sollmann-Straße 107	5000 Köln-Weidenpesch
Alexandridis, Prof. Evangelos	Univ.-Augenklinik	69 Heidelberg
Allmaras, Peter	Isartalstraße 8/6	8000 München
Allmaras, Wolfgang	Starleiten 4	8192 Geretsried-Gartenberg
Althaus, Helmut	Vor dem Leetor 12	5460 Linz
Alt-Stutterheim, Annette v.	Marienweg 297	2000 Hamburg 63
Amann, L.	Obermünsterstraße 9	8400 Regensburg
Amara, Widad	Erich-Oldenhauer-Str. 5	4000 Düsseldorf-Garath
Amend, Werner	Wiesenstr. 14	3040 Soltau
Andree, Günther	Bundeswehrzentral-krankenhaus	5400 Koblenz-Metternich
Angele, Josef		7958 Laupheim Wtb.
Antoniadis, A.	Burghofstr. 12	4 Düsseldorf
Apetz, Heinrich	Eichhornstraße 28	8700 Würzburg
Appel, H.	Werlestr. 16	6148 Heppenheim
Appel, Nikolaus	Jungfernstieg 38	2000 Hamburg 36
Arens, Claus-Donat	Uhlandstr. 8	567 Opladen
Arens, Heinz Paul	Sülzgürtel 29	5000 Köln-Klettenberg
Aretz, Herbert	Königsberger Str. 108	4400 Münster
Armbrust, Michael	Bincknerstr. 8	6650 Homburg
Arndt, Gerhard	Wallstr. 16	2370 Rendsburg
Arnold, Marlies	Torstraße 21	7860 Schopfheim
Aryus, Karl	Pielsticker Straße 7	4300 Essen-Altenessen
Aryus, Walter	Max-Halbach-Straße 196	4330 Mülheim
Asmus, Joachim	Altenhagener Str. 2	5800 Hagen
Atzler, Peter	Kaiser-Wilh.-Straße 37	6700 Ludwigshafen
Aub, W.	Karlsplatz 4	800 München 2
Auert, Kurt	Weststr. 49	4700 Hamm
Augstein, Eva-Maria	Am Kloster 413	8762 Amorbach
Aulhorn, Prof. Elfriede	Univ.-Augenklinik	7400 Tübingen
Aust, Prof. Wolfram	Stadtkrankenhaus	3500 Kassel
Austermann, Gertrud	Ostallee 60	4816 Senne
Axt, Eva	Landauer Straße 8	6747 Annweiler

Baasner, Helga	Altenderner Str. 12	4600 Dortmund-Derne
Baberowski, W.	Stolbergstraße 3	4300 Essen-Borbeck
Babnik, Gisela	Klaus-Groth-Weg 30	3340 Wolfenbüttel
Bach, Ernst J.	Eichenstraße 5	8011 Kirchseeon
Bach, Jochen	Bahnhofstr. 5	821 Prien
Bahr, Felicitas	Bundesplatz 8	1000 Berlin 31
Ball W.	Walkürenallee 4	5600 Wuppertal-Elberfeld
Balmes W.	Niederstraße 79	4040 Neuß
Barkhoff, E. R.	Egbertstr. 12	4400 Münster
Barmeyer, H.	Köln-Straße 52	5040 Brühl
Barsewisch, B. v.	Universitäts-Augenklinik	8 München 2
Barth, Ingeburg	Wilhelm-Allee 124	3500 Kassel
Barthelmeß, G.	Flurstr. 17	85 Nürnberg
Bartikowski, R.	....	
Bartsch, Christine	Kellinghusenstr. 18	2 Hamburg 20
Bassenge, W. L.	Zaubzerstraße 41	8000 München 8
Basten, W.	Saaruferstr. 10	66 Saarbrücken 1
Bauer, Bernd	Hans-Thoma-Weg 8	7600 Offenburg
Bauer, Eduard	Hauptstraße 229	5650 Solingen
Bauer, Hans	Setzbergstraße 4	8182 Bad Wiessee
Bauer, Horst	Große Bleiche 12	6500 Mainz
Bauer, Rosemarie	Bismarckstraße 75	5650 Solingen
Bauereiss, H.	Königstraße 85	8500 Nürnberg
Bauke, Walter	Moselpromenade 7	5590 Cochem
Baumann	Bahnhofstraße 37-39	8783 Hamelburg
Baumann, F. J.	Günther-von-Maltzahn-Str. 3	808 Fürstenfeldbruck
Baumert, O. H.	Brunnenallee 35	3590 Bad Wildungen
Baumgärtner, F.	Muthstraße 15	7573 Sinsheim
Baumsteiger, L.	Steege 12	4902 Bad Salzuflen
Baurmann	Mühlenstraße 16	5305 Alfter-Odekoven
Bär-Lau, E.	Bendesdorfer Str. 100	2110 Buchholz
Bäßler, Horst	Rosengarten 3	2000 Wedel
Baßler, H.	Rosengarten 3	2000 Wedel
Bätke, H.	Marktstr. 9	3380 Goslar
Bäumges, Wolfgang	Sanderstraße 180	5600 Wuppertal-Barmen
Bayer, Wolfgang	Holtenauer Str. 3	2300 Kiel
Bäz, Detlef	Kuenstraße 78	5000 Köln-Nippes
Beaumont, Klaus	Keplerstraße 39	7990 Friedrichshafen
Becker, Günter	Obere Königstr. 9	3500 Kassel
Becker, Karl	Höninger Weg 204	5000 Köln-Zollstock
Becker, Margit	Promenade 109	6380 Bad Homburg
Beckershaus, F.	Rheinstr. 65	2940 Wilhelmshaven
Beckmann, Ferdinand	Kurfurstenallee 26	2800 Bremen
Beckmann, Victor	Alicenstr. 18	6300 Gießen
Beel, Fr. Th.	Paulusstr. 43	4350 Recklinghausen
Begall, E.	Kohlmarkt 7-15	2400 Lübeck
Begall, J.	Kohlmarkt 7-15	2400 Lübeck
Behme, Harald	Steinweg 16	3300 Braunschweig
Behrens, Ingeborg	Max-Eydt-Str. 42	3000 Hannover
Behringer, Hedwig	Voltastraße 1	8500 Nürnberg
Beier, Hilde	Widenmayerstraße 25	8000 München 22
Breuer, Kurt	Gerh.-Hauptmann-Weg	7290 Freudenstadt
Belger, Helmut	Göttinger Str. 3	3410 Northeim
Belina, Miroslav	Josef-Schneider-Straße	8700 Würzburg
Belling, Franz	Sullinger Str. 14a	2830 Bassum
Benkendorf, Kurt	Steinbrückstr. 9	2210 Itzehoe

Benn-Kluge, Karin	Am Heesberg 4	4131 Rheink.-Baerl
Bensel, Ursula	Zöllnerstr. 2a	2000 Hamburg-Bahrenfeld
Bentele, Bruno	Friedrichstraße 15	7990 Friedrichshafen
Benthien, Horst	Altonaer Bahnhofspl. 24	2000 Hamburg 50
Bentz, K. H.	Rich.-Wagner-Straße 31	6750 Kaiserslautern
Berbeck, Bärbel	Westring 15	4400 Münster
Berger, Arthur	Kortumstr. 19-21	4630 Bochum
Berger, A.	Karlstraße 37	7972 Tettnang
Berghöfer, H. U.	Löhrstraße 135	5400 Koblenz
Bergler sen., Karl	Holzgasse 16	8832 Weißenburg
Bergler jun., Karl-A.	Holzgasse 16	8832 Weißenburg
Bergmann, Hedwig	Wiehagen 44	4650 Gelsenkirchen
Bergmann, Ursula	Stadtkirchenplatz 4	7140 Ludwigsburg
Bernd, Willy	Ludwigstraße 54	6700 Ludwigshafen
Berneaud-Kötz, G.	Hahneberger Straße 77	5600 Wuppertal 31
Berners, F.	Hub.-Roggendorf-Str. 3	5353 Mechernich
Berthold, Wiltrud	Ohmstraße 7	8000 München 23
Bertram, Hans	Löhergraben 30	5100 Aachen
Bertram, R.	Kurfürstendamm 186	1000 Berlin 15
Beschließer, W.	Karlstraße 5	7418 Metzingen
Besser, Bernhard	Lüneburger Str. 30	2000 Hamburg-Harburg
Best, Prof. W.	Univ.-Augenklinik	53-Bonn-Venusberg
Bettinger, F.	Augensanatorium	7821 Hochenschwand
Beuningen, E. G. A. van	Max-Beckmann-Str. 14	6 Frankfurt 70
Beyer, Jürgen	Bongardstr. 21	4630 Bochum
Beyer, L.	Königsplatz 7-9	8710 Kitzingen
Beyer, W.	Holtenaustr. 3	Kiel
Beyer-Krause, A.	Wilhelmstr. 7	76 Offenburg
Beyhoff	Kieler Straße 5	5650 Solingen-Ohligs
Beyhoff, Helmut	Beethovenstraße 53	5320 Bad Godesberg
Bialasiewitsch, A.	Kurt-Schumacher-Str.	3000 Hannover
Bialluch, Jürgen	Ziegelstr. 26	2400 Lübeck
Bickel, C.	Alter Heuweg 17a	89 Augsburg
Biechele, H.	Obere Bachstraße 16	8440 Straubing
Biedermann, Viktor	Gugelstraße 136	8500 Nürnberg
Biedermann, L.	Elsässer Str. 27	2000 Hamburg 43
Bieger, Hans	Emser Straße 284	5400 Koblenz-Horchheim
Bieler, Rudolf	Bahnhofstraße 3	4060 Viersen
Bieling, Gerhard	Hauptstr. 34	4650 Gelsenkirchen
Bier, Gerda	Lenbachstr. 10	2000 Hamburg 52
Bierbrauer, Ruth	Am Rebenberg 9a	6621 Köllerbach
Biller, M.	Rosenheimer Straße 40	8202 Bad Aibling
Billing, Günther	Planie 10	7410 Reutlingen
Bischoff, Barbara	Düppelstr. 24	5800 Hagen
Bischoff, Hildegard	Zum Sebaldsbhf. 49	2800 Bremen
Bissing-Härtel von	Grunewaldstraße 10	1000 Berlin 41
Blachnitzky, Otto	Kopernikusplatz 17	8500 Nürnberg
Blaicher, Grete	Gartenstraße 14	7972 Isny
Blankenagel, Anita	Landfriedstraße 4	6900 Heidelberg
Blasel, Berthold	Schulstr. 3	3057 Neustadt
Blieffert, Irmgard	Südstr. 6-8	3300 Braunschweig
Blobner, Ferdinand	Klosterstraße 5	8640 Kronach
Blonski, Verena	Mittelring 9	3500 Kassel
Blum, Otto	Untere Nabburger Str. 38	8450 Amberg
Boateng, Asa	Westring 15	4400 Münster
Bock, Friedrich		3551 Michelbach-Marburg

Bock, Dietrich	Wolfsgraben 6	3440 Eschwege
Bock, Heinrich	Bahnhofstr. 3	4967 Bückeburg
Bockberg, Horst	Fuhlsbutteler Str. 94	2000 Hamburg 33
Boddin, Hans-Jürgen	Gartenstraße 48	7410 Reutlingen
Bodeewes, Dirk	Ittenbachstraße 15	4300 Essen
Boden, Friedrich	Berliner Str. 16	3360 Osterode
Boedecker, Ute	Ohkampring 9	2000 Hamburg 63
Boente, Franz	Große Str. 57	4500 Osnabrück
Boeschl, W.	Quirinstraße 30	5300 Bonn-Dottendorf
Boguth, Birgit	Josef-Stelzmann-Straße 9	5000 Köln-Lindenthal
Bohnen, Karl	Wilhelmstraße 4	5100 Aachen
Bokermann, Ludwig	Hochstr. 74	4660 Gelsenkirchen-Buer
Bollbach	Wilhelmstr.	6690 St. Wendel
Bolle, Franz	An der Marienkirche 3	2370 Rendsburg
Bolz, W. K.	Kasseler Str. 8	3580 Fritzlar
Bommer, Georg	Swolinkystr. 15	5800 Hagen-Haspe
Borchart, H.	Duisburger Straße 333	4100 Duisburg-Huckingen
Borgmann, Hans	Augenklinik Brüderkrankenhaus .	55 Trier
Borgmann, Hilde	Osterfelder Str. 1	4250 Bottrop
Bormacher, Hans	Grasshoffstraße 111	4300 Essen
Bornemann, E.	Freiheitsstr. 2a	4640 Wattenscheid
Bourwig, Hermann	Domagweg 17	3000 Hannover
Bovers, Erich		5223 Nümbrecht-Benrath
Böckenhoff, Irmgard	Ostwall 4	4290 Bocholt
Böckenhoff, Wenzel	Ostwall 4	4290 Bocholt
Böckenhoff, W.	Ostwall 4	4300 Essen-Holsterhausen
Böcker	Am Kloster 3	3030 Walsrode
Böger, Reinhard	Mundsburger Damm 60	2000 Hamburg 22
Bögel	Herzogswall 55	4350 Recklinghausen
Böhle, Günther	Massenbergstr. 26	4630 Bochum
Böhm, Heinz-Werner	Unkeler Straße 9	5000 Köln-Sülz
Böhme, H. J.	Ostfriesland	298 Norden
Böhme, Gert	Gartenstr. 66	6000 Frankfurt
Böhmer, Fritz	Gutenbergplatz 39	5770 Arnsberg
Böke, Prof. W.	Univers-Augenklinik	2300 Kiel
Börsch, Egon	Friedrichstr. 4	4390 Gladbeck
Bös, Rolf	Im Wohnpark 21	5159 Ahe
Brab, Wilhelm	Aachener Straße 17	5102 Würselen
Brachmann, Uwe	Wallstr. 16	7057 Winnenden
Brandes, Rolf	Mühlenstr. 10	3100 Celle
Brandis, Heinz	Berliner Str. 6	4830 Gütersloh
Brauer, Werner	Rübenacher Straße	5400 Koblenz
Brauer, Werner	Yorckstr. 7	3000 Hannover
Braun, Prof. Reinhard	Gildemeisterstraße 4	2850 Bremerhaven 2
Braun, W.	Ludwigstr. 9	823 Bad Reichenhall
Brauns, Karlrobert	Jahnring 4a	2000 Hamburg 39
Braunsburger, Egon		2130 Rotenburg/Han
Braus, Wolfgang	Mühlenstraße 12	7770 Überlingen
Brechtken, Anne	Logenstraße 10	6750 Kaiserslautern
Bredel, Eckhard	Mühlstr. 66	6100 Darmstadt
Bredner-Hirr, Almut	Neckarstraße 71	7300 Eßlingen
Bredner, Fritz	Neckarstraße 71	7300 Eßlingen
Breinlich, Richard	Bahnhofstraße 4	7120 Bietigheim
Bremer, Gisela	Gersthofer Str. 6	623 Frankfurt – Höchst
Brenig, Heinrich	Alhausstraße 6	5600 Wuppertal 2
Brennecke, Walter	Eichendorfstr. 9	3301 Wenden

Brentano, Hermann	Bundesallee 61/62	1000 Berlin 41
Bekuhrs, H.	Ostwall 79	4150 Krefeld
Brewitt, Horst	Röntgenstr. 1	3012 Langenhagen
Briel, Ilse	Bürresheimer Straße 10	5440 Mayen
Brinkman, H. J.	Neußer Straße 10	5000 Köln
Bröse, E.	Carl-Schurz-Straße 41	1000 Berlin 33
Brockmeier	Hinter dem Salze	3327 Salzgitter-Bad
Brohr, Adolf	Barbarinostraße 1	8263 Burghausen
Brossoy, Eva	Hauptstraße 77	5063 Overath
Broy, Roman	Dülferstraße 14	8000 München 45
Bruch, P. M.	Univ.-Augenklinik	6650 Homburg
Bruens, Hedwig	Limbecker Platz 7	4300 Essen
Bruhn, A.	Stadtweg 62	238 Schleswig
Bruncken-Seitz, Eva	Nebsallee 15	2930 Varel
Brunke, Helmut	Lange Reihe 39	2000 Hamburg 1
Brunn, Jürgen von	Kölner Str. 47	4600 Dortmund-Aplerbeck
Brunner, Horst	Chemnitzer Weg 2	7032 Sindelfingen
Bruns, Christoph	Fritz-Reuter-Str. 2	2350 Neumünster
Bruns, Karl-Heinz	Beim Ohlenhof 15	2800 Bremen
Bruns-Wolff, H.	Luisenstr. 6	757 Baden-Baden
Brust, K.	Mainzer Straße 187	6580 Idar-Oberstein
Brücker, Agnes	Ottostraße 80	8012 Ottobrunn
Brüning, Albert	Grafenberger Allee 67	4000 Düsseldorf
Buchholz, Ch.	Marktstraße 27	7107 Neckarsulm
Buchholz, Eckhard	Ludwigstraße 13	8530 Neustadt/Aisch
Buchler, Ivan	Görlitzer Str. 2	3014 Misburg
Buchmann, H. H.	Parkweg 3	3430 Witzenhausen
Budde, E.	Bolkerstraße 56	4000 Düsseldorf
Budde, Hans	Sonnenwall 19	4100 Duisburg
Budde-Irmer	Sonnenwall 19	4100 Duisburg
Buhmann, Gunther	Diekmoorweg 14	2000 Hamburg 62
Bullerdieck	Tübinger Straße 92	7000 Stuttgart-S
Bullerschen, H. H., II	Krefelder Straße 17	4140 Rheinhausen
Bumiller, Ernst	Steinstraße 85	8000 München 8
Bungart, Klemens	Moltkestraße 23	5180 Eschweiler
Bunge, Eduard	Niemannsweg 59	2300 Kiel
Bunge, H.	Hasselbreite 5	2400 Lübeck-Moisling
Burhans, Magdalena	Baustraße 32	4100 Duisburg-Meiderich
Burk, Arnold	Falkenburgsweg 1	2000 Hamburg 92
Burk, Martin	Chrysander Str. 32	2050 Hamburg-Bergedorf
Burkhard, D.	Salzdahlumer Str. 90	33 Braunschweig
Burmeister, Heinrich	Rauschener Ring 17a	2000 Hamburg 70
Burmester, Fr.	Marktplatz 10-12	7410 Reutlingen
Burstin, Dorothea v.	Zähringer Straße 2	7600 Offenburg
Buschbaum, F.	K.-Lang-Str. 25	6208 Bad Schwalbach
Buse, Franz	Saarlandstr. 56	4600 Dortmund
Busse, Frowald	Eisenbahnstraße 40	7613 Hausach
Busse, Ortwin	Trierer Str. 24	3000 Hannover S 12
Butscher, Paul	Ringstraße 80	6780 Pirmasens
Bücking, Willi	Schonnebeckhöfe 164	4300 Essen-Katernberg
Bücking, L.	Schonnebeckhöfe 164	4300 Essen-Katernberg
Bühring, Kamilla	Kantstraße 64	1000 Berlin 19
Büning, K. Anton	Kesterkamp 35	4630 Bochum-Linden
Bürck, K. H.	Gartenstr. 22	6101 Groß-Bieberau
Büsing, Helmut	Königstr. 50	2200 Elmshorn
Büthe, Friedrich	Moerser Straße 220	4132 Kamp-Lintfort

Büttner-Wobst, W.	Heckinghauserstr. 57	56 Wuppertal-Barmen
Cause, Ludwig	Gutenbergplatz 1	6500 Mainz
Chamrad, Hans	Heußnerstraße 40	5600 Wuppertal-Barmen
Christ, F.	E.-Schmiewind-Straße 22	5604 Neviges
Chudzinski, Lothar	Rembrandtstraße 24	4300 Essen
Cimbal, Otto	Holsteinstr. 32	2400 Lübeck
Cizel, Vilim	Joh.-Philipp-Straße 3-4	5500 Trier
Claas, Werner	Prinzipalmarkt 11	4400 Münster
Clad, Renate	Ungsteiner Str. 12	67 Ludwigshafen
Claus, Siegfried	Wilhelmstr. 35	3070 Nienburg
Claussen, Joh.	Sievekingallee 76	2000 Hamburg 26
Clemente, Paul	Nymphenburger Str. 43	8000 München 2
Colditz, Heinz	Harkotstr. 60	4600 Dortmund-Hombruch
Comberg, D.	Wolfenbütteler Str. 82	33 Braunschweig
Commichau, F.	Pleugestr. 2a	3000 Hannover-Rickling- hausen
Condereit, J. Maria	Dechaneistr. 1	4400 Münster
Conrad, Dora	Friedrichstraße 7	7580 Bühl
Conrad, Friedrich	Kieler Str. 71	2330 Eckernförde
Conrads, Hans	Markt 4	4440 Rheine
Cordes, Reinhard	Lavaterweg 15	2000 Hamburg 52
Cramer, Agnes	Husaner Wald 83	7290 Freudenstadt
Cremer, G. G.	Gottorpstr.	2900 Oldenburg
Cremer, Max	Hermannstraße 15	7200 Tuttlingen
Cruse, Claus	Bismarckstr. 92-94	2390 Flensburg
Cullmann, B.	Schillerstr. 7	6202 Wiesbaden-Bieberich
Cuntz-Schüßler, E.	Burgstr. 3	62 Wiesbaden
Curschmann, Volker	Wredestraße 55	6700 Ludwigshafen
Custodis, Prof. E.	Berliner Allee 61	4000 Düsseldorf
Custodis, Michael	Laufener Straße 3	7800 Freiburg
Cüppers, Prof. C.	Friedrichstr. 13	6300 Gießen
Dahlström	Hauptstr. 70	6603 Sulzbach
Dahmann, F.	Bahnhofspl./Losseaustr. 5	8630 Coburg
Dalheimer	Goethestraße 15	4020 Mettmann
Dalhoff, Ernst	Katharinenstr. 6	4500 Osnabrück
Damaske, Eckart	Westring 15	4400 Münster
Damm, Josef	Königsallee 22	4000 Düsseldorf
Dammers, M.	Bismarckstr. 11	694 Weinheim
Dangschat, Klaus	Bahnhofstraße 40	5050 Porz
Dannheim, Helmut	Daimlerstraße 11	7000 Stuttgart-Bad Cann- statt
Dannheim, Reinhard	Univ. Augenklinik	74 Tübingen
Dardenne, Prof.	Graf-Stauffenberg-Str. 36	5300 Bonn
Darrelmann	Husemannstr. 77	4650 Gelsenkirchen
Daus, M.	Marktstraße 30	8170 Bad Tölz
Davids ....: ...	Pius-Allee 4	4400 Münster
Davids, Jürgen	Am Nachtigallen-wäldchen 21 ..	4053 Süchteln
Dähler, Herbert	Wechselpfad 7	4300 Essen-Heisingen
Däumer, Wilhelm	Berliner Straße 91	1000 Berlin 27
Debes, M.	Ebert-Pl. 17	5090 Leverkusen
Decker, Franz de	Knulsbarg 30	2000 Hamburg 55
Deckner, Siegfried	Steinweg 2	6000 Frankfurt
Deecke, Rüdeger	Hansastr. 18	2000 Hamburg 13
Dehe, Karl-Heinz	Hilbertstraße 4	1000 Berlin 49
Dehler-Birkholz, Herta	Mariengasse I	7570 Baden-Baden
Deicke, Hertmann	Dirolfstraße 18	6520 Worms

Deinhard-Sommerlad, U. ..	Bahnhofstr. 1	287 Delmenhorst
Deinlein, Hans	Obere Karl-Straße 16	8520 Erlangen
Deitmar, Lidger	Im Bockeloh 4	5870 Hemer
Demeler, U.	Univ.-Augenklinik	2 Hamburg 20
Demeler, Walter	Bahnhofstraße 31	7140 Ludwigsburg
Demmler, N.	Augenklinik der Techn. Hochschule R.d.I.	8 München
Denden, A.	Univ.-Augenklinik	3400 Göttingen
Denzer, G.	Weserstraße 58	1000 Berlin 44
Deppner	Trierer Str. 11	6602 Dudweiler
Dereskewitz, Johannes	Münchener Straße 116	2800 Bremen
Derkmann, Karl	Hauptstraße 26	7230 Schramberg
Derksen, Gisela	Bornheimer Landstr. 73/II	6000 Frankfurt
Dettmann, Heti-Ruth	Albrecht-Dürer-Straße 14	4006 Erkrath
Dettmering, M.	....	3513 Vaake-Süd
Dettmering, Wolrad	Rothenburger Str. 2a	6000 Frankfurt/M.NO. 14
Deuchler	Kaiserstr. 136	6670 St. Ingbert
Didion, Hans	Jahnstr. 3	3558 Frankenberg
Dieckhues, Prof. B.	Univ.-Augenklinik	44 Münster
Diehl, K. E.	Bergerstr. 85	6000 Frankfurt
Diehn, J.	Promenade 37	6380 Bad Homburg
Diener, Fritz	Goldstr.	4400 Münster
Dietrich, Gerhard	Kaiser-Max-Straße 44	8950 Kaufbeuren
Dietrich, Herbert	Markt 7	3370 Seesen
Dietze, H. H.	Königstr. 20	5760 Neheim-Hüsten
Dillschneider	Picardstr. 48	6610 Lebach
Dinger, G.	Frankfurter Str. 56	5 Köln-Mülheim
Dinter, Eva	Koblenzer Straße 14	5430 Montabaur
Dinter, Wolfgang	Koblenzer Straße 14	5430 Montabaur
Dippel	Markusallee 39a	2800 Bremen
Distelmaier	Münsterplatz 22	5300 Bonn
Dittmann, A.	Frankfurter Str. 2	5960 Olpe
Dittmann, M.	Ostertorwall 14	3250 Hameln
Dix, Ursula	Gildenstraße 7	4200 Oberhausen
Doden, Prof.	Ludwig-Rehn-Str. 14	6000 Frankfurt 70
Dodt, Prof. E.	W.-Kerckhoff-Institut	635 Bad Nauheim
Doelle, Hans	Marienstr. 8	3000 Hannover
Doemens, Karl	Barmbecker Str. 36	2000 Hamburg 39
Doerr, Guido	Bismarckstraße 4	7440 Nürtingen
Doerth, Fr.-Aug.	Kl. Salinenstr. 7	2060 Bad Oldesloe
Dohme, Bruno	A. Bernauer Straße	8000 München-Laim 42
Dohmes, Heinz-Bernd	Ernst-Sievers-Str. 13	4500 Osnabrück
Dolgner, Brigitte	Neuburger Straße 26	8900 Augsburg 10
Doremieux, Iris	Hauptstraße 13	7640 Kehl
Dorff, Wilhelm	Bismarckstraße 7	7550 Rastatt
Dorlöchter, Günther	Auf dem Damm 64	4100 Duisburg-Meiderich
Döderlein, Annemarie	Winterthurstraße 3	8000 München 49
Döhmen, Hellmut	Ostwall 152	4150 Krefeld
Döring, Franz	Marktplatz 30	8948 Mindelheim
Döring, Lore	Landsberger Straße 16	8948 Mindelheim
Dörnhöfer, A.	Elisabethstraße 1	8593 Tirschenreuth
Drabik, Klaus	Bergmannstraße 51	4330 Mülheim
Draeger, Prof. J.	St.-Jürgen-Straße	2800 Bremen
Dragutin	Augenkl. Brüderkrankenhaus ...	5500 Trier
Drechsel-Foerster	Elberfelder Straße 44	5630 Remscheid
Dreher, H.	Wolfg.-Wilh.-Platz 171	8858 Neuburg

Dreisel, Günther	Bernstr. 10	3000 Hannover
Drenkhahn	Kleinflecken 37	2350 Neumunster
Drescher Helga	Monbachweg 1	7220 Schwenningen
Duesberg, Hilda	Sonnenallee 47	1000 Berlin 49
Dunker, Werner	Aberstraße 2	4000 Düsseldorf
Duntze, J.	Oswaldstraße 29	8220 Traunstein
Dunzer	Mainzer Str. 28	6600 Saarbrücken
Durchschlag, Gert	Wundsb.-Marktstr. 69/71	2000 Hamburg 70
Dutescu, Mircea	Josef-Ponten-Straße 15	5100 Aachen
Düll, Ch.	Rügshöferstraße 24	8723 Gerolzhofen
Dünbier, Hermann	Markt 1-7	4040 Neuß
Dünkel, Elisabeth	Moorstr. 3	4490 Papenburg-Bokel
Düring, W. G.	Altstadtmarkt 13/14	3300 Braunschweig
Dyck-Denkhaus, G.	Brünckenstr. 14	2210 Itzehoe
Dyckerhoff, D.	Adolfsallee 27/29	62 Wiesbaden
Echte, Walter	Hugo-Preuß-Str. 9	3500 Kassel
Eckert, Jörg	Wölblinstraße 33	7850 Lörrach
Eckert-Harries, Lotte	Lockst. Steindamm 1	2000 Hamburg-Lockstedt
Eckhardt, Rolf	Richard Kirchner Str. 35	359 Bad Wildungen
Eckhardt, Ruth	Kölnische Str. 4	3500 Kassel
Eckold, Kurt	Niederstraße 22	1000 Berlin 41
Ederer-Wiegmann, J.	Regener Straße	8372 Zwiesel
Edler, Günter	Schillerplatz 6	6750 Kaiserslautern
Edlich, Helmut	Grüne Str. 7	5970 Plettenberg
Eggers, J. W.	Siebenbuchen 16a	2000 Hamburg 55
Eggert, W.	Konstanzer Straße 37	6900 Heidelberg
Ehrengard v. Lympius	Stollmannplatz 1	4830 Gütersloh
Ehrich, Prof. W.	Univ.-Augenklinik	6650 Homburg
Eichholtz, Wolfg.	Bühlstr. 21	3400 Göttingen
Eichhorn, K.	Triebstraße 18	8450 Amberg
Eickemeyer	Alte Landstraße 116	5090 Leverkusen 3
Eilers, H.	Schillerstraße 6	8672 Selb
Einhauser, C.	Waldfriedhofstraße 92	8000 München 55
Eisfeld, Max	Dom-Pedro-Straße 8	8000 München 19
Elben, Adolf	Hohenzollernring 2-10	5000 Köln
Elbrechtz, Johann	Leineweberstraße 33	4330 Mülheim
Eller, Bernd	Kurfurstenstraße 4	4300 Essen
Ellerhorst, M. J.	Hauptmarkt 17	5500 Trier
Ellermann, Maria	Degerstraße 50	4000 Düsseldorf
Ellgering, Eva-Maria	Markt 5	5340 Bad Honnef
Elling, Ilse	Lindwurmstraße 203	8000 München 15
Elschnig, H.	Hauptbahnstr. 20	75 Karlsruhe-Durlach
Elshorst, Karl	Weichselstraße 14	4000 Düsseldorf-Lierenfeld
Elsken, B.	Schuldstr. 3-4	4600 Dortmund-Hörde
Elster, Wolfgang	Obere Königstr. 20	3500 Kassel
Elze, Karl	Mühlenstr. 28	2950 Leer
Emmel, Gerhard	Lessingstr. 4	6420 Lauterbach
Emmerich, R.	Wenzelgasse 16	5300 Bonn
Encke, K. J.	Bockstr. 93a	4350 Recklinghausen
Engel, Gerd	Eschersheimer Landstr. 273	6000 Frankfurt
Engel, H. J.	Ostpreußenweg 2a	3260 Rinteln
Engel, W.	A.-Ladebeckstr. 6	4800 Bielefeld
Engelbrecht, Dieter	Schloßstr. 66b	6100 Darmstadt
Engelbrecht, Gisela	Buchauer Straße 17	8000 München 71
Engelbrecht, W.	Frankfurter Str. 41	6100 Darmstadt
Engelking, Prof. Ernst	Bergheimer Straße 20	6900 Heidelberg

Engelking, L.	Fasanenstr. 32	506 Bensberg-Frankenhorst
Engelmann, Margot	Albrechtstraße 132	1000 Berlin 41
Engelbrecht, Dieter	Voigtelstraße 23	5000 Köln 41
Epphardt, Christa	Ploener Str. 19a	2420 Eutin
Erben, Wilh.	Starenweg 7	8033 Krailling
Erdmann, Joachim	Hans-Böckler-Straße 17	4140 Rheinhausen
Erdmann, L.	Marienstraße 1	5160 Düren
Erdmann, Rudolf	Rennbahnstr. 28	2000 Hamburg 34
Erdniss, Helga	Mainkai 36	6000 Frankfurt
Ernst, Karl	Essenweinstraße 6	7500 Karlsruhe 1
Ernst, W.	Opferstr. 4	4950 Minden
Ertel, Rolf	Barmbecker Str. 191	2000 Hamburg 39
Esser, Hans	Nordstraße 90	4000 Düsseldorf
Esser, J.	In den Höfen 14	585 Hohenlimburg
Esser, Lucie	Albrechtpl. 11	4150 Krefeld
Esser, Rolf	Lambertistr. 16	4390 Gladbeck
Etscheit, Hans	Nikolausstr. 18	6228 Eltville
Euler, H. H.	Nienburger Str. 10	3000 Hannover
Ewald, Paul	Drosselweg 6	5043 Erftstadt
Ewen, Kurt	Schwabstraße 56	7000 Stuttgart
Eychmüller, W.	Wagnerstraße 10	7900 Ulm
Eyer, A.	Bahnhofsallee 3	635 Bad Nauheim
Fabian, Dietrich	Weulbrandtsweg	2861 Werschenrege
Fahr, Hans	Rotbühlplatz 19	7000 Stuttgart-S
Fahrnholz, Otto	Halserstraße 30	8390 Passau
Falkenroth	Hansaplatz 2	4600 Dortmund
Fangmann, Paul	Goebenstraße 47	4200 Oberhausen
Farkas, Ladislaus	Severinstraße 83	5000 Köln
Fassin, W.	Ostwall 209	4150 Krefeld
Faulborn	Universitäts-Augenklinik	78 Freiburg
Faulhaber, Werner	Rahd. Str. 9	4992 Espelkamp-Mittwald
Faust, Paula	Hohe Str. 29	4408 Dülmen
Fauth, Ernst	Moltkestr. 10	2300 Kiel
Fechner, D. U.	Georgstr. 6	3000 Hannover
Fecht	Parkstraße 15	4048 Grevenbroich
Fecht, W.	Behringstr. 3	6600 Saarbrücken
Fehmann, Wolfgang	Hansastr. 20	4600 Dortmund
Feireiss, D.	Breste Straße 16	1000 Berlin 33
Feldmann, Ernst	Rheinallee 50	5320 Bad Godesberg
Feldmann, Ina	Dr.-Julius-Leber-Str. 13	2400 Lübeck
Feller, Hans	Reichsstr. 5	3340 Wolfenbüttel
Fendel, H.	Pfuhlgasse 28	5400 Koblenz
Fenner, E.	Gasstraße 1a	6750 Kaiserslautern
Fenner, Klaus	Grabenseestr. 13	3100 Celle
Fenstermann-Harms, H.	Reichsb. Str. 7	2000 Hamburg-Eidelstedt
Fertl, Walter	Hohenzollernstraße 88	8000 München 13
Feuersenger, Chr.	Paschestr. 40	5800 Hagen
Feurig, Günter	Bismarckstraße 104-106	5630 Remscheid
Fickenday, Gisela	Neugrabener Bhfstr. 14a	2104 Hamburg 92
Fiedler, Ursula	Rahlstedter Str. 165	2000 Hamburg 73
Fiedler, W.	Rahlstedter Str. 165	2000 Hamburg 73
Filbry, G.	Hans-Gentner-Straße 2	8570 Pegnitz
Fingskes, B.	Lange Str. 126	2870 Delmenhorst
Fischbach	Rob.-Koch-Straße 7	8903 Haunstetten
Fischer, A.	August-Ruf-Straße	7700 Singen
Fischer, A.	Birkhahnweg 14	8000 München 13

Fischer, A.	Sanderstraße 50	8900 Augsburg
Fischer, F. W.	Marktplatz 25	7407 Rottenburg
Fischer, G.	Gruberzeile 69	1000 Berlin 20
Fischer, H.	K.-Wilhelm-Straße 84	1000 Berlin 46
Fischer, Heinz	Bahnhofstr. 47	4590 Cloppenburg
Fischer, H.	Kochberg 8	2350 Neumünster
Fischer, J.	Gr.-Flottb.-Str. 2a	2000 Hamburg-Großflottb. 1
Fischer, Lisa	Fabrikstraße 8	6750 Kaiserslautern
Fischer, M.	Marktplatz 61a	8833 Eichstädt
Fischer, S.	Gr.-Flottb.-Str. 2a	2000 Hamburg-Großflottb. 1
Fischer, Ulrich	Altheimer Eck 3	8000 München 2
Fischer, W.	Suchardstraße 18	5600 Wuppertal
Fischer-Geiger, Ingeborg	Carl-Schurz-Straße 33	1000 Berlin 20
Fischer-Wasels, C.	Eidelstedter P.	2000 Hamburg-Eidelstedt
Fischer-Wingendorf, H.	Thomasstraße 17	4152 Kempen
Fitz, H.	Oberhausenerstr. 166	433 Mühlheim-Styrum
Flamm, P.	Mittelstr. 19	2000 Norderstedt 2
Flamm, Peter	Mittelstr. 19	2000 Norderstedt 2
Flamminger, Jörg	Pettenkofer Straße 2	6700 Ludwigshafen
Fleck, Dieter	Westl. K.-Friedr.-Str. 70	7530 Pforzheim
Fleckner, W.	Im Ilmenautal 5	3118 Bevensen
Fleischer, E.	Jochensteinstraße 3	8500 Nürnberg
Fleischer, F.	Brandenburg 22	5583 Zell
Fleischer, H. P.	Hospitalstr. 39b	3560 Biedenkopf
Fleischhauer, H.	Elisabethstraße 25	4000 Düsseldorf
Fleischhauer, H. D.	Moltkestr. 4	4600 Dortmund
Flick, H.	Am Jägergarten 4	6650 Homburg
Flux, R.	Univ.-Augenklinik	7400 Tübingen
Foerst, Jürgen	Luisenstraße 3	5270 Gummersbach
Foerster-Fahnenbrock, Sybille	Grünstr. 76	4320 Hattingen
Förster, M.	Kaiserstr. 16	6000 Frankfurt
Förster, Walter	Frankfurter Str. 6	6233 Kelkheim
Franceschi, Nada	Klosterstraße 37	5000 Köln 41
Francu, Viorel	Wenzelstraße 6	5100 Aachen
Frank, Hans	Sandstr. 47	5900 Siegen
Frank, Kurt	Fürther Straße 176	8500 Nürnberg
Franke, J.	Uferstraße 12	5600 Wuppertal-Barmen
Franke, Rolf	Friedrichstr. 3	6070 Langen
Frehse, Karl-Dietrich	Heidelberger Straße 34	5000 Köln-Buchforst
Freier, Sigried	Wanheimer Straße 74	4100 Duisburg
Freigang, Manfred	Josephsplatz 20	8500 Nürnberg
Frerk, H.	Simeonstraße 8	5500 Trier
Fressel, A.	Am Kreuze 51	3400 Göttingen
Freund, Jochen	Univ.-Augenklinik	3550 Marburg
Freundorfer, A.	Fürstenr.-Straße 8	8000 München 42
Frey, Erna	Agnesstraße 53/II	8000 München 13
Frey, L.	Rathausplatz 11	8070 Ingolstadt
Freyberg, Hartmut	Berliner Str. 31-35	6236 Eschborn
Fricke, T.	Süder von Bentheimstr. 4	Bremen
Friedburg, Prof. D.	Moorenstraße 5	4000 Düsseldorf
Friederich	Friedrichstr. 43	5860 Iserlohn
Friedrich, Hermann	Neuhauser Straße 14	8000 München 2
Friedrichs, W.	Rossdörfer Str. 71	6100 Darmstadt
Frisch, Reimar	Wilhelm-Raabe-Str. 3	2970 Emden
Fritz, A.	Lange Str. 4	3257 Springe

Frohmann, C.	Maximilianstraße 47	8900 Augsburg
Fromberg, Günter	Hulser Straße 6-8	4150 Krefeld
Fröhner-Leidig, J.	Bohnstr. 21	2208 Glückstadt
Fröschel, Josef	Meichelbeckstraße 7	8952 Marktoberdorf
Früh, D.	Bahnhofstr. 19	64 Fulda
Frydrychowicz, G.	Bergerstr. 218	6000 Frankfurt/M.N.O. 14
Fuchs, Prof. J.	Am Eichenhain 38	7000 Stuttgart-Sillenbuch
Fuchs, Rudi	Karl-Janssen-Str. 7	6620 Völklingen
Fuchs, R.	Knappsch.-Krankenhaus	6603 Sulzbach
Fuhler, A.	Schützenstr. 23	4470 Meppen
Fuhler, Vera	Schützenstr. 23	4470 Meppen
Fung, Reginald	Am Heidenbaum	4401 Laer
Funke, Ruprecht	Goebenstraße 73	4200 Oberhausen
Funke, V.	Viktoriastraße 5	7520 Bruchsal
Funken-Orlowski, M.	Beseler Str. 461	2000 Hamburg-Großtlottb. 1
Fuß, W.	Ziethenstraße 4	5000 Köln-Weidenpesch
Füchte, H.	Hagsche Straße 68	4190 Kleve
Gaab, R.	P 6, 22	6800 Mannheim
Gabel, V. P.	Univ.-Augenklinik	8 München 15
Gaedertz, Prof. A.	Kisslinger Straße	8183 Rottach-Egern
Gärtner, J.	Univ.-Augenklinik	65 Mainz
Gaigl, A.	Eltinger Straße 9	7250 Leonberg
Galanski, W.	Kurfürstendamm 117	1000 Berlin 31
Galitionow, Alexand.	Gerberweg 18	5238 Hachenburg
Ganescu, Georg	Lindenstraße 48	5205 St. Augustin 2
Gareis, R.	Rich.-Wagner-Straße 66	8580 Bayreuth
Garreis-Helferich, E.	Marienkrankenhaus	6 Frankfurt
Gasteiger, Prof. H.	Hohenzollerndamm 112	1 Berlin 33
Gauß, H.	Silberburgstraße 168	7000 Stuttgart-S
Gebauer, P. C.	Brückenweg 1	5678 Wermelskirchen
Gebb, H.	Mainzer Landstr. 127	6000 Frankfurt
Gebhardt, Bärbel	Münchener Straße 46	8025 Unterhaching
Gehrig, H.	Altstadt 260	8300 Landshut
Geib, H.	Augustiner Straße 1	6720 Speyer
Geilenbrügge, A.	Lessingstr. 9	5880 Lüdenscheid
Geisel, H.	Brückenstraße 47	6900 Heidelberg
Geißendörfer, Erwin	Schonlinderweg 1	8592 Wunsiedel
Geller, F.	Schenkelstraße 13	5160 Düren
Geller, P.	Wilhelmstraße 111	5100 Aachen
Gembusch, G.	Kleinbahnstr.	459 Cloppenburg
Genée, E.	Univ.-Augenklinik	852 Erlangen
Gensler, Heinz	Unterl. Straße 49	7000 Stuttgart-Zuffenhausen
Gerhard, H.	Wasserhohl 8	6702 Bad Dürkheim
Georg, F.	Bergstr. 1	4502 Bad Rothenfelde
Georgi	Gmünder Straße 10	7060 Schorndorf
Georgiadis, Petros	Hohfuhrstr. 11A	5880 Lüdenscheid
Gerhard, H.	Wasserhol 15	Bad Dürkheim
Gerl, Rolf-Hellmar	Frankenstraße 304	4300 Essen-Bredeney
Gerlach, Knut	Marienstr. 14a	4450 Lingen
Gerloff, K.	Gartenstraße 6	6540 Simmern
Gerloff, W. D.	Bahnhofstraße 19	8450 Amberg
Gernet, Prof. Hermann	Westring 15	4400 Münster
Gesche, Rosemarie	Deutzer Freiheit 8	5000 Köln-Deutz
Geserick, Heinz	Hannoversche Str. 2	3100 Celle
Geusen, L.	Karlplatz 5	4000 Düsseldorf
Geyer, O. C.	Bahnhofstr. 12	633 Wetzlar

Geyer, Paul	Hopfgartenstr. 5	6202 Wiesb.-Bieberich
Giede, H.	An der Ochsenwiese	6450 Hanau
Giering-Gunkel, M.	Lindensteige 57	7972 Tettnang
Gieschen, A.	Gr. Bäckerstr. 15	314 Lüneburg
Gillert-Grüber, J.	Rüdesheimer Straße 6	1000 Berlin 31
Glaessgen, H. K.	Untere Schildwache 3	3380 Goslar
Glage, E.	Hagenmarkt 18	33 Braunschweig
Glasmacher, H.	Bundeskanzlerplatz	5300 Bonn 1
Glaßer, W.	Castroper Str. 30	4600 Dortmund-Mensede
Glatzel, B.	Univ.-Augenklinik	65 Mainz
Glauert, Gerda	Tulpenstraße 5	1000 Berlin 45
Glees, Prof. M.	St.-Elisab.-Krankenhaus	5000 Köln-Hohenlind
Glissmann, Volker	Londoner Straße 2	5300 Bonn-Auerberg
Glück, A.	Grabenstraße 1	7320 Göppingen
Goebl, E.	Luisenstraße 4	6520 Worms
Goecke, M.	Augenabteilung St. Josefsstift	28 Bremen
Goede, Martin	Wandelfeld 22/24	3141 Deutsch-Evern
Goetze, Ingeborg	Wiesenstraße 116	8500 Nürnberg
Goldschmidt, W.	Max-Fiedler-Str. 1a	43 Essen
Gondessen, H.	Pferdemarkt 17	2400 Lübeck
Gonnermann, H.	Bahnhofstr.	3578 Treysa
Gonschorek, G. H.	Fischerstraße 63	4100 Duisburg-Wanheimerort
Gorbahn, Fritz	Nordstr. 16	5810 Witten
Gorzny, Fritz	Hohenstaufenring	5400 Koblenz
Gottesbüren, B.	Univ.-Augenklinik	74 Tübingen
Gottesleben, H. U.	Vesenbergerstraße 634	7832 Kenzingen
Gottwald, Helmut	Kopbacherweg 29a	6300 Gießen
Goy, E.	Eschersh. Landstr. 415	6000 Frankfurt
Göb	Klöttschen 59	4330 Mülheim
Göldner, E.	Alfred-Brehm-Platz 14	6000 Frankfurt
Görtz, Prof. Heinz	Phillipstr. 2	5880 Lüdenscheid
Görtz, Gisela	Königstraße 41	4050 Mönchengladbach
Göß, H.	Campestraße 3	8500 Nürnberg
Gößling-Ebhardt, E.	Leher Heerstraße 11a	2800 Bremen 17
Götz, W.	Brauerei Götz	7487 Scheer
Graat, W. de	Kasinostraße 13-15	4100 Duisburg
Graeber, Prof. W.	Salzdahlumer Str. 90	3300 Braunschweig
Graefe, Ekkehardt	Kefersteinstr. 9	3140 Lüneburg
Graefe, H. J.	Welserstraße 10	1000 Berlin 30
Graepel, Hartwig	Schutzenstraße 18	8600 Bamberg
Graetz, W.	Schloßstraße 93	1000 Berlin 41
Graf, F.	Kaiserstraße 34	7520 Bruchsal
Graf, M.	Engelfriedhalde 9	7400 Tübingen
Grafer, K. F.	Ostwall 212	415u Krefeld
Graft, Gerd	Kilianstraße 2	7100 Heilbronn
Gramberg-Danielsen	Hallerstr. 25	2 Hamburg 13
Grasbon, W.	Univ.-Augenklinik	8 München 15
Grasser, E.	Altstadt 18	83 Landshut
Graßner, E.	Altstadt 18	8300 Landshut
Graupner, K. C.	Briennerstraße 44	8000 München 2
Graus, Adolf	Merziger Str. 50	6683 Dillingen/Saar
Greber, K. H.	Lenauplatz 3	5000 Köln-Ehrenfeld
Grefe, K. J.	Kleekamp 4	2000 Hamburg-Fuhlsbüttel
Greiner, Karl	Kronacher Straße 19	8620 Lichtenfels
Greite, H. J.	Univ.-Augenklinik	8 München 15
Grembusch, G.	Kleinbahnstr.	4590 Cloppenburg

Gresch, Wolfgang	Holm 70	2390 Flensburg
Grethe, Heinz	Gymnasiumstraße 31	7100 Heilbronn
Grevsmühl	Schießgraben 10	3140 Lüneburg
Grewe, J. F.	Kaiserstraße 44	6660 Zweibrücken
Grewe, Rolf	Frauenburgstr.	4400 Münster
Grimm, Ursula	Textorstr. 17	6000 Frankfurt
Gritzmann, A.	Hussenstraße 34	7750 Konstanz
Gröger, H.	Am Drosteipark 5	2080 Pinneberg
Gröger, H.	Goethestr. 41a	208 Pinneberg
Grohmann, R.	Lorenzstraße 64	1000 Berlin 45
Grohmann, Ulrich	Kurt-Schumacher-Str. 4	3300 Braunschweig
Gros, G.	Südanlage 11	6300 Gießen
Gross, Felix	Trützschlerstraße 8	6800 Mannheim
Gross, P.	Univ.-Augenklinik	8 München 15
Groß, G.	Münchener Str. 17	6000 Frankfurt
Groß, Ruth	Teltower Damm 33	1000 Berlin 37
Große-Ruyken, F. J.	Kaiser-Josef-Straße 180	7800 Freiburg
Großmann, S.	Hellweg 105	4600 Dortmund-Brackel
Grote, S.	Roßmarkt 9	8720 Schweinfurt
Grube, Johannes	Mendelsohnstraße 11	7000 Stuttgart-Sillenbuch
Gruber, Christian	Bahnhofstraße 24	8220 Traunstein
Gruber, I.	Rüdesheimer Str. 6	1 Berlin 33
Grubert, Harro	Auguststraße 37	5000 Köln-Nippes
Grümer, Gertrud	Königswall 16	4350 Recklinghausen
Grünenthal, Horst	Markt 5	1000 Berlin 20
Grunwald, Hartmut	Am Waldrand 53	2401 Groß-Grönau
Grüning, Heinz	Univ.-Augenklinik	6650 Homburg
Grüninger, Waltraud	Bahnhofstr. 74	4540 Lengerich
Grüninger, W.	Bahnhofstr. 72	4540 Lengerich
Grüterich, E.	Lohfeldstr. 3	4650 Gelsenkirchen
Grützner, Prof. Peter	Univers.-Augenklinik	7800 Freiburg
Gscheidel, E.	Elisabethenstraße 15	7000 Stuttgart
Gscheidel, S.	Myliusstraße 6	7140 Ludwigsburg
Guhl, H. A.	Bahnhofstraße 1	7460 Balingen
Guhr, Albert	Farmsener Landstr. 193	2000 Hamburg-Volksdorf
Guizetti, G.	Ostwall 3	4600 Dortmund
Gummert, Hans	Heinr.-Welt-Allee 88	2800 HB-Huchting
Gust, A.	Burgstr. 1	699 Bad Mergentheim
Gustav, Alice	Herm.-Löns-Str. 6	6650 Homburg-Altstadt
Gutsch, R.	Kleinschmidstr. 7	6000 Frankfurt-Eschersheim
Guttenberg	Habsburgerstraße 10-12	8000 München 13
Guttw.-Malagurski, L.	Schwabstraße 87	7012 Fellbach
Gutzeit, Heinz	Neutorstr. 89	2970 Emden
Gutzeit, Klaus	Wilhelmitorwall 17	3300 Braunschweig
Gülzow, E. S.	Holstentor 11	2370 Rendsburg
Güntsche, Joachim	Am Hexempfad 28	6450 Hanau
Günkel, M.	Kaiserstraße 20	5200 Siegburg
Gürich, H.	Kölner Straße 95/97	4047 Dormagen
Gütl, Walter	Kirchröder Str. 84	3000 Hannover-Kleefeld
Gütle-Nückel, B.	Stockmannstraße 104	4200 Oberhausen
Haack, Ruth	Kölner Tor 32	4000 Düsseldorf-Gerresheim
Haase, Adolf	Kisseleffstr. 11	6380 Bad Homburg
Haase, W.	Bramkoppel	2000 Hamburg 68
Haass, Karl	Bahnhofstraße 18	4060 Viersen
Habernoll-Klüner	Bahnhofstr. 55	4710 Lüdinghausen
Hackelbusch, K.	Dr.-Wilh.-Klingh.-Str. 16	2840 Diepholz

Hacker, Gisela	Bonner Talweg 53	5300 Bonn
Hadamzyck-Kaiser, E. M.	Neugrabener Bhfstr. 8b	2104 Hamburg 92
Haellmigk, Christian	Sandburgsteige 4	7100 Heilbronn
Haellmigk, C.	Kilianstr. 2	71 Heilbronn
Hagen, D. von	Erkstraße 1a	1000 Berlin 44
Hager, Prof. H.	Univ.-Augenklinik	1 Berlin Steglitz II
Hager, Ilse	König-Wilh.-Straße 1	7900 Ulm
Hahn, Helmut	Frankfurter Str. 48	6300 Gießen
Hahne, Rolf	Schlieffenstraße 84	5600 Wuppertal-Vohwinkel
Haist, Helmut	Kirchstraße 31	7320 Göppingen
Halbauer, J.	Breite Str. 25	3000 Hannover-Kleefeld
Hallermann, Lieselotte	Soleanderstraße 28	4000 Düsseldorf
Hallermann, Prof. W.	Univ.-Augenklinik	34 Göttingen
Halmai, Zoltan	Grabenstr. 7	2223 Meldorf
Hamann, Hans	Mülheimer Straße 58	4100 Duisburg
Hammer, K.	Karlstr. 95	6100 Darmstadt
Hammers, H.	Kalker Hauptstraße 194	5000 Köln-Kalk
Hamzei, Drawad	Frankenheimstraße 1	5000 Köln 41
Hanney, F.	Kaiser-Friedrich-Straße 46	1000 Berlin 12
Hanrath, Eva-Maria	Hohenstaufenallee 18	5100 Aachen
Hanssen, G.	Hopfengarten 19	3340 Wolfenbüttel
Hanxleden, Ursula v.	Staufenstraße	7812 Krozingen
Harder, Siegfried	Westfalenstr. 16	4660 Gelsenkirchen-Buer
Harff, Fritz	Marktstr. 48	4800 Bielefeld
Harms, Prof. H.	Schleichstraße 12	7400 Tübingen
Hart, A.	Münsterplatz 32	7900 Ulm
Harth	Hainstraße 9	8600 Bamberg
Hartleb, R.	Klusestr. 4	4780 Lippstadt
Hartleio, Norbert	Gasselstiege 196	4400 Münster
Hartmann, A.	Residenzstraße 128	1000 Berlin 51
Hartmann, R.	Münchener Straße 35	8120 Weilheim
Hartmann, F.	Jakobiwall 4	4420 Coesfeld
Hartmann, Heinz	Browerskamp 7	4530 Ibbenbüren
Hartwig, H. F.	Neckarstraße 23	7240 Horb
Haselbeck, J.	Bachstraße 5	8430 Neumarkt
Haselmann, G.	Augenklinik Städt. Krkh. St. Jügenstr.	28 Bremen
Hasenbein, Editha	Bartensteiner Straße 2	2800 Bremen
Hassel, R.	Bergstr. 99	5800 Hagen
Hasslinger, Claus	Leutstettenstraße 1	8130 Starnberg
Hasslinger, K.	Außere Maximilianstr. 1	8100 Garmisch-Partenkirchen
Hassovna, J.	Große Str. 31	4503 Dissen
Hauck, Doris	Hagener Allee 87	2070 Ahrensburg
Haugwitz, M. v.	Univ.-Augenklinik	6 Frankfurt
Haugwitz, Thilo v.	Kabelstieg 2	2000 Norderstedt 1
Haupeltsnofer, H.	Promenade 7	8800 Ansbach
Hauschild, E.	Seestr. 17	6460 Gelnhausen
Hausknecht, C.	Alter Fischmarkt 8	4400 Münster
Haussmann, W.	Grabenstraße 1	7312 Kirchheim-Teck
Hauß, H.	Karlsgasse 2	6720 Speyer
Havenstein, F.	Talbahnstraße 16	5190 Stolberg
Havers, Joseph	Kopernikusstraße 6	5320 Bad Godesberg
Häckl, F.	Rathausstraße 3	8200 Rosenheim
Heberer, Rosemarie	Biebricher Allee 109	6202 Wiesbaden-Bieberich
Heberling. K.	Wielandstraße 17	6900 Heidelberg
Heck, Joachim	Weender Str. 31	3400 Göttingen

Heckenhahn, K. H.	Augenklinik	6603 Sulzbach
Hecking, Eugen	Am Hauptbahnhof 10	4300 Essen
Heckmann, Bernd	Hohenzollernstr. 51	3000 Hannover-Kleefeld I
Heckmann, Christa	Fregestraße 58	1000 Berlin 41
Heckmann, D.	Appelstr. 15	3000 Hannover-Herrenhausen
Heckmann, Karl-Heinz	Schierker Straße 29	1000 Berlin 44
Heckmann, Klaus	Irenenstr. 1	62 Wiesbaden
Hegler, Hans	Glockengießerwall 6	2 Hamburg 1
Heilmann, Klaus	Augenklinik Rechts der Isar	8 München
Heimann, Klaus	Univ.-Augenklinik	5 Köln-Lindenthal
Heimburg, A. v.	Bei der Doppeleiche 3a	2 Wedel
Hein, H. J.	Badstr. 53	1 Berlin 65
Heinemann, K.	Humperdinckstr. 6	4 Düsseldorf-Benrath
Heinen, H.	Aachener Str. 631	5 Köln-Braunsfeld
Heinhold, P.	Ringstr. 13	7238 Oberndorf
Heinmüller, G.	Königsau 6	4780 Lippstadt
Heinrich, I.	Univ.-Augenklinik	65 Mainz
Heinrich, K.	Feldstr. 5	4830 Gütersloh
Heinrichs	Parlamentstr. 1	5600 Wuppertal
Heinrici, U.	Hauptstr. 39	2 Hamburg-Billstedt
Heinsius, Prof. E.	Rathenaustr. 35	2 Hamburg 39
Heintz, G.	Gerh.-Rohlf-Str. 35	28 HB-Vegesack
Heinze, K.	F 1. 1	Mannheim
Held, A.	Bahnhofstr. 15	44 Münster
Helferich, L. H.	Fürther Freiheit 12	8510 Fürth
Hell, G.	Allersbergerstr. 61	85 Nürnberg
Helldörfer, F.	Obere Hauptstr. 18	805 Freising
Hellmich, H. R.	Bahnhofstr. 12	352 Hofgeismar
Hellner	Martinistr. 52	2 Hamburg 20
Hengst, W.	Münsterstr. 7	483 Gütersloh
Henneberger, Ch.	Landshuter Str. 17	8493 Kötzting
Hennig, D.	Am Marktplatz	6798 Kusel
Hennighausen, H.	Schellengasse 4	632 Alsfeld
Henrich, C.	Kurfürstenstr. 19	53 Koblenz 32
Henssler, E.	Lassbergstraße 2	7710 Donaueschingen
Hentschel, E. M.	Eschersheimer Landstr. 9	6 Frankfurt
Hentschel, F.	Kronbergerstr. 5	6 Frankfurt
Herbst, W.	Alte Holsten Str. 9	2000 Hamburg-Lohbrügge
Hermann, D.	Brienner Straße II/II	8000 München 2
Hermann, F. K.	Viersener Straße 15	4052 Dülken
Hermann, H.	Hermannstraße 27	5450 Neuwied
Hermann, Irene	Bergweg 28	8172 Lenggries
Hermann, Klaus	Arndtstr. 2c	4800 Bielefeld
Herminghausen, Tewes	Kirchhofallee 56	2300 Kiel
Herrich-Schäfer, Käthe	Landshuter Straße 51a	8400 Regensburg
Herrlein, E.	Stuttgarter Straße 65	7000 Stuttgart-Feuerbach
Herzog, F.	Kammgasse 7	1000 Berlin 28
Herzum, Herwig	Bergstr. 9	6651 Schwarzenacker
Herzum, K.	Sallinger Straße 16	8340 Pfarrkirchen
Hesse, W.	I, 16-17	6800 Mannheim
Hetsch, Fritz	Osterstr. 161	2000 Hamburg 19
Heuberger	In der Vahr 65	2800 Bremen
Heydorn, R. J.	Mülheimer Straße 60	4300 Essen-West
Heyer, Herbert	Arsenalstraße 2	7140 Ludwigsburg
Heyer, M.	Augusta Anlage 49	68 Mannheim
Heykes, M.	Roonstr. 25	2350 Neumünster

Heymann, H.	Prinzregentenufer 3	8500 Nürnberg
Heymann-Behm	Bruchfeldstr. 34	6000 Frankfurt-Niederrad
Heymann-Nowarra, E.	Reichsstraße 84	1000 Berlin 19
Heyn, H.	Königsberger Straße 7	8312 Dingolfing
Hickisch, W. D.	Luitpolsplatz 2	858 Bayreuth
Hildebrand, L.	Mitterweg 8	8302 Mainburg
Hildebrandt, Peter	Untere Bahnhofstraße 55	8034 Germering
Hildenbrand, Th.	Ludwigstraße 6	8730 Bad Kissingen
Hilgenfeld, H. A.	Bahnhofstr. 50	3548 Arolsen
Himmelmann, H.	Knapper Str. 61	5880 Lüdenscheid
Hinkel, Jutta	In der Wehrhecke 110	5300 Bonn
Hintermayer, Klaus	Nibelungenallee 37	6000 Frankfurt
Hintethaner, Manfred	Mannheimer Str. 136	6550 Bad Kreuznach
Hinz, Otto Süel	Sudeckstr. 2	2000 Hamburg 20
Hinzpeter, E. N.	Tangstedter Landstr. 400	2 Hamburg 62
Hirsch, Paul	Bahnhofstraße 16	8970 Immenstadt
Hirschberg, H.	Zur dicken Linde 46	4740 Oelde
Hirte, Hans	Hansastr. 1	5952 Attendorn
Hjort, Heinrich	Grubesallee 4	2000 Hamburg-Rahlstedt
Hoch, Hermann	Schmiedstraße 23	8120 Weilheim
Hochgesand, H.	Mainzerstr. 11	609 Rüsselsheim
Hochgesand, P.	Univ.-Augenklinik	6500 Mainz
Hochgürtel, M.	Schwannstraße 11a	4040 Neuß
Hochrein, P.	Schillerpl. 6	3170 Gifhorn
Hodum-Röhm	Wolboldstraße 6	7032 Sindelfingen
Hoede, C.	Univ.-Augenklinik	65 Mainz
Hoehne, H.	Osterstr. 24	2000 Hamburg 19
Hof, L.	August Bebel Str. 64	48 Bielefeld
Hoffmann, Alfred	Kaiserstraße 22	8700 Würzburg
Hoffmann, C.	M.-Luther-Straße 27	6740 Landau
Hoffmann, Dietrich	Königstraße 84	7000 Stuttgart-N
Hoffmann, E. A.	Wolfenbüttler Str. 82	3300 Braunschweig
Hoffmann, E. R.	Markt 5	4131 Rheink.-Repelen
Hoffmann, F. W.	Evinger Dzr. 204	4600 Dortmund-Ewing
Hoffmann, H.	Münsterstr. 12	4620 Castrop-Rauxel
Hoffmann, R.	Bohlweg 64/65	3300 Braunschweig
Hoffmann, T.	Schillerstr. 12	2407 Bad Schwartau
Hoffmann, Th.	Hagener Str. 92	5868 Letmathe
Hoffmann-Conrads, E.	Königstraße 84	7000 Stuttgart-N
Hoffsümmer	Bremer Str. 14	2100 HH.-Harburg
Hohlbaum, R.	Marienstraße 48	8670 Hof
Holl, Josef	Wrangelstraße 8	4000 Düsseldorf
Holland, Prof. Gerhard	Fahnerstraße 135	4100 Duisburg 11
Holler, Christoph	A.-Ladebeck-Str. 64a	4800 Bielefeld
Hollmann, M.	Richmondstraße 1-5	5000 Köln
Hollwich, Prof. F.	Westring 15	4400 Münster
Holscher, Dagmar	An der Spiele 6	4770 Soest
Holscher, E. K.	An der Spiele 6	4770 Soest
Holst, G.	Sand 2	2100 Hamburg-Harburg
Holst, G.	Neue Str. 25	2100 Hamburg-Harburg
Holste, A.	Hölderlinweg	7518 Bretten
Holstege, K. H.	Betlehemstraße 45	5150 Bergheim
Holstein, A.	Geibelstr. 41	3000 Hannover-Buchholz
Holtermann, W.	Kaiserstr. 3	2300 Kiel-Gaarden
Holtgrave, B. A.	Dobler Str. 11	74 Tübingen
Holtmann, Horst	Ippendorfer Weg 32	5300 Bonn

Holtz, M.	Hohle Gasse 2	2250 Husum
Holzapfel, Marie-Elis.	Kölnische Str. 157	3500 Kassel
Holzhauer, Ursula	J.-Krämer-Straße 30	7000 Stuttgart-Sonnenberg
Homuth, Joh.-Carl	Schienenstraße 3	6800 Mannheim
Honegger, Prof. H.	Augenklinik Med. Hochschule	3 Hannover
Hoof, Doris	Keltenweg 6	6202 Wiesbaden-Bieberich
Hoops, Peter	Köln-Berliner-Str. 21	4600 Dortmund-Aplerbeck
Hoops, Renate	Obermassener Kirchweg 11	4750 Unna
Hopf, Werner	Brüggemannstraße 13	5100 Aachen
Horn, Brigitte	Hainallee 53	4600 Dortmund
Horn, F.	Wilhelminenstr. 5a	6100 Darmstadt
Hornung, G.	Borriesstraße 4	2850 Bremerhaven
Horstmann, Heinz	Schubertstraße 50	2800 Bremen 1
Hoyer, Elke	Hamburger Str. 23	2000 Hamburg 22
Höft, Uwe	Friedrichstr. 44	2240 Heide
Högel	Poststr. 8	6670 St. Ingbert
Höhn, Christa	Friedrichstraße 36	5300 Bonn-Beuel
Höller, Valentin	Freislebenstraße 9	7920 Heidenheim
Hölscher	Postplatz 3	5840 Schwerte
Höpping, W.	Rüttenscheider Straße	4300 Essen-Rüttenscheid
Hörstgen, W.	Duisburger Straße 237	4100 Duisburg-Hamborn
Hötte, E.	Markt 4	8630 Coburg
Hötte, Hubert	Weseler Straße 43	4100 Duisburg-Hamborn
Hövelmann, O.	Gartenstraße 41	5180 Eschweiler
Huck, Karl	Pirkheimer Straße 11	8500 Nürnberg
Hueck, G.	Hauerstr. 16	3540 Korbach
Hueck, H.	Russelstr. 19	4490 Papenburg
Huerkamp, Prof. B.	Liebermannstr. 5	3000 Hannover
Hufnagel. G.	Viktoriastraße 20-22	4330 Mülheim
Humburg, E. H.	Reeperbahn 114	2000 Hamburg 4
Hummelt, Klaus	Bahnhofspl. 17	2000 Hamburg 55
Huneus, G.	Bismarckstraße 72	4050 Mönchengladbach
Hungerland, Jürgen	Bremer Str. 26	2830 Bassum
Huppertz, Helga	Kaiserdamm 5	1000 Berlin 19
Husen, H. van	Ostwall 36	4150 Krefeld
Huth, K.	Kluse 10	5860 Iserlohn
Hutt, Ursula	Marktplatz 3	7250 Leonberg
Hübner, Erdmann	Ochsenzollerstr. 181	2000 Norderstedt
Hübner, E.	Ochsenzoller Str. 181	2000 Norderstedt
Hülsken, Dieter	Gahlener Str. 9	4270 Dorsten-I.
Hülsmann, F.	Stöckstr. 30	4680 Wanne-Eickel
Hüsch, L.	Artilleriestraße 8	5170 Jülich
Hütteroth, Heinz	Univ.-Augenklinik	6650 Homburg
Ibrahim, G.	Rumburgstr. 6	8458 Sulzbach-Rosenberg
Illert, Paul	Hüttenstraße 6	4000 Düsseldorf
Illgner, U.	Bremer Str. 42	2940 Wilhelmshaven
Iltgen, Gertrud	Tegenseer Landstraße 55	8000 München 90
Immand, H.	Propsteistraße 10	4300 Essen-Werden
Immendörfer, Irene	Seetalbachstraße 88	7343 Kuchen
Irlbacher, Brigitte	Bellinzonastraße 45	8000 München 49
Isenbeck, K.	Bahnhofstr. 14	4750 Unna
Issa, Anton	Westring 15	4400 Münster
Itschner, G.	Wormserstr. 59	6504 Oppenheim/Rhein
Ivanoff, Nikolaus	Wilhelmstraße 111	5100 Aachen
Iven, J.	Freiligrathstraße 19a	4000 Düsseldorf
Jablonka, Erich	Kaiserstraße 25	6500 Mainz

Jacobi, Karl-Wilh.	Friedrichstr. 18	6300 Gießen
Jacobsehn, F. B.	Ziegelhäuser Landstr. 39	69 Heidelberg
Jaeger, Prof. W.	Univ.-Augenklinik	69 Heidelberg
Jaensch, Roland	Viehofer Pl. 3	4300 Essen 1
Jahn, H.	Ainmillerstraße 1	8000 München 13
Jahn, O.	Elbinger Straße 50	8500 Nürnberg
Jahnel, Alfred	Vierhausstraße 25	4070 Rheydt
Jahnke, R.	Augenabt. d. Rudolf-Virchow-Krankenhauses	1 Berlin 65
Jakob, Elisabeth	Unterländer Straße 43	7000 Stuttgart-Zuffenhausen
Jakob, Klaus	Wagner Str. 3	5900 Siegen
Jakusen, Ch.	Mitlerweg 37	7186 Crailsheim
Jancke, Gerhard	Stephanstr. 9	3500 Kassel
Jancke, G.	Deisterallee 16	3250 Hameln
Janert, H.	Ob. Herrngasse 14	7170 Schwäb.-Hall
Jansen, Ingeborg	Alleestraße 43	5630 Remscheid
Jansen, R.	Bismarckstr. 29	6100 Darmstadt
Jansen, Wilfried	Schillerstraße 53	4050 Mönchengladbach
Janus, K.	Weidenbaumsweg 13	2000 Hamburg-Bergedorf
Januschowski, G.	Kortumstr. 93	4630 Bochum
Jauernig, G.	Bahnhofstraße 32	8360 Deggendorf
Jäger, Prof. A.	Goethestrßae 27/29	5100 Aachen
Jäger, A.	Karl Hintze Weg 73	33 Braunschweig
Jähner, Heinz	Kupferdreher Straße 114	4300 Essen-Kupferdreh
Jendralski, H. J.	Alt-Mariendorf 32	1000 Berlin 42
Jensen, S.	Holtenauer Str. 154	2300 Kiel-Gaarden
Jess, Prof. A.	Taunusstr. 2	62 Wiesbaden
Jess, R.	Schulstr. 11	6300 Gießen
Jessen, K. H.	Westl. Ringstraße 8	6710 Frankenthal
Jochmus, H.	Schloßstraße 53a	7000 Stuttgart
Joest, Dieter	Hailerer Str. 4	6460 Gelnhausen
John, Rolf-Dieter	Tempelhofer Damm 145	1000 Berlin 42
Jonas, A.	Grünstr. 48	3160 Lehrte
Joos, H.	Kaiser-Josef-Straße	7800 Freiburg
Jordan, H.	Friedrichstraße 7	8510 Fürth
Jordan, M.	Sternstraße 58	6700 Ludwigshafen
Jordan, S.	Bei der John.-Kirche 20	2000 Hamburg-Altona
Josten, K.	Salierring 64	5000 Köln
Jörg, H.	Viktoriastraße 24	7500 Karlsruhe
Jung, H.	Hohenzollernring 22-24	5000 Köln
Jung-Schulte, C.	Gartenstr. 13	649 Schlüchtern
Jungbluth, Hilde	Mittelstraße 105	4010 Hilden
Junghannß, K.	Kriegsbergstraße 60	7000 Stuttgart-N
Junker, F. K. .,.........	Karl-Marx-Straße 29	6750 Kaiserslautern
Junker, H.	Moorgärten 18	2848 Vechta
Justen, M.	Bahnhofstraße 44	5200 Siegburg
Jünemann, G.	Westring 15	4400 Münster
Jürgens, Vera	Schloßwall 20	4500 Osnabrück
Kaden, R.	Meerwiesenstr. 29	68 Mannheim 1
Kager, S.	Äuss. Lauferplatz 19	8500 Nürnberg
Kahlheyss, Belinde	Heemstr. 33	2878 Wildeshausen
Kallenberg, K.	Bezoldweg 3	8803 Rothenburg/Tauber
Kalthoff	b. Stuttgart	7251 Hemmingen
Kalthoff, H.	Kottbusser Damm 67	1000 Berlin 61
Kammann, Jochen	Baeumer Str. 26	4600 Dortmund
Kammann, P.	Alfred Trappenstr. 4	4600 Dortmund-Hörde

Kammeier, Heinz	Heinestr. 7	4680 Wanne-Eickel
Kampik, Gerda	Stauffenbergstraße 1	8000 München 13
Kaniuth, Ursula	Ringstraße 6b	8184 Gmund/Tegernsee
Kanther, Ilse	Hubertusstraße 3	8033 Planegg
Kapp, Jörg	Neuberger Straße 18	8700 Würzburg
Kappe, Rainer	Donhoffstraße 55b	5090 Leverkusen
Kapune, Stefi	Dorotheenstraße 4	5601 N.-Dönberg
Karasek, O.	Humboldtstraße 24	7600 Offenburg
Karges, E.	Ewaldstr. 91	4352 Herten
Karstien, H.	Hauptstraße 122	5070 Berg.-Gladbach
Karsch, Joh.	Merkurstraße 66	7560 Gaggenau
Karsch, Paul	Mittelstr. 32	4920 Lemgo
Karsch, Thomas	Kringel-Krugweg 19	2000 Norderstedt 1
Kasch, Friedrich	Nibelungenstraße 32	5030 Hermülheim
Kaskel, D.	Inst. f. Experimentelle Ophthalmologie	53 Bonn
Kasperek, Theresia	Heubnerweg 2	1000 Berlin 19
Kassner, G.	Stöckstr. 25	4680 Wanne-Eickel
Kastner, W.	Fr.-Ebert-Straße 5	6718 Grünstadt
Kattiofsky, W.	Hostatostr. 2	623 Frankfurt a.M.-Höchst
Katz, Rudolf	Sofienstraße 3	7570 Baden-Baden
Kaufmann, H.	Univ.-Augenklinik	5300 Bonn
Kaufmann, H.	Wilhelmstraße 30	5200 Siegburg
Kauke-Utermann, I.	Brunwardinger Str. 8	4784 Rüthen/Möhne
Käding, Klaus	Hindenburgstraße 7	6730 Neustadt
Käfer, Otto	Zähringer Straße 14	6900 Heidelberg
Kämmerling, F.	Dieckerstraße 60	5657 Haan
Kämpf, R.	Bahnhofstraße 13	8580 Bayreuth
Kämpf, Wilhelm	Bahnhofstraße 19/I	7340 Geislingen
Kästner, Maja	Leopoldstraße 67	8000 München 23
Keding, L.	Obere Königstr. 45	3500 Kassel
Keerl, Gerhard	Bahnstraße 58	4000 Düsseldorf
Kehl, Friedrich	Friedrichstr. 43	586 Kassel
Keidel, B.	Landsb. Straße 494	8000 Münden-Pasing
Keil, J.	Blanchardstr. 8	6000 Frankfurt
Keim, Eugen	Schwedenstraße 16	8510 Fürth
Keller, Paul	Sternstr. 6	4720 Beckum
Kellermann, H. W.	Uerdinger Straße 2	4130 Moers
Kellermann, V.	Tegeler Weg 4	1000 Berlin 10
Kellnar, W.	Bahnhofstraße	8100 Garmisch-Partenkirchen
Kemp, R.	Bocholter Str. 8	4280 Borken
Kemper, J.	Zingel 17	3200 Hildesheim
Kern, Arnold	Frauenbergweg 10	7060 Schorndorf
Kernbach, H. F.	Kölner Straße 34	5140 Erkelenz
Kerrinnes, E.	Aggertalklinik	525 Engelskirchen
Kerstan-Thies, Ch.	Liebfrauenstr. 11	637 Oberursel
Kessler, W.	Eisenbahnstr. 15	6650 Homburg
Kienecker, R.	Hindenburgstr. 9	4980 Bünde
Kienow, H. U.	Leineweberstraße 21-25	4330 Mülheim
Kiesel, R.	Hauptstraße 16	6780 Pirmasens
Kieslich, G.	Bürgerm.-Renz-Straße 21	6950 Mosbach
Kieslich, Gaby	Univ.-Augenklinik	6900 Heidelberg
Kiggen, R.	Buchstraße 36	7120 Bietigheim
Kimpel, Werner	Robert-Koch-Str. 14	4650 Gelsenkirchen
Kipper, Horst	Univ.-Augenklinik	6650 Homburg
Kiraly, Fernandine	Untere Hauptstraße 25	8050 Freising

Kirbach, Udo	Holtenauer Str. 182	2300 Kiel
Kirchener	Wandsb. Chaussee 112	2000 Hamburg 22
Kircher, H.	Körtlinger Str. 25	4354 Datteln
Kirst, G.	Benrodestraße 68	4000 Düsseldorf-Benrath
Kirsch, H.	Schillerstr. 19	3220 Alfeld
Kirschbaum, A. H.	Hegelstraße 46	6500 Mainz
Kistenmacher, D.	Kerperner Straße 93	5000 Köln 41
Klar, R.	Kurfürstenstraße 39	5400 Koblenz
Klaus, E.	Breite Str. 8	3380 Goslar
Klaus, Peter	Bahnhofstr. 9	2910 Westerstede
Klaus, W.	Friedr.-Ebert-Str. 48	3500 Kassel
Kleberger, Prof. E.	Cimbernstr. 16	1 Berlin 38
Klecker, Wilhelm	Ovelacker Str.	4630 Bochum-Langendreer
Kleckow, A.	Christ.-Blank-Str. 19	3428 Duderstadt
Kleifeld, Prof. O.	Nordallee 16	5500 Trier
Kleiminger, H.	Johannisstr. 130	45 Osnabrück
Klein, Michael	Berliner Str. 61	5804 Herdecke
Klein, R.	Am Kirchplatz 1	5892 Meinerzhagen
Klein, W.	Schubertstr. 60a	63 Gießen
Kleine, H.	Benderstraße 10	4000 Düsseldorf
Kleine, R.	Löwenstr. 64	4442 Bentheim
Kleinebrecht, W.	Am Bahnhof	5282 Dieringhausen
Kleinhaus, Klaus	Bebbelsdorfstr. 16	5810 Witten
Kleinkempel, H.	Nordwall 58	4170 Geldern
Kleintges, Heinrich	Bahnhofstr. 13	3100 Celle
Klemm, Otto	Poststraße 6	6900 Heidelberg
Klemme, Gisela	Wenckebachstraße 23	1000 Berlin 42
Klett, W.	Ganssweg 24	7320 Göppingen
Klier, Anton	Landshuter Straße 9	8400 Regensburg
Klier, Margarete	Bismarckstr. 1	6360 Friedberg
Klinge, Sigurd	Badstraße 23	1000 Berlin 65
Klinghardt, H. Ch.	Solmitzstr. 35	2402 Lübeck-Küchnitz
Klingner, Eva	Erikastr. 4	3422 Bad Lauterberg
Klinke	Feldbergstr. 60	637 Oberursel
Klitzsch, H.	Berkenstraße 16	8580 Bayreuth
Klock, Th.	Bahnhofstraße 58	4070 Rheydt
Klomp, G.	Berliner Str. 80	3320 Salzgitter-Lebenstedt
Klotzky	Kapuzinergraben 5	5100 Aachen
Klör, S.	Limitenstraße 86	4070 Rheydt
Kluxen, Marita	Rockumstraße 84	5300 Bonn
Kment, Marion	Marienplatz 9	8920 Schongau
Knauer, R.	Darmstädter Str. 30B	6140 Bensheim
Knepper, W.	Huskenbörde 22	4300 Essen
Knippschild, J.	Bergenthalstr. 22	4788 Warstein
Knüpfer, N.	Rottenb. Chaussee 58	2000 Hamburg 13
Kober, M.	Venloer Straße 338	5000 Köln-Ehrenfeld
Kober	Hauptstr. 85	5830 Schwelm
Koch, Eckhardt	Bergmannstraße 1	6700 Ludwigshafen
Koch, H.	Wartenau 1	2000 Hamburg 29
Koch, H. R.	Kaiser-Otto-Pl. 9	4300 Essen-Steele
Koch, Hans-Reinhard	Fasanenweg 18	5300 Bonn-Ippendorf
Koch, Karl	Neue Hochstraße 39	1000 Berlin 65
Koch, L.	Waldfrieden 19	4530 Ibbenbüren
Koch, Peter	Schottmüllerstr. 28	2000 Hamburg 20
Kochs, H.	Wilhelm-Leuschner-Str. 33	Viernheim/Hessen
Kodolitsch, F. X.	Holtzmarkt 11	8532 Bad Windsheim

Koegell, Hanns	Kapellenweg 3	6901 Waldhilsbach
Kohlhaas, E.	Denglerstraße 10	5320 Bad Godesberg
Kohlhaas, W.	Alleestraße 6	5350 Euskirchen
Kohlhagen, W.	Bismarckstraße 1	7110 Öhringen
Kohlhoff-Funke, A.	Jacob-Stafan-Str. 14	65 Mainz
Kohor, Josef	Schmalzingerweg 1	8070 Ingolstadt
Kokott, Irmgard	Rohrbacher Straße 9	6900 Heidelberg
Kolb, Alice	Funkenstraße 68	5020 Frechen
Kolb, Herbert	Enscheder Str. 19	4432 Gronau
Koletzko, G.	Emsstr. 7	4440 Rheine
Koll, Werner	Friedrich-Ebert-Straße 33	5600 Wuppertal-Elberfeld
Kolshorn, Hans	Karlstal 32	2300 Kiel-Gaarden
Kolshorn, Hans	Marktstatte 26	7750 Konstanz
Kommerell, G.	Univ.-Augenklinik	78 Freiburg
Kommerell, L.	Bahnhofstr. 2c	8013 Haar
Konen, Walter	Cheruskerstraße 101	4000 Düsseldorf-Oberkassel
Konrad, Annemarie	Berner-Heerweg 159	2000 Hamburg-Farmsen
Korff, Evelyn	Hegaustraße 15	7700 Singen
Korff, Jürgen	Marienhaus	7880 Säckingen
Korsten, H. B.	Eduard-Istas-Straße 18	4054 Lobberich
Korte, W.	Sedanstr. 11	4700 Hamm
Korthäuer, H.	Königstraße 52	4100 Duisburg
Kotowski, Hartmut	Friedrichring 16/18	7800 Freiburg
Köcher, Hildegard	Hermannstraße 14	4000 Düsseldorf
Köhl-Hoffmann	Am grünen Ring 21	4103 Walsum
Köhler-Rönnberg	Rathenaustr. 13/14	3000 Hannover
Köhn, J.	Schütt 22	673 Neustatdt/Weinstr.
Kölbl	Christian-Jorhan-Str. 10	8300 Landshut
Kölgen, Gudrun	Frauenstraße 17	8000 Munchen 5
Kölle, Kuno	Clay-Allee 341	1000 Berlin-Zehlendorf
Kölln, Lore	M.-Louisen-Str. 92a	2000 Hamburg 39
König, Dietr.-Peter	An der Stadtmauer 1	6700 Ludwigshafen
König, D.	Rolfinckstr. 10	2000 Hamburg-Wellingsb.
König, Odilia	Wunderstr. 36	3400 Göttingen
Könsgen, Roswitha	Oskar-Orth-Str. 35	6650 Homburg
Kössendrup, Th.	Schillstraße 20	4230 Wesel
Köster, Hans	Venloer Straße 389	5000 Köln-Ehrenfeld
Kraffel, G.	Kantstraße 75	1000 Berlin 12
Krahnert, E.	Waldhausenstr. 25	3000 Hannover-Kleefeld
Krahnert, Ernst-J.	Kiefernhalde 14	4300 Essen
Kranke, Dieter	Münsterplatz 10	6500 Mainz
Krannıg, H. D.	Marktstr. 2	6300 Gießen
Krastel, H.	Univ.-Augenklinik	69 Heidelberg
Kraus, Ellen	Univ.-Augenklinik	6900 Heidelberg
Krause, Andrea	Wilhelmstraße 7	7600 Offenburg
Krause, E. H.	Luisenstraße 8	7730 Villingen
Krause, G.	Hohfuhrstr. 11a	5880 Lüdenscheid
Krause, Gebhard	Dammtorstr. 27/II	2000 Hamburg 36
Krause, J.	Schloßstraße 26	4330 Mülheim
Krause, J.	Straßburger Straße 17	7290 Freudenstadt
Krause, Justus	Augsburger Straße 80	8958 Füssen
Krause, Renate	Scharnweher Straße 41	1000 Berlin 52
Krauseneck, Egon	Karlstraße 38	7480 Sigmaringen
Krebs, Emmy	Schloßstraße 112	1000 Berlin 41
Kreibig, Prof. W.	Univ.-Augenklinik	665 Homburg
Kreissig, I.	Univ.-Augenklinik	53 Bonn

Krekeler, Elmar	von-Eyß-Straße 17	5400 Koblenz-Horchheim
Kremers, Horst	Prümburgstr. 1	6613 Eppelborn
Kress, A.	Eggepfad 5	5980 Werdohl
Kressl, Günther	Obernstr. 42	2807 Achim
Kreuzer, Wolfgang	Arsenalstraße 2	7140 Ludwigsburg
Krey, Hauke	Friedrichstr. 18	6300 Gießen
Kropf, H.	Moosacker 23	8000 M.-Milbertshofen
Kropp, Rudolf	Rotthof 10	3530 Warburg
Krueger, Rudolf	Schützenstraße 63	8600 Bamberg
Krugel, K.	Bornheimer Landstr. 1	6000 Frankfurt
Krumeich, J.	Saarlandstr. 9	4640 Wattenscheid
Kruse, Fr.	Bayrischer Pl. 9	1000 Berlin 30
Kruse, F. W.	Hindenburgstr. 7	5800 Hagen
Kruse, Hermann	Paulinenstr.	4930 Detmold
Kruse, W.	Grabenstr. 29	5800 Hagen
Krückels, H.	Albertusstraße 15	4050 Mönchengladbach
Krümmel, Prof. H.	Langenstr. 17	44 Münster
Krysta, F.	Westliche 56	7530 Pforzheim
Kubert, K.	E, 3, 14	6800 Mannheim
Kuborn, J. P.	Kirchenstraße 1	8132 Tutzing
Kugler, A.	Wemdinger Straße 5	8860 Nördlingen
Kuhlgatz, W.	Goethestr. 51	3180 Wolfsburg
Kuhn, Peter	Lyserstr. 34 VI	2000 Hamburg 50
Kuhnhardt, G.	Krummacher Str. 3	4530 Ibbenbüren
Kujus, H.	Goerdeler Str. 21	6400 Fulda
Kumm, Günter	Bayreuther Straße 28a	8500 Nürnberg
Kunde, Gerd	Grabenstr. 4	4902 Bad Salzuflen
Kunkel, Hans	Gangolfplatz 3a	8600 Bamberg
Kunz, E.	Leopoldstraße 7	7530 Pforzheim
Kunzendorf, Götz	Johannesstraße 37	7014 Kornwestheim
Kurus, Carola	Friedrichsring 10	6800 Mannheim I
Kurus, E.	Friedrichsring 10	6800 Mannheim I
Kurz, H.	Frühlingstr. 1	808 Fürstenfeldbruck
Kutscher, F.	Freytagstraße 29-35	4300 Essen
Küchle, Prof. H. J.	Rochusstraße 2	4000 Düsseldorf
Kühnlein	Mohrenstraße 5	8630 Coburg
Küllenberg, E.	Dorpeshof 111	5650 Solingen
Küper, Jochen	Bismarckstr. 6	4730 Ahlen
Kürschner, D.	Pfeilschitterstr. 5	8905 Mering
Küster, Albert	Friedenstrasse 3	4812 Brackwede
Kyrieleis, E.	Univ.-Augenklinik	5000 Köln 41
Lack, A.	Fürst-Adolf-Str. 4	4963 Bad Eilsen
Lackner, Fritz	Gebhardstraße 8	8190 Wolfratshausen
Ladeburg, Friedrike	Hermannstraße 4	1000 Berlin 37
Ladwig, K. H.	Kirscherstraße 58	4019 Monheim
Laffers, Z.	In der Schornau 23-25	463 Bochum-Langendreer
Lahusen, Arnold	Klosterplatz 2	5358 Bad Münstereifel
Landenberger, F.	Paracelsusstraße 34	7300 Eßlingen
Landgraf, Sieglinde	Luisenstraße 25	7630 Lahr
Landwehr, U.	Nenndorfer Str. 2	3013 Barsinghausen
Lang, Fritz	Kaiserstraße 2a	6780 Pirmasens
Lange, C.	Buggenbeck 41	433 Mülheim/Ruhr
Lange, F.	Sophienblatt 47/51	2300 Kiel 1
Lange-Wühlisch, Joach.	Karl-Marx-Str. 204/206	1000 Berlin 44
Langenbeck, B.	Max-Säumestr. 1	28 Bremen
Langmann, K.	Saarnerstraße 497	4330 Mülheim

Langner, K.	Fixheiderweg 22	5000 Köln-Höhenhaus
Langschmidt, K.	Münsterstraße 16	5300 Bonn
Lappe, Anne-Margret	Luisenstraße 21	5100 Aachen
Lappe, G.	Ganderhofstraße 8	6700 Ludwigshafen V
Larsen, E.	Hemeling. Bahnhofstr. 15	2800 Bremen
Lassen, Wilhelm	Gronerstr. 28	3400 Göttingen
Lattermann, Dieter	Bischof-Meiser-Straße 2a	8800 Ansbach
Lattermann, U.	Alt Moabit 68a	1000 Berlin 21
Laue, Hanfried	Nußbaumstraße 14	8000 München 15
Lauer, H. J.	Univ.-Augenklinik	69 Heidelberg
Lautsch, Johannes	Brandenburgische Str. 69	1000 Berlin 31
Läufer, Hans-Joachim	Homberger Straße 49	4130 Moers
Lege, Jürgen	Parkstr. 21	6350 Bad Nauheim
Lehmut-Schonert, R.	Altenessener Straße 454	4300 Essen-Altenssen
Lehn, J.	Roonstraße 2	7550 Rastatt
Lehners, Dietrich	Claustorwall 30	3380 Goslar
Lehringer, F. E.	Eberhardstraße 47	7000 Stuttgart-S
Leidig, Ida Maria	Bahnhofstraße 7	8540 Schwabach
Leifeld, Heinz	Robert-Koch-Str. 7	5810 Witten-Annen
Leipert, Gotth.	Rathausplatz 19	8960 Kempten
Leiter, Stephan	Bahnhofstraße 14	7000 Stuttgart-Cannstatt
Leithäuser, U.	Petersstr. 3	2420 Eutin
Lemle, Ernst	Burgstraße 1	6990 Bad Mergentheim
Lemmen, Günther	Am Markt 4	6620 Völklingen
Lemmer, Klaus	Berliner Straße 185	5600 Wuppertal 2
Lemmingson, W.	Augenabt. Diakonissenanstalt	75 Karlsruhe-Rüppurr
Lempp	Frankfurter Straße 14	8752 Kleinostheim
Lengerken, Maja v.	Marienplatz 79	7980 Ravensburg
Lenne, Heinz	Rochusstraße 2	5300 Bonn-Duisdorf
Lenthe, Hilde-Rose	Dorfener Straße 7	8058 Erding
Lenz, Josef	Wasserb. Landstraße 234	8000 München 59
Lenzen, H.	Mittelstraße 71	4010 Hilden
Leo, M.	Hauptstraße	7742 St. Georgen
Leonhardt	Mainzer Straße 10	6530 Bingen
Lerche, W.	Martinistr. 52	2 Hamburg 20
Lersch, S.		8671 Selbitz
Lessel, Josef	Baumkirchener Straße 3	8000 München 8
Letschert, A.	Markenbildchenweg 3	5400 Koblenz
Leuwer, K. H.	Beethovenplatz 15	5300 Bonn
Leydhecker, Prof.	Univ.-Augenklinik	8700 Würzburg
Leykauf, G.	Bahnhofstraße 25	8670 Hof
Lieb. Prof. W.	Augenklinik Städt. Krkh. Höchst.	6 Frankfurt 80
Liebke, Ingeborg	Nestlestraße 64	6500 Mainz-Mombach
Liebsch	Maximilianstraße 48/1	8900 Augsburg
Liebsch, Dieter	Theresienstraße 5	8390 Passau
Liedke, W.	Kölner Straße 231	4000 Düsseldorf
Liegl, Otmar	Grünlingweg 6	1000 Berlin 47
Lienert, H.	Gust.-Vorst-Str. 5	5802 Wetter
Liesen, Werner	Gezelinallee 13	5090 Leverkusen
Liesenhoff, Claus	Ludwiggasse 77	6650 Homburg
Liesenhoff, Prof. H.	Adalbert-Stifter-Str. 12	6909 Walldorf
Linde, L.	Roßmarkt 9	6 Frankfurt 1
Lindemann, Olaf	Nansenstraße 1	7850 Lörrach
Linden, F.	Bahnhofstr. 18	4712 Werne
Linkenbach, Heinz	Wilhelmstr. 1b	4800 Bielefeld
Lindenberg, D.	Prinzenstr. 3	3400 Göttingen

Linnen, Prof. H. J.	Rich.-Wagner-Str. 14	6000 Frankfurt
Lippmann, H.	Dotzheimer Str. 65	62 Wiesbaden
Lisch, H.	Mainzer Str. 36	62 Wiesbaden
Littann, K. E.	Bahnhofsallee 3	3200 Hildesheim
Littig, M. G.	Nördl. Stadtgraben	8360 Deggendorf
Locht, H. van de	Fuhlsb. Str. 125	2000 Hamburg 33
Loew, Prof. F.	Univ.-Augenklinik	6650 Homburg
Lohlein, H.	Clarenstr. 3	4900 Herford
Lohoff, W.	Friedrichstr. 5	4790 Paderborn
Loos, Fritz	Bürstädter Str. 11	6840 Lampertheim
Lorenz, Roland	Kl. Grottenau 1	8900 Augsburg
Lorenz, Willi	Kölner Straße 226	5275 Bergneustadt 1
Lorenzen, V. K.	Kappelner Str. 14	2300 Kiel
Lose, Peter	Hafenstraße 66	2850 Bremerhav.-Lehe
Lossagk, H.	Pettenkoferstr. 33	43 Essen
Loth, Arthur	Kohlbrandstr. 14	6000 Frankfurt
Lotholz, Karl	Am Weserturm 7	2900 Oldenburg
Loula, Louise	Zeisstr. 31	4920 Lemgo
Löhlein, B.	Bahnhofstr. 17	4933 Blomberg
Löhlein, H.	Clarenstr. 13	49 Herford
Löhr, Klaus	Kirchenstr. 9	2308 Preetz
Löpping, Bernd	Friedr.-Ebert-Str. 15	4570 Quakenbrück
Lösche, W.	Robert-Koch-Straße 5	4200 Oberhausen-Sterkrade
Löw, Rainer	Krawigstr. 10	6618 Wadern
Lucas-Kremer, M.	Rüttenscheider Straße 163	4300 Essen
Lucassen, Marianne	Eppendorfer Landstr. 7	2000 Hamburg 20
Luce, I.	Riehestr. 10	4402 Greven
Ludwig, A.	Ringweg 2	8950 Kaufbeuren
Lund, Prof. Otto Erich	Mathildenstraße 8	8000 München 15
Lunecke, Hartmut	Arndtstr. 1	4900 Herford
Luntz, G.	Hinter den Höfen 13	3450 Holzminden
Luntz, Peter	Dürerweg 5	3450 Holzminden
Lux, P.	Kaiserstr. 112	75 Karlsruhe
Lübben, Karl	Parkstr. 8	4628 Lünen
Lübs, Gisela	Schülerstr. 41	4902 Bad Salzuflen
Lübs, Gisela	Lange Str. 51	4903 Schötmar
Lüdicke, Christa	Argent. Allee	1000 Berlin 31
Lüllwitz, W.	Univ.-Augenklinik	2 Hamburg 20
Lüpke, C. M.	Nonnendamm-Allee 96	1000 Berlin 13
Lüssem, Engelbert	Rheinallee 20	5407 Boppard
Lüssen, Peter	Rauschenerring 10a	2000 Hamburg 70
Lympius, E. v.	Eickhoffstr. 1	483 Gütersloh
Maag, Berthold	Körner Hellweg 81	4600 Dortmund-Körne
Maass, Ingeburg	Klingsorstraße 3/77	8000 München 81
Maass, Karl	Blanken. Bhfstr. 29	2000 Hamburg-Blankenese
Mackensen. Prof. G.	Lugostraße 7	7800 Freiburg
Maesse, W.	Seilerstr. 11	3180 Wolfsburg
Mai, Walter	Hasenweg 9	4044 Kaarst
Maier-Pfeiffer, J.	Florianstraße 19	7000 Stuttgart 13
Makabe, R.	Univ.-Augenklinik	6 Frankfurt
Malsen-Waldkirch, B. v.	Nordallee 22	5420 Oberlahnstein
Manger, J.	Werner-Siemens-Straße	8580 Bayreuth
Marckwort	Seminarweg 2	2418 Ratzeburg
Marckwort, F.	Bahnhofstr. 45	4980 Bünde
Markowsky, W.	Hindenburgstraße 2	7118 Künzelsau
Marquardt, C.	Friedrichstraße 6	7840 Müllheim

Marquardt, L.	Christianstr. 20	2350 Neumünster
Marquardt, Prof. R.	Baldingerweg 8	79 Ulm
Martens, G.	Waldgrenzweg 17	6904 Ziegelhausen
Martin, R.	Käthe-Kollwitz-Straße 7	7500 Karlsruhe
Marx, G.	Elisabethstr. 53	2300 Kiel 14
Marx, Josef	Poststr. 37	6640 Merzig
Marx, K. Uwe	Reinpfad 28	4750 Unna
Marx, W.	Kaiserstr. 39	4352 Herten
Maschke, K.	Richard-Bertram-Str. 12	504 Brühl
Maschmeyer, Klaus	Dreiringser Weg 10a	4770 Soest
Mathyl, Johannes	Schönbornstraße 7	8700 Würzburg
Matthes, K.	Mülheimer Straße 129	4200 Oberhausen
Mau, G.	Bismarckstraße 24	1000 Berlin 12
Mayer-Böricke, E.	Römerstraße 10	5170 Jülich
Mayer, H.	Seb. Graben 33	7090 Ellwangen
Mayer, Karl-Heinz	Marktstraße 16	7320 Göppingen
Mayer, K.	Theresienstraße 3	8070 Ingolstadt
Mayer, Ursula	Schenkstraße 57	8520 Erlangen
Mayr, G.	Friedrichstraße 3	5550 Bernkastel-Kues
Märker, Werner	Martinistr. 5	4350 Recklinghausen
Meder, Erich	Weingut-Annaberg	6701 Leistadt
Medicus-Lux, Luise	Roßmarkt 11	6508 Alzey
Medler, Adalbert	Gartenstr. 24	6413 Hünfeld
Meerbeck, A.	Karolingerweg 11-15	5000 Köln 1
Mees, G.	Kampstr. 12	4620 Castrop-Rauxel
Meesmann, K.	Bismarckstr. 8	592 Berleburg
Mehlhose	Bayerischer Platz 9	1000 Berlin 62
Mehlhose, Ute	Schloßstraße 59	7857 Haagen
Mehlitz, Hartmut	Heiligendammerstraße 18	1000 Berlin 33
Mehrle, Georg	Sautierstraße 58	7800 Freiburg
Meierhoffer, Josef	Katharinenhospital	7000 Stuttgart 1
Meineth, Rolf	Am Natruper Holz 69	4500 Osnabrück
Meinhardt, E.	Mommsenstraße 67	1000 Berlin 12
Meiser	Th.-Heuss-Pl. 1	4040 Neuß
Meisinger, J.	Frühlingstraße 8	8060 Dachau
Meisner, Gerhard	Elisabethstraße 90	8000 München 13
Meisner, Toni	Sonnenstr. 22	8 München
Meissner, F. M.	Herdweg 41	7000 Stuttgart
Meister, Ch.	Offenbacher Str. 21	6078 Neu-Isenburg
Meitinger, A.	Ahornstraße 3	4300 Essen
Meixner, H.	St. Bonifatiusstraße	8000 München 9
Mellin, A. v.	Provinzialstr. 54	6623 Altenkessel
Menk, Walter	Tituscorso 5	6000 Frankfurt/NO-Zentrum
Mennerich, Konrad	Schweinfurthstraße 43	1000 Berlin 33
Mentz, Otto	Kleiner Sand 1	2082 Uetersen
Merk, Hans	Univ.-Augenklinik	8700 Würzburg
Merkel, F.	Kirchowstraße 27	8500 Nürnberg
Merkel, S.	Fürstenrieder 32/I	8000 München 42
Merschmann, W.	Röntgenstraße 15	8560 Lauf
Merté, Prof. H. J.	Ismaninger Straße 22	8000 München 80
Mertens, H.	Hohe Str. 61 1/2	4600 Dortmund
Mertz, M.	Augenklinik R.d.I.	8 München
Mertz, O.	Albert-Schweitzer-Str.	3320 Salzgitter-Lebenstedt
Metten-Zeck, Ch.	Bahnhofstraße 6	6500 Mainz
Metzger, Benno	Heilmannstraße 7	8000 München 71
Metzler, Ursula	Büchelstraße 53a	5300 Bonn

Meves, H.	Veerser Str. 40	3110 Uelzen
Meves, Peter	Bei den Blöcken 6	2160 Stade
Mewes, Marlies	Moorhof 12	2000 Hamburg 65
Meyer	Schwachhs. Heerstraße 46	2800 Bremen
Meyer, Prof.	Johannisfreiheit 2/4	45 Osnabrück
Meyer, F. W.	Adolf-Schweer-Str. 4	4960 Stadthagen
Meyer, Gunnar	Hauptstraße 113	5020 Frechen
Meyer, Günther	Plochinger Straße 6	7300 Eßlingen
Meyer, G.	Graf-Adolf-Straße 86	4000 Düsseldorf
Meyer, H.	Große-Bergstr. 219	2000 Hamburg-Altona
Meyer, Klaus	Oddenskamp 17	2000 Hamburg 54
Meyer, K. H.	Grindel-Allee 157	2000 Hamburg
Meyer-Gotsch, L.	Duisburger Straße 218	4330 Mülh.-Speldorf
Meyer-Lau, M.	Residenzstraße 123	1000 Berlin 51
Meyer-Stoll, Ingo	Marienstraße 8	5159 Keppen
Meyer-Schwickerath, Prof.	Vossbusch 28	4300 Essen-Bredeney
Meyerratken, Edwin	Kronprinzenstr. 38	469 Herne
Meyhöffer, Klaus	Wittener Str. 5	5820 Gevelsberg
Meythaler, F.	Zeppelinstr. 4	852 Erlangen
Michtl, Arno	Kumpfmühlerstraße 41	8400 Regensburg
Mielke, S.	Johannesstr. 10	333 Helmstedt
Miessner, Eckhard	Sternwartstraße 21	4000 Düsseldorf
Mieth, Otto	Viehofer Pl. 9	4300 Essen
Miethke, Harro	Sonnenallee 68	1000 Berlin 44
Milanow, M.	Westfalenstraße 53	4000 Düsseldorf-Rath
Mildenberger, Arne	Hainbrunnstraße 5	8550 Forcnheim
Mildenberger, W.	Hainbrunnstraße 4	8550 Forchheim
Mildner, Ingrid	An der Kappe 91	1000 Berlin 20
Minges, A.	Exterstraße 1	6730 Neustadt
Minor, Hans	Mainstr. 30a	6202 Wiesbaden-Biederich
Misic, Dragoslav	Stein	5372 Schleiden
Mittelstaedt, Joach. v.	Hauptstraße 16	8990 Lindau
Moers-Messmer, H. v.	Hagellachstraße 54	6900 Heidelberg
Moghadam, Reza	Schoonebeekstr. 10-12	4504 Georgsmarienhütte-Oesede
Momcke-Bruhn, Anna	Stadtweg 62	2380 Schleswig
Monje, M.	Waldblick 21	2370 Molfsee/Rendsburg
Moog, E.	Mühlenstr. 85	2400 Lübeck
Moog, E.	Univers.-Augenklinik	2300 Kiel
Morgenthaler, W.	Hauptstraße 31	7602 Oberkirch
Moritz, Eugen	Am Schanzl 8	8390 Passau
Moritz, Karla	Am Schanzl 8	8390 Passau
Motzet, Dieter	Münchener Straße 4	8060 Dachau
Mödden, H.	Fr.-Ebert-Straße 9	8594 Arzberg
Möller, Reinhard	Engelbert-Kämpfer Str. 32	4920 Lemgo
Möller, Werner	Am Markt 20	4960 Stadthagen
Mössner, Franz	Kirchenlamitzer Straße 6	8660 Münchberg
Mrodzinsky, jr. K.	Talstraße 11	6730 Neustadt
Mrowietz, A.	In den Blumentriften 10	3320 Salzgitter-Lebenstedt
Mueller, F. O.	Josef-Schneider-Straße 11	8700 Würzburg
Mulzer, J.	Bahnhofstraße 6	8940 Memmingen
Mundschenck, A.	Siegfriedstraße 24	6520 Worms
Mutschler, J.	Wiedstraße 3	5230 Altenkirchen
Mügge, F.	An der Lachebrücke 12	6450 Hanau
Mühl, Norbert	Jahnstr. 21	6482 Bad Orb
Mühlendyck, H.	Augenklinik am Marienkrankenhaus	6 Frankfurt

Mühr, Adalbert	Rich.-Wagner Str. 14	6000 Frankfurt
Müller, Clemens	Rothenburg 46	4400 Münster
Müller, Ernst	Tegernseer Landstr. 154	8000 München 9
Müller, F. O.	Städt. Krankenanst.	6600 Saarbrücken
Müller, Prof. H.	Holzhausenstr. 75	6000 Frankfurt
Müller, H.	Cronestr. 6	4420 Coesfeld
Müller, Klaus	Marktstraße 39	7927 Giengen
Müller-Jensen, K.	Gustav-Schiefer-Str. 6/7	8000 München 54
Müller, M.	Holzhausenstr. 75	6000 Frankfurt
Müller, O.	Bergstraße	7777 Unterruhlingen
Müller, Peter	Waldstr. 47	5880 Lüdenscheid
Müller, Rosa	Sanderstraße 3	8700 Würzburg
Müller, R.	Engelbert-Kämpfer Str. 32	4920 Lemgo
Müller, Reinhard	Moritzplatz 4	8900 Augsburg
Müller, S.	Hindenburgstr. 18	4504 Georgsmarienhütte
Müller, Ulrich	Gudula-Straße 22	4300 Essen
Müller, Werner	Rudolfstraße 9	2850 Bremerhaven
Müller, W.	Schießgrabenstraße 21	8900 Augsburg
Müller, Prof. J. K.	Am Paulshof 7	5300 Bonn
Müller, W. A.	Isestr. 61	2000 Hamburg 13
Müller-Loeffelholz, Christoph	Hofackerstr. 18	7801 Neuershausen
Müller-Reisbrod, R.	Schnurgasse 20	6710 Frankenthal
Müllmerstadt, H.	Meyerstr. 62	2100 Hamburg-90
Münchow, R. von	Dilsb. Straße 3-5	6800 Mannheim-Freudenheim
Münich, Prof. W.	Neutorstr. 12	87 Würzburg
Münthen, Theo	Theaterplatz 6	4300 Essen
Mylius, Prof. Karl	Agnesstr. 31	2000 Hamburg 39
Nachtigäller, H.	Hammerweg 216	4050 Mönchengladbach
Nachtigäller, P.	Feldbrunnenstr. 23	2000 Hamburg 13
Nadler, A.	Hohenzollerndamm 7	1000 Berlin 31
Namislo, Joachim	Am Park 7	4151 Willich
Nagel, Robert	Rottstraße 12	8260 Mühldorf
Napp, Hans-Ulrich	Am Brink 3	2000 Hamburg-Bergedorf
Nase, Friedhelm	Waldrandstr. 19	5750 Menden
Nattenberg	Amtsgerichtstraße 26	4100 Duisburg
Nathrath, Paul-Dieter	Gartenstraße 2	5300 Bonn-Beuel
Naumann	Martinistr. 52	2000 Hamburg 20
Neeße, H.	Bliebtreustraße 33	1000 Berlin 15
Nehm, Otto	Beethovenstr. 33	5810 Witten
Neu, Hans Joachim	Deutsche Str. 2	6630 Saarlouis
Neubauer, Prof. Helmut	Josef-Stelzmann-Straße 9	5000 Köln-Lindenthal
Neubauer, K.	Luisenstraße 165	4050 Mönchengladbach
Neubner, H.	Jean-Paul-Straße 12	8730 Bad Kissingen
Neues, K. G.	Quiddestraße 41	8000 München 83
Neugebauer, Roman	Marktstr. 16	6400 Fulda
Neugschwender	Nr. 116	8871 Ellzee
Neuhann, H.	Corveyer Allee 5	3470 Höxter
Neuhann, Th.	Univ.-Augenklinik	69 Heidelberg
Neuhann, W.	Leopoldstraße 58	8000 München 23
Neuhaus, Burchard	Hohenburgstr. 21	6651 Kirrberg
Neukamm, H.	Cacilienstraße 62	7100 Heilbronn
Neumann, L.	Immermannstraße 10	4000 Düsseldorf
Neundörfer, Hans	Dominikanerplatz 9	8700 Würzburg
Neuner, H. P.	Univ.-Augenklinik	53 Bonn

Neuse, Dieter	Hauptstraße 11	7768 Stockach
Neyen	Ravensburger Straße 30	4100 Duisburg-Buchholz
Nickl, H.	Kohlenmarkt 5	8860 Nördlingen
Niedermeier, Prof.	Städt. Krankenanst.	4150 Krefeld
Niederstadt, F. A.	Badweg 4	6990 Bad Mergentheim
Niemz, Gisela	Battinger Straße 21	7889 Grenzach
Niermann, Herbert	Springer Str. 17	4660 Gelsenkirchen – Buer
Niessen, V.	Humboldstraße 57	4050 Mönchengladbach
Niethe, Ulrich	Tappenbeckstr. 4	2900 Oldenburg
Nietschmann, Armin	Stadtplatz 33	8260 Mühldorf
Nippels	Fürstenplatz 4	4000 Düsseldorf
Nitschke, Ernst	Kaiser-Josef-Straße 217	7800 Freiburg
Nitzsche, E.	Gelbinger Gasse 42	7170 Schwäb.-Hall
Nockemann, G.	Am Wehrenbeil 20	5270 Gummersbach
Nocken, Hans	Bahnhofstr. 1	4800 Bielefeld
Noll, Gert	Königsteiner Str. 17a	6000 Frankfurt-Höchst
Noll, Peter	Am Neutor 9	4220 Dinslaken
Nolte, Wilhelm	Geismar Landstr. 5	3400 Göttingen
Nonnemacher, H.	Zentmarkweg 18	6 Frankfurt 90
Notter, Helma	Münzplatz 9	5400 Koblenz
Nover, Prof. A.	Univ.-Augenklinik	65 Mainz
Novak, Alexander	Joh.-Müller-Str. 9	3350 Marburg
Nowak, G.	Kuhtorstr. 28	2240 Oldenburg
Nowak, K. H.	Kuhtorstr. 28	2240 Oldenburg
Nowak, Werner	Peutinger Straße 3	8900 Augsburg
Nürnberger, Kurt	Tempelhofer Damm 185	1000 Berlin 42
Obal, A.	Mansfelderstr. 15	1 Berlin-Wilmersdorf
Obens, Werner	Hölteweg 5	4400 Münster
Oberschulte, H. W.	Rheinische Str. 36	4600 Dortmund
Oblak, Maria	Wörthstraße 43	8000 München 80
Odefey, R.	Moenckebergstr. 5	2000 Hamburg 1
Oelker, Karl	Bahnhofstr. 16	4802 Halle
Oertel, H.	Friedberger Landstr. 103	6000 Frankfurt
Oettingen, H. v.	Frankfurter Str. 7	5900 Siegen
Ohm, Ph.	Kirchheller Str. 14	4250 Bottrop
Ohnsorge	Bahnhofstr. 7	4790 Paderborn
Ohse, Gisela	Bahnhofstraße 64	4200 Oberhausen
Ohse, H.	Bahnhofstraße 64	4200 Oberhausen-Sterkrade
Olbrich, F.	Nicolaistraße 4	8068 Pfaffenhofen
Olfs-Leineweber	Berliner Allee 61	4000 Düsseldorf
Olivier, W.	Hauptstraße 48	7812 Bad Krozingen
Ong, Keny Siong	St.-Jürgen-Straße	2800 Bremen
Onken, K.	Adalbertstr. 9	2940 Wilhelmshaven
Onken, Niels	Bödekerstr. 27	4500 Osnabrück
Oppel, Prof. O.	Heusnerstr. 40	Wuppertal
Ortbauer, R.	Im Sommwerwind 13a	7 Stuttgart-Vaihingen
Ortmann, W.	Mörickestraße 7	7142 Marbach
Oser, Wolfgang	Burgnindeckstraße 5	7580 Bühl
Ossendorff, Ingo	Eichenhofstraße 21	5253 Lindlar
Osswald, Robert	Königstraße 61	4100 Duisburg-Neudorf
Ostenried, Hans	Leopoldstraße 3	7530 Pforzheim
Ostwald, Henny	Kriegsstrasse 178	7500 Karlsruhe
Oswald, Alois	Geheimrat-Isl-Straße 12	8058 Erding
Ott, Carl	Brönner Str. 15	6000 Frankfurt
Overdick, H.	Kurfürstenstraße 16	5170 Jülich
Overhoff, W.	Friedr.-Ebert-Straße 27	2800 Bremen

Özer-Arrasti, M.	Römerstr. 5	6508 Alzey
Paasl, W.	Schulstr. 36	4690 Herne
Pabst, Rose	Lucas-Cranach-Straße 68	8640 Kronach
Paeper, F. J.	Georgstr. 15	309 Verdem am der Aller
Pahlitzsch, J.	Potsdamer Straße 154	1000 Berlin 30
Palucki, W.	Martin-Luther-Straße 65	1000 Berlin 30
Pape, H.	Am Dobben 100	2800 Bremen
Pape, Helmut	Holländische Str. 71	3500 Kassel
Pape, Rolf	In der Wann 16	7600 Offenburg
Papst, Prof. W.	Rübenkamp 148	2000 Hamburg 33
Paque	St.-Veith-Straße 7	5440 Mayen
Pasch, Elfriede	An der Golzheim-Heide	4000 Düsseldorf
Pasler, H.	Schillerstraße 12	7170 Schwäb.-Gmünd
Passow, Arnold	Seestraße 29	8036 Herrsching
Pau, Prof. Hans	Moorenstraße 5	4000 Düsseldorf
Paul	Wandrahmstr. 40	3140 Lüneburg
Paul, Ludwig	Gerstenstr. 4	4600 Dortmund
Paulsen, Heinz	Parkstraße 49	2800 Bremen
Paulus, E.	Bramfelder Ch. 281	2000 Hamburg 71
Pauly, Erich	Meckenheimer Allee 133	5300 Bonn
Paust, Eckhard	Hammer Str. 165	4403 Hiltrup
Pecking, Engelbert	Osterwall 20	4290 Bocholt
Peiker, F.	Hoher Weg 4	3200 Hildesheim
Penkert, H.	Gartenstr.	3352 Einbeck
Peny, Janina	Grillostr. 51	4650 Gelsenkirchen – Schalke
Peppinghaus, Jochen	Marienstr. 5-7	5800 Hagen
Peppmüller-Frotscher, H.	Düsseldorfer Straße 29	4020 Mettmann
Pernice, E.	Dudenstr. 16	6430 Bad Hersfeld
Pesch, K. J.	Vahrenwalder Str. 83	3000 Hannover
Pesendorfer, Ilse	Waldackerweg 82	7300 Eßlingen
Peters, H.	Ludwig-Nissen 38	2250 Husum
Peters, Willi	Bahnhofstr. 2	2900 Oldenburg
Peters-Tillmann, B.	Georgstr. 4	3000 Hannover
Pflanz, Waldemar	Sulzbacher Straße 66	8500 Nürnberg
Pfeifer, D.	Werner-Senger-Str. 7	6250 Limburg
Pfeifer, M.	Gymnasiumstr. 13	6253 Hadamar
Pfeiffer, Gerhard	Dingstatte 18	2980 Pinneberg
Pfeiffer, Hans	Ostbahnstraße 17	6740 Landau
Pfeiffer, Hermann	Seckendorfstraße 10	8820 Gunzenhausen
Pfirrmann, K.	Nobelring 23a	3000 Hannover-Kleefeld
Pfisterer, W.	With. Erb. Straße 4	6900 Heidelberg
Pfretzschner-Mayer, G.	Augsburger Straße 10	7910 Neu-Ulm
Pfriem, Walburga	Am Hofgut 4	6700 Ludwigshafen
Pförtner, H. G.	Marktgrafenstraße 20	7830 Emmendingen
Pfuhl, Emil	Am Postmoor 42	2800 Bremen
Pfund, W.	W. Ulmer Straße 10	8562 Hersbruck
Pfülb, Udo	Friedenstraße 57	4054 Nettetal
Pietsch, Susanne	Hohen Zollerinring 14	4400 Münster
Pildner von Steinburg, H.	Badstr. 10 1/2	817 Bad Tölz
Pilke, A. Marg.	Gartenstr. 31	5800 Hagen
Piper, Prof. H. F.	Ratzeburger Allee 160	2400 Lübeck
Pippow, G.	Grünstraße 2	5620 Velbert
Pisarek, Georg	Teltower Damm 33	1000 Berlin 37
Piwanke, Hans-Jürgen	Bismarckstraße 27	1000 Berlin 12
Plange, Manfred	Friedrichstr. 2	4400 Münster
Plate, F.	Kölner Straße 40	5630 Remsch.-Lennep

Platen-Velz, M.	Wilhelmstraße 35a	5100 Aachen
Plattner, H.	Kurfürstendamm 139	1000 Berlin 31
Plaul, H. W.	Linnebrink 6	4904 Enger
Plettenberg	Frühlingstraße 30	8160 Miesbach
Plitt, B.	Rich.-Wagner-Str. 3	4680 Wanne-Eickel
Plitt, W.	Königstraße 76	8500 Nürnberg
Plogas, Karin	Schulstr. 25	2200 Elmshorn
Plötz, Heinz	Alter Markt 17	2942 Jever
Plump, W.	Hans-Hacker-Straße 1	8650 Kulmbach
Podesta, H.	Poststr. 31	2000 Hamburg 1
Podszus, D.	Offerstraße 36	5620 Velbert
Poeplau, G.	Rheinstr. 12%.	6100 Darmstadt
Pohle, Günter	Bahnhofstraße 21	8122 Penzberg
Pohle, Hans	Haumannstr. 20	4600 Dortmund-Marten
Pohle, H.	Nevigesstraße 9	4000 Düsseldorf-Gerresheim
Pohlenz, Philipp	Marktstr. 40	2940 Wilhelmshaven
Pohlenz, S.	Gr. Allee 1	2000 Hamburg 1
Pohlig, G.	Matth.-Kirchplatz	5000 Köln-Bayenthal
Poppert	Am Karlsbrunnen 1	6350 Bad Nauheim
Porkert, R.	Bahnhofstraße 53	7130 Mühlacker
Posseleke, Lieselotte	Wandsb. Marktstr. 19	2000 Hamburg-Wandsbeck
Posselt, E.	Große Bergstr. 261	2000 Hamburg-Altona
Pörtel, E.	Burgmaierstraße 4	8000 München
Prettin, H.	Fuhlsbütt. Str. 326	2000 Hamburg 33
Preuß, Werner	Königstraße 23	8500 Nürnberg
Preuß, Wulfbert	Lenzhahner Weg 62	6272 Niedernhausen
Preysing, Joh. v.	Lederer Zeile 44	8090 Wasserburg
Prigge, G.	Graffring 31	4630 Bochüm
Priggert, W.	Castroper Hellweg 434	4630 Bochum-Gerthe
Priklonski, M.	Martin-Luther-Pl. 3	3327 Salzgitter-Bad
Probst, A.	Hasenstraße 23	8510 Fürth
Probst, Erwin	Stahlstraße 26	8000 München-Obermensing
Protzer, J.	Bismarckstr. 18	6100 Darmstadt
Pruggmayer, W.	Breite Str. 52	3150 Peine
Prumbs, Leo	Obere Borngasse	5429 Weyer
Prünte, Alfred	Westwall 19	5750 Menden
Puder, Reinhard	Geisbachstraße 63	5400 Koblenz
Pumptow, J.	Berliner Straße 1a	1000 Berlin 27
Purper	Romanplatz 5	8000 München
Putzmann, Lieselotte	Unter den Eichen 93	1000 Berlin 45
Pünder, Hermann	Winckelm. Str. 5b	2000 Hamburg-Nienstedten
Pürkhauer, W.	Parkstraße 19	5650 Solingen-Ohligs
Quednau, H. O.	Jürgensplatz 72	4000 Düsseldorf
Quint, Klaus	Marktstraße 2	7260 Calw
Quosdorf, U.	Pommernstr. 47	68 Mannheim
Raab, Oskar	Kraussoldstraße 22	8590 Marktredwitz
Raabe, Andreas	Heckerstr. 53	3500 Kassel
Raaf, M.	Marktplatz 18	7417 Urach
Raber, Felix	Bahnhofstr. 46	6680 Neunkirchen
Racenberg, Hana	Univ.-Augenklinik	6650 Homburg
Radetzky, Wolfgang	Langendörfer Str. 127	5450 Neuwied
Raffin, Ernst	Heinrichstr. 20	4690 Herne
Rahäuser, H. G.	Weinheimer Straße 12	6800 Mannheim-Käfertal
Rall, Alfred	Oststraße 32	7100 Heilbronn
Rammler, H.	Schellingstraße 20	8000 München 13
Raptis, N.	Baseler Str. 26	788 Säckingen

Rauhut, Heinz	Am Karl-Peter-Pl. 22	3000 Hannover
Raum, Karl	Löpsinger Graben 4	8860 Nördlingen
Raupp, Walter	Bismarckstr. 15	6360 Friedberg
Raykowski, Jürgen	Zwischen d. Brücken 5	2150 Buxtehude
Räppe, S.	Brehmstraße 2	8500 Nürnberg
Reccius, Wilhelm	Münsterstr. 36	4600 Dortmund
Rech, Heinz	Benediktusstraße 78	4000 Düsseldorf-Heerdt
Rechl, Herbert	Frauenstraße 2	8000 München 5
Reckmann	Kirchstr. 1	4250 Bottrop
Regel, Erich	Herforder Str. 50	4970 Bad Oeynhausen
Regenbrecht, U. Th.	Martin-Luther-Straße 76	1000 Berlin 62
Reger	Maximilianstraße 11	8240 Berchtesgaden
Reh, Hildegard	Waldseeweg 43	1000 Berlin 28
Reichel, Fr.	Bürgm.-Schmidt-Straße	2850 Bremerhaven
Reichel, Gottfried	Markt 4	5300 Bonn
Reichert, Walter	M.-v.-Schenckendorff 11	5050 Porz
Reidel, Hans	Univ.-Augenklinik	6650 Homburg
Reim, Martin	Univ.-Augenklinik	3550 Marburg
Reimer, L.	Osterstraße 77	2800 Bremen
Reimers, Otto	Monckebergstr. 17	2000 Hamburg 1
Rein, G.	Luneburger Straße 11	2800 Bremen
Reinfeld, Antje	Eggerscheidter Str. 27/15	4033 Hösel
Reinke, Dagmor	Blankensteiner Str. 5	4600 Dortmund
Reinke, Dirk	Sonnleite 1	8702 Lengfeld
Reinthaler, G.	Weißenburger Straße 34a	8750 Aschaffenburg
Reinwein, Irene		7888 Rheinfelden
Reiser, Prof.	Meckenheimer Allee 50	5300 Bonn
Reiter, Alfred	Wittelsbacher Straße 9	8230 Bad Reichenhall
Remé, Charlotte	Bosselweg 92a	2000 Hamburg 54
Remky, Prof. H.	Arabellastr. 5	8 München 81
Remler, Oskar	Hugenotten-Allee 116	6078 Neu-Isenburg
Renelt, Peter	Terstegenweg 22	4300 Essen
Rentsch, I.	Haldenstraße 62	7291 Garrweiler
Renz, Walter	Bustellistraße 8	8000 München
Requardt, Peter	Wiesenstr. 25	3030 Walsrode
Reschop, Ernst	Birkenweg 4	3004 Isernhagen
Rettelbach, E.	Henkestraße 9	8520 Erlangen
Rettinger, E.	Marktstr. 1	4780 Lippstadt
Reuling, F.	Prinz-Friedrich-Karl-Str. 2	655 Bad Kreuznach
Reusch, Ernst	Basaltweg 72	2000 Hamburg-Poppenb.
Reuscher, Bernhard	Bahnhofstr. 6	2190 Cuxhaven
Reuter, Fritz	Roonstraße 16	5400 Koblenz
Rey, Diether van	Theaterstraße 78	5100 Aachen
Rey-Kokett, Ute van	Theaterstraße 78	5100 Aachen
Reznicek, Leonh.	Auf der Schanze 5	8490 Cham
Richard, L.	Kurfürstenstraße 35	4150 Krefeld-Uerdingen
Richert, H. G.	Usedomer Straße 31	1000 Berlin 65
Richert, Jochen	Öjendorfer Damm 50	2000 Hamburg 70
Richert, Sibylle	Schloßstraße 25	1000 Berlin 27
Richter, G.	Marktstätte 28	7750 Konstanz
Richter, H.	Ludwigstr. 5	6350 Bad Nauheim
Richter, Werner	Schützenstraße 1	8000 München 2
Riedel	Pelkovenstraße 17	8000 München 54
Rieder, Helmut	Bahnhofstraße 7	5530 Gerolstein
Riegel	Viktoriastr. 13	6690 St. Wendel
Riegel, Dietrich	Rochusstraße 4	4000 Düsseldorf

Riegel, Hermann	Bahnhofstr. 38	6600 Saarbrücken
Rieger, Horst	Rhabanusstr. 21	6400 Fulda
Riehm, E.	Tangstedter Landstr. 400	2 Hamburg 62
Riehm, Herbert	Hohenellernweg 35	2950 Leer
Rieland, Fritz	Weidenauer Str. 168	5930 Hüttental
Riese, Wolfgang	Husener Str. 62	4790 Paderborn
Riester, Manfred	Obertorpl. 8	7450 Hechingen
Rilling, Franz	Goethestraße 44	7800 Freiburg
Rimele, Bruno	Buchnerstraße 20	7750 Konstanz
Rix, Jürgen	Dr.-Geiger-Straße 1	8200 Rosenheim
Roberg, Manfred	Möhlenring 55	4152 Kempen
Rochels	R.-Wagner-Straße 24a	5090 Le.-Waldsiedlung
Rockert, Helmut	Langenbeckstraße 1	6500 Mainz
Rodenroth, S.	Univ.-Augenklinik	69 Heidelberg
Roeder, H. v.	Lindwurmstraße 52	8000 München 15
Roesch, E.	Rathausstr. 6	82 Rosenheim
Roese, Hans	Lange Str. 13	2838 Sulingen
Roesen, K. D.	Friedrich- Eigenbrod-Str. 8	354 Korbach
Roesen, U.	Urbanstr. 12	78 Freiburg
Rogahm, E. J.	Alt Tegel 9	1000 Berlin 27
Roggenkämper, Peter	Hochkalter Straße 12	8000 München 90
Rohr, Peter	Hauptstraße 16	6900 Heidelberg
Rollin, J.	Rhathausmarkt 19	2000 Hamburg 1
Rom, D. von	Hauptstraße 48	8990 Lindau
Romahn, J.	Karlstr. 37	7992 Tettnang
Rommel, A.	Pfarrgasse 32	703 Böblingen
Roos, Herbert	Gorresstraße 12	8000 München 13
Rosch, Adolf	Bahnhofstr. 35	6640 Merzig
Rosch, Eckhard	Bandholzstraße 10	6902 Sandhausen
Rosehr, Klaus	Rathausstr. 2	2300 Kiel
Rosenberg, Michael	Windeckstr. 33	6000 Frankfurt
Rosenkötter, Hans	Schurthplatz 4	7828 Neustadt
Rosner, Eberhard	Fröbelstraße 1	8228 Freilassing
Roßberger, Anneliese	Klotzbahn 30	5600 Wuppertal-Sonnborn
Roßmann. Hermann	Klaus-Groß-Weg 22	2000 Norderstedt
Rostosky, E.	Bahnhofstraße 7	7050 Waiblingen
Rothhan, Dieter	Talstr.	6650 Homburg
Rothhan, Evelyn	Talstr.	6650 Homburg
Rott, Gerhard	Maxstraße 25	8400 Regensburg
Rottenburg, Günther	Salzmarkt 5	8950 Kaufbeuren
Röhlmann, G.	Kinderheimstr. 26	4370 Marl-Hüls
Röhrs, Klaus	Knochenhauerstraße 26	2800 Bremen
Römer, Klaus	Alte Holstenstr. 42	2050 Hamburg-Bergedorf
Römer, Manfred	Denksteinweg 3a	2000 Hamburg 70
Römmelt, Josef	Marktplatz 8	7080 Aalen
Rörig, E.	Amtstraße II	6967 Buchen
Rörig, Otto	Pfinztalstraße 71	7500 Karlsruhe-Durlach
Rösch, Olaf	Luisenstraße 44	5340 Bad Honnef
Ruckdeschel, Gerold	Bahnhofstraße 10	5320 Bad Godesberg
Rudolph, Günther	Uhlandstraße 11	7400 Tübingen
Rudolphi, H.	Seetorstraße 2	7760 Radolfzell
Ruehe, Gerald	Küntzelstraße 38	4300 Essen
Ruhberg-Wittig, H.	Brunnenallee 33	359 Bad Wildungen
Rummeld, Rosvita	Schichtheider Straße 70	5605 Hochdahl
Rump, K. H.	Nibelungenpl. 10	3300 Braunschweig
Rumpelhardt, Konrad	Alpenstraße 4	7700 Singen

Rupprecht, K.	Univ.-Augenklinik	2 Hamburg-Eppendorf
Russer, Hans	Eselbräustraße 1	8070 Ingolstadt
Rustler, G.	Postgartenstraße 7	8460 Schwandorf
Rüdinger, Otto	Eisenbahnstraße 23	6750 Kaiserslautern
Rüger, Gisela	Petritorwall 31a	3300 Braunschweig
Rüger, Klaus	Kirchplatz 6	3510 Hannover-Münden
Rühl, Werner	D 25	8420 Kelheim
Rüter, Jens-Jürgen	Thesdorfer Weg 190	2080 Pinneberg-Thesdorf
Rüttenauer, H.	Post Aschau	8213 Stocka
Rütter, Hans Heinrich	Brückenstraße 12	5242 Kirchen
Rüping, H.	Sandkuhle 3	2210 Itzehoe
Rüping, L.	Industriestr. 45	4650 Gelsenkirchen-Horst
Rüßmann, Walter	Nauheimer Straße 11	5000 Köln 41
Rzehulka, Gertraud	Friedrichstraße 21	6700 Ludwigshafen
Sachtleben, H.	Koblenzer Str. 21	5900 Siegen
Sack, Hans	Kantstr. 18	3150 Peine
Saleski, August	Hammerstr. 19	4760 Werl
Salm-Salm, E. zu	Theresienstraße 72	5000 Köln-Lindenthal
Salomon, H.	Ottenser Hauptstr. 3	2000 Hamburg 50
Salzmann, Helga	Im Erlenbusch 10	5300 Bonn
Samland, Helmut	Bahnhofstr. 2	3000 Hannover
Samon, Johanna	Westring 15	4400 Münster
Samson, Gerhard	Postdamm 3	4460 Nordhorn
Samson, Paul	Gerstenblöcken 16	2057 Geesthacht
Saretz, S.	Bruchstr. 34	4930 Detmold
Sartori, Carl	Max-Weber-Platz 11	8000 München 8
Sartori, Carlheinz	Max-Weber-Platz 11	8000 München 8
Sass, J. von	Königstr. 123-125	2400 Lübeck
Sasse, Carl	Luxemb. Straße 293	5000 Köln Klettenberg
Sattler, K. R.	Posener Str. 59a	2940 Wilhelmshaven
Sattler, Olga	Karl-Marx-Straße 80	1000 Berlin 44
Sattler, Rudolf	Fennstraße 4	1000 Berlin 65
Sauer, Heinz	Neustr. 1	4290 Bocholt
Sauerteig, Jürgen	Erdkampsweg 27	2000 Hamburg 63
Saul, Hugo	Brückenstr. 21	6000 Frankfurt
Sautier, Hans	Nibelungenstraße 12	8000 München 19
Sautter, Prof. H.	Martinistr. 52	2000 Hamburg 20
Sauvant, J.	Haus Nr. 80a	2951 Timmel
Sbaiti, Ali	Sebastianstraße 85	5300 Bonn
Schaaf, G.	Alt-Griesheim 22a	623 Frankfurt-Griesheim
Schack, Ernst	Brunnenstr. 16	6208 Bad Schwalbach
Schad, M.	Schönleinstr. 11	7 Stuttgart 1
Schad, W.	Lammstraße 7	6660 Zweibrücken
Schade, Dorothea	Bahnstr. 72	6070 Langen
Schaefer, Bertram	Gerstenblöcken 16	2057 Geesthacht
Schaefer, R.	Felix-Dahm-Straße 6	8700 Würzburg
Schaeffer, Oswald	Nassauische Straße 64	1000 Berlin 31
Schäfer, Elisabeth	Am Haberhof 13	3000 Hannover
Schäfer, G.	Hauptstraße 95	6972 Tauberbischofsheim
Schäfer, W. D.	Univ.-Augenklinik	87 Würzburg
Schäffer, H.	Regenwalder Str. 6	4520 Melle
Schaffer, Heinrich	Köln-Straße 433	5300 Bonn
Schafhausen, G.	Am Burgacker 14	4100 Duisburg
Scharf, H.	Gesandtenstraße 6	8400 Regensburg
Scharf-Mayweg, S.	Bahnhofstr. 36	58 Hagen-Haspe
Scharff, Prof. J.	Liebfrauenplatz 10	6500 Mainz

Scharnke, W.	Vordere Halde II	7032 Sindelfingen
Schaper, R.	Tempelhofer Damm 1	1000 Berlin 42
Scharl-Mayweg, S.	Römerstr. 16	5800 Hagen-Haspe
Scheele, Monika	Augustastraße 20	5650 Solingen
Scheffel, P. D.	Hainstraße 21	8600 Bamberg
Scheffer, W.	Linscheidstr. 2	5990 Altena
Scheffler, Ingeborg	Steindamm 28	2000 Norderstedt 1
Scheffler, Ingeborg	Kurt-Schumacher-Str. 12	3300 Braunschweig
Schell-Wölker, H.	Schleiermacherstraße 4	8500 Nürnberg
Schelle, Harald	Schildergasse 105a	5000 Köln 41
Scheer, L.	Bergstr. 1	6600 Saarbrücken
Schemuth, H.	Wiesenstraße 45	4180 Goch
Schenck, A.	Kriegstraße 191	7500 Karlsruhe
Schenck, A.	Pforzheimer Straße 46	7505 Ettlingen
Schenkel, R.	Landr.-Christian-Str. 98	2820 Bremen-Blumenthal
Scheppach, Peter	Uhlandweg 1	2000 Norderstedt 3
Scherer, Heinrich	Deutsche Str. 2	6630 Saarlouis
Scherz, W.	Hofeichenweg 4	4800 Bielefeld
Scherz, Wolfgang	Tiergarten 16	4300 Essen-Werden
Scheuch, R.	Hochstraße 47	5290 Wipperfürth
Scheuermann, Kl.	Moltkestraße 17a	6740 Landau
Scheyhing, H.	Untere Königstr. 83	35 Kassel
Schicke, H.	Marktplatz 9	8940 Memmingen
Schicketanz, Herbert	Segringer Straße 34	8804 Dinkelsbühl
Schilder, K.	Im Mühlenwinkel 33	4320 Hattingen
Schiller, B.	Spielleutestr. 24	2820 Bremen-Vegesack
Schimkat, E.	Venloer Straße 1	4000 Düsseldorf
Schimmelpfennig, W.	Augenklinik Steglitz	1 Berlin 45
Schindera, Horst	Danziger Straße 21	7033 Herrenberg
Schindler, H.	Walderdorffstraße 12	5415 Engers
Schindler, H.	Sofienstr. 23	757 Baden-Baden
Schinke, I.	Feuerbachstr. 21	6000 Frankfurt
Schippmann, H.	Mühlenstr. 85	24 Lübeck
Schlegel, Prof. H. J.	Univ.-Augenklinik	6650 Homburg
Schlemmer, W.	Rheinstr. 59	6200 Wiesbaden
Schley, H.	Alicestraße 20	6501 Budenheim
Schlicht, G.	Louisenstr. 63	638 Bad Homburg v.d.H.
Schlichting, B.	Karlstraße 22	7210 Rottweil
Schlichting, H.	Frohnhauser Straße 231	4300 Essen
Schliebs, J.	Apfelstr. 23a	4800 Bielefeld
Schloßhardt, H.	Camperstr. 14	2160 Stade
Schmack, E. N.	Wermingserstr. 47	586 Iserlohn
Schmack, Werner	Stiftstr. 5	4950 Minden
Schmans, Malte	Breslauer Str. 1	2260 Niebüll
Schmedes, R.	Barnestr. 26	3050 Wunsdorf
Schmelzer, Prof. H.	Herzog-Max-Str. 13	86 Bamberg
Schmerer, O.	Sulzbacher Straße 29	7150 Backnang
Schmid, Ernst	Untere Vorstadt 5	7470 Ebingen
Schmidt, A.	Ringstraße 8-10	5047 Wesseling
Schmidt, A.	Beethovenstraße 10	8000 München 15
Schmidt, B.	Doblerstraße 6	7400 Tübingen
Schmidt, B.	Josef-Schner-Str. 11	87 Würzburg
Schmidt, Dieter	Neubergweg 32	7800 Freiburg
Schmidt, Horst	Eigelstein 125	5000 Köln
Schmidt, H.	Herwarthstraße 12a	1000 Berlin 45
Schmidt, Joachim	Robert-Koch-Straße 22	5000 Köln-Lindenthal

Schmidt, Margarete	Bahnhofstr. 18	4790 Paderborn
Schmidt, K.	Ehrenstraße 15-17	5000 Köln
Schmidt, Prof. R.	Salinenstraße 55a	6550 Bad Kreuznach
Schmidt, R.	Univers.-Augenklinik	5000 Köln 41
Schmidt, W.	Bahnhofstraße 12	8960 Kempten
Schmidt-Mumm, E.	Lavesstr. 6	3000 Hannover
Schmidt-Schlegel, J.	Bergstr. 95a	4630 Bochum
Schmilewski, Walter	Wilhelmstraße 14	6502 Mainz-Kostheim
Schmitt, A.	Friedrichstraße 9	7980 Ravensburg
Schmitt, H.	Breite Straße 52	5470 Andernach
Schmitt, Heinspeter	Augenklinik	4600 Dortmund
Schmitt, H.	Heidengäßle 7	7980 Ravensburg
Schmitt, Wolfgang	Hofstraße 166	4010 Hilden
Schmitter-Westermann, G.	Grünewaldstr. 7	2880 Brake
Schmittmann, A.	Oberkasseler Str. 125a	1000 D-Oberkassel
Schmitz, Elmar	Marsiliusstraße 72	5000 Köln-Sülz
Schmutter, Jürgen	Goldstr. 7	4400 Münster
Schnabel, G.	Weinsenerstr. 12a	2000 Hamburg-Harburg
Schneider, Alfred	Berggärtenstraße 36	5450 Neuwied
Schneider-Sauvant, C.	Brühlstraße 1	7310 Plochingen
Schneider, H.	Erchenstraße 14	7920 Heidenheim
Schneider, H.-Henning	Bahnhofstr. 3	2930 Norden Süderneul. I
Schneider, H. L.	Erfurter Straße 21	7260 Calw
Schneider, M.	Schloßstr. 1	6308 Butzbach
Schneider, Peter	Erchenstraße 20	7920 Heidenheim
Schneider, Waltraud	Dorfstraße 3	4005 Büderich
Schneider, W.	Kaiser-Wilhelm-Ring 42	5000 Köln
Schneider, Yoerk	Nördl. Stadtgraben 6	7080 Aalen
Schnell, Dieter	Univers.-Augenklinik	5000 Köln-Lindenthal
Schoenberg	Wiesenstr. 10	3103 Bergen
Schoeneck, W.	Adalbertsteinweg 52	5100 Aachen
Schoenknecht, Elf.	Konrad-Beste-Str. 4	3457 Stadtoldendorf
Schoenknecht, L.	Neue Str. 1	3450 Holzminden
Scholz, W.	Wiener Straße 21	1000 Berlin 36
Scholz-Stammer, W.	Arndtpl. 4	2300 Kiel
Schornstein	Friedr.-Engels-Allee 289	5600 Wuppertal-Barmen
Schott, A.	Krummbogen 82	2300 Kiel
Schott, Chr.	Jahnstraße 2	7332 Eislingen
Schott, Klaus	Plattbergstraße 1-3	4300 Essen-Werden
Schoyerer, R.	Kasernenstraße 17	7910 Neu-Ulm
Schönewald, Kurt	Kreuzstraße 4	2850 Bremerhaven
Schöninger, L.	Charlottenstraße 21a	7000 Stuttgart
Schöpfer, O.	Hamburger Str. 80	2240 Heide
Schrader, Prof. K. E.	Kriegsbergstraße 60	7000 Stuttgart 1
Schreck, Prof. E.	Univ.-Augenklinik	852 Erlangen
Schreiber, A.	Annastraße 39	8900 Augsburg
Schreiber, A.	Bahnhofstraße 7	6252 Diez
Schreiber, F.	Rechtenbacher Straße 478	8770 Lohr
Schrick, Agnes	Dannekamp 18	2000 Hamburg 53
Schriever, Dietmar	An der Turnhalle 14	6500 Mainz
Schröder, E.	Dürkheimer Str. 41	6 Frankfurt 80
Schröder, Hans	Sieghartstr. 4	8019 Ebersberg
Schröeder, H.	Markt 10	3508 Melsungen
Schröter, M.	Lerchenstraße 67	7100 Heilbronn
Schubert, H.	Friedrichstraße 10	8510 Fürth
Schuck, S.	Main-Taunus-Zentrum	6231 Sulzbach

Schuler, H.	Schopenhauer 28	7000 Stuttgart-Vaihingen
Schulkamp	Mühltorstr. 5	6470 Büdingen
Schulte, G.	Friedrichstr. 22	4700 Hamm
Schulte, Prof. Dieter	von-Graefe-Straße 37	4330 Mülheim
Schulte, L.	Haus 10	5481 Rolandseck
Schulte, R.	Bahnhofstraße 34c	5420 Niederlahnstein
Schulten, Friedr.-W.	Niederstraße 68	4150 Krefeld-Uerdingen
Schultheiß, Klaus	Moorenstraße 5	4000 Düsseldorf
Schultz-Zehden	Nehringdamm 40	1000 Berlin 61
Schultze, Hans	Juvenellstraße 45	8500 Nürnberg
Schulz, Helga	Katharinenstraße 9b	8910 Landsberg
Schulz, Joachim	Katharinenstraße 9b	8910 Landsberg
Schulz, Rudolf	Kölner Landstraße 174	4000 Düsseldorf
Schulze, Gero	Eisenacher Straße 2	5400 Koblenz
Schulze, Joachim	Augustastr. 2	4900 Herford
Schulze, Wilfried	Kilianstraße 70	5400 Koblenz 32
Schum, R.	Dr.-Robert-Koch-Straße	5070 Bergisch-Gladbach
Schum, U.	Tappenstr. 1-3	338 Goslar
Schumacher, C.	Overwegstr. 8	4650 Gelsenkirchen
Schumacher, Chr.	Bahnhofstr. 6	5790 Brilon
Schumacher, H.	Friedrichsplatz 6	3500 Kassel
Schumacher, Heinz	Worringer Straße 85	4000 Düsseldorf
Schumacher, H.	Markt 8/9	2400 Lübeck
Schumacher, Ingrid	Rosenheimer Straße 2	8000 München 80
Schumacher, J.	Bergstraße 7	4200 Oberhausen-Osterfeld
Schumann, Brigitte	Hauptstr. 23	3052 Bad Nenndorf
Schumann, Ch.	Moerser Straße 275	4102 Homberg
Schuppe, H.	Zindelstr. 3	34 Göttingen
Schuwicht, E.	Brückenmüllerstr. 6	6430 Bad Hersfeld
Schübsgen, Arnold	Untere Straße 10	5290 Wipperfürth
Schüller, Erwin	Gertenstraße 11	4000 Düsseldorf
Schümann	Bahnhofstr. 1	3110 Uelzen
Schüren, O.	Weber Koppel 63	2400 Lübeck
Schütte, E.	Univ.-Augenklinik	355 Marburg
Schütz, Klaus	Zeller Straße 97	7600 Offenburg
Schwab, Berthold	Südring 94	6500 Mainz 22
Schwab, Erika	Lienhartstraße 6	8120 Weilheim
Schwaeppe, Cl.	Fr.-Ebert-Straße 45	4220 Dinslaken
Schwägerle, G.	Am Holzmarkt 7	74 Tübingen
Schwagmeyer	Münsterstr. 119	4600 Dortmund
Schwaiger, S.	Im Rothschild 14	6720 Speyer
Schwaiger, Sigurd	Burgenlandstraße 72	7000 Stuttgart-Feuerbach
Schwamborn, O.	Bahnhofstr. 1	5308 Rheinbach
Schwaner	Bahnhofstr. 13	3550 Marburg
Schwarz, K.	Holtenauer Str. 114a	2300 Kiel
Schwarze, Ursula	Sachsenstraße 15	5600 Wuppertal 2
Schwarzenburg, Prof. C.	Börsenbrücke 4	2000 Hamburg 11
Schwarzenburg, Lothar	Börsenbrücke 4	2000 Hamburg 11
Schwebel, F. K.	Devarannestraße 5	5650 Solingen-Wald
Schwiebert, Ernst	Kammanstr. 34	5800 Hagen
Schwiedessen, Uwe	Erwinstraße 81	7800 Freiburg
Schwind, Bernd	Gartenstr. 8	6231 Altenhain/Frankfurt-Höchs
Schwitalla, H.	Neue Straße 71	7900 Ulm
Schwoerer, Gudrun	Walderseestr. 29	3000 Hannover
Seefried, J.	Neustraße 43	5350 Euskirchen

Seidel John.	Oberntorwall 23	4800 Bielefeld
Seiler, Anton	Humboldtstraße 32	8000 München 8
Seißinger	Keesburgstraße 30	8700 Würzburg
Seitz, Prof. R.	Augenabt. d. Alten Vincentius-krankenhauses	75 Karlsruhe
Selan, Edvard	Schloßparkstraße 52	5105 Laurensberg
Selle, H.	Sedanstr. 28	3 Hannover 1
Sellerbeck, S.	Musterbahn 1	2400 Lübeck
Seraphin, R.	Landteilstraße 16	6800 Mannheim-Lindenhof
Serr, Prof. H.	Leoprechtingstraße 16	8000 München 67
Severin, B. D.	Rennstr. 49	4900 Herford
Severin, Maria	Mayener Straße 9	5000 Köln-Sülz
Seydewitz, R.	Fritz-Geige-Straße 22	7800 Freiburg
Siedenbiedel, H.	Bismarckstr. 49a	3388 Bad Harzburg
Siebel, U.	Graf-Edzard-Str. 14	2960 Aurich
Sieben, H.	Sternstraße 19	4150 Krefeld
Siebert, Wolfgang	Rheinstr. 5	6100 Darmstadt
Siegert, P.	Lichtwartstr. 7	2 Hamburg 20
Siegfried, H.	Eschenbruchstraße 1	5000 Köln-Dellbrück
Sievers, T.	Carl-Schinz-Straße 20	2800 Bremen
Sigmund, Erika	Goethestraße 18	7800 Freiburg
Sigmund, Rudolf	Sperberweg 6	6950 Mosbach-Waldstadt
Simon, O.	Friedr.-Ebert-Straße 132b	5600 Wuppertal-Elberfeld
Simon, W.	Marienstraße 36b	7000 Stuttgart-W.
Simons, Karl-Josef	Theaterstraße 96	5100 Aachen
Sint, Michael	König-Heinrich-Weg, 118	2000 Hamburg 61
Sinz, Dieter	Manfrd-v.-Richth.-Str. 8	1000 Berlin 42
Sippl, Florian	Bahnhofstraße 29	7080 Aalen
Skrljac, Dragutin	Trierer Straße 70	5508 Hermeskeil
Skutscheck	Gollierstraße 5	8000 München 12
Slanddorf, H.	Sandufer 4	4407 Emsdetten
Smetmans, F. K.	Kneippweg 11	7988 Wangen
Sobdermann, G.	Sautierstraße 83	7800 Freiburg
Soenning, R.	Hallhof 8	8940 Memmingen
Sommer, Lothar	Jasperallee 17	3300 Braunschweig
Sommerland, Deinhard	Humboldtstr. 2	2870 Delmenhorst
Sonntag, A.	Peterstr. 28	2910 Westerstede
Soyka, Hans	Holm 17	2390 Flensburg
Söllner, Prof. Friedrich	Augustenburger Pl.	1000 Berlin 65
Specht	Marktstraße 70	5450 Neuwied
Speicher, H.	Louise-Dumont-Straße 1	4000 Düsseldorf
Spiecker, J.	Lindenstr. 9a	2830 Bremen-Aumund
Spiegeler, Friedr.	Wilhelmstr. 10	4550 Bramsche
Spiess, Kurt	Oranienstraße 10-11	1000 Berlin 36
Spelsberg, E.	Kaiser-Max-Str. 11	895 Kaufbeuren
Spir, E.	Birkenau 4	2000 Hamburg 22
Spira, K.	Heimannstraße 221	1000 Berlin 44
Sprecher, F.	Anzengruberstraße 7	1000 Berlin 44
Sprenger, Hermann	Scharnhorst 90	4400 Münster
Sprenger, K. H.	Frankfurterstr. 22	605 Offenbach
Springob, Fr.	Neckarstraße 55	7300 Eßlingen
Sradj, Nadim	Am unteren Rain 11	6300 Gießen
Stache-Schenk, Ingrid	Hogenfelde 31a	2000 Hamburg-Norderstedt 2
Staenglen, K.	Wolfertweg 9	7930 Ehingen
Staffeldt, M.	Klosterstraße 34	1000 Berlin 20

Staiger, Guntram	Odenwaldstr. 5	6110 Dieburg
Stamer, O.	Frickenhäuser Str. 19	8703 Ochsenfurt
Stange, R.	Krayer Straße 197	4300 Essen-Kray
Stanjek, Wolfgang	Wasserstraße 18	7600 Offenburg
Stanka, Rudolf	Reichsstraße 31	8850 Donauwörth
Stark, Hilmar	Grüner Weg 43	2400 Lübeck
Starke, H.	Stadtweg 27a	2380 Schleswig
Stausberg, G.	Werderstr. 55	67 Ludwigshafen 28
Stäbler, W.	Hindenburgallee 13	3042 Munster-Lager
Stärk, N.	Egelbacher Str. 20	6 Frankfurt
Steck, Klaus	Margaretengasse 8	5500 Trier
Steden, E.	Moltkestr. 24	4930 Detmold
Stefani, F.	Richard-Strauss-Str. 107	8 München 80
Steffen, Rüdiger	Suhrfeldstr. 61	28 Bremen
Steffen, R.	Moltkestr. 32	2870 Delmenhorst
Stegmaier, J.	Lindenweg 3	7000 Stuttgart-Vaihingen
Stegmann, H.	Benekestr. 13	4930 Detmold
Steiger, R. M.	Kurfürstenstraße 49	4300 Essen
Stein, Arno	Snadenort 6	4600 Dortmund
Stein, H. J.	Eligersweg 73	2000 Hamburg 33
Stein, R.	Renate-Priv.-Straße	1000 Berlin 42
Stein, R.	Am Hauptbahnhof 12	6000 Frankfurt
Stein, W.	Am Staugraben 9	29 Oldenburg
Steinbach, P. D.	Tucholskyweg 49	6500 Mainz
Steinborn, J.	Hans-Fluck-Straße	6507 Ingelheim
Steinhoff, Wolf-Dieter	Dudenstr. 5	4600 Dortmund
Steinmetz, Bernhard	Stadtplatz 43	8260 Mühldorf
Steinmetz, W.	Gesandtenstraße 6	8400 Regensburg
Steinvorth, E.	Löpentinstr. 29	3000 Hannover-Kleefeld
Stemmermann, W.	Mulwald 38	8520 Erlangen
Stewens, H.	Markt 4	4600 Dortmund
Stephan	Gartenstraße 17	7410 Reutlingen
Stiebritz, Jutta	Elisabethstraße 144	4150 Krefeld
Stief, K.	Bahnhofsplatz 10	4630 Bochum
Stiefbold, E.	Aulberstraße 10	7410 Reutlingen
Stiefenhofer, C.	Beyerstraße 18	7900 Ulm
Stiehler, Dagmar	Annastraße 27	8000 München 22
Stiller, Fritz G.	Am Markt 12	2240 Heide
Stiller, Gerhard	Stiftstr. 5	4950 Minden
Stiller, W.	Rothenfelder Str. 25	3180 Wolfsburg
Stockhousen, P.	Gartenstraße 2	7050 Waiblingen
Stodtmeister, R.	Herzogstr. 62	6078 Neu-Isenburg
Stoewer, E.	Grumatten 25	7813 Staufen
Stoffel, Peter	Möbeck 57	5600 Wuppertal 11
Stolpmann, Elisabeth	Meraner Straße 42	1000 Berlin 62
Stolze, Elisabeth	Kaiserdamm	1000 Berlin 19
Stolzenburg, G.	Eppend. Baum 35	2000 Hamburg 20
Storp, Hermann	Darler Heide 14	4660 Gelsenkirchen-Buer
Stöhr, Carola	Südl. Münchener Straße 3	8022 München-Grünwald
Straub, R.	Geländeweg 6	7831 Kollmarsreute
Straub, Prof. Wolfg.	Rob.-Koch-Str. 4	3550 Marburg
Strauch, Barbara-Ursula	Robert-Koch-Str. 1-3	2300 Kiel
Strecker, Adolf	Haugener Straße 17	7850 Lörrach
Streißle, K.	Gartenstraße 6	7980 Ravensburg
Streitenberg, H.	Ettlinger Straße 9	7500 Karlsruhe
Strietzel, H. N.	Steinweg 76	5290 Stolberg

Stromb.-Kleinholz, E. v. ...	Schillerstraße 7	8788 Bückenau-Stadt
Stromburg, G.	Weender Str. 46	3400 Göttingen
Stroucken, M.	Colmanstraße 11	5300 Bonn
Strunden, D.	Germanicusstraße 2a	5000 Köln-Marienburg
Struve, Barbara	Sachsenwald Theater	2057 Reinbeck
Strüngmann, E.	Riedersteinstraße 39	8180 Tegernsee
Stryz, R.	Stadtamthof 3	8400 Regensburg
Stueke, F. W.	Bödekerstr. 102	3000 Hannover
Stumpf, F.	Theatinerstraße 44	8000 München
Stumptner, H.	Kisslingweg 5	7950 Biberach
Stümpel, W.	Ludwigstraße 79	8500 Nürnberg-Langwasser
Stürmer, W.	Kaplanstr. 12	3 Hannover-Linden
Sulima, Peter	Marienstr. 9	4950 Minden
Sumfleth, Hellmut	Hoheluftchaussee 15	2000 Hamburg 20
Sunder-Plassmann, Martin ..	Westring 15	4400 Münster
Süchting, Peter	Wilhelmstr. 26	3070 Nienburg
Süße, Ursula	Wilh.-Busch-Str. 39	6000 Frankfurt
Szegedi, Uwe	Kleistr. 6	3180 Wolfsburg
Szillinsky, R.	Karenweg 8	5520 Bitburg
Szopa, Rudolf	Brandanlage 10	8740 Bad Neustadt
Tacke, H.	Brunnenstraße 8	4000 Düsseldorf
Tams, G.	Univ.-Augenklinik	2 Hamburg 20
Taubitz, W.	Herm.-Balk-Str. 137	2000 Hamburg-Rahlstedt
Taubmann, W.	Städt. Augenklinik	76 Offenburg
Täumer, R.	Univ.-Augenklinik	78 Freiburg
Tegtmeier, Klaus	Herwigstr. 20a	6340 Dillenburg
Tehrani, Iradi	Habichtspl. 8	2000 Hamburg 33
Teichelmann	Senffenberger Ring 13	1000 Berlin 26
Tenner, Alfons	Bergheimer Straße 20	6900 Heidelberg
Terhorst, Theo	Josef-Schregel-Straße 30 ...,...	5160 Düren
Tertsch, R.	Homburger Straße 68	4130 Moers
Teping, Heino	Schönforster Straße 8	4108 Monschau
Teupel, Elisabeth	Fahrhaustr. 28	2000 Hamburg 22
Teutrine, Dieter	Westernstr. 6-8	4790 Paderborn
Thaden, F.	Mühlenstr. 72	2950 Leer
Thelen, E.	Wilhelmstr. 16	6200 Wiesbaden
Thesen, Ernst	Dorotheenstr. 176	2000 Hamburg 39
Thiel	Univers.-Augenklinik	2300 Kiel
Thiel, L.	Städt. Krankenhaus	67 Ludwigshafen
Thiele, H.	Wursterstr. 49	285 Bremerhaven
Thielmann-Grieger, M.	U 3, 19	6800 Mannheim
Thier, C. J.	Wilhelmstraße 58	5100 Aachen
Thierfelder, Ludwig	Ziegelgasse 1	8450 Amberg
Thies, F. C.	Beim Strohhause 34 II	2000 Hamburg 1
Thimme, Erich	Meitnerstr. 2	3000 Hannover 1
Thomann, Prof. Heinrich ..	Im Sonnenwinkel 2	5850 Hohenlimburg
Thommsen, Jens	Ringstr. 3	3301 Cremlingen
Thranberend, Ch.	Univ.-Augenklinik	6 Frankfurt
Thumm, H. W.	Augustenburger Platz, Städt. Rudolf-Virchow-Krankenhaus	1 Berlin 65
Thurm, Klaus	Frühlingsanger 7	8000 München 45
Thurn, Gisela	Taunusstraße 17	6500 Mainz-Hechtsheim
Thuss, J.	Lavesstr. 6	3 Hannover 1
Thyavorabun, Vorachal ...	Thomastr. 8	6300 Gießen
Tiburtius, Prof. H. F.	Hindenburgdamm 30	1 Berlin 45
Tiedan, Joachim	Lippestr. 10	4270 Dorsten

Tiedtke, H.	Im Neuwerk 24	2160 Stade
Tienss, K. H.	Hindenburgstr. 7	4910 Lage
Tielmann, L.	Hochstraße 19	4030 Ratingen
Tietmeyer, J.	Zeppelinstraße 8	4000 Düsseldorf
Tietze, Guntram	Morillenhang 4	5100 Aachen
Tilling, Gudrun	Paradeplatz 5	6728 Germersheim
Tillmann, W.	Bertoldstraße 6	4300 Essen
Tominschek, Viktor	Frankenwaldstraße 4	8674 Naila
Toppel, L.	Gabriel-Max-Str. 27	8 München 90
Tosch, C.	Gutschmidtstraße 7	1000 Berlin 47
Traub, H.	Ratiborstraße 31	8500 Nürnberg
Träm, Otto	Aachener Straße 326	5000 Köln-Braunsfeld
Trehkopf-Voicu, G.	Skalitzer Straße 74	1000 Berlin 36
Treschkow, E. von	Bonner Talweg 23	5300 Bonn-Endenich
Treumer, Karl-Heinz	Marienhölzungsweg 7	2390 Flensburg
Triebe, Ingrid	Hindenburgstr. 9	4980 Bünde
Triller, M.	Schimperstraße 10	6800 Mannheim
Troubal, R.	Siegfriedstraße 23	6520 Worms
Trödtmann, M.	Wittekindstr. 5	4990 Lübecke
Tröndle, W.	Lameystraße 8	7500 Karlsruhe
Trübenbach, F.	Tempelhofer Damm 139	1000 Berlin 42
Trümper, G.	Werner-Senger-Str. 14	6250 Limburg
Tschoepke, M.	Ringstr. 6	Landsthul/Pfalz
Turss, Rüdiger	Berliner Str. 7	3550 Marburg
Twelmeyer	Am Ring 4	325 Hameln
Uckely, W.	Marktplatz 15	3440 Eschwege
Ufer, E.	Brehmstraße 19	4000 Düsseldorf
Uhl, H. K.	Plenganserstraße 36	8000 München
Uhlenbrock, J.	Weststr. 27	4700 Hamm
Ullerich, Prof. Klaus	Beurhausstr. 40	4600 Dortmund
Unger, Prof. H. H.	Karlstraße 65	7800 Freiburg
Unger, L.	Altendorfer Straße 288	4300 Essen
Uniereiner, H. G.	Adam-Rauch-Str. 13	6030 Groß-Gerau
Unhhür, Uwe	Kriegsbergstraße 60	7000 Stuttgart 1
Urbahn, H.	Graf-Adolf-Str. 36	4628 Lünen
Utermann, Dieter	Saturnweg 32	2000 Hamburg 64
Utermann, H.	Beethovenstr. 14	5810 Witten
Utke, F.	Klosterkamp 2a	2360 Bad Segeberg
Vatteroth, K. L.	Gerichtsstraße 31	4300 Essen-Borbeck
Veit, E.	Wehmenkamp 4	4300 Essen-Rüttenscheid
Veit, R.	Herman-Lans-Str. 2	6308 Butzbach
Venz, M.	Kurfürstendamm 69	1000 Berlin 15
Vetter, G.	Im Fange 75	4500 Osnabrück
Vettin, Günther	Rothschildallee 6	6000 Frankfurt
Viedebandt, A.	Lesserstr. 158	2000　Hamburg-Wandsbeck
Viefhues, T. K.	Carolinenstr. 10	4450 Lingen
Vieweger, Konrad	Metzmacher Straße 11	4018 Langenfeld
Villinger, Helga	Schwarzwaldstraße 4	7800 Freiburg
Vilmar, K. F.	Obere Königstr. 51	3500 Kassel
Voelkel, R.	Unterstraße 24	7737 Bad Dürkheim
Vogel	Niendorfer Marktpl. 22	2000 Hamburg-Niendorf
Vogel, F.	Erichsenweg 25	2250 Husum
Vogel, K.	Schwicheldtstr. 6	31 Celle
Vogel, M.	Augenklinik Klinikum Essen	43 Essen
Vogel, Rudolf	Parkstr. 3	6368 Bad Vilbel
Vogel, W.	Münchener Straße 25/I	8200 Rosenheim

Vogelsang, K.	Hohenzollerndamm 34	1 Berlin Grunewald 33
Vogt, M.	Friedrichstr. 1	69 Heidelberg
Voigt, C.	Krögerskamp 47	4424 Stadtlohn
Voit, H.	Fürther Straße 17a	8500 Nürnberg
Volkmann, G. von	Friedenstr. 1	4800 Bielefeld
Volkmer, G.	Hermannstr. 53/57	4600 Dortmund-Hörde
Volkner, O.	Drawehner Str. 14	3130 Lüchow
Volmer, D. E.	Kirchstr. 7	4690 Herne
Vonnegut-Witzel, K.	Hopmannstraße 4	5320 Bad Godesberg
Voss, H. J.	Kirchenstraße 2	8510 Fürth
Voth, J. A.	Ottenser Hauptstr. 13	2000 Hamburg-Altona
Völger, Peter	Bremer Str. 1	Buchholz i.d. Nordheide
Vüllers, Th.	Städt. Krankenhaus	7500 Karlsruhe
Wachholz, Ernst-A.	Seestr. 63	6901 Eppelheim
Wagner, Anneliese	Gellerstraße 48	5000 Köln-Nippes
Wagner, E.	Standeplatz 11	3500 Kassel
Wagner, Prof. F.	Kapellenstr. 42	6200 Wiesbaden
Wagner, Gerhard	Filandastraße 11	1000 Berlin 41
Wagner, Georg	Heinr.-Koch-Str. 61	6600 Saarbrücken
Wagner, Georg	Im Drachenfeld 5	6122 Erbach
Wagner, Gunter	Fürstenbergstraße 7	5670 Opladen
Wagner, Knut	Domhof 4a	4500 Osnabrück
Wagner, Michael	Moltkestr. 4	2380 Schleswig
Wagner, Otto	Osterholzstr. 27	4600 Dortmund
Wagner, Wigand	Am Eichenwald 18	6651 Jägersburg
Wahl, H.	Westliche 96	7530 Pforzheim
Waibel, B.	Königsberger Straße 13	7990 Friedrichshafen
Wak, Helmut	Gänsemarkt 13	4832 Wiedenbrück
Wallenstern, L. v.	Waldachstraße 5	7270 Nagold
Waller, Wolfgang	Bäumlstraße 8	8450 Amberg
Wallmann, E.	Nobistor 34	2000 Hamburg 50
Wallow, Ingolf	Ebersberger Straße 30	8000 München 80
Walser, Prof. Erwin	Theatinerstr. 23	8 München 2
Walser-Körner, G.	Nds. Landeskrankenhaus	3405 Tiefenbrunn
Walter, Mathias	Mühlenstraße 29	7505 Ettlingen
Walter, R.	Menzelstraße 7	8000 München 27
Walther, D.	Sonnenplatz 6	8670 Hof
Walther, W.	Zobelreuther Straße 35	8670 Hof
Wanckel, E.	Ronnstraße 12	5270 Gummersbach
Waubke, Prof. Theo	Lürsweg 9a	4300 Essen-Werden
Weber	Spitalstraße 7	8720 Schweinfurt
Weber, Bernd	Sandberggäßchen 44 IV	6000 Frankfurt
Weber, Bruno	Bahnhofstr. 15	633 Wetzlar
Weber, Daniel	Obere Grabenstraße 34	5470 Andernach
Weber, Günter	Duisburger Straße 229	4100 Duisburg-Hamborn
Weber, Hans	Walsroder Str. 48	3012 Langenhagen
Weber, H. Chr.	Graf-Gessler-Straße 8	5000 Köln-Deutz
Weber, Hans	Bergstr. 387	4370 Marl
Weber, Joachim	Buchheimer Straße 61	5000 Köln-Mülheim
Weber, Karl-Heinz	Schwindstr. 3	6000 Frankfurt
Weber, Margarete	Hauptstr. 55	6140 Bensheim
Weede, Wolfhart	Billstedter Pl. 7	2000 Hamburg 74
Wegerhoff, Heinz	Binzengrün 24	7800 Freiburg
Wegerhoff, Heinz	Augenklinik	4330 Mülheim
Wegener, Klaus	Kafkaweg 6	7000 Stuttgart-Freiberg
Wegner, E.	Stephanienstr. 38	78 Freiburg

Wehner, Frank	Am Schiefen Berg 46	3340 Wolfenbüttel
Wehner, H.	Ernst-Bode-Str. 17	2140 Bremervörde
Wehrmann, M.	Hildehardstraße 31	1000 Berlin 31
Weichert, H.	Bleichertwiesen 10	3150 Peine
Weiden, Helmut	Kalker Hauptstraße 141	5000 Köln 91
Weigelin, Prof. E.	Univers.-Augenklinik	5300 Bonn
Weil, Klaus	Siegfriedstraße 16	6520 Worms
Weil, R.	Siegfriedstraße 16	6520 Worms
Weimar, H.	Kaiserstraße 65	5220 Waldbröl
Weimershausen, H. J.	Augenklinik	5600 Wuppertal-Barmen
Weinand, Klaus	Soesfeldweg 20	4400 Münster
Weinbeck, Wilh.	Plinganser Straße 124	8000 München 25
Weinges, Gabriele	Am Kehrberg 10	6650 Homburg
Weintz, Fritz	Juvenellstraße 23	8500 Nürnberg
Weirauch, Sigrun	Evang. Krankenhaus	4300 Essen-Werden
Weissbach, Isolde	Bahnhofstraße 97	7160 Gaildorf
Weisner	Kronshagener Weg 29	2300 Kiel 1
Weiß, Hans	Beiertheimer Allee 3	75 Karlsruhe
Weiß, Norbert	Hittorfstr. 40	4400 Münster
Weiße, Ursula	Europa-Center	1000 Berlin 30
Weitz, G.	Hs. Kirchberg	5171 Kirchberg
Welge-Lüßen, Lutz	Univ.-Augenklinik	3550 Marburg
Weller, Joachim	Steinstr. 29	4970 Bad Oeynhausen
Wellern	Hochstraße 9	4030 Ratingen
Welsch, M.	Judithstraße 10	8720 Schweinfurt
Welt, Rüdiger	Paul-Reiss-Straße 1	6232 Bad Soden
Wendt	Gütersloher Str. 14	4840 Rheda
Wendt, W.	Bäckerstr. 39	3250 Hameln
Wening, Elmar	Alleestraße 89	5630 Remscheid
Wenzel, Sabine	Grunewaldstraße 25	1000 Berlin 62
Werb	Theresienstraße 5	8730 Bad Kissingen
Wermbter, Uwe	Eckermannstr. 10	2102 Hamburg 93
Wertheimer, E.	Kegelfeldstraße 22	8019 Glonn
Wesselmann, Dietrich	Oststr. 22	4410 Warendorf
Wessely, E. O.	Romanstraße 26a	8000 München 19
Wessing, Prof. Achim	Hufelandstraße 55	4300 Essen-Holsterhausen
West, K. H.	Am Rathaus 15	5628 Heiligenhaus
Westholt, H. G.	Wickeder Hellweg 81	4600 Dortmund-Wickede
Westphal, P.	Bahnhofsallee 18	3200 Hildesheim
Wethmar, Armin	Wesereschstr. 39	4500 Osnabrück
Wetzel, Wilfried	Im Beismar 18	4690 Herne
Wichert, H. G.	Nürnberger Straße 37	8542 Roth
Wick, J.	Promenade 6	7900 Ulm
Wieber, H.	Waldesruh 33	6401 Döllbach
Wiebusch, D.	Buchenweg 18	5301 Röttgen
Wiegand, Ingeborg	Frankfurter Str. 77½	3500 Kassel
Wiegang, W.	Hagsche Straße 46	4190 Kleve
Wieland, R.	Vogelsangstraße 12	7300 Eßlingen
Wielgoss, H.	Pforzheimer Straße 368	7000 Stuttgart-Weilimdorf
Wienhues, A.	Hauptstr. 82	4812 Brackwede
Wilbrand-Bützow	Detmolder Str. 24	4800 Bielefeld
Wilcke, F.	Andreaswall 8	3090 Verden
Wildt, Maria	Wiesenweg 10	3280 Bad Pyrmont
Wilke, Armin	Möllmansweg 31	4400 Münster
Wilke, H. J.	Grandweg 15	2 Hamburg 54
Wilkening, D.	Kaiserdamm 27	1000 Berlin 19

Will, Heino	Ruhrstr. 2	5800 Hagen
Willkommen, Heidi	Kapuzinerstraße 26	6530 Bingen
Willkommen, Wilfried	Kapuzinerstraße 26	6530 Bingen
Wilmes, J.	Bahnhofsallee 1	32 Hildesheim
Windrath, E.	Donnersberger Straße 8	8000 München 19
Wink, Bernhard	Univers.-Augenklinik	5300 Bonn
Winkler, Gerhard	Porta-Nigra-Platz 2/I	5500 Trier
Winkler-Franke, H.	Lennestr. 17	4940 Altenhundem
Winter, Almuth	Meppener Str. 17	4500 Osnabrück
Winter, R.	Am Dobben 87	2800 Bremen
Winter, Wigbert	Delbrücker Hauptstr. 94	5000 Köln
Wintzer, Ursula	Amalienstraße 4	5000 Köln-Zollstock
Wirsing, G.	Wurthembergische Straße	1000 Berlin 31
Wirt, J.	Luruper Hauptstr. 109c	2000 Hamburg-Lurup
Wirthgen, Hartmut	Leipziger Str. 65	6000 Frankfurt W 13
Wirz, Elmar	Lange Straße 33	7570 Baden-Baden
Witt, Gerhard	Gudower Weg 5	2410 Mölln
Wittich, K.	Frohsinnstraße 21	8750 Aschaffenburg
Wittmer, H.	Holm 12	2390 Flensburg
Wittmer, H.	Anzinger Straße 4	8000 München 8
Wittwer, Klaus	Goebenstr. 30	4400 Münster
Witzell, Heinrich	Bahnhofstr. 54	2150 Buxtehude
Woelcke, H.	Hamburgerstr. 7	207 Ahrensburg
Wolandski, Hedwig	Reypl. 12	5112 Baesweiler
Woock, R.	Neuer Pferdemarkt 23	2000 Hamburg 6
Wolf, Hans	Walderdorff-Str. 1	6250 Limburg
Wolf, Manfred	Lenaustraße 12	8440 Straubing
Wolf, Walter	Bahnhofstr. 30	6680 Neunkirchen
Wolff, R.	Wilhelmstraße 85	5100 Aachen
Wollensack, Prof.	Spandauer Damm 130	1000 Berlin 19
Wollnik, Magdalene	Jungfrauenthal 13	2000 Hamburg
Wörner, Gerhard	Wilmesdorfer Straße 52	1000 Berlin 12
Wulle, Klaus-Günther	Honiggasse 41	6200 Wiesbaden-Bierstadt
Wulzinger, Max	Maximilianstraße 54/III	8000 München 22
Wülfing-Lienemann, E.	Am Sternenfeld 13	4070 Rheydt
Wünsch, E.	Rich.-Wagner-Str. 31	3000 Hannover
Wüseke, W.	Marienplatz 15	4790 Paderborn
Wüstenberg, W.	Hauptstraße 60	5060 Bensberg
Wychgram, Hayo	Obermarkt 48	8110 Murnau
Zanleck, C.	Admiralstraße 157	2800 Bremen
Zapp, Franz Josef	Bahnhofstr. 51	6600 Saarbrücken
Zarrinnam, Abolgh.	Schützenstraße 112	4030 Ratingen
Zdravkovic, Miodrag	Schunterstr. 2	3300 Braunschweig
Zeep, Klaus R.	Wakenitzufer 56	2400 Lübeck
Zemke	Ackerstraße 20	5419 Dierdorf
Zenker, C.	Nymphenburger Str. 43	8000 München 2
Zentgraf, H.	Kortumstr. 45	4630 Bochum
Zesch, Gerlinde	Rauroggener Straße 36a	1000 Berlin 10
Zetsche, C.	Klosterstraße 12	7730 Villingen
Zetsche, K.	Allersberger Str. 76	8500 Nürnberg
Zettl, W. R.	Viktoriastr. 11	8000 München 23
Zeyen	Vierhausstraße 15	4070 Rheydt
Zielinski, H. W.	Weigelstr. 3	3500 Kassel
Ziemsen, R.	Rheinische Str. 141	4600 Dortmund
Zillessen, G.	Seestraße 98	1000 Berlin 65
Zillmann, Dietrich	Goerdeler Straße 51	5650 Solingen

Zillmann, Günther	Gartenstr. 16	2900 Oldenburg
Zimmer, J.	Haußmannstraße 186	7000 Stuttgart 13
Zimmermann, J.	Wirtelstraße 22	5160 Düren
Zinsser, F.	Wilhelmstraße 49	7140 Ludwigsburg
Zintz, Prof.	Augenabt. St. Josephsstift	28 Bremen
Zitzlaff, E.	Grünbauerstraße 1	8000 München-Solln
Zschosche, C.	Grabenstraße 24	5608 Radevormwald
Zumbansen, Heinz	Luitpoldstraße 3	8750 Aschaffenburg
Zuschlag, H. G.	Friedr.-Ebert-Damm 93g	2000 Hamburg 70
Zwanzig, Mechtild	Scharnweber Straße 41	1000 Berlin 52
Zwecker, Peter	Leipziger Str. 115	3500 Kassel

NOSOCOMIA QUIBUS OCULIS AEGRI CURANTUR

Universitäts-Augenkliniken

Aachen   Bettenzahl·

Augenklinik der Techn. Hochschule, 51 Aachen, Goethestr. 27/29. Direktor: Prof. Dr.
M. Reim 42

Berlin-West

Univ.-Augenklinik der Freien Universität, 1 Berlin 19, Spandauer Damm 130. Direktor:
Prof. Dr. J. Wollensak 80

Augenklinik des Klinikum Steglitz der Freien Universität Berlin, 1 Berlin 45, Hindenburgdamm 30. Direktor: Prof. Dr. H. Hager ......,........................... 84

Bonn

Univ.-Augenklinik, 53 Bonn-Venusberg. Direktor: Prof. Dr. W. Best 140

Institut für experimentelle Ophthalmologie, 53 Bonn-Venusberg. Director: Prof. Dr. E.
Weigelin 24

Düsseldorf

Univ.-Augenklinik, 4 Düsseldorf, Moorenstr. 5, Direktor: Prof. Dr. H. Pau 100

Erlangen-Nürnberg

Univ.-Augenklinik, 852 Erlangen, Universitätsstr. 27. Direktor: Prof. Dr. E. Schreck 120

Essen

Augenklinik des Klinikum Münster, 43 Essen, Hufelandstr. 55. Direktor: Prof. Dr. G. Meyer-
Schwickerath 120

Frankfurt/Main

Univ.-Augenklinik, 6 Frankfurt/M., Ludwig-Rehnstraße. Direktor: Prof. Dr. W. Doden 88

Freiburg/Br.

Univ.-Augenklinik, 78 Freiburg/Br., Killianstraße. Direktor: Prof. Dr. G. Mackensen 140

Giessen

Univ.-Augenklinik, 63 Giessen, Friedrichstr. 18. Direktor: Prof. Dr. C. Cüppers 103

Göttingen

Univ.-Augenklinik, 34 Göttingen, Gosslerstr. 12. Direktor: Prof. Dr. W. Hallermann 102

Hamburg

Univ.-Augenklinik, 2 Hamburg 20, Martinistr. 52. Direktor: Prof. Dr. H. Sautter 110

Hannover
Augenklinik der Medizinischen Akademie, 3 Hannover, Haltenhoffstr. 41. Direktor: Prof.
Dr. B. Huerkamp 66

Heidelberg
Univ.-Augenklinik, 69 Heidelberg, Bergheimerstr. 20. Direktor: Prof. Dr. W. Jaeger 120

Homburg/Saar
Univ.-Augenklinik, 665 Homburg/Saar. Direktor: Prof. Dr. H. J. Schlegel 103

Kiel
Univ.-Augenklinik, 23 Kiel, Hegewischstr. 3. Direktor: Prof. Dr. W. Böke 100

Köln
Univ.-Augenklinik, 5 Köln-Lindenthal. Direktor: Prof. Dr. H. Neubauer 127

Lübeck
Augenklinik der Medizinischen Akademie, 24 Lübeck, Ratzeburgerallee 160. Direktor: Prof.
Dr. H. F. Piper 36

Mainz
Univ.-Augenklinik, 65 Mainz, Langenbeckstr. 1. Direktor: Prof. Dr. A. Nover 92

Mannheim
Univ.-Augenklinik, 68 Mannheim, Theodor-Kutzer-Ufer. Direktor: Prof. Dr. H. Liesenhoff . 31

Marburg
Univ.-Augenklinik, 355 Marburg/Lahn, Robert-Kochstr. 4. Direktor: Prof. Dr. W. Straub .. 80

München
Univ.-Augenklinik, 8 München 15, Mathildenstr. 8. Direktor: Prof. Dr. O. E. Lund 217
Augenklinik der Technischen Universität München, 8 München 80, Ismaningerstr. 22.
Direktor: Prof. Dr. H. J. Merté 93

Münster
Univ.-Augenklinik, 44 Münster/Westfalen, Westring 15. Direktor: Prof. Dr. F. Hollwich 80

Tübingen
Univ.-Augenklinik, 74 Tübingen. Direktor: Prof. Dr. H. Harms 143

Ulm
Univ.-Augenklinik, 79 Ulm, Prittwitzstraße. Direktor: Prof. Dr. R. Marquardt 48

Würzburg
Univ.-Augenklinik, 87 Würzburg, Röntgenring 12. Direktor: Prof. Dr. W. Leydhecker 105

Augenkliniken Ausserhalb der Universitäten

Bettenzahl

Berlin/Tempelhof
Augen-Abteilung Städt. Krankenhaus, Wenckebachstr. 23. Direktor: Dr. G. Fischer 60

Berlin/Neuköln
Augen-Abteilung Städt. Krankenhaus, Rudower Str. 56. Direktor: Dr. O. Liegl 60

Augen-Abteilung Rudolf-Virchow-Krankenhaus, Augustenburger Platz. Direktor: Prof. Dr.
F. Söllner 55

Braunschweig
Städt. Augenklinik, Salzdahlumer Str. 90. Direktor: Prof. Dr. W. Graeber 46

Bremen
Augenklinik d. Zentralkrankenhaus, St. Jürgenstraße. Direktor: Prof. Dr. J. Draeger 105

Augen-Abteilung St. Joseph-Stift, Schwachhauser Heerstr. 54. Direktor: Prof. Dr. R. Zintz . 34

Dortmund
Augenklinik d. Städt. Krankenanst., Beurhausstr. 40. Direktor: Prof. Dr. K. Ullerich 90

Düsseldorf
Augen-Abteilung Marien-Hospital, Rochusstr. 2. Direktor Prof. Dr. H. J. Küchle 45

Duisburg/Hamborn
Augenklinik Evangel. Krankenhaus. Direktor: Prof. Dr. G. Holland 80

Essen/Werden
Augen-Abteilung Evangel. Krankenhaus. Direktor: Dr. K. Schott 35

Frankfurt/M.
Augenklinik St. Marien-Krankenhaus, Richard Wagnerstr. 14. Direktor: Prof. Dr. H. J.
Linnen 60

Augenklinik am Bürgerhospital, Holzhausenstr. 75. Direktor: Prof. Dr. H. Müller 54

Augenklinik Städt. Krankenhaus Hoechst, Gotenstr. 6/8. Direktor: Prof. Dr. W. Lieb 58

Hagen
Augenklinik St. Joseph-Hospital, Friedenstr. 24. Direktor: Prof. Dr. H. Thomann 42

Hamburg
Augen-Abteilung Allgem. Krankh. Barmbek, Rübenkamp 148. Direktor: Prof. Dr. W. Papst . 90

Augen-Abteilung Allg. Krankh. Heidberg, Landstr. 400. Direktor: Dr. Riehm 72

Augen-Abteilung Allgem. Krankh. St. Georg, Lohmühlenstr. 5. Direktor: Prof. Dr. H. D.
Utermann 50

Allgem. Krankenhaus Orthmarschen, 50 Holmbrook. Direktor: Dr. B. Gramberg-Danielsen . 40

Karlsruhe
Augenklinik St. Vincentius-Krankenhaus, Kriegsstr. 49/51. Direktor: Prof. Dr. R. Seitz 78

Augen-Abteilung Diakonissenkrankhaus, Diakonissenstr. 28. Direktor: Dr. W. Lemmingson . 40

Kassel
Augenklinik Stadtkrankenhaus, Mönchenbergstraße. Direktor: Prof. Dr. W. Aust 56

Köln
Augen-Abteilung St. Elisabeth-Krankhaus, Hohenlind. Prof. Dr. M. Glees 50

Krefeld
Augenklinik d. Städt. Krankenanstalten, Marianne Rhodiusstr. 20. Direktor: Prof. Dr.
S. Niedermeier 70

Ludwigshafen
Augenklinik d. Städt. Krankenanstalten. Direktor: Prof. Dr. H. L. Thiel 92

Lüdenscheid
Augen-Abteilung Städt. Krankenhaus, Philippstr. 2. Direktor: Prof. Dr. H. Görtz 40

Mühlheim/Ruhr
Augenheilanstalt, von Graefestr. 37. Direktor: Prof. Dr. D. Schulte 100

München
Augenklinik Herzog Carl Theodor, Nymphenburger Str. 43. Direktor: Dr. C. Zenker   60

Nürnberg
Augenklinik d. Städt. Krankenanstalten, Flurstr. 17. Direktor: Dr. G. Barthelmeß   60

Offenburg
Augen-Abteilung Städt. Krankenhaus, In der Wann 16. Direktor: Prof. Dr. R. Pape   54

Osnabrück
Augen-Abteilung Marien-Hospital, Johannisfreiheit 2/4. Direktor: Prof. Dr. H. J. Meyer . . .   40

Saarbrücken/Winterberg
Augen-Abteilung d. Städt. Krankenanst. Direktor: Dr. F. Mueller   36

Stuttgart
Augenklinik d. Katharinen-Hospitals, Kriegsbergstr. 60. Direktor: Prof. Dr. K. E. Schrader .   62

Charlottenheilanstalt f. Augenkranke, Elisabethenstr. 15. Direktor: Dr. E. Gscheidel   52

Sulzbach
Augenklinik d. Saarknappschaft. Direktor: Dr. K. Heckenhahn   45

Trier
Augen-Abteil, Krankenh. d. Barmherzigen Brüder, Nordallee 1. Direktor: Dr. Borgmann. . . .   40

Wiesbaden
Augenheilanstalt, Kapellenstr. 42. Direktor: Prof. Dr. F. Wagner   60

Wuppertal
Städt. Augenklinik, Barmen Heusnerstr. 40. Direktor: Prof. Dr. O. Oppel   76

INSTITUTA SCHOLAEQUE CAECIS DESTINATAE

Organisationen des Blinden- und Sehbehindertenwesens

Verein zur Förderung der Blindenbildung e.V. 3 Hannover-Kirchrode, Bleekstr. 26.
Deutscher Blindenverband e.V. 53 Bonn-Bad Godesberg, Bismarckstr. 30.
Bund der Kriegsbilden Deutschlands e.V. 53 Bonn, Schumannstr. 35.
Bund zur Förderung sehbehinderter Kinder e.V. 41 Duisburg-Rahm-West, Ahrenstr. 7.

Blindenschulen   Schülerzanı

Blindenbildungsanstalt, 1 Berlin 41 (Steglitz) Rothenburgstr. 14   31

Rheinische Sonderschule für Blinde, 516 Düren, Meckerstr. 1-3   146

Landeswohlfahrtsverband Hessen, Johann-Peter-Schäfer-Schule für Blinde, 636 Friedberg,
    Mainzer Toranlage 6   93

Blindenschule und Sehbehindertenschule, 2 Hamburg 39, Borgweg 17a   271

Niedersächsische Landesblindenschule, 3 Hannover-Kirchrode, Bleekstr. 22   190

Private Heimsonderschule für blinde und sehbehinderte Kinder, St. Franziskus, 7231
    Schramberg-Heiligenbronn   75

Umschulungsstätten für Späterblindete

mit
Zweigstelle in 8111 Saulgrub/Obb.
und
Zweigstelle für Industrieausbildung in 87 Würzburg, Franz-Ludwig-Str. 19-21

Deutsches Taubblindenwerk G.m.b.H.

Blindenstudienanstalt

Selbständige Sehbehindertenschulen

GRAECIA

SOCIETATES OPHTHALMOLOGICAE

Nationalis

Hellenic Ophthalmological Society
President: Ch. Topalis
Vice-President: N. Brissimis
General Secretary: G. Chilaris, 14 Navarinou St., Athens 144
Treasurer: P. Protonotarios
Members of the council: D. Nikolaou, A. Malevitis
Assistant Secretary: J. Koliopoulos
Number of members: (Titular and Associate) 270

Regionalis

Ophthalmological Society of Northern Greece
President: Prof. G. Georgiades
General Secretary: A. Argalias, 71 Fr. Rousvelt St., Thessaloniki
Number of members: 64

NOMINA ET DOMICILIA MEDICORUM AB OCULIS

Aggelakis, E.	Damareos 19	Athens-506
Aleksakis, N.	Stournara 23	Athens-147
Alexiades, Theodoros		Drama
Alimicis, Sotirios	B' Parodos Omonias	Kavala
Anastaciadis, Anastasios	6 Aristotelous	Thessaloniki
Anastasopoulos, N.	Solomou 58	Athens-147
Anastopoulou, A.	Skiathou 70-72	Athens-806
Andriopoulos, Th.	Kolokotroni 54	Piraeus
Andreanos, D.	Dodekanisou 31	Athens-811
Aposkitis, K.	Akadimias 35	Athens-135
Argalias, Achilleus	71, Fr. Rousvelt	Thessaloniki
Atsalis, E.	Alkiviadou 118	Piraeus
Avlidou, Anna	B33 Ag. Paulou	Thessaloniki
Bairaktaris, A.	I. Drosopoulou 64	Athens-803
Baltatzis, S.	Arrianou 25	Athens-501
Batsolas, Vasilios	67 M. Alexandrou	Thessaloniki
Bazeou, S.	Alkiviadou 115	Piraeus
Bechrakis, E.	Karneadou 22	Athens-139
Bessas, Christos		Kojani
Bisogianis, Zisis	Plapouta 9	Tripolis
Bitsas, Chr.	Solonos 80	Athens-144
Bogdanits, A.	Al. Soutsou 20	Athens-134
Bouzas, A.	Skoufa 59	Athens-135
Brisimis, N.		Volos

Chachamidis, Dimitrios	69 Egnatia	Thessaloniki
Charamis, Prof. J.	Licabette 1	Athens-135
Chatzialexiadis, K.	Flemig 2	Ilioupolis-Athens
Chatzis, Periklis	Patision 59	Athens
Chaviaras, S.		Kiaton, Korinthias
Chilaris, G.	Navarinou 14	Athens-144
Chilas, Stelios	7 Egnatia	Thessaloniki
Chiliadakis, Chr.	Kantanoleon 6	Iraklion, Kritis
Chimonidou, E.	Spartis 95	N. Ionia-Athens
Chlorokostas, V.	Solonos 140	Athens-141
Chouliaras, N.	Matsou 5	Arta
Chrisafis, Vasilios	22 Pr. Nikolaou	Thessaloniki
Christakis, Chr.	Karneadou 9	Athens-139
Chronakis, J.		Agios Nikolaos, Kritis
Chronis, J.	Anagnostara 65	Kalamata
Chronopoulos, D.	Stournara 23	Athens-147
Daskalopoulos, A.	Patision 50	Athens-147
Daskalopoulos, G.	Navarinou 17	Athens-145
Daskalopoulos, K.	Solonos 26	Athens-136
Daskalopouios, N.	Patision 50	Athens-147
Deligiannis, Armandos	83 Leof. Kennedy	Thessaloniki
Diafas, G.		Edessa
Diamantakos, P.	Skoufa 52	Athens-135
Diamantis, Victor		Komotini
Dimitriou, T.	Skoufa 11	Athens-135
Diamantopoulos, P.	Kanakari 160	Patrai
Drakontaidis, K.	Thiseos 94a	Kallithea, Athens
Doris, M.	Koumpari 5	Athens-138
Dougas, Charisis		Serrai
Efkarpidis, A.	Stournara 32	Athens-103
Efkarpidis, Ch.	Patision 53	Athens-147
Evageliou, E.	Damareos 29	Athens-506
Fountis, A.	Kritis 30	Athens-109
Fountoulakis, Th.	Konstantinou 33	Chania, Kritis
Fouskakis, S.	Mayrommataion 9	Athens-147
Frangopoulos, Gikas	62 M. Alexandrou	Thessaloniki
Frangoulis, Christos	5 P.P. Germanou Str.	Thessaloniki
Friderikos, E.	Alopekis 50	Athens-140
Fronimopoulos, J.	N. Vamva 6	Athens-138
Gabriil, L.	Alexandrou Soutsou 20	Athens-134
Galanou-Kontaxi, E.	Patision 135	Athens-814
Georgalas, G.	Frinis 6	Athens-503
Georgariou, P.	Licabette 5	Athens-135
Georgiadis, Georgios	15 Karolou Dil	Thessaloniki
Giannousis, Ion	29 Egnatia	Thessaloniki
Gillas, K.	Solonos 39	Athens-135
Glykos, G.	Vouliagmenis 153	Athens-454
Grigoratos, N.	Sekeri 4	Athens-138
Grigoropoulos, G.	Akadimias 16	Athens-134
Ignatiadis, A.	Solonos 113	Athens-142
Ioannidis, Orestis	97 Egnatia	Thessaloniki
Ismiridis, I.	Koumbari 10	Athens-138
Kachrimanides, Constantinos	1 Vikella	Veria
Kalaitjis, Apostolos		Serre
Kalampokas, Constantinos .		Alexandroupolis
Kaliolias, P.		Arta

Kalofonos, D.		Rethimmon, Kritis
Kaloudis, K.	Sevastoupoleos 76	Athens-608
Kambitsopoulos, G.	Akadimias 28	Athens-134
Kandilakis, I.	Veikou 87	Athens
Kappa, A.	Acharnon 296	Athens-816
Karagianis, A.	Skoufa 16	Athens-136
Karagounidis, Alexandros ..	30 Aristotelous	Thessaloniki
Karakitsos, G.	Eptanissou 73	Athens-804
Karakostas, S.	Averof 5	Athens-103
Karantinos, D.	Vas. Konstantinou 59	Piraeus-37
Karavias, E.	Panormou 81	Athens-605
Kariophillis, Constantinos ..	7 Carolou Dil	Thessaloniki
Kariotis, Constantinos	73 Ermou Str.	Thessaloniki
Karkazis, L.	Skoufa 19	Athens-136
Karkoulis, D.	Danaou 12	Argos
Karveleas, M.	Patr. Ioakim 3	Athens-136
Karvounidis, Charalampos .	11 Dimitriou Karaoli	Xanthi
Karvounis, P.	George 3	Athens-147
Kasimati-Mazaraki, V.	Midias 7	Athens-805
Kastanas, David	16 Bijaniou	Thessaloniki
Kastrantas, A.	Patision 52	Athens-147
Katikos, Georgios		Ferre
Katsantonis, Z.	Evmenous 17	Pagrati, Athens
Katsaras, Nik.		Karditsa
Katsikinis, A.	Bouboulinas 28	Athens-147
Katsourakis, N.	Akadimias 19	Athens-134
Katopodis, E.	Stournara 25a	Athens-147
Kavounidou, K.	Solonos 52	Athens-135
Ketseas, Th.	Alopekis 42	Athens-140
Kefalianos, N.	Chr. Enoseos 16	Peristeri, Athens
Kinnas, J.	Adamantou 34	Korinthos
Kipiotis, N.	Vasil. Sofias 62a	Athens-612
Kipourgos, N.	Vasil. Irakliou 20	Athens-147
Kiriakou, Kiriakos		Kojani
Kirimis, Ioannis	1 Venijelou	Kavala
Kiroplastis, Christos		Serre
Kokkonis, M.	Sof. Venizelou 54	Chalandrion, Athens
Koliopoulos, J.	Omirou 21	Athens-135
Koliopoulos, X.	Omirou 21	Athens-135
Korillos, K.	Merlin 3	Athens-135
Kosionis, Ch.	Chalkokondili 54	Athens-102
Kotrozos, K.	Char. Trikoupi 25	Athens-145
Kounezis, J.	Vas. Konstantinou 6	Piraeus
Kourinos, E.	3rd Septemvriou 54	Athens-103
Koutouzis, A.		Agion
Koutroulis, P.	Amalias 30	Amalias
Kofinas, I.	Stournara 57	Athens-102
Konstantinidis, Nikolaos ...		Florina
Konstantopes, K.	Bouboulinas 28	Piraeus
Konstas, Constantinos	23 Ag. Sofias	Thessaloniki
Konstas, Panagiotis	6 P.P. Germanou Str.	Thessaloniki
Kosmetatos, Prof. G.	Sina 64	Athens-135
Kremoutis, F.		Tripolis
Lambrakis, G.	Massalias 10	Athens-144
Lambrou, N.	Massalias 20	Athens-144
Latousakis, J.		Chios

Leanis, Dimitrios	75 Ermou Str.	Thessaloniki
Leontaris, Chr.	....	Arginion
Liarikos, S.	Vasol. Sofias 60	Athens-612
Ligopsichakis, S.	....	Siros
Louletzoglou, M.	Omirou 46	Nea Smirni, Athens
Maggos, K.	Efpalinou 21	Athens-815
Maglousidis, Stilianos	....	Kilkis
Magouritsas, N.	Stournara 21	Athens-147
Makris, G.	Zalokosta 6	Athens-134
Malamas, Athanasios	....	Veria
Malevitis, A.	Bouboulinas 8	Athens-147
Mandras, Gr.	Vasil. Sofias 37	Athens-139
Manoliadis, E.	3rd Septemvriou 54	Athens-103
Markakis, G.	Pasaromiligou 11	Iraklion, Kritis
Markomichalakis, M.	....	Iraklion, Kritis
Marsan, P.	Al. Soutsou 15	Athens-134
Mavropoulou-Kolokitha, Sofia	16 Aristotelous	Thessaloniki
Minas, Vasilios	112 Egnatia	Thessaloniki
Moraitis, G.	Pindarou 23	Athens-136
Moschos, M.	Acti Moutsopoulou 12	Piraeus
Moustakas, A.	Kolokotroni 54	Piraeus
Natsouli-Kalianidou, V. ...	Solonos 45	Athens-134
Negris, M.	Solonos 54	Athens-135
Nikolakis, S.	Solonos 73	Athens-143
Nikolakopoulos, J.	P. Ioakim 19	Athens-139
Nikolaou, D.	Akadimias 32	Athens-135
Nikolinakos, Georgios	20 Carolou Dil	Thessaloniki
Nychas, G.	Ipirou 6	Athens-103
Palimeris, Gerasimos	Sina 32	Athens-135
Panousakis, Ch.	Bizaniou 13	Komotini
Papavlasakis, J.	Skaltsa 11	Athens-709
Papadopoulos, Dim.	Loukianou 7	Athens-139
Papageorgiou, Al.	Solonos 46	Athens-135
Papageorgiou, Theofanis ..	....	Serre
Papakonstantinou, K.	Boufidou 27	Levadia
Papakonstantinou, S.	Vironos 40	Lamia
Papamattheakis, Nic.	Dimokritou 6	Athens-134
Papapanos, Gr.	....	Korinthos
Papastilianos, Stilianos	Leof. Paralias	Kavala
Papastratigakis, B.	Asklipiou 6	Athens-144
Papathanasiou, Andreas ...	147 Egnatia	Thessaloniki
Papoulis, Athanasios	93 Fr. Rousvelt	Thessaloniki
Papazoglou, E.	Omirou 24	Athens-135
Paterakis, Em.	Voukourestiou 27	Athens-136
Pelagidis, Avaggelos	66 M. Alexandrou	Thessaloniki
Perifanis, Al.	J. Drosopoulou 48	Athens-802
Petridis, Ioannis	34 M. Alexandrou	Thessaloniki
Petrochilos, Manousos	Akadimias 41	Athens-135
Palekis, Nikolaos	Skoufa II	Athens-135
Pichion, An.	Eftichidou 6	Athens-502
Pitias, J.	....	Agrinion
Pollalis, Sp.	N. Vamba 4	Athens-138
Polikratis, A.	Patision 61	Athens-103
Polichronakos, Dimitrios ..	12 Aristotelous	Thessaloniki
Polichroniadid, F.	Mérlin 8	Athens-134

Pountzas, D.	....	Patras
Profilis, K.	....	Bizaniou, Pirgos Illias
Protonotarios, Petros	P. Ioakim 45	Athens-140
Rajoglou, Christos	22 Aristotelous	Thessaloniki
Rangabi, Ourania	George 5	Athens-147
Raptis, V.	Egnatias 74	Thessaloniki
Rodopoulos, Stelios	Pl. Eleutherias	Katerini
Roulias, E.	....	Larissa
Roussos, A.	....	Siros
Roussos, J.	Pindarou 26	Athens-136
Sarafianos, K.	Acharnon 35 ·.............	Athens-109
Savas, Periclis	Patision 113	Athens-813
Saltikis, D.	Spiridi 58	Volos
Sarakotsis, Georgios	77 Egnatia	Thessaloniki
Sevastakis, Th.	3rd Septemvriou 35	Athens-102
Simonetos, G.	P. Ioakim 58	Athens-140
Soulas, Sp.	....	Chalkis
Souliotis, K.	Marni 11	Athens-103
Soureas, G.	Pindarou 11	Athens
Spanopoulos, A.	Saripolou 10	Athens-147
Spiratos, S.	Pindarou 17	Athens-136
Stamatinis, Chr.	Skopelou 1	Athens-809
Stamelos, Chr.	Vas. Sofias 50	Athens-612
Stangos, Nikolaos	3 Despere	Thessaloniki
Stavropoulos, A.	....	Larisa
Stianidis, Aristotelis	21 Egnatia	Thessaloniki
Stathaki, I.	Sisini 35	Athens-612
Sfalagakou-Tranou, L.	Ir. Attikou 5	Athens-138
Taktikos, A.	Asklipiou 7	Athens-143
Taktikos, G.	Asklipiou 7	Athens-143
Theodoridis, A.	Karneadou 4	Athens-139
Theodosiadis, G.	Omirou 54	Athens-135
Theodoropoulos, Th.	Venizelou 40	Alexandroupolis
Theophilaktou, Anna	97 Ag. Dimitriou	Thessaloniki
Tigas, K.	....	Trikala
Topalis, Chr.	Dimokritou 9	Athens-134
Torolopoulos, P.	Navarinou 12	Athens-144
Trantas, N.	3rd Septemvriou 48	Athens·103
Trikoulis, D.	Ferron 6	Athens-104
Tsamparlakis, J.	Omirou 39	Athens-135
Tsannidis, Prof. Th.	Raviné 24	Athens-140
Tsapakis, M.	Zalogou 5	Iraklion, Kritis
Tsiantis, E.	Stournara 17a	Athens-148
Tsigdinos, Charalampos ...	75 Egnatia	Thessaloniki
Tsilivakos, Ksenofon	Kountouriotou 189a	Pireus
Tsimpidas, P.	Skoufa 41	Athens-134
Tsinopoulos, Theodoros ...	16 P. Mela	Thessaloniki
Tsipas, Dimitrios	M. Alexandrou	Thessaloniki
Tsitros, Antonios	....	Serre
Tsolakis, P.	Solonos 42	Athens-135
Tsoumis, Pavlos	13 Papakiriaji	Larissa
Tzakos, K.	Sina 34	Athens-135
Tzanis, A.	Solonos and Sina 7	Athens-135
Tzatzari, M.	E. Benaki 57	Athens-145
Tzavalas, Ch.	....	Patras
Vagiatis, Georgios	7 Tsontjou	Kojani

Vamvakidis, Ioannis	45 E. Venijelou	Kavala
Vartzelis, A.	Voukourestiou 25a	Athens-135
Varvitsiotis, P.	Sapfous 172	Kallithea, Athens
Vasiliou, G.	Amerikis 15	Athens-135
Velissaropoulos, Prof. P.	Akadimias 37	Athens-135
Vikas, G.		Ioannina
Vlachos, J.	Solonos 51	Athens-135
Vloumidis, A.	Vissarionos 3	Athens-135
Vogiatjis, Constantinos	90, M. Alexandrou	Thessaloniki
Voureksakis, A.	Skoufa 23	Athens-136
Voutsas, Stayros	14, Aristotelous	Thessaloniki
Xatzhs, A.	E. Venizelou 128	Kallithea, Athens
Xirokostas, Chr.	Skoufa 79	Athens-144
Zagoras, A.	Pindarou 18-20	Athens
Zervakakos, Constantinos	16 Egnatia	Thessaloniki
Zervanos, P.	Ammochostou 11	Rodos
Zisiadis, Constantinos	1 Seleukou	Thessaloniki
Zisis, G.		Argos
Zitonoulis, A.	Metaxas 30	Larisa
Zografos, I.	Akadimias 34	Athens-135
Zografos, Paulos	61 Ermou Str.	Thessaloniki
Zoidis, Ch.	Laskaridou 110	Kallithea, Athens

NOSOCOMIA QUIBUS OCULIS AEGRI CURANTUR

	No. of Beds
National Ophthalmological Centre. Dir.: Prof. P. Velissaropoulos	220
Ophthalmiatrion (Athens). Dir.: Ass. Prof. J. Tsambarlakis	62
General National Hospital Athens. Dir.: Ass. Prof. C. Topalis	20
General Hospital 'Kings Paul'. Dir.: Ass. Prof. N. Katsourakis	27
Neas Ionias General Hospital. Dir.: Dr. J. Ismiridis	12
Hippokration (Athens). Dir.: Ass. Prof. P. Protonotarios	27
'Elpis' General Hospital Athens. Dir.: Ass. Prof. D. Nikolaou	8
'Evangelismos' (Athens). Dir.: Dr. M. Petropoulos	32
Red Cross Hospital (Athens). Dir.: Dr. K. Coryllos	29
Children's Hospital 'Agia Sophia'. (Athens). Dir.: K. Aposkitis	20
Hospital 'Agios Savas' (Athens). Dir.: Dr. G. Chilaris	15
General National Hospital of Piraeus. Dir.: Ass. Prof. G. Mandras	26
Tzanion Hospital (Piraeus). Dir.: Ass. Prof. L. Tranou	20
Pammakaristos Hospital (Athens). Dir.: Ass. Prof. I. Fronimopoulos	40
University Clinic of Salonika. Dir.: Prof. G. Georgiadis	42
Hippokration Hospital of Salonika. Dir.: Ass. Prof. K. Kostas	42
Municipal Hospital of Salonika (Ag. Dimitrios). Dir.: Ass. Prof. D. Polichonakos	26
General Central Hospital of Salonika. Dir.: Ass. Prof. A. Argalias.	20
General Hospital of 'Agios Nikolaos Crete	10
General Hospital of Agrinion	9
General Hospital of Arta	5
General Hospital of Volos	10
General Hospital of Drama	10
General Hospital of Agios Nikolaos Crete	4
General Hospital of Ioannina	10
General Hospital of Iraklion	10
General Hospital of Kavala	10
General Hospital of Keffalinias	8
General Hospital of Corfu	7

INSTITUTA SCHOLAEQUE CAECIS DISTINATAE

No of pupils

Institute for the Blind of Kallithea (Ikos, Tyflon), El. Veniselou 210, Kallithea, Athens ... 35
Institute for the Blind 'Pharos', Doiranis 198, Kallithea, Athens 35
Institute for Protection of the Blind of Northern Greece 'Ilios', Vasil. Olgas 32, Thessaloniki 38
Institute for the Blind, Patras 50
Institute for the Blind, Heraklion, Crete 50

HELVETIA

SOCIETATES OPHTHALMOLOGICAE

Nationalis

Schweizerische Ophthalmologische Gesellschaft; Société suisse d'Ophtalmologie
Präsident: Dr. Hans Ruedi Bonringer
Ständiger Sekretär: Dr. Franz Della Casa, Kreuzgraben 12, Burgdorf
Mitgliederzahl: 192

Regionales

Vereinigung Basler Augenärzte
Präsident: Prof. Roland Brückner, Basel

Vereinigung Bernischer Augenärtze
Präsident: Dr. Hans Heinrich Rickli, Thun

Zürcher Augenärtze Gesellschaft
Präsident: Dr. Jean Paul Arbenz, Zürich

NOMINA ET DOMICILIA MEDICORUM AB OCULIS

Achermann, Emil	Morgartenstr. 11	6003 Luzern
Ackermann, Henriette	Av. des Alpes 51	1820 Montreux
Aebli, Leo	Hauptstrasse 97	9400 Rorschach
Ammann, Paul B.	Oberstadtstr. 4	8500 Frauenfeld
Anderes, Willi	Obergrundstr. 3	6003 Luzern
Arbenz, Jean Paul	Schaffhauserstr. 340	8050 Zürich
Atar, Zeev	Birsigstrasse 4	4054 Basel
Audeoud-Naville, Anne	Rue Bellot 10	1206 Genf
Augustin, Marius	Posthörnli, Gurzelngasse	4500 Solothurn
Babel, Prof. Jean	Rue A. Jentzer 22	1205 Genève
Balavoine, Colette	Rue E. Yung 1	1205 Genève
Bamert, Werner	Veresiusstr. 13	2502 Biel
Bangerter, Prof. Alfred	Rorschacherstr. 95	9006 St. Gallen
Bangerter-Blaser, Katharina	General Guisan Strasse 4	3800 Interlaken
Barth, Jost	Ottostrasse 4	7000 Chur
Baumann, Heinz	Alpenstrasse 1	6004 Luzern
Baumberger, Arthur	Lerchenfeldstr. 16	9500 Wil SG
Bedö-Donath, Natasa	Greifengasse 1	4000 Basel
Bernoulli, René	Rheinsprung 1	4051 Basel
Bianchetti, Mario	Bahnhofstr. 56	8001 Zürich
Bianchi, Giorgio	Via Canova 18	6900 Lugano
Bischler, Vera	Plateau Champel 16	1206 Genève
Bischoff, Ulrich	Haus du Lac, Merkurstrasse 3	8820 Wädenswil

Bleiker, Hans	Unterer Zielweg 91	4143 Dornach
Blum, John D.	Boulevard des Tranchées 44	1206 Genève
Böhringer, Hans Rudolf	Oberstadt 12	8200 Schaffhausen
Bourquin, André	Richemont Petit Chêne 18	1003 Lausanne
Bozin, Ivo	Rue du concert 6	2000 Neuchâtel
Bracher, Hans Rudolf	Junkerngasse 61	3011 Bern
Brändle, Karl	Badenerstrasse 681	8048 Zürich
Breitenmoser, Rudolf	Badstrasse 17	5400 Baden
Brückner, Prof. Arthur	Oberer Batterie-weg 74	Basel
Brückner, Prof. Roland	Dufourstrasse 5	4052 Basel
Bühler, Enrico	Castelsplatz	7320 Sargans
Burger, Paul	Henzmannstrasse 7	4800 Zofingen
Bürki, Prof. Ernst	Arnold Böcklinstr. 15	4051 Basel
Cagianut, Bernard	Freiestr. 76	8032 Zürich
Chomé-Bercioux, Noelle	Rue Maupas 1	1003 Lausanne
Cometta, Fernando	Via G.B. Pioda 8	6900 Lugano
Compassi-Faoro, Natalina	Zentralstrasse 14	6000 Luzern
Cuendet, Prof. Jean François	Av. Rumine 31	1005 Lausanne
Cuendet, Madeleine	Rue Mathurin Cordier 12	1005 Lausanne
Delaloye, Jean	Av. de Beaulieu 19	1004 Lausanne
Della Casa, Franz	Vorderer Kreuzgraben 12	3400 Burgdorf
Deller, Maurice	Av. Schnetzler 2	1003 Lausanne
Del Notaro-Stauffenegger, Ursula	Piazza Grande	6600 Locarno
Diallinas, Nicos	Av. Krieg 11	1208 Genève
Dieterle, Peter	Av. de Champel 6	1206 Genève
Doret, Michel	Boulevard James Fazy 2	1201 Genève
Dubler, Hans	Zentralstr. 21	5610 Wohlen AG
Dufour, Prof. Rene	Rue du Midi 7	1003 Lausanne
Eisner, Georg	Univ.-Augenklinik, Freiburgstrasse 8	3008 Bern
Eisner-Guggenheim, Irma	Nonnenweg 20	4055 Basel
Fabiny C. E.		Porrentruy
Frankhauser, Prof. Franz	Bremgartenstrasse 117	3012 Bern
Favre, Maurice	Rue Abbé, Bovet 12	1700 Fribourg
Fellmann-Wey, Eleonore	Seehofstrasse 9	6004 Luzern
Forgacs, Joseph	Rue de Saint Jean 34	1203 Genève
Forni, Sergio	Viale Stazione 30	6500 Bellinzona
Frydman, Rachel	Place Claparède 7	1205 Genève
Gafner, Erich	Oristalstrasse 21	4410 Liestal
Gafner, Frank	Oristalstrasse 21	4410 Liestal
Girardet, Maurice	Av. de la Gare 1	1003 Lausanne
Goldmann, Prof. Hans	Humboldstrasse 39	Bern
Graf, Hans Peter	Zeitglocken 1	3011 Bern
Grämiger, Albert	Bahnhofplatz 1	9000 St. Gallen
Gränicher-Frick, Denise	Aebistrasse 9	3012 Bern
Gruber, Max	Fraumünstergasse 11	8001 Zürich
Gut, Adolf	Löwenstrasse 59	8001 Zürich
Gut, Edwin	Alpenstrasse 11	6300 Zug
Haefliger, E.		Zürich
Haldimann, Carl	Kramgasse 16	3011 Bern
Haldimann, Rudolf	Kramgasse 16	3011 Bern
Hediger, Karl	Grossmünsterplatz 8	8001 Zürich
Hegner, Hansjörg	Weseminstr. 2	6000 Luzern
Heim, Max	Boulevard Pérolles 19	1700 Fribourg
Hermann, Charlotte	Av. Rumine 38	1005 Lausanne

Hof, Walter	Kornhausstrasse 3	9000 St. Gallen
Hoffmann-Egg, Lilly	Minervastrasse 149	8032 Zürich
Hotz, Gerhard	Spalenring 138	4055 Basel
Hotz, R.		Winterthur
Houber, H. P.		Nyon
Huber, Prof. Alfred	Stadelhoferstr. 42	8001 Zürich
Huber, Paul	Ringstrasse 4	4900 Langenthal
Huber, Peter	Dorfplatz	7503 Samedan
Jenny, Eduard	Ländliweg 7a	5400 Baden
Jöhr, Pierre	Frutigenstrasse 8	3600 Thun
Itin, W.		Genève
Kalberer, Max	Augenabteilung des Bezirksspirals	3800 Interlaken
Karbacher, Paul	Sihlporteplatz 3	8001 Zürich
Keller, Hans	Seilerstrasse 3	3011 Bern
Keller, Hans H.	Bahnhofstr. 27	8280 Kreuzlingen
Kern, Rudolf	Augenklinik des Kantonsspitals	6000 Luzern
Kessler, Emma	ob. Bahnhofstrasse Stadthofplatz	8640 Rapperswil SG
Kessous-Odermatt, Franziska	Rue Caroline 3	1003 Lausanne
Koenig, Fritz, jr.	Theaterstrasse 18	8001 Zürich
Koenig, Heinrich	Seilerstrasse 22	3011 Bern
Korff, Jürgen		Wetzikon
Krassai, A.		Basel
Kretzschmar, Serge, jr.	Av. de la Gare 7	2502 Bienne
Kull, Jenny	Ringstrasse 22	4600 Olten
Laer, Peter, van	Bahnhofstr. 43	3400 Burgdorf
Landolt, Prof. Ernst	Kantonsspital, Augenklinik	8400 Winterthur
Lang, Josef	Freiestrasse 47	8032 Zürich
Lanini, Paolo	Piazza Fontana Pedrazzini	6600 Locarno
Luder, Paul	Bubenbergplatz 8	3011 Bern
Maeder, Guy	Rue E. Yung 1	1205 Genève
Marty, Franz	Rue des Vergers 6	1950 Sion
Marxer, Jutta	Leonhardstr. 31	9000 St. Gallen
Meier, Elisabeth	Schafmattweg 23	4102 Binningen
Menestrier, André	Place des Charmilles 1	1203 Genève
Messikomer, Werner	Genferstrasse 3	8002 Zürich
Meyer, Gerhard	Untertor 4	8400 Winterthur
Meyer-Steineg, Nora	Morgartenstrasse 3	6003 Luzern
Mittelholzer, Kurt Walter	Schwamendingenstrasse 5	8050 Zürich
Moeschlin-Sandoz, Yvonne	Lunaweg 22	4500 Solothurn
Moginier-Forel, Ariane	Rue Centrale 9	1110 Morges
Moretti, Giuliano	Piazza Stazione	6600 Muralto-Locarno
Moser-von Arx, Renée	Jurastr. 9	4600 Olte:.
Müller, Alfred	Neugasse 49	9000 St. Gallen
Müller, Paul	Poststrasse 18	9000 St. Gallen
Neuenschwander, Max	Kopfsteig 15	Zürich
Niesel, Prof. Peter	Freiburgstrasse 8	Bern
Nouri, A.		Sierre
Ochsner, Heinz	Dufourstrasse 5	4052 Basel
Otto, Prof. Joachim	OPOS, Rorschacherstrasse 103	9006 St. Gallen
Payer, Helmut	Quaderstrasse 2	7000 Chur
Pestalozzi, David	Baslerstr. 44	4600 Olten
Petrovic, D.		Schwytz
Piffaretti, André	Chemin du Vorbourg 1	2800 Delémont
Portmann, Urs Peter	Dornacherhof	4500 Solothurn
Regamey, Elisabeth	Cours des Bastions 15	1205 Genève

Rentsch, René	Zugerstr. 30	8810 Horgen
Ricci, A.		Genève
Richner, Hermann	Bahnhofstrasse 53	Aarau
Rickli, Hans Heinrich	Bahnhofstrasse 8	Thun
Rintelen, Prof. Friedrich	Mittlere Strasse 91	Basel
Rohner, Margrit	Septerstrasse 16	4056 Basel
Rosen, Lucien	Av. Léopold Robert 70	2300 La Chaux-de-Fonds
Rosselet, Edy,	Place Benjamin Constant 2	1003 Lausanne
Rumpf, Jean	Rue du Clos 5	1800 Vevey
Rusca-Scendrowitz, Polia	Via Ramogna 4	6600 Locarno
Sandoz, Jean-Daniel	Rue St. Honoré 2	2000 Neuchâtel
Schafroth, Peter	Aarefeldstrasse 3	3600 Thun
Schläpfer, Hans	Bahnhofstrasse 40	8001 Zürich
Schläppi, Victor	Place Pury 4	2000 Neuchâtel
Schmid, H. P.		Biel
Schmidt-Berghofer, Silvia	Kornhausplatz 11	3011 Bern
Schmidt, Theodor	Kornhauspl. 11	3000 Bern
Schnyder, Walter, F.	Werkhofgasse 59	4500 Solothurn
Schönbrunn, Mirla	Bachstr. 40	5000 Aarau
Schönenberger, Hans, sen.	Schafthauserplatz 3	8006 Zürich
Schönenberger, Hans, jun.	Alpenstr. 1	6004 Luzern
Schorr, Marianne	Untere Rebgasse 22	4058 Basel
Schwarz, Alfred	St. Urbanstr. 3	4900 Langenthal
Seddik, N.		Martigny
Senn, Hans	Spital	Laufen
Siegwart, Benno	Konradstrasse 1	Aarau
Siegwart, Karl	Steinenvorstadt 79	Basel
Sinzig, Hanspeter	Hirschengraben 10	Bern
Smolik, Henri	Av. du Casino 13	Montreux
Speiser, P.	Triemlispital	Zürich
Stadlin, Walter	Kronenhof, Hirschenplatz	6300 Zug
Stampfli-Glockner, Beatrice	Kapellstrasse 33	2540 Grenchen
Starobinski, Jacqueline	Rue de Candolle 12	1205 Genève
Steiger, Max E.	Schwanengasse 6	3011 Bern
Stoeckli-Bay, Verena	Rue Pestalozzi 1	1400 Yverdon
Streiff, Prof. Bernardo	Av. de France 15	Lausanne
Streuli, Heinrich	Bahnhofstr. 12	3600 Thun
Stucchi, Carlo A.	Corso Bello	6850 Mendrisio
Studer-Salzmann, Ulrike	Steinwiesstrasse 2	8032 Zürich
Tissières, Pierre	Av. Justé Olivier 2	1006 Lausanne
Tosello, Albert	Av. de Tivoli 5	1700 Fribourg
Vacharidis, Georges	Av. Montchoisi 14	1000 Lausanne
Verrey, Prof. Florian	Rämistrasse 23	8001 Zürich
Vicari, Sergio	Via Nassa 7	6900 Lugano
Vogelsanger, Walter	Vordersteig 3	8200 Schaffhausen
Wagner, Prof. Hans	Asylstrasse 82	8032 Zürich
Wagner, Paul	Burgstrasse 12	8750 Glarus
Waldvogel, Milda	Aeschengraben 6	4051 Basel
Weber, Ernst	Bahnhofstrasse 13	2502 Biel
Werner, Heinrich	Oberwies Platz	7270 Davos-Platz
Wettler, Heinrich	Neue Jonagasse 85	8640 Rapperswil SG
Wiesli, Paul	Uraniastrasse 9	8001 Zürich
Witmer, Prof. Rudolf	Kantonsspital, Rämistr. 100	8006 Zürich
Wolf, Hans	Pilatusstrasse 24	6003 Luzern
Wyss, Kurt	Unterer Quai 25a	2502 Biel
Younessian, S.		Genève

Zehnder-Albrecht, Susy ...	Waldeggstrasse 71	3097 Liebefeld
Zenklusen, Guido	Stadthausstrasse 71	8400 Winterthur
Zollinger, Rudolf	Bankstrasse 39	8610 Uster
Zuccoli, Aldo	Via Nassa, 'Pax'	6900 Lugano

NOSOCOMIA QUIBUS OCULIS AEGRI CURANTUR

Universitäts-Augenkliniken		**Betten**
Basel, Dir.: Prof. F. Rintelen		110
Bern, Dir.: Prof. P. Niesel		65
Genève, Dir.: Prof. J. Babel		63
Lausanne, Dir.: Prof. B. Streiff		66
Zürich, Dir.: Prof. R. Witmer		85

Kantonale Augenabteilungen		
Aarau, Dir.: Dr. H. Richner		50
Luzern, Dir.: Dr. R. Kern		59
St. Gallen, Dir.: Prof. A. Bangerter	Klinik	79
	Opos	58

INSTITUTA SCHOLAEQUE CAECIS DESTINATAE

Blindenschulen		**Plätze**
Kinderstation für Sehbehinderte, Clarahofweg 47, Basel		7
Schule für blinde und hochgradig sehschwache Kinder, Weiherweg 48, Basel		4-5
Schulheim für Blinde u. Sehschwache, Zollikofen		72
Blindeninstitut Sonnenberg, Fribourg		75
Asile des Aveugles, av. de France, Lausanne		30
Blindenschule Stadt Zürich, Arbentalstr. 28, Zürich .... pro Abt.		10

Blindenheime, Werkstätten u. Eingliederungszentren		
Blindenheim Basel, Kohlenberggasse 20, Basel .... Wohnpl..		21
	Arbeitspl.	30
Blindenheim d. bernischen Blindenfürsorgevereins, Neufeldstraße 97, Bern		46
Vereinigte Blindenwerkstätten, Neufeldstr. 31, Bern		109
Luzernisches Blindenheim, Waldegg, Horw		26
Ostschweizerisches Blindenheim, St. Gallen		50
Berufliche Schulungsstätte für Blinde und Sehschwache, Bruggwaldstraße 37, St. Gallen ...		40
Werkstäte für selbständige Blinde, Austr. 18, St. Gallen		4
Blindenheim Boningen, Boningen SO		20
Home Recordon pour femmes, 15, av. de France, Lausanne		29
Home Dufour pour hommes, 30, av. de France, Lausanne		26
Arbeitsheim Wangen ZH, Wangen b. Dübendorf		6
Blindenarbeitsheim f. Männer, St. Jakobsstr. 7, Zürich		48
Blinden-Leuchtturm Zürich, Leonhardstr. 14, Zürich		20
Blindenwohnhaus des Vereins Blindenhaus Zürich, Seefeldstr. 65, Zürich		12
Frauen-Blindenheim Dankesberg, Bergheimstr. 22, Zürich		21
Werkstätte für Blinde und Gebrechliche Oerlikon, Wehntalerstraße 294/296, Zürich		2

Blinden-Altersheime

Heime für mehrfachgebrechliche Blinde

HIBERNIA (Eire)

SOCIETATES OPHTHALMOLOGICAE

Nationales

The Irish Ophthalmological Society (founded 1917)
President: V.A.F. Martin
Secretary: G.P. Crookes, 18 Fitzwilliam Place, Dublin 2
Number of members: 137

The Irish Faculty of Ophthalmology (founded 1958)
President: J.L. Ryan
Secretary: F. D. McAuley, 45 Upper Leeson Street, Dublin 4
Number of members: 67

Regionalis

The Munster Ophthalmological Society
President: J. V. O'Sullivan
Secretary: D. J. Wilson, 23a St. Patrick's Hill, Cork
Number of members: 20

NOMINA ET DOMICILIA MEDICORUM AB OCULIS

Archer, Desmond	6, Quarry Court	Helen's Bay, Co. Down
Arkins, Evelyn	21, St. Mary's Road	Galway
Baird, R. H.	20, Broomhill Park	Belfast 9
Ball, J. E.	11, Beechwood Park	Strathfoyle, Derry
Blake, John	14, Ailesbury Road	Dublin 4
Bolton, S. E.	Chilcot, Prelin Woods	Derry
Bolton, S. M.	Strandmore House	Portrush, Co. Antrim
Bowell, Roger	Regional Hospital	Sligo
Campbell, B. J.	11, Dealfield, Limavady Road	Derry
Campbell, Mary	33, John Street	Omagh, Co. Tyrone
Cantillon, C. J.	17, St. Patrick's Hill	Cork
Collum, L. M. T.	9, Fitzwilliam Place	Dublin 2
Condon, R. A.	128, The Quay	Waterford
Connolly, Dorothy	45, Fitzwilliam Square	Dublin 2
Corkey, J. A.	67, University Road	Belfast 7
Counahan, Gloria	3, Rus-in-Urbe	Lr. Glenageary, Co. Dublin
Cowan, E. C.	23, Wellington Park, Malone Road	Belfast
Crookes, G. P.	18, Fitzwilliam Place	Dublin 2
Crookes, Jean	Ashton, 6, Martello Tce.	Dun Laoghaire
Cullen, B. T.	5, Farnham Street	Cavan
Douglas, D. H.	31, Upr. Fitzwilliam Street	Dublin 2
Eustace, J. A.	92, West Street	Drogheda, Co. Louth

Fenton, Maurice	18, Fitzwilliam Place	Dublin 2
Finan, C. F.	10, Montpelier Tce.	Galway
Fitzpatrick, Catherine	16, Fitzwilliam Square	Dublin 2
Fleming, P.	2, Munster Tce.	Sandycove, Co. Dublin
Gormley, P.	23, Windsor Park, Malone Road	Belfast
Guinan, Philomena	36, Fitzwilliam Place	Dublin 2
Hewson, G. E.	The Crescent	Galway
Hickey, J. B.		Letterkenny, Co. Donegal
Horan, E. C.	21, St. Patrick's Hill	Cork
Hurley, T.	15, St. Patrick's Hill	Cork
Johnston, S. S.	43, Adelaide Park	Belfast
Joyce, Anna	49, Upr. Drumcondra Road	Dublin 9
Joyce, P. Dwyer	11, Merrion Square	Dublin 2
Keane, Monica	Verelands, Garden Vale	Athlone
Kelly, Geraldine	Brookvale	Stillorgan, Co. Dublin
Kelly, Margot	Glebelands	Warrenpoint, Co. Down
Kennedy, Eileen	Rathfeigh	Ennis, Co. Clare
Kilkelly, Ethel	Lydican, Ballymahon Road	Athlone
Lavery, F. J.	Sorrento House	Dalkey, Co. Dublin
Lavery, F. L.	54, Fitzwilliam Square	Dublin 2
MacAuley, Anna	33, Stewartstown Road	Belfast
McAuley, F. D.	45, Upr. Leeson Street	Dublin 2
McConn, J. D.	Cloonfadda House	Killaloe, Co. Clare
MacMahon, Anna	2, The Crescent	Galway
MacMahon, S. T.	Montpelier, The Crescent	Galway
McWilliams, E. H.	Woodgreen, Ballymacvea	Ballymena, Co. Antrim
Macdougald, T. J.	94, Upr. Leeson Street	Dublin 2
Mackey, E. C.	12, Merrion Square	Dublin 2
Madden, J. G.	21, St. Patrick's Hill	Cork
Mahon, D	Doonard, The Mall	Sligo
Martin, V. A. F.	13, Adelaide Park	Belfast
Mathews, P	20, Fitzwilliam Place	Dublin 2
May, Margaret C.	Glengesh, Howth Road	Dublin 3
Monahan, Sarah	Moatlands	Navan, Co. Meath
Mooney, A. J.	33, Fitzwilliam Place	Dublin 2
Mooney, David	33, Fitzwilliam Place	Dublin 2
O'Byrne, J	44, O'Connell Street	Limerick
O'Connell, Sr. R.	Our Lady of Lourdes Hospital	Drogheda
O'Connor, Ina	7, Camden Place	Cork
O'Donnell, P. J.	16, Denny Street	Tralee, Co. Kerry
O'Donoghue, D.	14, Nutley Ave.	Dublin 4
Ogilvie, K. R.	17, St. Patrick's Place	Cork
O'Malley, C. C.	County Club	Galway
O'Malley, Sarah	4, Pery Square	Limerick
O'Reilly, G. A.	34, Fitzwilliam Square	Dublin 2
O'Sullivan, J. V.	11, Sidney Place	Cork
Phelan, F. G.	7, The Crescent	Galway
Quinn, Catherine	17, Fitzwilliam Place	Dublin 2
Robinson, W. L.	Ardbeara	Fahan, Co. Donegal
Ryan, J. L.	13, Parnell Street	Waterford
Shorten, D.	24, Upr. Mallow Street	Limerick
Smith, F. P. E.	Bunraskin, Casement Street	Cavan
Smith, F. W. G.	Merton	Cobh, Co. Cork
Solan, E. M.	50, O'Connell Street	Clonmel
Tierney, P. I.	Fairy Hill	Clonmel, Co. Tipperary
Tomkin, A.	1, Fitzwilliam Square	Dublin 2

Tomkin, H.	1, Fitzwilliam Square	Dublin 2
Walsh, Alphonsus	Department of Health, Custom House	
Walsh, Joseph	25, Fitzwilliam Place	Dublin 2
Walshe, M. M.	Woodmice, Freshford Road	Kilkenny
Werner, L. E.	94, Upr. Leeson Street	Dublin 2
Wilson, D. J.	23a, St. Patrick's Hill	Cork

NOSOCOMIA QUIBUS OCULIS AEGRI CURANTUR

	No. of beds
Altnagelvin Hospital, Derry	30
Belfast City Hospital, Belfast	14
Eye & Ear Hospital, Adelaide Road, Dublin 2	112
Eye, Ear & Throat Hospital, Western Road, Cork	27
Galway Regional Hospital, Galway	18
Jervis St. Hospital, Jervis Street, Dublin 1	6
Mater Infirmorum, Crumlin Road, Belfast	18
Mater Misericordiae Hospital, Eccles St., Dublin 7	17
Newtownards Hospital, Newtownards, Co. Down	4
Our Lady's Childrens' Hospital, Crumlin, Dublin 12	6
Royal Victoria Hospital, Belfast	77
St. Vincent's Hospital, Dublin 4	16
South Charitable Infirmary & County Hospital, Old Blackrock Road, Cork	7
Ulster Hospital for Children & Women, Dundonald, Belfast	4
Waveney Hospital, Belfast	4

INSTITUTA SCHOLAEQUE CAECIS DESTINATAE

		Inmates
Institution for the Industrious Blind, Infirmary Road, Cork	Men	15
	Women	19
Rochfort Wade Hostel for Blind Women, 33, Moyne Rd., Rathmines, Dublin 6		12
The Molyneux Home for the Blind, Leeson Park, Dublin 6		31
Board for the Employment of the Blind, Workshops, Ardee Road, Rathmines, Dublin 6		70
St. Joseph's School for Blind Boys, Gracepark Road, Drumcondra, Dublin 9	Boys	95
	Men	35
St. Mary's Home & School for the Blind & Partially Sighted, Merrion, Dublin 4	Children	82
	Adults	97
Irish Association for the Blind, 8, Nth. Great Georges St., Dublin 1		
Irish National League of the Blind, 35, Gardiner's Place, Dublin 1		
National Council for the Blind of Ireland, 10, Lr. Hatch Street, Dublin 2 (affiliated with the International Society for the Prevention of Blindness)		
Royal National Institute for Blind, Bryson House, Bedford St., Belfast 1		
Workshops for the Blind, Lawnbrook Ave., Belfast	Workers	65
	Trainees	9
Jordanstown Schools, 85, Jordanstown Rd., Newtownabbey, Co. Antrim (for children with auditory or visual handicaps)	Blind	30
	Part sight	70
Home for the Blind, Cliftonville Road, Belfast 14		19

HISPANIA

SOCIETATES OPHTHALMOLOGICAE

Nationalis

Sociedad Española de Oftalmología

Presidente: Dr. Carlos Costi Garcia de Tuñón
Vicepresidente: Dr. Alejandro Palomar y Palomar
Secretario general: Dr. Gustavo Leoz de la Fuente, Clinica de N.S. de la Concepcíon, Avenida Reyes Catolicos, 2, Madrid 3
Secretario 1: Dr. Pedro Tena Ibarra
Vocal 1: Dr. Nicolás Belmonte González
Vocal 2: Dr. Fernando Palomar Petit
Vocal 3: Dr. Emilio Gil del Río
Vocal 4: Dr. Antonio Piñero Carrión
Vocal 5: Dr. Jaime Péraz-Llorca Rodrigo
Vocal 6: Dr. Luis Dolcet Buxeres
Vocal nato como Director de Archivos: D. Jóse M.ª Aguilar Bartolomé
Ex presidentes consejeros: Dr. Galo Leoz Ortín, Dr. José Pérez Llorca, Dr. José Casanovas Carnicer, Dr. Juan Arjona Trapote, Dr. Diego Díaz Dominguez
Presidente de Honor: Dr. Galo Leoz Ortin

Regionales

Asociación Catalana de Oftalmología

Secretary: Dr. L. A. Noguer, C. Manuel Gironés, 11, Barcelona 17

Sociedad Oftalmológica de Madrid

Secretary: Dr. Del Rio Cabañas, Avenida de Felipe II, 4, Madrid, 9

Sociedad Andaluza y Extremeña de Oftalmología

President: Dr. Caballero del Castillo, General Moscardó, 5, Sevilla

Sociedad de Oftalmología de Galicia

President: Prof. M. Sanchez Salorio, Compostela, 6, Santiago de Compostela

NOMINA ET DOMICILIA MEDICORUM AB OCULIS

Abad Montaño, Cándido ...	Paseo Alfonso XIII,7	Cartagena (Murcia)
Abraldes Puertolas, Maximino	República de El Salvador, 3	Santiago de Compostela (La Coruña)
Achúcarro Ylund, Severino de	Navarro, 6	Bilbao-1

Adán Gonzalvo, José Pablo . Avda. Jaime I, 63, pral. . . . . Gerona
Agua López, Eduardo del . . Correo Viejo, 8 . . . . Lérida
Aguilar Bartolomé, José
  María . . . . Alcalá Galiano, 8 . . . . Madrid-4
Aguilar Rico, Mariano . . . . . Cátedra de Optica, Facultad de
  Ciencias . . . . Valencia
Albelda Gliment, Carlos . . . San Francisco, 16 . . . . Carcagente (Valencia)
Albisúa Elcoro, Enrique . . . Buen Pastor, 7, 2.º . . . . San Sebastián
Alcala Fernández, Antonio . Liborio García, 3 . . . . Málaga
Alcalá López, Antonio . . . . Liborio García, 3 . . . . Málaga
Alemán Hernández-Ros,
  Antonio . . . . Pl. Fuensanta, Edificio Banco
  Vitalicio . . . . Murcia
Alemán Hurtado, E. José . . Infanta Carlota, 100, 2.º 2.ª Barcelona-15
Alemán Picatoste, Fulgencio Pl. Fuensanta, Edificio Banco
  Vitalicio . . . . Murcia
Alemany Gutiérrez, Alfonso. Calvo Sotelo, 29 . . . . Zaragoza
Alfonso González, Miguel . . Méndez Núñez, 1 . . . . Santa Cruz de Tenerife (Ca-
  narias)
Alomar Más, Rafael . . . . . . Obispo Perelló, 18 . . . . Palma de Mallorca
Alonso Bañuelos, José Anto-
  nio . . . . Espolón 2, 2.º . . . . Burgos
Alonso Bañuelos, Lorenzo . Espolón, 2.2.º . . . . Burgos
Alonso Castellano, Mariano . Arnuces, 4 . . . . Las Palmas
Alonso Caviedes, Santiago . Isabel II, 16 . . . . Santander
Alonso De Medina y Bono,
  Francisco . . . . Castaños, 16 . . . . Alicante
Alonso Santos, Francisco . . Gran Vía Vallellano, 17 . . . . Hellín (Albacete)
Altes Pineda, José . . . . Mallorca, 330 . . . . Barcelona-9
Alvarez Alvarez, Maria Jesús. Toledo, 137, 7.º A . . . . Madrid
Alvarez Elosua, Emilio . . . . Toreno, 5 . . . . Oviedo
Alvarez Garcia, Manuel . . . . Hilarión Eslava, 55 . . . . Madrid-3
Alvarez Hevia, Isidro . . . . . . Jerónimo Ibrán, 9 . . . . Mieres (Asturias)
Alvarez Lledó, Javier . . . . . . General Mola, 207 . . . . Madrid
Alvarez Suárez, Roberto . . . Góngora, 9, 5.º . . . . Córdoba
Alvarez Torre, Julio . . . . . . Arquitecto Reguera, 6 . . . . Oviedo
Amaro Cabera, Augstín . . . General Mola, 31 . . . . Santa Cruz de la Palma
  (Tenerife)
Amer Fiol, Antonio . . . . . . Angel Guimerá, 28 . . . . Manresa (Barcelona)
Amer Fiol, Bartolomé . . . . . Jaime I, 13 . . . . Manresa (Barcelona)
Amías Menchaca, Pedro . . . Ibáñez de Bilbao, 17 . . . . Bilbao-9
Amigo Cuevas, María Dolo-
  res . . . . Lucas de Tuy, 1, 8.º izqda. . . . . . León
Amigó Mañé, Salvador . . . . Plaza Mosén Jacinto Verdaguer,
  10 . . . . Tarragona
Amo Molina, Antonio . . . . . Sevilla, 17 . . . . Córdoba
Andrés Soraluce, José Maria . Carlos III, 11 . . . . Pamplona
Angulo Cuellar, Luis Ismael . Juan S. Bach, 28, 2.º . . . . Barcelona
Aparisi Gijón, Tomás . . . . . Colón, 50 . . . . Valencia-4
Aráez Pacheco, Rafael . . . . General Segura, 4 . . . . Almería
Aragón Ruiz, Pablo . . . . Pilar de Zaragoza, 104 . . . . Madrid-28
Aranda Latorre, Fermín . . . Pedro Alonso, 66 . . . . Jerez de la Frontera (Cádiz)
Arechaga Vázquez, Francis-
  co . . . . Doctor Teijeiro, 14 . . . . Monforte de Lemos (Lugo)
Arias López, M.ª del Carmen Paseo Ribalta, 10, 6.º . . . . Castellón
Arias Moreno, Antonio . . . . Santa Tomé, 9 . . . . Toledo

Ariza Cardenal, José M.ª ..	Balmes, 163-3.º	Barcelona-8
Arjona Santos, Juan José ..	Av. Generalísimo, 34	Madrid-16
Arjona Trapote, Juan	Avda. José Antonio, 65	Madrid-13
Arnalot Sansa, Ignacio	Viladomat, 55	Barcelona-15
Arostegui Salaverri, Jesús de.	Ercilla, 30, 2.º izqda...........	Bilbao
Arques Girones, Emilio	Imagen, 6	Sevilla
Arrazola Garicano, Luis ...	Oquendo, 13	San Sebastián
Arriaga Cantullera, José ..	José María Osborne, 7	Sevilla
Arribas Bensusan, José Maria	Génova, 1, 1.º B.	Sevilla
Arrola y Noriega, Luis Maria	Velázquez, 22	Madrid-1
Arruga Forgas, Alfredo	Pasaje Méndez Vigo, 3	Barcelona-9
Arruga Liró, Ricardo	Paseo de Gracia, 52	Barcelona-7
Artajo Arana, José María ..	Colón de Larreátegui, 30	Bilbao-9
Arumi Bonet, Joaquín	Via Augusta, 241, 2.º	Barcelona-6
Asenjo Rodriguez, Julia ...	Paseo de la Habana, 14, 5.º D ...	Madrid-16
Azadeh, Modebbollah	Instituto Barraquer	Barcelona
Azcoaga Arana, José María .	Av. Sancho el Sabio, 15	San Sebastián
Aznárez Cocho, José Manuel	Virgen de Luján, 3, 1.º	Sevilla
Aznárez Cocho, María del Pilar	Avenida de Cádiz, 4, 6.º B	Sevilla
Aznárez García, José :....	Virgen de Luján, 3, 1.º B.	Sevilla
Baamonde Ferreiro, Carlos .	G. Franco, 101	El Ferrol (La Coruña)
Baamonde Ferreiro, Diego .	Langreo, 13	Gijón (Asturias)
Bajo Fernández, Antonio ..	Melquiades Alvarez, 3	Oviedo
Baldoví Morales, Mariano ..ᶜ	Plaza de Roca, 19	Játiva (Valencia)
Ballester Bernial, Arturo ...	Carniceros, 13	Valencia
Bañuelos Achiaga, Gregorio .	Plaza José Antonio, 2	Burgos
Barahona Hortelano, José María	C. M. Fonseca	Salamanca
Barahona Martín, Benito ..	Plaza del Doctor Laguna, 2	Segovia
Barberá Carré, José	Rambla Caudillo, 63	Villanueva y Geltrú (Barcelona)
Barcena De La Calzada, Ramón	Hernán Cortés, 23	Santander
Barcia Goyanes, Juan José .	Gran Via Marqués del Turia, 62 .	Valencia-5
Barja Diéguez, Gonzalo	Parque de San Lázaro, 16	Orense
Barraquer Cerezo, Tomás ..	Plaza de las Salesas, 10	Madrid-4
Barraquer Monter, Joaquín .	Muntaner, 314	Barcelona-6
Barreda Espinosa, Marino de la	General Mola, 98 ....·....	Santa Cruz de Tenerife
Barreiro Saavedra, Manuel .	Eduardo Pondal, 19	Santiago de Compostela (La Coruña)
Barroso Estrada, José María	Donoso Cortés, 7	Don Benito (Badajoz)
Barry Rodríguez, Julio	Viera y Clavijo, 19	Las Palmas (Canarias)
Bartolozzi Sánchéz, Rafael .	Avda. Alemania, 20, 7.º A	Salamanca
Bascarán Asunsolo, Antonio.	Fruela, 4	Oviedo
Bascarán Collantes, Antonio.	Uría, 21	Oviedo
Basterra Ibarra, Alberto ...	Cronista Carrere, 4	Valencia-3
Basurte De Cisneros, José Luis	Espinel, 84-86	Ronda (Málaga)
Bautista Vázquez de Parga, José M.ª	Claudio Coelo, 128	Madrid-6
Becerra Caballero, Emilio ..	Guillermo Nicolau, 2	Zafra (Badajoz)
Belmonte García, Juan	Mayor, 31	Albacete
Belmonte González, José ..	San Fernando, 21	Alicante
Belmonte González, Manuel	Tinte, 26	Albacete

Belmonte González, Nicolás.	Gamazo, 24	Valladolid
Belmonte Martínez, José	San Fernando, 21	Alicante
Beltrán Moreno, Fernando .	Av. Tenor Fleta, 3	Zaragoza
Beltran Pareja, Enrique	Martínez Campos, 7	Andújar (Jaén)
Benavente Campos, José ...	Plaza del Ecuador, 7	Madrid-16
Benítez del Castillo, José Manuel	Plaza Monti, 11-13	Jerez de la Frontera (Cádiz)
Benjumeda Salinas, Alfredo .	Pedro Pérez Fernández, 7	Sevilla
Bernabéu, Rafael	Conde de Peñalver, 68, 6.º izqda.	Madrid-6
Bertrán Castellví, Francisco .	Av. Puerta del Angel, 40	Barcelona-2
Betancourt Ramos, Raúl ...	Av. de Betanzos, 17	Madrid-20
Birba Cordomi, Sebastián ..	Muntaner, 31	Barcelona-11
Blanch Martí, Luis Fernando	Paseo Manuel Girona, 78, 8.º 2.ª .	Barcelona-17
Blas Mantecón, Carmen de .	Avda. Rey Don Jaime I, 56	Castellón de la Plana
Bobes Naves José	Cristóbal Bordíu, 10	Madrid-3
Boldu Bobin, Enrique	Despuig, 26	Tortosa (Tarragona)
Bonilla de Mingo, Julián ...	Ramón y Cajal, 6	Ciudad Real
Bouvier Ferir, Jorge	San Elías, 37, 5.º, 1.ª	Barcelona-6
Bovis Bermúdez, José	Carlos Cañal, 23	Sevilla
Branco Pereira Marouco, Francisco	Avda. Cruz Campo, 35	Sevilla
Bruix Solanes, Jorge	Londres, 188	Barcelona-11
Buigues Carrio, Vicente ...	Av. Generalísimo, 43	Denia (Alicante)
Burch Y de Barraquer, Manuel	Gerona, 18	Barcelona-10
Burgo Fernandez, Felipe ...	San Vicente Ferrer, 6	Granada
Caballero Cabañero, Francisco	General Franco, 43	Zaragoza
Caballero Carretero, Francisco	Av. Generalísimo, 4	Melilla
Caballero Del Castillo, Daniel	General Moscardó, 5	Sevilla
Cabré Garriga, Juan	Via Layetana, 151	Barcelona-9
Cabrera López, José M.ª ...	Correos, 10	Valencia
Cabrera Pérez, Antonio	Canalejas, 63	Las Palmas de Gran Canaria
Cadenas Ugidos, Cesáreo ...	Buen Suceso, 14	Madrid-8
Calafat López-Figueredo, José M.ª	General Mola, 99	Madrid-6
Calbo de Castro, Juan M. ..	Queipo de Llano, 22	Elda (Alicante)
Calderón Allúe, Jorge	Diagonal, 558	Barcelona-11
Calandria Posada, Adolfo ..	San Francisco, 28	Cádiz
Calvet, Josefina	Barón de Cárcer, 34	Valencia-1
Calvet Fontova, Antonio ..	Mayor, 41	Lérida
Calvo García, Luis A.	General Franco, 1, 1.º Izqda ...	Las Palmas de Gran Canaria
Calvo Picó, José	Compositor Bach, 24	Barcelona-6
Cámara Hermoso, Julio	Carlos III, 63-Bis, 5.º-2.ª	Barcelona-17
Cámara Solís, Ezequiel	Plaza de San Martín, 19	Plasencia (Cáceres)
Camíns Ribera, José	Conde Vallellano, 119	Tarragona
Camíns Ribera, Juan	Ingeniero, 7 y 9, 10, 3.º	Granollers (Barcelona)
Campo Balboa, José Antonio	Moral, 2	Villanueva de Córdoba (Córdoba)
Campos Paz, José M.ª	S. Moreno, 29	Pontevedra
Campos Pérez, Salvador ...	Plaza de Santiago, 2	Villena (Alicante)
Candina Aguirremota, Vicente	Marqués del Puerto, 9	Bilbao-8
Canduela Company, Victor .	Queipo de Llano, 4	

Capelastegui Herrero, Alberto	Plaza de Navarra	Abadiano (Vizcaya)
Carrancio De La Plaza, Flaviano	Arcipreste de Hita, 3	Madrid-15
Carreras Matas, Buenaventura	Recogidas, 39	Granada
Carreras Matas, Marcelo	Hernán Cortés, 24	Valencia
Carretero Garcia, Margarita	Altamira, 47	Almería
Carrilero de La Torre, Julio	Tinte, 15	Albacete
Carrillo Nieves, Antonio	General Bravo, 42	Las Palmas de Gran Canaria
Carrió Caballero, Joaquín	Cervantes, 20	Denia (Alicante)
Casado González, Miguel	República Argentina, 6	Valencia
Casado Rosa, Alfonso	Virgen de la Antigua, 9	Sevilla
Casado Sañudo, José	Yanguas y Miranda, 7	Tudela (Navarra)
Casanellas Ybarz, José	Pelayo, 43	Barcelona-1
Casanovas Carnicer, José	Freixá, 46	Barcelona-6
Casanovas La Rosa, Román	Lauria, 77, 1.º, 1.ª	Barcelona-9
Casero Fernández, Luis	Av. Nazaret, 8	Madrid-7
Castanera Pueyo, Alfonso	Via Augusta, 20	Barcelona-6
Castañeda Chornet, Luis	Plaza del Castillo, 7	Valencia
Casteños Uriarte, José M.ª	Anunciación, 10	Madrid-9
Castiella y Maíz, José M.ª	Berástegui, 1	Bilbao-1
Castiella Zalba, Francisco	Zapatería, 36	Pamplona
Castresana y Alonso De Prado, José Ignacio	Marqués del Puerto, 10	Bilbao-8
Castresana Guinea, Angel	Gran Vía Lope de Haro, 43	Bilbao
Casulleras Gil, Valentín	Puigdorfila, 4	Palma de Mallorca
Catarinéu Nieto, Alvaro	Rafalafena, 1	Castellón
Cea Gil, Anastasio	Avda. República Argentina, 13, 1.º B	Sevilla
Ceara Viñas, Ernesto Zenón	Martín de los Heros, 80, 3.º C, 'Casas de Ana Josefa Garrido'	Madrid-8
Ceci Alzamora, Rolando Arturo	República Argentina, 6, 2.º B	Santiago de Compostela (La Coruña)
Celis Herencia, Agustín	General Aguilera, 5	Ciudad Real
Centeno Martínez, M.ª Josefa	Batalla de Belchite, 12	Madrid-7
Ceres Frías, M.ª Josefa	Dr. Severo Ochoa, 1, 4.º B	Granada
Cerezo Abad, Teófilo	Calle Madrid, 3	Burgos
Cervantes Párraga, Manuel	Carretera de Garrucha, 11	Huércal-Overa (Almería)
Cervera Alpera, Manuel	Av. Marqués de Sotelo, 9	Valencia-2
Cervero Fernández, José Antonio	Uría, 15	Oviedo
Cisneros Mesa, Angel Luis	Plaza de la Seo, 15	Tarazona de Aragón (Zaragoza)
Clement Casado, Francisco	Fuencarral, 90	Madrid-4
Cobanera Alcalde, José Luis	Pl. Zabalburos, 2, 3.º Izqda	Bilbao, 3
Coll Taverner, Antonio	General Mola, 10	Huelva
Collado Hornillos, José Antonio	Institución Valdecilla	Santander
Collado Soto, José	Mártires, 2	Torrelavega (Santander)
Corcóstegui Moliner, José Luis	Gran Vía, 74, 3.º izqda.	Bilbao-11
Corcóstegui Moliner, Rafael	Bidebarrieta, 1, 3.º	Bilbao-5
Cordoves Pérez, Luis	Jesús Maria, 23	Santa Cruz de Tenerife

Coret Novoa, Andrés	San Bruno, 44	Badalona (Barcelona)
Cortes de Los Reyes, Hernán	Paseo al Mar, 26	Valencia-10
Costi García de Tuñón, Carlos	Alfonso XII, 46	Madrid-14
Cotanda García, M.ª del Pilar	Lérida, 20	Mollet del Vallés (Barcelona)
Crespi Cascar, Federico	Cea Bermúdez, 34	Madrid-3
Crespi Jaume, Gonzalo	García de Paredes, 66	Madrid-3
Cuadrado González, Miguel .	Santiago, 17	Portugalete (Vizcaya)
Cuéllar Vaca, Roger	Santa Cruz, Casilla 677	Bolivia
Cuello Salamero, Miguel Angel	José María Osborne, 3	Sevilla
Cuenca García, Rafael	Avda. Cataluña, 1	Valencia-10
Cuenca Trenco, Rafael	Avda. Cataluña, 1	Valencia-10
Cuervo Arango, José	Plaza de San Miguel, 11	Gijón (Asturias)
Cumplido Fernández-Salguero, José A.	Juan XXIII, 5	Las Palmas
Chabas Martí, Josefa	Colón, 3	Madrid-10
Chaguaceda Romero, Ricardo	Virgen de la Antigua, 2	Sevilla
Chaguaceda Villabrille, Juan.	Duque de Alba, 8	Avila
Chavarría Iriarte, Félix Angel	Doctor Chavarría, 21	Calahorra (Logroño)
Chavarría Iriarte, José M.ª .	San Pablo, 42	Figueras (Gerona)
Chavarría Iriarte, Ricardo ..	Doctor Chavarría, 21	Calahorra (Logroño)
Chunliá Mallol, Vicente ...	En Sanz, 12, 10.º	Valencia-1
Dalmáu Jover, José	Avda. Generalísimo Franco, 449, 2.º	Barcelona-8
Damborena Terroba, Antonio de	Gran Via, 46, 1.º	Bilbao-11
Dapena Crespo, M.ª Teresa .	Buen Suceso, 8, 5.º	Madrid-8
Delgado Espinosa, Juan ...	José Antonio, 55	Madrid-13
Delgado Vera, Juan B.	Medieras, 6	Cartagena (Murcia)
Delsors Pujol, José Luis ...	Avda. Generalísimo, 99, 2.º izqd.	Tortosa (Tarragona)
Deo Ridruejo, José M.	Paseo de Gracia, 20	Barcelona-7
Díaz-Caneja Bustamante, Arturo	General Mola, 20	Castro Urdiales (Santander)
Díaz-Caneja Bustamante, Emilio	Lealtad, 8	Santander
Díaz Estévez, Diego	Pl. Alonso el Magnánimo, 5, 4.º .	Valencia
Díaz y García Del Viso, Gregorio	Espalter, 5	Madrid-4
Díaz Maíllo, Luis	Avda. José Antonio, 4, 1.º	Zamora
Díaz Martínez, Manuel	Pl. de San Agustín, 3	Valencia-6
Díaz Rodríguez, José F. ...	Albareda, 32	Las Palmas
Díez del Corral Angulo, Pablo	San Marcos, 2	Lugo
Díez del Corral Cerón, Salvador	Corrida, 64	Gijón (Asturias)
Díez del Corral Ramírez, Pablo	Pradillo, 15	Madrid-2
Díez Feijoo, Elio	José Antonio, 38, 2.º	Ponferrada (León)
Díez García, Juan J.	Viera y Clavijo, 16	Las Palmas (Canarias)
Díez Lage, Andrés	Reina, 13	Lugo
Dios Ortiz, Enrique	Michelena, 10, 2.º	Pontevedra

Dolcet Buxeres, Luis	P. Valle Habrón, s/n. Residencia General Ciudad Sanitaria Francisco Franco	Barcelona-6
Domingo Pérez, José	Policarpo Sanz, 22, 3.º	Vigo (Pontevedra)
Domínguez Casal, Tomás ..	Real, 65	El Ferrol (La Coruña)
Domínguez Collazo, Alfredo	Velázquez, 75, 4.º	Madrid-6
Domínguez Fernández, Ramón	Fivasa, 4	Avila
Dou Mas-De-Xexás Manuel .	Londres, 35	Barcelona-15
Duch Bordás, Francisco ...	Via Augusta, 63	Barcelona-6
Durban Benito, Joaquín ...	Rambla de Cataluña, 37	Barcelona-7
Ellacuria Larrauri, Ildefonso.	General Castaños, 2	Portugalete (Vizcaya)
Encinas García, Antonio ...	....	Guadramino-Vitigudino (Salamanca)
Encinas Martin, José Luis ..	Clinica Puerta de Hierro, Servicio de Oftalmología, San Martín de Porres, 4	Madrid
Encinas Sanz, Jacinto D. ...	Avda. del Generalísimo, 4, 5.º ..	San Sebastián
Escolá Caus, Ramón	Paseo de Gracia, 76, 3.º, 2.ª	Barcelona-8
Escolar González, José A. ...	Gallos, 25	Sevilla
Espalza Sagarminaga, Ignacio	Gardoqui, 4	Bibao-8
Espasa Molina, Juan A.	Mayor de Gracia, 47	Barcelona-12
Espejo Camacho, Manuel ..	Colonia S. Rafael, 15	Ubeda (Jaén)
Espejo Escribano, Domingo .	Requeté de España, 1, 4.º B	San Fernando (Cádiz)
Esteban de Antonio, Mario .	Paseo de la Habana, 184	Madrid-16
Esteban Monteleón, Miguel .	Gran Vía Fernando el Católico, 5.	Valencia-8
Fabón Barco, Gabriel	Pío XII, 1, 2.º	Logroño
Faci Muñoz, Angel	Alfonso I, 10	Zaragoza
Faci Paricio, Angel	Alfonso I, 10, 1.º	Zaragoza
Fandino Martínez, José ...	Fuentes San Antonio, 17, 2.º ...	Santiago de Compostela (La Coruña)
Fariza Martín, Leandro	General Mola, 9	Castellón de la Plana
Fernández Aldave, Leandro .	P. Castellana, 51 bis	Madrid-1
Fernández Carvajal, Emilio .	Cuatro Calles, 5	Ciudad Rodrigo (Salamanca)
Fernández Contra, Gonzalo .	Paseo de las Acacias, 5	Madrid-5
Fernández Díaz, José	Vallehermoso, 100, piso 4.º C ..	Madrid-3
Fernández Fernández, Maximiliano	Muro, 10	Valladolid
Fernández Garcia, Julio ...	Conde de Peñalver, 17	Madrid-6
Fernández González, Angel .	Balmes, 349	Barcelona-6
Fernández González, Miguel	Pl. Santocildes, 16	Astorga (León)
Fernández de La Fuente, Pedro J.	Fuente del Hierro, 2, 4.º B	Pamplona
Fernández Mendiola, Soledad	Reyes, 13	Madrid-8
Fernández Muñoz, Eduardo	Jaime I el Conquistador, 3, 1.º B	Murcia
Fernández de Ortega Fernández de Bretoño, José Ramón	Gral. Alava, 28, 2.º dcha.	Vitoria
Fernández Ortiz, Jesús	Avda. Lugo, 17	Avilés (Asturias)
Fernández Pacheco, Ramiro.	Paseo de la Estación, 1	Manzanares (Ciudad Real)
Fernández Ramírez, Octavio	Fajardo, 1	Arrecife-Lanzarote (Canarias)
Fernández-Repeto y Repeto, Santiago	Valverde, 5	Cádiz

García García, Jesús	Mesón de Paredes, 86	Madrid-12
García Gil, José Luis	R. Convento, 1	Jumilla (Murcia)
García Gómez, Salvador ...	Peñuelas, 20	Madrid-5
García de la Infanta Peinado, Francisco	Av. Doctor Federico Rubio, 123 .	Madrid-20
García Iñíguez, Juan	Travesía Andrés Mellado, 5, 3.º izqda.	Madrid
García Junceda, Eladio	Principado, 7	Oviedo (Asturias)
García de Leaniz García, Alfonso	Panamá, 12	Madrid-16
García Madruga Valcarce, Virgilio	República Argentina, 22	León
García Mansilla y de la Mesa, Luis	Lagasca, 16	Madrid-1
García Marco, Tomás	Joaquin Arnáu, 16	Teruel
García Márquez, Emilio ...	D/particular, J. Flórez, 19	La Coruña
García Miranda, Ramón ...	Independencia, 1	León
García Montes, Manuel	Avda. Rey Don Jaime I, 56	Castellón
García Montoro, Inocente .	Garrigues, 8	Valencia-1
García Oncins, José M.ª ...	Av. del Generalísimo, 79	Madrid-16
García de Oteyza, Juan A. .	Av. de José Antonio, 31	Lérida
García Pérez, Antonio	José Antonio, 15, 5.º izqda	Salamanca
García Sánchez, Julián	Plaza de la Mina, 12, 1.º	Cádiz
García Santa Cruz, Salvador.	Rafael Calvo, 40	Madrid-10
García Sesma, José M.ª	Generalísimo, 4	Murcia
García Sinova, Acacio	Claudio Moyano, 5	Valladolid
García Soldevilla, José	San Vicente, 16	Gandía (Valencia)
García Suarez, José L.	Francisco Mariño, 5	La Coruña
García Valdecasas, Pedro .	Rivero, 3	Ecija (Sevilla)
García Valdecasas Soler, Rafael	Miguel de Cervantes, 1, 1.º	Ecija, Sevilla
García Vidal, Antonio	Linares Rivas, 52	La Coruña
Garmendía Duinat, Enrique.	Plaza de Colón, 7	Irún (Guipúzcoa)
Garnica, Lina	Cruz, 63	Badalona (Barcelona)
Gasalla Rivero, María Paz ..	Santo Domingo, 10	Lugo
Gázquez Gómez, Manuel ..	Méndez Nuñez, 17, 2.º	Almería
Gázquez Martínez, Manuel .	Martinez Campos, 1	Almería
Genís Gálvez, José M.ª	Santiago Ramón y Cajal, 15	Salamanca
Gil Fernández, Ambrosio ..	Andújar, 5	Ubeda (Jaén)
Gil Gibernáu, Juan J.	Juan Sebastián Bach, 10, 2.ª	Barcelona-6
Gil Del Río, Emilio	Olaguibel, 19	Vitoria
Gimbert Routra, José	Ronda del General Mitre, 214 ...	Barcelona-6
Giménez Alvarez, Manuel ..	Amado Nervo, 5	Madrid
Giménez Cánovas, Juan ...	Pl. Vicente Iborra, 3, esc. B.	Valencia-3
Giménez Guerra, Luis	P.º de la Habana, 52, 7.º	Madrid
Giménez Mirabet, Rafael ..	Poeta Querol, 10, 7.º	Valencia-2
Gómez Casa, Germán	Urbieta, 43	San Sebastián
Gómez Larrañaga, Jesús ...	Bidebarrieta, 14, 2.º	Eibar (Guipúzcoa)
Cómez de Liano Cobaleda, Fernando	Núñez de Balboa, 39	Madrid-1
Gómez Naval, José Luis ...	José Antonio, 44, 1.º	Vigo, Pontevedra
Gómez Pardo, Manuel	Loaces, 9	Orihuela (Alicante)
Gómez Torre, Rafael	Francisco Lozano, 5, 6.º dcha. ..	Madrid-8
Góngora y Rivero, José de .	San Cristóbal, 7	Valencia-3
Gonzalo Gadalda, Vicente .	Colón, 76, 2.º B	Castellón

González de Audicana, Manuel	Plaza de Indauchu, 1	Bilbao-11
González Carbajo, Félix ...	Puente Castañeda, 5, 2.ª	Granada
González Cervantes, José ..	Duque, 21	Cartagena (Murcia)
González Costa, José Alberto	Jaime I, 5, 1.º	Murcia
González Díaz, Luis	Sagasta, 21, 1.º D	Madrid
González Fernandez, Tomás.	Av. de España, 12	Cáceres
González Garra, Francisco .	Uruguay, 15	Vigo (Pontevedra)
González Gutiérrez, Félix ..	Alcalá, 348	Madrid-17
González Hubertas, Francisco	Juan Jiménez Cuenca, 10	Lucena (Córdoba)
González Marín, Pascual ...	Santa Gertrudis, 8, 6.º	Murcia
González Martin, Demetrio .	General Franco, 7	Arévalo (Avila)
González Martín, Juan A. ...	Fortuny, 29	Sabadell (Barcelona)
González Moldes, Elías	Bravo Murillo, 200 bis, 3.º E. ...	Madrid-20
González Muñoz, Franscisco	Gran Vía, 12, 3.º dcha.	Huelva
González Pacheco, Plácido .	Calatrava, 10	Badajoz
González del Rio, Pedro ...	Capúa, 4	Gijón (Asturias)
González Soler, Fernando ..	Mayor, 19	Tarrasa (Barcelona)
González-Sierra Padin, Ramón	Capitan Carreró, 4	Vigo (Pontevedra)
Gonzalo Platero, José A. ...	C. de Toro, 14	Algeciras (Cádiz)
Gras Salas, Fransico	Llovera, 35, 1.º	Reus (Tarragona)
Guasp Taverner, Ramón P. .	Convento de Santa Clara, 11	Valencia-2
Guerrero Cano, Pedro	General Primo de Rivera, 5	Huelva
Guijarro Ortiz de Zárate, Pedro	San Francisco, 30	Aranda de Duero (Burgos)
Guillén Madriñán, Alejandro	Feijoo, 9	La Coruña
Gullón Walker, Alfonso ...	Españoleto, 5	Madrid-4
Gutiérrez Mazeres, Carlos ..	Francisco Mariño, 3, 3.º dcha. ..	La Coruña
Gutiérrez Meca, Ginés	Alfonso XII, 2	Los Dolores - Cartagena (Murcia)
Gutiérrez Velarde, Rafael ..	Julián Ceballos, 21, 3.º	Torrelavega (Santander)
Hera Gutiórrez, José M.ª ...	General Franco, 128, 1.º	Zaragoza
Heras Aguilar, Angel de las .	Calvo Sotelo, 45	Reus (Tarragona)
Heras Hercilla, José	Pl. N. Granados, 8	Soria
Heredia García, Carlos D. ..	Paseo Manuel Girona, 15, 1.º 2.ª .	Barcelona-17
Hernández Benito, Emiliano.	Pl. Gabriel y Galán, 1, 1.º	Salamanca
Hernández Botejera, Fulgencio	Trajano, 14	Azuaga (Bajajoz)
Hernández Gómez, Angel ..	Pl. Gabriel y Galan, 1	Salamanca
Hernández Hernández, José L.	Tomás Morales, 40	Las Palmas
Hernández López, Pablo ...	Barceló, 13	Madrid-4
Hernández Vallejo, J.	Castelló, 102	Madrid-6
Hernández Velasco, Emilio .	P.º Isabel la Católica, 5, 8.º izqda	Valladolid
Hernández Viera, Celso	Córdoba, 11	Málaga
Hernanz Cano, Jesús	Av. Fernández Ladreda, 18	Segovia
Herrero Saura, José A.	Pl. Obispo Berenguer de Palou ..	Palma de Mallorca
Herrero Zapatero, Vidal ...	Av. de Cádiz, 4, 6.º B	Sevilla
Higueras Palacios, Basilio ..	Tablerón, 2	Jaén
Hita Caballero, Vicente de .	José Antonio, 5	Baena (Córdoba)
Höhr Castán, José M.ª ...	San Miguel, 16	Cadiz
		Ronda (Málaga)
Honrubia López, Francisco M.	Cirilo Amorós, 42, 1.º 1.ª	Valencia-4

Iboleón Hurtado, Francisco .	Cuadro San Vicente, 13, 3.º	Granada
Iglesias García de Vicuña, José A.	Córcega, 216	Barcelona-11
Iglesias Gomá, José M.ª ...	General Aranda, 19	Castellón de la Plana
Illueca Domenech, Enrique .	Gran Via Marqués del Turia, 2 ..	Valencia-5
Intante Nieto, Cleto	Eduardo Lucena, 5	Córdoba
Iñigo, Santiago	Laín Calvo, 17	Burgos
Iñigo del Cerro, Luis	Paseo de Pereda, 1	Santander
Iribas de Miguel, Gregorio ..	Francisco Silvela, 55	Madrid-6
Iturralde Goñi, Rafael	Sarasate, 6	Pamplona (Navarra)
Ivorra Lahuerta, Pilar	Colón, 72	Valencia-4
Jareño Paricio, Carmen	Hospital Provincial de Valencia ..	Valencia
Jarreño Paricio, Manuel ...	Manuel Luna, 1, 2.º A	Madrid
Javaloy Lizón, Andrés	José Antonio, 2	Orihuela (Alicante)
Jimena Sánchez, César	Gran Capitán, 19 dpdo.	Córdoba
Jiménez Almenara, Julián ..	José Cruz Conde, 8	Córdoba
Jiménez Almenara, Guillermo	Claudio Marcelo, 11	Córdoba
Jiménez Cazorla, Luis	Juan Bravo, 51, 4.º izqda	Madrid-6
Jiménez Colmenero, Rafael .	Colón, 13	Peñarroya-Pueblonuevo (Córdoba)
Jiménez Muñoz, Ramón ...	J. Navarrete, 62	Puerto de Santa Maria (Cádiz)
Jiménez Sindreu, José	Queipo de Llano, 47	San Juan de Aznalfarache (Sevilla)
Jinot Cutchet, Andrés	San Ramón, 5	Barbastro (Huesca)
Jofre Martínez, José	Plaza del Caudillo, s/n.	Cúllar-Baza (Granada)
Jordano, José	Duque de Fernán Núñez, 4	Córdoba
Jordano Pérez, José	Recogidas, 45, 4.º A	Granada
Jove Arechandieta, Rogelio .	Generalísimo, 30	Avilés (Asturias)
Junceda Avelló, Júan M. ...	Principado, 7	Oviedo
Labella Marina, Fernando ..	Hnos. González Murga, 10	Córdoba
Laiseca Negro, Juan	Francisco Silvela, 54	Madrid-6
Lamas Castro, Gustavo M. .	Av. Buenos Aires, 42	Orense
Latorre Morasso, Salvador .	Alberto Aguilera, 3	Madrid-15
Lattur Montón, Manuel ...	Marqués de Campos, 20	Denia (Alicante)
Lavers Pérez, Francisco	General Franco, 48	La Laguna (Tenerife)
Legeren Campos, Rafael ...	Av. José Antonio, 32, 1.º	Vigo (Pontevedra)
Legeren Buceta, Rafael	Montero Ríos, 4	Vigo (Pontevedra)
Leiva Alvarado, Modesto ..	San Quirico, 34, 3.º	Sabadell (Barcelona)
Leoz de la Fuente, Gustavo .	Cadaceros, 9	Madrid-14
Leoz Ortin, Galo	Cedaceros, 9	Madrid-14
Liébana Angeles, José	Martín Belda, 17, pral.	Cabra (Còrdoba)
Lillo Florit, Juan	Aragón, 298, Clínica Quirurgica .	Barcelona-9
Linares Montes, José	Queipo de Llano, 16	Huelva
Loidi Arrasate, Luis M.ª ...	Fuenterrabía, 15	San Sebastián
Loidi Arrasate, Manuel M.ª .	Fuenterrabía, 15	San Sebastián
Lon Teller, Manuel	Los Olmos, 94	Palma de Mallorca
López Alfaro, Juan Francisco	San Vicente de Paúl, 1.	Zaragoza
López Carreño, Manuel	José Antonio, 55	Bullas (Murcia)
López Conejos, Mercedes ..	San Vicente de Paúl V. Esperanza, 15	Sevilla
López Checa, Francisca ...	Virgen de Luján, 3, 1.º B	Sevilla
López Domínguez, Bernabé .	Mesa y López, 8	Las Palmas
López Gurpegui, Félix T. ..	San Vicente Ferrer, 6	Granada

López García, Agustín	Caldereros, 6	Valdepeñas (Ciudad Real)
López Luque, José Luis ...	Ibiza, 30. 2.º D	Madrid
López Marín, Ignacio	Gran Vía, 33	Granada
López Muñoz, Daniel José .	Gregorio Espín 4, 3.º	Granada
López Nieto, Carlos	Avda. de Lugo, 2	Santiago de Compostela
López Oliveros, Miguel	Trinidad, 1	Motril (Granada)
López Ramos, Pedro	Doctor Esquerdo, 1 26. 5.º F. ..	Madrid-30
Lorente Buesa, Marcelo ...	Postas, 17, pral	Vitoria (Alava)
Lorente Talamas, José	Plaza de Santa Ana, 2	Valladolid
Lorente Zuzaga, Juan I. ...	Fueros, 15 C	Vitoria (Alava)
Lorenzo Díaz Cortés, José .	San Bernardo, 122	Madrid-8
Lorenzo Inglés, José	Valverde, 8	Madrid-13
Losada García, Jesús	General Mola, 116	Madrid-2
Losada García Ontiveros, Gonzalo	Avda, General Franco, 23	Las Palmas
Losada Suevos, Jesús	Rue Nueva, 19	La Coruña
Loscos Piñol, Francisco ...	Balmes, 217	Barcelona-6
Lozano Rodríguez, Antonio.	Gabriel y Galán, 43	Navalmoral de la Mata (Cáceres)
Luelmo Román, Santiago ..	Rubén Darío, 19, 1.º	Palma de Mallorca
Luengo Sanz, Isidoro	Plaza de España, 1	Don Benito (Badajoz)
Llamas Larruga, Juan	Generalísimo, 9	Melilla
Llarenas Codecido, Guzmán .	San Ficente Ferrer, 21	Santa Cruz de Tenerife (Canarias)
Lledó Carreres, Manuel	Castaños, 22, 3	Alicante
Lloberas Camino, José	Lauria, 117	Barcelona-9
Llovera Alvarez, Pedro	Bruch, 75	Barcelona-9
Llopis Escrivá, José	Roger de Lauria, 22	Valencia-2
Llopis Palares, M.ª Dolores .	Plaza San Agustín, 3	Valencia-2
Magdalena Castiñeira, Jaime.	Daniel de la Sota, 9, 3.º	Pontevedra
Mairlot Nieto, Roberto	Av. Granada, 10	Jaén
Mallén Ramón, Marina	Paz, 34	Valencia-3
Malvar Senra, Manuel	García Borbón, 1	Vigo (Pontevedra)
Manzanares López, Miguel .	Góngora. 7	Córdoba
Maraña González, Manuel ..	Mariano Maspons, 6, 3.º	Granollers (Barcelona)
Marco Martín, Marina	Ciscar, 55. 4.º	Valencia
Marcos Holgueras, Angel de .	Av. del Generalísimo, 31	Alcázar de San Juan (Ciudad Real)
Marcos Villa, Luis	Uria, 27	Oviedo
March Comas José Gerardo .	Costa y Llobera, 5	Palma de Mallorca
Marí Castelló, Mariano	Conde de Sallent, 75	Palma de Mallorca
Marieges Corbo, Joaquín ..	Av. del Generalísimo 418	Barcelona-9
Marín Aguirregomezcorta, Mariano	Consejo de Ciento, 299	Barcelona-7
Marín Blanco, Diego	Santa Clara, 5	Sevilla
Marín Enciso, Enrique	Av. Imperio, 5	Ciudad Real
Marín Enciso, Manuel	Conde de Xiquena, 13	Madrid-4
Marín Lillo, Alejandro	General Martínez Campos, 39 ...	Madrid-10
Marín Mancebo, Juan de Mata	Comedias, 11-13	Málaga
Márquez Gómez, Luis	Murcia, 22	Madrid-7
Martín García, Miguel	Almirante Cadarso, 5, 5.ª	Valencia-5
Martín Sánchez, José A. ..	Julián Sánchez, 11	Ciudad Rodrigo (Salamanca)
Martín Valverde, José Antonio	Juan Urosa, 10	Madrid-19
Martínez Alegría, Gerardo	Victor Pradera, 6, 1.º	Logroño

Martínez García, José Luis .	Calle Muro, 16, 2.º G	Valladolid
Martínez Garchitorena, Juan	General Perón, 25, 8.º G	Madrid-20
Martínez Crisolla, Miguel ..	G. Ruiz Chorro, 2, 1.º C.	Elche (Alicante)
Martínez Güimil, Alfonso ..	Calle Prosperidad	Villagarcía de Arosa (Ponte-vedra)
Martínez León, Fernando ..	Conde Vallellano, 124	Tarragona
Martínez Mínguez, Miguel .	....	Lorca (Murcia)
Martínez Nevot, Enrique ..	Molina Larios, 4	Málaga
Martínez de Pinillos Pena, Manuel	Calvo Sotelo, 12	Logroño
Martínez Román, José	Cuesta del Rosario, 7	Sevilla
Martínez Urcaregui, Javier .	Ercilla, 42, 4.º F	Bilbao-6
Mata López, Pedro	Hermanos Miralles, 50	Madrid-1
Mateos Herrera, José L. ...	Gran Vía, 14	Salamanca
Maza de Lizana, Rafael	Alfonso XI, 10	Algeciras (Cádiz)
Mazuelos Vela, Carlos	Avda. Reina Mercedes, 19 C, escal. A, 6.º, 4.ª	Sevilla
Mazuelos Vela, Manuel	San Pedro, 32	Osuna (Sevilla)
Medina Medina, José	Parque de San Julián, 5, 3.º	Cuenca
Medina Villapalos, Jesús ...	Avda. Felipe II, 15	Madrid-9
Medrano y Ruiz del Arbol, F. Javier	General Mola, 5	Valladolid
Megías Hinojosa, José	Regino Martínez, 20	Algeciras (Cádiz)
Menacho García Menacho, Rafael	Avda. José Antonio, 646	Barcelona-7
Menacho Moner, Eduardo ..	Avda. José Antonio, 646	Barcelona-7
Méndez González, Julio ...	Perdomo, 45	Las Palmas de Gran Canaria
Menéndez Vallejo, José A. .	Carlos Maurrás, 5, 6.º A	Madrid-16
Menezo Alvarez, José Maria	General Aranda, 4	Castellón de la Plana
Menezo Rozalén, José L. ..	Huerto Sogueros, 6	Castellón de la Plana
Menezo Rozalén, Victor M. .	Huerto Sogueros, 6	Castellón de la Plana
Mengual Guijarro, Rafael ..	Calderón de la Barca, 2	Alicante
Merono Oñate, Juan	Bruch, 151	Barcelona-9
Mesa Galarreta, J. M.	Chalet Santa Alicia, El Piles	Gijón
Mestre Espinach, Juan	Balmes, 266	Barcelona-6
Miguel Alvarez, Daniel	Gran Vía Santos Patronos (Edifi-cio Avenide), 3.º B.yC.	Alcira (Valencia)
Mikhael, Halabi, Nicolás ...	Lope de Haro, 5, 1.º C	Madrid
Millan Hernández, José	Infanta María Teresa, 13, 4.º, izqda	Madrid
Mingo González, Luis A. ...	Santiago, 31	Valladolid
Mohedano Iglesias, José A. .	Cardenal González, 87	Córdoba
Moncada Frías, José M. ...	Moreno Nieto, 4	Almendralejo (Badajoz)
Monmany Magnet, Ramón .	San Quirico, 13	Sabadell (Barcelona)
Monsalve Aguilar, José	Diego de León, 58	Madrid-6
Montanary Hurtado, Francis-co	Pza. Poniente, 2, 7º	Valladolid
Montañes Gutiérrez, Joaquin	P.º Fernando el Católico, 18 ...	Zaragoza
Montaño Montaño, Isidoro .	Eduardo Dato, 37	Sevilla
Monteagudo López, José Maria	Gran Vía Fernando el Católico, 62	Valencia-8
Montero Marchena, Jesús ..	Imagen, 9	Sevilla
Montserrat Cavaller, José ..	Argentina, 8...............	Tortosa (Tarragona)
Mora Calvo-Flores, Francisco	José Antonio, 40, Hotel Bristol .	Madrid 19
Morales Cortes, Fermín ...	....	Alcañiz (Teruel)

Morales Muñoz, Antonio ..	Av. del Ejército, 17	Bilbao-14
Moratal Gisbert, Antonio ..	San Nicolás, 67	Alcoy (Alicante)
Moratal Pedrós, Antonio ...	San Nicolás, 67	Alcoy (Alicante)
Moreno Cadierno, Manuel ..	Horno de los Bizcochos, 14	Toledo
Moreno Casanovas, Federico	Real, 13	Aranjuez (Madrid)
Moreno Castaño, Ignacio ..	Gravina, 8	Sevilla
Moreno Igual, Ramón	Cordonería, 10	Toledo
Moreno Lupiáñez, Ernesto .	Coblas, 18	Granada
Moreno Pirla, Júan	Fernando IV, 36	Sevilla
Morilias Soriano, José Maria.	San Eloy, 31	Sevilla
Morón Salas, José	Turia, 11	Sevilla
Mosquera Arroyo, Vicente .	Juan Flórez, 18	La Coruna
Muiños Simón, Alfredo	Angli, 60	Barcelona-17
Munguía Argüelio, Roger ..	Laforja, 88	Barcelona-6
Munoa Roiz, José Luis	Hernani, 2, 1.º	San Sebastián
Muñoz, Leonardo	Calvo Sotelo, 9	Mieres (Asturias)
Muñoz Lucas, Rafael	Miguel Fluiters, 19	Guadalajara
Muñoz Pato, Felipe	Arenal, 8	Madrid-13
Muñoz Poy, Francisco	Fresca, 12	Málaga
Muro Perez, Tomás	Generalísimo, 31	Sama de Langreo (Asturias)
Muro Sánchez, Juan Ignacio.	Gral. Franco, 41, 5.º D	Sama de Langreo (Asturias)
Murube Del Castillo, Juan ..	Avda. Candelaria, 29	La Laguna (Tenerife)
Nadal Abella, José Maria ...	Bruch, 44	Barcelona-10
Navarro Menéndez, Baldo- mero	Altamira, 1	Alicante
Navio Lantada, Maravillas ..	Ayala, 152	Madrid-9
Negrete Rojas, Octavio	Mariano de Lucas, 12	Pozuelo de Alarcón (Madrid)
Nieto Montero, José	Díaz Calvo, 4	Villanueva de la Serena (Badajoz)
Noguer Rodríguez, Luis A. .	Manuel Gironés, 11	Barcelona-17
Nubiola Cunill, Jorge	Provenza, 330	Barcelona-9
Núñez Salas, Antonio	Viriato, 4	Sevilla
Ojeda Villarejo, Manuel ...	Plaza de José Antonio, 1	Málaga
Olazaguirre y Gorostiaga, José María	Alameda de Urquijo, 66	Bilbao
Olivella Casals, Antoniu ...	Av. Generalísimo, 606	Barcelona-15
Orbegozo Eguiguren, Fran- cisco J.	Fábrica Orbegozo	Zumárraga (Guipúzcoa)
Orduña Otero, Gemma	Conde Duque, 44	Madrid-8
Orellana Toledano, Fernan- do	Marqués de Larios, 5	Málaga
Ormaechea Iraizoz, Jaime ..	Plaza de Zaragoza, 2	San Sebastián
Oroz Zabaleta, Hilario	Rodríguez Arias, 4	Bilbao-8
Ortega Andréu, M.ª Luisa ..	Escritor Sánchez Moreno, 1, 3.º .	Murcia
Ortega García, Juan M.	O'Donnell, 49	Madrid-9
Ortega Tartas, Ignacio	Joaquín García Morato, 138	Madrid-3
Orti Palanca, Ramón	Guillén de Castro, 79	Valencia-8
Ortiz Lama, Angel	Gran Capitán, 6	Montilla (Córdoba)
Ortiz de Lanzagorta, José Maria	Larios, 3	Málaga
Ortiz Mitterer, Germán	José Picón, 28	Madrid-2
Ortuño Lloréns, Vicente ...	Plaza del Generalísimo, 10	Orihuela (Alicante)
Pablo Ramón, Manuel	Aribau, 123, 1.º 1.ª	Barcelona-11
Padín Botana, Manuel	Puerta del Sol, 9	Vigo (Pontevedra)
Padín Botana, Pablo	Plaza de la Constitución, 1-2	Vigo (Pontevedra)
Padrón Mauricio, Juan	Santa Rosa de Lima, 5	Santa Cruz de Tenerife

Palazón Godínez, Alfonso .	Bartolomé, 4	Murcia
Palomar Gómez, Alejandro .	San Clemente, 25, 1.º	Zaragoza
Palomar y Palomar, Alejandro	San Clemente, 25	Zaragoza
Palomar Petit, Fernando ...	Mallorca, 314	Barcelona-9
Palomares Cortes, Juan A. .	José Antonio Primo de Rivera, 17	Jerez de la Frontera (Cádiz)
Pallarés Lluesma, Juan	Jorge Juan, 24	Valencia-4
Pallarés Ortuño, Gaspart ...	Béjar, 28	Huelva
Pardo Bedia, Jaime	Fernando Villaamil, 69, 1.º	El Ferrol del Caudillo (La Coruña)
Pardo Vega, Pablo	Av. de Baviera, 16	Madrid-2
Parra Cascón, José M.ª	Joaquin García Morato, 119.....	Madrid-3
Parrado Ramos, Antonio ...	Doctor Chil, 10	Las Palmas de Gran Canaria
Pascual Jover, Narciso	Espalter, 3	Madrid-14
Pascual Martí, Vda. de José .	Convento de Santa Clare, 7	Valencia-2
Pascual Trébol, Gonzalo ...	Treviana, 6, 3.º D	Madrid-27
Pastor Moltó, Jorge	General Tovar, 2, 2.º	Valencia-3
Pastor Olmedo, José M. ...	Avda. D. Antonio Alonso, 2	Zamora
Pastor Vallvé, Salvador	Paulino Caballero, 6	Pamplona
Peiró Artal, José	Islas Filipinas, 40	Madrid-3
Peiró Ibáñez, Jose Félix ...	Avda. Islas Filipinas, 40, 1.º	Madrid
Peña y de Andrés-Moreno, Adolfo de la	Rúa Nueva, 57	Santiago de Compostela (La Coruña)
Peña Carrillo, Juan A.	Peña del Mar, 15	Málaga
Peña Carrillo, Jesús Francisco	Paseo de Ronda, 12	Granada
Perarnau Gorgas, Benito ...	Paseo de Pedro III, 11	Manresa (Barcelona)
Perea Garcia, José	Jardines, 14, 2.º	Toledo
Pérez Albert, Guillermo ...	Alfonso I, 28	Zaragoza
Pérez Avilés, Ricardo	San Miguel, 139	Palma de Mallorca
Perez-Bufill Pitchot, Gabriel.	Valencia, 247	Barcelona-7
Pérez Chiscano, Daniel	San Francisco, 8, bajo dcha.	Villanueva de la Serena (Badajoz)
Pérez Fuentes, M.ª Fernanda	Avda. Miraflores, 64, 1.º	Sevilla
Pérez Hernández, Francisco .	León y Castillo, 51	Las Palmas
Pérez Irisarri, Javier	Alicante, 27	Barcelona-6
Pérez Jiménez, Juan R.	Martínez de Villena, 11	Albacete
Pérez López de la Hoz, Diego	Ganivet, 6	Granada
Pérez Lucas Izquierdo, Eleuterio	Federico Tapia, 49 2.º	La Coruña
Pérez Llorca, José	Juan Bravo, 21	Madrid-6
Pérez Llorca Rodrigo, Jaime.	Alameda, 12	Cádiz
Pérez Macías, José	Colonia Militar Cuatro Vientos, Chalé 26	Madrid
Pérez Martín, Fidel	Residencia de Posgraduados, Espejo, 12	Salamanca
Pérez Martín, Julián	Vara de Rey, 18	Ibiza (Baleares)
Pérez Martínez, Valentín ..	Suárez de la Riva, 7	Oviedo
Pérez Moreda, Florencio ...	Avda Héroes de Brunete, 1, 7.º D	Salamanca
Pérez Pérez, Telmo	Marqués de Valladares, 35, 3.º ..	Vigo (Pontevedra)
Pérez Rodríguez, Domingo..	General Mola, 8	Pontevedra
Pérez Salvador, José L.	Avda, Pío XII, 1, 4.ª, 18	Valencia-9
Pérez Santalla, Guillermo ..	General Franco, 102	El Ferrol del Caudillo (La Coruña)

Pérez Tomás, Augustín	Nicolás Rabal, 5	Soria
Pérez Vera, Eugenio	Lancia, 1, 4.º	León
Pérez Villanueva, Jesús	P.º Germanías, 28, 2.º	Gandía (Valencia)
Perpiñá Mas, Ramón	Provenza, 185	Barcelona-11
Piera Cebriá, Carmen	Virgen, 84	Sueca (Valencia)
Pinos Roldán, José A.	Alcoy, 7	Valencia-4
Piñero Carrión, Antonio ...	Ciudad de Ronda, 4	Sevilla
Pita Salorio, Demetrio	República de El Salvador, Edificio Apolo II, 7.º D	Santiago de Compostela
Planas Salud, Juan	Rosellón, 232	Barcelona-8
Planelles Lazaga, Juan	García de los Herrán, 11 y 13 ...	San Fernando (Cádiz)
Plasencia Muñoz de Lucas, Ricardo	Avda. Reyes Católicos, 10	Burgos
Pons Ibáñez, Alejandro	Av. J. Benavente, 22	Valencia-5
Poveda Pagán, Eduardo	Riquelme, 1	Murcia
Power Alesson, Rafael	Rocha, 14	Algeciras (Cádiz)
Payales Ureña, Alvaro	Olózaga, 3	Madrid-1
Poyatos Goiri, José	Avda. José Antonio, 8	Valencia-5
Pozueta Jaén, Julio	Mayor, 37	Estella (Navarra)
Prado Moreno, Angel	Relatores, 10	Madrid-12
Pueyo Pujol, Alberto	Caspe, 30	Barcelona-10
Pujol Borrás, Amadeo	Balmes, 306	Barcelona-6
Pujol Canicio, Alberto	Plaza Verdaguer, 8	Tarragona
Quer Falgueras, Ramón ...	Pl. Santa Clara, 7	Vich (Barcelona)
Quero González, José	Ramón Gordillo, 5	Valencia
Quesada Domínguez, José M.ª	Regimiento de Infantería de Granada número 34	Huelva
Quesada Moya, Francisco ..	Av. Doctor Gálvez Ginachero, 17	Málaga
Quintana Casany, Manuel ..	Bruch, 93	Barcelona-9
Quintana Románs, Juan ...	Bruch, 93	Barcelona-9
Rabadán, Fernández, Pedro .	Plaza de los Mártires, 13	Crevillente (Alicante)
Rabinal Martínez, Angel ...	Fernando el Católico, 14	Zaragoza
Raduán Boronat, Miguel ...	San José, 27	Alcoy (Alicante)
Rafat Selga, Juan	Cra. Cardona, 62	Manresa (Barcelona)
Ramón Roda, José	Pza. del Pintor Pinazo, 1, 4.º ...	Valencia-4
Ramón de Prat, Fernando ..	Plaza Pintor Pinazo, 1	Valencia
Ramos Ortiz, Baltasar	C. Santa Lucía, 2, 2.º	Málaga
Ramos de la Sierra, Félix ..	Rafael Villa, 2	El Plantío (Madrid)
Recalde Larre, José L.	Fundidores, 2	Eibar (Guipúzcoa)
Redondo Delgado, Agustín .	Jacinto Benavente, 6	Pozoblanco (Córdoba)
Regúlez Molina, Eladio ...	Jesús y María, 11	Madrid-12
Regurera Fernández, Ricardo	Pza. Alfalfa, 3 y 5	Sevilla
Regueras Flores, Angel L. ..	Narváez, 15	Madrid-9
Reig de Argüeso, León	Paseo de la Victoria, 43	Córdoba
Renedo Sampedro, Enrique .	Marqués de Urquijo, 24	Madrid-8
Rey Giménez, José del	Pérez Pujol, 4	Valencia-2
Riaza y Peña, Manuel	Cea Bermúdez, 41	Madrid-3
Ribas Clotet, Francisco	Regas, 3	Barcelona-6
Ribas Montobbio, Juan B. .	Rambla de Cataluña, 11	Barcelona-7
Ribes Castelló, Vicente	Mayor, 19	Gandía (Valencia)
Riera Domenech, Antonio .	Mayor de Gracia, 107	Barcelona-12
Río Cabañas, José L. del ...	Av. Felipe II, 4	Madrid-9
Ríos Sasiain, Manuel	Ibiza, 56	Madrid-9
Ripoll Ruiz, Juan	San Ildefonso, 4	Alicante

Riquelme Saguier, Benigno .	Fernando Agulló, 10, 4.º, 2.ª ...	Barcelona-6
Riscos Valencia, Regino ...	Busto Tavera, 21, bajo	Sevilla
Ribas Valero, Ramón	Canalejas, 2	Sevilla
Rivera Moreno, Antonio ...	Herrería del Rey, 1	Málaga
Rivilla Vidaurre, Antonio ..	Pl. Guipúzcoa, 2	San Sebastián
Robles Oñate, Emilio	Avda. José Antonio, 42, 1.ª Escal. 1.º B	Murcia
Robles Sánchez-Cortes, Miguel	Gómez Jordana, 1, Clínica de Oftalmología	Caravaca de la Cruz (Murcia)
Roca Berga, Guillermo	San Rafael, 10	Olot (Gerona)
Roca Bonet, Francisco	Valero, 2	Palma de Mallorca
Rodríguez Alvarez, Manuel .	Plazuela de Fuente Viejo, 1	Luarca (Asturias)
Rodríguez Caballero, Maria Luisa	Colegio Mayor Arzobispo Fonseca, Fonseca, 4	Salamanca
Rodríguez Campoamor, José M.ª	Plaza de España, 4	Zaragoza
Rodríguez Carrascal, Julio .	Prado, 6, 5.º	Talavera de la Reina (Toledo)
Rodríguez Cons, Emilio Santiago	Marco Aurelio, 9, 3.º	Barcelona
Rodríguez Galan, Enrique .	San Francisco, 16-18	Ribadeo (Lugo)
Rodríguez Galván, Corviniano	18 de Julio, 1	Santa Cruz de Tenerife
Rodríguez López, Corviniano	18 de Julio, 1	Santa Cruz de Tenerife
Rodríguez Martínez, Pedro .	Doctor Palanca, 10	La Bañeza (León)
Rodríguez Montes, Jesús ..	Paloma, 1, 1.º A	Ciudad Real
Rodríguez Montes, Oscar ..	Avda. Mártires, 29	Ciudad Real
Rodríguez del Rio, José ...	Glorieta del Comandante Ayuso, 1	Ceuta
Rodríguez Rivas, José	Primo de Rivera, 36	Ceuta
Rodríguez Salmones, Luis .	Ruiz Tagle, 4	Torrelavega (Santander)
Román Arroyo, Petra	Fray Luis de Granada, 2	Salamanca
Romero Galán, Victor	Clavellina, 13	Cáceres
Romero Romero, Arístides .	Calvo Sotelo, 4	Salamanca
Romero Romero, Manuel ..	Ximénez de Enciso, 8	Sevilla
Romo Ocaña, Angel	Can Menor, 10	Madrid-30
Ros Alférez, Rafael	Angustias, 4	Torre del Mar (Málaga)
Ros González, Fernando ...	Glorieta de Bilbao, 4	Madrid-10
Ros Peña, Rafael	Plaza de Queipo de Llano, 3 ...	Málaga
Rosado Rodríguez, Enrique .	Alarcón Luján, 6	Málaga
Rozaut Garbayo, Francisco J.	Chapitela, 21	Pamplona
Rubiales Campos, Carlos ...	Linarejos, 9	Linares (Jaén)
Rubio Berrio, Roque	Zaragoza, 11, 1.º A	Huesca
Rubio Carlos, Salvador	Valencia, 292	Barcelona-9
Rubio García Agustín	Menéndez Pelayo, 3	Cartagena (Murcia)
Ruiz Barranco, Francisco ..	Kansas City, 4	Sevilla
Ruiz Bulumar, Atilano	Universidad, 3	Valencia-3
Ruiz Camacho, Gregorio ...	Ramón y Cajal, 15	Antequera (Málaga)
Ruiz Galán, Augusto	Calvo Sotelo, 2-3	Calatayud (Zaragoza)
Rutllán Juliá, Joaquín	Plaza de Níez de Arce, 1	Barcelona-6
Sabala Durán, Antonio	Aribau, 5	Barcelona-11
Sabater Guarneiro, Vicente .	Hernández Velasco, 64	Motril (Granada)
Sáenz Alonso, Roberto	Guetaria, 2	San Sebastián
Sagasti Bengoa, Joaquín ...	Alameda de Recalde, 72	Bilbao

Salado Marín, Francisco ...	Alameda Moreno Guerra, 3	San Fernando (Cádiz)
Salaverri Soriano, Fermín ..	Pl. San José, 2	Bilbao-9
Salcedo de Miguel, José ...	Santuchu, 28, 4.º	Bilbao-4
Salgado Benavides, Enrique .	Ordoño II, 19	León
Salgado Gómez, Fernando .	Ordoño II, 7	León
Salinas Llopis, José Elías ..	Castaños, 1	Alicante
Salmerón Bermudez, Bayar-		
do	Camp, 68, 2.º D	Barcelona
Salom Vidal, Jaime	Mallorca, 279	Barcelona-9
Salvá Mulet, Juan	Játiva, 17	Valencia-2
San Martín Alonso, Ricardo .	José Antonio, 48	Vigo (Pontevedra)
Sánchez Agesta, Ricardo ...	Almona de San Juan de Dios, 13 .	Granada
Sánchez Agesta Ortega, Ri-		
cardo	Av. de Andaluces, 14	Granada
Sánchez Arcilla de la Pascua,		
Agustín	Alcalá, 117	Madrid-9
Sánchez Baños, Mariano ...	Conde de Peñalver, 17	Madrid-6
Sánchez-Jara Luengo, Juan .	Monroy, 4, 1.º	Salamanca
Sánchez-Palencia, Angel ...	Obispo Enstúñiga, 5, chalé	Jaén
Sánchez-Palencia, Ramón ..	Av. del Generalísimo, 2	Jaén
Sánchez Payo, Jesús	José Antonio, 1	Orense
Sánchez Peña, Ulpiano	Gaspar Duque, 6	Talavera de la Reina (Tole-
		do)
Sánchez Piñel, Aniceto	Colón del Salvador, 32	Béjar (Salamanca)
Sánchez Ruiz, Julio	Hurtado de Amézaga, 32, 1.º ...	Bilbao-8
Sánchez Salorio, Manuel ...	Compostela, 6, 1.º	Santiago de Compostela (La
		Coruña)
Sandez Figueras, Manuel ...	Reina, 9	Lugo
Sánchez Macho, Manuel ...	República Argentina, 6, 3.º B ...	Santiago de Compostela (La
		Coruña)
Sandoval García. Ernesto ..	Manuel de Falla, 10, 3.º dcha. ..	Granada
Santalices Muñiz, Faustino .	Raimundo Fernández Villaverde, '	
	19	Madrid-3
Santamaría Rodríguez, José.	General Franco, 1	Jerez de la Frontera (Cádiz)
Santamaría Urízar, María		
Luisa	Santuchu, 28	Bilbao-4
Santamarina Rodero, Jesús .	Elcano, 2, 2.º dcha.	Mondragón (Guipúzcoa)
Santolaria Rosel, Mariano ..	Córcega, 272-274, 3.º 2.ª	Barcelona-8
Santos Pérez, Marino	Pza. de Alemania, 3	Zamora
Sanz Sanz, Priscili	Lope de Haro, 15	Madrid-20
Saracíbar Alonso, José M.ª .	Marina de Escobar, 4	Valladolid
Sarriá Solá, Mariano	Arrieta, 2	Pamplona
Sastre Martí, Fernando	Velázquez, 59	Madrid-1
Sayás Gómez, Juan A.	Avda. de Madrid, 22	Avila
Sebastián Sáenz, Francisco .	Bailén, 2	Valencia-7
Seoane López, Pedro	Pza. Generalísimo, 6	Pontevedra
Serra Ferrer, José	Caballero, 5	Valencia-1
Serrano Gonzalo, José L. ...	Paseo María Agustín, 37	Zaragoza
Serrano Maestro, Pedro J. ..	Joaquín Arnau, 12	Teruel
Sifré Pasqual, Bernardo	Moncada, 15	Játiva (Valencia)
Silva Ciliberto, Juan	San Martín de Porres, 41, 5.º, 'i',	
	buzón 46	Madrid
Silván López, Fernando ...	Arrieta, 18	Pamplona
Simón Muñoz, Elías	Alba, 7	La Línea (Cádiz)
Simón Tor, José M.ª	Mayor de Gracia, 13	Barcelona-12
Simón Zapater, Vicente ...	José Antonio, 4, 2.º	Castellón de la Plana

Sociats Pozo, Juan	p⁰ de la Florida, 3, 1.⁰	Vitoria
Soler Poré, Carlos	Eduardo Dato, 11	Elche (Alicante)
Soler Sala, José M.ª	Mallorca, 333	Barcelona-9
Solsona Llansama, José	Sans, 71-73	Barcelona-14
Sosa Tolosa, Antonio	Calvo Sotelo, 9	Villagarcía de Arosa (Pontevedra)
Sofo Faure, Luis	Av. Generalísimo, 28, 6.⁰	Madrid-16
Suárez López, Jesús	Dr. Teijerio, 20, 4.⁰izqda	Santiago de Compostela (La Coruña)
Suoro Mazariegos, Angel ...	General Sanjurjo, 12	Tetuán
Súñer Sanchiz, Rafael	Gómez Ulla, 8	Madrid-28
Susín de Caso, Ramón	Pza. de Navarra, 2	Huesca
Sust Mir, Feliciano	Ausías March, 56	Barcelona-10
Tarrús Estechs, Francisco ..	Jaime I, 16	Gerona
Taverna Avila, Antonio	Escuelas Pías, 24	Barcelona-17
Tellechea Urtizberrea, Jesús M.ª	Paseo de Colón, 10	Irún (Guipúzcoa)
Tello Fernández, Carlos ...	Gral. Moscardó, 28	Madrid-20
Temprano Acedo, José	Infanta Carlota, 114, 4.⁰ 4.ª	Barcelona-15
Tena García-Arevalo, José ..	General Franco, 8	El Ferrol del Caudillo (La Coruña)
Tena Ibarra, Pedro	Serrano, 17	Madrid-1
Terol Altet, José M.ª	San Vicente, 16	Valencia-3
Tibáu Pagés, Juan	General Primo de Rivera, 53	Gerona
Torre Bononnto, Manuel de la	General Sánchez Mira, 4	Jerez de la Frontera
Torrent Faiges, Ramón	Quemada, 29	Tarrasa (Barcelona)
Torrente Gallar, Carmen ...	San Pedro, 98	Badalona (Barcelona)
Torres Lucena, Miguel de ..	Ximénez de Enciso, 2	Sevilla
Torres Sánchez Pallasar, Juan	Avda. del General Rodrigo, 6, 3.⁰	Badajoz
Torriente Rivas, Julio de la .	Amós de Escalante, 6	Santander
Trigueros Pacheco, Miguel .	Ramón y Cajal, 18	Jumilla (Murcia)
Turati Alvarez, Eduardo ...	Regás, 16	Barcelona-6
Ulloa Fariña, Castor	Av. Menéndez Pelayo, 11, dpdo. .	Madrid-9
Ulloa Garmendia, Armando .	Carmen, 14	Madrid-13
Unamuno Lizárraga, Raimundo Rafael de	Generalísimo Franco, 21	Salamanca
Uribarrena Berrecheguren, Javier	Fernando el Católico, 1	Guernica (Vizcaya)
Urquiola Permisán, Javier ..	Eduardo Dato, 8	Vitoria
Uson Lozano, Edmundo ...	Andrés Baquero, 5	Murcia
Valaer Ramallo, Angel	Pl. Tres Carabelas, 1	Cádiz
Valbuena Artolozábal, Fernando	Reina, 15	Zamora
Valbuena Morán, Luis	República Argentina, 8	Ponferrada (León)
Valcarce Abelló, Joaquin ..	Núñez de Balboa, 84	Madrid-6
Valcarce Alvarez, Joaquin ..	Ordoño II, 15	León
Valcárcel Burgos, Luis	Octavio Picón, 40	Pedregalejo (Málaga)
Valdivia Del Castillo, Carlos .	Pza. Iglesias	Ugijar (Granada)
Valentín-Gamazo Fernández, Ignacio de	Orellana, 1	Madrid-4
Valentín-Gamazo Fernández de la Hoz, José M.ª	Alférez Provisional, 5, 1.⁰	Toledo
Vázquez y Aragon, Saúl ...	Reyes Magos, 30	Madrid-30

Vázquez de Parga y Jorge, Antonio	Generalísimo Franco, 127	Orense
Vázquez de Parga Santamarina, Antonio	Generalísimo Franco, 127	Orense
Vazquez de Parga Santamarina, M.ª del Rosario	General Franco, 127	Orense
Vega Díaz, Cayetano de la	Real, 1	Charches (Granada)
Vega Monroy, Francisco	Real, 29	Santa Cruz de la Palma (Tenerife)
Vela Barca, Antonio	República Argentina, 4, 1.º	Cádiz
Velarde Cañuelo, Manuel	Zaragoza, 15	Sevilla
Vélez Esparano, Manuel	José Antonio, 27, 2.º	Guadix (Granada)
Vélez Medina, José	Héroes del Baleares, 3	San Fernando (Cádiz)
Velilla del Campo, Enrique	Gran Vía, 6	Logroño
Velilla Mateo, Enrique	Vara del Rey, 36, 3.º	Logroño
Vena Rodríguez, Antonio	Avda. Generalísimo. 23, 1.º	Jaén
Ventosa Echevarría, José	Comandante Baiget, 1	Lérida
Ventura Baztán, Saturnino	Sandoval, 6	Pamplona
Vercet Pastor, Antonio	Generalísimo, 3	Alcoy (Alicante)
Vicente Esquinas, Andrés de	O'Donnell, 30, pral.	Sevilla
Vicente Isasi, José Luis	Dos de Mayo, 2	Miranda de Ebro (Burgos)
Vidaechea Erausquin, Domingo	Pl. de la Merced, 4	Segovia
Vigil González Cutré, Manuel	Uria, 45	Gijón (Asturias)
Vila Coro, Antonio	Muntaner, 573	Barcelona-6
Vila Mascarell, Emilio	Av. Barón de Cárcer, 38	Valencia-1
Vilaplana Ríus, Alvaro	San Cucufate, 117	Sabadell (Barcelona)
Vilar Sanz, Gèrardo	P. San Cristóbal, 6	Toledo
Vilella Pérez Albéniz, Antonio	Meléndez Valdés, 41, 2.º	Badajoz
Villa Olmedo, Aurora	Lagasca, 11	Madrid-1
Villafranca Díaz de Rábago, Jorge M.	Calle Armaña, 9, 2.º	Lugo
Villamor Roldán, Eduardo	Don Ramón de la Cruz, 66	Madrid-1
Villar de la Fuente, Miguel	República Argentina, 22	Córdoba
Villasante Velázquez, Luis Eulogio	Concepción, 730	San Salvador (El Salvador)
Villegas del Cubillo, Carlos	Jesús y María, 9, 2.º C	Córdoba
Villegas Laguna, Enrique	Jesús y María, 9, 2.º C	Córdoba
Villén Diéguez, Francisco	Conde Romanones, 12	Madrid-12
Viñas Rosés, Jorge	Valencia, 376	Barcelona-13
Viñuela Valiente, José	Pl. del Alcázar, 7, 'Villa Bego'	Zafra (Badajoz)
Wieden Navarro, Eduardo	Plaza del Caudillo, 21	Valencia
Wieder Palomir, Eduardo	Almenara, 20	Sagunto (Valencia)
Yagües García, José	Avda. de Valladolid, 73	Madrid-8
Zaragoza García, Pablo	Arturo Soria, 310	Madrid-33
Zbirowski Balbontín, Enrique de	Torneo, 36	Sevilla

NOSOCOMIA QUIBUS OCULIS AEGRI CURANTUR

Madrid:
Department of Ophthalmology, Faculty of Medicine. Prof. R. Bartolozzi
Barcelona:
Department of Ophthalmology, Faculty of Medicine. Prof. J. Casanovas
Sevilla:
Department of Ophthalmology, Faculty of Medicine. Prof. A. Piñero
Granada:
Department of Ophthalmology, Faculty of Medicine. Prof. Buenaventura Carreras
Zaragoza:
Department of Opthalmology, Faculty of Medicine. Prof. A. Palomar
Valladolid:
Department of Ophthalmology, Faculty of Medicine. Prof. N. Belmonte
Valencia:
Department of Opthalmology, Faculty of Medicine. Prof. Marcelo Carreras
Santiago de Compostela:
Department of Ophthalmology, Faculty of Medicine. Prof. M. Sánchez Salorio
Cadiz:
Department of Ophthalmology, Faculty of Medicine. Prof. J. García Sánchez
Pamplona:
Department of Ophthalmology, Faculty of Medicine. Prof. D. Diaz Dominguez
Salamanca:
Department of Ophthalmology, Faculty of Medicine. Prof. Adj. Hernández Benito
Madrid:
Instituto Oftalmico Nacional, Director: Dr. Pedro Tena Ibarra
Madrid:
Servicio de Oftalmologia, Hospital del Niño Jesús. Director: Dr. Carlos Costi
Madrid:
Servicio de Oftalmologia, Instituto Jimenez Diaz. Director: Dr. G. Leóz
Barcelona:
Servicio de Oftalmologia, Hospital de San Pablo. Director: Dr. M. Burch
Barcelona:
Servicio de Oftalmologia, Hospital de la Cruz Roja. Director: Dr. A. Vila Coro
Barcelona:
Servicio de Oftalmologia, Hospital de San Juan de Dios. Director: Dr. A. Castanera
Barcelona:
Servicio de Oftalmologia del, Hospital de N. S. del Sagrado Corazón. Dirección Dres: A. Arruga
y F. Palomar
Barcelona:
Instituto Barraquer. Director: Prof. J. Barraquer

In each one of the Capitals of 'Provincia' there are Departments of Ophthalmology in the Hospital
Residencia and Seguro Obligatorio de Enfermedad.

INSTITUTA SCHOLAEQUE CAECIS DESTINATAE

Colegio de la Inmaculada Concepción. Boys department: Pº de la Habana nº 208, Madrid 16.
Residential School for 220 pupils. Girls department: C/ Nuria nº 42, Madrid 34. Residential
School for 100 pupils.

Colegio Santiago Apostol. C/ Luis Braille n⁰ 5, Pontevedra. Residential School for 130 pupils, only boys.

Colegio Espiritu Santo. Carretera Murcia-Valencia, km. 85.400. Vistahermosa. Alicante. Residential School with two units: one for 100 boys, the other for 100 girls.

Colegio San Luis Gonzaga. Carretera de Alcala de Guadaira, km. 4. Sevilla. Residential School with two departments: one for 150 boys, the other for 100 girls.

Servicio Educativo De La Delegación de Barcelona. (Educational Service of the Barcelona Delegation). Non residential School for about 30 pupils of both sexes.

Centro de Formación y Rehabilitación Profesional Industrial. (Vocational Rehabilitation Industrial Training Centre). Residential Centre for 20 trainees, who will work later in open industry.

Escuela de Fisioterapia. (Physiotherapy School for the Blind). Non residential school for 35 students of both sexes.

Escuela de Telefonia. (Telephony School) Non residential school. Ten girls in each training course.

Centro de Rehabilitación Social Para Ciegos Adultos. (Social Rehabilitation Centre for Blind Adults), Residential centre with two departments: one for 20 males and the other for 12 females.

HOLLANDIA

SOCIETATES OPHTHALMOLOGICAE

Nationalis

Netherlands Ophthalmological Society
Chairman: Dr. J. E. Winkelman
Vice-President: Prof. Dr. N. M. J. Schweitzer
Secretary: Dr. P. P. H. Alkemade, Sweelinckplein 83, den Haag
Ed. Secretary: A. J. Otto
Treasurer: H. de Jong
2nd. Vice-President: Dr. A. M. Leeman
Assessor: K. L. J. Hoefnagels
Number of members: 371

Regionales

Oostelijk Oogheelkundig Gezelschap
Secretary: Dr. A. C. Copper, Coehoornsingel 42, Zutphen
Number of members: 84

Zuid-Westelijk Oogheelkundig Gezelschap
Secretary: Dr. P. P. H. Alkemade, Sweelinckplein 83, den Haag
Number of members: 100

Zuidelijk Oogheelkundig Gezelschap
Secretary: Dr. A. A. J. J. van der Eerden, Oliemolenstraat 1, Heerlen
Number of members: 33

NOMINA ET DOMICILIA MEDICORUM AB OCULIS

Acker, J. A. J. v.	Henri Heimanspark 3	Maastricht
Agsterstibbe-Luning Prak, M. D.	Garstenstraat 21	Nigtevegt
Alkemade, Dr. P. P. H.	Sweelinckplein 83	Den Haag
Alphen, Dr. G. W. H. M. v. .	van Alkemadelaan 354	Den Haag
Antic, V.	Oogziekenhuis, Leyweg 293	Den Haag
Apituley, H. Z. M.	de Breekstraat 55	Amsterdam-N.
Arnoldus, Mej. M.	Louis Davidsstraat 155	Den Haag
Assen, E. C. v.	Laan van Meerdervoort 410	Den Haag
Aten, Mej. Dr. A. H.	van Swietenstraat 62	Tilburg
Aukes, G. N. L. J.	van Meursstraat 49	Eindhoven
Baas, J.	Want 41	Huizen
Bakker, N. J. A.	Larixlaan 187	Rotterdam

Balen, Dr. A. Th. M. van ...	C. N. A. Looslaan 70	Rotterdam-13
Bastiaensen, L. A. K.	Nw. Bosscheweg 17	Tilburg
Beek, Dr. C. J. van	Ter Borchstraat 16	Zwolle
Begheyn, J. M. A. A.	Boerhaavestraat 7	Weert
Beintema, D. K.	Bilderdijkstraat 46	Leeuwarden
Beintema, Mej. M. R.	Vreewijkstraat 19	Leiden
Berg, Mej. G. A. v.d.	Molenwater 129	Middelburg
Berghuis, G.	Diakonessenhuis	Groningen
Bergh, Jhr. E. O. van den ..	Fransestraat 69	Nijmegen
Biesheuvel, K.	Beneden Krolendijk 1	O. Beijerland
Binkhorst, Dr. C. D.	Axelsestraat 54	Terneuzen
Binkhorst, Dr. P. G.	Sweelincklaan 20	Bilthoven
Birkenfeld-Tierie, Mevr. D. A.	Gerbrandylaan 44	Delft
Blanksma, L. J.	Kamperfoelieweg 8	Paterswolde
Bleeker, Prof. Dr. G. M. ...	Muzenplein 1	Amsterdam
Boelsma, S. H. F.	Rapenburg 96	Leiden
Boen-Tan, Mevr. T. N.	Kathl. Ferrierlaan 34	Amstelveen
Boet, Dr. D.,J.	Groot Hertoginnelaan 19	Den Haag
Bolmers, D. J. M.	Wilhelminastraat 5	Breda
Boon, J.	Singravenlaan 16	Enschede
Booy, D.	H. Gorterstraat 253	Capelle a/d IJssel
Bos, H. J. v.	v. Hogendorplaan 22	Huizen N.H.
Bos, P. J. M.	De Lairessestraat 6	Amsterdam
Bos, J. van den	Beethovenstraat 115 II	Amsterdam
Botermans, C. H. G.	Soestdijksestraatweg 113	Bilthoven
Boucher, H. T.	Maliesingel 33	Utrecht
Bouma, G. N.	Z-O Singel 11	Harlingen
Bouws, G. P.	Koninglaan 1	Stiphout gem. Helmond
Brakelé, J. C.	Wierdensestraat 120	Almelo
Breebaart, Dr. A. C.	Willem Royaardsstraat 6	Amsterdam
Breebaart-de Miranda, Mevr. J. G.	W. Royaardsstr. 6	Amsterdam
Brenkman, Dr. R. F.	Sweilandstraat 11	Warmond
Breukink, Dr. E. W.	Hogelandsingel 57	Enschede
Bruggen, J. van	Wendeling 90	Emmen
Bruyn, J. P. F. M. de	Burg. Schrevensingel 6	Veghel
Bryne, D. C. de	Weteringpark 1	Zwolle
Buitenhuis, H. J.	Amsterdamseweg 42	Amstelveen
Butler, Dr. I.	Noordeinde 15	Delft
Bijll Nachenius, D. W. de ..	Wilhelminastraat 32	Haarlem
Bijnen, Dr. A. B.	Wilhelminastraat 15	Breda
Bijnsdorp, B. A.	Brediusweg 21	Bussum
Bijsterveld, Dr. O. P. van ...	Pr. Marijkeweg 4	Houten (U)
Calcar, J. W. van	Bergweg 179	Rotterdam
Colenbrander, J. A.	Zusterstraat 26	Gorinchem
Colenbrander, Prof. Dr. M. C.	Oude Vest 105	Leiden
Colombijn, R. J.	Heemst. Dreef 307	Heemstede
Copper, Dr. A. C.	Coehoornsingel 42	Zutphen
Cozijnsen, Dr. M.	Kerkewijk 42	Veenendaal
Craandijk, A.	van Alkemadelaan 86	Den Haag
Cremers, A. H. J. A.	Schoolstraat 6	Utrecht
Crone, Prof. Dr. R. A.	Henr. Bosmanstraat 34	Amsterdam-Z
Dake, Dr. C. L.	Jan van Eyckstraat 12	Amsterdam
Dekkers, N. W. H. M.	Gaspeldoorn 3	Krimpen a/d IJssel

Delleman, J. W.	ws. Jono, Zijkanaal F	Halfweg
Dethmers, H.,W.	Jupiterstraat 61	Groningen
Deursen Jr., Fr. v.	Aristotelesstraat 6	Amsterdam-W
Deutman Sr., Dr. A. F.	Stationsweg 23	Meppel
Deutman Jr., Prof. Dr. A. F..	Bovenste weg 21	Mook
Doesschate, Prof. Dr. J. ten .	Lindenlaan 30	Zeist
Doesschate, Mej. Dr. J. ten .	van Kettwich Verschuurlaan	
	153A	Groningen
Doesschate, Mej. M. J. L. ..	Leyweg 293, Oogziekenhuis	Den Haag
Dols, R. C. I. M.	Kummenaedestraat 15	Geleen
Donders, H. L. Th. C. M. ..	Wilhelminapark 24	Venlo
Donders, Dr. P. C.	Hondsruglaan 11	Groningen (Helpman)
Dongen, C. J. van	Ravetsmaer 13	Nieuwenhage
Donick, J. van	Kwendelhof 251	Tilburg
Driessen-Khouw, Mevr. T. H.	Soesterbergstraat 120B	Soest-Zuid
Drift, J. van der	Stationsweg 102	Ede
Dubois, Dr. H. F. W.	Mariannelaan 18	Apeldoorn
Dunnewold, Dr. C. J. W. ...	Sweelinckstraat 3	Heemskerk
Duurtsema, E. G.	Vondellaan 84	Beverwijk
Duijff, A. G.	Waalsdorperweg 111	Den Haag
Duijster, Dr. C. B.	Burg. Gülcherlaan 26	Hilversum
Dijk, J. R. van	Middenweg 106	Amsterdam-O
Edens, Dr. W. J.	Burg. Wuilweg 14	Drachten
Eerden, Dr. A. A. J. J. v.d. .	Oliemolenstraat 1	Heerlen
Eerden, A. H. A. M. v.d. ...	Molenberglaan 34	Heerlen
Eerden, J. J. J. M. v.d.	Aldenhof 61-91	Nijmegen
Egger, E. G. E.	Diepenbrockstraat 10	Amsterdam
Eggink, Dr. E. D.	Herenplein 12	Groningen
Ekelmans, L.	Wermerlaan 12	Hilversum
Ennema, Dr. M. C.	Minister Hartsenlaan 4	Hilversum
Ermers, H. J. M.	Nieuwe Binnenweg 114	Rotterdam
Eykenboom, Mej. G. J. M. .	Essenburgsingel 97	Rotterdam
Faber, H. H.	Beneluxlaan 12	Harderwijk
Falger, E. L. F.	Kozakkenweg 15	Putten
Fast, R.	Ieplaan 73	Den Haag
Feenstra, G. A. T.	Stolberglaan 43	Utrecht
Feenstra, W. H. A.	Nrd. Houdringelaan 2	Bilthoven
Fernandes, Dr. A.	de Mildestraat 11	Den Haag
Fesevur-van Bart, Mevr. A. .	Benoordenhoutseweg 255	Den Haag
Fischer-von Bünau, Mevr. Dr. H.	Verhulstlaan 18	Bilthoven
Flieringa, Prof. Dr. H. J. ...	Vijverlaan 22	Rotterdam
Flohil, J. W.	's-Gravendijkwal 24	Rotterdam
Franken, Dr. S.	Hofstede de Grootkade 36	Groningen
Gadroen, I.	Amerbos 3	Amsterdam
Galema, D. H.	"De Eekhof", Arnhemseweg 16A.	Leusden-Z
Gier, D. L. de	Schubertlaan 130	Leiden
Gier, Mej. M. F. de	St. Odastraat 23	Eindhoven
Go-Sennema, Mevr. A. A. ..	Rijnsburgerweg 296	Leiden
Gobin, Dr. M. H. M. A.	p/a Oogh. Kliniek, Acad. Ziekenh.	Leiden
Goedbloed, Dr. J.	Schouwweg 38	Wassenaar
Goekoop, G. J.	Kanaalweg 44	Leiden
Goettsch, F. J. B.	Veerallee 7	Zwolle
Gommers, P. A. M.	Einsteinstraat 20	Nijmegen
Gortzak-Moorstein, N.	Cannenburg 72	Amsterdam
Gouvernante, J.	Kathleen Ferrierlaan 26	Amstelveen

Greve, E. L.	Rupel 13	Amstelveen
Haan, A. B. de	Willemsparkweg 101	Amsterdam-Z
Haas, Dr. H. L. de	Schellardweg 19	Oosterbeek
Haas, Dr. J. P. de	Prinses Christinalaan 2	Vlaardingen
Hagedoorn, Prof. Dr. A.	Apollolaan 129	Amsterdam-Z
Hamburg, Dr. A.	's Jacoblaan 28	Bussum
Hamzaruddin, L. S.	's Gravenlandseweg 489	Schiedam
Hartman-Visser, S. R.	Briljantstraat 361	Groningen
Hartogs, J.	Ds. van Dijkweg 16	Doetinchem
Haveman, J.	Coronastraat 60	Groningen
Haye, O. W.	Ruusbroeclaan 6	Eindhoven
Heer, L. J. de	Mussetstraat 11	Rotterdam-24
Heer-Ancona, Mevr. S. de	Jac. Catslaan 7	Eindhoven
Helm, Dr. F. G. M. van der	Molenberglaan 98	Heerlen
Henkes, Prof. Dr. H. E.	's Lands Werf 70	Rotterdam-16
Henry, P.	Stationsweg 23	Leiden
Herwaarden, Dr. A. van	Vondelstraat 7a	Amsterdam-W
Heuvel, Prof. Dr. J. E. A. van den	Rijksweg 191	Mook
Heuvel-Aghina, Mevr. J. W. M. Th. van den	Rijksweg 191	Mook
Heuven, Dr. G. J. van	Frans van Mierisstraat 133	Amsterdam-Z
Heysser, G.	Randweg 84 b	Rotterdam
Hilbert, Dr. B.	Nieuwe Binnenweg 174	Rotterdam
Hilgers, Dr. J. H. C.	G. Washingtonlaan 10	Rijswijk
Hoefnagels, K. L. J.	Burg. v.d. Mortelplein 49	Tilburg
Hoeksema, B. L.	Bosscheweg 41	Vught
Hogeweg, Mej. M.	Reguliersgracht 32	Amsterdam
Holthuis, P.	Singel 26	Deventer
Hooftman-Timmers, Mevr. S. E.	Dr. Beguinlaan 10	Voorburg
Hoogerheide, J.	Naarderstraat 184	Huizen
Hoppenbrouwers, R. W. J. N.	F. C. Dondersstraat 65	Utrecht
Hora Adema, J. H.	de Lairessestraat 59	Amsterdam-Z
Horst, R. I.	Goereesestraat 8	Rotterdam-Z
Hötte, F. A.	Dr. de Weverlaan 12	Heerlen
Hötte, Dr. H. H. A.	Nassaulaan 45 b	Baarn
Houtman, W. A.	Wijde Begijnestraat 25 a	Utrecht
Huberts, J. J.	Draafsingel 32	Hoorn
Humme, E. L.	Velperweg 121	Arnhem
Hupsel, Dr. O.	Barchman Wuytierslaan 20	Amersfoort
Huysmans, E. G.	Joh. Verhulststraat 79	Amsterdam
Hylkema, Dr. B. S.	Zuidersingel 47	Assen
Idema, W. P. R.	Dr. Schaepmanstraat 7	Tiel
Imhof-Revers, Mevr. C. M.	Borgesiuslaan 15	Amersfoort
Janse-Stuart, Mevr. Dr. C.	Nic. Maesstraat 84	Amsterdam-Z
Jansen, Dr. L. M. A. A.	Burg. van Rijnsingel 3	Venlo
Jansonius, D.	St. Geertruidenziekenhuis	Deventer
Janssen, J. A. M. J.	Beemdenlaan 12	Roermond
Janssens Capriles, Dr. G. J. A.	Zonneweilaan 2	Vught
Japing, H. K.	Landréstraat 293	Den Haag
Jap Tjong, K. R. O.	Sint Josephstraat 9	's-Hertogenbosch
Jockin, R.	Spiegelenburghlaan 29	Aerdenhout
Jong, H. de	Oosterhoutlaan 5	Haarlem

Jong-Busnac, Mevr. M. de ..	Oosterhoutlaan 5	Haarlem
Jong, P. T. V. M. de	Joh. Huizingalaan 320 I	Amsterdam
Jonkers, Dr. G. H.	Burg. Knappertlaan 90-92	Schiedam
Junge, Dr. J.	Haerstraat 6	Oldenzaal
Kats, A.	Churchilllaan 7	Axel
Keiner, E. C. J. F.	Burg. van Rooyensingel 1	Zwolle
Kerlen, C. H.	Albertus Perkstraat 50	Hilversum
Keur, J. H. W.	Boerhaavelaan 36	Zwolle
Khohonggiem, A. B.	Eikstraat 22	Hoorn
Kiewiet de Jonge, J.	Oranje Nassaulaan 18	Warmond
Knegt, J. C. de	Crabethstraat 73	Gouda
Kogel, G. de	Uranusstraat 7	Aalsmeer
Kok-van Alphen, Mevr. Dr. C. C.	Warmonderweg 12	Oegstgeest
Kooyman, M.	Gen. Foulkesweg 99	Wageningen
Korver, C.	Bosseweg 8	Best
Koster, M. S.	Thorbeckelaan 3	Reeuwijk
Kristiansen, O.	Damsterdiep 237	Groningen
Kroonenberg, S.	Fr. den Hollanderlaan 31	Goes
Krouwels, A. G.	Emmastraat 27	Alkmaar
Kuik, D. J. v.	Nic. Moensstraat 40 II	Amsterdam-Z
Kuiper, J. H. E.	Lankforst 10-14	Nijmegen
Kurstjens, Dr. J. H.	Wassenaarseweg 29	Den Haag
Lamers, Dr. W. P. M. A. ...	St. Lambertuslaan 10 a	Maastricht
Landvreugd, A. L. O.	Jamaicadreef 63	Utrecht
Leeman, Dr. A. M.	van Hogendorplaan 1	Amersfoort
Leenaars-van Driest Dr. E. .	Frederik Hendriklaan 44	Den Haag
Leeuwen-de Boer, Mevr. M. v.	De Weer 19	Zaandam
Leffertstra, Dr. L. J.	Harlingerstraat 11	Leeuwarden
Legein, Dr. Ch. P. J. J. M. M.	....	Eindhoven
Lekkerkerker, J.	Singel 16	Deventer
Lettinga, Dr. Tj. W.	Enschedesestraat 114	Hengelo (O.)
Ley, J. D. van der	Schuttersweg 6	Hilversum
Lie, K. L.	Stationsstraat 10	Winschoten
Liem, H. G.	Harpstraat 15	Nijmegen
Lim, H. J.	Cannenburg 14	Amsterdam-Buitenveldert
Lindenburg, P. A. W.	Prinses Marielaan 4	Amersfoort
Lith, Dr. G. H. M.	's Gravesandestr. 82	Rotterdam-14
Loenen Martinet, A. H. J. v..	C.N.A. Looslaan 56	Rotterdam-13
Loewer-Sieger, Mevr. Dr. D. H.	De Sav. Lohmanlaan 1	Amstelveen
Ludwig, H. H. H.	Heresingel 4	Groningen
Manen, Prof. Dr. J. G. van .	Woelwijklaan 11	Voorschoten
Manschot, Dr. W. A.	Nieuwe Binnenweg 157	Rotterdam-3
Marchie Sarvaas, G. J. du ..	van Deldenweg 5	Hattem
Maren, J. G. van	Sav. Lohmanstraat 11	Woerden
Massaro, R. G.	Heresingel 4	Groningen
Matusz, L.	Tafelbergdreef 204	Utrecht
Meer, Dr. B. C. J. v.d.	Sint Lambertuslaan 46	Maastricht
Melchers, Dr. M. J.	Nieuwe Heescheweg 25	Oss
Melles, J.	Ursulaland 8 ,..............	Den Haag
Mertens, Mej. Dr. D. E. A. .	De Lairesselaan 71	Rotterdam
Mesker, Dr. R. P.	Minervaplein 44 I	Amsterdam-Z
Meyer, Th. M. A.	Haydnlaan 39	Enschede

Middelhoven, Mej. Dr. C. W. C.	Memlingstr. 15	Amsterdam-Z
Mierlobensteyn, Mevr. M. K. Th. v.	H. v. Spangessingel 17	Rotterdam
Möller, J. H.	van Foreestlaan 16	Heiloo
Mosselman, G. C.	Meidoornlaan 8	Zuid Laren (Dr.)
Mulock Houwer, Prof. A. W.	Arnh. Bovenweg 12	Zeist
Nanninga, H. D.	Noordeinde 10	Monnickendam
Napel, J. A. ten	Gliphoeve 809	Amsterdam
Nieuwenhuis-Koster, Mevr. B. H. C.	Koningstr. 19	Leiderdorp
Nieuwenhuis, E. A.	Koningstraat 19	Leiderdorp
Nordheim, Dr. R. W. von ..	Maliesingel 16 b	Utrecht
Nordlohne, M. E.	Vrijdomweg 18	Vlissingen
Notting, J. G. A.	Weezenhof 83-04	Nijmegen
Notting, J. A.	Parklaan 50	Eindhoven
Nijland, R.	Rijksstraatweg 233C	Haren (Gr.)
Nijs, Mej. A. M. de	Jacob Catskade 60 III	Amsterdam-W
Nijs, A. A. M. de	Argonautenstraat 23 I	Amsterdam
Obbink, Dr. J.	Woestenbergweg 6	Emst (gem. Epe - Gld.)
Odijk, E. J. A. van	Boerhaavelaan 216	Leiden
Oei, T. H.	Koninginneweg 257	Amsterdam
Oey, J. K. D.	Burg. le Fèvre de Montignylaan 26	Rotterdam-13
Ooms, P. F.	Frissenstein 283	Amsterdam
Oosterhuis, Prof. Dr. J. A. .	Prinsenweg 57	Wassenaar
Oostingh, F. F.	Statenlaan 87	Den Haag
Os, R. S. van	Schiedamseweg 104	Vlaardingen
Otto, A. J.	Papenbergseweg 11	Mook
Ouborg, P. E. J.	Kruisstraat 1	Haarlem
Ouwejan, Dr. A. J.	van Heemstralaan 28	Arnhem
Pala, Mevr. M. M. S.	Boslaan 3	Schaesberg (L.)
Pannevis, Dr. M.	Mathenesserlaan 268	Rotterdam
Parren, H. G.	Herenlaan 7	Zeist
Pas, J. W. M. v.d.	De Willemskamp 2	Hengelo (O)
Peeters, H. J. F.	Ruimzicht 322	Torenwijk Osdorp, Amsterdam
Philipsen, W. M. J. G.	Eikenlaan 24	St. Michiels Gestel
Pinckers, Dr. A. J. L. G. ...	Hylekamp 10	Mook
Planten, Dr. J. Th.	Harlingerstraatweg 6B	Leeuwarden
Poppel, A. L. A. van	Graaf Hendrik-III-Laan 2	Breda
Post, H. J.	Schansweg 35	Rotterdam-8
Pot-Meekhof, Mevr. M. W. .	Loolaan 27, flat 3	Apeldoorn
Prins, A.	van Boetzelaerlaan 171	Den Haag
Prins-Berkhemer, Mevr. E. .	van Boetzelaerlaan 171	Den Haag
Quartero-van der Starp, Mevr. A. E.	Burg. Diepenhorstlaan 20	Epe (Gld)
Raemakers, Dr. Ch. L.	Huygensweg 17	Nijmegen
Regensburg, Mevr. N. I. ...	Oogziekenhuis	Rotterdam
Rempt, Dr. F.	Frans Halsstraat 29	Utrecht
Renardel de Lavalette, J. G. C.	de Lairesselaan 90	Rotterdam-16
Reynvaan, M. J.	Nachtegaallaan 20	Den Haag
Reijntjes, G. A.	Genistalaan 17	Apeldoorn
Riaskoff, Dr. S.	Willemsplein 13 d	Rotterdam
Roesink, W. J.	Velperweg 34a	Arnhem

Romunde, Mevr. S. A. van	Willemplantsoen 1	Utrecht
Rooy, Dr. A. J. P. M. de ...	Wilhelminasingel 3	Nijmegen
Rozemeyer, J. A.	Roosendaalseweg 29	Etten-Leur (N.Br.)
Rümke, A. M. L.	Prof. Lorentzlaan 105	Zeist
Rutgers van der Loeff-Manschot	G. Voethstraat 2	Arnhem
Rutten, H. J.	Looxmagracht 24	Sneek
Ruijs, Th. C.	Alg. Ziekenhuis, Röpke Zweers-stichting	Hardenberg
Rijnders, J.	v. d. Waalslaan 21	Enschede
Sampimon, Dr. R. L. H. ...	Oudwijk 37	Utrecht
Sande, H. M. van der	Brugstraat 73	Roosendaal
Sanders, B. G. H. M.	Burg. Damstraat 33	Tilburg
Sandifort Westhof, A. J. ...	Comm. Cramerlaan 11	Coevorden
Sauter, J. J. M.	Nyenoertweg 139	Leek
Schappert-Kimmijser, Mevr. Dr. J.	Flat Waalsdorp 313	Den Haag
Scheffer, C. H.	T. Brandsmalaan 14	Vleuten
Schilt, P. D.	Biesboschstraat 5	Amsterdam
Schnitker, A.	Monnikensteeg 30	Arnhem
Scholten, Mej. E. J. M.	Graafschap Hornelaan 30a	Weert
Schreinemachers, H. P.	Bowlingstraat 66	Oosterhout
Schröder, J. E.	Fruinplantsoen 19	Utrecht
Schubert, Dr. H. C. P. M. ..	Nic. Beetsstraat 31	Assen
Schweitzer, Prof. Dr. N. M. J.	De Esstukken 22	Haren (Gr.)
Sedney, S. C.	Aert van Neslaan 425	Oegstgeest
Seepers, F. A.	Helmondseweg 20	Deurne
Senus, Dr. A. H. C.	Straatweg 15	Rotterdam
Sie, S. H.	Lokhorst 123	Leiderdorp
Siersema, J. A.	Oostzeestraat 13	Kampen
Sloot, Dr. G. H. W. L.	Oude Dijk 23	Rotterdam
Smals, A. J. M.	Grote Spie 54	Breda
Smit, D. H.	Zevenwoudenlaan 28	Heerenveen
Smit, Dr. J. A.	Kromhout 217	Amsterdam
Smit, P.	Groeneveen 241	Haarlem
Smith, G. N.	W. Boothstraat 30	Amsterdam
Smulders, F. M.	Sinjeur Semeynsstraat 25	Amstelveen
Sonnega, H.	Beneluxlaan 172	Utrecht
Speckman, H. M.	Crabethstraat 71	Gouda
Staalman, J. H.	Nassaulaan 43	Schiedam
Stapper, M.	Obbinklaan 2	Utrecht
Steenbeek, R. V. F.	Vondellaan 17	IJsselstein
Stegewerns, J.	Hillevliet 20 B	Rotterdam
Steinmeyer, J. H. C.	Min. van Houtenlaan 29	Velsen (Z.)
Stenger-Muller, Mevr. M. A. H.	Voorstraat 65	Delft
Sterk, C. C.	Wagnerplein 72	Leiden
Stoltz, W. P.	B. Zweerskade 2	Amsterdam-Z
Stoutenbeek, P.	Jisperveldstraat 71	Amsterdam-N
Straaten-Hage, Mevr. D. C. van	Scherpenzeelseweg 56	Leersum
Supicić, R. D. M.	Dovenetelweg 20	Den Haag
Swart, H. J.	Wilhelminastraat 5	Breda
Swelheim, Dr. I.	Koninginneweg 146	Amsterdam-Z
Taams, Dr. G.	Singel 323	Dordrecht

Tamboenan, K.	Burg. v. Necklaan 197	Leidschendam
Tan, Dr. K. E. W. P.	F. C. Dondersstraat 65	Utrecht
Tan, S. T.	Jisperveldstraat 28	Amsterdam
Tengkey, B.	Groeneveen 171 II	Bijlmermeer
Tenpierik, J. C. J.	Wickenburglaan 56	Utrecht
Tillema, Dr. A.	Elzentlaan 19	Eindhoven
Timmerman, G. J. M. E. N. .	Groot Ziekengasthuis	Den Bosch
Timmerman, Mej. Z.	Zaagmuldersweg 342	Groningen
Tjan, T. T.	Kempenaerstraat 88	Oegstgeest
Tjoa, S. T.	Burg. Hogguerstraat, flat 617 ...	Amsterdam-W
Treffers, W. F.	Breitnerweg 10	Groesbeek
Umar-Firtiwa, Mevr. S. K. ..	Pr. Mauritssingel 10	Nieuwerkerk a/d IJssel
Vader, J.	Staten Bolwerk 8	Haarlem
Valk, L. E. M.	Pres. Rooseveltlaan 20	Helmond
Valk, W. G. M. van der	Noordzijde Zoom 7	Bergen op Zoom
Veelen, Dr. A. W. C. van ...	Maliesingel 33	Utrecht
Velzeboer, Prof. Dr. C. M. J.	Oranje Nassaulaan 18 II	Amsterdam-Z
Verduin, Mej. P. C.	's Landswerf 72	Rotterdam
Verduyn Lunel, H. F. E. ...	Pampus 11	Amstelveen
Verhey, H. W. J.	Prins Bernhardstraat 4	Nijmegen
Versteegh, W. A.	Salvia 11	Dordrecht
Vierhout, H. C.	Ootmarsumsestraat 76	Almelo
Visser, Dr. G. J.	Jansbinnensingel 25	Arnhem
Vogelaar, J. J.	Hoogstraat 8	Bergen op Zoom
Voldere, A. J. de	Pinksterbloemweg 7	Zaandam
Volmer, Ch.	Amersfoortseweg 5	Apeldoorn
Völker-Dieben, H. J. M. ...	ws. "Akka", Morskade t/o 7	Leiden
Vos, J. L.	Stationslaan 16	Harderwijk
Vos, Dr. Tj. A.	Laan van Meerdervoort 394	Den Haag
Vries, A. J. de	Valkenburgplein 6	Heemstede
Vries, Dr. S. de	Willem Pijperstraat 35	Amsterdam
Vroom, Mej. M. de	Rietzangerlaan 5	Den Haag
Waardenburg, Dr. P. J.	de Valkenburch. A 21	Oosterbeek
Wagenaar, Dr. J. W.	Catharijnesingel 80	Utrecht
Walbeek, Dr. K. van	Vinkenstraat 22	Zaandam
Walburg Schmidt, J. F.	Javastraat 64	Den Haag
Waveren, Ch. W. van	Middenweg 96	Den Helder
Waveren, H. F. van	De Spanring 14	Heiloo
Werf, D. I. A. van der	Parklaan 25	Sittard
Werf, P. J. P. v. d.	Julianasingel 26	Venray
Westrhenen, D. W. van	Planetenbaan 547	De Bilt
Weyden, P. C. R. v. d.	Min. Kanstraat 30	Emmen
Wezer, C. P.	Venloseweg 491	Tegelen
Wiel-de Jong, Mevr. C. Ch. v. d.	Koornmarkt 45	Delft
Wielick, Mej. Z.	Joh. Bosboomstraat 16	Amersfoort
Winkelman, Dr. J. E.	De Lairessestraat 67	Amsterdam-Z
Winning, Jhr. Dr. C. H. O. M. von	Wassenaarseweg 29	Den Haag
Wismans, Th. M. J.	Oyen 4	Kessel (L.)
Witkam, W. G. M.	Weverslaan 37	Voorburg
Witte, M. de	Anna van Burenlaan 11	Alphen a/d Rijn
Wolff-Rouendaal, Mevr. D. de	Koekoekstraat 77	Leiderdorp
Worst, Dr. J. G. F.	de Sav. Lohmanlaan 62	Groningen
Wyers, J. G.	Boterdiepstraat 57 II	Amsterdam

Wijnen, W. G. van	Jasmijnstraat 6	Winsum-Obergum
Wijngaarde, Mej. R.	Schiedamse Vest 180, Oogzieken-huis	Rotterdam
Zahn, Dr. K. J.	Fred. v. Eedenplaats 67	Capelle a/d IJssel
Zandbergen, H.	Talmastraat 14	Winterswijk
Zivojnovic, R.	Vredeman de Vriesstraat 26	Rotterdam

Antillae

Blommestein, Dr. J. D. A. v..	Bernhardstraat 310	Aruba
Bochove, J. v.	Arikokweg 18	Curaçao
Spierenburg, P. J.	Taubergeb. k 33	Willemstad, Curaçao

Suriname

Komproe, Mej. Dr. C. C. ...	Zwartenhovenbrugstraat 143	Paramaribo
Themen, Dr. Ch. W. G.	Prinsessestr. 39	Paramaribo
Wijngaarde, Prof. Dr. E. G. .	A. Dragtenweg K 17	Paramaribo

NOSOCOMIA QUIBUS OCULIS AEGRI CURANTUR

No. of beds

Oogheelkundige Kliniek der Universiteit van Amsterdam. Wilhelmina Gasthuis, Amsterdam-W. Head: Prof. Dr. R. A. Crone 105

Oogheelkundige Kliniek der Rijksuniversiteit te Groningen. Academisch Ziekenhuis, Groningen, Head: Prof. Dr. N. M. J. Schweitzer 60

Oogheelkundige Kliniek der Rijksuniversiteit te Leiden. Academisch Ziekenhuis, Leiden. Head: Prof. Dr. M. C. Colenbrander en Prof. Dr. J. A. Oosterhuis 52

Oogheelkundige Kliniek der R.K. Universiteit te Nijmegen, St. Annastraat 313, Nijmegen. Head: Prof. Dr. J. E. A. v. d. Heuvel en Prof. Dr. A. F. Deutman jr. 50

Koninklijk Nederlandsch Gasthuis voor Behoeftige en Minvermogende Ooglijders, tevens Oogheelkundige Kliniek der Rijksuniversiteit te Utrecht. Head: Vacant 100

Oogziekenhuis, Schiedamsevest 180, Rotterdam. Oogheelkundige Afdeling Erasmus Universiteit Head: Prof. Dr. H. E. Henkes 158

Oogheelkundige Kliniek van het Academisch Ziekenhuis der Vrije Universiteit, Amsterdam. Head: Prof. Dr. C. M. J. Velzeboer 38

Oogziekenhuis, Leyweg 295, den Haag. Head: Jhr. Dr. C. H. O. M. von Winning 72

INSTITUTA SCHOLAEQUE CAECIS DESTINATAE

General information:

Algem. Ned. Vereniging ter voorkoming van blindheid. Secr.: Mej. Dr. J. ten Doesschate. c/o Oogziekenhuis, Leyweg 295, den Haag.

Stichting 'Algemene en Individuele Blindenbelangen', Vondelstraat 128, Amsterdam-W.

Vereniging 'Het Nederlandse Blindenwezen', Vondelstraat 146, Amsterdam-W.

Blind children
Koninklijk Instituut tot Onderwijs van Blinden, Amersfoortsestraatweg 189, Huizen N.-H., post Bussum.
Chr. Instituut voor Blinden 'Bartiméus', Utrechtseweg 84, Zeist.
'Sint Henricus', Katholiek instituut voor visueel gehandicapten, Nijmeegselaan 61, Nijmegen.
'De Wijnberg', Katholiek instituut voor visueel gehandicapten. Kleuters en meisjes, Elisabethstraat 4, Grave N.Br.

Bad sighted children
School voor kinderen met beperkt gezichtsvermogen, 'Prins Alexander Stichting', Huis ter Heide.
School voor kinderen met beperkt gezichtsvermogen, 'Prinses Magriet Francisca', Heindijk 4, Rotterdam 21.
School voor kinderen met beperkt gezichtsvermogen 'Comeniusschool', Bilderdijkkade 61, Amsterdam 14.
Chr. Instituut voor kinderen met beperkt gezichtsvermogen, 'Bartiméus', Utrechtseweg 84, Zeist.
'St. Henricus', Nijmegen.
'De Wijnberg', Grave (N.Br.)
'Lichtklas' verbonden aan de 'Stichting Werkplaats Kindergemeenschap', Kees Boekelaan 10, Bilthoven.

Mentally defective and visually handicapped children.
'Mr. H. P. van Heukelomstichting', Rijksstraatweg 286, Haren (G).
Stichting 'de Brink', Groningerstraat 15, Vries (Dr.).
'De Springplank', afd. Chr. Instituut Bartiméus, Wrangelaan 9, Doetinchem.
'De Hondsberg', R.K. Observatiecentrum, Hondsbergselaan 5, Oisterwijk (N.Br.).
'De Binckhorst', R.K. Instituut voor jongens, Waterleidingstr. 2, Rosmalen (N.Br.).
'De Blauwe Kamer', R.K. Instituut voor meisjes, Galderseweg 65, Breda.
'De Wijnberg', Grave, N.B.
'Bartiméushage', O. Arnhemse Bovenweg 3, Doorn.

Revalidation of adults:
'De Schansenberg', Beekbergerweg 46, Loenen (Gld).

Homes for the blind aged:
Huize 'Het Schild', Wolfheze.
Stichting 'Finspong', Boulevard 24, Zeist.
Chr. Blindentehuis 'Sonneheert', Putterweg 140, Ermelo (Gld).
'Adriaan Moonenstichting', Pr. Bisschopsingel 20, Maastricht.

HONG KONG

SOCIETATES OPHTHALMOLOGICAE

The Hong Kong Ophthalmological Society
Chairman: Dr. Lawrence T. S. Leong
Honorary Secretary and Treasurer: Dr. Timothy Kai-ching Liu, Yaumatei Ophthalmic
  Centre, Knowloon, Hong Kong
Number of members: 41

NOMINA ET DOMICILIA MEDICORUM AB OCULIS

Au-Yeung, S. M.	c/o Yaumatei Ophthalmic Centre	Hong Kong
Chan, S. C.	313 Nathan Rd., 2nd Floor	Hong Kong
Chan, W. K.	Rm. 1606, Hang Seng Bank Building	Hong Kong
Chang, John	148, Prince Edward Rd., 3rd floor	Hong Kong
Chen, Y. P.	41, Conduit Rd., 13th floor, Rome Court, Flat C	Hong Kong
Chew, L. G.	337-339 Nathan Rd., 3rd floor, Flat B	Hong Kong
Ching, Ronald	20, Kennedy Terrace, Top floor .	Hong Kong
Chow, K. C.	c/o Violet Peel Ophthalmic Centre	Hong Kong
Chow, S. N.	c/o Violet Peel Ophthalmic Centre	Hong Kong
Chow, Stephen W. C.	c/o Yaumatei Ophthalmic Centre	Hong Kong
Chun, M. L.	2B, King Tak Street, 1st floor ...	Hong Kong
Feng, Marie	221D, Nathan Rd., 2nd floor ...	Hong Kong
Foo, C. C.	c/o Yaumatei Ophthalmic Centre .	Hong Kong
Lam, T. K.	1Q, Avenida Almeida Ribeiro ...	Macau
Leong, Lawrence T. S.	335, Nathan Rd., 4th floor	Hong Kong
Leung, Colin M. Y.	c/o Yaumatei Ophthalmic Centre .	Hong Kong
Ling, Mabel	c/o Yaumatei Ophthalmic Centre .	Hong Kong
Ling, M. W.	c/o Yaumatei Ophthalmic Centre .	Hong Kong
Liu, Timothy K. C.	c/o Yaumatei Ophthalmic Centre	Hong Kong
Lor, K. H.	Rm. 315, Edinburgh House	Hong Kong
Lou, J. T.	Nathional Court, Nathan Rd., 2nd. floor	Hong Kong
Sheung, Mak	c/o Yaumatei Ophthalmic Centre .	Hong Kong
Mok, C. H.	404, Regent House, Queen's Rd. Central	Hong Kong
Ng, Rita	Rm. 105, Pedder Bldg., Pedder Street	Hong Kong
Ng, Y. H.	c/o Yaumatei Ophthalmic Centre .	Hong Kong
Poon, K. Y.	c/o Yaumatei Ophthalmic Centre .	Hong Kong
Raj, B.	c/o Arran Street Eye Clinic	Hong Kong
Singh, Mahan	Rm. 102, Pedder Bldg., Pedder Street	Hong Kong
So, Eugene M.	238, Nathan Rd., 2nd floor	Hong Kong
Sousa, O, de	China Building, Pedder Street ...	Hong Kong
Tang, C. T.	Rm. 411 Shaw's Bldg., Nathan Rd.	Hong Kong

Tham, M. H.	c/o Violet Peel Ophthalmic Centre	Hong Kong
Toh, David	48, Kennedy Rd., F2	Hong Kong
Wong, Francis K.	308, Hing Wai Bldg., Queen's Rd., Central	Hong Kong
Wong, W. T.	Milton Mansion, 3rd floor, 96, Nathan Rd	Hong Kong
Woo, C. P.	c/o Yaumatei Ophthalmic Centre .	Hong Kong
Yang, Judy Y.	232, Nathan Rd., 3rd floor	Hong Kong
Young, Wilson	753, Nathan Rd., 6th floor	Hong Kong
Yiu, Alex.	10, Wang Fung Terrace, Flat I, Tai Hange Rd	Hong Kong
Yung, Y. F.	Flat 6, Honour House, 4th floor, 379, Nathan road	Hong Kong

NOSOCOMIA QUIBUS OCULIS AEGRI CURANTUR

Government Hospitals with eye beds:	No. of beds
Queen Mary Hospital	10
Queen Elizabeth Hospital	18
Kowloon Hospital	8
Kwong Wah Hospital	8

Consultant Ophthalmologist in-charge: Dr. Timothy K. C. Liu.
Consultant Ophthalmologist: Dr. M. H. Tham.

INSTITUTA SCHOLAEQUE CAECIS DESTINATAE

	No. of pupils
Canossa School for the visually disabled	107
Ebenzer School and Home for the Blind	113

HUNGARIA

SOCIETATES OPHTHALMOLOGICAE

Hungarian Society of Ophthalmology
President: Prof. Magda Radnót
Secretary: Dr. A. Medgyaszay
Bureau: First Eye Clinic, University Medical School, VIII Tomo utca 25-29, 1083 Budapest

NOMINA ET DOMICILIA MEDICORUM AB OCULIS

Aczél, György	Szilágyi E. fs. 4	1125 Budapest
Agg, Zoltán	Tanácsház u. 7	7700 Mohacs
Alberth, Béla	Szemklinika	4012 Debrecen
Alföldy, Arpád	Ady E. u. 12	1165 Budapest
Altorjay, Aladár	Béke sug. ut 12	5700 Gyula
Anda, Lujza	Tárogató u. 42	1021 Budapest
Annau, Ella	Füge u. 4	1022 Budapest
Arató, Mária	Zalatnai u. 6. 1.6	1125 Budapest
Aszalós, Imre	Deák F. u. 10	6500 Baja
Ábrahám, Sándor	Lőwy S. u. 5	3100 Salgotarjan
Ágoston, Irén	Tompa u. 18	7623 Pécs
Áhi, Olga	Asztalos J. u. 8	1016 Budapest
Bagóczky, Lajos	Szécheny uti sarokházak, E 30	2700 Cegled
Baja, József	Somorjai u. 10/a	1124 Budapest
Baján, Miklós	Bem J. u. 29/c	9700 Szombathely
Bajka, Ágnes	Uzsoki u. 56. II.4	1145 Budapest
Bajnok, Györgyi	Himfy u. 5	1118 Budapest
Balassa, Miklós	Vöröshadsereg u. 17. III. 3	3529 Miskolc
Balaton, Csilla	Rózsa F. u. 7	1074 Budapest
Balázs, Erzsébet	Baross u. 75	1082 Budapest
Bali, Brigitta	Mária u. 39	1085 Budapest
Balogh, Judit	Ménesi U. 18. mf. 2/b	1118 Budapest
Balthazár, Erzsébet	Esze T. u. 77	1196 Budapest
Barabás, Zsuzsanna	Tarr I. ut 4/c., f. 3	7633 Pécs
Baranyai Miklós	Mező I. u. 19. 1. 1	3000 Hatvan
Barcza, Ida	Budakeszi u. 46/a	1121 Budapest
Barta, Erzsébet	Egészségház u. 2	3300 Eger
Bartha, Elamér	Ady E. u. 8	2600 Balassagyartmat
Barthos, Erzsébet	Hámán K. u. 22. II. 1	4027 Debrecen
Bartl, V. Ferenc	Megyei Kórház	8900 Zalaegerszeg
Bartók, Imre	Lovag u. 16	1066 Budapest
Bausz, Mária	Kinizsi u. 2-6	1092 Budapest
Bauer, Nándor	Kórház, Szemészet	2862 Ajka
Bazsika, Mária	Május u. 67	7400 Kaposvár
Bánfalvi, Mária	Elek u. 9/B	1113 Budapest
Bálint, Julia (Juhászné)	Perczel M.u. 49	7250 Bonyhád
Bánkuti, Hedvig	C/2-E/2 III. L. II. 5	7100 Szekszárd
Bárdos, Márta	Lenin krt. 70	1066 Budapest

Bárdy, Károly	Megyei Kórház	9002 Gyór
Bártfay, Klára	Alkotás u. 25	1123 Budapest
Báthory, Zoltán	Mártirok u. 29	1024 Budapest
Bednár, János	Dob u. 87. f. 17	1077 Budapest
Bellák, Ervin	Dagály u. 8	1138 Budapest
Bencsik, Rózsa	Böszörmény ut 9-11	1126 Budapest
Bendenritter, Ferenc	Sollner u. 26/c	1131 Budapest
Benkő, Éva	Irinyi J. u. 32/b	1117 Budapest
Beöthy, Klára	Kórház, Szemészet	2660 Balassagyarmat
Bertényi, Anna	Pozsonyi ut 12	1137 Budapest
Betkó, János	Pasaréti u. 179/181	1026 Budapest
Biró, András	Bugát Pál Kórház, Szemészet	3200 Gyöngyos
Biró, Imre	Sallai I. u. 5/D	1136 Budapest
Boér, Ildikó	Kehely u. 4	1221 Budapest
Bohár, Anna	Logodi u. 51. I. 10	1012 Budapest
Borbás, Alujzia	Szalay u. 10/B. V. 20	7623 Pécs
Boros, Béla	III. Épitők u. I/B	7633 Pécs
Boros, Mária	Pf. 407	6701 Szeged
Bozsó, Etelka	Csabai kapu 9. Kórház	3501 Miskolc
Böcskey, Anna	Rottenbiller u. 6/a	1074 Budapest
Bögi, Julia	Kresz G.u. 29	1132 Budapest
Bölcs, Sándor	Tömő u. 25-29	1083 Budapest
Brand, Imre	Mátyás kir. u. 17	9400 Sopron
Brooser, Gábor	Ráday u. 34	1092 Budapest
Buzsáky, Katalin	Jókai u. 13	8900 Zalaegerszeg
Borbély, Judit	Vöröshadsereg u. 85	1021 Budapest
Czigány, Attila	Kórház, Szemészet	9700 Szombathely
Czudor, Edit	Dozsa Gy. u. 77	2800 Tatabánya
Csaba, Ágnes	Kórház, Szemészet	3000 Hatvan
Csaba, Zsuzsa	Szemklinika	4012 Debrecen
Csanádi, Lászlóné	Olympia u. 11. I. 3	3200 Gyöngyös
Csapody, István	Szilágyi E. fasor 27	1026 Budapest
Csernák, Lajos	Városmajor u. 76	1126 Budapest
Csillag, Ferenc	Ady E. u. 60	6800 Hódmezővásárhely
Csüllög, Ferenc	Kórház, Szemészet	4400 Nyiregyháza
Csolák, Magdolna	Rossenberg hp. u. 19	1054 Budapest
Csoma, Éva	Márvány u. 25	1126 Budapest
Dajnits, Rózsa	Szentpéteri u. II. Orvosi 1	3526 Miskolc
Danielisz, Ernő	Rákóczi u. 1	8200 Veszprém
Darabos, György	Kórház	8000 Székesfehérvár
Deák, György	Kut u. 5	1024 Budapest
Deckmann, Erzsébet	Kulich Gy. u. 4/a	7621 Pécs
Deutsch, Stefánia	Kossuth u. 7-9. II. lp. 3	2700 Cegléd
Dérczy, Sarolta	Széchenyi város C. ép. VII. 1	6000 Kecskemét
Dienes, Gábor	V. T. Kórház, Szemészet	4700 Mátészalka
Dóczy, László	Dáni I. u. 7	6722 Szeged
Domokos, Márta	Attila u. 69. fsz. 2	1013 Budapest
Dózsa, György	Legénybiró u. 17. VIII. 26	1157 Budapest
Dömsödy, Vilma	Dózsa Gy. u. 13	4027 Debrecen
Egres, Jenő	Kossuth tér 7-9	3000 Hatvan
Elek, József	Széchenyi u. 3	6500 Baja
Endrei, Ágnes	Hajnóczi J. u. 10	1122 Budapest
Erdei, Zoltán	Szemészeti Klinika	6701 Szeged
Ernyei, Alice	Belgrád rkp. 27	1056 Budapest
Ernyei, István	Gyarmat u. 80	1147 Budapest
Eröss, Sándor	Mária u. 39	1085 Budapest

Eszes, Ilma	Széchenyi u. 5	6900 Makő
Emődy, Judit	Bartók B. u. 4	4043 Debrecen
Ébner, Béláné	Rendelóintézet	3300 Eger
Farkas, Ágnes	Mária u. 39	1085 Budapest
Farkas, Éva	Bagoly u. 2 IV	2030 Érd IV
Farkas, Julianna	Kelenhegyi u. 81	1118 Budapest
Farkas, Zita	Üllői u. 66/a	1082 Budapest
Fazekas, Ilona	Megyei Kórház	4400 Nyiregyháza
Fehér, János	Tömő u. 25-29	1083 Budapest
Fehér, Lajos	Lenin krt. 70. I. 2	1066 Budapest
Fejér, Gyula	Béke tér 3	2890 Tata
Felden, Éva	Erkel u. 22	8360 Keszthely
Ferencz, Mária	Dohány u. 30/b. III. 6	1077 Budapest
Ferenczy, Zoltán	Bán Tibor u. 53	1041 Budapest
Fischer, Matild	Mátyás kir. u. 5	7621 Pécs
Fisi, Gabriella	Liezen-Mayer u. 57	9021 Győr
Fodor, Mária	Üllői u. 126. 1. L. 1.2	1107 Budapest
Follmann, Piroska	Zápor u. 59. III. 17	1032 Budapest
Födő, Vilma	Mozsár u. 10	1066 Budapest
Fátrai, Attila	Szakasits Á. u. 66/a	1115 Budapest
Frivaldszky, Kornélia	Pázmány P. u. 5	9400 Sopron
Galli, Lóránt	Semmelweis Kórház, Szemészet .	3501 Miskolc
Garai, László	Csanády u. 12	1132 Budapest
Gazdag, Imre	Pozsonyi u. 40	1137 Budapest
Gál, Zsuzsanna	Árpád fejedelem u. 49. III	1036 Budapest
Gáll, János	Orló u. 3/a	1026 Budapest
Gát, György	Szenpéteri kapu Kórház	3501 Miskolc
Gát, László	TBC Klinika	4012 Debrecen
Gonda, Gyula	Ihász köz 4. VIII. 47	1105 Budapest
Gödry, Enikő	Tanács Kórház	8900 Zalaegerszeg
Grósz, István	Erőmü u. 4	1117 Budapest
Gruber, Mária	Kórház, Szemészet	9700 Szombathely
Gulyás, Ibolya	Dagály u. 6	1138 Budapest
Gyöngyösi, Margit	Ifjusági ut 3. D. I. 1	1181 Budapest
Győrffy, István	Bródy S. u. 10	1088 Budapest
Gaál, Csilla	Retek u. 22	1024 Budapest
Gulás, Judit	Kórház, Szemosztály	7701 Mohács
Giesel, Vilmos	Semmelweis u. 3	8400 Ajka
Glóner, Bernadette	Szentpéteri kapu Kórház	3501 Miskolc
Hajda, Márta	Sobieski J. u. 28	1096 Budapest
Halda, Tamás	Zetkin K. u. 2	7621 Pécs
Halmai, Ottó	Kórház	2500 Esztergom
Hammer, Helga	Bocskay u. 11	6701 Szeged
Hanisch, József	Baross u. 43	1088 Budapest
Hank, Csilla	Üllői u. 59. I. 5	1091 Budapest
Hatvani, István	Simonyi u. 15	4028 Debrecen
Hegedüs, Jolán	Ady E. u. 43	1203 Budapest
Hegyi, Mária	Zrinyi u. 1	8900 Zalaegerszeg
Hegyi, Márta	Tusnádi u. 28/a	1125 Budapest
Horváth, Lajos	Seregélyisi u. 3	8000 Székesfehérvár
Horváth, Miklós	Kórház, Szemészet	3300 Eger
Hudomel, József	Hankóczy u. 20	1022 Budapest
Horváth, Józsefné	Végh D. u. 17	4027 Debrecen
Hutás, Imre	Tanácsköztársaság u. 45. I. 5 ...	9022 Győr
Imre, György	Süveg u. 14/a	1112 Budapest
Jakab, Terézia	Mártirok utja 32	1043 Budapest

Jobbágyi, Péter	Eperjes u. 90. III. 11	1201 Budapest
Joó, Mária	Ősz Szabó János u. 67	1204 Budapest
Juhász, Gabriella	Rudas L. u. 31	7626 Pécs
Juhász, Ludmilla	Batthyány u. 5	4024 Debrecen
Juhos, Piroska	Ady E. u. 5	1211 Budapest
Janáky, Márta	Pf. 407	6701 Szeged
Járfás, Katalin	Visegrádi u. 47/c	1132 Budapest
Kahán, Ágoston	Jókai u. 4	6720 Szeged
Karádi, Ágnes	Köbölkut u. 13	1118 Budapest
Katsányi, Olga	József u. 4	2081 Piliscsaba
Kálmán, Zsuzsa	Rajk L. u. 36. IV. 4	1136 Budapest
Kántor, Géza	Hevesi Gy. u. 24	1156 Budapest
Károlyi, Katalin	II. Borbély S. u. 59	2800 Tatabánya
Kelemen, Vera	Lágymányosi u. 26. IV. 39	1111 Budapest
Kenyeres, Borbála	Hetény Géza Kórház	5000 Szolnok
Kerek, Andrea	Róbert K. krt. 44	1134 Budapest
Kerek, Sándor	Dózsa Gy. u. 8	7400 Kaposvár
Kereszturi, István	Kórház, Read. Int.	5900 Orosháza
Kerty, Emilia	Magyar u. 8	1053 Budapest
Kettesy, Aladár	Nagyerdei krt. 78	4032 Debrecen
Keve, Mária	Felszabadulás u. 103	9024 Győr
Kincses, Éva	Ujkert u. 17	4027 Debrecen
Kiss, F. Hilda	József A. u. 1	6640 Csongrád
Kiss, Jolán	Köbölkut u. 13. f. 3	1118 Budapest
Kiss, Gabriella	Mártirok u. 1/A	6100 Kiskunfélegyháza
Koleszár, Gyula	Kórház, Szemészet	8600 Siófok
Kollányi, Miklós	Bartók B. u. 4	6500 Baja
Kolozsvári, Csenge	Kórház, Szemészet	3700 Kazincbarcika
Kolozsvári, Lajos	Simonyi u. 24	4028 Debrecen
Korchmáros, Imre	Somlói u. 22	1118 Budapest
Korecz, Károly	Kinizsi u. 16. I. 3	1092 Budapest
Kormos, Katalin	Madách tér 2	1075 Budapest
Kóródi, Mária	Váci u. 4. III. 1	1132 Budapest
Korompay, Edith	Wartha V. u. 22	8200 Veszprém
Korondi, István	Szilágyi E. fasor 13-15	1024 Budapest
Kovács, Bálint	Tompa M. u. 18	7623 Pécs
Kovács, Katalin	Bezerédy u. 18	7100 Szekszárd
Kovács, Margit	Széchenyi u. 84/a	4031 Debrecen
Kováth, Mária	Megyei Kórház, Szemészet	9700 Szombathely
Kozma, Ilona	Garai u. 1	7623 Pécs
Kozma, Zsuzsanna	Csermák A. u. 1	8200 Veszprém
Kő, Judit	Jókai u. 13-17. I. 1	9021 Győr
Könyves, Kolonics Lászlóné	Kórház Rendelőintézet, Szemészet	3300 Eger
Kőszegi, György	Korház, Szemés zet	7200 Dombóvár
Koronkai, Ildikó	Ferenc krt. 3. 4. 24	1094 Budapest
Krassói, Erzsébet	Kórház, Szemészet	8900 Zalaegerszeg
Kugler, Stefánia	Erdőkerülő ut 13. IX. 29	1157 Budapest
Kuhár, Gabriella	Pozsonyi u. 40	1137 Budapest
Lakatos, István	Lágymányosi ut 14/a	1111 Budapest
Láng, Zsuzsanna	Kruspér u. 5-7	1111 Budapest
Lányi, Zsuzsa	Megyei Kórház, Szemészet	9700 Szombathely
László, Zsófia	Megyei Rend. Int. Szemo	9700 Szombathely
Lehrer, Judit	Tolbuchin ut 88-90/b	6725 Szeged
Liszauer, Dezsőné	Madách I. u. 7	1057 Budapest
Littmann, Judit	Rajk L. u. 36	1136 Budapest

Lovas, Béla	Honvéd u. 22-24	1055 Budapest
Lovas, Edit	Ady E. u. 122-124	1194 Budapest
Lovász, Sára	Széchenyi u. 21	3525 Miskolc
Ludvig, Irén	Ady E. u. 17	1024 Budapest
Lugossy, Gyula	Mecset u. 9	1023 Budapest
Lehner, Aladárné	Beloiannisz u. B/5. sz. 2	7100 Szekszárd
Lenkefi, Ferenc	Zrinyi u. 22	8500 Pápa
Madarász, Márton	Árpád u. 75	1042 Budapest
Magossy, Edit	Tolbuchin sgt. 53/55 A/A	6725 Szeged
Mailáth, László	Bessenyei u. 4	4032 Debrecen
Majláth, Gabriella	Bartók B. u. 19	1114 Budapest
Majoros, János	Székely u. 5	6400 Kiskunhalas
Makrai, Erzsébet	Pf. 188	3501 Miskolc
Marek, Péter	Vörösvári u. 7	1035 Budapest
Marsovszky, László	Kossuth L. u. 34	6300 Kalocsa
Martoni, Győző	Kossuth u. 1	8300 Tapolca
Mayer, Katalin	Bem J. u. 29/c	9700 Szombathely
Mákos, Ilona	Pécskő u. 10 fsz. 3	3100 Salgótarján
Mándy, Erzsébet	Ugocsa u. 8/b	1126 Budapest
Márton, Dezső	Martós Flóra u. 1. I.3	8200 Veszprém
Medgyaszay, Attila	Ajtósi Dürer sor 27/b. II. 2	1146 Budapest
Mezey, Pál	Szabolcska M. u. 7. II. 2	1114 Budapest
Mező, Lajos	Zrinyi tér 15	4600 Kisvárda
Miklós, Andor	Köztársaság tér 17	9700 Szombathely
Milcsák, Ágnes	Vörösmarthy u. 13	1074 Budapest
Milecz, Tihamér	Kispest, Thököly u. 9	1192 Budapest
Moldoványi, Antal	Lenin u. 9	8800 Nagykanizsa
Moll, Ágnes	Sziv u. 34·	1063 Budapest
Molnár, Kálmán	Orló u. 3/b	1026 Budapest
Molnár, Klára	Jókai u. 33	3980 Sátoraljaujhely
Molnár, Lajos	Simonyi u. 36	4028 Debrecen
Mónay, Tibor	Eötvös L. u. 8	1053 Budapest
Móri, Edit	Széplak u. 16	1026 Budapest
Mucsi, Gabriella	Megyeri u. 19	1044 Budapest
Mócsy, Ágnes	Mária u. 39	1085 Budapest
Nagy, Ágnes	Hegyalja ut 1	1016 Budapest
Nagy, Erzsébet	Thököly u. 15	1076 Budapest
Nagy, Julia	Mártirok u. 8/10	1027 Budapest
Nagy, Ferenc	Tarcali u. 15	1113 Budapest
Nagy, Margit	Vasvári P. u. 83. III. 11	4400 Nyiregyháza
Nagy, Márta	Arany J. u. 10. IV. 30	6000 Kecskemét
Nádrai, Ágnes	Orló u. 3/b	1026 Budapest
Nagy, Anna	V. Kilián krt. 6	2800 Tatabánya
Nécsei, Pál	Baross u. 10. I. 3	1088 Budapest
Németh, Béla	Ady E. u. 17	1024 Budapest
Németh, Edit	Üllői u. 60-62	1082 Budapest
Németh, Lajos	Üllői u. 60. II. 16	1091 Budapest
Nikolaeva, Mária	Kun Béla u. 1. III. 2	3527 Miskolc
Novák, Erna	Batthyányi u. 26	6722 Szeged
Nyitrai, Ildikó	VI. Ösz u. 6	2700 Cegléd
Oláh, Imre	Zsámbéki u. 1	1124 Budapest
Oláh, Katalin	Gvadányi u. 4	3528 Miskolc
Oláh, Miklós	Vedres u. 8. A. I/3	6726 Szeged
Opauszki, Anna	Szilágy E. fasor 43/b	1026 Budapest
Orbán, Gyöngyi Jolán	Mártirok tere 8	9700 Szombathely
Orbán, Tibor	Ferenczy u. 28	1053 Budapest

Orosz, Sándor	Benczur u. 10. I	1068 Budapest
Osgyán, István	Gutenberg tér 2. II. 2	5000 Szolnok
Orosz, István	József A. u. 4	5400 Mezotur
Papp, Dezső	Aradi u. 52/b	1062 Budapest
Papp, Ágnes	Bolyai u. 38	9700 Szombathely
Papp, Dezsó	Szabadság u. 6	7623 Pécs
Papp, Erzsébet	Idegklinika	7600 Pécs
Papp, László	Vas Gereben u. 28	1124 Budapest
Papp, Terézia	Bástya u. 12	3000 Hatvan
Papp, Zoltán	Kórház, Szemészet	4043 Debrecen
Patai, Dorottya	Üllői u. 30. IV. 4	1085 Budapest
Pál, Magdolna	Tétényi uti Kórház	1115 Budapest
Pálfalvi, Mária	Testvériség u. 5	1155 Budapest
Pálfia, Ernó	Mátray u. 5-7. fsz. 1	1012 Budapest
Pánczél, Ibolya	Lenin u. 11. I. 9	1155 Budapest
Pánczél, Márta	Petőfi u. 35	6800 Hodmezővásárhely
Pápai, Ibolya	Aradi vértanuk tere 3	6720 Szeged
Pék, László	Lumumba u. 89	1149 Budapest
Pénzes, Tibor	Kórház, Szemosztály	8500 Pápa
Péterfy, Margit	Kun u. 12	1081 Budapest
Pétery, Miklós	Puskás tér 12. fsz. 1	1119 Budapest
Pilaszanovich, Ildikó	Münnich G. u. 16/c	7633 Pécs
Pintér, Erzsébet	Münich F. u. 16/b	7633 Pécs
Pintér, Éva	Ső u. 5	1056 Budapest
Pintér, László	Kórház, Szemészet	3200 Gyöngyös
Pirityi, Károly	Gyulai u. 1	5600 Békéscsaba
Podhorányi, György	Tömő u. 25-29	1083 Budapest
Pohli, Ferenc	Pécsi u. 45	7300 Komlo
Polgár, József	Szemklinika	6701 Szeged
Pré, Magdolna	Mártirok u. 61-63	1024 Budapest
Prohászka, Mária	V. Felszabadulástér 3	2800 Tatabánya
Puskás, Mária	Szőllőhegy	8600 Siófok
Pusztai, Lenke	Attila u. 15	6722 Szeged
Raák, Endre	Geisler u. 1	7625 Pécs
Rácz, József	Városi Kórház	3700 Kazincbarcika
Rácz, Péter	Geisler E. u. 9	7625 Pécs
Radnót, Magda	Rákóczi u. 27/b	1088 Budapest
Radó, István	János u. 4	2132 Felsőgöd
Rávnay, Márta	Petőfi u. 75	7623 Pécs
Regéci, Mária	Szaboles köz 4A 1h. II	3600 Ozd
Rehák, Ágnes	Hunyadi J. u. 1	7400 Kaposvár
Remenár, László	Jagello u, 13	1124 Budapest
Rénes, Margit	Pf. 187	3501 Miskolc
Réthy, István	Árpád fej. u. 49. III	1036 Budapest
Réz, Flóra	Damjanich u. 28/b	1071 Budapest
Salacz, György	Erkel u. 20	1092 Budapest
Sallai, Sándor	Kórház, Szemészet	8900 Zalaegerszeg
Sas, Gizella	Katona J. u. 28	1137 Budapest
Sáfrán, Stefánia	Sztahanov u. 8	3100 Salgótarján
Sármány, Judit	Lepke Köz 4	1026 Budapest
Schnitzler, Ágota	Szemklinika	4012 Debrecen
Sebestyén, János	János u. 6	7621 Pécs
Seres, Géza	Széchenyi u. 27	4025 Debrecen
Séthy, Viktor	Hollósi Simon u. 38	1126 Budapest
Singer, Gyula	Madách I. tér 7	1075 Budapest
Sipos, Irma	Pálu. 2	1085 Budapest

Solymos, Gizella	Kárpát u. 5	1133 Budapest
Somody, Lászlóné	Semmelweis u. 4	7623 Pécs
Somogyi, Ilona	Rendelőintézet	3780 Edelény
Somogyi, Zoltán	Hatvan u. 12	4025 Debrecen
Somogyvári, Éva	Királyhágó u. 5/a	1126 Budapest
Sternberg, Alice	Garibaldi u. 3	1054 Budapest
Strenger, János	VT. Kórház, Szemészet	7901 Szigetvár
Süveges, Ildikó	Dóczi J. u. 26	4032 Debrecen
Szabó, György	Guszev u. 7	1215 Budapest
Szabó, György	Szegedi u. 24/b	6900 Mako
Szabó, Gyula	Horváth Z. u. 2	6100 Kiskunfélegyháza
Szabó, Károly	Bajcsy Zs. u. 27	6800 Hodmezővásárhely
Szabó, Márto	Ady E. u. 43	1203 Budapest
Szabó, Zoltán	Baross u. 19. I. 1	1088 Budapest
Szalay, Edit	Attila u. 79	1012 Budapest
Szalay, Judit	Tanács krt. 8	1052 Budapest
Szalőczi, Károly	Tanácsköztársaság u. 42	8360 Keszthely
Szatmáry, Sándor	Sallai Imre u. 33/b	1136 Budapest
Szegedi, László	Rend. Int. Szemészet	9200 Mosonmagyarovár
Szeghy, Gergely	Beloiannisz u. 12. I. 1	5000 Szolnok
Szekeres, Márta	Szász K. u. 1	1027 Budapest
Szendrey, Gábor	Hurok u. 13	1091 Budapest
Szerneva, Evelina	Szlovák ut 7	1162 Budapest
Székely, István	Eötvös u. 40	1153 Budapest
Szigeti Zoltán, Tibor	Hunyadi u. 51/a, B/4	9700 Szombathely
Sziklai, Árpád	Baross tér 20	1077 Budapest
Szilvássy, Ildikó	Jókai u. 51	7622 Pécs
Szirmák, Éva	Trombitás u. 27	1026 Budapest
Szitás, Márta	Olympia u. 11. I. 3	3200 Gyöngyös
Szivák, Kunigunda	Deák F. u. 8	6500 Baja
Szlamka, Klára	Földmüves u. 22	6725 Szeged
Sztrilich, Lajos	Arany J. u. 2	7150 Bonyhád
Szabó, Márta	Balfasor 34	6701 Szeged
Szakolczay, Zita	Kórház, Szemészet	3700 Kazincbarcika
Szalay, Eszter	H. Fő u. 92	8600 Siófok
Szalay, László	Pf. 407	6701 Szeged
Szarvas, Éva	Rómer Fl. u. 34	1020 Budapest
Szaniszló, Angela	Pf. 407	6701 Szeged
Szentes, Emese Ildikó	Liptó u. 9/a	1124 Budapest
Sziklai, Pál	Pf. 407	6701 Szeged
Takács, Edit	Ferenczy I. u. 28	1053 Budapest
Takáts, István	Athinay u. 6. A/1	7623 Pécs
Takó, Károly	Szekfü u. 2/a	2230 Gyömrő
Tamási, Stefánia	Pf. 188	3501 Miskolc
Tapasztó, István, Imre	Villám u. 8	6000 Kecskemét
Tapasztó, István András	Villám u. 8	6000 Kegskemét
Tarnóctzky, Klára	Megyei Kórház, Szemészet	3501 Miskolc
Tátrai, Katalin	Csengery u. 25	1074 Budapest
Thész, László	Munkácsy M. u. 9	7100 Szekszárd
Técsy, Sára	Könyves K. u. 25	3534 Miskolc
Timár, Mária	Középfasor 13/c	6726 Szeged
Tóth-Bagi, Zita	Nagyerdei krt. 98	4032 Debrecen
Tóth, Berenc	Lenin krt. 93	1067 Budapest
Tóth, Jusztinia	VT. Kórház, Szemészet	5301 Karcak
Tóth, Margit	Kacsóh P. u. 5	1146 Budapest
Tóth, Zoltán	Népköztársaság u. 6	1061 Budapest

Tóth, Pál	8 Pf. 7	1428 Budapest
Tóthkomlósy, Sarolta	Benczur u. 35/c	1068 Budapest
Tötök, Éva	Dagály u. 6	1138 Budapest
Török, Irén	Megyei Kórház, Szemo	9700 Szombathely
Török, Magdolna	Egyetem tér 1	4032 Debrecen
Törs, Eszter	József u. 9	1084 Budapest
Trux, Erzsébet	Karinthy F. u. 16. VI. 62	1111 Budapest
Turbucz, Irma	Rendelőintézet	9600 Sárvár
Turi, Károly	Dohány u. 12	1077 Budapest
Tihor, János	Pf. 19	3001 Hatvan
Tokaji, Ida	Megyei Kórház, Szemészet	4043 Debrecen
Török, Ildikó	Kórház, Szemészet	4100 Berettyoujfalu
Takáts, Éva	Attila u. 31	1013 Budapest
Tasnádi, Ilona	Rendelőintézet, Szemészet	2000 Szentendre
Uhrin, Mária	Paulay E. u. 57	1061 Budapest
Uzonyi, György	Semmelweis u. 4	1052 Budapest
Vadász, Zsuzsa	Kresz G. u. 26	1132 Budapest
Vajda, Péter	Városi Kórház	5900 Orosháza
Valenta, Andtás	Táncsics tér 3	3980 Sátoraljaujhely
Val kó, Éva	Balassa u. 6	1083 Budapest
Valu, László	Megyei Kórház, Szemészet	9700 Szombathely
Varga, Béla	Pf. 15	3300 Eger
Varga, Margit	Victor Hugó u. 36	1132 Budapest
Vargha, Emilia	Henvéd u. 3	7624 Pécs
Vass, Zoltán	Partizán u. 16. I. 3	6722 Szeged
Vastag, Oszkár	Epitők utja 1	7633 Pécs III
Várhegyi, Zoltán	Szentpéteri kapu	3526 Miskolc
Váry, István	Pasaréti u. 32	1026 Budapest
Vereb, Katalin	Frankel L. u. 88-90	1023 Budapest
Vermes, Elly	Majakovszkij u. 43/45	1072 Budapest
Véli, Margit	Szüret u. 23. I. 1	1118 Budapest
Vén, Rezső	Sztahanov u. 8	3100 Salgótarján
Vigváry, László	Kórház, RTG Osztály	4400 Nyiregháza
Villányi, Mária	Irottkő park 8. I. 6	1142 Budapest
Virág, Márta	Fodor u. 7	1126 Budapest
Vogt, Ferenc	Szepesi u. 136	1161 Budapest
Vönöczky, Katalin	Szentpéteri kapu 72	3526 Miskolc
Vörös, Márta	Szabolcs u. 33-35	1135 Budapest
Vörösmarthy, Dániel	Rákóczi u. 4	2092 Budkeszi
Walawka, Joanna	Béke u. 10	3900 Szerencs
Weinstein, Pál	Balassi B. u. 9. /11	1055 Budapest
Winkler, Mária	Győri u. 15	9400 Sopron
Zajácz, Magdolna	Szemklinika	4012 Debrecen
Záborszky, Judit	Pozsonyi u. 82	3526 Miskolc
Zájer, József	Németvölgyi u. 13	1126 Budapest
Zolnai, Antal	Petőfi u. 24	4220 Hajduböszörmeny
Zoltán, Katalin	Róbert K. krt. 44	1134 Budapest

NOSOCOMIA, INSTITUTA, SCHOLAEQUE

No data received.

INDIA

SOCIETATES OPHTHALMOLOGICAE

Nationalis

All-India Ophthalmological Society

Bureau: Sarojini Sadan, Congress House, V. Patel Road, Bombay 400 004
President: Dr. M. Sengupta
Vice-Presidents: Dr. M. C. Misra, Dr. B. D. Telang
Hon. Gen. Secretary: Dr. D. G. Mody
Jt. Hon. Secretary: Dr. R. P. Dhanda
Hon. Treasurer: Dr. A. G. Sardesai
Jt. Hon. Treasurer: Dr. J. Agarwal
Editor-Journal: Dr. S. R. K. Malik

Regionales

Bihar Ophthalmological Society
New Area (Near Blind School), Kadamkuan, Patna – 3
Secretary: Dr. Gopal Prasad
Number of members: 57

Ophthalmological Society of West Bengal
94, Chittaranjan Avenue, Calcutta – 12
Secretary: Dr. P. Mondal
Number of members: 175

Bombay Ophthalmologists' Association
c/o T.N. Medical College Staff Room, A. Nair Road, Bombay – 8
Secretary: Dr. P. Dikshit
Number of members: 60

Darbhanga Ophthalmological Society
Darbhanga Medical College, P.O. - D.M.C., Darbhanga (Bihar)
Secretary: Dr. Basantkumar Singh
Number of members: 41

Delhi Ophthalmological Society
B–2, Bhagwandass Nagar, New Delhi – 26
Secretary: Dr. A. C. Chadha
Number of members: 93

Gujarat Ophthalmological Society
M & J Institute of Ophthalmology, Civil Hospital, Ahmedabad – 16
Secretary: Dr. V. Kalevar
Number of members: 60

Hyderabad Ophthalmological Association
Sarojini Devi Eye Hospital, Hyderabad (Andhra)
Secretary: Dr. N. Subramanya Reddy
Number of members: 99

Madya Pradesh State Ophthalmological Society
Medical College, Jabalpur
Secretary: Dr. S. C. Batalia
Number of members: 54

Madras City Ophthalmological Association
155/1, Lloyd Road, Madras – 14
Secretary: Lt. Col. V. Rangachari
Number of members: 45

The Madras State Ophthalmological Association
48, Puthna High Road, Puthur, Tiruchurapalli
Secretary:
Number of members: 150

Mysore State Ophthalmological Society
127/1, Bull Temple Road, Bangalore – 19
Secretary: Dr. K. Eswar
Number of members: 45

Orissa State Ophthalmological Society
S.C.B. Medical College Campus, Cuttack
Secretary: Dr. B. Rajguru
Number of members: 26

U.P. State Ophthalmological Society
J.N. Medical College, Muslim University, Alirgarh
Secretary: Dr. O. P. Ahuja
Number of members: 106

NOMINA ET DOMICILIA MEDICORUM AB OCULIS

Abdul Sathar, A.	218, West Masi Street	Madurai (Madras State)
Abraham, John Edwin	Schell Eye Hospital	Vellore (S.I.)
Abreau, R.	May Villa, Victoria Rd.	Bombay-27
Acharya, Chandidas	C-2/8, Gangail Road	Agartala P.O. (Tripura)
Acharya, Dhirendra N.	Q. No. SD9 – Medical College,	
	Burla P.O.	Sambalpur (Orissa)
Adhvaryoo, B. G.	C.M.O., Sausrashtra, C. Hosp.	Virnagar (Saurashtra)
Adrianwalla S.	Tafti Mansion, Kohimoor Rd.,	
	Dadar	Bombay-14

Agarwal, D. C.	E.1. Medical Enclaves	Patiala (Punjab)
Agarwal, D. P.	Dept. of Ophthalmology, Medical College	Panaji
Agarwal, Gokuldas	Central Hosp., Jawahar Marg 3rd floor	Indore (M.P.)
Agarwal, Gyanchand	M.. D. Eye Hospital	Allahabad (U.P.)
Agarwal, G. K.	A.M.O. N.E.Rly. Hospital	Bareilly (U.P.)
Agarwal, Hari Shanker	18/IE, Jamir Lane	Calcutta-19
Agarwal, Jaiveer	29-C, Edward Elliots Rd.	Madras-4
Agarwal, Lalit P., Prof.	R.P. Centre for Ophth. Sc. A.I.I.M.S.	New Delhi - 16
Agarwal, Prof. Mohanial ...	Medical College	Gwalior (M.P.)
Agarwal, R. C.	26-D, Connaught Place	New Delhi
Agarwal, Ram Prakash	Barabanki Eye Hospital, Munsiganj	Barabanki (U.P.)
Agarwal, Tahira	29-C Edward Elliots Rd.	Madras-4
Ahikrishna, Rednam	Rednam Gdns., Jail Road P.O. Waltair R.S.	Vishakhapatnam-4 (A.P.)
Ahluwalia, Charanjitsingh ..	A.K. Hospital	Beawar (Rajputana)
Ahluwalia, P. P.	495, Napier Town	Jabalpur (M.P.)
Ahmed, Amiruddin T.	A/17, Nasehmum, S. Thillai-Nagar	Tiruchirapalli-3 (Madras State)
Ahmed, Bashiruddin	M. D. Road	Nowgong (Assam)
Ahmed, Ema juddin	3-A, Congress Exhib. Road	Calcutta-17
Ahmed, Sayed Hafiz	Med. College	Jabalpur (M.P.)
Ahuja, Bulchand	Jawahar Nagar	Raipur (M.P.)
Ahuja, O. P.	M.U.I.C. Gandhi Eye Hosp.	Aligarh (U.P.)
Albal, Madhusudan V.	'Padma', Hotgi Road	Sholapur (M.S.)
Ambeker, Dinkar A.	Vaibhav, Post Office Rd.	Jalna (Maharashtra)
Angra, Surendra Kumar ...	R.P. Centre for Ophth. Sc. A.I.I.M.S.	New Delhi-16
Anklesaria, E. D.	Railwaypura	Ahmedabad-2 (Gujarat)
Anklesaria, S. D.	53, Katrak Parsi Colony	Karachi (Pakistan)
Annaswami, Subbier	5, Hanumantha Rao St. T. Nagar .	Madras - 17
Ansari, Abid M. Hussain ...	At & Post	Hasua, Dist. Gaya (Bihar)
Apte, Chandrakant S.	217, Goldenfinch Peth	Sholapur (Maharashtra)
Arora, Geeta	398, Napier Town	Jabalpur (M.P.)
Arya, Raghuvir Singh	Raghuvir Nursing Home	Chandpur, Dist. Bijnor (U.P.)
Arya, Yogesh B.	Eye Hosp., P.O.	Unjha, Dist. Mehsana (Gujarat)
Ashraf, Prof. Md. Hassan ..	Rajendra Med. College	Ranchi - 9
Athavle, Sadashiv D.	Navipeth	Jalgaon (Khandesh)
Avadesh, Prasad	Dehri-on-Sone	Dehri (Bihar)
Avasthy, P.	Medical College	Agra (U.P.)
Ayachit, S. D.	Dist. Hospital	Satna (M.P.)
Badlani, H. G.	Office Bldg. No. 6 Plant Nagar, Ghatkopar	Bombay-75
Bagchi, S. K.	Chatterji Memorial Eye Hosp. Upper Circular Rd.	Calcutta-9
Bagmar, Madanchand	K.C.P. Hospital, P.O.	Khetrinagar (Rajasthan)
Baijal, Girish Chandra	6, Shanti Nagar, Nai Sarak	Gwalior - 1 (M.P.)
Bajaj, M. S.	S/195, Gr. Kailash No. 1	New Delhi
Bajaj, Prakash Kumar	Tilak Nagar, Main Rd.	Balispur (M.P.)
Bakre, H. Y.	Rukmini Nivas	Jaljaon (Khandesh)
Baldev, Singh	Astley Hall	Dehra Dun (U.P.)
Baldha, Chunilal R.	Jubilee Chowk	Rajkot-1 (Saurashtra)

Bhave, L. S.	1476, Sadashiv, Opp. S.P. College, Tilak Rd.	Poona-4
Bhide, Ashok Vishnu	5, Shraddhanand Peth	Nagpur - 3
Bhide, Madhukar G.	619, Budhwar Peth	Poona-2
Bhide, Nandkumar	Bokaro Gen. Hospital P.O.	Bokaro Steel City (Dhanbad)
Bhinder, Gurbax Singh	Dept. of Ophthalmology M.A. Medical College	New Delhi
Bhiwapurkar, K. B.	Ramdas Peth	Nagpur
Bhor, Ananth Bandhu	Lal Baghan	Post Chandanwal, Dist. Hugli
Bhura, Prabhavati	770, Sarafa	Jabalpur (M.P.)
Bhutani, J. C.	B/8, Rajori Gardens	New Delhi-27
Billimoria, N. P.	61, Burns Way, Heston	Middlesex (England)
Bishnu, Anilkumar	Military Hospital	Jhansi (M.P.)
Biswas, Samir K.	18/8, Ballygunge Place East	Calcutta-19
Bodiwalla, Govindlal R. ...	Govind Niwas, Maninagar	Ahmedabad-8
Bokil, Madhav D.	Arogyadarshan, 3 Yadav Gopal Peth	Satara City
Boparai, Manjit Singh	Military Hospital	Jullunder Cantt
Bose, Dhrub Kumar	Road 6−B, Rajendra Nagar	Patna-4
Bose, Jyotimoy	Flat 2, Block D, Govt. Emp. Hsg. Estate, 82, Belgachia Road ..	Calcutta-37
Bose, Nilamdhab	34−Harish Mukerjee Road	Calcutta-25
Brahmbhatt, Thakorlal	Brahmpuri, Dandia Bazar	Baroda (Gujarat)
Brij, Mohanlal	Ripon Hospital	Simla (H.P.)
Bupathy, Radhakrishnan ..	7, Marslvalls Road, Egnore	Madras-8
Bujarborua, Dhirendranath .	Eye Dept., Assam Med. College ...	Dibrugarh (Assam)
Byramji, Tehmas D.	127, M.G. Road	Secunderabad (A.P.)
Candamurty, S.	182, Barathiar Road, Karaikel P.O.	Pondicherry
Chacko, P. T.	Puthenpurayil, Kalamsery Ernakulam Univ. Centre P.O.	Cochin-22 (Kerala)
Chadda, M. R.	C−2, Medical Enclave, Circular Road	Amritsar (Punjab)
Chahwala, Jitendra C.	Chandulal Seth's St., Sayedpura .	Surat (Gujarat)
Chakraborty, J. N.	33, Bhupen Bose Avenue	Calcutta-4
Chakravarti, I. B.	Jubilee Mission Hospital	Trichur-5
Chakaraborty, Susanta	14/2 Girish Bidhyananda Lane ..	Calcutta-9
Chakraborti, Susilkumar ...	63 K.C. Sen Road, Morepukur ..	Rishra, Dist. Hoogaly
Chakravarty, G. R.	Jalpaiguri Hospital	Jalpaiguri (W.B.)
Chanda, Nagendra Nath ...	73, Rishi Bankimchandra Rd. ...	Calcutta-34
Chandra, D. B.	M.D. Eye Hospital	Allahabad (U.P.)
Chandra, Giriah	Dept. of Ophthalmology, K.G. Med. College	Lucknow (U.P.)
Chandra, N. K.	76, Bipin Bihari Ganguly Street .	Calcutta-12
Chandra, Sekaran T. S......	Madurai Med. College	Madurai Tamil Nadu
Charegaonkar, S. M.	Uma Nivas, D.L. Vaidya Rd. Dadar	Bombay-28
Chaudhry, Jagdish Lal	V.P.O.-Dhankot	Dist. Gurgaon (Haryana)
Chaudhuri, Sucheta	321/11, Russ Rd. South	Calcutta-33
Char, V. A.	69, Pritam No. 7, 11th Road, Khar	Bombay 52 AS
Chatterjee, A.	Eye Services to Villages C.M.C. ..	Ludhiana (Punjab)
Chatterjee, A.	Christian Medical College	Ludhiana (Punjab)
Chatterjee, Bankim C.	SSLNT Eye Hospital	Dhanbad (Bihar)
Chatterjee, Brojo M.	53, Chittaranjan Avenue	Calcutta-12

Chatterjee, Sakti Pada	Asansol Optical, G.T. Road	Asansol (W.B.)
Chaudhar, O. P.	Chowk Ghantaghar	Sirsa (Haryana)
Chaudhury, C. D.	Type 4–94, P.O.	Baravani Urwarak Nagar, Dist. Monghyr (Bihar)
Chaudhury, Chandra Mohan.	66 H.O.R., P.O. Darbhanga Medical College	Dist. Darbhanga (Bihar)
Chaudhuri, P. Mohan	5/1/2, Cornfield Row	Calcutta-19
Chaudhuri, P. N.	56, Dharamtolla St.	Calcutta
Chaukar, A. R.	Post - K.H.I.	Ghataprabha, Dist. Belgaum
Chhabra, B. S.	Jivan Hosp. & Mat. Home	Bharatipur, Jabalpur (M.P.)
Chhabra, H. N.	Ophthalmic Dept., S.M.S. Med. College	Jaipur (Rajasthan)
Chhabra, O. P.	Blind Relief Association, Dhantoli	Nagpur
Chhadha, A. C.	B/2, Bhagwandas Nagar	Delhi-26
Chug, Kuldeepsingh	House No. 38, Public Park	Shriganganagar (Rajasthan)
Chhapan, Rasiklal J.	190/B, Opp. Nehru Nagar S.M.Rd., Ambawadi	Ellis Bridge, Ahmedabad-15
Chhaya, Sukhwantarai	c/o Dr. D. P. Chhaya, Tilak Road	Bulsar (W. Rly.)
Chitale, A. S.	C/9, Med. College Campus	Jamnagar (Saurashtra)
Chitnis, V. K.	Krishna Nivas, Queens Rd.	Bombay-4
Cholia, Paritosh R.	'Urmi' 10th Road, Khar	Bombay-52
Chopra, Suresh Kumar	Eye Dept., Christian Med. College	Ludhiana (Punjab)
Chowdhari, Naresh S.......	12, Ravikunj, Jawahar Nagar, Coregagon	Bombay-62
Chowdhary, Chhedi	12, Radhika Inst. Road	Padna - 1 (Bihar)
Chowdhary, Badalkanti ...	76, Acharya Prafullachandra Road	Calcutta-9
Chowdhary, O. P.	Balkrishna Hospital, Krishnan Nagar	Hoshiarpur
Chudasama, V. A.	Eye Clinic, Ranjit Road	Jamnagar (Saurashtra)
Coapullai, J. A.	Arogyacaram Hospital	Somapeta, Dist. Srikakulam (A.P.)
Consul, Prof. B. N.	Nehru Inst. of Ophthalmic Research, Eye Hospital	Sitapur (U.P.)
Cooper, S. N.	21, Queen's Road	Bombay-4
Daljit, Singh	Med. College	Amritsar (Punjab)
Dandekar, B. M.	....	Aurangabad (Marathwada)
Daniel, Richard	C.M.C. & Hospital	Ludhiana (Punjab)
Das, A.B.	A.F.M.C.	Poona-1
Das, Amarkumar	18, Rajvallabh Saha Lane	Howrah-1
Das, Bibhudatta	Q. No. 3R/3	Dist. Sambhalpur (Orissa)
Das, Brajnand	Medical College	Berhampur-4 (Orissa)
Das, Chandi	S.C.B. Med. College	Cuttack-7 (Orissa)
Das, N. C.	113/168, Swarup Nagar	Kanpur 2 (U.P.)
Das, P. C.	B. R. Singh Hospital	Calcutta-14
Das, Panani Shanker	Kopil Pharmacy 3, Gharga Lane .	Calcutta-32
Das, Santosh Kumar	Radhakrishna Sebayatan P.O. ...	Mondir Bazar, 24 Parganas
Day, Subhas Chandra	21, Shahitiya Parishad Street ...	Calcutta-6
Day, Shrimati	21, Shahitiya Parishad Street ...	Calcutta-6
Das, Subarata	27, Cantonment	Shillong (Assam)
Dastoor, Adi H.	375, D. Maorojo Rd., Fort	Bombay-1
Dastoor, H. D.	375, D. Naoroji Road, Fort	Bombay-1
Dastur, K. J.	Ferena, Behind Telephone Bhavan, Colaba	Bombay-5
Datta, Chandidas	33/70, Nabinchandra Das Rd. Baranagar	Calcutta-50

Datta, Kanak Ranjan	Civil Hospital	Mokochung (Nagaland)
Dave, Devendra H.	A/4, Daulat Vihar Co-op. Hsg. Secty. 57/58, Dadabhai Road, Vile Parle	Bombay-56
Dave, Rasiklal D.	....	Rajkot (Saurashtra)
Dave, S. A.	Ramkuver Eye Hospital	Veraval, Dist. Junagadh (Saurashtra)
Dave, V. P.	Dr. Karachiwala Eye Clinic	Dhrangadhra (Gujarat)
David, Daniel	c/o Mr. D. Williams, Palani Gowader St.	Coimbatore-9
Daval, Y.	A.I.I.M.S.	New Delhi-16
Desai, C. B.	Ashvini Prasad	Miraj Dist. Sangli
Desai, Jayendra C.	Eye Clinic, Pragnath Rd.	Sihor (Saurashtra)
Desai, Krishnamurari K. ...	Near Post Office Restampura ...	Surat-2 (Guj.)
Desai, Meenakshi R.	Aditya Ambawadi, Ellis Bridge ..	Ahmedabad (Guj.)
Desai, P. L.	Tanksali Bhuvan, Opp. City Courts, Bhadra	Ahmedabad (Gujarat)
Desai, Ramesh J.	Ramnivas No. 2, Khanpur	Ahmedabad (Guj.)
Desai, Rameschandra M. ...	Mani Mahetwad	Bulsar (Gujarat)
Desai, Ratilal G.	Shraddha Eye Hospital, Nagarwad	Navsari (Guj)
Desai, Rohiniben	Ramnivas No. 2, Khanpur	Ahmedabad-1
Desai, Vishnubhai K.	'Jyoti' Pratap Road	Baroda-5 (Guj.)
Deshmukh, L. N.	1204/2, Ghole Road Shivaji Negar	Poona-5
Dhanda, R. P.	Inst. of Ophthalmology, New Civil Hospital	Ahmedabad-16
Dhanwant, Singh	Govt. Medical College	Patiala (Punjab)
Dhir, Balraj K.	Gandhi Eye Hospital	Aligarh (U.P.)
Dhruv, Hasmukh J.	Devlatta, 10 Panchnath Plot	Rajkot (Gujarat)
Dhurandhar, C. B.	112, Habib Bldg., Girgaon	Bombay-4
Dikshit, P. A.	Above Eastern Stores Stn. Rd., Santa Cruz (West)	Bombay-54
Doctor, Jayesh N.	Spenta Mansion, S.V. Road, Andheri	Bombay-58
Dongre, Ramesh Chandra ..	Nehru Medical College	Raipur (M.P.)
Dordi, H. K.	Dhun House, 4, Tejpal Rd.	Bombay-7
Doshi, Devendra M.	Opp. R. R. Girls' School	Surendranagar (Saurashtra)
Dishi, Kishor J.	Himanshu, 15, Ramkrishna Nagar	Rajkot-2 (Guj.)
Doshi, Ramniklal R.	Station Rd.	Anand (Gujarat)
Dubere, A. V.	Eye Hosp., Opp: Oil Industries ..	Latur, Dist. Oosmanabad
Dudhia, R. L.	Raipur	Ahmedabad (Gujarat)
Dukhan, Ram	Exhibition Road	Patna (Bihar)
Duraiswami, T. S.	Rajeshwari Gardens, Madeley Rd.	Madras-17
Dutta, Anutosh	1/26, Rupchand Muganjee Lane .	Calcutta-25
Dutta, Lakshman C.	Medical College	Gauhati (Assam)
Dwivedi, D. N.	Western Ry. Hospital	Rajkot (Guj.)
Dwivedi, Prakash Chandra .	N.E.Ry.	Gorakhpur (U.P.)
Eswara, Kalasa	127/1, Bell Temple Road	Bangalore-19
Fernandez, T. Simon	Little Flower Hospital	Angamally (Kerala)
Ferreira J. F.	Largo De Igrefa	Goa
Firdosi, A. H.	M-ah Fooz Manzil Kampoo	Gwalior (M.P.)
Gajaria, A. T.	96/3383, Nehru Nagar Kurla (East)	Bombay-70
Gambhir, Narendra Kumar .	M. G. Hospital	Bhidwara (Rajasthan)
Ganadhikam, R. L.	9–B, Birds Road	Trichy (Tamil Nadu)
Gandhewar, Ramakrishna ..	Med. College Colony, Q. No. B/1/2, Ajni	Nagpur

Ghandi, A. H.	ESI Disp. No. 25, Near Hathikai Garden, Gomtipur	Ahmedabad-21
Ghandi, O. M.	Near Lal Gate	Surat (Gujarat)
Gandhi, V. H.	Sonawala Bldg.. Tardeo	Bombay-7
Ganga, Roa M.	Shr Venkateshrwara	Tanuku (W. Godaveri Dist)
Ganguli, Debaprased	4, Maharaja Kumar Road	Calcutta-29
Gangully, Ardhendu K.	14/3, Gariahat Road	Calcutta-19
Gantayet, S.	Town Hall Rd.	Berhampur, Dist. Ganjam
Gantayet, Usharani	Town Hall Rd.	Berhampur, Dist. Ganjam (Orissa)
Garg, Bhim Sain	Eye Dept., P.G. Institute	Chandigarh (E.P.)
Garg, Ghanashyamdas	c/o M/s. Jairaj Ghanashyamdas, Hospital Road	Bhatinda (Punjab)
Garg, Kailash Chandra	K.G. Medical College	Lucknow (U.P.)
Garg, M. P.	Eye Hospital	Sitapur (U.P.)
Garkal, Reghubir Singh	40, Hanuman Road	New Delhi
Garla, Ramiah Chetty	Andhra Medical College	Vishakhapatnam (A.P.)
Ghai, K. R.	c/o A.O.C. Hospital	Digboi (Assam)
Ghaswalla, K. S.	Nr. Govt. of India Offices 97, Karve Rd.	Bombay-20
Ghate, M. L.	Cama Plots	Akola (Vidarbha)
Ghose, Nirmal K.	99, Park Street	Calcutta-16
Ghose, Gopi Krishna	34/B, B.K. Pal Aveneu	Calcutta-5
Ghose, C. K.	12, Bhupendra Bose Avenue	Calcutta-4
Ghosh, Aloke	26, Chowringhee Road, Room No. 34	Calcutta-13
Ghosh, Prakash Chandra	28/1-A, Garihat Road	Calcutta-19
Ghosh, Pratike	Plot No. 404, Block G, New Alipur	Calcutta
Ghosh, Ramchandra	44/14/1, Brindadan Mallick Lane, Kadamtola	Howrah (W.B.)
Ghosh, Swetketu	12, Bhupen Bose Avenue	Calcutta-2
Ghosh, Tushar Kanti	C/70, Sector 19	Rourkela - 22 (Orissa)
Ghulam, Nabi	Khanquahi – Mualla	Shinagar (Kashmir)
Gian, Singh Raikhi	Civil Hospital	Moga (Punjab)
Giridhar, N. D.	K. J. Free Eye Hospital	Bhiwani, Dist. Hissar
Girdhar, P. D.	K. J. Free Eye Hospital	Bhiwani, Dist. Hissar
Girdhar, R. D.	K. J. Free Eye Hospital	Bhiwani, Dist. Hissar
Gnandikam, R. J.	Swedish Mission Hosp.	Tiruputtur, Dist. Ramnad
Goel, Baldev Kishen	Ripon Hosp.	Simla (H.P.)
Goel, B. S.	206, Greater Kailash	New Delhi-48
Goel, D. N.	Eye Clinic, Davendra Bazar	Jammu (Kashmir)
Goei, Indubhushan	Medical College	Indore (M.P.)
Gogoi, Padamkumar	Jorhat Civil Hospital	Jorhat-1
Gokhale, A. M.	380, N.C. Kelkar Road	Bombay-28
Gokhale, S. A.	A/4, Sahaker Nivas, Off Gokhale Road South	Bombay-28
Gopalan Nair, K. N.	Tirur, Kozhikode Dist.	Kerala
Gopalkrishna, Rao B.	145, Broadway	
Goswami, Anirudha	23/10, Gariahat Road	Calcutta-19
Goswami, A. P.	Goswami Sadan 15/210, Dudwala Bungalow, Civil Lines	Kanpur (U.P.)
Goswami, B. L.	Dist. Hosp.	Saugor (M.P.)
Goswami, Subhash	R.P. Cent. of Ophth. Sc. A.I.I.M.S.	New Delhi-16
Govindrajulu, N.	23/B, Sterling Road	Madras-34

Grewal, Surjutsingh	Gurudev Nagar	Ludhiana (Punjab)
Growar, S. S.	150, General Hospital	C/o 56 A.P.O.
Guha, Ajit Kumar	Dak Bungalow Road	Patna-1 (Bihar)
Guha, Dangobinda	Qr. G5, Uluberia Sub Div.	Dist. Howrah (W.B.)
Guha, D. N.	M. R. Bangur Hospital	Calcutta-33
Guha, P. K.	8, N.C. Mitter Road	Calcutta-28
Guha, S. K.	184, S.P. Mukherjee Rd.	Calcutta-26
Gulati, G. C.	Med. College & Hosp., Kankarbagh Rd.	Patna-1 (Bihar)
Gunaji, Satchidanand	Military Hospital, Eye Department	Jabalpur (M.P.)
Gupta, Amiya Kumar	28, Apurkia Mitra Rd.	Calcutta-26
Gupta, A. K.		Jipmer (Pondicherry-6)
Gupta, Babulal	Civil Hospital	Jhabua (M.P.)
Gupta, B. S. I.	Anandram Jaipuria Hosp.	Nawalgarh (Raj)
Gupta, Chandra P.	50, Santhome High Rd.	Madras-28
Gupta, D. P.	Civil Hospital	Hissar (Haryana)
Gupta, Daulal		Jhabua (M.P.)
Gupta, G. P.	Inst. of Ophthalmology, Gandhi Eye Hospital	Aligarh (U.P.)
Gupta, Kaulendra Kumar	L. 27. Medical College Campus	Kanpur-2
Gupta, Madan Gopal	c/o M/s. Krishna Med Hall, Palace Road	Jammu (Kashmir)
Gupta, P. C.	Bachelor's Quarters, Patna Med. Coll. Hosp.	Patna-4 (Bihar)
Gupta, Prakash Chand	Prem Eye Hosp., G. T. Road	Jullunder City (E. Punjab)
Gupta, Prabhansu K.	1, Rammoy Road	Calcutta-25
Gupta, Ram Kumar	M.E.S. Hospital	Kota (Rajasthan)
Gupta, S. D.	P.G.I. Sector	Chandigarh (Punjab)
Gupta, S. K.	Military Hospital	Bareilly (U.P.)
Gupta, Surendra D.	Gupta Clinic	Bhagalpur (Bihar)
Gupta, Prof. S. P.	Rana Pratap Marg, Opp. Shahnazaf	Lucknow (U.P.)
Gupta, Sushil Kumar	Civil Hospital, P.O. Bagha Purana	Faridkot (Punjab)
Gupta, Tej. Bahadur	Road No. 7, Rajendranagar	Patna-16 (Bihar)
Gupta, T. N.	1/25, Sector IX	Bhilainagar (M.P.)
Gupta, U. C.	Trachoma Control Project, Gandhi Eye Hospital	Aligarh (U.P.)
Guptarye, M. C.	P.O.	Sasaram (Bihar)
Gurubatham, K. G.	Subramaniam Nagar	Salem-5 (Madras)
Gurubax, Singh	Rly. Rd. Nawanshahr	Doaba, Dist. Jullunder
Gyasuddin, S.	S. D. Eye Hosp.	Hyderabad (Andhra)
Hans, Raj	Vidhan Sabha Marg	Lucknow
Hari, Charan	Laxmi Kunj, Malavia Marg, Ashok Nagar	Jaipur-1 (Rajasthan)
Harinandan, Yadav	Darbhanga Medical College	Laheria Sarai, Darbhanga (Bihar)
Hariprased, Rao G.	Bose Road Tenali Post	Tenali Post Guntur (A.P.)
Harnandha, Banu N.	Bose Rd. Tenali Post	Tenali Post Guntur (A.P.)
Hasem, S. M. H.	R.M.O. Minto Hospital	Bangalore-2
Hathi, H. J.	Hathi Cottage, Sardarpura	Jodhpur (Raj)
Hardia, Pratap Singh	68, Hardia Compound	Indore-1 (M.P.)
Hebbar Kattingeri, Indira.	Dr. Hebbar's Eye Clinic, Trunk Rd.	Nellore (Andhra)
Harshadkumar, R.	Desai Bldg., Station Road	Nadiad (Gujerat)
Hatim, D. M.	Mahatma Gandhi Road	Dohad, Dist. Panchamahal
Hazari, K. K.	9, Jatindra Mohan Ave	Calcutta-6 (W.B.)

Hazarika, K. Hussain	B 4131, Safdarjang Enclave	New Delhi-16
Hebbar, K. Sheshgiri	Dr. Hebbar's Eye Clinic, Trunk Road	Nellore (A.P.)
Hedge, Balkrishna	25, Rly. Parallel Road, Nehru Nagar	Bangalore-20
Hoonka, Govind Das	F-1444, Nehru Nagar, Near Rly. Station	Jabalpur (M.P.)
Husein, S. E.	Court Regal, Christ Church Road, Byculla	Bombay-8
Hussain, Md. Atiqul	Gauhati Med. College	Gauhati (Assam)
Hussein, Yousuf	11/5/338, Red Hills	Hyderabad (Andhra)
Irani, A. B.	16, Cumbala Hill Road	Bombay-36
Irani, B. H.	16, Cumbala Hill Road	Bombay-36
Irani, Daryush A.	19, Framrose Court, Marine Drive	Bombay-20
Ishwarchandra	Med. College Hospital	Nagpur
Isloor, Suresh D.	Sahydri Hospital	Shimoga (Mysore)
Jadeja, Rudrasingh J.	Mayur Bhuwan, Adresh Society	Bhuj Kutch (Gujarat)
Jagannath, Rao H. M.	Med. Officer, S.C.Co. Ltd	Belampalli P.O. (Andhra)
Jagdish, Raj	Civil Hosp.	Hoshiarpur (Punjab)
Jain, Devendra Kumar	F.C.I. Hospital, P.O.	Sindri, Dist. Dhanbad
Jain, Inder Sen	63/1034 - Sector 24 B	Chandigarh (Punjab)
Jain, Janeswar Das	Zilaparishad Eye Hospital	Bulandshar (U.P.)
Jain, M. R.	Head of Eye Dept., Med. College, Christianganj Main Road	Ajmer (Raj)
Jain, Narendra Singh	Kucha Mahajani, Chandni Chowk	Delhi
Jain, O. P.		Mainpuri (U.P.)
Jain, Surendra Kumar	D.M.C.H.	Laheriasarai (Bihar)
Jain, Surendra	I.N.H.S., Sanjivani	Cochin-4 (Kerala)
Jaiwal, Hari Narain	80, H.O.R., D.M.C.H. P.O. Laheriasarai	Darbhanga (Bihar)
Janneswami, Krishnamurthi.	Kamal Bhuvan, Budhapura	Raipur (M.P.)
Jayakrishna, K.	9, Tank Bund Road, Nungamnakkam	Madras-34
Jayaram, Rao G.	Janata Hospital, M. Gandhi Rd.	Kothagudem P.O. (Andhra Pradesh)
Jena, Braj Gopal	H.Q. Hospital, Baripada	Dist. Mayurbhunj (Orissa)
Jhaveri, B. N.	Jai Hind Estate Bldg., Bhuleswar .	Bombay-2
Jogalekar, M. D.	Talshella, 4th floor Bhandarwada Road, Shivaji Park	Bombay-28
Joseph Rajasekharan	Dr. Joseph's Eye Hospital	Tiruchirapalli (Madras)
Joseph, Prof. F. A.	College Hospital	Kottayam-1 (Kerala)
Jehangir, Rumi Pesi	'Commonwealth', Nariman Point .	Bombay-20 BR.
Jithendra, Arikeri	Med. College	Kurnool (A.P.)
Joshi, B. K.	Imli Bazar	Indore (M.P.)
Joshi, Chandrashanker	Subhanpura Road, Race Course Circle	Baroda-7
Joshi, Dwarkadas S.	Vadnagar Eye & Gen. Hosp.	Vadnagar (N. Gujarat)
Joshi, M. H.	510, Kalbadevi Road 1st floor ..	Bombay-2
Joshi, M. M.	15/1, New Javali Bazar	Hubli-20 (Mysore)
Joshi, M. P.	Waniwad	Bhuj (Kutch)
Joshi, Mahebdra V.	Joshi Nivas, Fata Talao	Broach (Gujarat)
Joshi, Mihir D.	Jyoti Hospital	Visnagar (N. Gujarat)
Joshi, P. D.	Harihar Nivas, Sadar	Rajkot (Saurashtra)
Joshi, Shreesh K.	Gadikhana Subhedar Lane	Nagpur-2

Joshi, Streekrishna C.	C-3, BARC Bldg., Agra Road, Ghatkopar	Bombay-77
Joshi, Sukhlal U.	Central Bazar Road, Ramdas Peth	Nagpur
June ja, B. M.	No. 426, 10th Road, Chembur ..	Bombay
Kadam, Subhas P.	Kusum Kunj, Vithal Sty. Nava-pura	Baroda (Gujarat)
Kailash, Nath	Gandhi Eye Hospital	Aligarh
Kalewar, V. K.	Dept. of Ophth. New Civil Hospi-tal	Ahmedabad-16
Kalidasan, C. S.	14, Mukhtial St.	Madras-7
Kalita, S. N.	P.O. Assam Med. College	Dibrugarb (Assam)
Kamath, C. P.	Sri Ramkrishna Eye Hosp.	Mangalore (S.I.)
Kamath, C. Ramkrishna ...	Temple Square	Mangalore (S.I.)
Kamdar, Arvind J.	Premji Ladha Bldg., 357, Bhan-darkar Road	Bombay-19
Kameshwar, Rao K.	Main Road	Vishakapatnam-2 (Andhra)
Kanchan, Hari Shanker	P-24, Gariahat Road	Calcutta-29
Kandaswami, N.	M. G. Eye Hospital, Big Bazar Street	Coimbatore (S.I.)
Kane, Suresh Keshao	c/o Dr. H. Y. Bakre, Station Road	Jalgaon (E.K.)
Kanwar, S. N.	Armed Forces Med. College	Poona
Kapalmit, Singh	P.G.I. of Med. Education	Chandigarh (Punjab)
Kapathia, G. C.	155, General Hospital	C/o 99 A.P.O.
Kapoor, B. L.	Dist. Hospital	Chamba (H.P.)
Kapoor, Rajendra K.	Jagjivan Ram Hospital, Club Road	Bombay-8
Kar, Sashisekhar	Capital Hospital	Bhubaneswar (Orissa)
Karmarkar, B. R.	2912, Subhash Road	Ratnagiri-1
Karyekar, Sharad D.	Madhavi Co-op. Housing Society, Bldg. No. 2, Block No. 25 IInd floor, Mogul Lane, Matunga (W.Rly.)	Bombay-16
Kaul, S. M.	27, Karjan Road	New Delhi
Kaulgud, Mukund R.	1698, Ramdeo Gulli	Belgaum (Mysore)
Kayarkar, Vasant	Bel Haven, 1st floor Flat 4, 23 New Marine Lines	Bombay-20
Khajgicala	Snehlate, ESI, Dispensary Rakhial	Ahmedabad
Khan, Gulam Mustafa	Alamchand Bazar	Cuttack-2 (Orissa)
Khanna, B. N.	6395, Katra Baryan Fatehpuri ..	Delhi
Khanra, Chittaranjan	Eye Dept. M.R. Cir Med. College & Hosp. 138, Archarya J. Bose Rd.	Calcutta
Khanuja, Pritam Singh	Military Hospital	Meerut (U.P.)
Kher, Narendra N.	Civil Hospital	Ujjain (M.P.)
Khedgikar, Dilip Bhimrao ..	Eye Clinic, Near Bank of Maha-rashtra, Ambajogai	Dist. Bhir (Marathwada)
Khetrapal, Ramesh	99/XI, Brahmapuri	Ajmer (Rajasthan)
Kinariwalla, Uma Lalit-Mohan	Gosmos Circular Rd., Ville Parle West	Bombay-56
Kishore, Lal	M.O. I/C, KDD Eye Hosp. Civil Lines	Rampur (U.P.)
Kohli, Harnam Singh	Bharat Nagar Chowk, Opp: ESI Hospital	Ludhiana (Punjab)
Kolhatkar, Priyamvada	P.O. Box No. 6 Eye Hospital ...	Mahuva, Dist. Bhavnagar
Koppikar, V. R.	94, Khanapur Road	Camp Belgaon (Mysore)

Kothari, Ramanlal C.	Raopura Tower	Baroda (Gujarat)
Kotnis, Ramakant V.	19, Pushpa Nagri Stn. Road	Aurangabad
Krishna, Kumar	House No. 1089, Section 19–B .	Chandigarh (Punjab)
Krishnamurthy, A.	1661, Laxmipuram	Mysore-4
Krishnamurthy, S.	....	Vijayawada-2
Krishnamurthy, V.	59, Seetharam Nagar	Cuddalore-1 (South Arcot Dist.)
Krishmoorthy, H.	Prabha Eye Clinic, V. Puram	Bangalore
Krishmurthy, P.	43/6, E. Narasinghrao Pet	Kurnool (A.P.)
Kulkarni, G. S.	....	Gadag (New Mysore)
Kulkarni, Madhukar	B.M.S. Quarters J. J. Hospital ...	Bombay-8
Kulshekharan, P.	Sarojini Devi Eye Hospital	Hyderabad (A.P.)
Kulshrestha, Prof. O. P. ...	Sawai Mansingh Hosp.	Jaipur (Rajasthan)
Kulshresta, Ramesh C.	Ramkrishna Mission Hosp.	Vrindaban (Mathura)
Kumar, Rajendra	At & P.O. Banarjhula, Dist. Muzaffarpur	Bihar
Kumar, S. P.	G/62, Connaught Circus	New Delhi-14
Kumarswami, T. M.	No. 10, Bharathi Road 1st street, Perambur	Madras-11
Kundu, M.	160/2, Upper Circular Rd.	Calcutta-5
Krupashankar, Y. V.	Minto Opth. Hospital	Bangalore
Kulkarni, Rangnath G.	At & Post – Kini Yelladevi	Tel. Udgir, Dist. Osmanabad
Kundu, R. R.	AMO, (Eye), SERY. Hospital, P.O.	Adra, Dist. Purulia (W.B.)
Kundu Sisir Kumar	Apcar Gardens	Asansol (W.B.)
Kundu, Tarapade	34, R.B. Ghose Road C.978, Khorahghar	Burdwan (W. Bengal)
Kuriakose, E. T.	Netra Bhavan, Karkat Road, Ernakulam	Cochin-16
Krishna, Lal	Opp: Chaman Hotel	Kota-1 (Rajasthan)
Ladani, Givindbhai T.	Patel Nayan Hospital, Sodha Sheri, Bhadar Rd.	Upleta (Gujarat)
Lakhanpal, V.	746, Sector 22–1	Chandigarh (Punjab)
Lall, James S.	Buty Bldg., 1st floor Variety Square, Sitabardi	Nagpur-12
Lal, Moti	Godanlia Crossing	Varanasi (U.P.)
Limaye, S. P.	Eye Hospital, Vishrambag	Sangli (Maharashtra)
Lalaji, N. M.	Balaji Road	Surat (Gujarat)
Laliyanaik, R.	8th Main Road	Yadagari
Lamba, P. A.	Govt. Med. College	Panaji (Goa)
Lakshmidas, D.	40/440, Bhaskar Nagar	Kurnool (A.P.)
Laxmi, Narain	Central Hospital, P.O. Jagjivan Nagar	Dhanbad (Bihar)
Lele, B. N.	Okha Charity Trust Bldg., Wright Town	Jabalpur (M.P.)
Limaye, Suresh R.	Jai Nivas, 5th Road Ghatkopar ..	Bombay-86
Luong, Mongkol, Bhaedykom	281/31 (Swadi), Sukumint Road	Bangkok (Thailand)
Luthra, C. L.	Military Hospital	Dehradun (U.P.)
Luthra, J.	Military Hospital	Ranchi (Bihar)
Madan, Gopal A. V.	Irwin Hospital	Amaravati (Vidarpha)
Madan, Mohan N. B.	9, Patel Road	Dehradun (U.P.)
Madan, Mohan	RP. Cent. for Ophth. Sc. AIIMS. .	New Delhi-16
Madhav, Rao G. S.	62, Girundappa Road, Baswangudi	Bangalore-4
Mahadevan, K.	1st Agraharam	Salem - 1 (Madras)

Mahashabde, J. S.	284, Samyogitaganj Murai Mohalla	Indore (M.P.)
Mahen, P. D.	INHS 'Asvini' Colaba	Bombay-5
Mahendra, P. M.	13, Mall Road	Sitapur Cantt. (U.P.)
Mahendra, Ramesh C.	Govt. Hospital, Miryalguda	Dist. Nalagonda (A.P.)
Maitra, Ajoy Kumar	Kishanganj, Dist. Purnia	Bihar
Majumdar, Asish Kumar ...	15/B, Gangadhar Sen Lane	Calcutta-36
Majumdar, Nirad Bhusan ..	43/3, Mahatma Gandhi Road ...	Calcutta
Makhija, J. M.	PWD, 12/C, Kothi Baug Residency, ...	Udaipur (Rajasthan)
Malik, Shivraj K.	Dept. of Ophth., M. A. Medical College	New Delhi
Malleswara, Rao D.	Siddharth Nursing Home	Rajahmundry-1
Mandal, Jibananda	Villa-Silla, P.O. Ramgopalpur ...	Dist. Burdwan (W.B.)
Mandrekar, D. J.	Laud Mansion, 3rd floor Queen's Road	Bombay-4
Mane, B. V.	Post Kadpur, Via Chakur	Dist. Usmanabad
Mankodi, Mahendrarai C. ..	Irwin Group of Hospitals	Jamnagar (Saurashtra)
Mansharamani, P. P.	Qr. No. M.D./560 A, Opp. Rly. Hospital	Kota (Rajasthan)
Marathy, S. H.	3, Metropolitan Bldg., Fort	Bombay-1
Maria, Devendra Pal	Medical College	Aurangabad (Marathwada)
Maskati, B. T.	1, Shiv Tirth, 4/6, Bhulabhai Desai Road	Bombay-26
Maskati, N. T.	Nawapura Street	Surat (Gujarat)
Master, Darius R.	2040 South, Jan Mohamed St. ..	Poona
Manthalkar, R. Rao	Opp. Govt. College, Station Road	Gulbarga
Mathur, Jagdish Saran	1, Doctor's Enclave, B.H.U.	Varanasi-5
Mathur, Rajendra Nath	C/22, M. Shah Med. College	Jamnagar (Saurasthtra)
Mathur, S. B. L.	Shappawalla Kua Karolbagh	Delhi
Mathur, Saran P.	156/X, Civil Lincs	Ajmer (Rahasthan)
Mathur S. S.	A.M.O., N.Rly. Hospital	Muradabad (U.P.)
Mazumdar, A. M.	Ramgiri, Ist Road, Chembur	Bombay
Mehkri, M. B.	59, Lalbaug Road	Bangalore
Mehkri, Mohamed S.	59, Lalbaug Road	Bangalore
Mehra, Krishna S.	College of Med. Sciences B.H.U. .	Benares-5
Mehrotra, A. S.	c/o Sri R.N. Malvia, I.A. Road, Sardarpura	Jodhpur (Rajasthan)
Mehta, Hemendra Kumar ..	Metha Eye Hospital	Rajot (Gujarat)
Mehta, Kaikhusru R.	Sea Side, Ist floor, 147, Miodle Colaba	Bombay-5
Metha, Keshavlal N.	Eye Hospital	Rajkot (Gujarat)
Metha, Natvarlal A.	Kansada Darwaja	Patan (N. Gujarat)
Metha, Rameshclandra N. d	Sardar Patel Road	Godhra, Dist. Panchmahal
Metha, Shreenarayan	73, House Off. Residence D.M. College	Dist. Darbhanga (Bihar)
Metha, Umedrai Lallubhai .	Mody Bldg. Nanbha Road	Bhavnagar (Saurashtra)
Menon, Prof. Gopinath	Medical College	Kottamyam-1 (Kerala)
Mishra, Anil Kant.	CD/218, Sector II	Ranchi-4
Mishra, Prof. Kulmani	MKCG. Medical College	Berhampur (Orissa)
Mishra, Mahendra Chandra .	Mahateb Road, Dolmundei	Cuttack (Orissa)
Mishra, Mahesh C.	5, B.C. Road	Jamshedpur (Bihar)
Mishra, Nirmal Chandra ...	R.M.O. (Eye) Darbhanga, Medical College, P. O.	Laheriasarai (Bihar)
Mishra, Prof. R. K.	Medical College	Jabalpur (M.P.)
Mishra, S.	Medical College	Darbhanga (Bihar)

Mishra, Sachidanand	ESI. Hosp., Brajraj Nagar	Dist. Sambhalpur (Orissa)
Mishra, Shambu	80, H.O.R., DMCH	Laheriasarai (Bihar)
Mistry, J. P.	S.K. Verma Road	Mandvi (Kutch)
Mistry, Purshottam T.	c/o Mascati Eye Hospital, Navapura	Surat (Gujarat)
Mitra, Amal	4, Hospital Road, Asansol	Burdwan (W.B.)
Mitra, B. K.	9, Chauringhee Road	Calcutta-13
Mitra, Prasant K.	8, Ramanand Chaterjee Road ...	Calcutta-9
Mittal, Premanand	15/4, Doctor's quarters	Indore (M.P.)
Mitter, Surendra Nath	11/B, Gangaram Hosp. Marg	New Delhi-60
Mokadam, Prafulla J.	Mokadam Clinic, New Ramdas Peth	Nagpur-1
Mondal, Baidynath	138, Mahatma Gandhi Road	Calcutta-7
Mondal, Prayagraj	53, Chittaranjan Ave.	Calcutta-12
Moody, Jack C.	Shanti Bhuvan Hospital Box 252 .	Khatmandu (Nepal)
Modi, Rasiklal A.	Govt. Med. College	Surat (Guj.)
Modi, Shantilal J.	Ras Kunj, 4, Jagannath Plots ...	Rajkot (Saurashtra)
Mody, Mansukhlal	Malifalia	Surat (Gujarat)
Mody, D. G.	Congress House, V. Patel Rd. ...	Bombay-4
Mohamed, Salik	....	Buldana (M.P.)
Mohan, Hari	3778, Subhash Marg Daryaganj ..	Delhi-6
Mohan, Rao K. R.	....	Nandyal, Dist. Kurnool (A.P.)
Mohan, Singh	Harbhajan Md. Hall, Jullunder Road	Hoshiarpur (E.P.)
Mohanlal, Jareth	Gandhi Chowk	Kota (Rajasthan)
Mohapatra, Laxmikant	Med. College	Berhampore, Dist. Ganjam (Orissa)
Mohindranath	Jeewan Nursing Home 28, Russa Road	New Delhi
Mrechea, Manmohan	16, Pratap Chowk	Delhi Cantt - 10
Mukerjee, Ajay Kumar	12, Bidhan Street	Calcutta-6
Mukherjee A. K.	Block I, Flat 6, M.I.G. Hsg. Estate, 37, Belgachia Road	Calcutta-37
Mukherjee, Arun Kumar ...	S.C.B. Med. College	Cuttack (Orissa)
Mukherjee, G. N.	295/2B, Upper Cir. Road	Calcutta-9
Mukerjee, Haraprased M. ..	Villa Barset	Chandernagoré, Dist. Hooghly
Mukherjee, P. C.	B.R. Singh Hospital	Calcutta-14
Mukherjee, P. K.	3/747, Shanti Nagar	Raipur (M.P.)
Mukherjee, Paresh N.	D.S.P. Hospital	Durgapur-4 (W.B.)
Mukherjee, Ranabir	79/D, Ekdalia Road	Calcutta-19
Mukherjee, Shiva D.	Kalibari Road, Seetla Gali	Agra (U.P.)
Mukherjee, Somesh	P.O. Jharia, Lalbazar	Dhanbad (Bihar)
Muljiani, R. H.	Abookkar Bldg., Colaba Causeway	Bombay-1
Mulik, J. S.	43/1, Jillah Peth	Jalgaon, Dist. Jalgaon
Munsi, Nihar K.	1/3, Dover Place	Calcutta-19
Murthy, A. S. R.	Old Govt. Hosp. Road	Rajamundry (A.P.)
Murthy, K. R.	Prabha Eye Clinic National High School Rd.	Bangalore-4
Murti, G. S.	Kaktives	Belgaum (Mysore)
Murti, K. B. K.	....	Kurnool (A.P.)
Mustafi, Pramode C.	Astarag, 28, Contractor's Area ..	Jamshedpur (Bihar)
Muthia, J.	Karunanidhi Med. Hall	Tanjore (S.I.)
Muthia, J.	Med. College Hosp.	Kottayam (Kerala)

Nagaraja, Row R. . . . . 'Retina' 55, Ist Main Road, Raja
                                 Addamalaipuram Madras-28
Nagpal, P. N. . . . . Inst. of Ophth. New Civil Hospital Ahmedabad-16
Nahar, Sohan . . . . 55 Prem Court, Peddar Road . . . Bombay-26
Nahata, M. C. . . . . 116, Jaora Compound . . . . Indore (M.P.)
Naidu Venkatiah . . . . Srinivas Nursing Home . . . . Narasarapet, Dist. Guntur
                                                                           (A.P.)
Nanavaty, J. N. . . . . Nanavaty Eye Hospital . . . . Junagadh (Saurashtra)
Narayan, Binod . . . . Swarajpuri Road, Opp. Fire Briga-
                                 de . . . . Gaya (Bihar)
Nanavaty, Jugalkishore . . . . Bhojeshwar Plot . . . . Porbandar (Saurashtra)
Narain, Pratap . . . . 1426, Chandni Chowk Delhi-6
Narang, S. K. . . . . Institute of Ophth., New Civil
                                 Hospital . . . . Ahmedabad
Narasimha, Rao N. V. L. . . . 16–2–13, Official Colony . . . . . Vishakhapatnam (A.P.)
Nargish, Patel . . . . Northcote Nursg. Home, Ormis-
                                 ton Rd. Bombay-1
Nath, N. L. . . . . Bhatia Hospital, Neeva Bazar . . . Amritsar (Punjab)
Nath, S. . . . . Lahurabir . . . . Benares (U.P.)
Nath, Subodh Chandra . . . . Belgachia Villa Block T/4 . . . . . . Calcutta-37
Natrajan, K. . . . . 30/2 Pilkinton Road Madras-23
Navmani, Doraiswamy . . . . 38 A Co-operative Colony . . . . . Thanjvur (Tamil Nadu)
Nema, H. V. . . . . Dept. of Ophthalmology, College
                                 of Med. Sciences B.H.U. . . . . Varanasi
Nicholson D. B. . . . . Wassiamul Bldg., 2nd floor 'D'
                                 Block, New Charoi Rd. Jn. . . Bombay-7
Nirankari, M. S. . . . . 14, Doctor's Avenue, Majitha Rd. Amritsar (Punjab)
Narayan, Atul . . . . 55, Garaichal Road Calcutta-19
Nisar, R. K. . . . . Mody Bhuvan, Phandita Ramabai
                                 Rd., Gamdevi Bombay-7
Nyaya, Saroj Kantilal . . . . . c/o Mr. Jitendra Shah, 6 Kirti
                                 Colony Ila Smruti Kunj, Islam-
                                 pura Ahmedabad-13
Oak, Shridhar V. . . . . Vijay Nagar, Block No. 72 Dadar . Bombay-28
Ohri, Ravinder Nath . . . . . . I-D Block . . . . Sri Ganganagar (Raj.)
Om, Prakash . . . . 42-A, The Mall . . . . Amritsar (E.P.)
Oomen, C. E. . . . . Sara Mem. Nursing Home, Fort
                                 Road . . . . Cannanore (Kerala)
Oza, Kiritkumar . . . . 2/22, D. N. Nagar, Varsova Rd.,
                                 Andheri (East) Bombay-58
Pabby, Vinod Kumar . . . . . Eye Dept., P.G.I. . . . . Chandigarh (Punjab)
Padhy, Krishna Charan . . . . P.G. Student, Eye Dept. SCB Me-
                                 dical College . . . . Cuttack-7 (Orissa)
Padmewar, B. U. . . . . Med. College Colony Quarter I,
                                 AIV/2 . . . . Nagpur
Pahwa, J. M. . . . . Eye Hospital . . . . Sitapur (U.P.)
Pal, S. N. . . . . 43, Peskar Lane, Salkia . . . . Howrah (W.B.)
Pal, Prasanta Kumar . . . . . . Rly. Qr. RB 1V-291/1, Central
                                 Rly. Hospital Compound, By-
                                 culla Bombay-27
Palit, M. G. . . . . HR – 154 G. H. . . . . C/o 99 A.P.O.
Panchal, Shanta Venilal . . . C/o 18/49 Venus Apartment
                                 Worli Sea Face Bombay-18
Pancholi, Chhabildas K. . . . P.O. – . . . . Sawar-Kundala (Gujarat)
Pande, B. L. . . . . Eye Clinic, Ry. Stn. Road . . . . . . Etawah (U.P.)
Pande, Mahendra P. N. . . . . Ispat General Hospital . . . . Rourkela-2 (Orissa)

Pande, Venkatesh S.	....	Yeotmal (Maharashtra)
Pandeya, Alak Nath	7, Med. Officer's Flat, P.M.C.H. .	Patna-4
Pandeya, Chhaya	7, Med. Officer's Flat, P.M.C.H. .	Patna (Bihar)
Pandit, Y. K. C.	Bombay Mutual Buiding, D. Naoroji Road	Bombay-1
Pandya, Mahesh C.	Rajada Road	Jam-Khambalia (Gujerat)
Panjiyara, Bindeshwar	80, H.O.R., D.M.C.H. P.O. Laheriasarai	Darbhanga
Paranjpe, B. Y.	24, New Queens Road	Bombay-4
Parekh, Harilal M.	Eye Hospital	Palanpur (Gujarat)
Parikh, Madanmohan V. ...	Opp. Municipal Clock Tower Near Lal Darwaja, Mirzapur Road .	Ahmedabad
Patel, Ashok R.	243–45, Walkeshwar Road	Bombay-6
Patel, Bhikubhai S.	535, Relief Road	Ahmedabad (Guj.)
Patel, Babaebhai C.	....	Miyagam - Karjan (Gujarat)
Patel, Chhotubhai K.	Hira-Kunj, Near Maharashtra Society, Netaji Rd., Ellis Bridge	Ahmedabad-6
Patel, Ganpatram G.	Gokul, Ashram Road	Ahmedabad-14
Patel, Gulcher	Northcole Nursing Home, Apollo Street	Bombay
Patel, Javerbhai D.	Opp: Kothi	Baroda (Gujarat)
Patel, Jitendra K.	Dr. 's Quarters, Behind Ward 15 S.S.G. Hospital	Baroda (Gujarat)
Patel, J. H.	Moli Salvivad, Saraspur	Ahmedabad
Patel, Praful H.	Jer Mansion, 5, New Queen's Road	Bombay-4
Patel, Prafulla Ambalai	M.P. Shah Med. College	Jamnagar (Gujarat)
Patel, Pravinchandra S.	Station Road	Raipur (M.P.)
Patel, Nalini M.	M.J.K. Inst. of Ophth., Civil Hospital	Ahmedabad-6
Patel, Ramesh Maranji	Chaitanya Nivas, Vaidya St.	Navsari (dist. Bulsar) (Gujerat)
Patel, Rustom J	21, Queens Road	Bombay-4
Pathak, K. L.	Dayanand Hospital Road	Ludhiana (Punjab)
Pathak, Narsinha A.	....	Miraj, Dist. Sangli
Pathak, Shyanrao	5/N-4, Habibganj H.E.I., Hospital Campus	Bhopal-24
Pati, Jyotirmoy	Eye Dept., G-11, Sector 2	Rourkela-2
Patil, Kishor Dattarao	Patil Clinic, Main Road	Wardha (Central Railway)
Patnaik, Bijoyananda	M. A. Med. College	New Delhi
Patnaik, S. P.	V.S.S. Med. College Qr. 3R/4 ...	Burla, Dist. Sambhalpur (Orissa)
Patney, S.	Patney's Eye Clinic Alanker, Gondal Rd., Near Gurukul	Rajkot-2
Patwardhan, A. D.	Saraswati Vilas, Laxmi Rd.	Poona-2
Patwardhan, D. G.	Deccan Gymkhana	Poona-4
Paul, Ajitkumar	Eye Hospital	Sitapur (U.P.)
Paul, D. N.	6, Mahendra Sarker Street	Calcutta-12
Paul, Radha Govind	21, Grey Street	Calcutta-5
Pendse, Padmakar V.	Raopura	Baroda (Gujarat)
Pickrd, Raleigh H.	Holston Hospital	Yadgiri (Mysore)
Prabhakar, Rao S.	S.E.Rly. Hospital	Bilaspur (M.P.)
Prabhakaran, M.	Medical College	Calicut-8
Pralhad, Rao D.	Krishna Kripa, Satyanarayan Pet .	Bellary (Mysore)
Prasad, Anjani Kishore	Jagat Narain Road	Patna-3 (Bihar)

Rao Ramnarayan, S. G. ...	29/1, K.H. Road	Bangalore-27
Rathi, O. L.	Nikalas Mandit Road, Itwari	Nagpur-2
Ratnaparkhi, K. G.	....	Dhulia (Khandesh)
Ratnaraj, Arthur	101, Mission Hospital	Pondicherry
Ray, Amalendu Mohan	S.E.Rly. Hospital	Kharagpur (W.B.)
Ray, Anand Mohan	3R/39, Doctor's Colony, V.S.S. Medical College	Burla, Dist. Sambhalpur (Orissa)
Ray, Narendra Nath	11/1, Central Road H.B. Town, Sodepur	24 Paraganas (W.B.)
Ray, Pinaki Ranjan	P.O. & Dist.	Malda (W.B.)
Ray, Samir	Kulti Hospital, P.O.	Kulti (Dist. Burdwan) (W.B.)
Ray, Satendra Nath	18/20, Ramchandra Sett Rd., Ranviraj Tala	Howrah-4
Reddi, P. Raghurami	Eye Clinic, Govt. Hq. Hospital ..	Nellore (A.P.)
Reddy, G. V. B. K.	Gangadhar Anand Nulayam, Begumpet	Hyderabad-16
Reddy, T. N. Krishna	Govt. General Hospital	Kurnool-2
Reddy, N. Subrananya	Sorojini Devi Eye Hosp.	Hyderabad (A.P.)
Robert, L. P.	25, Dr. Shivanand Nagar	Coimbatore-12
Rohatgi, J. N.	Khudabux Library Road	Patna-4 (Bihar)
Rohatgi, Rajendra	Civil Lines	Kanpur (U.P.)
Roy, Anand Prakash	6, M.G. Road	Poona-1
Roy, Chaudhary Kumudini .	213, Charni Road............	Bombay-4
Roy, Chaudhary Diptish ...	12, Gobinda Pal Lane	Calcutta-2 (W.B.)
Roy, P.	R.K. Mission Hospital, Luxa Road	Varanasi (U.P.)
Roy, S. C.	Hospital Road	Asansol (W.B.)
Roy, I. S.	15, Prafulla Sarkar St.	Calcutta-13
Roy, S. R.	Kadar Road	Gauhati (Assam)
Sabharwal, Satish	Shree Jeewan Hospital, 67/1, New Rohtak Road	New Delhi-5
Sabui, Narayan Chandra ...	Inchapore, Nawabganj	24 Parganas (W.B.)
Sah, Arun Prakash	Shamaram, Durgakund	Varanasi-5 (U.P.)
Saha, N. G.	Victoria Hospital	Darjeeling (W.B.)
Saha, Ramendra Lal	97, Akhil Mistri Lane	Calcutta-9
Saha, Upendra Chandra ...	Tikapara, P.O. Suri	Dist. Birbhun
Sahai, R.	112/10, Civil Lines, Govind Bhawan	Ajmer (Rajasthan)
Sahay, B. N.	Eye & ENT Dept. D.M.C.H. P.O. Laheriasarai	Dist. Darbhanga
Sahoo, Indramani	S.C.B. Medical College	Cuttack-7 (Orissa)
Sahu, Y.	Medical College, Berhampur	Dist. Ganjam (Orissa)
Saiduzzafar, H.	Gul Rana, Nr. Amir Nishan	Aligarh (U.P.)
Saikia, Gautam	Eye Care & Contact Lens Clinic, Danish Road ....,	Gauhati-1 (Assam)
Salunke, Arun Zulalrao	Lane 5, Home No. 1391	Dhulia (Maharashtra)
Samaddar, Prasoon K.	c/o Dr. S. Samaddar, Pataliapura	Patna-3
Samanta, Muktipada	Burnpur Road	P.O. Asansol, Dist. Burdwar
Sambandam, S. P. T.	C.M.C. Hospital	Chengalput (Tamil Nadu)
Sambamurthy, N. B.	Mettur Road	Erode Madras-3
Sampangay, Radha K.	16, Hospital Road	Bangalore Cantt-1
Samuel, Annamma	Emanuel Clinic, Mount Pleasant Road	Coonoor-2 (Nilgiries)
Sangle, Vasant R.	Lane No. 6	Dhilia (Khandesh)
Sankar, N. P.	I.A. Ramchander Iyer St., Perambur	Madras-11

Sankaran, V.	Parmani Road	Calicut
Sansar, Singh Sangha	Ram Lal Eye & ENT Hospital	Amritsar (Punjab)
Santhamani, Rajgopal	No. 10, Marshall's Road, Egmore	Madras-8
Santok, Singh	Hamida Hospital	Bhopal (M.P.)
Saradeshpande, H. V.	Dhanrajgiri Hospital	Sholapur (MRT)
Saraf, G. K.	4, Little Russel Street	Calcutta-16
Sarda, R. P.	39, Hospital Road	Jaipur (Rajasthan)
Sardesai, Arvind G.	Garden View, Parsi Colony, Dadar	Bombay-14
Sardesai, D. S.	213, Charni Road	Bombay-4
Sardeshpande, Y. H.	Eye Hospital, Gandhi Chowk	Chandrapur (Maharashtra)
Sareen, D. K.	Central Town	Jullunder City (Punjab)
Sarkar, Asutush	41/1/B, Ram Kanto Bose St.	Calcutta-3
Sarkar, Bharat Chandra	Vill. & P.O. Banitala	Dist. Howrah (W.B.)
Sarkar, Ranjit Kumar	23-A, Jitendranath Laheri Rd.	P.O. Serampore, Dist. Hooghly (W.B.)
Sarkar, Sukumar	c/o Shri J. C. Sen, Bakhrabad	Cuttack-2
Sarkar, Tarani Kumar	189-A, West Cotannagar	P.O. Gauhati-VV (Assam)
Sarma, C. Mangiah	Ophth. Dept. Govt. Hosp.	Machilipatnam (Dist. Kistna)
Sunder, Prof. Rama Sarma, C.	Gen. Hosp.	Kakinada (A.P.)
Saroya, Jaswin Singh	Guman Pura	(Kota) (Raj)
Sathe, S. M.	9, Sadanand Wadi, N.P. Road	Bombay-4
Satnam, Singh	C/o WHO office, P.O. Box 33	Kabul (Afghanistan)
Satpathy, Madhusudan	Sarojini Devi Eye Hospital	Hyderabad (A.P.)
Satpathy, Prasanne Kumar	5 Post-graduate Hostel, V.S.S. Medical College, P.O. Burla	Dist. Sambalpur (Orissa)
Satsangi, U. C.	13-B, Civil Lines	Bikaner (Rajasthan)
	107, Jorbagh	New Delhi-3
Satyanarayana, C.	Govt. Gen. Hospital	Kakinada (W. Godaveri)
Satyendran, G. M.	Sarojini Devi Eye Hospital	Hyderabad (A.P.)
Savla, Somchand K	Genesh Nivas, Near Kismat Cinema, Prabhadevi	Bombay-25
Saxena, Rameshchandra	G/19, Reserve Bank Colony	Lucknow (U.P.)
Saxena, R. C.	34, Meena Bazar, Court Rd.	Bilaspur
Saxena, S. N.	Shri Kamal Hospital	Rewari (E.P.)
Seal, Golak Nath	13-B, Durga Pithuri Lane	Calcutta-12
Sen, Amal Kumar	3, Lake View Road	Calcutta-29
Sen, D. K.	Eye Department, M.A. Medical College	New Delhi
Sen, Gopal Chandra	120-B, Lower Circular Rd.	Calcutta-14
Sen, Jagdish C.	B/5, Nimak Mahal Road	Calcutta-43
Sen, Santimoy	Bank Mor	Dhanbad (Bihar)
Sen, Satendra Nath	11, Fern Place, P.O. Ballygunge	Calcutta
Sen, Sisiransu Bhusan	157/2B, Acharya P.C. Road	Calcutta
Sen, Surendra Chandra	54, Government Colony	P.O. & Dist. Malda (W.B.)
Sengupta, M.	44, Lake Temple Road	Calcutta (W.B.)
Seshechari, Komandur S.	Stanley Medical College, 73, Audiappa Naick Street	Madras-1
Seth, K. J.	New Internee Hostel	Baroda (Guj)
Seth, Narendra Mohan	Eye Hospital	Gorakhpur (U.P.)
Setha, R. M.		Hoshangabad (M.P.)
Sethi, Amolak Ram	Dr. Sethi's Nursing Home, 74-F, Kamla Nagar	Delhi-6
Sethi, Jagdish Rai	Doctor's Bldg., Flat no. 4, Central Rly. Hospital, Byculla	Bombay-8
Sethi, J. R.	Shalimar Road	Jammu (Kashmir)

Sethi, Pradipchandra K. ...	Manik Bhavan, 26, Gukoganj ...	Indore (M.P.)
Setti, Ramkrishna	....	Raichur (C.Rly.)
Setty, A. M.	M.O. Primary Health Unit Malli-patna, Ankalgud Taluk	Dist. Hassan (Mysore)
Sevak, Mukundraj	Eye Hospital, Opp. Anupam Talkies	Jamnagar (Guj)
Shah, Gamanlal M.	Subhash Chowk	Nandurbar
Shah, Kirtikumar D.	8, Soman House, Chaupatty Sea Face	Nadiad (Gujarat) Bombay-7
Shah, Mayank Juthabhai ...	Behind Bank of Baroda	Mehsana (N. Gujarat)
Shah, Narendra R.	Eye Hospital, Nr. Gita Mandir, Santram Road	Nadiad, Dist. Kaira
Shah, Pravinkant C.	'Bachubhai Chamber', Baranpuri Bhagal, Bundelawed	Surat-1
Shah, Ramanlal Narottamdas	Eye Hospital, Tanshal Kalupur ..	Ahmedabad-1
Shah, Ramesh Ratilal	Shree Niwas	Rajkot (Gujarat)
Shah, Saroj J.	48, Prof. Quarters, Civil Hospital .	Ahmedabad-16
Shah, Suresh	Oholi Pole, Maliwad	Wadhwan City (Guj.)
Shah, Vadilal M.	Nagarwad, Hakim Street	Baroda (Gujarat)
Shah, Vipinchandra C.	'Shree' 23, S.V. Road, Santacruz (West)	Bombay-54
Shamsher, Singh	Eye & Gen. Hospital	Khanna, Dist. Ludhiana (Punjab)
Shanmugam, K. S.	11/94, Thiruvenkataswamy Rd. R.S: Puram	Coimbatore (S.I.)
Shanta, Ramiah	No. 3, Seetavilas, Agrahar	Mysore-1
Shantikumar, S. R.	Prakash Nagar	Rajahmundry-1 (A.P.)
Shariff, Md. Oosman	Chigtari Gen. Hosp.	Davengere-4 (S.I.)
Sharma, Amarnath	Hauz Katora, Barna Phatak	Benares (U.P.)
Sharma, A. N.	S. D. Marg	Alwar (Rajasthan)
Sharma, Bindeswar	Sitapur Eye Hospital	Bahraich (U.P.)
Sharma, Durga Prasad	D'Villa In front of Padam Hotel, Station Road	Japir (Rajasthan)
Sharma, K. M.	General Hospital	Udaipur
Sharma, R. G.	5 B 112 Dubey Bhovan, Lal Kothi	Jaipur
Sharma, P. C.	Sadar Hospital	Dholpur (Gujarat)
Sharma, Rudra Deo	House No. 25/93, Azad Chowk .	Raipur (M.P.)
Sharma, Satya Deo	S.P. Medical College	Bikaner (Rajasthan)
Sharma, Sohanlal	Rajendra Hospital	Patiala (Punjab)
Sharma, Vasudeo	V.P.B.	Jwalamukhi, Dist. Kangra (Punjab)
Shendurniker	(Kulkarni) Meenaxi D/30, Medical Campus	Jamnagar (Guj)
Shetgar, P. C.	Near Uppali Buruj	Bijapur (MRT)
Shiv, Prasad	M.O. Dist. Hospital	Etah (U.P.)
Shivalkar, Arunkumar	4A, Dhun Apartments, 66, Worli Hill Estate	Bombay-18 (W.B.)
Shrinivasan, Dwarka	T. Elliot Road, Mylapur	Madras
Shrinivastav, U. S. S.	Gandhi Eye Hospital	Aligarh
Shrivastava, K. P.	158, Base Hospital	C/o 99 A.P.O.
Shrivastava, Shyam	Budhari Bazar	Seoni (M.P.)
Shrivastava, S. P.	Shroff Eye Hospital, Daryaganj .	Delhi-6
Shrivastava, U. S.	Gandhi Eye Hospital	Aligarh (U.P.)
Shroff, Ashok C.	69, Marine Drive	Bombay-1
Shroff, C. N.	Round Bldg. Kalbadevi Road ...	Bombay-2
Shroff, Minoo S.	Daryagani	Delhi-6

Shukla, Bhartendu	Zanshi Road	Gwalior (M.P.)
Shukla, G. P.	Civil Hospital	Guna (M.P.)
Shukla, Prof. Indramani	I.N.M. Med. College	Raipur
Shukla, S. P.	c/o Shri B.S. Shukla MALLB, P.O. Bhatapara	Dist. Raipur (M.P.)
Sindhu, Pratap Sing	Marina Arcade	New Delhi
Sihota, G. S.	Army Hospital	Delhi Cantt-10
Silla, Bhimaratna	P.O. Behrampur	Dist. Ganjam (Orissa)
Singa, Basant Kumar	Barbhanga Med. College, P.O. Laheriasarai	Dist. Darbhanga
Singh, B. N.	30 R.M.C.H.	Ranchi (Bihar)
Singh, Chandra Bhan	235, Daula Kuan	New Delhi-10
Singh, Gurupratap	Sadar Hospital, Hazaribaug	Bihar
Singh, H. K.	R.S.O. Eye Department, Patna Med. College & Hospital	I.P.W. 8, (Patna) (Bihar)
Singh, Hari Charan	Military Hospital, St. Thomas Mount	Madras-16
Singh, N.	148, Adv. Base Hospital	C/o 56 A.P.O.
Singh, N. B.	Military Hospital	Firozpur (Punjab)
Singh, R.	22, Lytton Road	Dehradun (U.P.)
Singh, Raghubir	A.F.M.C.	Poona
Singh, Rajendra	17, Sankat Mochan Colony, Lanka	Varanasi-5
Singh, Ram Tirth	G.S.V.M. Med. College	Kanpur (U.P.)
Singh, Shivnandon P.	Sadar Hospital	Ranchi
Singh, Waikhom Jilangamba	Tuensang Civil Hospital	Tuensang (Naga Land)
Singhal, K. C.	Daresi No. 2	Agra (U.P.)
Singhal, N. C.	Safdarganj Hospital	New Delhi
Sinha, Arvind Kumar	c/o Prof. A. K. Sinha, Kadam Kaun, Opp: Dharmshala	Patna-3 (Bihar)
Sinha, Awadh Bihari	c/o Shri S. P. Sinha, Advocate	Aurangabad, Dist. Gaya (Bihar)
Sinha, Birendra M.	Jail Road	Arrah (Bihar)
Sinha, Chandradip	Darbahanga Medical College	Darbhanga (Bihari)
Sinha, N. K.	Darbhanga Med. College, Hospital Campus P.O. Laherisarai	Dist. Darbhanga
Sinha, P. N.	Hasan Imam Road	Patna (Bihar)
Sinha, Rajendra Nath	Hasan Imam Road	Patna (Bihar)
Sinha, Ramanuj	Reg. Dy. Dir. Health Services, Tirhut Divn.	Muzaffarpur (Bihar)
Sinha, Prof. R. H. P.	Rajendra Med. College	Ranchi-9 (Bihar)
Sinha, Rana Pratap	Bihari – Bihar Bldgs.	Patna-7 (Bihar)
Sinha, T. P.	Sadar Hospital	Muzaffarpur (Bihar)
Siva, Reddy P.	Sarojini Devi Eye Hospital	Hyderabad (A.P.)
Sivasubramaniam, P.	11/1, Cambridge Place	Colombo (Ceylon)
Soan, P. S.	Luchaki Para Chowk	Durg (M.P.)
Sodhi, A. S.	Eye Hospital	Pilphit (U.P.)
Sodhi, Narjit Singh	Eye & General Hospital, Khanna	Dist. Ludhiana (E.P.)
Sofar, Balaram Kumar	H.P. State Hospital	Snowdon (Simla-1)
Soni, P. N.	Eye Hospital	Basti (U.P.)
Soni, Swaraj Kumar	62/B, Rly. Hospital	Ferozpur, Cantt
Soni, Virendra Kumar	c/o Dr. K. L. Soni, Tilak Road	Dehradun (U.P.)
Sood, Prof. G. C.	H.P. Medical College	Simla-1 (H.P.)
Sood, N. N.	Cent. for Ophth. Sc. A.I.I.M.S.	New Delhi-16
Sood, Subhash Chander	c/o Shri. S.N. Sood, Morinda	Dist. Ropar (Punjab)
Soodan, Surinder Singh	Dist. Hosp.	Kathua (Jammu & Kashmir)

Sree, Rangnath H.	43–41, Narsing Rao Pet	Kurnool (A.P.)
Sreenivasan, N.	84, Pondy Bazar	Madras-17
Srinivas, Rao P. N.	Kasturba Hospital	Manipal (S.I.)
Srinivasan, K. R.	No. 80, Eddar Street	Tiruvannamalai (N. Arcot Dist.)
Srinivasmurthy, V.	8/101, Adimurththynagar	Anantpur P.O. (Andhra)
Srirammurthy, C.	Bapuji Nursing Home	Chilakaluriput, Dist. Guntur (A.P.)
Srirammurthy, K.	Dr. Butchiraju Mem. Hosp.	Rajahmundry-1 (S.I.)
Srivastava, S. P.	34, Civil Lines	Rewa (M.P.)
Subba Rao, B. N.	D.M.O., S.C.Rly. Rail Nilanam	Secunderabad-25
Subarao, Mogalsetty	Ramnaidupet	Masulipatam (S.I.)
Subramanayam, M. R.	D-97, Thirunagar P.O.	Madurai-6 (S.I.)
Subramaniam, G.	11 st. Melamangulam, Periakulam Taluk	Dist. Madura (Madras)
Subramaniam, K.	Dept. Of Ophthalmology, Karnatak Medical College	Hubli, Dist. Dharwar
Subramaniam, K. S.	Sri Krishna, 13/28, Carmel Road .	Trivandrum (Kerala)
Subramaniam, S.	198, Mint Road, George Town	Madras
Sudama, Mehboobani	General Hospital	Karauli, Dist. Sawaimadhopur (Rajasthan)
Sudhalker, M. S.	Pratap Ganj	Baroda (Gujarat)
Sudrik, G. S.	238, Chhatrapati Shivaji Maharaj Rd.	Ahmedabad
Sujir, Rabindra Nayak	866, J. Pai Lands, K.S. Rao Cross Road	Mangalore-1
Sule, Satish V.	933, Sunder Vilas Khare Town, Dharam Peth	Nagpur
Sundara, Rajan R.	67, Ponnuranga Mudliyar Rd., R.S. Puram P.O.	Coimbatore-2
Sundaram, C. Ramlingam	Govt. Hd. Qrs. Hospital	Anantpur (A.P.)
Sunderasen, K.	184, Commercial Street	Bangalore-1
Sundereswaran, D.	9/41, Sarojini Street, Ramnagar .	Coimbatore (S.I.)
Sudarsanam, V. C.	K.M.F. Hospital	Kotagiri (The Nilgiris)
Sunthankar, S. V.	Sunder Nivas, Hind Wadi Goa Ves	Belgaum (Mysore)
Surchand, Singh	Singjamei Thongam Leikai	Imphal (Manipur)
Suresh, K. Hansraj	Vidhansabha Marg, Mansorovar Eye Hospital	Lucknow (U.P.)
Surjan, Singh	Nimak Mandi	Amritsar (E.P.)
Surya Rao, S. V. M.	M.G.M. Hospital	Warnagal (A.P.)
Suryanarayan, Murthy M.	Andhra Medical College	Vishakhapatnam (A.P.)
Susheelamma, K.	1598, Hosakeri, IV. Cross Laxmipuram	Mysore
Sutaria, Kantilal C.	Haveli Mohalla	Navsari
Sutaria, Sudha, N.	Ramdas Peth, Canal Road	Nagpur-1
Swaminathan, P. M.	J. G. Chester House, 54, Pantheon Road, Egmore	Madras-8
Swaminathan, T. R.	No. 5, Palur Kanniappa Gramani St., Mylopore	Madras 600004
Swami Rao, Krishna	1598, Hosakeri, IV. Cross Laxmipuram	Mysore
Talwalkar, V. S.	153, B. Hindu Colony Matunga .	Bombay-19
Tambe, Dattatreya B.	Chowpatty, Karanja Road	Ahmednagar
Tandon, K. N.	Astley Hall	Dehra Dun (U.P.)
Tare, Suresh Vasant	3-A Gore Pet, West High Court Road	Nagpur

Tondon, Rajeshwar P.	58/B, Circular Road	Ranchi (Bihar)
Taneja, L. N.	Hari Subha Road	Muzaffarpur (Bihar)
Taterh, Dalpat Singh	Ketki Chowki	Kota (Rajasthan)
Tiwari, Prem Kant	E.S.I. General Hospital, Nanda Nagar	Indore (M.P.)
Tej, Pal Saini	Tulsidas Street N-4, Daryaganj ..	Delhi-6
Telang, B. D.	395, Dr. D. Bhadkamkar Marg ..	Bombay-4
Thakur, Vidyeswar	156/B, Durgakund Colony	Varanasi (U.P.)
Theakamuthu, Selvara ju ..	9, Marshall's Road, Egmore	Madras-8
Thiagarajan, S.	6, Nanmai Tharuvar Coil St., Near West Masi Street	Madurai-1 (S.I.)
Thomas, A.	Schell Eye Hospital C.M.C.	Vellore (S.I.)
Thomas, R.	National General Hospital	Khurai, Dist. Sagar (M.P.)
Thomas, T. M.	National General Hospital	Khurai, Dist. Sagar (M.P.)
Threhan, R. P.	Jain Hospital	Saharanpur (U.P.)
Tiwari, D. P.	7, Civil Lines	Sagar (M.P.)
Tiwary, R.	Swarajpuri Road	Gaya (Bihar)
Tiwary, Ramkeshwar	54–55, New S.O.P.O. Bldg., Patna Med. College Hosp. ...	Patna-4 (Bihar)
Tiwary, T. C.	Military Hospital	Roorkee (U.P.)
Tomar, V. P. S.	P. B. M. Hospital	Bikaner (Rajasthan)
Tonpay, Nagesh Damodar ..	Ramanuj Nivas, Opp. Arya Kanya Vidyalaya Luniapura	Mhow, Dist. Indore (M.P.)
Toshniwal, S. G.	428, Chatti Gulli	Sholapur-2
Tulsi, Das	207, Sector 16–1	Chandigarh (E.P.)
Urseker, T. N.	Krishna Nivas, Jn. Off Queen's Road & Charni Rd.	Bombay-4
Vaidya, V. B.	27, 'Roshni' Opp. Charoi-Road Station, Queen's Road	Bombay-4
Vakil, Hilla H.	Maison Belvedere, Queen's Road	Bombay-4
Valeeswaran, S.	First Agraharam	Salem (Madras)
Vani, Sonalal B.	....	Shirpur, Dist. Dhulia
Varma B. M. D.	L-21	Kanpur (U.P.)
Vasavada, D. M.	B.R. Eye Hospital, Sindhwai Road	Broach (Gujarat)
Vasavada, R. K.	Vasavada Khadki	Junagadh (Saurashtra)
Vaid, R. L.	Institute of Ophthalomology, Gandhi Eye Hospital	Aligarh
Vetath, Naomi J.	Medical Mission Hospital P.O.	Kulienchery, Dist. Earnakulam
Vasudevan, S. M.	D-48, S. Bhavnam Fair Lands ...	Salem-4 (S.I.)
Vaswani, V. G.	I/C Janta Eye Hospital, S.M.S. Highway	Jaipur (Rajasthan)
Vaze, R. K.	Kagalwalla Building, Dr. Ambedkar Road, Dadar	Bombay-14
Veerappa, T. S.	B-3, N.M.C. Campus Nehru Nagar	Belgaum 10
Veerbhadrappa, J. M.	Kappargal Road, Gandhi Nagar ..	Bellary (Mysore State)
Velankar, B. B.	Deshmukh Bldg., Deshmukh Road	Bombay-4
Venkata Rao, I	c/o I. M. Rao, Block-D, Flat-6, R.K. Nagar	Madras-28
Venkata Rao, V.	Powerpet	Eluru, Dist. W. Godaveri (A.P.)
Venkataswamy, G.	240, Naicker New St.	Madurai (Madras State)
Venkateswarlu	Armed Force Medical College ...	Poona-1
Venkateswara Rao, S.	Med. College	Kurnool (A.P.)

Venkatiswara Rao, G.	Eye Clinic Mallpet	Guntur-1 (Madras)
Verma Jagdish Chandra ...	Newyarpur Road	Patna-V (Bihar)
Verma, S. C.	Military Hospital	Jullunder Cantt (Punjab)
Verma Pursottam	Philadelphia Mission Hosp.	Ambala City (Haryana)
Verma Sushil Kumar	K.N. 225, Sector 16-A	Chandigarh (Punjab)
Vijay Kumar AMC	Military Hospital	Poona-20
Vindhyavalli, K.	People's Poly Clinic, Kasturi Devi Nagar	Nellore (A.P.)
Vora, Narendra Nagardas ..	c/o Dr. Mrs. Vora Bhagat Hosp. 267/269. Kalbadevi Rd.	Bombay-2
Wadhwanki, K. A.	2, Raj Mahal, Plot 185, Sion	Bombay-22
Wagle, G. S.	70, Race Course Road, North Tukoganj	Indore (M.P.)
Yadgir Rao	16-2-146/F, Malakpet	Hyderabad (A.P.)
Yash, Pal	Shri Ratnagarh Eye Hosp.	Ratnagarh, Dist. Churu (Rajasthan)
Zafrul, Islam	At & Post: Rafiganj	Dist. Gaya (Bihar)
Zaidi, Fatima Azra	Habibullah Manzil, La Diggi	Aligarh (U.P.)
Zunjarwad, Madhav Vyanka-tesh	953, North Sadar Bazar	Sholapur (Maharashtra)

NOSOCOMIA QUIBUS OCULIS AEGRI CURANTUR

No. of Beds

Andhra Pradesh

King George Hospital Vishakhapatinam	50
Sarojini Devi Eye Hospital & Institute of Ophthalmology	250

Assam

Shreemanta Sankar Mission Private High School, Nowgong	25
American Baptist Mission Private Hospital, Jorhat	15

Delhi & New Delhi

Safdarjang Hospital, New Delhi-16	28
Dr. Shroff's Charity Hospital Daryaguni, Delhi-6	214
Willingdon Hospital, Dept. of Ophthalmology, New Delhi	20
Sant Parmananda Eye Hospital, Rajpura Road, Delhi-6	25

Goa, Diu & Daman

Dr. Rajadhyaksha's Eye Hospital, Panjim.	20

Gujarat

Sheth Jagjivandas Visanji Trust Eye Hospital, Ahmedabad.	50
Sheth C. H. Nagri Eye Hospital, Ahmedabad.	85
Parvatibai Charitable Hospital, Opp. Dariapur Tower, Ahmedabad.	50
Rattanku Nathubhai Chausar Free Eye Hospital, Bulsar.	36
Civil Hospital, Ahmedabad.	54

Kerala

Ophthalmic Hospital, Trivandrum.	150
District Hospital, Ernakulam.	80

Madhya Pradesh

Christian Hospital, Mungeli, Dist. Bilaspur	50
Kirodimal Eye Hospital, Rajgarh	100
Shri Hukum Chand Eye Hospital, Indore	18
Hamidia Hospital, Bhopal	57

Maharashtra

Blind Relief Mission Free Eye Hospital, Dhantoli, Nagpur	40
Kankubai Eye Hospital, Sholapur	50
Khan Bahadur Haji Bachooali Free Ophthalmic Hospital, Parel, Bombay 12.	90
Shri C. J. Ophthalmic Unit, J. J. Group of Hospitals, Bombay-8	112
B. Y. L. Nair Charitable Hospital, Bombay.	18
Lokamanya Tilak Municipal General Hospital, Sion, Bombay	24
King Edward VII Memorial Hospital, Parel, Bombay	32
Mayo General Hospital, Napur	32
Sassoon General Hospital, Poona	50
Municipal Free Eye Hospital, Kamathipura, Bombay	40
Ramwadi Free Eye Hospital, Bombay-2	37

Mysore

Minto Ophthalmic Hospital, Bangalore	265
K.R. Hospital, Mysore	45
District Hospital, Chickmaglur	24

Punjab

Eye Hospital, Birgikalan	30
Krishan Lal Jain Free Hospital, Bhiwani	200
Civil Hospital, Jullundur	15
Dayanand Hospital, Ludhiana	36
M.D. Eye Hospital, Moga	36
Rajinder Hospital, Patiala	64
V.J. Hospital, Amritsar	64
Primary Health Centre, Malaudh	30

Rajasthan

Free Hospital, Ratangarh	50
Jaipur Eye Hospital, Nawalgarh	180
Surana Eye Hospital, Churu	50
Alexandra Eye Hospital, Alwar	24
M.B.S. Hospital, Kotah	20
S.K. Hospital, Sikar	25
General Hospital, Bharatpur	52
S.M.S. Hospital, Jaipur	83
M.G. Hospital, Jodhpur	62

Tamil nadu

Government Ophthalmic Hospital, Madras	326
Moses Gananabraham Eye Hospital, Coimbatore	60
Christian Medical College & Hospital, Vellore	80

Uttar Pradesh

M.D. Eye Hospital, Allahabad	72
B.S. Mehta Eye Hospital, Allahabad	100

Gandhi Eye Hospital, Aligarh 450
Hari Eye Hospital, Hathras, Dist. Aligarh 250
Sitapur Eye Hospital, (Branch), Bareilly 100
Kanpur Eye Hospital, Kanpur 70
Budhdha Devi Eye Hospital, Kanpur 45
Eye Hospital, Moradabad 37
Eye Hospital, Muzaffarnagar 32
Sitapur Eye Hospital, Sitapur 544
Eye Hospital, Khairabad, Dist. Sitapur 100
Sir Sunderlal Eye Hospital, Varanasi 300
Ursula Horsman Memorial Hospital, Kanpur 28
Lala Lajpat Rai Hospital, Kanpur 34
Balrampur Hospital, Lucknow 32

West Bengal

Dr. M. N. Chatterjee Memorial Hospital, Calcutta 54
Chittaranjan Hospital, Calcutta 25

INSTITUTA SCHOLAEQUE CAECIS DESTINATAE

Andhra Pradesh

Andhra Blind Model High School, Rayapet, Narsapur, West Godavari Dist.
Disabled Blind Children's Home & School, Anandanasamaj Buildings, Amravati Road, Guntur-2
Government School for the Blind, Cuddapah
'Jeevana Jyothi' C. S. I. Vidyanagar, Via Kondapalli, Penpaka Post, Krishna Dist.
Lutheran School for the Blind, Narsarapet, Guntur Dist.
National Association for the Blind (Andhra Pradesh State Branch), B6/F4, Vigyanpuri, Hyderabad-7
Society for Helping the Handicapped, Usmansahebpet, Nellore-2

Assam

Blind School attached to the Shreemanta Shankar Mission, P.O. Nowgong, New Gond Dist.

Bihar

Blind Relief Society, De Nobili School, P.O.F.R.I., Dist. Dhanbad
Home for the Blind, Muzaffarpur
Netraheen Chhatra Vidyalaya, Mudichak, Bhagalpur
Shree Kameshwari Priya Poor Home, Darbhanga
St. Michael's School for the Blind, P.O. Box No. 1, Ranchi

Delhi

Bharat Blind School, 510-A Circular Road, Shahdara, Delhi-32
Blind Social Welfare Society, 96, Panchkuin Road, New Delhi
Delhi Public Library (Braille Section) 425, Lakshmibai Nagar, New Delhi-5
Institution for the Blind, Panchkuin Road, New Delhi
National Society for the Prevention of Blindness, c/o Department of Ophthalmology, all-India Institute of Medical Science, Ansari Nagar, New Delhi-16
Rashtriya Virja Nand Andh Kanya Vidyalaya, New Rajinder Nagar, Shankar Road, New Delhi-60
Training & Rehabilitation Centre for the Blind, C-20 Model, Town, Delhi-9

Gujarat

Adult Training Centre for the Blind, Near A.T.I.R.A., Vastrapur Road, Ahmedabad-15
Ambaben Maganlal Andhjanshala, Race Course, Athwa Lines, Surat-1
Andh Abhyudaya Mandal, c/o Lions Club of Bhavnagar, Bhavnagar
Andh Kanya Prakash Griha (Light House for Blind Girls), Memnagar, Navrangpura, Ahmedabad-9
Andha Mahila Vikas Griha, Gondal Road, Near Swaminarayan Gurukul, Rajkot
Andh Sarvodaya Mandal, Dhebar Road, Rajkot 2
Baroda Association for the Blind, Mahajans Lane, Raopura, Baroda
Blind Men's Association, Near A.T.I.R.A., Vastrapur Road, Ahmedabad-15
Blind Physiotherapist Association, Bajrang Kruper, L.I.C. Society, Rajkot
Government School for the Blind, Madan Zanpa Road, Baroda
Gujarat Rajya Nayanjyot Raksha Samiti, Opp. R.C. High School, Dr. Tankaria Road, Ahmedabad 1
Krishnakumarsinhji School & Home for the Blind, College Road, Takhteshwar Plot, Bhavnagar
M.T. Doshi Andhvidyalaya, Near Kasturba Society, Surendranagar
Meghji Pethraj Blind School, Mahatma Gandhi Road, Junagadh
Mohanben Bhavanilal Jain Andh Jan Vidyalaya, Dohad
National Association for the Blind (Gujarat State Branch), Near A.T.I.R.A., Vastrapur Road, Ahmedabad-15
School for the Blind, Ellis Bridge, Ahmedabad
School for the Blind, Visavadar, Dist. Junagadh
Shri Bharatiya Pragna Chakshu Gurukul, Porbunder
Tata Agricultural & Rural Training Centre for the Blind, Phansa

Haryana

Blind relief Section, District Red Cross Society, Hissar
Government Institute for the Blind, Panipat
S.D. Institute for the Blind, Ambala Cantt
Training Centre for the Adult Blind, Sonepat

Jammu-Kashmir

Abhedananda Home, Home for Blind & Handicapped, Modern School for Integrated Education, Silk Factory Road, Shrinagar
Akhil Bharatiya Netrahin Society, Jammu Branch, Ved Mandir, Jammu-1
Residential School for the Blind, Ved Mandir, Jammu

Kerala

Government School for the Blind, Kasargod
Kerala Blind Welfare Association, Mankadapallippuram, Angadipuram
Light to the Blind, Varkala, L.M.S. Compound, South Kerala Diocease, Trivandrum P.O.
School for the Blind, Kunnamkulam, Talpally Trichur District
School for the Blind, Thottumugham P.O., Alwaye-5

Madhya Pradesh

Blind Relief Association, 72/13-14 South T.T. Nagar, Bhopal
Deaf, Dumb & Blind School, Bada Rawla, Juni Indore, (Opp. Gira Mandir), Indore-4
Madhav Andh Ashram, Jhansi Road, Lashkar, Gwalior
Madhya Pradesh Welfare Association for the Blind, 84, Veer Savarkar Market, Indore-4

Maharashtra

Bassein Blind Relief Association, Eye Hospital, Azad Road, Bassein, Thana Dist.
Blind Men's Association, 81-A, Jaldarshan, L. Jagmohandas Marg, Bombay-6
Blind Relief Association, Botawala Building, 475–83, Kalbadevi Road, Bombay-2
Blind Relief Association, South Ambazari Road, Nagpur-3

Blind Welfare Association, Housing Colony, Amravati-2
Dadar School for the Blind, 160, Dadasaheb Phalke Road, Dadar, Bombay-14
Government School for the Blind, Nasik
Haji Allarakhia Sonawala Andh and Anath Stree Ashram, 37, Gilbert Hill, Dadabhai Road, Andheri, Bombay-58
Happy Home & School for the Blind, Dr. Annie Besant Road, Worli, Bombay-18
Industrial Home for Blind Women, 160, Dadasaheb Phalke Road, Dadar, Bombay-14
Krishanlal Jalan Charity Trust, 339, Kalbadevi Road, Bombay-2
M. N. Banajee Industrial Home for the Blind, 280, Swami Vivekanand Road, Jogeshwari, Bombay-60
Maharogi Seva Samiti Warora, P.O. Anandvan, Dist. Chanda
National Association of the Instructors of the Blind, 22, Jal Bungalow, Arab Lane, Corner Grant Rd., Bombay-8
National Christian Council, Nagpur-1
N.S.D. Industrial Home for the Blind, 52, B.D.D. Chawls, Worli, Bombay-18
Poona Blind Men's Association, 82, Rasta Peth, Poona
Poona School & Home for the Blind, Koregaon Park, Poona
Pragati Andh Vidyalaya, 18, Narayan Niwas, Ghantali Colony, Nowpada, Thana
Ramabai Mukti Mission, Khedgaon, Poona District
Sanjivani Arogya Sanakari Sanstha Ltd., Virar, Thana Dist.
School for the Blind, Bodadi (Both Road) Taluka Kinwat, Dist. Nanded
School for the Blind, Deopur, Dhulia
Victoria Memorial High School for Blind, 73, Tardeo Road, Bombay-34
Workshop for the Blind, Dr. Annie Besant Road, Prabhadevi, Bombay-25

Mysore

Blind Relief Association, Bijapur
Government School for the Blind, Hubli, Dharwar District
Government School for Deaf & Blind Boys, Mysore
Mysore Welfare Association for the Blind, 1623, 17th Cross (Upstairs), IInd Main Road, Malleswaram, Bangalore-3
School for the Blind, Institute of Social Service, Department of Social Work, Roshni Nilaya, Fr. Muller Road, Bangalore-2
Shri Ramana Maharishi Academy for the Blind, 511, Garutman Park, East End Road, Bangalore-4

Orissa

Orissa State Council for Child Welfare, Raj Bhuvan, Bhubneshwar

Punjab

Andh Vidyalaya (Institution for the Blind), Amritsar
Bharatiya Andth Hitakarini Sabha 212–13, Gurudwara Building, Inside Lohgarth Cate, Amritsar
District Council for the Welfare of the Handicapped, Home for the Blind, 1, Maheshchand Library Road, Ferozepur City
Surma Singh Ashram, G.T. Road, Amritsar

Rajasthan

Government School for the Blind, Adarshnagar, Ajmer
Pragya Chakshu Sikshan Shansthan, (Andh Vidyalaya) Udaipur
Rajasthan Netrahin Kalyan Sangh Farsoia Market, Bapu Bazar, Jaipur-3

Tamil Nadu

Bishop Diehl Rehabilitation Home for the Blind, Tranguebar House Compound, Tiruchirapalli-1
Blind Relief Association, 17, Gang Shala, Pondicherry
Blind Relief Association, Fort Round Road, Vellore, North Arcot District

Government School for the Blind, Shivpet, Salem-2
Government School for the Blind, Poonamallee
Madras Christian College (Students' Service for the Blind), Tambaram, Chingleput District
Government School for the Blind, Sir T. Desikachariar Buildings, Puthur, Tiruchirapalli
National Association for the Blind (Tamil Nadu State Branch) Y.M.C.A. College of Physical
    Education Campus, Nandanam, Madras-35
Pilot Demonstration Rehabilitation Centre for the Blind, Madurai Medical College, Madurai-13
School for the Blind, Palayamkottai, Tirunelvelli-2
School for the Blind, Swedish Mission Hospital, Tirupattur, Ramnathpuram District
School for the Blind & Deaf, Cathedral Post, Madras-6
Society for Aiding the Handicapped, 'Kamakoti', 37, VI, Main Road, R.A. Puram, Madras-28
St. Louis Institute for the Deaf and Blind, Madras-20
Telc Home & School for the Blind, Moses Gnabaram Eye Hospital, Coimbatore-1
'The Blind' Society, 'Jamadhagni', 10, Telegraph Office Lane, Ootacamund-1

Uttar Pradesh

Ahmedi School for the Blind, Civil Lines, Aligarh
Blind School, Bhadaini, Varanasi
Blind Welfare Society, B1/152, Assi Ghat, Varanasi-5
Indumati Andh Shishu Sharanalaya, P.O. Tehri, Dist. Tehri Garhwal
Kashi Seva Samiti, Varanasi
Netraviheen Kalyan Sangh, 9-C, Civil Lines, Gorakhpur
School & Home for the Blind, Naini, Allahabad
School for the Blind attached to the Eye Hospital, Sitapur
School for the Blind, Deaf & Dumb, 110/241, Nehru Nagar, Kanpur
Sharp Memorial School for the Blind, Rajpur Road, Dehra Dun
Shree Ajara Nand Andh Vidyalaya, Sapt Sarovar, Hardwar, Dist. Saharanpur

West Bengal

Blind Boys' Academy, Ramkrishna Mission, P.O. Narendrapur, District 24 Parganas
Blind Persons' Association, Bapujinagar Society, Jadarpur, Calcutta-32
Light House for the Blind (Society), c/o Mrs. S.N. Ghosh, 6, Old Post Office Street, Calcutta-1
Mary Scott Home for the Blind, Kalimpong, Darjeeling District
National Association for the Blind (West Bengal State Branch), c/o Union Paper and Board Mills
    Ltd., 18, Netaji Subhash Road, Calcutta-1
School for the Blind, Swedish Mission, Cooch Behar

IRAN

SOCIETATES OPHTHALMOLOGICAE

Société Iranienne d'Ophtalmologie
Secrétaire: Prof. G. Sadoughi, Av. Chah Reza en face Villa, Téhéran
No data received.

IRAQ

SOCIETATES OPHTHALMOLOGICAE

Ophthalmological Society of Iraq
Secretary: Dr. A. M. Abutrah, Al Ramad Eye Hospital Uarkh, Baghdad
No data received.

ISRAELIA

SOCIETATES OPHTHALMOLOGICAE

Nationalis

Israel Ophthalmological Society
(Igud rol'ey ha'eynayim be–Israel)
Chairman: Prof. E. Neumann
Vice-Chairman: Dr. R. Sachs
Board-members: Dr. A. Avshalom, Dr. E. Aviel, Dr. S. Barkai, Dr. H. Ben-Moshe, Dr. M. Blumenthal, Dr. D. Berson, Dr. W. H. Felsenthal, Prof. O. Kurz, Dr. M. Lazar, Prof. J. Landau, Prof. I. C. Michaelson, Prof. L. Nawratzki, Dr. E. Sinai, Dr. H. Spier, Prof. R. Stein, Dr. S. Sonis, Dr. M. Romem, Prof. H. Zauberman
Secretary: Dr. A. Lavyel, 3 Disraeli St., Haifa
Treasurer: Dr. V. Sachs
Number of members: 195

Regionales

Jerusalem Ophthalmological Society
Chairman: Prof. I. C. Michaelson, 19 Balfour St., Jerusalem

Tel-Aviv Ophthalmological Society
Chairman: Prof. R. Stein
Secretary: Dr. R. Sachs, 67 Arlosrov St., Tel Aviv

Haifa Ophthalmological Society
Chairman: Prof. E. Neumann
Secretary: Dr. A. Lavyel, 3 Disraeli St., Haifa

NOMINA ET DOMICILIA MEDICORUM AB OCULIS

Aizikov, Itzhak	14 Uziel Str., Bat Yam	Tel Aviv
Antel, Yehudith	19/23 Moldet Str.	Kfar Saba
Arnold, Hedda	Bath Oren Str., Yad Eljahu	Tel Aviv
Arsler, Gabriel	Shderot Hayeled	Ramat Gan
Auerbach, Edgar	27 Matolda Str.	Jerusalem
Aviel, Eliezer	Ashkelon Hospital	
Avramovic, Fanny	106/2 Lehman Str., Kiryat Bialik	Haifa
Avshalom, Asher	Sheshet Hayamin Str.	Kefar Sava
Bar-Am, Yehuda	8 Einstein Str.	Affula
Bar-Itzhak, Robert	Shikun Roffim	Tel Hashomer

Barkai, Shoshana	Poria Hospital	Tyberias
Baruch, Haim	91 Ben Yehuda Str.	Tel Aviv
Ben-Bassat, Jacob	14 Melchett Str.	Tel Aviv
Ben-Dor, D	4 Mane Str., Talbia	Jerusalem
Ben-Ezra, David	30 Haarav Berlin Str.	Jerusalem
Ben Mosh, Hayim	21 Hanita Str., Neveh Shanan Str.	Haifa
Berach, Rivka	13 Amsterdam Str.	Tel Aviv
Berar, Ladislav	9 Shderot Chen	Tel Aviv
Berke, Zeev	25 Bin Nun Str.	Tel Aviv
Bialik, Magdalene	30/6 Hagiborim Str.	Haifa
Belkin, Michael	17 Island Str.	Jerusalem
Belkind, Haya	70 Rothchild Str.	Petha Tikva
Berson, David	12 Hameshoreret Str.	Jerusalem
Blumenthal, Michael	Beth Cholim Hamerkazi Lanegev	Ber Sheva
Blumenthal, Ruth	18 Elchanan Str.	Haifa
Brand, Laskin Eva	9 Harofe Str.	Haifa
Brener, Itzhak	35 Ben Yehuda Str.	Jerusalem
Bukshpan, Olla	34 King George Str.	Tel Aviv
Cohen, Hilda	10 Hatommer, Str.	Jerusalem
Cohen, Miriam		Affula
Cohen, Nissim	6 Gretz Str.	Tel Aviv
Davidson, Alexander	5 Yesheyahu Str., Ramat Gan	Tel Aviv
Derbaum, Yeshayahu	15 Yackob Str.	Rehovot
Deuel, Fanny	24 Bari Str.	Tel Aviv
Eckstein, Meir	12/a Wedgwood Str.	Haifa
Ehrlich, Brand	100 Arlosorof Str.	Tel Aviv
Eibschitz, Naomi	74 Moriah Str.	Haifa
Elenbogen, Paul	28 Shapira Str.	Petah Tikva
Erez, Ruth		Kefar Sava
Estricher, K.	5 Herzel Str.	Ramat Gan
Farber, Binyamin	8/3 Malther Str.	Rehovot
Farber, Lidia	8/3 Malther Str.	Rehovot
Feiler, Ofri, V.	113 Yehuda Hammcabi Str.	Tel Aviv
Feitlberg, Israel	10 Jabotinsky Str.	Jerusalem
Felichenfeld, Margaretta	13 Bialik Str.	Tel Aviv
Felix, Juster	15 Hahistadrut Str.	Petah Tikva
Felix, Mendel	4/4 Aba Hillel Silver Str.	Haifa
Felsenthal, W. H.	6 Shderoth Hanassi Str.	Haifa
Fleischer, Alexander	8 K.K.L. Str.	Jerusalem
Fodor, Josef	Ulpan Ben Yehuda	Natania
Folman, Wanda	42/a Tel Manne	Haifa
Freudenthal, E.	25 Ben Josef Av.	Tel Aviv
Freund, Michael	1 Bilu Str.	Kfar Saba
Fridlich, Cheslava	21 Harava Str.	Holon
Friedmann, G. Ludvik	103/7 Hameshahrerim Str.	Ber Sheva
Friedman, Guttman H.	55 Tchernichovsky Str.	Haifa
Friedman, Thea	20 Shaanan Str.	Ramat Gan
Friedman, Zvi	13 Shimshon Str.	Haifa
Fuchs, Kivo		Ashdod
Gabby, Anuar	Beth Haroffim, Beilinson	Tel Aviv
Gdal On, Mordechai	843 Str. No. 4	Haifa
Glikson, Josf	40 Meir Rutenberg Str.	Haifa
Godel, Victor	8 Krause Str.	Natania
Goldstein, Chana	7 Bialik Str.	Holon
Gotthelf, Ernest	17 Hanoter Str., Affeca	Tel Aviv
Gottlieb, Rachel	7 Ben Ami Str.	Jerusalem

Gross, Berli Doba	6 Massada Str.	Haifa
Grun, Esperina	28 Ben Zion Str.	Tel Aviv
Ginor, Arie	42 Shinkin Str.	Tel Aviv
Hyams, Stenli	8 Yochvet Str.	Haifa
Harel, Itzhak	15 Herzel Str.	Haifa
Hass, H.	279 Hayarkon Str.	Tel Aviv
Hayt, Chava	47/2 Vurborg Av., Kiriat Yam	Haifa
Heller, Emanuel	2 Gordon Str., Kiriat Yovel	Jerusalem
Herzberg, Fritz	56 Herzel Str.	Haifa
Hirschberg, Frida	50 Gordon Str.	Tel Aviv
Karib, Georg	116 Shderot Um	Haifa
Keroub, K.	Simtat Abanon 8	Haifa
Klevid, Stefan	23 Haavoda Str., Herzlia	Tel Aviv
Krakovsky, David	66 Krinizi Str., Ramat Gan	Tel Aviv
Kropivnicka, A.	19 Josef Haglili Str, Ramat Gan	Tel Aviv
Koni, Mary	9 Shul Hamelech Str.	Tel Aviv
Kanner, Samuel	19 Shapira Str.	Petah Tikva
Kurz, Otto	11 Jonah Hanavy Str.	Tel Aviv
Landau, Jacob	20 Hahistadrut Str.	Jerusalem
Landau, Louis	26 Hameshoreret Str.	Jerusalem
Lavyel, Amos	6 D'israeli Str.	Haifa
Lazar, Hari	Ulpan Yarkon	Natania
Lazr, Moshe		Tel Hashomer
Levy, Josef	1 Smolensky Str.	Natania
Lieberman, Ritta	9 Habanim Str. Neveh Sranan	Haifa
Liebling, Sabina	29 Eidilson Str.	Tel Aviv
Liechtanberg, Gabriela	133 Shderot Rothchild	Tel Aviv
Littman, Shoshana	1 Bilu Str.	Kffar Saba
Lobel, David	16 Mishmar Hagvul Str., Affeka	Tel Aviv
Loebel, Emanuel	40 Tchernichvsky Str.	Jerusalem
Lombrozo, J.	Iben Gvirol 74	Tel Aviv
Loven, David	10 Jerusalem Str.	Haifa
Luger, David	9 Hamatmid Str.	Natania
Mahlin, Michael	11 Hatzalvnim Str.	Haifa
Malmud, Sharon	Hatzvi Str.	Beer Sheva
Mandel, Itzhak	90 Hashalom Rd.	Tel Aviv
Manor, Dori	72 K.K.L. Str.	Tel Aviv
Marcus, M.	226 Shderot UM	Haifa
Merin, Shaul	11 Hameshoreret Str.	Jerusalem
Meyer, Eva	6 Margalit Str.	Haifa
Mishali, Itzhak	10 Leon Blum Str.	Haifa
Mishouri, Miriam	36 Bari Str.	Tel Aviv
Mecklin, Zvi	9 Hateena Str.	Tel Aviv
Michaelson, I. C.	19 Balfour Str.	Tel Aviv
Mirovski, Avraham	40 Moriah Str.	Haifa
Muller, Ahcer	40 Shderot Hatzvi	Haifa
Maythar, Batia	54a Hanavyim Str.	Jerusalem
Navratzki, Ilse	17 Keren Hayessod Str.	Jerusalem
Nelken, Edith	20a, Harrav Berlin Str.	Jerusalem
Neumann, Eliyahu	4 Dauns Str.	Haifa
Ninsenkorn, Ilana		Affula
Nissan, Teu	174 Moddien Str., Givataim	Tel Aviv
Nissan, Ezra	86 Herzel Str.	Ramat Gan
Oliver, Moshe	18/a Hapalman Str.	Jerusalem
Ostfeld, Samuel	23/5 Hagalil Str., Kiryat Bialik	Haifa
Paggy, Yeshaya	3 D'israeli Str.	Haifa

Pasco, Michael	137 Shlomo Hamelech Str.	Tel Aviv
Perlman, Tova	72 Sheinkin Str.	Tel Aviv
Pechner, Arthur	24 Herzel Str.	Hedera
Perlman, G.	20a Lochamei Hagetaot Str.	Haifa
Pinhas, Albert	5 Dizingof Str.	Tel Aviv
Politi, Fredy	115 Yosefftal Str., Bat Yam	Tel Aviv
Psemnic, Shaul	24 Tirtza Str.	Ramat Gan
Psiga, Frieda	147/3 Allenby Str.	Haifa
Rachmann-Hoop, R.	1 Gan Rechavia	Jerusalem
Rasiar, Jacob	45/6 Jerusalem Str., Bat Yam	Tel Aviv
Reif, Josef	14 Feivel Str.	Tel Aviv
Regenbogen, L.	16 Bloch Str.	Tel Aviv
Rosenbaum, Sophia	1 Elisha Str.	Haifa
Rosenberg, Hilda	22 Hapoalim Str.	Jerusalem
Rosenberg, Liza	15 Balfour Str.	Tel Aviv
Rosenberg, Milla	52 Golomb Str., Givataiim	Tel Aviv
Rom, Jacob	7 Hemelech Shlomo Str.	Tel Aviv
Romen, Miriam	15 Kdusey Kahir Str., Holon	Tel Aviv
Rozenet, Thamara	30 Herzlia Str.	Haifa
Rozsansky, Miriam	13/8 Kdusey Kahir Str.	Holon
Rubilovicz, M.	1 Golomb Str.	Haifa
Rubinfeld, Gideon	7 Haporcim Str.	Rishon Lezion
Sachs, Rudolf	67 Arlosrov Str.	Tel Aviv
Sachs, Willy	6/a Mappu Str.	Haifa
Savir, Hanna	5 Haddera Str.	Tel Aviv
Salmon, Marcel	62/71 Hanita Str.	Haifa
Schonfeld, K.	110 Arlozorof Str.	Haifa
Scholl, Adalbert	18 Balfour Str., Bat Yam	Tel Aviv
Schwartz, Vili		Affula
Shaulson, L.	87/9 Heinkin Str.	Holon
Shabatai, Henric	46 Jerusalem Str.	Jaffa
Shalom, Elijahu	53 Pinsker Str.	Tel Aviv
Sheratzki, Zeev	29 Herzel Str.	Naharia
Sherf, Jehudith	2 Dolfin Str.	Haifa
Shiber, Moshe	131 Ben Yehuda Str.	Tel Aviv
Shifmenovich, B.	5 Sharret Str.	Tel Aviv
Shifrin, Olga	13 Haatzmaut Str., Bat Yam	Tel Aviv
Shilo, Zeeb	27 Thon Str., Holon	Tel Aviv
Shiloach, Or G.	Ramot	Hashavim
Shlamovits, Arnold	46 Haroe Str., Ramat Gan	Tel Aviv
Shmukler, William	14 Jabutinsky Str.	Natania
Shmilovic, Eva	10/7 Shikun Haroffim	Tel Hashommer
Shpeler, Leon	24 Rambam Str.	Ber Sheva
Sinai, Ephraim	19 Hayotman Str.	Tel Aviv
Safra, Doris	4 Hovevei Zion Str.	Jerusalem
Singer, Bardov L.	11 Jabutinski Str.	Holon
Slowes, Miriam	98 Allenby Str.	Tel Aviv
Sohar, Hanannel	18 Pombdita Str.	Tel Aviv
Sommer, Zvi	20 Ben Yehuda Str.	Haifa
Smilovici, A.	14/5 Marsille Str.	Haifa
Spier, Hanna	229/32 Haalia Str.	Ber Sheva
Stein, Richard	20 Hess Str.	Tel Aviv
Streich, Arthur	9 Ahrav Kuk Str.	Tel Aviv
Stern, Reich R.	Shalag Str.	Tel Aviv
Syrkin, Norman	11a Einstein Str.	Haifa
Szonis, Shlomo	70 Margalit Str.	Haifa

Traister, Gyora	12 Jabutinski Str., Givataim	Tel Aviv
Tweig, Nissim	1 Shprinzak Str.	Tel Aviv
Unger, Elchanan	128 Dizingof Str.	Tel Aviv
Valner, Clara	45 Degania Str., Kiriat Haim	Haifa
Wapner, Brach	45 Bialik Str., Ramat Gan	Tel Aviv
Wehena, Jacob	7/1 Shikun Roffim Yashan	Haifa
Weinstein, Rifka	94 Arlosorof Str.	Tel Aviv
Weiss, Yehuda	138/a Jabutinski Str.	Tel Aviv
Wender, Tamara	11 Asaf Shimshoni Str., Petach Tikva	Tel Hashomer
Windman, Abraham	39 Hakeshet Str.	Ramat Gan
Wollstein, Josef	27 Urugvay Str.	Tel Aviv
Yadlin, Ephraim	126 Ahad Ha'am Str.	Tel Aviv
Yarmilovic, Natalia	89 Ben Yehuda Str.	Tel Aviv
Yassur, Yuval		Kibutz Zova
Yavorski, Miriam R.	Hannasi, 24 Eli Cohen, Bat Yam .	Tel Aviv
Youster, Felix	Rechov Hahistadrut	Tel Aviv
Zadok, Josef	1 Ehaad Haam Str.	Holon
Zar, Ilana	79 University, Ramat Gan	Tel Aviv
Zauberman, Hanan	26 Ben Maymon Str.	Jerusalem
Zeifrani, Shaul	24 Aliya Str.	Haifa
Zivoni, Sara	31 Maaze Str.	Tel Aviv

NOSOCOMIA QUIBUS OCULIS AEGRI CURANTUR

	No. of beds
Eye Dept., Afula Sick-Fund Hospital (Head: Dr. W. Sachs)	18
Eye Dept., Assaf Harofe Sarafand, Government Hospital (Head: R. Sachs)	33
Eye Dept., Ashkelon. Sick-Fund Hospital. (Head: Dr. E. Aviel)	15
Eye Dept., Belinson. Petah-Tiqva University Sick-Fund Hospital Tel-Aviv, Med School. (Head: Prof. O. Kurz)	22
Eye Dept., Beer-Sheva. Government Hospital (Head: Dr. H. Speier)	20
Eye Dept., Donolo. Jaffa University Government Hospital Tel-Aviv Med School (Head: Dr. M. Romem)	18
Eye Dept., Hadassah. University Med School Hospital Jerusalem (Head: Prof. H. Zauberman)	26
Eye Dept., Ichilov. Tel-Aviv Municipal Hospital (Head: Dr. M. Lazar)	25
Eye Dept., Kfar-Saba. Sick-Fund Hospital (Head: Dr. A. Avshalom)	24
Eye Dept., Naharia. Government Hospital (Head: Dr. H. Ben-Moshe)	15
Eye Dept., Poriah. Government Hospital (Head: Dr. S. Barkai)	24
Eye Dept., Rothschild University Hospital, the Aba Khoushy School of Medicine (Head: Prof. E. Neumann)	22
Eye Dept., Rambam. University Hospital, the Aba Khoushy School of Medicine (Head: Dr. W. E. Felsenthal)	42
Eye Dept., Saarei-Zedek. Hospital Jerusalem (Head: Dr. D. Berson)	16
Eye Dept., Tel-Hashomer. Government Hospital. University Med. School Tel-Aviv (Head: Prof. R. Stein)	60

INSTITUTA SCHOLAEQUE CAECIS DESTINATAE

Israel Institute for the Blind (Beth Hinnuh Ivrim Livney Yisrael), Kiryat Moshe, Jerusalem.
Rehabilitation Center for the Blind, 'Migdal Or' P.O.B. 4775, Haifa.
Seeing Eye Dog School, Kiryat Haim.
Central Braille Library for the Blind, Nathania.

Society for the Care of the Blind and Prevention of Blindness, 19 Balfour St., Jerusalem.
Malben runs sheltered workshops.
Ministry for Social Welfare-Sherut Laiver, runs sheltered workshops.

ITALIA

SOCIETATES OPHTHALMOLOGICAE

Nationalis

Società Oftalmologica Italiana

Honorary President: Prof. Luigi Maggiore
President: Prof. G. Battista Bietti
Vice-President: Prof. Riccardo Gallenga, Prof. Benedetto Strampelli
Counsellors: Prof. Bruno Boles Carenini, Prof. Ivan Esente, Prof. Antonio Grignolo, Prof. Mario Maione, Prof. Guiseppe Scuderi, Prof. Angelo Vannini
Secretary: Prof. Ivan Esente, 2, Corso Italia, 50123 Firenze
Number of members: 836

Regionales

Associazione Lombarda

Clinica Oculistica Università di Milano
President: Prof. Carlo Toselli

Associazione Meridionale

Clinica Oculistica Università di Bari
President: Prof. Giuseppe Scuderi

Associazione Triventa

Clinica Oculistico Università di Padova
President: Prof. Franco D'Ermo

Circolo Oftalmico Romano

Address: c/o Clinica Oculistica Università di Roma

Bollettino di Oculistica

Edizione Cappelli di Bologna
President: Prof. G. Battista Bietti

Analisi di Oftalmologia e di Clinica Oculistica

Clinica Oculistica Università di Parma
President: Prof. Mario Marione

NOMINA ET DOMICILIA MEDICORUM AB OCULIS

Soci Onorari

Bencini, Prof. A.	Via Monna Agnese 8	Siena
Von Berger, Prof. F.	Via Ricasoli 11	Livorno
Caramazza, Prof. F.	Via Vallescura 12	Bologna
Cattaneo, Prof. D.	Viale della Selva 8	Tirrenia - Pisa
Favaloro, Prof. G.		Catania
Raverdino, Prof. E.	Via Verri 4	Milano
Santonastasio, Prof. A.	Via Gabelli 1	Padova
Sgrosso, Prof. S.	Salerno	Ravello

Soci Fonditori

Bietti, Giovan Battista	Direttore Clinica Oculistica Universitaria	Roma
Castelli, Adolfo	Primario Ospedale Maggiore	Bergamo
Cristini, Giuseppe	Direttore Clinica Oculistica	Bologna
De Conciliis, Nicola	Corso Vittorio Emanuele, 670	Napoli
De Vincentiis, Giuseppe	Via Pessina, 90	Napoli
Di Ferdinando, Renato	Primario Oculista Ospedale Civile	Pesaro
Focosi, Marcello	Direttore Clinica Oculistica Universitaria	Firenze
Galeazzi, Cesare	Via Boccaccio, 45	Milano
Gallenga, Riccardo	Direttore Clinica Oculistica Universitaria	Torino
Grancini, Enrico	Primario Ospedale Circolo	Varese
Leonardi, Epimaco	Direttore Emerito Ospedale Oftal. Provinciale	Roma
Marucci, Luigi	Primario Oculista Ospedale Civile	Mantova
Menestrina, Gino	Via Weggenstein, 17	Bolzano
Moscardi, Paolo	Primario Emerito Oculista Ospedale Civile	Aquila
Motolese, Alfonso		Martina Franca (Taranto)
Nichelatti, Paolo	Via Moretto, 84	Brescia
Orzalesi, Francesco	Direttore Clinica Oculistica Universitaria	Milano
Pagani, Mario	Primario Oculista Ospedale Maggiore	Novara
Santoni, Armando	Direttore Clinica Oculistica Universitaria	Napoli
Scullica, Francesco	Direttore Clinica Oculistica Universitaria	Messina
Spinelli, Francesco	Corso Magenta, 31	Milano
Strampelli, Benedetto	Corso d'Italia, 33	Roma
Valerio, Mario	Primario Oculista Ospedale Croce Rossa Italiana	Milano
Venco, Luigi	Primario Ospedali Civili	Brescia
Zoldan, Luigi G.	Via Altinate, 69	Padova

Soci Ordinari

Alagna, Gaspare	Via Giuseppe Natoli, Isolato 196 .	Messina
Alajmo, Arnaldo	Ospedale Riuniti	Venezia
Aliquò, Mazzei Alessandro .	Viale Ledra, 1	Udine
Ambrosio, Andrea	Via Ponte di Tappia, 47	Napoli
Amidei, Bruno	Primario Oculista Ospedale Civile.	Vicenza
Angelini, Alessandro	Via Dante, 2	Bologna
Angelone, Luigi		Frosinone
Angius, Tullio	Via S. Frola, 4	Torino
Apollonio, Alfonso	Via Magenta, 12	Varese
Apponi, Giovanni	Via Annibale Vecchi, 240	Perugia
Arnone, Guido	Clinica Oculistica Universitaria ..	Palermo
Attanasio, Vito	Via Morello, 4	Licata
Aulizio, Bartolomeo	Via Carducci, 56	Venezia-Mestre
Aureggi, Dario		Carimate (Como)
Auricchio, Giacinto	Clinica Oculistica Universitaria ..	Palermo
Avanza, Carlo	Via Venezuela, 3	Milano
Avola, Salvatore	Piazza C. Rizzone, 140	Modica (Ragusa)
Bagolini, Bruno	Clinica Oculistica Universitaria ..	Sassari
Balcet, Carlo	Via Vescovado, 16	Biella
Baquis, Mario	Via Cavour, 60	Firenze
Baratta, Orazio	Via Parmigianino, 8	Parma
Barraquer, Josè	Apartado Acreo, 11056	Bogota
Battistini, Antonio	Viale Damiano Chiesa, 26	Pavia
Bauman, Adamo	Via Giuseppe La Farina, 3	Palermo
Bellomio, Salvatore	Via Giordano Bruno, 82	Catania
Bentivoglio, Marco	Piazzale San Francesco, 154	Modena
Berardi, Mario	Via Bicchierai, 129	Montecatini Terme
Beretta, Francesco	Via Benedetto Marcello, 30	Milano
Berger, Gian Pietro von	Via Ricasoli, 11	Livorno
Bertoldi, Maria	Via Montebello	Tortona
Betetto, Giovanni	Piazza Stanga, 3	Padova
Biancacci, Attilio	Via Rivareno, 6	Bologna
Bianchi, Giorgio	Via Canova, 18	Lugano
Biffis, Andrea	Via F. Filzi, 20	Treviso
Blanchi, Guido	Via A. Rosmini, 5	Torino
Bocci, Giorgio	Piazza Europa, 20	Cuneo
Boles, Carenini Bruno	Clinica Oculistica Universitaria ..	Cagliari
Bolettieri, Daniele	Ospedale Civile	Matera
Bonavalontà, Aldo	Clinica Oculistica Universitaria ..	Napoli
Bonardi, Mauro Rina	Viale Sarca, 85	Milano
Borioni, Domenico	Via Menicucci, 3	Ancona
Borsellino, Gaspare	Via XX Settembre, 8	Palermo
Borsello, Giuseppe	Corso Torino, 84	Pinerolo
Bosa, Filippo	Primario Ospedale Civile	Ragusa
Bassalino, Giuseppe	Via Moscova, 18	Milano
Bosso, Gian Carlo	Corso Mazzini, 29	Navara
Bottasso, Giovanni	Via Gropello, 2-bis	Torino
Bottoni, Angelo	Piazzetta Guastalla, 5	Milano
Bozzoni, Giovanni	Viale Trieste, 2	S. Benedetto del Tronto
Bozzoni Pantaleoni, Filippo .	Piazza Winkelmann, 5	Roma
Bozzoni Pantaleoni, Giulio .	Viale Trieste, 71	Ascoli Piceno
Brognoli, Carlo	Corso Martiri Libertà, 14	Brescia
Bruno, Franco	Corso Trieste, 42	Roma
Busti, Angelo	Piazza Martiri, 4	Novara

Caffi, Mariuccia	Viale Partigiani, n. 109	Pavia
Calamandrei, Giorgio	Via Lorenzo il Magnifico, 72	Firenze
Calogero, Nicola	Viale Giusti, 8	Firenze
Cambiaggi, Amerigo	Lungoparco Gropello 4/10	Genova
Canepa, Nicolò	Via Cavour, 309	La Spezia
Capaccini, Alberto	Via Pier Capponi, 54	Firenze
Capra, Piera	Via Claudio Monteverdi, 18	Roma
Caprara, Maria Rosa	Via S. Caterina da Siena, 41	Ferrara
Capucci, Mario	Viale Cassiodoro, 20	Milano
Cardello, Giovanni	Corso Alfieri, 63	Asti
Cardi, Gabriella	Via Modena, 154	Ferrara
Carelli, Benedetto	Via Orazio, 145	Napoli
Carlevaro, Gianfrancesco	Via Ponzio, 82	Milano
Carmi, Alberto	Via Farini, 43	Parma
Carones, Alessandro Valerio.	Corso Porta Romana, 6	Milano
Carra, Giorgio	Via Boncompagni, 61	Roma
Carusillo, Mario	Ospedale Civile	Mantova
Casà, Girolamo	Viale Vittoria, 97	Agrigento
Casati, Emanuele	Via Donatello, 37	Roma
Cascio, Giuseppe	Via Salvatore Meccio, 25	Palermo
Caselli, Francesco	Clinica Oculistica Universitaria	Palermo
Casini, Francesco	Viale Trieste, 58	Rovigo
Caso, Giuseppe	Piazza di Portanuova, 1	Salerno
Catalino, Pietro	Via Martelli, 3	Roma
Cati, Paolo	Via S. Pietro Martire, 40	Rieti
Cavallacci, Giulio	Via L. Papi, 11	Lucca
Cavalli, Ettore	Piazza Duomo, 5	Lucera (Foggia)
Celotti, Mario	Via Bronzino, 6	Milano
Centanni, Leonardo	Clinica Oculistica Universitaria	Bologna
Cerabolini, Ernesto	Viale Libertà, 111	Pavia
Chieppa, Franco	Piazza Imbriani, 3	Andria (Bari)
Chinaglia, Vincenzo	Primario Ospedale Civile	Treviso
Ciotola, Guido	Viale Mazzini, 33	Roma
Ciserani, Cesare	Via Parini, 5	Milano
Citroni, Mario	Clinica Oculistica Universitaria	Pavia
Clerici, Antonio	Piazza S. Maria Beltrade, 1	Milano
Collevati, Umberto	Via Adelardi, 15	Ferrara
Colombi, Carlo	Via Magnacavallo, 22	Casale Monferrato
Colombo, Giuseppe	Via Libertà, 10	Palermo
Contarini, Loris	Via Pani, 1	Rimini
Contini, Poli Ornella	Via Vitali, 2	Milano
Contino, Filippo	Via Lago di Nicito, 19	Catania
Cordella, Marco	Viale Partigiani d'Italia, 4	Parma
Cordero, Celso	Primario Oculista Ospedale S.M.N.	Reggio Emilia
Coriglione, Giuseppe	Primario Ospedale M. Paternò Arezzo	Ragusa
Cornalba, Nino	Via XX Settembre, 17	Lodi
Corrado, Mario	Via Peschiera, 17	Genova
Crepaldi Antonio	Via Pio X, 19	Padova
Cricchi, Marcello	Primario Ospedale S. Maria del Prato	Feltre
Croci, Luigi	Via degli Scipioni, 265	Roma
Cucchia, Alberto	Piazza Nichelotti, 4	Perugia
Cucco, Giovanni	Via di Villafranca, 22	Palermo
D'Agostino, Aldo	Via G. D'Annunzio	Salice Salentino

Dal, Dosso Raffaele	Via F. Caroto, 1	Verona
Dal, Fiume Egidio	Clinica Oculistica Universitaria ..	Ferrara
Danielli, Castellazzo Olga ..	Via Cantore, 47-4	Genova (Sampierdarena)
Da Pozzo, Ezio	Via Zanon, 16	Udine
D'Arrigo, Pasquale	Via Santa Marta, 27	Messina
De Berardinis, Elio	Via Tasso, 480	Napoli
De Concilis, Ugo	Via Pacuvio, 21	Napoli
De Crecchio, Antonio	Piazza S. Pasquale a Chiaia, 10 ..	Napoli
De Ferrari, Gastone	Via Torlonia, 39	Roma
De Gennaro, Giuseppe	Via Mergellina, 169	Napoli
De Leonibus, Fernando ...	Via Bernini, 64	Napoli
Dell'Aquila, Antonio	Via Marini, 19	Faenza
Delle Grottaglie, Bruno	Piazza Argentina, 1	Milano
Delogu, Antonio	Clinica Oculistica Universitaria ..	Perugia
Del Zoppo, Italo	Via Cantore, 50	Genova (Sampierdarena)
Demajo, Francesco	....	Rignano Garganico (Foggia)
De Michele, Tullio	Via Nizza, 56	Roma
De Paolis, Luigi	Via Luce, 57	Galatina (Lecce)
De Poli, Attilio	Via Lamarmora, 20	Milano
D'Ermo, Franco	Clinica Oculistica Universitaria ..	Padova
De Rosa, Carlo	Via Guglielmo Sanfelice, 33	Napoli
De Rosa, Luigi	Via Guglielmo Sanfelice, 33	Napoli
De Santis, Gaspare	Via G. Leopardi, 9	Ascoli Piceno
De Simone, Silvio	Via Broggia, 11	Napoli
D'Esposito, Mario	Via Cassano, 16	Piano di Sorrento (Napoli)
De Vincentiis Mario	....	Camerino
Di Luca, Giuseppe	Via della Liberazione, 1	Chieti
Diotallevi, Mario	....	Fermo
Di Pietro, Guido	Via Borghi Mamo, 2	Bologna
Donazzan, Sante	Via Druso, 43	Bolzano
Dorello, Ugo	Clinica Oculistica Universitaria ..	Modena
Dotti, Mariuccia	Via S. Caterina, 27/5	Merano
Dugnani, Emilio	Clinica Rovera	Varese
Durando, Francesco	Via Legnano, 16	Alessandria
Errani, Francesco	Via Beatrice Alighieri, 15	Ravenna
Esente, Ivan	Ospedale Oftalmico Fiorentino ..	Firenze
Etienne, Raymond	Hôpital Edouard Herriot	Lyon
Fabozzi, Mario	Via Vittorio Emanuele, 10	Bari
Fadda, Antonio	Via Matris Domini, 9	Bergamo
Fallica, Giuseppe	Via Fogliano, 10	Roma
Fascinelli, Nino	Via Volto Cittadella, 16	Verona
Fazio, Francesco	Via Vittorio Emanuele, 24	Caltagirone
Fedrizzi, Giuseppe	Via Goccia d'Oro, 4	Trento
Ferraboschi, Corrado	Via Lamberti, 1	Reggio Emilia
Ferrante, Angelo	Via Belzoni, 6	Padova
Ferrara, Aristide	Piazza Municipio, 4	Napoli
Ferrari, Aldo	Via Trinchese, 46	Lecce
Ferrata, Luigi	Primario Ospedale Civile	Lecco
Fioretti, Enrico	Corso Vittorio Emanuele, 192 ..	Avellino
Foppiano, Pier Lorenzo ...	Corso A. Giannelli, 14/4	Chiavari
Forlani, Delvino	Via Albergati, 19	Bologna
Forni, Sergio	Palazzo Giumini, Viale Stazione, 30	Bellinzona (Ticino)
Foroni, Gian Maria	Via XX Settembre, 2-16	Genova
Francia, Corrado	Via Gazzata, 16	Reggio Emilia
Frasca, Gennaro	Via Dante, 6	Bologna

Frezzotti, Renato	Via XXIV Maggio, 23	Siena
Gaipa, Marcello	Via Posillipo, 56/A	Napoli
Galante, Calogero	Via Candia, 22	Lido di Venezia
Galbiati, Luigi	Via L. Angelini, 6	Voghera
Gallo-Basteris, Alessandro	Via Paleocapa, 6-6	Savona
Gandolfi, Carlo	Viale Regina Elena, 68	Pescara
Gargioni, Ettore	Viale Piave, 9	Macerata
Garigali, Francesco	Via Uruguay, 14 F	Milano
Garsìa, Gio. Battista	Via Verdi, 6	Trapani
Garzino, Mario	Via Mazzini, 2	Torino
Gasparri, Franco		Palombina Nuova (Ancona)
Gattini, Enrico	Via Buonarroti, 8	Pesaro
Gemolotto, Guglielmo	Piazza San Cristoforo, 1	Udine
Gerhardinger, Rodolfo	Via S. Nicolò, 72	Treviso
Germani, Aurelio	Via Montebello, 21	Voghera
Giacomelli, Giulio	Via Cavour, 71	Roma
Giacomelli, Piero	Via A. Mangini, 41	Livorno
Giancipoli, Ermete	Via Matteotti, 10	Ginosa (Taranto)
Giardini, Aniceto	Primario Ospedale S. Anna	Como
Giuffrè, Vincenzo	Via delle Croci, 47	Palermo
Grande, Gian Tommaso	Clinica Oculistica Universitaria	Ferrara
Grasso, Cannizzo Emanuele	Via Magenta, 121	Vittoria
Grignolo, Antonio	Clinica Oculistica Universitaria	Genova
Grilli, Franco	Via Chieti, 5	Pescara
Guadalupi, Ugo	Via Bertoloni, 47	Roma
Guaschino, Angelo	Via Meilana, 2	Casal Monferrato
Guffanti, Adele	Via Campini, 1	Monza
Guzzinati, G. Carlo	Via Monteverde, 31 bis	Carrara
Heer, Giuseppe	Corso Casale, 170	Torino
Isola, Raffaele	Via Sonnino, 142	Cagliari
Joli, Giovanna	Clinica Oculistica Universitaria	Roma
Jorio, Sergio	Viale Mazzini, 5	La Spezia
Juglio, Nicola	Via Tino da Camaino, 9	Napoli
Lampis, Raffaele	Viale Gramsci, 63	Firenze
Lanzieri, Mario	Clinica Oculistica Universitaria	Padova
Latte, Bachisio	Primario Ospedale S. Francesco	Nuoro
Leccisi, Antonio	Corso Garibaldi, 22	Brindisi
Leonardi, Filippo	Ospedale Oftalmico Provinciale	Roma
Licheri, Giovanni	Via Cavour, 40	Sassari
Ligorio, Amerigo	Via Lamarmora, 6	Torino
Lo Cascio, Girolamo	Via G. Verga, 3	Bagheria
Longhena, Luisa	Via Marconi, 6	Bologna
Luciani, Erasmo	Via S. Michele alla Porta, 3	Verona
Magnasco, Mario	Via Fiasella, 3/8	Genova
Magni, Sallustio	Primario Ospedale Civile	Forlì
Maione, Mario	Clinica Oculistica Universitaria	Parma
Mammarella, Ennio	Clinica Oculistica Universitaria	Parma
Manconi, Giovanni	Ospedale Civile	Pordenone
Marchi, Federico	Via del Gesù, 89	Roma
Marconcini, Eraldo	Ospedale Lotti	Pontedera (Pisa)
Marinosci, Alessandro	Corso Umberto I, 114	Taranto
Marsico, Vincenzo	Largo Barbelli, 1	Potenza
Massimeo, Angelo	Via di Vagno, 10	Mola di Bari
Mastrangeli, Wilfredo	Via F. Fabrizi, 7	Città di Castello (Perugia)
Mathis, Giovanni	Via Madama Cristina, 9	Torino
Mecca, Mario	Via Nizza, 5	Verona

Mega, Amedeo	Via Pennino, 28	Matera
Melenchi, Orazio	Corso Trieste, 124	Caserta
Melodia, Corrado	Via Frattini, 12	Verona
Menna, Francesco	Via S. Lucia, 173	Napoli
Merlin, Umberto	Via Altinate, 71	Padova
Messina, Luigi	Primario Ospedale Trigona	Noto
Miani, Paolo	Ospedale Civile	Udine
Miglior, Mario	Corso di Porta Romana, 123	Milano
Milano, Achille	Via Luca Giordano, 56	Napoli
Milano, Carlo	Clinica Oculistica Universitaria	Roma
Missiroli, Giuseppe	Primario Ospedale San Camillo	Roma
Montanelli, Mario	Via Galilei, 7	Mantova
Montresor, Dante	Viale della Repubblica, 39	Verona
Morelli, Enrico	Corso Amedeo, 70	Livorno
Moro, Ferruccio	Clinica Oculistica Universitaria	Catania
Morone, Giulio	Clinica Oculistica Universitaria	Pavia
Morpurgo, Fabio	Corso Magenta, 43	Milano
Mosci, Lamberto	Via Mura dello Zerbino, 18/10	Genova
Musini, Attilio	Via S. Sofia, 12	Milano
Napoleoni, Valerio	Via Roma, 49	Grottamare (Ascoli Piceno)
Nastri, Francesco	Via Alessandria, 160	Roma
Navarra, Rosita	Via Garibaldi, 139	Ferrara
Neuschüler, Ignazio	Via Monte Zebio, 37	Roma
Nicolato, Vincenzo	Viale Albertoni, 6	Mantova
Nigro, Laetitia	Via Nicola Fabrizi, 189	Pescara
Orsoni, Josè	Canareggio, 4504	Venezia
Pagliarani, Nicola	Via S. Giuliano, 1	Bologna
Palamà, Giovanni	Piazza Angeli, 31	Brindisi
Palmieri, Leopoldo	Via Righi, 34	Bologna
Palmieri Luciano	Clinica Oculistica Universitaria	Modena
Panico, Emanuele	Piazza Minicio, 2	Roma
Panzardi, Domenico	Primario Ospedale Civile	Cosenza
Pasino, Luigi	Ospedale Maggiore	Cremona

Soci Corrispondenti

Accardi, Antonio	Via Dancalia, 21	Roma - 00161
Adami, Marco	Via Cadlolo, 118	Roma
Agugini, Giovanni	Via Anfossi, 19	Milano
Alfano, Gaetano	Ospedale Civile	Avellino
Alfieri, Giorgio	Via Peitro Giuria, 20	Torino
Alfonso, Gian Franco	Via Baracchini, 10	Milano
Altieri, Alfredo	Via Mercantile, 24	San Severo (Foggia)
Anastasi, Giovanni	Via XX Settembre, 67	Palermo
Andreani, Domenico	Clinica Oculistica Universitaria	Pisa
Andreano, Giuseppe	Via Zuppetta, 34	Foggia
Andreocci, Manlio	Strada Sanmartinese Km. 3°	Viterbo
Andreoletti, Agostino	Via Guglielmo D'Alzano, 10	Bergamo
Anselmi, Paolo	Via Costa, 73	Bologna
Antonibon, Arrigo	Centro Traumatologico I.N.A.I.L.	Padova
Arcangeli, Giuseppe	Largo Goldoni, 41	Terni
Ascolani, Enzo	Corso Mazzini	S. Benedetto del Tronto
Asperti, Giacomo	Via Parco Vecchio, 7	Pavia
Balacco, Gabrieli Corrado	Via Putignani, 128	Bari
Balestrazzi, Emilio	Via Mauro Amoruso, 19 B	Bari
Baquis, Giulio	Via Cavour, 60	Firenze

Bardeli, Anna Maria	Clinica Oculistica Universitaria ..	Siena
Barlotta, Francesco	Clinica Oculistica Universitaria ..	Catania
Basenghi, Giovanni	Clinica Oculistica Universitaria ..	Modena
Bassani, Alfio	Via Apuana, 2 bis	Ferrara
Battignani, Agostino	Via Stalloreggi, 38	Siena
Battista, Ugo	Via 4 Novembre, 2	Termoli (Campobasso)
Beccaria, Francesco	Via Cesare Battisti, Is. 83	Messina
Belci, Corrado	Via Prati, 24	Vicenza
Bellan, Bruno	Via Juvara, 19	Torino
Bellone, Giorgio	Clinica Oculistica Universitaria ..	Torino
Belmonte, Michele	Via Conti, 41	Sergnano (Cremona)
Benine, Paolo	Molinetto, 51	Ravenna
Bernabei, Maria	Via Amici, 5	Forlì
Bernardotti, Piero	Ospedale Civile	Vigevano
Bertoncini, Giovanni	Clinica Oculistica Universitaria ..	Firenze
Bertoni, Giancarlo	Università Cattolica del S. Cuore .	Roma
Bertotto, Pier Giorgio	San Luca, 4038	Venezia
Bettini, Luigi	Piazza Vittoria, 7	Brescia
Bianchi, Costantino	Via Masone, 1	Bergamo
Billardello, Cesare	Via Messina, 36 A	Palermo
Biondi, Bruno	Via Capo d'Istria, 6	Roma
Bisantis, Cesare	Viale Regina Margherita, 269 ...	Roma
Blumenthal, Oreste	Lungodora Firenze, 119	Torino
Bonaccorsi, Antonino	Via Francesco Riso, 74	Catania
Bondi, Pasquale	Via del Rizzani, 17	Roma
Bonanni, Raffaele	Clinica Oculistica Universitaria ..	Siena
Bongiorno, Angelo	Via Bonito, 27	Napoli
Bonomi, Luciano	Via Paoletti, 3	Padova
Bonora, Franco	Via Casiraghi, 39	Sesto San Giovanni
Borello, Carlantonio	Ospedale Mauriziano	Aosta
Bottino, Carlo	Via Ippolito d'Asti, 8-2	Genova
Bozzini, Sandro	Clinica Oculistica Universitaria ..	Milano
Bracaglia, Renato	Viale delle Milizie, 114	Roma
Bracciolini, Matteo Renato .	Via Sagarriga Visconti, 73	Bari
Braggio, Franco	Via Vigorelli, 22	Domodossola
Brancato, Rosario	Clinica Oculistica Universitaria ..	Firenze
Brignola, Domenico	Corso Trieste, 121	Caserta
Brogi, Mario	Piazza Giotto, 13	Firenze
Bruno, Giovanni	Via Toschi, 8	Reggio Emilia
Bucalossi, Antonio		Vercelli
Buonfiglio, Rosa	Via Nizza, 11	Roma
Busacca, Annibale	Via Dante, 14	Milano
Caccese, Alfonso	Corso Vittorio Emanuele, 128 ..	Napoli
Calabria, Giovanni	Clinica Oculistica Universitaria ..	Genova
Calabrò, Saverio	Via Brunamonti, 51	Perugia
Calandra, Salvatore	Via Favara Nuova	Agrigento
Calogero, Rino	Clinica Oculistica Universitaria ..	Padova
Calvi, Zampetti Aurelio ...	Via San Senatore, 6/3	Milano
Cameo, Dario	Via Terni, 48	Roma
Camici, Agostino	Via Garofani, 8	Pisa
Campana, Giuseppe	Clinica Oculistica Universitaria ..	Firenze
Canali, Dante	Via Cantore, 8	Brescia
Candian, Bianca	Via Appiani, 19	Milano
Canova, Roberto	Viale dei Caduti, 31	Mantova
Capalbi, Stefano	Via A. Volta, 15	Piombino
Capone, Pasquale	Ospedale Civile	Chieti

Cappelli, Lello	Clinica Oculistica Universitaria ..	Firenze
Caramazza, Roberto	Clinica Oculistica Universitaria ..	Bologna
Carbone-Fossa, Angel Osval- do	Avenida Bolivia, 591	Lima (Perù)
Cardeti, Pietro	Via Gaeta, 15	Piombino
Cardia, Luigi	Clinica Oculistica Universitaria ..	Bari
Carella, Giuseppe	Via Genova, 32	Piacenza
Carinci, Lorenzo	Via Umberto I, 29	Adria
Carli, Antonio	Corso Milano, 82	Padova
Carlucci, Pasquale	Via Principe Amedeo, 145	Taranto
Carta, Francesco	Clinica Oculistica Universitaria ..	Parma
Casellato, Luciano	Viale Umbria, 83	Milano
Castellazzo, Renato	Viale Cambiaso, 1/18	Genova
Castellino, M. Paola	Ospedale Oftalmico	Torino
Catanese, Rosario	Via Fratelli Bandiera	Bovalino Marino (R.C.)
Cattani, Fulvio	Piazza Ospedale Maggiore, 3	Milano
Cavallaro, Nicola	Via dello Stadio, 6	Catania
Ceri, Anna Maria	Via S. Giorgio, 31	Prato
Cerulli, Luciano	Via Lovanio, 11	Roma
Casa, Raffaele	Reparto Oculistico Ospedale Civile	Lucca
Cetrullo, Bruno	Via Piacenza, 25	L'Aquila
Chiaravalloti, Francesco ...	Clinica Oculistica Universitaria ..	Ferrara
Chiavazza, Giorgio	Corso Francia, 15	Torino
Chicco, Giuseppe	Villa Marciano, 47	Siena
Chiriaco, Giorgio	Viale Miramare, 37	Trieste
Ciacciarelli, Filippo	Viale del Flavi, 20	Rieti
Ciboldi, Annibale	Viale Italia, 77	Lodi
Ciucci, Bruno	Via Farnesina, 322	Roma
Ciurlo, Giuseppe	Corso Buenos Aires, 2/7	Genova
Cocco, Greca	Clinica Oculistica Universitaria ..	Cagliari
Colaci, Cosimo	Piazza Eritrea, 30	Napoli
Colombo, Bolla Mario	Via Isonzo, 1	Castellanza (Varese)
Consoli, Francesco	Servizio di Oculistica Ospedale Civile	Vibo Valentia
Coslovich, Eugenio	Via Crispi, 5	Trieste
Crety, Edoardo	Viale Don Minzoni, 13	Lecce
Cusumano, Vincenzo	Via Nicolò Orsini, 3-bis	Padova
D'Amato, F. J.	38, Arcade Street	Paula (Malta)
D'Ambrosi, Dario	Via Madonna del Riposo, 46	Roma
D'Ambrosi, Mario	Corso Vittorio Emanuele, 203 ..	Salerno
Damiani, Alessio	Via Alessi, 27	Perugia
Daniele, Salvatore	Clinica Oculistica Universitaria ..	Perugia
D'Aponte, Raffaele	Via Cilea, 145	Napoli
D'Aprile, Vincenzo	Ospedale Civile	Brindisi
De Giovanni, Luigi	Via San Antonio	Maglie
Del Buono, Gilberto	Via Matteotti, 8	Firenze
Della Porta, Vittorio	Via Durini, 23	Milano
Della Valle, Adolfo	Corso Francia, 3	Torino
Della Valle, Ciro	Corso Vittorio Emanuele, 6	Campobasso
Della Joio, Giovanni	Via Denza, 21	Castellammare di Stabia
Del Re, Mario	Viale 24 Maggio, 1	Foggia
Del Zoppo, Italo	Via Cantore, 50	Genova Sampierdarena
De Marco, Dario	....	San Martino di Castrozza (Trento)
De Molfetaa, Vito	Via Murat, 8	Milano
De Negri, Tullio	Via Sartori, 73	Roma

Detti, Silvano	Ospedale Civile	Grosseto
De Vecchi, Ido	Corso Fogazzaro, 24	Vicenza
Di Comite, Piero	Clinica Oculistica Universitaria	Padova
Di Giacomo, Camillo	Clinica Oculistica Universitaria	Catania
Di Giulio, Ferruccio	Corso Umberto, 64	Brindisi
Di Martino, Cosimo	Via 24 Maggio, 13, Is. 245	Messina
Dionisio, Pasquale	Via Pupino, 10	Taranto
Diotti, Giorgio	Via Vico, 2	Torino
Di Santo, Gino	Via Roma, 14	Pederobba (Treviso)
Di Tizio, Antonio	Ospedale Oftalmico Provinciale	Roma
Dossi, Fabio	Via Governolo, 28	Torino
Dragoni, Paolo	Ospedale Civile	Macerata
Errico, Salvatore	Via Pendino, 47	Tricase (Lecce)
Fabris, Antonio	Via Manin, 57	Treviso
Fabbri Guido	Via Andrea Doria, 32	Milano
Faggioni, Ruggero	Via Guicciardini, 9	Firenze
Faieta, Elio	Ospedale Civile	Pescara
Falagario, Matilde	Via di Venere, 14	Ceglie di Campo (Bari)
Falcinelli, Gian Carlo	Ospedale S. Camillo	Roma
Faldi, Silvano	Via Custavo Modena, 19	Firenze
Falomo, Irene	Via Franco Martelli, 7	Pordenone
Fanciullo, Alberto	Via Cavour, 21	Lecce
Faraldi, Italo	Clinica Oculistica Universitaria	Torino
Fauci, Antonio	Corso Garibaldi, 33	Salerno
Ferraris De, Gaspare Paolo	Via S. Fermo, 9	Padova
Ferreri, Giuseppe	Via Galileo Galilei, 75	Reggio Calabria
Filippone, Antonio	Via Dante, 206	Cremona
Filippone, Carlo	Clinica Oculistica Universitaria	Siena
Fini, Anna Maria	Via Sabotino, 10	Bologna
Fiorini, Giorgio	Viale Oriani, 33	Bologna
Foà, Raffaele	Via G. Lanza, 16	Casal Monferrato
Fogliati, Romano	Via P. Boselli, 13/10	Genova
Fornaro, Luigi	Viale Virgilio, 59	Taranto
Foroni, Oliviero	Via Principe Amedeo, 14	Mantova
Fortunato, Francesco	Viale Regina Margherita, 159	Roma
Foti, Antonio	Via De Nava, 78	Reggio Calabria
Franceschetti, Alberto	Le Grand Maney	Vésenaz (Genève)
Franchino, Maria	Via Cenischia, 50	Torino
Frazetto, Francesco	Piazza Europa, 1	Catania
Fregnan, Ettore	Via Pescatori, 36	Treviso
Frosini, Riccardo	Clinica Oculistica Universitaria	Firenze
Fusco, Giuseppe	Via Annella di Massimo, 75	Napoli
Gallenga, Pier Enrico	Clinica Oculistica Universitaria	Ferrara
Garavaglia, Luigi	Via XX Settembre, 47	Busto Arsizio
Gargiulo, Antonio	Via Col. De Bartolomeis, 11	Salerno
Gasparri, Tullio	Via Manin, 69	Roma
Gastaldi, Gian Marco	Ospedale Oftalmico	Torino
Gelanzè, Amedeo	Via Affaccio, 103	Vibo Valentia
Gelmi, Pier Angelo	Via Trento, 15-D	Brescia
Genovesi, Elio	Viale Italia, isolato 197	Messina
Germani, Luciano	Santa Croce, 21	Venezia
Ghibellini, Mario	Via Calliera, 70	Bologna
Giannussis, Jon	Via Egnatia, 29	Thessaloniki (Grecia)
Giordano, Pietro	Via Centonze, 137	Messina
Giovannella, Giuseppe	Via Crocefisso, 58	Reggio Calabria
Gorgone, Giovanni	Clinica Oculistica Universitaria	Catania

Gracis, Giuseppe	Via L. Coletti	Treviso
Gramoli, Alberto	Via Battaglione Toscano, 1	Reggio Emilia
Graziani, Walter	Via Spadari, 3	Ferrara
Graziano, Francesco Maria	Via Savioli, 3	Bologna
Greco, Salvatore	Via Vittorio Emanuele, 438	Biancavilla (Catania)
Gualdi, Giovanni	Clinica Oculistica Universitaria	Modena
Guerra, Roberto	Clinica Oculistica Universitaria	Siena
Inserra, Énrico	Via Nocero, 60	Castellammare di Stabia (Napoli)
Jura, Vincenzo	Viale Poggio di Capodimonte, 29.	Napoli
Kastanas, David	Via Bizaniou, 12	Salonicco, Grecia
Kriznic, Marisa	Via dei Bersaglieri, 5	Bologna
Lamberti, Onofrio	Via Fucilari, 9	Nocera Inferiore
Lasagni, Franca	Via Emanuele Filiberto, 2	Milano
Laverone, Ferruccio	Ospedale Oftalmico Fiorentino	Firenze
Leonardi, Achille	Ospedale Oftalmico Provinciale	Roma
Leonardi, Elvio	Circonvallazione Appia, 101	Roma
Lepri, Luciano	Ospedale Oftalmico Provinciale	Roma
Linciano, Raffaele	Via Dosa, 5	Lecce
Lodato, Gaetano	Largo Degli Abeti, 16	Palermo
Lodato, Giuseppe	Via Liberta, 18	Palermo
Lodi, Menestrina Paola	Via Mannelli, 13	Firenze
Loffredo, Antonio	Clinica Oculistica Universitaria	Napoli
Longo, Francesco	Via Roma, 171	Palermo
Lugli, Luigi	Via Tempio, 34	Piacenza
Lumbroso, Bruno	Via Brofferio, 7	Roma
Lupis, Giuseppe	Via Dante Alighieri, 51	Bari
Maestrelli, Will	Via Borgognissanti, 16	Firenze
Maffei, Sigismondo	Via Cernuschi, 35	Varese
Maggi, Achille	Via Rismondo, 12-1	Trieste
Maggi, Carlo	Via Latina, 8	Roma
Magistretti, Alessandra	Via Cola di Rienzo, 212	Roma
Magistretti, Fulvio		Piverone (Torino)
Magnasco, Agostino	Via Domenico Chiodo, 28	Genova
Magno, Pietro	Via Buonarotti, 1	Martina Franca (Taranto)
Magris, Tullio	Via Nincis, 43	Udine
Manes, Lino	Via Manzoni	S. Giorgio a Cremano
Manfredini, Umberto	Clinica Oculistica Universitaria	Pavia
Manuelli, Gian Franco	Clinica Oculistica Universitaria	Pavia
Manusia, Mario	Clinica Universitaria	Bari
Maraini, Giovanni	Clinica Oculistica Universitaria	Parma
Marchesini, Ettore	Ospedale Sampierdarena	Genova
Marchi, Vincenzo	Via Vasi, 18	Roma
Marin, Severina	Via Sisenatore, 2	Milano
Marinelli, Luisa	Clinica Oculistica Universitaria	Bologna
Marinosci, Francesco	Clinica Oculistica Universitaria	Roma
Marsile, Gian Franco	Via Palmanova, 133	Milano
Marsili, Maria Teresa	Via Goldoni, 27	Monza
Marucchi, Mario	Via Guglielmo Silva, 33	Milano
Masci, Ezio	Clinical Oculistica Universitaria	Roma
Maselli, Eduardo	Clinica Oculistica Universitaria	Milano
Mastronardi, Vito	Via Emilia S. Stefano, 13	Reggio Emilia
Mauceri, Francesco	Viale Montedoro, 54	Siracusa
Mazza, Carlo	Viale Muratori, 185	Modena
Mazzantini, Luigi	Clinica Oculistica Universitaria	Pisa
Mazzeo, Gabriele	Via San Felice, 79	Nola

Mazzilli, Giorgio	Clinica Oculistica Universitaria ..	Modena
Meduri, Renato	Via Gandino, 57	Bologna
Melchionda, Costanzo	Ospedale Oftalmico Provinciale .	Roma
Meli, Calogero	Piazza Europa, 6	Caltanissetta
Melillo, Ignazio	Via G. Pecchio, 1	Milano
Menestrina, Fabrizio	Via Mannelli, 13	Firenze
Mercurelli, Salari Domenico .	Via V. Cialdini, 50	Fabriano (Ancona)
Micati, Francesco	Via 95° Fant., 9	Lecce
Milano, Luigi	Via Luca Giordano, 56	Napoli
Milito, Pagliara Roberto ...	Via Velia, 15	Salerno
Minazzi, Piero	Salita S. Anna, 123	Casale Monferrato
Minini, Filippo	Via Cavour, 11	Brescia
Miorin, Giorgio	Via Giacosa, 15	Vicenza
Miranda, Maria	Circonvallazione Appia, 97	Roma
Missiroli, Alberto Maria ...	Via Carlo Fea, 15	Roma
Modugno, Giacomo Carlo ..	Via Adelaide Ristori, 21	Roma
Molinari, Italo	Via Murri, 45	Bologna
Molinelli, Giorgio	Via Bruno Bonci, 39	Siena
Morano, Massimo	Clinica Oculistica Universitaria ..	Bologna
Morra, Mario	Dirigente Consultorio Oculistico .	Marostica
Moschimi, Giovanni Battista.	Viale Bruno Buozzi, 18	Roma
Murialdo, Antonino	Via dei Tassorelli, 13	Genova
Muzzi, Marco	Viale Bovio, 29	Teramo
Negro, Pier Giovanni	Via San Secondo, 22	Torino
Nervi, Italo	Clinica Oculistica Universitaria ..	Genova
Nicodemi, Vinci	Via Ascoli	Marina di Massa
Nicosia, Armando	Via Porto Salvo, 9	Messina
Novati, Mario	Clinica Oculistica Universitaria ..	Cagliari
Noventa, Emilio	Viale Venezia, 130	Brescia
Nucci, Ettore	Ospedale Civile	Arezzo
Nuti, Ferruccio	Via del Rossi, 67	Siena
Nuvoloni, Antonio	Ospedale Maggiore	Novara
Orzalesi, Nicola	Clinica Oculistica Universitaria ..	Cagliari
Ottaviano, Aristide	Via Giusti, 8	Ragusa
Padoa, Sergio	Via Besana, 10	Milano
Paganoni, Camillo	Via Giorgio Paglia, 33	Bergamo
Paliaga, Gian Paolo	Via Rosselli, 17	Como
Palmieri, Carlo	Via Castello, 6213	Venezia
Pandolfi, Maurizio	Allmänna Sjukhuset	Malmö (Svezia)
Pandolfo, Giuseppe	Viale Cadorna, 14	Messina
Pannarale, Carlo	Via Sparano, 149	Bari
Pannarale, Mario Rosario ..	Clinica Oculistica Universitaria ..	Roma
Pansini, Tommaso	Via M. Vittoria, 56	Torino
Pantalone, Tommaso	Via Vittorio Emanuele, 126	Firenze
Parducci, Francesco	Via Masaccio, 102	Firenze
Parducci, Mario	Via Marradi, 83	Livorno
Parodi, Dino	Via Teodoro II di Monferrato, 2/5	Genova-Pegli
Pasculli, Pasquale	Ospedale Di Venere	Bitonto
Pastore, Vito	Via Principe di Napoli, 12	Gioia del Colle (Bari)
Pecori, Giraldi Josè	Via Tortolini, 29	Roma
Pellegrini, Mario	Via S. Lucia, 107	Napoli
Pellutié, Giovanni	Corso Nizza, 13	Cuneo
Peralta, Sergio	Clinica Oculistica Universitaria ..	Parma
Perelli, Piero	Via Vecchia S. Marco	Lucca
Piccinelli, Bruno	Clinica Oculistica Universitaria ..	Padova
Pieracci, Vincenzo	Via Maestro da Castello, 11	Città di Castello

Pietracaprina, Gherardi Laura	Via delle Rose, 18	Lucca
Pirri, Angela	Via Madonna dei Cieli, 12	Catanzaro
Pistocchi, Paolo	Viale Crucioli, 72	Teramo
Pivetti, Paola	Via Cavallini, 24	Roma
Polenghi, Francesco	Corso di Porta Romana, 116	Milano
Pollini, Sergio	Corso Garibaldi, 25	Pordenone
Polzella, Abner	Via Orsi, 6	Napoli
Proto, Franco	Via Grossi Gondi, 54	Roma
Pruneri, Franco	Via Trieste, 27	Sondrio
Puddu, Piero	Via Irnerio, 6	Bologna
Pupi, Flavio	Via Francesco Flamini, 7	Pisa
Ragni, Guido	Via Appia Nuova, 71	Roma
Rama, Giovanni	Ospedale Civile	Mestre
Ranieri, Francesco	Ospedale Di Venere	Bari - Carbonara
Ranieri, Guglielmo	1ª Traversa Interna Orazio Flacco, 30	Bari
Rapaccini, Giorgio	Corso Tacito, 93	Terni
Rapizzi, Albino	Ospedale Civile	Mestre
Ravalico, Giuseppe	Clinica Oculistica Universitaria ..	Sassari
Revoltella, Roberto	Prato della Valle, 29	Padova
Riggio, Tommaso	Piazza Verdi, 3	Ribera (Agrigento)
Rinaldi, Ernesto	Via Portalba, 30	Napoli
Rizzini, Vittorio	Via Martelli, 8	Firenze
Roghi, Bonella	Via Acquarone, 48/A	Genova
Romani, Enrico	Clinica Oculistica Universitaria ..	Roma
Rossini, Angelo	....	Attigliano (Terni)
Russo, Ernesto	Corso Roma, 71	Foggia
Sabbadini, Arnaldo	Via Cicognara, 3	Milano
Saccol, Giuseppe	Via Gobetti, 46	Ferrara
Salvatori, Luciano	Viale N. Sauro, 19	Rimini
Sabbadini, Arnaldo	Piazza Conciliazione, 1	Milano
Sanna, Gavino	Ospedale Civile S. Paolo	Savona
Santillo, Clemente	Via Panciroli, 7	Roma
Santino, Domenico	Via Sciuti, 79	Palermo
Santori, Giuseppe	Via Ingegneri, 2	Cremona
Santori, Mario	Via Robelotti, 14	Cremona
Saviotti, Giuseppe	Via Cura, 60	Ravenna
Sbordone, Antonio	Via Filangieri, 72	Napoli
Sbordone, Girolamo	Clinica Oculistica Universitaria ..	Napoli
Sborgia, Gianfranco	1ª Trav. Int. O. Flacco, 12	Bari
Scardovi, Carlo	Viale Oriani, 2	Bologna
Schillaci, Carmine	Piazza San Domenico, 30	Catania
Schirru, Mario	Via del Corso, 504	Roma
Sciaccaluga, Pier Luigi	Via Damiano Chiesa, 1/4	Genova-Sampierdarena
Scialfa, Aldo	Via Firenze, 194. doni, 41	Catania
Scollo, Giovanni	Clinica Oculistica Universitaria ..	Catania
Scorsonelli, Mirella	Via Canestro, 14	Parma
Scotti, Luciano	Corso Campi, 36	Cremona
Scuderi, Alfio	Viale Sicilia, Palazzo Serpente ..	Caltanissetta
Secchi, Antonio	Clinica Oculistica Universitaria ..	Padova
Semeraro, Franco	Via Bascio, 14	Martina Franca (Taranto)
Serafini, Sergio	Corso Umberto, 56	Pescara
Settimo, Enrico	Via Cavour, 4	Alba (Cuneo)
Shtylla, Ylli	Spital Klinik N. 1 Universitit Shteteror	Tirana (Albania)
Sighinolfi, Giuseppe	Via Garibaldi, 23	Camposanto (Modena)

Simonetti, Antonio	Corso Francia, 3	Torino
Sisti, Alberto	Viale della Vittoria, 6	Ancona
Sisto, Alberto	Via Calefati, 80	Bari
Sodaro, Francesco	Via Onorato, 52	Palermo
Sola, Mauro	Via del Pozzo, 156	Modena
Spadaro, Luigi	Clinica Oculistica Universitaria	Bari
Spina, Pietro	Via Renato Imbriani, 222	Catania
Spinelli, Demetrio	Corso Magenta, 31	Milano
Stirpe, Mario	Via Pasubio, 4	Roma
Stolfi, Angelo Vito	Via Due Torri, 33	Potenza
Stradolini, Luigi	Via Rossetti, 14/A	Genova Quarto
Striano, Luigi	Via De Simone, 4	Torre Annunziate (Napoli)
Tabacchi, Giovanni	Via Cavedomi, 41	Modena
Tamborini, Angelo		Tremate (Varese)
Tarricone, Michele	Via Pio XI, 11	Segnano (Milano)
Tavolara, Luigi	Via Mercato, 3	Sassari
Tedesco, Nicola	Via Carlo Poma, 4	Roma
Terrana, Carlo	Via Roccantica, 9	Roma
Testa, Michele	Clinica Oculistica Universitaria	Palermo
Tinelli, Francesco	Via Vecchini, 1	Ancona
Tota, Amodio	Via Cavour, 2, (Villino Spetrino)	Campobasso
Travia, Antonio	2ª Traversa Interna Orazio Flacco, 38/9	Bari
Trerotoli, Pompilio	Corso Vittorio Emanuele, 78	Bari
Tripodi, Giuseppe	Piazzale Stadio, Traversa 1ª, 14	Reggio Calabria
Trillo, Michele	Corso Magellano, 11/8	Genova
Trimarchi, Fernando	Clinica Oculistica Universitaria	Pavia
Trivelato, Alberto	Via Canove, 8	Vicenza
Trombetta, Giuseppe	Via Pracchiuso, 16	Udine
Tucci, Francesco	Via Moena, 33	Roma
Tusa, Enzo	Via Panama, 26	Roma
Ubaldino, Vito	Via del Giardino, 5	Palermo
Urbani, Giancarlo	Castello S. Lio, 5448	Venezia
Urso, Giuseppe	Clinica Oculistica Universitaria	Bari
Vallavanti, Cesare	Via Vincenzo Porri, 16	Piacenza
Valvo, Giuseppe	Ospedale Trigona	Noto (Siracusa)
Verdi, Gian Paolo	Clinica Oculistica Universitaria	Milano
Verraz, Romano	Via Begetti, 27	Torino
Verzella, Franco	Corso Porta Mare, 11	Perrara
Viale, Carlo	Via Grimani, 9	Venezia-Lido
Vigna, Luigi	Corso Umberto, 61	Torino
Vigorelli, Enrico	Via Solferino, 7	Milano
Vinciguerra, Enrico	Strada n. 1 di Via Lagrola, 5	Parma
Vitali, Giovanni	Clinica Oculistica Universitaria	Sassari
Vittadini, Angelo	Via Boldrini, 7	Vigevano
Vittone, Paolo	Via Lungoparco Gropallo, 4/16	Genova
Vollaro, Achille	Via Torricone, 102	Reggio Calabria
Volpones, Vladimiro	Via Milazzo, 39	Rimini
Zavarise, Giancarlo	Via Solitro, 11	Padova
Zeppa, Rosario	Via Caggiano	Benevento
Zigliara, Emerico	Via Fiume, 6/8	Chiavari (Genova)
Zingirian, Mario	Clinica Oculistica Universitaria	Genova
Zucchini, Girolamo	Clinica Oculistica Universitaria	Firenze
Zucchini, Raffaele	Viale Bertacchi	Lugo (Ravenna)

NOSOCOMIA QUIBUS OCULIS AEGRI CURANTUR

Ospedale Oftalmico Provinciale Di Roma   No. of beds
Director: Prof. Filippo Leonardi, Piazza degli Eroi, 11-00136 Roma 140

Ospedale Oftalmico Fiorentino
Director: Prof. Ivan Esente, Via Masaccio, 213-50132 Firenze 80

Ospedale Oftalmico Torinese
Director: Prof. Angelo Vannini, Via Juvara, 19-10122 Torino 80

Ospedale Oftalmico di Milano
Director: Prof. Cesare Galeazzi, Prof. Riccardo Vozza, Via Boccaccio, 34-20123 Milano ... 140

INSTITUTA SCHOLAEQUE CAECIS DESTINATAE

Ardenza (Livorno), Via del Mare, 90-c.a.p. 57100 – (Ist. Liedin Nina Frediani)
Assisi (Perugia), Istituto Serafico per Ciechi dei PP. Rogazionisti – Via Marconi, 6-06081
Assisi (Perugia), Istituto P. Ludovico da Casoria per Cieche – Via Frate Elia, 1-812541
Brescia, Istituto Professionale per Ciechi 'Carlo e Giulia Milani' – Via Divisione Tridentina, 54-25100
Bologna, Istituto per Ciechi 'Francesco Cavazza' – Via Catiglione, 71-40124
Bologna, Istituto delle Canossiane – Via S. Isaia, 63-40100
Cagliari, Istituto per Ciechi – Via Aurelio Nicolodi, 100-09100
Catania, Istituto per Ciechi 'Ardizzone Gioeni' – Via Etnea, 595–95100
Citta 'Di Castello (Perugia) – Istituo per Ciechi 'Beata Margherita', 06012
Cremona, Istituto 'Margherita', per Ciechi – Via Cesari, 9-26100
Genova, Istituto per Ciechi 'David Chiossone' – Corso Armellini, 11-16122
Firenze, Istituto Nazionale dei Ciechi 'Vittorio Emanuele II' – Via Aurelio Nicolodi, 2
Firenze, Istituto Procfessionale di Stato per l'Industria o l'Artigianato per Ciechi – Via Aurelio Nicoloci, 2-c.s.
Lecce, Istituto per Ciechi 'Anna Antonacci' – Via Scipione di Summa, 1-73100
Milano, Istituto dei Ciechi – Via Vivaio, 7-20122
Napoli, Istituto Professionale di Stato per l'Industria e l'Artigianato per Ciechi – 'Paolo Colosimo' – Via S. Teresa degli Scalzi, 36-80135
Napoli, Istituto per Ciechi 'Domenico Martuscelli' – Largo Martuscelli al Vomero – 80127
Napoli, Scuola-Convitto per Cieche 'Strachan Rodinò' – Via Filippo Rega, 17-80100
Padova, Istituto per Ciechi 'L. Configliachi' – Via Sette Martiri, 33-35100
Palermo, Istituto per Chiechi 'Florio e Salamone' – Via Angiò, 27-90142
Placenza, Istituto per Cieche 'Madonne della Bomba' – Pubblico Passaggio, 52-29100
Reggio Emilia, Istituto Regionale per Ciechi 'G. Garibaldi' – Via Franchetti n. 3-42100
Roma, Istituto Statale 'Augusto Romagnoli' di Specializzazione per gli Educatori dei minorati della Vista – Via Casale S. Pio V°, 60-00165
Roma, Istituto per Ciechi 'S. Alessio' – Viale C. T. Odescalchi, 38/A-00147
Rutigliano (Bari), Istituto Provinciale per Ciechi 'Gino Messer i Localzo' – 70018
Sassari, Istituto dei Ciechi – Via Armando Diaz, 25-07100
Spoleto, Istituto Nazzareno per Ciechi – 06049
Torino, Istituto Regionale dei Ciechi – Via Nizza, 151-10126
Trieste, Istituto 'Rittmeyer' per Ciechi, Viale Miramare, 119-3416
Villa Rivalta (Reggio Emilia), Scuola Elementare per Ciechi – Via Pascal – 42020

Presso alcuni degli Istituti sopra indicati (Milano-Padova-Genova-Napoli 'Martuscelli') funzionano anche Scuole Musicali non statali. Al Convitto di questi quattro Istituti possone essere ammessi anche giovani ciechi che frequentano la Scuola Pubblica.

L'Istituto 'F. Cavazza' di Bologna – ospita giovani ciechi che frequentano la Scuola Pubblica. Presso di esso funziona un pensionato per studenti universitari privi di vista nonchè una Scuola Musicale non statale.

L'Istituto 'S. Alessio' di Roma ospita giovani ciechi che frequentano la Scuola Pubblica. Ad esso sono altresi annesse una Scuola Elementare non statale, una Scuola musicale non statale, una Scuola Media parificata.

L'Istituto di Firenze oltre all'Istituto Professionale, comprende anche la Scuola Media la Scuola Elementare Statale per Ciechi Adulti e la Stamperia Nazionale Braille.

JAPONICA

SOCIETATES OPHTHALMOLOGICAE

Japanese Ophthalmological Society (Nippon Ganka Gakkai)

Address: c/o Nippon Ishikaikan, No. 5, 2-chome, Kanda-Surugadai, Chiyoda-ku, Tokyo 101
President: Shikano, Shinichi
Director of publication: Otsuka, Jin
General secretary: Kato, Ken, Dept. of Ophthalmology, School of Medicine, Nihon University, Surugadai Hospital, Kanda-Surugadai, Chiyoda-ku, Tokyo 101
Director of foreign affairs: Nakajima, Akira
Treasurer: Matsuo, Harutake
Members: Sugiura, Seiji; Mizuno, Katsuyoshi; Hayano, Saburo; Mizukawa, Takashi; Okuda, Kanji; Ikui, Hiroshi; Kishimoto, Masao; Kirisawa, Naganori; Komoto, Shoichi; Hagino, Ryutaro; Mita, Hiroshi
Number of members: 3659

Affiliated societies

Association of Japanese Ophthalmologists
Hioki Bldg., 1-Sugamachi Shinjuku-ku, Tokyo 160
Number of members: 4800

Japanese Contact Lens Society
c/o Department of Ophthalmology, Osaka University Medical School, Fukushima-ku, Osaka 553
Number of members: ca. 500

Japanese Society of Ophthalmic Optics
c/o Tokyo Kogaku Co., 75-1, Hasunuma-cho, Itabashi-ku, Tokyo 174
Number of members: ca. 100

NOMINA ET DOMICILIA MEDICORUM AB OCULIS

Abe, Fusako	2-15 Higashi 1-chome, Kunitachi-shi	Tokyo 186
Abe, Tetsuo	4-8-28 Higashi 1-bancho	Sendai-shi 980
Aihara, Yasushi	Hachiman-cho 1-12, Hanno-shi	Saitama-ken 357
Aizawa, Futaba	Dept. of Ophthalmology, Sapporo Medical College, South 1, West 16	Sapporo-shi 060
Aizawa, Seishi	2700-13, Katayama, Niizamachi, Kitaadachi-gun	Saitama-ken 352
Akagi, Goro	1070-10, Maruyama	Okayama-shi 700
Akiya, Nobuo	27-5, Chuo 1-chome	Aomori-shi 030
Akutagawa, Seiji	23-14, 3-chome, Kita Nishiogi, Suginami-ku	Tokyo 167

Goto, Hideo .... 1-5-1, Tōkaichi-cho, Hiroshima-
                       shi .... Hiroshima-ken 733
Goto, Nobu .... 508, Ohme, Ohme-shi .... Tokyo 198
Hachiya, Teiji .... 1, Araikuta-machi, Yahata-ku ... Kitakyushu-shi 805
Hadeyama, Tōru .... 1-5, Iizuka, Iizuka-shi .... Fukuoka-ken 820
Hagino, Ryutaro .... 1-25, Matsukaze-cho, Showa-ku . Nagoya-shi 466
Hagino, Yutaka .... 1-8-6, Midori-cho .... Chiba-shi 280
Hagihara, Takako .... 13-20, Shimotatsuo-cho .... Kagoshima-shi 892
Hagihara, Masayuki ...... 3-147, Miyauchi-cho .... Amagasaki-shi 660
Hamada, Shinobu .... 2-14-24, Miyakojimaminami-dori
                       Miyakojimaku .... Osaka-shi 534
Hamada, Toyosuke .... 3-18, Osatoharamachi, Moji-ku .. Kitakyushu-shi 800
Haniu, Takaaki .... Nakanouchi, Ishioka-shi .... Ibaragi-ken 315
Hanyuda, Susumu .... 2-10-13, Chiyoda-cho .... Maebashi-shi 371
Hara, Atsushi .... 5-15, Minamihanabatake, Aizuwa-
                       kamatsu-shi .... Fukushima-ken 965
Hara, Keizo .... 1-9-19, Hon-machi, Toyonaka-shi. Osaka-fu 560
Hara, Sunao .... 3-5, Shimanose-cho, Sasebo-shi .. Nagasaki-ken 857
Hara, Tōa .... ōte-machi 135, Nano-shi .... Ishikawa-ken 926
Hara, Yoshiaki .... 26-28, Masamune, Momoyama-
                       cho, Fushimi-ku .... Kyoto-shi 612
Harada, Hideko .... 1-50-16, Gotokuji, Setagaya-ku . Tokyo 154
Harada, Kiyoshi .... 17-13, Shojihigashi, 3-chome,
                       Ikuno-ku .... Osaka-shi 544
Harada, Masami .... 26-1, Sekimae 3-chome, Musa-
                       shino-shi .... Tokyo 180
Harada, Michiyuki .... 1-39-15, Morino, Machida-shi ... Tokyo 194
Harada, Sumie .... 1-26-10, Kitamachi, Kichijoji,
                       Musashino-shi .... Tokyo 180
Harada, Yasuharu .... 624, Minato-machi, Mihara-shi .. Hiroshima-ken
Haruta, Chosaburo .... 3-8, Matsunouchi-cho, Ashiya-shi. Hyogo-ken 659
Hasegawa, Jun .... 1437, Higuchi, Mizumaki-machi,
                       Onga-gun .... Fukuoka-ken 807
Hasegawa, Yōko .... 452, Hiranonodōcho, Sumiyoshi-
                       ku .... Osaka-shi 546
Hashimoto, Hiroshi .... 2-13-11, Kaguike, Kōriyama-shi . Fukushima-ken 563
Hashimoto, Keikichi ...... C-53 101, 1410, Sakae-cho, Soka-
                       shi .... Saitama-ken 340
Hashimoto, Yoshikuni .... 5-22, Ōido-cho, Wakamatsu-ku .. Kitakyushu-shi
Hata, Katsutada .... 2-3, Tenjin-cho .... Okayama-shi 700
Hatakeyama, Yasushi ..... 421, Nakaminatomachi, Yaizu-shi . Shizuoka-ken 425
Hatano, Tsuneo .... 2-13 Shintomi-cho, Chuo-ku .... Tokyo 154
Hatsuda, Hiroshi .... 4-24-7, Honkomagome, Bunkyo-
                       ku .... Tokyo 113
Hatta, Yoshikatsu .... 5-10, Koshomachi .... Kanazawa-shi 920
Hattori, Jiryu .... 25-12, Yaesaki-cho .... Hiratsuka-shi 254
Hattori, Masayoshi .... Sugawara, Tanushimaru-machi,
                       Ukiha-gun .... Fukuoka-ken 839-12
Hattori, Sadao .... 1-2, Tohatacho, Showa-ku ..... Nagoya-shi 458
Hayakawa, Kōgaku .... 4-36, Minamidōri Kameno-cho .. Akita-shi 010
Hayano, Saburo .... 1980, Masaki-cho .... Gifu-shi 500
Hayashi, Bōzō .... 1-3-1, Kagoikedori, Fukiai-ku ... Kobe-shi 651
Hayashi, Hirofumi .... Hayashi Ophthalmic Clinic. No.
                       5-10, 3-chome, Konan-cho,
                       Higashinada-ku .... Kobe-shi 658

Ishikawa, Yuichiro	78, Shojima-machi	Kurume-shi 830
Ishikawa, Satoshi	Dept. of Ophthalmology, Kitasata University School of Medicine, 1 Asamizodai	Sagamihara-shi 228
Ishizaki, Tadahiko	142, Hishiya-nishi	Higashiosaka-shi 577
Isogai, Atsushi	2-335, Sekiyahonson-cho	Niigata-shi 951
Itabashi, Yoshinori	5, Sakura, Iwanuma-machi, Nato-rigun	Miyagi-ken 989-24
Ito, Hisako	1-2-16, Nagadohei	Kanazawa-shi 920
Ito, Kenichi	4-3, Tanakamachi	Shimonoseki-shi 751
Ito, Kimiko	5-1-20, Minami Aoyama, Minato-ku	Tokyo 107
Ito, Masaaki	4-13-8, Tafuse, Saga-shi	Saga-ken 840
Ito, Reiko	12-11-19, Tamagawa, Denencho-fu, Setagaya-ku	Tokyo 158
Ito, Tsune	920 Otsu, Toyomi, Kase-machi, Higashikanbaragun	Niigata-ken 959-43
Ito, Yasuko	1-7, Kameicho	Okazaki-shi 444
Itoi, Motokazu	2-6-1, Kunitachi	Tokyo 186
Itotagawa, Yoshio	Kamojimacho, Oegun	Tokushima-ken 776
Iyoda, Tadashi	785, Tuyoda	Shizuoka-shi 420
Iwasawa, Takeshi	82, Takasukamachi, Nakamura-ku	Nagoya-shi 453
Iwashige, Yozo	Shibushi-cho, So-gun	Kagoshima-ken 899-71
Iwata, Masashi	3323, Daigyoji, Ōaza, Otomachi, Takawagun	Fukuoka-ken 824-05
Izutsu, Hatsuko	1-1-5, Higashi, Kumano-cho, Sakai-shi	Osaka 590
Kabayama, Hisao	211, Kanayama-cho	Kawaguchi-shi 332
Kaji, Riichi	1-449, Totsukacho, Shinjuku-ku .	Tokyo 160
Kajigaya, Yasuichi	2-5-4, Ichibancho	Matsuyama-shi 790
Kajimoto, Yoshinori	511 Howaito Hause, 1-4-15 Yamanone	Zushi-shi 249
Kajiwara, Seiichi	2-61, Ōtemachi, Kudamatsu-shi .	Yamaguchi-ken 744
Kajiura, Mutsuo	Dept. of Ophthalmology, Fuku-shima Medical College, 4-45, Sugitsuma-cho	Fukushima-shi 960
Kakisu, Yoneo	716-2, Iwasakishimo, Togano-shi .	Chiba-ken 283
Kamata, Takeshi	5-7, Hinode-cho, Tagawa-shi	Fukuoka-ken 825
Kaminaga, Seishi	3-14-10, Kyodo, Setagaya-ku ...	Tokyo 156
Kamisawa, Kookichi	1-14, Murakami-cho, Mizuho-ku .	Nagoya-shi 467
Kamiya, Sadayoshi	108, Sakura-honmachi, Minami-ku	Nagoya-shi 457
Kanazawa, Takumi	589-6, Fuchu-cho, Fuchu-shi ...	Hiroshima-ken 726
Kandori, Fumio	226-4, chome, Bakuromachi	Yonago-shi 683
Kaneda, Shoshige	Kyumichi, Kawasaki-machi, Taga-wa-gun	Fukuoka-ken 827
Kano, Masaya	4-7, Chu-cho, Tsukumi-shi	Ōita-ken 879-24
Kansaku, Toshio	1390, Funakata, Tateyamashi ...	Chiba-ken 294
Karino, Toshiyuki	21-14, Honmachi, Himi-shi	Toyama-ken 935
Kashiwai, Tetsuro	5, Naiki	Fukutiyama-shi 620
Katayama, Taro	172-12, Monden	Okayama-shi 700
Kato, Akinobu	1-5, Shin-oto-cho, Atsuta-ku	Nagoya 456
Kato, Ken	3-10-17, Yagisawa, Hoya-shi	Tokyo 188
Kato, Kinkichi	2-778, Soshigaya, Setagaya-ku ..	Tokyo 157
Kato, Masakazu	52-55, Inoue-cho, Yamashina-Higashino, Higashiyama-ku ..	Kyoto-shi 607

Kumanomido, Mamoru	5-18-9, Nakano, Nakano-ku	Tokyo 164
Kume, Itsuro	49-3, Asahi-cho, Seto-shi	Aichi-ken 489
Kunii, Hikojyu	1-5-27, Chūō, Sagae-shi	Yamagata-ken 991
Kunitomo, Noboru	1235, Yamanouchi	Kamakura-shi 247
Kuniya, Nobuko	4-11-2, Nishiochiai, Shinjuku-ku .	Tokyo 161
Kurachi, Yoshi	2-9-35, Kikugawa	Kanazawa-shi 920
Kurakazu, Masao	1-39, Bandamachi	Tagawa-shi 825
Kurao, Joo	4-13, Heiandori, Kitaku	Nagoya-shi 462
Kurimoto, Ei	B8-306, Shirasagi-danchi, Nojiri, Sakai-shi	Osaka 591
Kusuhara, Hideo	2164, Tsuruga-tamachi	Nagano-shi 380
Kuwabara, Tadasu	3-27-15, Shimoigusa, Suginami-ku	Tokyo 167
Kuwahara, Susumu	4-14-3, Fukuokacho, Takamatsu-shi	Kagawa-ken 770
Kuwahara, Yasuharu	27, Shinanomachi, Shinjuku-ku .	Tokyo 160
Kuwajima, Jisaburo	1-2-38, Katahira	Sendai-shi 980
Kuwajima, Makoto	Hon-cho, Nagai-shi	Yamagata-ken 993
Kuwano, Fujie	Tsuchiana, Munakata-machi, Munakata-gun	Fukuoka-ken 811-41
Kuzuya, Hiroshi	3-16-10, Nishiki, Nakaku	Nagoya-shi 460
Kyoka, Yo	3-23-3, Nishi-azabu, Minato-ku ..	Tokyo 106
Maeda, Koichi	1-1-8, Omachi	Aizuwakamatsu-shi 965
Maekawa, Yūsei	1-5-28, Kawara- machi	Sendai-shi 982
Maeda, Sadayoshi	81, Namimatsu-cho	Kishiwada-shi 596
Majima, Takashi	Nagoya City University Medical School, 1-Kawasumi Mizuho-cho, Mizuho-ku	Nagoya-shi 467
Majima, Yoshinori	1-138, Shimoshakujii, Nerima-ku .	Tokyo 177
Maki, Tetsuo	53, Ryogaemachi	Kurume-shi 830
Makiuchi, Shōichi	3-3, Minami-cho, Sakuragaoka ..	Takatsuki-shi 569
Makino, Keigo	1-25-10, Shakujimachi, Nerima-ku	Tokyo 177
Manabe, Seizo	2-3-30, Minami-cho, Dogo-cho ..	Matsuyama-shi 790
Maruyama, Kazuo	694, Annaka, Annaka-shi	Gunma-ken 379-01
Maruo, Hikaru	7690, Shingū, Shingū-shi	Wakayama-ken 647
Maruo, Takeshi	8-19, Yaotomi-cho	Gamagori-shi 443
Masuda, Osamu	3355, Teidaimae-machi, Hakosaki	Fukuoka-shi 812
Masuda, Shigeru	2-14-1, Nakamachi	Musashino-shi 830
Masuko, Fumiko	5-117, Kohamahigashi, Sumi-yoshi-ku	Osaka-shi 558
Mashiko, Yōtarō	23, Shozan-cho, Ōmuta-shi	Fukuoka-ken
Masuda, Yoshiya	Dept. of Ophthalmology, Fukuoka University, School of Medicine, Nishi-ku	Fukuoka-shi 814
Masuya, Giichi	3, Chuō-cho	Muroran-shi 051
Matsubara, Toshimaro	2-4-3 Higashi, Nuttari	Niigata-shi 950
Matsubara, Tadahisa	38-75, Yagoto Omoteyama, Tempakucho, Showa-ku	Nagoya-shi 468
Matsuda, Hiroko	5-29-205, Tsurukabuto, 3-chome, Nada-ku	Kobe-shi 657
Matsuda, Kazuo	5-6, Nishiyama-cho, Koyoen	Nishinomiya-shi 662
Matsuda, Kumiko	176, Kariyado	Kawasaki-shi 211
Matsuda, Naoya	4-13-3, Ishibiki, Kanazawa-shi ..	Ishikawa-ken 920
Matsuda, Yoshimi	24-400, Aza Higashinagamine, Myodaijicho	Okazaki-shi 444

Matsui, Mizuo	Dept. of Ophthalmology, Suruga-dai-Hospital of Nihon University 1-8, Surugadai, Kanda, Chiyoda-ku	Tokyo 101
Matsui, Shosaku	1-13-3, Teramachi	Kanazawa-shi 921
Matsumoto, Kazuro	1521-3, Shironomae, Mikage-cho, Higashinada-ku	Kobe-shi 658
Matsumoto, Tadatsugu	1-3-3, Higashiōme, Ōme-shi	Tokyo 198
Matsumoto, Takahisa	3-23, Kikawa-higashinocho, Higashiyodogawa-ku	Osaka-shi
Matsunaga, Tsutomu	326-2, Misono-cho, Kodaira-shi	Tokyo 187
Matsuo, Harutake	Dept. of Ophthalmology, Tokyo Medical College Hospital, 6-7-1, Nishi-Shinjuku, Shinjuku-ku	Tokyo 160
Matsuo, Hidehiko	Dept. of Ophthalmology, Kawasaki Medical College, 577, Matsushima	Kurashiki-shi 701-01
Matsuoka, Hideo	646, Yashiro Higashino-cho	Himeji-shi 670
Matsusaka, Toshihiko	Ophthalmic Circulation Clinic, The Center for Adult Diseases, Osaka Higashinari-ku.	Osaka-shi 537
Matsushita, Kazuo	49-66, Yamanotecho, Korien	Hirakata-shi 573
Matsutaka, Mitsuo	171 Sakuragicho, Ueda-shi	Nagano-ken 386
Matsuura, Masaaki	20-4, Tōbo, Taishi-machi, Ibogun.	Hyogo-ken 671-15
Matsuyama, Teruya	1243 Tonomachi	Matsuzaka-shi 515
Matsuyama, Michiro	4-10. Minamimachi	Kurashiki-shi
Matsuzaki, Hiroshi	1-6-10, Nakamagome, Ota-ku	Tokyo 143
Matsuzaki, Yo	1-6-7 Sengoku, Bunkyo-ku	Tokyo 112
Mikami, Shoji	1-6-18, Yanagi-machi, Mutsu-shi	Aomori-ken 035
Miki, Wataru	1-10-7, Midorimachi	Hofu-shi 347
Mikuni, Masakichi	1-14-504, 4-chome, Minami-Azabu, Minato-ku	Tokyo 106
Mikuni, Sukemori	1-4-16, Nishiasabu, Minato-ku	Tokyo 106
Mimura, Morichika	1-chome, Kanada-machi, Kokura-ku	Kitakyushu-shi 803
Mimura, Yasuo	Dept. of Ophthalmology, Osaka University Medical School, Fukushima-ku	Osaka-shi 553
Minami, Kumata	492, Higashi-machi	Kurume-shi 830
Minami, Mitsu	492, Higashi-machi	Kurume-shi 830
Minato, Toshio	2-4-1, Maruyama, Isogoku	Yokohama-shi 235
Mine, Hajime	Ekidōri, Shiroishi-cho, Kishima-gun	Saga-ken 849-11
Mine, Tōru	19-5, Daigo-kokocho, Fushimiku	Kyoto-shi 612
Mishima, Koichi	570, Yanaitsu, Yanaishi	Yamaguchi-ken 742
Mita, Hiroshi	7-9-14, Kishi-machi, Urawa-shi	Saitama-ken 336
Mita, Masac	37, Oaza Yashio, Kurobane-machi, Nasugun	Tochigi-ken 324-02
Mitamura, Kyozo	2-4-27, Nakaochiai, Shinjuku-ku	Tokyo 161
Mitamura, Toyoki	10 kumi, Sakuragaoka, Kasuga-machi, Chikushigun	Fukuoka-ken 816
Mitani, Kie	396, Nakano-cho	Itami-shi 664
Mitani, Michio	8-49, Maruhashicho, Nishinomiya-shi	Hyogo-ken 662

Mitarai, Genyo	145-78, Aza Kobayashi, Iwasaki, Nisshin-cho, Aichi-gun	Aichi-ken 470-01
Mitsui, Yukihiko	4-2-1-4, Kitayaso-cho	Tokushima-shi 770
Miura, Jun	2-8-8, Miyagino	Sendai-shi 983
Miura, Kanichi	148 Kashiramachi, Shinkarasuma-ru, Kamikyo-ku	Kyoto-shi 602
Miwa, Haruo	62, Aza Yamazuka, Oaza Shino-da, Miwa-cho, Amagun	Aichi-ken 490-12
Miyake, Hideji	2625, Kita Arima-machi, Minami-takaki-gun	Nagasaki-ken 859-23
Miyake, Torazo	2758-576, Obata-kitayama, Mori-yama-ku	Nagoya-shi 463
Miyamoto, Michi	429, Tukaba, Iwase, Matsudo-shi .	Chiba-ken 271
Miyasaka, Shizuko	898, Tanoura-machi, Ashikita-gun	Kumamoto-ken 869-53
Miyashita, Tadao	5-10-7, Matsubara, Satagaya-ku .	Tokyo 156
Miyata, Goro	1-18-26 Minami, Meguro-ku	Tokyo 152
Miyata, Seiko ....·....	Johen-cho, Minami-uwagun	Ehime-ken 798-41
Miyatani, Naofumi	Onmaedori, Imakojidori, Kami-gyo-ku	Kyoto-shi 602
Miyazaki, Shigeo	2-1-7, Sakae-cho	Odawara-shi 250
Miyazaki, Tamotsu	4-21-9, Kamikitazawa, Seta-gaya-ku	Tokyo 156
Miyazawa, Akimasa	4708, Toyoshina-machi, Minami-azumigun	Nagano-ken 399-82
Miyazawa, Minoru	7-100, Minami, Yamamoto-cho .	Yao-shi 581
Mizukawa, Takashi	5-18, Muromachi, Ikeda-shi	Osaka 563
Mizuki, Takashi	10-41, Chuo-machi, Tonami-shi .	Toyama-ken 939-13
Mizuno, Hideo	805, Koban No. 2, Hichihonmat-su, Nakaku	Nagoya-shi 460
Mizuno, Katsuyoshi	5-23, Kameoka-juutaku, 68, Kameoka, Kawauchi	Sendai-shi
Mizuta, Atsumasa	156, Nishicho, Taishogun, Kita-ku	Kyoto-shi 603
Mizutani, Yutaka	Nippon Contact Lens Research Institute, Shin-Nagoya Bldg, Minami-kan, Nakamura-ku ..	Nagoya-shi 450
Mogi, Shigeru	350, Noda, Noda-shi	Chiba-ken 278
Momose, Mitsuko	2-5-5, Shimizu, Suginami-ku	Tokyo 167
Mori, Katsusaburo	Aza Higashihama, Minamihama, Naruto-shi	Tokushima-ken 772
Mori, Naoyuki	1-19, Chitose-cho	Nishinomiya-shi 662
Mori, Shigetomo	8-3 chome, Nishi Terashima, Honcho	Tokushima-shi 770
Mori, Shinnosuke	347, Ichiraku, Ishii-cho, Myozai-gori	Tokushima-ken 779-32
Morikawa, Midori	2-632, Hondori, Higashi-ozone-cho, Kitaku	Nagoya-shi 462
Morikawa, Shuichi	ru 6, Kitamorimoto-machi, Kana-zawa-shi	Ishikawa-ken 920-01
Morikawa, Tsugako	Onmaedori, Imakojidori, Kami-gyoku	Kyoto-shi 602
Morinobu, Iwa	878-1, Hirotani-cho, Fuchu-shi ..	Hiroshima-ken 726
Morinobu, Takayoshi	2-7, Tsurumi-cho	Hiroshima-shi 730
Morishige, Shiro	1-6-28, Uemachi, Ube-shi	Yamaguchi-ken 755
Morita, Shiro	1-4-4, Minamirinkan, Yamato-shi	Kanagawa-ken 242
Moriyama, Takeshi	4-88, Tamagawa-cho, Fukushima-ku	Osaka 553

Motegi, Tsutomu	3-12-12, Minami-ikebukuro, Toshima-ku	Tokyo 171
Motegi, Matsujiro	2-2-73, Matunami	Chikugaki-shi 253
Mukaiyama, Masanobu	8-9-1, Goko-dori, Fukiai-ku	Kobe-shi 651
Munakata, Takumi	1-8-36, Higashi Honcho, Kashiwazaki-shi	Niigata-ken 945
Murai, Genhachi	5, Sakae-machi, Konakano-machi, Hachinohe-shi	Aomori-ken 031
Murai, Masajiro	3-2, Zaimokucho, Morioka-shi ..	Iwate-ken 020
Muraji, Yoneko	3-55, Abiko Nishi, Sumiyoshi-ku	Osaka-shi 558
Murakami, Hajime	1-91, Rikyumae, Sumaku	Kobe-shi 654
Murakami, Masuji	11-12, Asahimachi	Suita-shi 564
Murakami, Mitsuma	587, Sukumo, Sukumo-shi	Kochi-ken 787
Muromoto, Kamekichi	2-5-3, Daikan	Utsunomiya-shi 320
Murata, Shinroku	22-21, Hiranomachi	Nagasaki-shi 852
Murayama, Kenichi	757-58, Katakura-cho, Kanagawa-ku	Yokohama-shi 221
Muto, Kiyo	2-10-11, Kashiwa, Kashiwa-shi ..	Chiba-ken 277
Nabeshima, Taneyuki	75, Takaramachi, Kokura-ku ...	Kitakyushu-shi 802
Nagahashi, Ichiji	22, Shoji, Hanawamachi, Katsuno-gun	Akita-ken 018-52
Nagai, Teiko	1-19, Kyoshincho, Minami-ku ...	Yokohama-shi 233
Nagamata, Hiroyuki	2-585, Nagaoyama, Kirihata	Takarazuka-shi
Nagasawa, Hiroshi	2-26-1, Daikokumachi	Omuta-shi 836
Nagashima, Kohji	62 Miyagawa-cho, Shimogamo Sakyo-ku	Kyoto 606
Nagata, Makoto	Houren Yamazoe-nishi-machi, 818-3	Nara-shi 630
Nagayama, Chikuro	163, Maruyamacho, Miyazaki-shi .	Miyazaki-ken 880
Nagayama, Kōhei	1-7, Yamato-cho, Takahagi-shi ..	Ibaraki-ken 318
Nagayama, Shohei	1015, Honkan, Sadorihaitu, 1-4-20, Nakameguro Meguro-ku	Tokyo 153
Nagayama, Shigeyuki	31-11, Takaramachi	Kochi-shi 780
Nagayoshi, Sanemitsu	5-4, Himegi-cho, Miyaonojo-shi .	Miyazaki-ken 885
Nakada, Hajime	2-2-14, Asahi, Kisarazu-shi ...	Chiba-ken 292
Nakagaki, Hisao	Azumacho, Tanushimaru-machi .	Fukuoka-ken 839-12
Nakagawa, Junichi	1890-59, Asahigaoka	Sapporo-shi 060
Nakagawa, Keikō	Suginacho, Toyosaka-shi	Niigata-ken 950-33
Nakaizumi, Yukimasa	5-7-25, Minami-aoyama, Minato-ku	Tokyo 107
Nakajima, Akira	1-41-14, Miyasaka, Setagaya-ku .	Tokyo 156
Nakajima, Motoi	15, Tadodai	Yokosuka-shi 238
Nakajima, Yoshie	Nishi-iru, Imakumano Dentei agaru, Higashiyama-ku	Kyoto-shi 605
Nakakura, Ichiro	1-78, Higashi-toyonakamachi ...	Toyonaka-shi 560
Nakamura, Akira	2-22-1 Nakano, Nakano-ku ...	Tokyo 164
Nakamura, Kazuo	3409, Sawara, Sawara-shi	Chiba-ken 287
Nakamura, Masanao	Yobuko-machi, Higashimatsuura-gun	Saga-ken 847-03
Nakamura, Osamu	4-28, Tezukayama Higashi, Sumi-yoshi-ku	Osaka-shi 558
Nakamura, Shigeru	2-22-14, Chidori, Ōta-ku	Tokyo 144
Nakamura, Yukichi	5-6-9, Amakawacho	Tsuchiura-shi 300
Nakamura, Yoshiko	69 Aza Minamihoribata, Oaza Yōfu, Yokosukacho, Chitagun	Aichi-ken

Oshima, Sukeyuki	5-7-213, Harumi 3-chome, Chuo-ku	Tokyo 104
Oshio, Sadao	1-5-16, Jigyo	Fukuoka-shi 810
Ōsumi, Kametaro	2-33-1 Eitai, Fukagawa, Koto-ku	Tokyo 135
Otsuka, Jin	Minami-1-12, Ebisu, Shibuya-ku .	Tokyo 150
Otsuka, Katsushiro	1-3408, Sawara, Sawara-shi	Chiba-ken 287
Otsuka, Takuzo	1-1967, Sawara, Sawara-shi	Chiba-ken 287
Otsuka, Tokuhei	30, Hama-machi, Akune-shi	Kagoshima-ken 899-16
Otsuki, Yorio	90, Aza Tamachi, Kakuda, Kakuda-shi	Miyagi-ken 981-15
Ouchi, Entaro	4-8-12, Ifukucho	Okayama-shi 700
Oyamada, Kazuo	2-91, Kitaikuno-cho, Ikuno-ku ..	Osaka-shi 544
Oyama, Noburo	1159, Kitatanaka-cho, Nerima-ku	Tokyo 177
Ozasa, Hayao	548, Totsukamachi, Totsuka-ku .	Yokohama-shi 244
Ozeki, Sumiko	Aza Tomita, Tachiarai-cho, Mimui-gun	Fukuoka-ken 830-12
Ozima, Hideyuki	20, Kakinoki-cho, Takahashi ...	Okayama-ken 716
Ryu, Junichiro	5, Nikawatori, Hagashi, Kure-shi .	Hiroshima-ken 737
Ryu, Motoki	36, Dekimachi, Yanagawa-shi ...	Fukuoka-ken 832
Saeki, Hidemasa	6-21, Uehonmachi, Minamiku ...	Osaka 542
Sagae, Kazuo	10-1654, Nishiborimaedori	Niigata-shi 951
Saigo, Takakazu	1-7-10, Nishiazabu, Minato-ku ..	Tokyo 106
Saito, Hatsue	2-6-11, Tani	Fukuoka-shi 810
Saito, Osamu	91 Hatago, Ōnomachi, Tokoname-shi	Aichi-ken
Saito, Saburo	24, Aioicho, Sano-shi	Tochigi-ken 327
Saito, Shigehiro	5-15, Saiwaicho, Kuroiso-machi, Nasugun	Tochigi-ken 325
Saito, Toshio	1-1, Shinjukucho	Numazu-shi 410
Saito, Zenpei	1-4-25, Senjuji-machi, Furukawashi	Miyagi-ken 989-61
Sakai, Heihachiro	3297, Toide, Takaoka-shi	Toyama-ken 939-11
Sakai, Shinichi	870-4, Nanukamachi, Amagi-shi .	Fukuoka-ken 838
Sakai, Toshihiko	19 Nishihiromi, Chiryucho, Hekikaigun	Aichi-ken 472
Sakamoto, Masatoshi	2422, Seya-cho, Totsuka-ku	Yokohama-shi 246
Saishin, Mototsugu	1-15-25, Hannancho, Abeno-ku ‚‚	Osaka-shi, 545
Sakamoto, Rinpei	1-28-11, Minowa, Taito-ku	Tokyo 110
Sakanashi, Michi	21-16, Kiyamacho, Nichinan-shi .	Miyazaki-ken 887
Sakanoue, Toshihiko	5-13-5 Nishi-Ikebukuro, Toshima-ku	Tokyo 171
Sakatani, Shinji	221-4, Matogata, Matogata-cho ..	Himeji-shi 671-01
Sakaue, Ei	3-20, Umegaoka, Ngaokakyo-shi .	Kyoto-fu 617
Sakimoto, Yukio	4-12, Higashisengoku-cho	Kagoshima-shi 892
Sakka, Masao	1-chome, Anoomachi, Yahata-ku .	Kitakyushu-shi 806
Sako, Tsunenori	2-26, Kamocho	Yonago-shi 683
Sakuma, Katsuyoshi	3-9-5, Nukui, Nerima-ku	Tokyo 176
Sano, Kuniyoshi	1-13, Monzencho	Okazaki-shi 444
Sano, Taiko	71, Ichibacho, Atsuta-ku	Nagoya-shi 456
Sano, Toyoko	1-14-4, Ekota, Nakano-ku	Tokyo 165
Sano, Yotsumi	Nishiojioike agaru, Nakakyo-ku .	Kyoto-shi 604
Sasakawa, Reiko	3-6-27, Kasugashinden, Naoetsushi	Niigata-ken 942
Sasaki, Shigeru	2043-13, Higashinocho	Akashi-shi 673
Sasaki, Tamio	5-9-17, Hagoromo, Takaishi-shi .	Osaka 592

Shinoda, Sugao	1-chome, Shirakawa-machi, Yaha-taku	Kitakyushu-shi 805
Shinohara, Masatoshi	9-6, Nishi 1-jo Minami	Obihiro-shi
Shinozuka, Seishi	Takanawa Ganka Eye Clinic, 2-16-36, Takanawa, Minato-ku	Tokyo 108
Shintaku, Nobuo	8-32, Takatacho, Nagahama-shi .	Shiga-ken
Shinya, Shigeo	98, Kazusauchi, Matsuda-shi	Chiba-ken
Shinzato, Kotoku	2-7, Miebashi-cho, Naha-shi	Okinawa
Shoji, Isao	1-12-14, Higashihara-machi	Yamagata-ken
Shoji, Yoshiharu	3-20-19, Inokashira	Mitaka-shi
Shirai, Nakaba	Takase-cho, Mitoyogun	Kagawa-ken 767
Sonoda, Kunizo	13-1, Higashioji-cho, Yahata-ku .	Kitakyushu-shi 806
Sonoda, Saneharu	124, Midori-cho, Makurazaki-shi .	Kagoshima-ken 898
Sonoda, Shigeru	4642, Shimokorimoto-cho, Miya-konojō-shi	Miyazaki-ken 885
Sueyoshi, Toshizo	Nishi 25, Minami 7	Sapporo-shi 060
Suda, Akira	1-9-1, Haruyama	Fukui-shi 910
Suda, Eiji	1-9-15, Hashimoto	Aomori-shi 030
Suda, Ikkaku	133 Jōroku	Sakai-shi 588
Suda, Keiu	Suda Glaucoma Clinic, R-413, Co-op Olympia, 6-35-3, Jingu-mae, Shibuya-ku	Tokyo 150
Suda, Tadashi	1-33-12, Hongo, Bunkyo-ku	Tokyo 113
Suga, Kazuo	132-3, Otani-cho, Tsu-shi	Mie-ken 514
Sugahara, Atsushi	1-5, Kankōdōri	Takamatsu-shi 760
Sugahara, Kazuhiko	2-15-5, Sakaigawa, Tobataku ...	Kitakyushu-shi 804
Sugai, Hiroshi	4839, Miyada, Miyada-machi, Kurate-gun	Fukuoka-ken 823
Sugai, Masao	Miyada-machi, Kurate-gun	Fukuoka-ken 823
Sugamata, Osamu	Ichibancho, Higashinakatori	Niigata-shi
Sugano, Tadao	1-17-10, Sumiyoshi-cho	Maebashi-shi 951
Sugasawa, Narahiko	4-6-5, Naka-cho, Uozaki, Uozaki-cho, Higashinadaku	Kobe-shi 658
Sugasawa, Tokusaburo	6-11, Higashinodamachi, Miyako-shima-ku	Osaka
Sugimoto, Shigenori	3-13-31, Ōtemachi	Hiroshima-shi 730
Sugita, Aiko	4-4, Egawacho, Nishi-ku	Nagoya-shi
Sugita, Masaomi	3-2-30, Tachibanadori-higashi ...	Miyazaki-shi 880
Sugita, Shinichiro	5-1-30, Sakae, Naka-ku	Nagoya-shi 460
Sugiura, Seiji	Nishi 6, Kita 16jo	Sapporo-shi 065
Sugiura, Shoji	20, Kitamachi, Heisaka-cho	Nishio-shi 444-01
Sugiyama, Katsumi	1-5, Honmachi, Ono-shi	Fukui-ken 912
Sumida, Yoshikane	1-chome, Minami, Engaricho 1-jōdori, Monbetsugun	Hokkaido 099-04
Suzaki, Fumihiko	10-3728, Kōrigaoka	Hirakata-shi 573
Suzawa, Mitsuo	86, Motoishishita, Ishige-machi, Yuki-gun	Ibaraki-ken 300-27
Suzue, Tadashi	5-1-8, Takanodai	Suita-shi 565
Suzuki, Hideo	1-158, Sawara, Sawara-shi	Chiba-ken 287
Suzuki, Isaku	1288, Takaida	Higashi-osaka-shi
Suzuki, Kōdō	6-40-3, Yahiro, Sumida-ku	Tokyo
Suzuki, Kunihiko	4-40-8, Honcho, Funabashi-shi ..	Chiba-ken 273
Suzuki, Murako	4-20, Nishimiyamachi, Nakatsuga-wa-shi	Gifu-ken 508

Suzuki, Norio	2, Terakoji, Mizusawa-shi	Iwate-ken 023
Suzuki, Shinsuke	4-9, Matsubara-cho	Gamagori-shi 443
Suzuki, Toshio	3-7, Chihaya-cho, Toshima-ku	Tokyo 171
Suzuki, Yasuko	2-11-15, Higashi-kaigan, Kita, Chigasaki-shi	Kanagawa-ken
Suzuki, Yoshitami	4-8, Higashihoncho	Chiba-shi 280
Suzumura, Akihiro	1-4, Namiuchi-cho, Kita-ku	Nagoya-shi 462
Tabata, Shizue	2-5-14, Suido, Bunkyo-ku	Tokyo 112
Tada, Hidekazu	4-19, Echizenmachi	Toyama-shi 930
Tanoue, Sadako	145, Higashimachi, Nishino-omote-shi	Kagoshima-ken 891-31
Tagawa, Sadatsugu	Nishi 4, Minami 2	Sapporo-shi 060
Tawara, Tatsuhiko	2151, Kashii	Fukuokashi 813
Tahara, Yoshiaki	1444-7, Ōaza Shime, Shimemachi, Kasuyagun	Fukuoka-ken 811-22
Tajino, Masateru	57, Shimo-gionmachi, Hyogo-ku	Kobe-shi 652
Takata, Kaoru	3-3-22, Ōmiya-cho	Mishima-shi 411
Takata, Miyo	582, Sugita-cho, Isogo-ku	Yokohama-shi 235
Takagaki, Masuko	4-10, Kamidori, Shibuya-ku	Tokyo
Takagi, Yoshihiro	1271-1, Ōsone-kō, Nankoku-shi	Kochi-ken 783
Takahashi, Fujie	415, Tsuruhakicho, Kaminoyama-shi	Yamagata-ken 991-31
Takahashi, Haruo	24-8, Aza Machi-higashi, Harano-machi, Wakata-ku	Sendai-shi 983
Takahashi, Hiroshi	Kado, Sakae-cho, Takoyakushi-dori, Nakagyo-ku	Kyoto-shi 604
Takahashi, Kenji	2-13-6, Sakuragaoka, Setagaya-ku	Tokyo 156
Takahashi, Kiyoshi	4-43-7, Higashi Tateishi, Katsushi-ka-ku	Tokyo 124
Takahashi, Mamoru	4-147, Kurume, Koriyama-shi	Fukushima-ken 963
Takahashi, Masuo	4668, Totsuka-cho, Totsuka-ku	Yokohama-shi 244
Takahashi, Rihei	3-63-2, 4-chome, Kosanomachi, Kamaishi-shi	Iwate-ken 026
Takahashi, Shigezo	4-2, Yanagimachi, Ichinomiya-shi.	Aichi-ken 491
Takahashi, Takeji	3-7-12, Dai	Kamakura-shi 247
Takahashi, Yoshinari	1-23, Sakae-machi, Soden	Gufu-shi 500
Takahashi, Yukio	27-15, Korien-cho, Hirakata-shi	Ōsaka 573
Takaki, Sueka	27-40, Kamegawa Higashimachi, Beppu-shi	Oita-ken 874-01
Takaku, Isao	Dept. of Ophthalmology, School of Medicine Nagasaki University, 7-1, Sakamotomachi	Nagasaki-shi 852
Takano, Fumio	403, Bididunsu, 1-1-14, Komika-fukuro	Sendai-shi 980
Takano, Toshio	1070, Miyamachi, Kumagaya-shi	Saitama-ken 360
Takano, Yasuo	1-3-9, Mejirodai, Bunkyo-ku	Tokyo 112
Takao, Noboru	2680, Kitashinkoji, Nobeoka-shi	Miyazaki-ken 882
Takao, Suketomo	948, Nakada-cho, Totsuka-ku	Yokohama-shi
Takashi, Tatsuko	1403-4, Minami-edomachi	Matsuyama-shi 790
Takatsuji, Masae	1-12, Daikokumachi, Fukuyama-shi	Hiroshima-ken 720
Takayasu, Akira	5-kumi, Soen-cho	Beppu-shi 874
Takazawa, Yutaka	4-21, Hirokoji, Kariya-shi	Aichi-ken 448
Takei, Hisashi	4-6-5, Katayama-cho, Suita-shi	Osaka 564
Takeda, Shizuka	100-11, Kariya, Ako-shi	Hyogo-ken 678-02

Takemura, Kei	708, Oaza, Himihama, Hama-cho, Miho-gun	Takamatsu-shi 769-16
Takemura, Toshiji	3-12-11, Minimidai	Kawagoe-shi 350
Takeo, Tsuneki	2-1, Yaga, Yamakita-machi, Ashi-gara-kamigun	Kanagawa-ken
Takeshita, Sachiko	Nakayama, Takashima-machi, Nishisonogigun	Nagasaki-ken 851-13
Takeshita, Shozo	3-7-13, Mizugae-machi	Saga-shi
Takeshita, Takeyoshi	5-6-21, Tagara, Nerima-ku	Tokyo 176
Takeuchi, Mitsuhiko	Minami 4, Nishi 15	Sapporo-shi 060
Takeuchi, Takahiko	13-15, Sakaemachi, Hondo-shi	Kumamoto-ken 863
Tamura, Shigemi	1-14-8, Beppu, Nishi-ku	Fukuoka-shi 814
Tanabe, Nobuyasu	53-4, Shimogawara, Tatsuno-shi	Hyogo-ken 679-41
Tanabe, Taro	1-613, Higashi-ozone, Hondori, Kitaku	Nagoya-shi 462
Tanabe, Taro	30, Higashi-kajiyamachi	Wakayama-shi 640
Tanahashi, Toichi	2-33, Oshiba-cho, Ichinomiya-shi	Aichi-ken 491
Tanaka, Hatsuo	3-491, Ukimachi, Isahaya-shi	Nagasaki-ken 854-01
Tanaka, Kiyoto	1-12-17, Chūo	Ishinomaki-shi 986
Tanaka, Masaji	1-1-8, Umegaoka, Setagaya-ku	Tokyo 154
Tanaka, Saburo	4-12-18, Mukonoso	Amagasaki-shi 661
Tanaka, Shigeyuki	1549, Midorimachi	Hiroshima-shi 734
Tanaka, Sonoko	2-645, Hakusanura	Niigata-shi 951
Tanaka, Tatsuya	4-16-9, Shimosuketo-cho, Toku-shima-shi	Tokushima-ken 770
Tanaka, Tomojiro	174, Minamitamachi, Matsue-shi	Shimane-ken 690
Tanaka, Yoshifumi	412, Nishikagiyacho, Fushimi-ku	Kyoto-shi 612
Tanaka, Yōtarō	8-20-2, Tateishi, Katsushika-ku	Tokyo 124
Tanaka, Yoshimatsu	1-10-18, Sanbonmatsu, Hida-shi	Ōita-ken 877
Tanamura, Etsuko	2-13-8, Fujimicho	Chiba-shi 280
Tane, Sadanao	Dept. of Ophthalmology, St. Marianne University, School of Medicine, 2095, Sugao, Takatsu-ku	Kawasaki-shi 210
Tani, Katsuo	10-7. Tashirocho	Nishinomiva-shi 662
Tani, Michiyuki	Dept. of Ophthalmology, Kyoto Prefectural University of Medicine, Kawaramachi, Hirokoji, Kamikyo-ku	Kyoto-shi 602
Taniguchi, Yoshiaki	Dept. of Ophthalmology, Faculty of Medicine, Kagoshima University, 8-3, Shiroyama-cho	Kagoshima-shi 892
Taniwaki, Takuma	Kiyomi-Tetsudo-Kansha 801, Hanayamadori-2, Moji-ku	Kitakyushu-shi 801
Tano, Yoshio	46, Wada-cho, Nishiwaki-shi	Hyogo-ken 677
Tasaka, Sumiyuki	18, Takanawa-cho, Shichiku, Kitaku	Kyoto-shi 603
Tashiro, Masamori	13-16, Hiranocho	Kagoshima-shi 892
Tazawa, Yutaka	Dept. of Ophthalmology, School of Medicine, Iwate Medical University	Morio-ka-shi 020
Terada, Yasuo	577, Fujishiro, Fujishiro-machi, Kitasōmagun	Ibaraki-ken 309-01
Terayama, Saiichi	1 Shinonomecho, Chtose-shi	Hokkaido 066
Toda, Shintaro	1-8-6, Matoba-cho	Hiroshima-shi
Togano, Nikyuji	2-6, Kanto-machi	Nagaoka-shi

Ueno, Tomoaki	132-2, Motoshirocho	Hamamatsu-shi
Uenoyama, Kenshiro	Wakayama Rosai Hospital, 435, Koya	Wakayama-shi 640
Ueoka, Terukata	4-14, Imagawacho, Hatano-shi	Kanagawa-ken 257
Uesugi, Moto	56, Kawanayama-cho, Showa-ku	Nagoya-shi 466
Uezono, Rinko	32, Kajiyacho	Akashi-shi 673
Ukari, Junichi	49, Miyanojocho, Satsumagun	Kagoshima-ken 895-18
Umazume, Kakichi	No. 605, Mansion Mejirogaoka, 3-12-28, Shimoochiai, Shimoochiai, Shinjuku-ku	Tokyo
Umazume, Yuzuru	1-1-20, Momoi, Suginami-ku	Tokyo
Umimura, Shiro	1-219, Suehirocho, Choshi-shi	Chiba-ken 288
Urabe, Kazutaka	1-6-21, Hujita, Yahata-ku	Kitakyushu-shi 806
Urayama, Akira	Dept. of Ophthalmology, School of Medicine, Akita University, 6-10, Senshu-Kubotamachi	Akita-shi 010
Urushihara, Shinkichi	5-11-1, Hatanodai, Shinagawa-ku .	Tokyo 141
Usuda, Hana	Konya-machi, Komoro-shi	Nagano-ken 384
Usui, Kunio	311, Nishinakanomachi	Toyama-shi 930
Utsumi, Ryuzo	15-1, Kitaguchicho, Nishinomiya-chi	Hyogo-ken 662
Utsumi, Yoshiharu	2-112, Hinodecho, Nakaku	Yokohama-shi 232
Utsunomiya, Kōji	3-52, Tsuruyacho, Kanagawa-ku .	Yokohama-shi 221
Uyama, Yasuo	6-24, Midorigaoka, Itami-shi	Hyogo-ken 664
Wada, Kesao	39, Tamaya-cho, Nakadachi-uri Senbon, Kamikyoku	Kyoto-shi 602
Wada, Nobuo	2-chome, Kumademachi, Yawata-ku	Kitakyushu-shi 806
Wada, Shiro	2-22, Konohanacho, Kitaku	Osaka 530
Wakahara, Hideo	11-23, Takatsuki-machi, Takatsuki-shi	Osaka 569
Wakao, Tōru	6530-31, Aza Maruyama, Unuma.	Kakumuhara
Wakatsuki, Haruo	10, Nakakachimachi	Wakayama-shi 641
Watanabe, Hirota	No. 20, Omachi, Shimodate-shi .	Ibaraki-ken 308
Watanabe, Osamu	Jizodo, Bunsuicho, Nishikanbaragun	Niigata-ken
Watanabe, Tatsuya	2564, Tomita, Sannanyo-shi	Yamaguchi-ken 746
Yachi, Michiko	2-1, Yoyogi, Shibuya-ku	Tokyo 151
Yagasaki, Kaoru	Kōgakubumae, Kamiube, Ube-shi.	Yamaguchi-ken 755
Yagasaki, Yoshiro	4 Yanagimachi	Ichinomiya-shi 491
Yagi, Michio	9-7, Tsutsumishitamachi, Koriyama-shi	Fukushima-ken 963
Yagi, Tokihiko	5-14-13, Shinden, Ichikawa-shi	Chiba-ken 272-00
Yamada, Hideyuki	11-12, 3-chome, Saburōmaru-cho, Kokura-ku	Kitakyushu-shi 802
Yamada, Kotaro	2-910, Ikebukuro, Toshima-ku	Tokyo 171
Yamada, Senichi	44-1, Egawa-yokomachi, Nishiku	Nagoya-shi 451
Yamada, Shigeko	1-24-9, Sako 7 Bancho	Tokushima-shi 770
Yamada, Shinsuke	1-11-12, Ekimae, Koriyama-shi	Fukushima-ken
Yamada, Takashi	2-48-3, Hatagaya, Shibuya-ku	Tokyo 151
Yamada, Yasuo	2-87, 5 Bancho, Koshien	Nishinomiya-shi 662
Yamaga, Isamu	3-8-13, Hanazono-cho	Otaru-shi 047
Yamagata, Torajiro	1-4-13, Chuō-cho	Ube-shi 755
Yamagishi, Hisao	2123, Tsurugatamachi	Nagano-shi 380
Yamagishi, Mutsuo	86, Shimochi, Shimoichi-machi, Yoshinogun	Nara-ken 638

Yoshida, Eiichi	Chiekoin-higashi, Marutamachi, Kamikyo-ku	Kyoto-shi 602
Yoshida, Shigeki	11, Umezonocho, Moriguchi-shi .	Osaka 570
Yoshida, Shoji	1-4-35, Honcho	Sendai-shi 980
Yoshida, Tei	6-chome, Nishi, 9-jo Minami	Sapporo-shi 060
Yoshidomi, Shinji	107, Nishijin-machi	Fukuoka-shi 814
Yoshie, Fumi	2-8-4, Okamoto	Ise-shi 516
Yoshimura, Ichiro	3-1-17, Nakadori	Akita-shi 010
Yoshimura, Yoshio	Kakuosan Mansion 4B, 1-71, San-moncho, Chikusa-ku	Nagoya-shi 464
Yoshino, Mieko	13, Kōgacho, Deguchi	Wakayama-shi 641
Yoshioka, Hisaharu	Dept. of Ophthalmology, Kurume University School of Medicine, Asahimachi	Kurume-shi 830
Yoshizawa, Kiyoshi	2-1229, Shimota-machi, Kanuma-shi	Tochigi-ken 322
Yotsukura, Nobuo	1-14-31, Sakae-cho, Odawara-shi	Kanagawa-ken 250
Yuge, Tsunekazu	51, Kitauracho, Kawashima, Ukyo-ku	Kyoto-shi
Yui, Naoyuki	2-22-13, Tsutsumi-cho	Aomori-shi 030
Yuki, Akira	Asahi-cho, Ojiya-shi	Niigata-ken 947
Yukino, Hiroyoshi	17 Machikumicho, Hachinohe-shi.	Aomori-ken 031
Yukisada, Noriko	4-15, Wakitahoncho, Kawagoe-shi	Saitama-ken 350
Yuri, Taro	1681, Shibukawa-shi	Gunma-ken 377
Yusa, Mitsuru	1-13-2 Honchodōri	Morioka-shi 020

NOSOCOMIA QUIBUS OCULIS AEGRI CURANTUR

University Eye-Departments in Japan

Hokkaido Univ. Nishi-5, Kita-14, Sapporo 060. Head: Prof. Seiji Sugiura
Hirosaki Univ. 2, Sagara-cho, Hirosaki. 036. Head: Prof. Kimiho Irinoda
Sapporto Med. College. Nishi-16, Minami-1, Sapporo 060. Head: Prof. Toshizo Sueyoshi
Iwate Med. College. 19-1, Uchimaru, Morioka, Iwate 020. Head: Prof. Kitetsu Imaizumi
Akita Univ. 6-10, Senshu-kubota, Akita, Akita 010. Head: Prof. to be appointed
Fukushima Med. College. Sugizuma, Fukushima 960. Head: Prof. Mutsuo Kajiura
Tokohu Univ. 1-1 Seiryo, Sendai, Miyagi 980. Head: Prof. Katsuyoshi Mizuno
Univ. of Tokyo. 7-3-1 Hongo, Tokyo 113. Head: Prof. Saiichi Mishima
Tokyo Med. and Dental Univ. 1-5-47, Yushima, Bunkyo-ku, Tokyo 113. Head: Prof. Jin Otsuka
Nihon Univ. 30, Ohtani-kojo-machi, Itabashi-ku, Tokyo 173. Head: Prof. Noboru Kunitomo
Nihon Univ. 1-8-13, Kanda-surugadai, Chiyoda-ku, Tokyo 101. Head: Prof. Ken Kato
Keio Univ. 35, Shinano-machi, Shinjuku-ku, Tokyo 160. Head: Prof. Yasuharu Kuwabara
Tokyo Womens Med. College. 10, Kawada-cho, Shinjuku-ku, Tokyo 162. Head: Prof. Kinkichi Kato
Juntendo Univ. 3/1/3, Hongo, Bunkyo-ku, Tokyo 113. Head: Prof. Akira Nakajima
Jikei Med. College. 3-25-8, Nishishimbashi, Minato-ku, Tokyo 105. Head: Prof. Tomoya Funahashi
Showa Univ. 1-5-8, Hatanodai, Shingawa-ku, Tokyo 141. Head: Prof. Shigeru Masuda
Toho Univ. 6-11-1, Nishiohmori, Ohta-ku Tokyo 143. Head: Prof. Yoshiko Ohoka
Tokyo Med. College. 1-53, Kashiwagi, Shinjuku-ku, Tokyo 160. Head: Prof. Harutake Matsuo
Nihon Med. College. 1-1-15, Sendagi, Bunkyo-ku, Tokyo 113. Head: Prof. Masami Oguchi
Kitazato Univ. Asamizodai, Sagamihara, Kanagawa 228, Head: Prof. Satoshi Ishikawa
Kyorin Univ. 6-20-2, Shinkawa, Kanagawa 228. Head: Prof. Hisaya Tokuda

Yokohama Med. College. 4-57, Urafune-cho, Minami-ku, Yokohama 232. Head: Prof. Tokuji Ohkuma
Chiba Univ. 313, Inohana, Chiba, Chiba 280. Head: Prof. Yoshitami Suzuki
Gumma Univ. Showamachi Maebashi, Gunma 371. Head: To be appointed
Shinshu Univ. Asahicho, Matsumoto, Nagano 390. Head: Prof. Seiichi Kato
Niigata Univ. Ichibancho Asahichodori, Niigata, Niigata 951. Head: To be appointed
Kanazawa Univ. 13, Takaracho, Kanazawa, Ishikawa 920. Head: Prof. Daizo Yonemura
Nagoya Univ. Tsurumaicho, Showaku, Nagoya, Aichi 466. Head: To be appointed
Nagoya Shiritsu Univ. Kawasumi, Mizuho, Mizuho, Nagoya Aichi 467. Head: to be appointed
Gifu Univ. 70 Tsukasacho, Gifu, Gifu 500. Head: Prof. Saburo Hayano
Kyoto Univ. Yoshidakonoecho, Sakyoku, Kyoto 606. Head: Prof. Masao Kishimoto
Mie Univ. 1-96, Sakaemachi, Tsu, Mie 541. Head: Prof. Kazuo Suga
Kyoto Furitsu Med. College. Kawaramachi Kamikyoku, Kyoto, Kyoto 602. Head: Prof. Michiyuki Tani
Osaka Univ. 3-1-2, Doshimahamadori, Fukushima-ku, Osaka, Osaka 553. Head: Prof. Takashi Mizukawa
Osaka Med. College. 2-7, Daigakumachi, Takatsuki, Osaka 530. Head: To be appointed
Osaka Shiritsu Univ. Asahicho, Abenoku, Osaka, Osaka. Head: Prof. Ichizo Ikeda
Kansai Med. College. Fumisonocho, Moriguchishi, Osaka 570. Head: Prof. Isamu Tsukahara
Wakayama Med. College. Shichibancho, Wakayama, Wakayama 640. Head: Prof. Iwao Iinuma
Kobe Univ. Kusunokicho, Ikutaku, Kobe, Hyogo 650. Head: Prof. Yuzuru Imachi
Nara Med. College. Shizyomachi, Kashiwarashi, Nara 634. Head: Prof. Shuichi Nakao
Okayama Univ. 2-5-1, Shikadamachi, Okayama, Okayama 640. Head: Prof. Kanshi Okuda
Kawasaki Med. 577 Matsushima, Kurashikishi, Okayama 700. Head: Prof. Kakuji Yamamoto
Hiroshima Univ. Kasumicho, Hiroshima, Hiroshima 734. Head: Prof. Tsugio Dodo
Tottori Univ. 36-1, Nishimachi, Yonago, Tottori 683. Head: Prof. Yutaka Fujinaga
Tokushima Univ. Kuramotocho, Tokushima, Tokushima 770. Head: Prof. Yukihiko Mitsui
Yamaguchi Univ. Ogushi Ube, Yamaguchi 755. Head: Prof. Shunsaku Kobayashi
Kurume Univ. Asahicho, Kurumeshi, Fukuoka 830. Head: Prof. Yoshiya Masuda
Kryushu Univ. Katakusu, Fukuoka, Fukuoka 812. Head: Prof. Hiroshi Ikui
Nagasaki Univ. 7-1, Sakamotocho, Nagasaki, Nagasaki 852. Head: Prof. Isao Takaku
Kumamoto Univ. 1-1-1 Honjo, Kumammotoshi, Kummamoto 860. Head: Prof. Jun Tsutsui
Kagoshima Univ. Shiroyama, Kagoshima, Kagoshima 892. Head: Prof. Yoshiaki Taniguchi
Teikyo Univ. 2-11-1, Kaga, Itabashi, Tokyo 173. Head: Prof. Toshio Maruo
Toyo Med. College. 2095. Kawasaki, Kanagawa 211. Head: Prof. Sadanao Tane

Eye departments of medical schools

School of Medicine, Hokkaido University. Kita-15-jo, Kita-ku, Sapporo-shi, Hokkaido 060. Head: Prof. Sugiura Seiji.
Sapporo Medical College, Minami-1-jo, Chuo-ku, Sapporo-shi, Hokkaido 060. Head: Prof. Tagawa Sadatsugu
School of Medicine, Hirosaki University. Zaifu-cho, Hirosaki-shi 036. Head: Prof. Irinoda Kimiho
Iwate Medical College. Uchimaru, Morioka-shi 020. Head: Prof. Imaizumi Kitetsu
School of Medicine, Akita University. Senshu-Kubota-cho, Akita-shi 010. Head: Prof. Urayama Akira
School of Medicine, Tohoku University. Seiryo-cho, Sendai-shi 980. Head: Prof. Mizuni Katsuyoshi
Fukushima Medical College. Sugizuma-cho, Fukushima-shi 960. Head: Prof. Kajiura Mutsuo
Jichi Medical School. Nakatomatsuri Utsunomiya-shi 320. Head: Prof. Shimizu Hiroyuki
School of Medicine, Dokkyo University. Mibumachi, Shimotsuga-gun, Tochigi-shi 321-02. Head: Prof. Seki Ryo.
Tokyo Medical and Dental University. Yushima, Bunkyo-Tokyo 113. Head: Prof. Otuska Jin
School of Medicine, University of Tokyo. Hongo, Bunkyo-ku, Tokyo 113. Head: Prof. Mishima Saiichi

School of Medicine, University of Tokyo (Branch Hospital) Mejirodai, Bunkyo-ku, Tokyo 112

School of Medicine, Keio University. Shinanomachi, Shinjuku-ku, Tokyo 160. Head: Prof. Uemura Yasuo

School of Medicine, Nihon University. Oyaguchimachi, Itabashi-ku, Tokyo 173. Head: Prof. Kitano Shunsaku

School of Medicine, Nihon University (Surugadai Hospital). Kanda-Surugadai, Chiyoda-ku, Tokyo 101. Head: Prof. Kato Ken

Jikei University School of Medicine. Nishi-Shinbashi, Minato-ku, Tokyo 105. Head: Prof. Funabashi Tomoya

Showa University School of Medicine. Hatanodai, Shinagawa-ku, Tokyo 141. Head: Prof. Masuda Shigeru

Tokyo Medical College. Nishi-Shinjuku, Shinjuku-ku, Tokyo 160. Head: Prof. Matsuo Harutake

School of Medicine, Teikyo University. Kago-cho, Itabashi-ku, Tokyo 173. Head: Prof. Maruo Toshio

Tokyo Women's Medical College. Kawada-cho, Ichigaya, Shinjuku-ku, Tokyo 162. Head: Prof. Kato Kinkichi

School of Medicine, Juntendo University. Hongo, Bunkyo-ku, Tokyo 113. Head: Prof. Nakajima Akira

Nippon Medical College. Sendagi-cho, Bunkyo-ku, Tokyo 113. Head: Prof. Oguchi Masami

Nippon Medical College, the 1st Hospital. Iidabashi, Chiyoda-ku, Tokyo 102

School of Medicine, Toho University. Omori, Ota-ku, Tokyo 143. Head: Prof. Ooka Ryoko

School of Medicine, Kyorin University. Mitaka-shi, Tokyo 181. Head: Prof. Tokuda Hisaya

School of Medicine, Kitazato University. Asamizodai, Sagamihara-shi, Kanagawa 228. Head: Prof. Ishikawa Satoshi

School of Medicine, Yokohama University. Urafune-cho, Minami-ku, Yokohama-shi 232. Head: Prof. Tanaka Naohiko

St. Marianna University School of Medicine. Nakahara-ku, Kawasaki-shi 210. Head: Prof. Tane Sadanao

School of Medicine, Chiba University. Inohana-cho, Chiba-shi 280. Head: Prof. Suzuki Yoshitami

Saitama Medical College. Moroyama-cho, Iruma-gun, Saitama 350-04. Head: Prof. Noyori Kimiharu

School of Medicine, Gunma University. Showamachi, Maebashi-shi 371. Head: Prof. Shimizu Koichi

School of Medicine, Shinshu University. Asahimachi, Matsumoto-shi 390

School of Medicine, Kanazawa University. Takaramachi, Kanazawa-shi 920. Head: Prof. Yonemura Diazo

Kanazawa Medical College. Uchinada-cho, Kawakita-gun, Ishkawa-ken 920-02. Head: Prof. Kurachi Yoshi

School of Medicine, Niigata University. Asahimachi, Nigata-shi 951. Head: Prof. Iwata Kazuo

School of Medicine, Nagoya University. Tsurumai-cho, Showa-ku, Nagoya-shi 466

School of Medicine, Nagoya University. (Branch Hospital). Higashi-Monzen-cho, Higashi-ku, Nagoya-shi 461

Nagoya City University Medical School. Mizuho-cho, Mizuho-ku, Nagoya-shi 467. Head: Prof. Majima Akio

Aichi Medical University. Moriyama-ku, Nagoya-shi 463. Head: Prof. Suzumura Akihiro

Gifu Prefectural Medical School. tsukasamachi, Gifu-shi 500. Head: Prof. Hayano Saburo

Faculty of Medicine, Mie Prefectural University. Sakae-cho, Tsu-shi 514. Head: Prof. Suga Kazuo

Osaka University Medical School. Dojimahamadori, Fukushima-ku, Osaka-shi 543. Head: Prof. Mizukawa Takashi

Osaka City University Meical School. Asahimachi, Abeno-ku, Osaka-shi 545

Osaka Medical College. Daigakumachi, Takatsuki-shi, Osaka-fu 569

Kainsai Medical College. Fumizono-cho, Moriguchi-shi, Osaka-fu 570. Head: Prof. Tsukahara Isamu

Faculty of Medicine, Kyoto University. Shogoin, Sakyo-ky, Kyoto-shi 606. Head: Prof. Kishimoto Masao

Kyoto Prefectural University of Medicine, Kawaramachi, Kamigyo-ku, Kyoto-shi 602. Head: Prof. Tani Michiyuki

Wakayama Medical College. 7-Bancho, Wakayama-shi 640. Head: Prof. Iimura Iawao
Hyogo College of Medicine. Mukogawa-cho, Nishinomuya-shi 663. Head: Prof. Imachi Jo
Nara Medical College. Shijo, Kashihara-shi, Nara 634. Head: Prof. Nakao Shuitsu
Nara Medical College, Nara Hospital. Nijo, Nara-shi 630
School of Medicine, Kobe University. Kusunoki-cho, Ikuta-ku, Kobe 650. Head: Prof. Isayama Yoshimasa
Okayama University Medical School. Shikada-cho, Okayama-shi 700. Head: Prof. Okuda Kanshi
Kawasaki Medical College. Nakayamashita, Okayama-shi 700. Head: Prof. Yamamoto Kakuji
School of Medicine, Tottori University. Nishimachi, Yonago-shi 683. Head: Prof. Fujinaga Yutaka
Hiroshima University School of Medicine. Kasumi-cho, Hiroshima-shi 734. Head: Prof. Dodo Tsugio
Yamaguchi Medical College. Nishi-ku, Ube-shi, Yamaguchi 755. Head: Prof. Kobayashi Shunsaku
School of Medicine, Tokushima University. Kuramotomachi, Tokushima-shi 770. Head: Prof. Mitsui Yukihiko
Kurume University School of Medicine. Asahimachi, Kurume-shi 830. Head: Prof. Yoshioka Hisahura
Faculty of Medicine, Kyushu University. Katakasu, Higashi-ku, Fukuoka-shi 812. Head: Prof. Ikui Hiroshi
Fukuoka University School of Medicine. Nishi-ku, Fukuoki-shi 814. Head: Prof. Masuda Yoshiya
Nagasaki University School of Medicine. Sakamotomachi, Nagasaki-shi 852. Head: prof. Takalu Isao
Kumamoto University Medical School. Honjomachi, Jumamoto-shi 860. Head: Prof. Tsutsui Jun
Faculty of Medicine, University of Kagoshima. Shiroyama-cho, Kagoshima-shi 892. Head: Prof. Taniguchi Yoshiaki
School of Health, Ryukyu University. Naha-shi, Okinawa 902. Head: Prof. Kiribuchi Mitsunori

INSTITUTA SCHOLAEQUE CAECIS DESTINATAE

National   Inmates
School for the Blind attached to Faculty of Education, Tokyo University of Education.
27-6, 3-chome, Mejirodai, Bunkyo-ku, Tokyo 112 282

Prefectural
Hokkaido Hakodate School for the Blind. 19-12, Tayamachi, Hakodate-shi 040 78
Hokkaido Otaru School for the Blind. 28-38, 4-chome, Iribune-cho, Otaru-shi 047 20
Hokkaido Asahikawa School for the Blind. 15-chome, 2-jo, Asahimachi, Asahikawa-shi 070 . 114
Hokkaido Obihiro School for the Blind. Minami-1-chome, Nishi, 24-jo, Obihiro-shi 080 ... 68
Hokkaido Sapporo School for the Blind. 1891, Motomachi, Chuo-ku, Sapporo-shi 060 271
Aomori Prefectural Hachinohe School for the Blind. 33-5, Aza-Genchuji, Oaza-Ruike, Hachinohe-shi 031 23
Aomori Prefectural Aomori School for the Blind. 24-1, Aza-Asai, Oaza-Yadamae, Aomori-shi 039-35 76
Iwate Prefectural School for the Blind. 10-1, 1-chome, Kitayama, Morioka-shi 020 182
Miyagi Prefectural School for the Blind. 5-1, 6-chome, Uesugi, Sendai-shi 980 153
Akita Prefectural School for the Blind. 2-72, 3-chome, Minami, Tsuchizaki-minato, Akita-shi 010 90
Yamagata Prefectural Yamagata School for the Blind. 1111, Aza-Kanegamine, Oaza-Kaneya, Kaminoyama-shi 999-31 211
Yamagata Prefectural Tsuruoka School for the Blind. 20-33, Inao-cho, Tsuruoka-shi 997 .. 91
Fukushima Prefectural Fukushima School for the Blind. 6-34, Moriai-machi, Fukushima-shi 960 99
Fukushima Prefectural Taira School for the Blind. 61, Aza-Umamezaki, Taira-Umame, Iwaki-shi 970-01 22

Shimane Prefectural School for the Blind. 468, Nishihamasada-cho, Matsue-shi 690-01   118
Okayama Prefectural Okayama School for the Blind. 799, Osunaba, Haraojima, Okayama-
shi 700   171
Hiroshima Prefectural School for the Blind. 2-1, 2-chome, Ushida-shinmachi, Hiroshima-shi
730   194
Yamaguchi Prefectural School for the Blind. 1, Higashi Otsubo-machi, Shimonoseki-shi 750.   144
Tokushima Prefectural School for the Blind. 1134, Mugizuka, Minami Nikenya-cho,
Tokushima-shi 770   183
Kagawa Prefectural School for the Blind. 9-12, 2-chome, Ogimachi, Takamatsu-shi 760   93
Ehime Prefectural Matsuyama School for the Blind. 112, Kumanodai, Matsuyama-shi 790 .   157
Kochi Prefectural School for the Blind. 90, Daizen-cho, Kochi-shi 780   116
Fukuoka Prefectural Yanagawa School for the Blind. 170, Imakoga, Mitsubashi-machi,
Mikado-gun, Fukuoka 832   121
Fukuoka Prefectural Fukuoka School for the Blind. No. 40, 14-Gai-ku, 2-chome, Shirogane,
Fukuoka-shi 810   171
Fukuoka Prefectural Kitakyushu School for the Blind. 7-jo, Yahata-ku, Kitakyushu-shi 805 . 150
Saga Prefectural School for the Blind. 8-5, 1-chome, Tenyu, Saga-shi 840   130
Nagasaki Prefectural School for the Blind. 10-47, Hashiguchi-cho, Nagasaki-shi 852   194
Kumamoto Prefectural School for the Blind. 3-7, Higashi-cho, Kumamoto-shi 862   217
Oita Prefectural School for the Blind. 1-75, 3-chome, Kaneike-cho, Oita-shi 870   153
Miyazaki Prefectural School for the Blind. 1390, Oaza-Shimanouchi, Miyazaki-shi 880-0 ...   137
Kagoshima Prefectural Kagoshima School for the Blind. 80, Shimoishiki, Kagoshima-shi 890   186
Okinawa Prefectural School for the Blind. 3-296, Sekirei-cho, Shuri, Naha-shi, Okinawa 903   107

Municipal
Yokohama Municipal School for the Blind. 26, 1-chome, Matsumi-cho, Kanagawa-ku,
Yokohama-shi 211   140
Osaka Municipal School for the Blind. 619, Toyozato-machi, Higashi-Yodogawa-ku, Osaka-
shi 533   235
Kobe Municipal School for the Blind. 4-1, Daikaidori, Hyogo-ku, Kobe-shi 652   122

Private
Kumagaya School for the Blind. 390, Hakoda, Kumagaya-shi, Saitama 360   26
Yokohama Kunmo Gakuin. 181, Takenomaru-cho, Naka-ku, Yokohama-shi 232   48

Branch School (Prefectural)
Maizuru Branch of Kyoto Prefectural School for the Blind. 83, Shimo-Ouchi-machi, Minami-
Tanabe, Maizuru-shi 624   9

Rehabilitation centers for visually handicapped

National
Inmates

Hakodate Rehabilitation Center for Visually Handicapped. 1-35, Yunokawa-cho, Hakodate-
shi 042   210
Shiobara Rehabilitation Center for Visually Handicapped. 21, Shimo-Fukuhara, Shiobara-
cho, Shioya-gun, Tochigi-ken 329-29   210
Tokyo Rehabilitation Center for Visually Handicapped. 2-34-18, Umezato, Suginami-ku,
Tokyo 166   300
Kobe Rehabilitation Center for Visually Handicapped. Yoshida, Tamatsu-machi, Tarumi-ku,
Kobe-shi 673   210
Fukuoka Rehabilitation Center for Visually Handicapped. 4820, Aza-Nagahama, Imazu,
Fukuoka-shi 819-01   210

Prefectural

Private

JUGO-SLAVIA

SOCIETATES OPHTHALMOLOGICAE

Nationalis

Udreženje oftalmologa Jugoslavije (Association Yugoslave d'Ophtalmologie)
Address: Očesna klinika, Zološka 2, 61000 Ljubljana
President: Prof. Dereani Carmen
Secretary: Dr. Kavčič Silvo
Treasurer: Dr. Videnšek Jože

The bureau consists of the following members:
First Vice-President: Prof. Miovski Dimitrije, Očesna klinika, 91000 Skopje
Second Vice-President: Prof. Dr. Postić Diode, Očesna klinika, 21000 Novi Sad
Dr. Sekolec Jože, Očesni oddelek, 62000 Maribor
Prof. Dr. Ferić, Seifert Feodora, Očesna klinika, 41000 Zagreb
Prof. Dr. Gligo Davor, Očesna klinika, 51000 Rijeka
Prof. Dr. Mastilović Borislava, Očesna klinika, 71000 Sarajevo
Dr. Parunović Aleksander, Očna klinika, 11000 Beograd
Dr. Budeć Ljubinko, Očno odelenje, 81000 Titograd
Dr. Kotevski Dimitar, Očno odelenje, 97000 Bitola
Dr. Hadžija Camil, Očno odelenje, 38000 Priština

Regionales

Oftalmološka sekcija Slovenije

President: Prof. Dr. Stergar Stane
Secretary: As. Dr. Kolar Gorazd, Zaloška 2, 61000 Ljubljana
Number of members: 54

Oftalmološka sekcija Hrvatske

President: Prof. Dr. Ljuština Nevenka
Secretary: Dr. Peić Mirko, Šubicava 29, 41000 Zagreb
Number of members: 115

Oftalmološka sekcija Srbije

President: Prof. Dr. Litričin Olga
Secretary: Dr. Popović, Očna klinika, 11000 Beograd
Number of members: 246

Oftalmološka sekcija Črne Gore

President: Dr. Budeć Ljubinko
Secretary: Dr. Jovović Miodrag, Očno Odelenje, 81000 Titograd
Number of members: 9

Oftalmološka sekcija Bosne i Hercegovine

President: Prof. Dr. Čavka Vladimir
Secretary: Prof. Dr. Bijedić Marjana, Očna klinika, 71000 Sarajevo
Number of members: 56

Oftalmološka sekcija Makedonije

President: Prof. Dr. Miovski Dimitar
Address: Očna klinika, 91000 Skopje
Number of members: 31

Oftalmološka sekcija Kosmet i Metohija

President: Prim. Dr. Hadžija Čamil
Address: Očno odelenje, 38000 Priština

NOMINA ET DOMICILIA MEDICORUM AB OCULIS

BOSNE I HERCEGOVINE

Adžović, Suada	Dom zdravlja	Novo Sarajevo
Akajbegović, Rizo	Gorica 37	Sarajevo
Alirejsović, Sehija	Djure Salaja 13	Sarajevo
Avdić, Tatjana		Tuzla
Bijedić, Mirjana	Maršala Tita 13/II	Sarajevo
Bilenjki, Vladimira	Nemanjina 39	Sarajevo
Blažanović, Ivo	Očna klinika	Sarajevo
Čavka, Prof. Vladimir	Očna klinika	Sarajevo
Ćupić, Slobodan	Rave Jankovića 31	Sarajevo
Ćurković, Erzamo	Zagrebačka 13	Sarajevo
Ćustović, Hasan	Dom zdravlja	Mostar
Defterdarević, Tehvida	Gor. Hajduk Veljka 4	Sarajevo
Djurović, Mileva	Marjana Baruna 1	Sarajevo
Godler, Boris	Očna klinika	Sarajevo
Godler, Zdenka	Očna klinika	Sarajevo
Gorobinski, Miroslav	Očna klinika	Sarajevo
Hadžiselimović, Nina	Augusta Cesarca 4	Sarajevo
Hlubna, Dragutin	Dom zdravlja	Mostar
Hodžić, Meho	Dom zdravlja Sarajevo, Vrazova 5	Sarajevo
Hodžić, Sabahudín	Sava Jankovića 31	Sarajevo
Janev, Kosta	Rave Jankovića 24	Sarajevo
Jovicević, Boško	Očno odelenje bolnice	Banja Luka
Kadijević, Vera	Očni odjel bolnice	Mostar
Kočović, Ljubica	Takovska 12	Sarajevo
Kojović, Vladimir	Nemanjina 23	Sarajevo
Kovačević, Slavica	Omladinsko šetalište 2	Sarajevo
Krajačić, Radmila	Očna klinika	Sarajevo
Kuštrić, Smail	Očni odjel bolnice	Banja Luka
Mastilović, Borislava	Stjepana Tomića 25	Sarajevo
Mičičević, Miroslava	Škerličeva 20	Sarajevo
Milanović-Ajhberger, Ljiljana	Save Jankovića 24	Sarajevo
Milošević, Gordana	Vuka Karadžića 131	Sarajevo

Milutinović, Zagorka	Jovana Cvijića 7	Sarajevo
Momčinović, Adela	Dom zdravlja Centar, Vrazova 5 .	Sarajevo
Novaković, Aleksandar	Skerličeva 15	Sarajevo
Perazić, Vera	Dom zdravlja	Novo Sarajevo
Pištèljić, Aleksander	Očno odelenje bolnice	Banja Luka
Plavšić, Vasilija	Vulka Karadžića 143	Sarajevo
Radosavljević, Petko	Nemanjina 57	Sarajevo
Resulbegović, Meliha	Dom zdravlja	Tuzla
Rosić, Ana	Dom zdravilja	Tuzla
Stolić, Vladimir	Rave Jankovića 24	Sarajevo
Sabolovljev, Zora	Dom zdravlja željezničara	Sarajevo
Savović, Ananije	Dom zdravlja Centar, Vrazova 5 .	Sarajevo
Sefić, Mustafa	Očni odjel bolnice	Banja Luka
Sladojević, Slobodan	Očno odelenje bolnice	Zenica
Smiljanić, Borislav	Očni odjel bolnice	Banja Luka
Sredanović, Ksenija	Očna klinika	Sarajevo
Stanek-Tankosić, Katarina	Očni odjel bolnice	Bilhać
Stanić, Rikard		Banja Luka
Stanković, Dragan	Očna klinika	Sarajevo
Šahović, Kanita	Dom zdravlja	Tuzla
Šehovac, Nada	Dom zdravlja Centar	Sarajevo
Šteinberger, Fridrich	Dom zdravlja Centar, Vrazova 5 .	Sarajevo
Vujica, Josip	Očna klinika	Sarajevo
Vujošević, Emira	Hajduk Veljka 2	Sarajevo

MAKEDONIJE

Aceski, Kiril	Medicinski centar očno odelenje .	Prilep
Babunski, Lazar	Medicinski centar	Titov Veles
Bužanovski, Zage	Očna klinika	Skopje
Čakar, Stefan	Očna klinika	Skopje
Delivanova, Stojka	Institut za medicina pri Rudnici i železarnica	Skopje
Dimitrova, Julijana	Vojna bolnica, očno odelenje ...	Skopje
Dučovski, Mitko	Opšta bolnica očno odelenje	Bitola
Georgievski, Dragi	Med. centar, očno odelenje	Kumanovo
Golev, Risto	Medicinski centar	Ohrid
Ivanov, Jovan	Očna klinika	Skopje
Janeva, Savica	Očna klinika	Skopje
Jovanovska, Elefterija	Medicinski centar	Struga
Kikerkov, Spase	Zdravstveni dom 'Skopje', Poliklinika 'Bukurešt'	Skopje
Konjanovski, Dragi	Opšta bolnica, očno odelenje ...	Bitola
Kotevski, Dimitar	Opšta bolnica, očno odelenje ...	Bitola
Krstevska, Ljupka	Očna klinika	Skopje
Malinov, Ilija	Medicinski centar, očno odelenje .	Strumica
Manajlovski, Krume	Medicinski centar, očno odelenje .	Tetovo
Milanov, Mile	Zdravstveni dom	Skopje
Miovski, Dimitar	Očna klinika	Skopje
Netkovski, Aleksandar	Vojna bolnica, očno odelenje ...	Skopje
Nošpal, Vladimir	Očna ambulanta pri ŽTP	Skopje
Ognjanova, Olga	Ambulanta pri DSVR	Skopje
Popovski, Trajko	Očna klinika	Skopje
Ristevski, Aleksandar	Medicinski centar, očno odelenje .	Prilep
Stojčevska, Vera	Očna klinika	Skopje
Stojčevski, Dimitar	Očna klinika	Skopje
Vasić, Dušan	Opšta bolnica, očno odelenje ...	Pirot

Veninova, Blagorodna	Vojna bolnica, očno odelenje ...	Skopje
Vesov, Ilija	Zdravstveni dom 'Skopje'	Skopje
Zeškova, Dominka	Zdravstveni dom 'Skopje', Poliklinika 'Bukurešt'	Skopje

KOSOVO

Čalil, Hadžija	Očno odelenje Gradske bolnice ..	Priština
Jovanović, Danica	Medicinski centar, očno odelenje .	Kosovska Mitrovica
Kalundžić, Aleksandar	Opšta bolnica, očno odelenje ...	Priština
Novaković, Miodrag	Medicinski centar, očno odelenje .	Kosovska Mitrovica
Orlić, Miodrag	Medicinski centar, očno odelenje .	Kosovska Mitrovica

SRBIJE

Batak, Emil	K. A. Petra Drapšina 21	Novi Sad
Bimoski, Nevenka	Dom zdravlja, Školska služba ...	Novi Sad
Božić, Branko	Vojna bolnica, Očno odelenje, Petrovaradin	Novi Sad
Brkić, Velimir	Opšta bolnica, Očno odelenje ...	Smederevska Palanka
Bukovala, Aleksandar	Opšta bolnica, Očno odelenje ...	Kraljevo
Crnijački, Milena	Pokrajinska bolnica, očno odelenje	Novi Sad
Cvetanović, Kosana	Opšta bolnica, ocno odelenje ...	Kragujevac
Cvetkov, Zoran	K. A. Cara Dušana 28	Zrenjanin
Cvetković, Jova	Vojvode Mišića 6	Niš
Cvetković, Milivoje	Rentgenova 9/a	Niš
Čupić, Rajko	Opšta bolnica, očno odelenje ...	T. Užice
Dabović, Branislav	Opšta bolnica, očno odelenje ...	Čačak
Dakić, Vojislav	Medic. centar, očno odelenje K. A. Djure Jakšića 1	Vršac
Dejanović-Djordjević Radmila	Opšta bolnica, očno odelenje ...	Kikinda
Djordjević, Ljubinko	Medic. centar, očno odelenje ...	Prokuplje
Dobošarević, Vladislav	Opšta bolnica, očno odelenje ...	Požarevac
Filimonović, Dragica	Opšta bolnica, očno odelenje ...	Zaječar
Ilić, Zoran	Pokrajinska bolnica, očno odelenje	Novi Sad
Ivković, Petar	Opšta bolnica, očno odelenje, K.A. Brače Taskovića 9	
Jakovljević, Milivoje	Medic. centar, očno odelenja ...	Cupriya
Jeličić, Sibin	Medic. centar, očno odelenje ...	Arandjelovac
Jerinić, Ljubomir	K. A., Daničićeva 16	Valjevo
Jonić, Ivo	K. A., Željezničak 4	Novi Sad
Josifov, Dobri	K. A., Lole Ribara 29	Sremska Mitrovica
Jovanović, Dušan	Sremska 13/9	Niš
Jovanović, Ljubica	Centar za majku i dete	Niš
Kapamadžija, Zarko	K. A., Zmaj Jovina 22	Novi Sad
Kapor, Milan	Zdravstveni centar, K.A., Trg M. Tita 3	Senta
Knežev-Jelić, Dobrinka	Medicinski centar 'Dr. Mihajlo Ilić', Oftalmoloska sluzba ...	Kragujevac
Kojić, Dragutin	Opšta bolnica, očno odelenje ...	Srem. Mitrovica
Kovačević, Tomislav	K.A., Karnedžijeva 103	Valjevo
Krstić, Radmila	Opšta bolnica, očno odelenje ...	Niš
Kupusarević, Slobodan	Opšta bolnica, očno odelenje ...	Sombor
Kutešić, Milorad	Vojna bolnica	Niš
Mačkatović, Duža	Opšta bolnica, očno odelenje ...	Subotica
Mandić, Dobrila	Opšta bolnica, očno odelenje ...	Pančevo
Mandić, Ljubiša	K.A., Knez Iveo od Semberije ...	Šabac

Manić, Miloš	Opšta bolnica, očno odelenje ...	Leskovac
Manić, Vojislav	Opšta bolnica, očno odelenje ...	Pančevo
Mašić, Vera	Opšta bolnica, očno odelenje ...	Kruševac
Mejedović, Smiljana	Očno odelenje bolnice	Užička Požega
Mešterović, Dušan	Opšta bolnica, očno odelenje ...	Sombor
Mičović, Vidak	Opšta bolnica, očno odelenje ...	Bor
Mihajlović, Branislav	Medicinski centar 'Dr. Mihajlo Ilić', Očno odelenje	Kragujevac
Milojković, Božidar	K.A., Despota Djurdja	Smederevo
Misajlović, Radojko	Opšta bolnica, očno odelenje ...	T. Užice
Mojsilović, Milenko	Opšta bolnica, očno odelenje ...	Kraljevo
Mortvanski, Dragutin	K.A., M. Stanivukovića 75	Zrenjanin
Nauparac, Blagoje	Medic. centar, očno odelenje ...	Kraljevo
Obrenović, Milojka	Opšta bolnica, očno odelenje ...	T. Užice
Panić, Ivanka	Opšta bolnica, očno odelenje ...	Požarevac
Pantić, Milanka	Opšta bolnica, očno odelenje ...	Kragujevac
Pataj, Aranka	Pokrajinska bolnica, očno odelenje	Novi Sad
Paunović, Dobrivoje	K.A., I. Proleterska 16	Zrenjanin
Paunović, Dušica	Opšta bolnica, očno odelenje ...	Zaječar
Pavlović, Nada	Opšta bolnica, očno odelenje ...	Pančevo
Perović, Bojko	Klinička bolnica, očno odelenje .	Niš
Perović, Miloš	Dom zdravlja željezničara	Niš
Pešić, Milivoje	Opšta bolnica, očno odelenje ...	Vranje
Petrović, Jordan	Opšta bolnica, očno odelenje ...	Niš
Petrović-Stevanović, Angelina	Opšta bolnica, os,cno odelenje ..	Valjevo
Popović, Jova	K.A., Brače Jugović 10	Zrenjanin
Popović, Predrag	Medic. centar, Očno odelenje ...	Svetozarevo
Poštić, Djordje	K.A., Željeznička 4	Novi Sad
Pušin, Stanko	Opšta bolnica, očno odelenje ...	Subotica
Radosavljević, Miloš	Opšta bolnica, očno odelenje ...	Čačak
Robert Mak, Klur	Opšta bolnica 'Dr. Voja Dulić', očno odelenje	Požarevac
Savić, Prof. Dušan	Higijenski zavod	Novi Sad
Simić, Hermina	Pokrajinska bolnica, očno odelenje	Novi Sad
Smiljković, Vlastimir	Klinička bolnica, očno odelenje .	Niš
Srajber, Zoltan	Opšta bolnica, očno odelenje ...	Subotica
Stankov-Tomić, Miroslava ..	K.A., Milana Petrovića 9/a	Novi Sad
Stefanović, Branka	Opšta bolnica, očno odelenje ...	Pančevo
Stefanović, Budimir	Psihiatrijska bolnica Topolnica ..	Niš
Stojanović-Balać, Mileva ..	K.A., Ruže Šulman 12/II ulaz I .	Zrenjanin
Tomašević, Milovan	Ul. Pobede 124/II ulaz	Niš
Trajković, Djordje	Vojna bolnica, očno odelenje ...	Niš
Turajlić, Miroslava	Medic. centar, očno odelenje ...	Čuprija
Tvrtković, Marin	K.A., Fruškogorska kula 56/II ..	Novi Sad
Vasović, Mihajlo	Opšta bolnica, očno odelenje ...	Šabac
Veselinović, Božidar	Zdravstveni dom željezničara ...	Niš
Zdravkovíx, Božidar	Zdravstveni dom željezničara ...	Niš
Zdravnković, Milan	K.A., Voždova 2	Niš
Zlatković, Živojin	Medic. centar, očno odelenje ...	Smederevo
Zrlić, Jovanka	K.A., Papa Pavla 2/III	Novi Sad
Zivković, Vojislav	Opšta bolnica, očno odelenje ...	Kragujevac

BEOGRAD

Baronija, Josip	Očna ambulanta Doma narodnog zdravlja 'Vračar', Proleterskih brigada br. 57	Beograd
Biga, Sofija	Očno odjelenje Gradske bolnice .	Beograd
Blagojević, Prof. Milan	Očno klinika, Džordža Vašingtona 19	Beograd
Bulić, Nikša	Majke Jevrosime 42, penzioner ..	Beograd
Cvetković, Dobrosav	Očna klinika, Džordža Vašingtona 19	Beograd
Čobeljić, Mirjana	Očna klinika, Višegradska 22 ...	Beograd
Čoratonović, Milorad	Zeleni Venac 4/III – penzioner .	Beograd
Damjanović, Vera	Dom nar. zdravlja 'Stari Grad' Očna ambulanta, Simina 27 ..	Beograd
Danić, Milovan	Makedonska 11 – penzioner	Beograd
Danilović, Jovan	Dom nar. zdravlja 'Stari Grad' Očna ambulanta, Simina 27 ..	Beograd
Dergenc, Slobodan	Očno odelenje Gradske bolnice ..	Beograd
Dimitrijević, Vojislav	VII Dom nar. zdravlja 'Dr. Sima Milošević' Očna ambulanta, Požeška 82	Beograd
Dobrojević, Dragutin	Ivana Milutinovića 48	Beograd
Dobrović, Dušan	Dom zdravlja	Novi Beograd
Dodić, Vera	Očna klinika, Džordža Vašingtona 19	Beograd
Dučić-Petrović, Milenija ...	Očna klinika, Džordža Vašingtona 19	Beograd
Djaković, Siniša	Očna klinika, Višegradska 22 ...	Beograd
Djurić, Angelina	VI Dom narodnog zdravlja Očna ambulanta, Krivolačka 4–6 ..	Beograd
Grbić, Ruža	Dom narodnog zdravlja 'Stari Grad', Očna ambulanta, Simina 27	Beograd
Ilić, Ružica	Očna klinika, Višegradska 22 ...	Beograd
Jagličić, Dragoslava	Očna klinika, Džordža Vašingtona 19	Beograd
Jelenković, Olga	Zemun Očna ambulanta, Gradska bolnica	Beograd
Joksimović, Ljiljana	Očna klinika, Džordža Vašingtona 19	Beograd
Jovanović, Aleksandar	Očna ambulanta, Dom narodnog zdravlja 'Stari Grad', Simina 27	Beograd
Jovanović, Slavoljub	Očna klinika, Višegradska 22 ...	Beograd
Jovčić, Olivera	Očna klinika, Džordža Vašingtona 19	Beograd
Kecmanović, Zlatimir	Gradska bolnica Očno odjelenje .	Beograd
Klisić, Leposava	Centralna specijalistička poliklinika Nemanjina ul.	Beograd
Kodžić, Jelena	Očna klinika, Dž. Vašingtona 19 .	Beograd
Kopša, Prof. Milan	Očna klinika VMA	Beograd
Kostić, Damjan	Centralna specijalistička poliklinika, Nemanjina ul.	Beograd
Kujačić, Bogdan	Očna klinika VMA, Pasterova 2 ..	Beograd
Litričin, Prof. Olga	Očna klinika, Višegradska 22 ...	Beograd
Livada, Vojislav	Očna klinika VMA, Pasterova 2 .	Beograd

Lozanić, Vojislav	Očna klinika, Dž. Vašingtona 19 .	Beograd
Luković, Božana	Esad Pašina 5	Beograd
Ljubovijević, Vera	Gradska bolnica Očno odelenje ..	Beograd
Mandić, Dragoje	Gradska bolnica, Očno odjelenje .	Beograd
Marušić, Kazimir	Očna klinka VMA, Pasterova 2 ..	Beograd
Milenković, Milivoje	Svetozara Markovića 2	Beograd
Milošević, Božidar	Hadži Djeriha 3 – penzioner	Beograd
Milošević, Vlada	Carli Ćaplina 10	Beograd
Nikolić, Anča	Očna klinika VMA, Pasterova 2 .	Beograd
Nikolić, Vlada	Hadži Milentijeva 23 – pensioner	Beograd
Novaković, Aleksandar	Nebojšina 14 – penzioner	Beograd
Pavičić, Jovan	Gradska bolnica Očno odelenje ..	Beograd
Pavković-Bugarski, Djordje .	Baba Višnjina 33	Beograd
Parunović, Aleksandar	Očna klinika, Višegradska 22 ...	Beograd
Petrović, Miodrag	Mirka Tomića 3	Beograd
Petrović, Radmila	Očna klinika, Višegradska 22 ...	Beograd
Petrović, Zoran	Očna klinika VMA, Pasterova 2 .	Beograd
Pišteljić, Dušan	Neuropsihijatrijska klinika Med. fakulteta, Višegradska 26 ...	Beograd
Popović, Dragiša	Očna klinika VMA, Pasterova 2 .	Beograd
Purković, Julijana	Očna ambulanta, Dom nar. zdravlja 'Vračar', Proleterskih brigada 57	Beograd
Savin, Ljiljana	III Dom narodnog zdravlja 'Boris Kidrič', Pasterova 1	Beograd
Savić, Slobodan	Institut za medicinu rada	Beograd
Savičević, Milograd	Očna klinika VMA, Pasterova 2 .	Beograd
Stanković, Prof. Ivan	Očna odjelenje Gradske bolnice .	Beograd
Stanković, Prof. Miodrag ..	Kosovska 35 – penzioner	Beograd
Steković, Predrag	VI Dom nar. zdravlja	Beograd
Stojanović, Branislav	Baltazara Bogišića 6	Beograd
Stojanović, Dušan	Očna klinika, Dž. Vašingtona 19 .	Beograd
Skondrić, Magdalena	III Dom nar. zdravlja Očna ambulanta 'Boris Kidrič', Pasterova 2	Beograd
Rajčević, Nebojša	Lole Ribara 49	Beograd
Stanisavljević, Mirjana	Očna ambulanta doma narodnog zdravlja, Kej oslobodjenja 29 .	Zemun
Stefanović, Sida	Sonje Marinkovića 4	Zemum
Rašković-Mijatović, Mirjana .	Bulevar revolucije 43/V	Beograd
Tomić, Nedelijka	Očna klinika, Višegradska 22 ...	Beograd
Tomić, Petar	Očna klinika, Dž. Vašingtona 19 .	Beograd
Velimirović, Mirjana	IV Dom narodnog zdravlja, Sredečka 2	Beograd
Veselinović, Živko	Dušanova 60	Beograd
Vukov, Borislav	II Dom narodnog zdravlja, Vojvode Vuka 10	Beograd
Zec, Bosiljka	Dom narodnog zdravlja 'Stari grad' Očna ambulanta, Simina 27	Beograd
Žanko, Ljerka	Očna odjelenje Gradske bolnice .	Beograd
Žugić, Olga	Poliklinika sekretarijata unutrašnjih poslova, Durmitorska 9	Beograd

576 JUGO-SLAVIA

HRVATSKE

Antolović, Marko	Očni odjel Opće bolnice	Osijek
Bacelj, Katica	Očni odjel Med. centra	Dubrovnik
Berak, Ksenija	Očna ambulanta Med. centar	Vinkovci
Biščan, Božidar	Očna ambulanta Med. centar	Bjelovar
Borčic, Božena	Krašova 12	Zagreb
Breitenfeld, Mira	Očna ambulanta DNZ Trnje, Kruge 44	Zagreb
Bublik, Marija	Očni odjel Opće bolnice	Osijek
Bujanić-Cuculić, Suzana	Očna klinika 'Boln. Braća Sabol' .	Rijeka
Car, Daina	Martićeva 21	Zagreb
Cvetnić, Bosiljka	Dom zdravlja željezničara, Grgureva 3	Zagreb
Ćelić, Marija	Braće Oreški 35	Zagreb
Čoti-Maurin Mira	Nova cesta 105	Zagreb
Čupak, Prof. Krešimir	Bulićeva 12	Zagreb
Devčić, Marija	Opća bolnica Gospić	Zagreb
Dobrić, Miroslav	Pavletićeva 16	Zagreb
Dokozić, Ivan	Boln. 'dr. Kajfeš', Pavleka Miškine	Zagreb
Domac, Blaženka	Nodilova 11	Zagreb
Džodžo-Kukoć, Radmila	Školska poliklinika	Split
Durić, Smilja	Očna klinika 'Boln. Braća Sabol' .	Rijeka
Feric, Prof. Feodora	Palmotićeva 18	Zagreb
Fulgozi Ante	Marinkovićeva 5	Zagreb
Gligo, Prof. Davor	Očna klinika 'Boln. Braća Sabol' .	Rijeka
Grgas-Bego, Mate	Očni odjel Opće bolnice	Šibenik
Grzunov, Eduard	Očni odjel Opće bolnice	Split
Hegeduš, Ivan	Očno odelenje Vojne bolnice JRM	Split
Henč, Ljerka	Bolnica 'dr. Kajfeš', Pavleka Miškine	Zagreb
Hofer, Želimir	Očna klinika 'Boln. Braća Sabol' .	Rijeke
Horvat, Stjepan	Očna klinika Rebro	Zagreb
Hrabar, Dalma	Domagojeva 21	Zagreb
Jug, Ivan	Zlatarska 9	Zagreb
Juretić, Silvije	Očni odjel Opće bolnice	Karlovac
Jurković, Sonja	Jakićeva b.b.	Zagreb
Jutruša-Koržinek, Blanka	Vlaška 92	Zagreb
Kalebić-Guglielmi, Mejra	Nazorova 2	Zagreb
Kargačin, Ante	Proleterskih brigad 43	Zagreb
Kovačević, Franc	Očna klinika 'Boln. Braća Sabol' .	Rijeka
Kovačević, Slavka	Očno odelenje Vojna bolnice, Vočarska	Zagreb
Kozulić, Blaženka	Očno klinika 'Boln. Braća Sabol' .	Rijeka
Krsnik, Mirko	Proleterskih brigad 235	Zagreb
Krstinić, Ivica	Očni odjel Opće bolnice	Split
Krstulović, Sonja	Očni odjel Opće bolnice	Split
Kušić, Vjekoslav	Martićeva 14	Zagreb
Laktić, Nikola	Gundulićeva 52	Zagreb
Lazić, Stojan	Očni odjel Opće bolnice	Split
Ledić, Ivo	Slovenska 4	Zagreb
Ljubibratić, Dora	Socijalističke revolucije 6	Zagreb
Ljuština-Ivančić, Prof. Nevenka	Novakova 9	Zagreb
Lukačić-Očak, Ruža	Vinkovićeva 25	Zagreb
Lutenberger, Igor	Očna klinika 'Boln. Braće Sabol' .	Rijeka
Maixner, Ivo	Gundulićeva 14	Zagreb

Mesarić, Branko	Boln. 'dr. Kajfeš', Pavleka Miškine	Zagreb
Mezulic, Čedo	Očni odjel Opće bolnice	Pula
Mihok, Inga	Dom zdravlja SUP, Šarengradska ul.	Zagreb
Mladinec, Margita	Očni odjel Opće bolnice	Osijek
Nadenčic, Lucija	Opća bolnica Med. centra	Pula
Nola, Borislava	Radnički dol 24	Zagreb
Ognjanovski, Olga	Očni odjel Opće bolnice	Zadar
Ozretić, Miljenko	Očni odjel Opće bolnice	Split
Padovan, Smilja	Vramčeva 13	Zagreb
Pajalić, Alenka	Amruševa 19	Zagreb
Panac, Vinko	Martićeva 35	Zagreb
Panian, Zdravko	Martićeva 19	Zagreb
Parfenjuk, Stjepan	Amruševa 5	Zagreb
Pavičić, Ankica	Očni odjel Opće bolnice	Karlovac
Pavišić, Prof. Zvonimir	Nazorova 13	Zagreb
Pavlović, Matilda	Očna klinika 'Boln. Braća Sabol' .	Rijeka
Peić, Milko	Mažuranićev trg 9	Zagreb
Petković, Vlado	Moše Pijade 168	Zagreb
Pinković, Marcela	Očna klinika Rebro	Zagreb
Polak-Poljak, Marija	Očna klinika	Zagreb
Posednik, Rikard	Očni odjel Opće bolnice	Pakrac
Prevedan, Franjo	Očni odjel Med. centra	Varaždin
Radončić, M. Rijeka	Očna klinika 'Boln. Braća Sabol' .	Rijeka
Raguš, Ivo	Crnčićeva 9	Zagreb
Rahelić, Vera	Očna klinika 'Boln. Braća Sabol' .	Rijeka
Raić, Nikola	Očna klinika Rebro	Zagreb
Rukavina, Olga	Očni odjel Med. centra	Varaždin
Sasso, Bogomir	Očni odjel Opće bolnice	Šibenik
Sebastijan, Mladen	Dom zdravlja željezničara	Zagreb
Sklepić, Ivan	Očna ambulanta Med. centra	Čakovec
Smrkinić, Bogoslav	Očni odjel Opće bolnice	Zadar
Sokolić, Prof. Petar	Petrova 138	Zagreb
Spevec, Jelka	Habdelićeva 2	Zagreb
Stojanović, Mato	Zavod za zaštitu zdravlja, Mirogojska 16	Zagreb
Sušić, Miro	Očni odjel Vojne bolnice JRM ..	Pula
Sviben, Marija	Očna klinika 'Boln. Braća Sabol' .	Rijeka
Szekler, Robert	Haulikova 1	Zagreb
Šakić, Prof. Dinko	Očni odjel Opće bolnice	Split
Šerman, Biserka	Očna klinika 'Boln. Braća Sabol' .	Rijeka
Šestić, Augusta	Trg M. Oreškovića 23	Zagreb
Šivački, Neda	Očni odjel Opće bolnice	Virovitica
Šoša, Tomislav	Očni odjel Med. centra	Dubrovnik
Špoljar, Ivan	Očni odjel Opće bolnice	Osijek
Šrenger, Željko	Bogovićeva 9	Zagreb
Štambuk, Vjera	Očni odjel Opće bolnice	Split
Štriga, Miladin	Jurišećeva 26	Zagreb
Šupe, Katica	Očni odjel Med. centra	Dubrovnik
Švalba, Velinka	Šetalište XIII, Divizije 58	Rijeka
Tiljak, Oto	Očna ambulanta DNZ	Osijek
Trajer, Dragan	Lašćinska 4	Zagreb
Trčak-Ocvirek, Vera	Očni odjel Opće bolnice	Osijek
Trogrlić, Kazimir	Vinkovićeva 16	Zagreb
Turčić, M.	Očni odjel Vojne bolnice JRM ..	Pula
Vedlin, Zdravko	Očni odjel Opće bolnice	Slav. Brod

Vidović, Nada	Hercegovačka 123	Zagreb
Vidulić, Izak	Očni odjel JRM, Vojna bolnica ..	Split
Vlašić, Ladislav	Očna ambulanta Zdr. centra	Osijek
Vondraček-Jambrenšić, Nada	Očna ambulanta Med. centra ...	Koprivnica
Vrančić, Jiržina	Dolac 31	Zagreb
Vraneš, Branko	Krapinska 4	Zagreb
Vrsalović, Melita	Palmotićeva 29	Zagreb
Zajec, Mira	Očni odjel Opće bolnice	Sisak
Zlatar, Ivo	Očni odjel Opće bolnice	Split
Zlatar, Pero	Očni odjel Opće bolnice	Split
Zuber, Branko	Boln. 'dr. Kajfeš', Pavleka Miškine	Zagreb

SLOVENIJE

Ankerst, Erik	Očesna klinika	Ljubljana
Benčan-Treppo, Darja	Šolska poliklinika	Maribor
Bidovec, Franc	Vojna bolnica 'Mladika' očesni oddelek	Ljubljana
Boljka-Kolar, Milica	Očesna klinika	Ljubljana
Bošković, Anton	Vojna bolnica 'Mladika' očesni oddelek	Ljubljana
Breznik, Marija	Splošna bolnica očesni oddelek ..	Maribor
Čačković, Josip	Zdravstveni dom očesni oddelek .	Ptuj
Černčec, Vera	Šolska poliklinika očesni oddelek .	Ljubljana
Dereani, Prof. Carmen	Očesna klinika	Ljubljana
Dolenc, Biljana	Splošna bolnica očesni oddelek ..	Maribor
Egger-Pfeifer, Mira	Šolska poliklinika očesni oddelek .	Ljubljana
Gračner, Bojan	Splošna bolnica očesni oddelek ..	Maribor
Hrovatin, Borut	Očesna klinika	Ljubljana
Jurekovic, Branimir	Splošna bolnica očesni oddelek ..	Novo mesto
Jeruc-Gruden, Milena	Ocesna klinika	Ljubljana
Jurko, Stane	Splošna bolnica očesni oddelek ..	Celje
Kalan, Anda	Zdravstveni dom očesni oddelek .	Kranj
Kavčič, Silvo	Očesna klinika	Ljubljana
Keše, Viktor	Zdravstveni dom očesni oddelek .	Kranj
Kobler, Metka	Železniški zdravstveni dom očesni oddelek	Ljubljana
Koklič, Ivan	Tavčarjeva 8	Ljubljana
Kolar, Gorazd	Očesna klinika	Ljubljana
Kristl, Vinko	Očesna klinika	Ljubljana
Kurelac, Zlatko	Splošna bolnica očesni oddelek ..	Maribor
Leskovšek, Marija	Splošna bolnica očesni oddelek ..	Celje
Morela, Vesna	Splošna bolnica očesni oddelek ..	Novo mesto
Novak-Modrijan, Neva	Splošna bolnica očesni oddelek ..	Maribor
Novak, Stane	Očesna klinika	Ljubljana
Oblak, Bogomir	Splošna bolnica očesni oddelek ..	Piran
Pavlović, Milorad	Vojna bolnica očesni oddelek ...	Ljubljana
Potrč, Iva	Splošna bolnica očesni oddelek ..	Maribor
Pregelj-Močnik, Elvira	Splošna bolnica očesni oddelek ..	Nova Gorica
Ramšak, Anica	Šolska poliklinika očesni oddelek..	Maribor
Rudolf-Vukan, Marija	Splošna bolnica očesni oddelek ..	Murska Sobota
Sevelj, Marta	Očesna klinika	Ljubljana
Sekolec, Jože	Splošna bolnica očesni oddelek ..	Maribor
Skočic, Snježana	Zdravstveni dom 'Zasavje' očesni oddelek	Trbovlje
Srebrnič, Julij	Splošna bolnica očesni oddelek ..	Nova Gorica
Stergar, Prof. Stane	Očesna klinika	Ljubljana

Strnad, Stanko	Očesna klinika	Ljubljana
Spicer, Vladimir	Vojna bolnica 'Mladika' očesni oddelek	Ljubljana
Svagelj, Igor	Očesna klinika	Ljubljana
Svarc, Aleksandar	Očesna klinika	Ljubljana
Talanyi, Lea	Splošna bolnica očesni oddelek ..	Murska Sobota
Trček, Alenka	Splošna bolnica očesni oddelek ..	Murska Sobota
Vastovec, Jože	Splošna bolnica očesni oddelek ..	Nova Gorica
Videnšek, Joža	Očesna klinika	Ljubljana
Vidović, Savo	Očesna klinika	Ljubljana
Vrevo-Eleršek, Marjeta	Očesna klinika	Ljubljana
Vrhovec, Janez	Splošna bolnica, očesni oddelek .	Celje
Zajc, Franc	Splošna bolnica očesni oddelek ..	Piran
Zeilhofer, Zlatko	Splošna bolnica, očesni oddelek .	Maribor
Zupan, Ciril	Očesna klinika	Ljubljana
Zupančič-Brovet, Irena	Očesna klinika	Ljubljana
Žel, Tone	Očesna klinika	Ljubljana

NOSOCOMIA QUIBUS OCULIS AEGRI CURANTUR

No. of beds

Bosne i Hercegovine

Banja Luka – Medicinski Centar, šef: Prim. dr. doc. med. soc. Aleksandar Pišteljić	65
Bihać – Medicinski Centar, šef: Dr. Stjepan Ban	29
Foča – Medicinski Centar, šef: Prim. dr. Milhajlović Srdjan	20
Zenica – Medicinski Centar, šef: Dr. Veljko Sladojević	50
Doboj – Medicinski Centar, šef: Dr. Pero Sredanović	20
Mostar – Medicinski Centar, šef:	55
Tuzla – Medicinski Centar, šef: Prim. dr. Ana Rosić	47
Trebinje – Medicinski Centar, šef: Prof. Azra Dordević	20
Brčko – Medicinski Centar (ambulatory), šef: Bogoljub Bošnjak	–
Sarajevo – Klinička Bolnica za Očne Bolesti Univerziteitskog Centra, šef: Prof. dr. Borislava Mastilović	250

Srbye

Bor, Očno odelenje , šef: Dr. Vidak Mičović	35
Cačak, Očno odelenje, šef: Prim. dr. Miloš Radosavljević	25
Kragujevac, Očno odelenje. šef: Dr. Knežev-Jelić, Dobrinka	32
Kruševac, Očno odelenje. šef: Prim. dr. Mašić Vera	27
Leskovac, Očno odelenje. šef: Prim. dr. Miloš Manić	21
Prokuplje, Očno odelenje. šef: Dr. Ljubinko Djordjević	20
Požarevac, Očno odelenje. šef: Dr. Robert Mak Klur	25
Pirot, Očno odelenje, šef: Dr. Dušan Vasić	18
Smed. Palanka, Očno odelenje. šef: Dr. Dušan Milhailović	25
Smederevo, Očno odelenje. šef: Dr. Božidar Milojković	12
Sabac, Očno odelenje. šef: Dr. Mihajlo Vasović	35
Tžužice, Očno odelenje. šef: Dr. Ćupić Rajko	32
Valjevo, Očno odelenje. šef: Dr. Angelina Petrović-Stevanović	24
Vranje, Očno odelenje. šef: Dr. Milivoje Pašić	21
Zaječar, Očno. šef: Dr. Dušica Paunović	28
Cuprija, Očno odelenje. šef: Dr. Milivoje Jakovljević	24
Kraljevo, Očono odelenje. šef: Dr. Blagoje Novotarac	30
Loznica, Očno odelenje. šef: Dr. Stajić Andjelić	23

Beograd, Očna klinika. šef: Prof. dr. Milan Blagojević 220
Beograd, Institut za oftalmologiju Kliničke bolnice. šef: Prof. dr. Zlatomir Kecmanović 85
Beograd, Inst. za zdravstv. zaštitu majke i deteta, Samost. očno odel. šef: Prim. dr. Boško
Jovičević (uskoro 26) 10
Beograd, Očna klinika VMA. šef: Doc. dr. M. Savičević .... –
Ozren – Sokobanja, Spec. bolnica za plučne i očne bol. i rehab. šef: Dr. Stojan Bogoj 100
Niš, Očna klinika. šef: Prof. dr. Tomašvić 70

INSTITUTA SCHOLAEQUE CAECIS DESTINATAE

Zemun, Zavod za slešu decu i omladinu ....
Beograd, Osnovna škola za zaštitu vida 'Dragan Kovačević". ....
Pančevo, Dom slepih ....
Beograd, 'Sloga' – Centar za zapošljavanje i rehabilit. slepih invalida. ....

KOREA MERIDIONALIS

SOCIETATES OPHTHALMOLOGICAE

Nationalis

The Korean Ophthalmological Society

President: Koo, Bon Sool
Vice-President: Yoon, Zeung Woc
Secretary General: Kim, Sang Min
Director of Scientific Activity: Shin, Tong Yoll
Director of Publication: Kim, Jae Ho
Director of Foreign Affairs: Kim, Hong Bok
Auditor: Im, Kyung Yul
Auditor: Cho, Byung Chai
Bureau: c/o Department of Ophthalmology, Han-Gang Sacred Heart Hospital, Chung-Ang University School of Medicine, 94-200, Yeongdeungpo-Dong Yeongdeungpo-Gu, Seoul
Number of members: 144
Number of associate members: 60

Regionales

The Seoul Regional Society

Secretary: Kim, Seong Deuk, M. D.; Secretary in General, c/o Department of Ophthalmology, Yonsei University School of Medicine and Hospital, San-15, Sinchon-Dong, Seodaemun-Gu, Seoul
Number of members: 126

The Busan Regional Society

Secretary: Choi, Sang Hae, M. D., Gu Se Eye Clinic, 159, 4 Ga, Dargyo-Dong, Yeongdo-Gu, Busan

The Gyeong Gi Regional Society

Secretary: Lee, Hong Kyo, M. D., Lee's Eye Clinic, 187, Nae-Dong, Incheon-Si, Gyeong-Gi-Do

The Chung Nam Regional Society

Secretary: Kim, Gun Yong, M. D., Gwang Myeong Eye Clinic, 65-1, Eunhaeng-Dong, Daejeon-Si, Chungcheong-Nam-Do

The Chung Bug Regional Society

Secretary: Lee, Eun Suk, M. D., Jung Ang Eye Clinic, 1-B, Bugmun-Ro, Cheongju-Si, Chungcheong-Bug-Do

The Gang Weon Regional Society

Secretary: Kim, Young Tack, M. D., Kim's Eye Clinic, 103, Joyang-Dong, Chuncheon-Si, Gang-Weon-Do

The Jeon bug Regional Society

Secretary: Yoo, In Sang, M. D., Jeon Ju Clinic, 69, 3 Ga, Jungang-Dong, Jeonju-Si, Jeonra-Bug-Do

The Jeon Nam Regional Society

Secretary: Hong, Seung Min, M. D., Hong's Eye Clinic, 50, Gung-Dong, Gwangju-Si, Jeonra-Nam-Do

The Gyeong Bug Regional Society

Secretary: Choi, Sung Koo, M. D., c/o Department of Ophthalmology, Patima Hospital, 302-1, Sinam-Dong, Daegu-Si, Gyeongsang-Bug-Do

NOMINA ET DOMICILIA MEDICORUM AB OCULIS

Ahn, Chung Sook	583-3, Changsin-Dong, Dong-daemun-Gu	Seoul
Ahn, Young Soon	111, Seorin-Dong, Jongro-Gu	Seoul
Bae, Dong Woo	30-8, Changcheon-Dong, Seodae-mun-Gu	Seoul
Byun, Jae Wuk	381, 2 Ga, Chungmu-Dong	Busan
Byun, Yong Soo	158, Dandae-Ri, Jungbu-Myeon, Gwangju-Guon	Gysong-Gi-Do
Cha, Ok Ja	88-345, Haweolgog-Dong, Seong-bug-Gu	Seoul
Chai, Byoung Sik	340, 5 Ga, Samseon-Dong, Seong-bug-Gu	Seoul
Chang, Bong Leen	65-17, Eungam-Dong, Seodaemun-Gu	Seoul
Chang, Chung Ok	80, 6 Ga, Yeongdeungpo-Dong, Yeongdeungpo-Gu	Seoul
Cho, Byung Chai	44-5 1 Ga, Jangchung-Dong, Jung-Gu	Seoul
Cho, Suk Ju	129, Gysong-Dong, Incheon-Si	Gyeong-Gi-Do
Cho, Jai Choon	266, Bujeon-Dong, Busanjin-Gu	Busan
Cho, Woo Jae	66-9, Mangweon-Dong, Mapo-Gu	Seoul
Choi, Chang Shoo	196-6, Gyeongun-Dong, Jongro-Gu	Seoul
Choi, Gee Yong	172, Dongseong-Dong, Jinju-Si	Gyeongsang-Nam-Do
Choi, Jong San	136, Seongnae-Dong, Seongdong-Gu	Seoul

Choi, Joon Kiu	San 8-2, Haengdang-Dong, Seong-dong-Gu	Seoul
Choi, Ouk	156, Gweonnong-Dong, Jongro-Gu	Seoul
Choi, Sook Kyoung	24-32, 1 Ga, Pil-Dong, Jung-Gu .	Seoul
Choi, Sung Koo	1989-13, Daemyeong-Dong, Daegu-Si	Gyeongsang-Bug-Do
Choi, Yu Keun	263-8, 3 Ga, Suseong-Dong, Dong-Gu, Daegu-Si	Gyeongsang-Bug-Do
Choo, Cha Hyon	226, Gyeong-Dong, Incheon-Si ..	Gyeong-Gi-Do
Chun, Jong Han	5, Munhwa-Dong, Jung-Gu, Dae-gu-Si	Gyeongsang-Bug-Do
Chung, Bong Jo	89-4, Haweolgog-Dong, Seongbug-Gu	Seoul
Chung, Soo Ja	249-6, Seogyo-Dong, Mapo-Gu ..	Seoul
Chung, Young Tai	192, 1 Ga, Junghwasan-Dong, Jeonju-Si	Jeonra-Bug-Do
Hah, Jae In	24, 1 Ga, Jongro, Jongro-Gu	Seoul
Hahn, Chun Suk	102-2, 2 Ga, Jongro, Jongro-Gu .	Seoul
Han, Duck Kee	39, Pojeong-Dong, Jung-Gu, Dae-gu-Si	Gyeongsang-Bug-Do
Han, Hong Joo	358, 37 Ban, Baegun-Dong, Gwangju-Si	Jeonra-Nam-Do
Han, Kyung Sik	9-1, Yongdu-Dong, Dongdaemun-Gu	Seoul
Han, Kyung Sook	102-16, Namgajwa-Dong, Seodae-mun-Gu	Seoul
Hong, Keh Hoo	170, Oncheon-Dong, Dongrae-Gu.	Busan
Hong, Kun Soo	10-70, Hongeun-Dong, Seadae-mun-Gu	Seoul
Hong, Seung Ho	195-346, Jeonnong-Dong, Dang-daemun-Gu	Seoul
Hong, Seung Min	50, Gung-Dong, Gwangju-Si	Jeonra-Nam-Do
Hong, Soon Kak	48-84, Hongeun-Dong, Seodae-mun-Gu	Seoul
Im, Kyung Yul	120-2, Gosa-Dong, Jeonju-Si	Jeonra-Bug-Do
Jung, Hai Ryun	128-69, Heangdang-Dong, Seong-dong-Gu	Seoul
Kang, Nae Youl	65-3, Seoseong-Dong, Masan-Si ..	Gyeongsang-Nam-Do
Kim, Byong Hong	88-36, 1 Imun-Dong, Dongdae-mun-Gu	Seoul
Kim, Chang Woo	104, Beomil-Dong, Dong-Gu	Busan
Kim, Choo Young	4, 1 Ri, Yeongju, Yeongju-Eub ..	Gyeongsang-Bug-Do
Kim, Choong Durk	286, Haengdang-Dong, Seong-dong-Gu	Seoul
Kim, Chung Whan	113, 1 Ga, Dongsomun-Dong, Seongbug-Gu	Seoul
Kim, Dong Won	196, Il-Dong, Euijeongbu-Si	Gyesong-Gi-Do
Kim, Gun Yong	65-1, Eunhaeng-Dong, Daejeon-Si	Chungcheong-Nam-Do
Kim, Gwang Yun	3-8, Daecheong-Dong, Jung-Gu ..	Busan
Kim, Hak Soo	203-169, Cheongryangri-Dong, Dongdaemun-Gu	Seoul
Kim, Hi Joon	62-14, 1 Ga, Chungcheong-Ro, Seodaemun-Gu	Seoul
Kim, Hi Soc	80, 6 Ga, Yeongdeungpo-Dong, Yeongdeungpo-Gu	Seoul

Kim, Hong Bok	24-253, Hwagog-Dong, Yeong-deungpo-Gu	Seoul
Kim, Hyung Jean	244-16, 6 Ga, Jongro, Jongro-Gu .	Seoul
Kim, In Soon	145-161, Seongbug-Dong, Seong-bug-Gu	Seoul
Kim, Jae Ho	16-206, Maensyon-Apt., Dong-buichon-Dong, Yongsan-Gu ..	Seoul
Kim, Jae Duk	172-59, Daejo-Dong, Seodaemun-Gu	Seoul
Kim, Jae Myung	338-432, Seoggwan-Dong, Seong-bug-Gu	Seoul
Kim, Joung Ja	8, 3 Ga, Donggwang-Dong, Jung-Gu	Busan
Kim, Kyung Ja	28-9, Ihwa-Dong, Jongro-Gu	Seoul
Kim, Kyung Sil	239, Yong-Dong, Incheon-Si	Gyesong-Gi-Do
Kim, Sang Ha	12, 4 Ga, Daecheong-Dong, Jung-Gu	Busan
Kim, Sang Min	312-15, Noryangjin-Dong, Yeong-deungpo-Gu	Seoul
Kim, Sang Yong	1030, Choryang-Dong, Dong-Gu .	Busan
Kim, Seong Deuck	260-17, 1 Yeonheui-Dong, Seo-daemun-Gu	Seoul
Kim, Soon Chang	2-39, Dasheung-Dong, Mapo-Gu .	Seoul
Kim, Tae Uck	51-39, Jangtae-Dong, Jinju-Si ...	Gyeongsang-Nam-Do
Kim, Won Seek	10-57, Haweolgog-Dong, Seong-bug-Gu	Seoul
Kim, Woo Kon	362-2, Choryang-Dong, Dong-Gu .	Busan
Kim, Yong Bok	968-27, Hawangsib-Ri, Seongdong-Gu	Seoul
Kim, Young Tack	103, Joyang-Dong, Chuncheon-Si.	Gang-Weon-Do
Ko, Chung Je	99-4, Itaeweon-Dong, Yongsan-Gu	Seoul
Ko, Jin Suck	24, Weolsan-Dong, Gwangju-Si ..	Jeonra-Nam-Do
Kong, Byung Woo	111, Seorin-Dong, Jongro-Gu ...	Seoul
Kong, In Ho	78-1, Gye-Dong, Jongro-Gu	Seoul
Koo, Kwang Il	18-79, 6 Ga, Eulji-Ro, Jung-Gu ..	Seoul
Koo, Bon Sool	144, 2 Ga, Samseon-Dong, Se-ong-bug-Gu	Seoul
Kwack, Young Sae	125-1, 4 Ga Chungmu-Ro, Jung-Gu	Seoul
Kwon, Dal Man	1792, 2 Gu, Daemyeung-Dong, Nam-Gu, Daegu-Si	Gyeongsang-Bug-Do
Kwon, Sang Kyu	2, Namseong-Ro, Daegu-Si	Gyeongsang-Bug-Do
Kwon, Yung Ho	561-8, Changsin-Dong, Dongdae-mun-Gu	Seoul
Lee, Bok Soon	312, Hagseong-Dong, Weonju-Si .	Gang-Weon-Do
Lee, Chang Sung	255, 2 Bujeon-Dong, Busanjeon-Gu	Busan
Lee, Dong Sick	664, Jangrae-Dong, Anyang-Eub .	Gyeong-Gi-Do
Lee, Eun Joo	114-2, Cheongun-Dong, Jongro-Gu	Seoul
Lee, Eun Suk	1-8, Bugmun-Ro, Chaongju-Si ...	Chungcheong-Bug-Do
Lee, Hae Sook	San 19-57, Mia-Dong, Seongbug-Gu	Seoul
Lee, Jae Heung	127-151, Jeonnong-Dong, Dong-daemun-Gu	Seoul
Lee, Jang Woo	1030-3, Seryu-Dong, Suweon-Si .	Gyeong-Gi-Do

Lee, Jong Goo	3-9, Namsan-Dong, Gimcheon-Si	Gyeongsang-Bug-Do
Lee, Ki Nam	120, Beomil-Dong, Dong-Gu	Busan
Lee, Ki Suk	26-16, Jung-Dong, Daejeon-Si ...	Chungcheong-Nam-Do
Lee, Kyung Cheul	43-9, Gwancheol-Dong, Jongro-Gu	Seoul
Lee, Kyung Soo	465, Sangweon-Dong, Pohang-Si .	Gyeongsang-Bug-Do
Lee, Myung Soo	278-4, Yeonheui-Dong, Seodaemun-Gu	Seoul
Lee, Ok Hi	208-35, Daejo-Dong, Seodaemun-Gu	Seoul
Lee, Pil Woong	47, 1 Ga, Jongro, Jongro-Gu	Seoul
Lee, Song Hee	28, Gaya-Dong, Busanjin-Gu	Busan
Lee, Soo Jik	Sogyeog-Dong, Yeongdeungpo-Gu	Seoul
Lee, Ya Chun	261, Bujeon-Dong, Busanjin-Gu .	Busan
Lee, Yong Hi	266-19, Eungam-Dong, Seodaemun-Gu	Seoul
Min, Byung Sam	43-9, Gwancheol-Dong, Jongro-Gu	Seoul
Moon, Haeng Ja	138-54, Donggyo-Dong, Mapo-Gu	Seoul
Oh, Junes Sup	78, 1 Ga, Seomun-Ra, Daegu-Si .	Gyeongsang-Bug-Do
Oh, Se Min	2-12, Nampo-Dong, Jung-Gu ...	Busan
Oh, Sung Kuen	1, Gu, Nae-Ri, Yesan-Eub	Chungcheong-Nam-Do
Oh, Tae Woong	402-3, Daebang-Dong, Yeongdeungpo-Gu	Seoul
Oh, Young Hwan	115, Hyoje-Dong, Jongro-Gu ...	Seoul
On, Byoung Jong	111, 1 Ga, Gyeangweon-Dong, Jeonju-Si	Jeonra-Bug-Do
Paek, Un Sang	11-1, Daeja-Dong, Seodaemun-Gu	Seoul
Park, Byong Gook	48, Amnam-Dong, Seo-Gu	Busan
Park, Byong Il	216, 5 Ga, Geumnam-Ro, Gwangju-Si	Jeonra-Nam-Do
Park, Byong Ki	159-2, Bujeon-Dong, Busanjin-Gu	Busan
Park, Eun Ho	162, Ilsan-Dong, Weonju-Si	Gang-Weon-Do
Park, Hong Kyun	149, Daein-Dong, Gwangju-Si ...	Jeonra-Nam-Do
Park, Jung Ja	408-2, Galhyeon-Dong, Seodaemun-Gu	Seoul
Park, Kun Soo	129, Jeonnong-Dong, Dongdaemun-Gu	Seoul
Park, Sang Yun	23-81, Sangweolgog-Dong, Seongbug-Gu	Seoul
Park, Won Teak	294, Gye-Dong, Yeosu-Si	Jeonra-Nam-Do
Park, Young Soon	111, Searin-Dong, Jongro-Gu ...	Seoul
Rhee, Sang Wook	2-301, Maensyeon Apt., 300-26, Dongbuichon-Dong Yongsan-Gu	Seoul
Rhym, Myung Hee	22-2, 2 Ga, Jongro, Jongro-Gu ..	Seoul
Sa, You Sup	11, 2 Ga, Sangrag-Dong, Mogpo-Si	Jeonra-Nam-Do
Shin, Han Ho	31-3, Choryang-Dong, Dong-Gu .	Busan
Shin, In Sun	314-4, Mangweon-Dong, Mapo-Gu	Seoul
Shin, Jong Sik	62, 5 Ga, Geumnam-Ro, Gwangju-Si	Jeonra-Nam-Do
Shin, Ne Yong	43-9, Gwancheol-Dong, Jongro-Gu	Seoul
Shin, Tong Yoll	141-1, Sinseol-Dong, Dongdaemun-Gu	Seoul
Shyn, Kyung Hwan	4-2, Gwansu-Dong, Jongro-Gu ..	Seoul
Soh, Kyung Sub	88, Yulmog-Dong, Incheon-Si ...	Gyeong-Gi-Do
Sohn, Chung Kyoon	6-80, Changjeon-Dong, Mapo-Gu .	Seoul

Sohn, Eui Sun	69-45, Galweol-Dong, Yongsan-Gu	Seoul
Sohn, Kyung Sup	6-80, Changjeon-Dong, Mapo-Gu .	Seoul
Sohn, Moo Shik	72, Insa-Dong, Jongro-Gu	Seoul
Song, Cho Young	12, 3 Ga, Dongseong-Ro, Daegu-Si	Gyeongsang-Bug-Do
Suhk, Jae Soo	38-4, Seongnam-Dong, Ulsan-Si .	Gyeongsang-Nam-Do
Yoo, In Sang	69, 3 Ga, Jungang-Dong, Jeonju-Si	Jeonra-Bug-Do
Yoon, Byung Joo	193-10, 2 Ga, Jangchung-Dong, Jung-Cu	Seoul
Yoon, Choong Hyun	136, Eunhaeng-Dong, Daejeon-Si .	Chungcheong-Nam-Do
Yoon, Soon Ja	188, 2 Ga, Myeongryun-Dong, Jongro-Gu	Seoul
Yoon, Zeung Woo	59-4, Gongpyeong-Dong, Jung-Gu, Daegu-Si	Gyeongsang-Bug-Do
Youn, Won Shik	70-2, 5 Ga, Sanseon-Dong, Seong-bug-Gu	Seoul
Yuk, Kang Woo	414-12, 3 Gu, Bisan-Dong, Seo-Gu, Daegu-Si	Gyeongsang-Bug-Do
Yun, Dang Ho	567-15, 1 Mia-Dong, Seongbug-Gu	Seoul
Yum, Teak Koo	101-2, 2 Ga, Eulji-Ro, Jung-Gu ..	Seoul

NOSOCOMIA QUIBUS OCULIS AEGRI CURANTUR

No. of beds

The Seoul National University Hospital, 28, Yeongeon-Dong, Jongro-Gu, Seoul. *Director of Dpt. of Ophthalmology:* Youn, Won Shik 446

The Yonsei University Hospital, San-15, Sinchon-Dong, Seodaemun-Gu, Seoul. *Director of Dpt. of Ophthalmology:* Hong, Soon Kak 616

Woo-Suk Hospital The Korea University, 4, 2 Ga, Myeongryan-Dong, Jongro-Gu, Seoul. *Director of Dpt. of Ophthalmology:* Kim, Chung Whan 280

St. Mary's Hospital Catholic Medical College and Center, 1, 2 Ga, Myeong-Dong, Jung-Cu, Seoul. *Director of Dpt. of Ophthalmology:* Rhee, Sang Wook 450

The Ewha Womans University Hospital, 72, 6 Ga, Jongro, Jongro-Gu, Seoul. *Director of Dpt. of Ophthalmology:* Lee, Myung Soo 150

Sacred Heart Hospital Chung-Ang University, 82-1, 2 Ga, Pil-Dong, Jung-Gu, Seoul. *Director of Dpt. of Ophthalmology:* Kco, Bon Sool 282

Han-Gang Sacred Heart Hospital, Chung-Ang University, 94-200, Yeongdeungpo-Dong, Yeongdeungpo-Gu, Seoul. *Director of Dpt. of Ophthalmology:* Kim, Sang Min 324

The Han Yang University Hospital, San 8-2, Haengdang-Dong, Seongdong-Gu, Seoul. *Director of Dpt. of Ophthalmology:* Ko, Chung Je 317

The Kyung Hee University Hospital, 1, Hoegi-Dong, Dongdaemun-Gu, Seoul. *Director of Dpt. of Ophthalmology:* Shin, Tong Yoll 200

The Busan National University Hospital, 10, 1 Ga, Ami-Dong, Seo-Gu, Busan. *Director of Dpt. of Ophthalmology:* Park, Beyong Gook 280

The Chung Nam National University Hospital, 22, 3 Daeheung-Don, Daejeon-Si, Chungcheong-Nam-Do. *Director of Dpt. of Ophthalmology:* Lee, Chong Won 192

The Cho Sun University Hospital, 375, Seoseog-Dong, Gwangju-Si, Jeonra-Nam-Do. *Director of Dpt. of Ophthalmology:* Kim, Hong Duk 227

The Chon Nam National University Hospital, 8, 1 Gu, Hag-Dong. Gwangju-Si, Jeonra-Nam-Do. *Director of Dpt. of Ophthalmology:* Park, Byong Il 344

INSTITUTA SCHOLAEQUE CAECIS DESTINATAE

Schools	Inmates
Seoul School for the Blind	278
Immanuel School for the Blind	32
Kyong-Ki School for the Blind	98
Kang-Won School for the Blind	65
Chong-Ju School for the Blind	90
Choong-Joo Sacred School for the Blind	47
Choong-Nam Sacred School for the Blind	71
Taegu Kwang Myung School for the Blind	116
Busan Kwang Myung School for the Blind	88
Iri School for the Blind	60
Mokpo School for the Blind	52
Chun-Nam School for the Blind	78
Bug-Je-Ju School for the Blind	25

Institutes & Homes	
Korea Dae Rim Home for the Blind	80
Immanuel Home for Blind Girls	65
Korea Rehabilitation Center for the Blind	80
Oh-Am Home for the Blind	20
Korea Rehabilitation Home for the Blind	30
Yung-Dong Vocational Training Home for the Blind	45
Yung-Sue Han-Kang Vocational Training Home for the Blind	16
Choong-Buk Kwang Hwa Home for the Blind	
In-Chun Kwang Myung Home for the Blind	98
Taegu Light House for the Blind	20
Busan Light House for the Blind	98
Chun-Kwang Home for the Blind	74
Chun-Nam Kwang Myung Home for the Blind	62

LEBANON

SOCIETATES OPHTHALMOLOGICAE

Lebanese Ophthalmological Society
Executive Secretary: Adnan H. Halasa, c/o American University of Beirut, Beirut
Treasurer: Husui Shams
Members: Antoine Esta, Munir Sultan
Number of members: 38

NOMINA ET DOMICILIA MEDICORUM AB OCULIS

Aboud, Edouard	....	Saida
Acra, Victor	Lebanon St., Akra Bldg.	Beirut
Anouti, Nabil	Bourj Abi Haydar	Beirut
Arrata, Moufi	Hotel Dieu	Beirut
Ashkar, Joseph	Gourau St., Gemayzeh Saint Famille	Beirut
Awad, Juan	Hotel Dieu St., Natafji Bldg.	Beirut
Baba, Abdel Rahman	Mohammad El-Hout Bldg.	Beirut
Baghdassarian, Sahag	American University Hospital	Beirut
Baloglou, Paul	American University Hospital	Beirut
Baz, Camille	Patriarche Hoyek St., Antoine Baz Bldg.	Beirut
Chemali, Michel	Bechara El-Khouri St.	Beirut
Cocony, George	139 Abdel Aziz St., British Bank Bldg.	Ras-Beirut
El-Khouri, Joseph	Hotel-Dieu Hospital	Beirut
El-Yafi, Nabila	Rue Amin Gemayel, Im. Zouein .	Beirut
Esta, Antoine	Badara St., Akar Bldg.	Beirut
Farhat, Yehia	P.O.B. 7270	Beirut
Faris, Bishara	American University Hospital	Beirut
Halasa, Adnan	American University Hospital	Beirut
Hasan, Melhem	Assour, Eseyli Bldg.	Beirut
Jaroudi, Nabil	American University Hospital	Beirut
Kamerman, Roger	Kantari St., Kamerman Bldg.	Beirut
Khaouam, Edward	American University Hospital	Beirut
Khouri, Antoine	Freij Bldg. Furn-El-Sheback	Beirut
Lawand, A. H.	Corniche El-Mazraa	Beirut
Majzoub, Husni	Rue Mother Gelas, Markaziyeh Bldg.	Beirut
Majzoub, Usama	Gefinor Medical Center	Ras-Beirut
Mamo, Jubra	American University Hospital	Beirut
Matta, Camille	American University Hospital	Beirut
Melki, Raymond	86, Rue Badaro	Beirut
Naccache, René	France St., Sandary Bldg.	Beirut
Salamoun, Samir	American University Hospital	Beirut
Salem, Jack	Ghandour Saad St., Moubayed Bldg.	Beirut
Saliby, Samir	Emir Bechir St.	Beirut
Salman, Kamal	Military Hospital	Beirut

Sayegh, Roger	American University Hospital ...	Beirut
Serhal, Philip	Damas St.	Beirut
Shams, Husni	287 Mohamad El-Hout St., Dr. Fouad Tabbara Bldg.	Beirut
Sinno, Wafic	Picot St., Hotel Omar Khayam Bldg.	Beirut
Sultan, Munir	American University Hospital ...	Beirut

NOSOCOMIA QUIBUS OCULIS AEGRI CURANTUR

All eye hospitals have eye departments.
Saleeby Eye Hospital is under construction.

INSTITUTA SCHOLAEQUE CAECIS DESTINATAE

The Lebanese Society for the Relief of the Blind runs a school with 125 inmates.

MAROCCO

SOCIETATES OPHTHALMOLOGICAE

Société Marocaine d'Ophtalmologie

Bureau: 6 Rue Mohamed Diouri, Casablanca
Président: Dr. Moh. Boutaleb
Vice Président: Dr. El Yacoubi
Secrétaire Général: Dr. Sekkat
Trésorier: Dr. Milosvich
Assesseurs: Dr. P. Laborde de Laulne, Dr. Fr. Noël
Membres: 33

NOMINA ET DOMICILA MEDICORUM AB OCULIS

Amour	5, Bd. Mohamed El Hansali	Casablanca
Benhamou	Rue Colona d'Ornano	Marrakech
Benjelloun-Mezzian	161, Avenue Hassan II	Casablanca
Berbeche	Centre Ophtalmologique	Salé
Boutaleb	8, Avenue Mohamed V	Casablanca
Chamih	Centre Ophtalmologique	Salé
Croce	Hôpital Omar Drissi	Fes
Durix	13, Rue des Terves	Casablanca
El Yacoubi	Centre Ophtalmologique	Salé
Franc	Hôpital el Antaki	Marrakech
Fruchon	96, Avenue Lyautey	Meknes
Gallet	49, Rue Poincarré	Casablanca
Guy	Immeuble Tuj	Marrakech
Laborde de Laulne	Hôpital el Antaki	Marrakech
Lafont	2, Avenue Pasteur	Rabat
Lahlou	28, Rue Allal Ben Abdallah	Rabat
Laurent	12, Rue Idriss Lahrizi	Casablanca
Magnon	3, Rue de Toulon	Meknes
Mohhieddine	Hôpital Omar Drissi	Fes
Milosevich	Hôpital du 20 Août 1953, Service Ophtalmologie	Casablanca
Oger	57, Rue du Prince Moulay Abdallah	Casablanca
Ouazzani	Hôpital Civil	Meknes
Perez Gonzalez, J.	35, Bd. Pasteur	Tanger
Polev, Léonide	16, Rue de la Saône	Salé
Pop Stefanov	19, Rue du Prince Moulay Abdallah	Casablanca
Roig	57, Rue du Prince Moulay Abdallah	Casablanca
Sakon	27, Rue Lacépède	Casablanca
Sasson	4, Rue de Mostaganem	Rabat
Sava, Cvetkovic	371, Avenue Mohammed V	Kenitra
Supelano, Sanchez	54, Bd. Pasteur	Tanger
Tazi	14, Rue de Champagne et de Constantinople	Casablanca

Torfeh	Hôpital Civil, Service Ophtalmo-logie	Safi
Ulrich	Hôpital el Antaki	Marrakech
Villard	2, Rue de Foucault	Fes

NOSOCOMIA QUIBUS OCULIS AEGRI CURANTUR

Casablanca   Lits
Hôpital du 20 Août 1953 — Service Ophtalmologie — Chef du Service: Dr. Mohammed
Boutaleb 120

Salé
Centre Ophtalmologique de Salé-Chef du Service: Dr. El Yacoubi 140

Marrakech
Hôpital El Antaki — Service Ophtalmologie — Chef du Service: Dr. Franc Noël 137

Fes
Hôpital Omar Drissi — Service Ophtalmologie — Chef du Service: Dr. Croce, Dr. Zouaoui .. 134

Oujda
Chef du Service: Dr. Veyrier, Dr. Christina 45

Meknes
Hôpital Civil — Service Ophtalmologie — Chef du Service: Dr. Ouazzani Moahtar 65

Safi
Hôpital Civil — Service Ophtalmologie — Chef du Service: Dr. Torfeh Hossein 26

Services Ophtalmologiques: Capacité
Agadir, *Chef:* Dr. Madelmo 68
Beni Mellal 22
Ouarzazate, *Chef:* Dr. Sipov 60
Tetouan, *Chef:* Dr. Anjel Souiro 35
Nador 6
Ksar-Es-Souk, *Chef:* Konaksas 35
Kénitra, *Chef:* Dr. Cvetkovic Sava 17

INSTITUTA SCHOLAEQUE CAECIS DESTINATAE

Organisation Alaouîte pour la Protection des Aveugles, 15, rue Canizarès, Casablanca
Association Hassan II pour la Sauvegarde de l'Aveugle, Rue 65, n° 3, Derb Chorfa, Casablanca
Association 'Les Amis des Aveugles' 218, Bd. de la Résistance, Casablanca
Institut des Aveugles 2, rue Saïd Hajji, Salé
Le siège Social de l'Organisation Alaoüite pour la Protection des Aveugles se trouve à Rabat, Rue
Hussein 1er.

Le Comité est présidé par Son Altesse la Princesse Lamia, assistée par Son Excellence le Ministre d'Etat, Mr. Haj M'Hamed Bahnini

Cette Association pour les Aveugles dispose de différents centres dans toutes les provinces du Royaume, composée par des Comités, qui à leur tour coiffent des Ecoles et Centres de formation. Ces Comités Siègent dans les provinces de: Marrakech – Agadir – Taroudant – Safi – Oujda – Taza – Meknès – Fès – Tetouan – Beni-Mellal

MEXICO

SOCIETATES OPHTHALMOLOGICAE

Nationalis

Sociedad Mexicana de Oftalmología
President: Prof. Roberto Wallentin
Vice-President: Prof. David Gutierrez
Secretario: Dr. Evaristo Guevara
Tesorero: Dr. Bernardo Bidart
Address: Teotihuacan # 17A, México D.F.
Number of members: 503

Regionales

Sociedad Oftalmológica Dr. Manuel Covarrubias de la Asociación para evitar la Ceguera en México
President: Dr. Raúl Santos Mazal
Vice-President: Dr. René O'kelard Conzález
Secreatrio: Dr. Rubén Arriaga Martinez
Tesorero: Dr. Virgilio Morales Ledezma

Sociedad Médica del Hospital Oftalmológico de Nuestra Señora de la Luz
Presidente: Dr. Guillermo Sánchez Flores
Vice-Presidente: Dr. Gustavo Berges Salgado
Secretario: Dr. Jaime Lozano
Tesorero: Dr. Héctor Leos

Sociedad Ergo Oftalmológica Mexicana
President: Dr. Enrique López Quiñones
Vice-Presidente: Dr. Carlos Noble Gutiérrez
Secretario: Dr. Alfonso Ahumada Beltrán
Tesorero: Dr. Bonfilio Cuevas Domínguez

Sociedad de Oftalmología del Centro A.C.
Presidente: Dr. Cecilio Páez Stille
Secretario: Dr. José Mendoza Arciga
Tesorero: Dr. José Arturo Ponce Arámbula
Vocal: Dr. Manuel Ulaje Medina

Pertenecen a la Sociedad del Centro:
Zacatecas, San Luis Potosi, Aguascalientes, Guanajuato, Queretaro, Michoacan

Sociedad Oftalmológica Centro Médico Nacional
Presidente: Dr. José Rojas Dorsal
Vice-Presidente: Dr. Francisco Martínez Castro
Secretario: Dr. Lucila Ramirez López
Tesorero: Dr. Juan Lara Mondragón

Sociedad de Oftalmología y Otorrinolaringología de Nuevo León
Presidente: Dr. Ezequiel Cavazos Treviño
Vice-Presidente: Dr. Armando Ibarra (Otorrinolaringologo)
Secretario: Dr. Alonso Mario Treviño
Tesorero: Dr. Luis Garza Treviño

Sociedad Oftalmologica de Yucatan
Presidente: Dr. Jose Gurrutia G.
Vice-Presidente: Dr. Fernando Rosas Marin
Secretario: Dr. Fernando Torres Gamboa

NOMINA ET DOMICILIA MEDICORUM AB OCULIS

Aboytes Patiño, Benjamin	Condominio Hidalgo desp. 204 ..	Léon, Gto.
Acosta Acosta, Efrain	Calle 57 # 503	Mérida, Yucatán
Acosta Cervantes, Pedro ...	Enrique González Martínez # 142 S.J.	Guadalajara, Jal.
Acuña del Villar, Rogelio ..	Ilefonso Vázques # 6, Lomas de Sotelo	Mexico 10 D.F,
Acuña Rosado, Carlos	Acatzingo # 20 desp. 101	Puebla, Puebla
Aguire Holguin, Carlos	Ojinaga # 205 desp. I	Chihuahua, Chih.
Aguirre Marquez, Martin ...	Altamira # 105 desp. 2	Tampico, Tamps.
Aguirre Valdez, Raymundo .	Zaragoza # 707 – A norte	Piedras Negras, Coah.
Agundis Anguiano, Teodulo M.	Campeche # 138	México, D.F.
Agundis Oliva, Rafael	Zaragoza # 210	San Luis Potosí, S.L.P.
Alamilla Gutierrez, Ruben ..	Tiber # 13-403, Col. Cuauhtemoc	México 5, D.F.
Alamillo Torres, Manuel ...	Citlaltepetl # 64	México 11, D.F.
Almada Pimentel, Jorge Rafael	Leopoldo Beristain # 10 Circ. Actores	Cd. Satélite, Edo. de México
Alegria Gonzalez, Javier ...	Zaragoza # 81 Ote	Tepic, Nayarit
Alvarado Areguin, Francisco	Guerrero # 2	Irapuato, Gto.
Allison Sierra, Pedro	2 Norte y 8 Oriente, Col. Obrera .	Poza Rico, Veracruz
Angel Placencia, Jose Guadalupe	Madero # 106-303, Edificio Drogueria Francesa	León, Gto.
Antillon Sanchez, Florencio.	Nogales # 28 'A'	México, D.F.
Aragon Martinzes, Oscar ...	Mariano Escobedo # 65 Pte	Culiacán, Sinaloa
Aranda Torres, Marco Antonio	Av. 20 de Enero # 412	León, Gto.

Arce Santamarina, Jose Luis.	Tuxpan # 16 desp. 303, Col. Roma	México 7, D.F.
Aregullin Garcia, Pedro	Washington Ote. # 546	Monterrey, N.L.
Arenas Bolaños, Francisco .	Monterrey # 147-201	México 7, D.F.
Argais Gamas, Jorge	Insurgentes sur # 421 'A' dpto. 206-1	México 11, D.F.
Arriaga Martinez, Rúben ...	Mar Blanco # 44, Col. Popotla ..	México 17, D.F.
Arroyo Damian, Agustin ...	Polanco # 94	México 5, D.F.
Aveleyra Fierro, Rafael	División del Norte # 143-10	México 12, D.F.
Avila Ramos, Hugo	Pino Suárez # W 446 2/o. piso desp. 5	Monterrey, N.L.
Aviña Zepeda, Jaime G. ...	Insurgentes sur # 1862 4/0. piso .	México 20, D.F.
Ayala Betancourt, Alberto .	Lic. Isidro Fabela # 210 Col. Morelos	Toluca, Edo. de México
Ayala Calvillo, Juan Manuel ·	José Maris Chévez # 201	Aguascalientes, Ags.
Babayan Mena, Juan Ignacio	Av. Amsterdam # 27 desp. 502 .	México 11, D.F.
Baca Castañeda, Carlos	Insurgentes sur # 421 'A' desp. 406	México 11, D.F.
Badillo Sevilla, Jose Francisco	Petén nte. # 224-4	México 12, D.F.
Barbiaux Hernandez, Marquez	Retorno 8 # 3 desp. 101, Fray santa teresa de mier	México, D.F.
Barbosa Horta, Sara	Silos # 10 desp. 104, Col. Cipreses	México 13, D.F.
Barojas Armiñom, Mario ...	Sur 3 # 255	Orizaba, Ver.
Barojas Weber, Everardo ...	Huatabampo # 64 bis, Col. Roma	México 7, D.F.
Barcelata Balladares, Filiberto	Insurgentes # 682 desp. 604, Col del Valle	México 12, D.F.
Barraza Ibarra, Alberto	Monterrey # 147 desp. 201, Col. Roma	México 7, D.F.
Barrenechea Ortuño, Teresa .	Santa María la Rivera # 82	México 4, D.F.
Bauza Gonzalez, Ignacio ...	13 sur # 301	Puebla, Pue.
Bazan Perez, Calixto	Puebla # 162 sur	Obregón, Sonora
Bazañez Galindo, Enrique ..	Edificio Juárez	Poza Rica, Ver.
Beathley Garcia, Ignacio ...	Juan Soto # 253-108	Veracruz, Ver.
Beck Carlos, Alberto	Florencia # 18, Col. Juárez	México, D.F.
Benavides Gonzallez, Jesus Maria	P. Mier # 321 dpto. 205	Monterrey, N.1.
Benavides Jacques, Christian	Víctor Hugo # 88, Col. Portales .	México 13, D.F.
Benavides Valazquez, Guillermo	Calle Regina # 24	México, D.F.
Benitez Flores, J. Ignacio ..	Tlaxcala # 177-901	México, D.F.
Berdala de Romero, Maria Teresa	Juan Ruíz de Alarcón # 99	Morelia, Michoacan
Berges Salgado, Gustavo ...	Insurgentes sur # 753 70. piso ..	México 18, D.F.
Berumen Lira, Francisco Julio	Lerdo # 101 sur desp. 504	Cd. Juárez, Chih.
Berrutia Manriquez, Antonio	Edif. Pons desp. 2	Irapuato, Gto.
Bek Beyer, Dieter Juan	Maria M. A. De Quevedo # 8 desp. 205	México 20, D.F.
Bidart Ramos, Bernardo ...	Zacatecas # 44 desp. 503, Col. Roma	México, D.F.
Biringer Esteban	San Juan de Letrán # 11-101 ...	México 1, D.F.
Bosque Romo, Manuel	Hidalgo # 211-213	Aguascalientes, Ags.

Brid Torres, Vicente	5 de Mayo # 225	Veracruz, Ver.
Buck Salazar, Nohemi	Jacarandes # 74-12, Santa María Insurgentes	México 4, D.F.
Bueno Ayala, Jesus Gerardo.	Central Médica	Cd. Juárez, Chih.
Caballero Herrera, Leandro .	Av. 1 # 518	Córdova, Ver.
Cabrera Rodriguez, Antonio.	Calle 55 # 511	Mérida, Yucatán
Cadena Cadena, Sergio	Morelos # 535 ote	Cd. Reynosa, Tamps.
Calderon Sanchez, Jose Maria	Ramón Corona # 128 nte	Cd. Juárez, Chih.
Camacho Guadarrama, Enriqueta	Oaxaca # 50-504	México 7, D.F.
Camacho Moreno, Humberto	Ac. Juárez y 13/a. # 171	Cd. Victoria, Tamps.
Campos Robledo, Heliodoro	Allende # 30	Irapuato, Gto.
Canudas Oreza, Eduardo ...	NNzcozari # 242 - Dpto. 1	Veracruz, Ver.
Carral Escalante, Manuel ...	Durango # 33-44	México 7, D.F.
Castañeda Humberto, Lucio.	Rivera de san Cosme # 134-104 Col. San Rafeal	México 4, D.F.
Castellanos Gutierrez, Angel.	Av. México # 120 nte	Tepic, Nay.
Castellanos Hernandez, Marco Antonio	División del Norte # 19-201, Col. del Valle	México, D.F.
Castillas Centeno, Carlos J. .	Calle 60 # 197	Mérida, Yuc.
Castilleja Buendia, Arturo ..	Av. Trujillo # 672-305	México 14, D.F.
Castillo Ramirez, Angelina .	Av. de los Pinos # 24, Col. Ampliación Providencia	México 4, D.F.
Castro Riddle, Guillermo ..	Tlaxcala # 177-601	México 7, D.F.
Carrillo Ballesteros, Luis Angel	16 de Septiembre # 103 altos ...	Toluca, México
Cavazos Gallardo, Angel ...	Cuauhtemoc # 105	Monclova, Coah.
Cavazos Treviño, Ezequiel .	Río Mocorito # 247, Col. México	Monterrey, N.L.
Cerna Martinez, Abel	Madero ote. # 560	Morelia, Mich.
Contreras Pliego, Joel Sergio	Medellín # 43-702, Col. Roma ..	México 7, D.F.
Correa Silva, Jose Luis	Coahuila # 159 Altos	México 7, D.F.
Contreras Garcia, Lizardo ..	Cuarto 403 residencia Médica, Av. Goyoacán # 1344	México, D.F.
Cruz Prieto, Mario	Insurgentes sur # 222-305	México 11, D.F.
Cruz Vega, Andres	Madero # 67-501	México 1, D.F.
Guagliotti Perez, Elizabeth .	San Borja # 633-205	México 12, D.F.
Cuevas Cancino, Diego	Eugenio Sué # 555	México 5, D.F.
Colmenero Tarin, Victor ...	Av. 5 de Mayo # 625	Tijuana, B.C.
Chacon Chavez, Manuel ...	Hospital Civil # 278	Guadalajara, Jal.
Chacon Mendoza, Arcadio .	Av. Madero # 557 altos	Mexicali, B.C.
Chacon Torres, Edmundo ..	Medellín # 94	México, D.F.
Chantiri Perez, Jorge Nicolas	Arista # 1020 altos	Veracruz, Ver.
Chavez Anaya, Eugenio ...	Pedro Moreno # 1348 S.J.	Guadalajara, Jal.
Chavez Morfin, Fernando ..	Ezequiel Montes # 135, Hospital de Nuestra Señora de la Luz .	México, D.F.
Chávez Taboada, Emma ...	Hamburgo # 302	México 7, D.F.
Chavez Anaya, Francisco ..	Benjamin Romero # 65, Arcos Sur	Guadalajara, Jal.
Chavira Diaz, Sergio Raul ..	Regina # 7-8	México 1, D.F.
Chayet Wolchansky, Jose ..	Madero # 3340 pte	Monterrey, N.L.
Dalma Kende, Alejandro ...	Paseo de las Palmas # 745-1202 .	México, D.F.
De Buen L. de H., Sadi	Zompatilla # 45, Coyoacan	México, D.F.
De Neira Laporte, Eduardo .	Campeche # 46, Col. Roma	México 7, D.F.

De Nigris Albricci, Buena Ventura	Clínica de Diagnóstico, Allende # 700 ote	Torreón, Coah.
De Noriega Garcia, Juan ...	Durango # 193-304	México 7, D.F.
De Tuono Zorzatto, Vinivio.	Durango # 213, Col. Roma	México 7, D.F.
Del Bosque Uribe, Sergio ..	Oriente # 2 # 10	Orizaba, Ver.
Del Castillo Fernandez, Gustavo	25 ote. # 1014	Puebla, Pueb.
Desentis Lezama, Agustin ..	Plaza de la Republica # 1 ote ...	Cd. Delicias, Chih.
De La Mora, Jorge	Republica del Salvador # 96-200 .	México 1, D.F.
De La O Almazan, Mario ..	Miguel Alemán # 211-401	Acapulco, Gro.
Diaz Aranda, Carlos Fernando	Angel Urraza # 206-1, Col. Vertiz noroeste	México 13, D.F.
Dominguez Cuevas, Bonfilio.	Vertiz # 184 dpto. 3	México, D.F.
Dominguez Villalpando, Eduardo	Av. Madero pte. 94-2	Querétaro, Qro.
Dorcich Miranda, Ernesto ..	Av. Aguilares # 219, Col. Libertad San Salvador, el Salvador .	Centroamérica
Duran Moisen, Salvador ...	Chilpancingo # 71	México, D.F.
Elizondo Cardenas, Arnoldo	Xicotencatl sur # 216	Saltillo, Coah.
Equihua Hernandez, Carlos .	Chihuahua # 3, Col. Roma	México 7, D.F.
Escalente Lozano, Victor Manuel	Londres y Berlín, Col. Andrade .	León, Gto.
Escalante Padilla, Jorge Antonio	San Luis Potosí # 126	México 7, D.F.
Escudero Bachè, R. Eduardo	Morelos y Garizuruta	Tuxpan, Ver.
Espinoza Gamez, Alberto ..	Homero # 411 1/er. piso, Col. Polanco	México, D.F.
Espinoza Bernal, Gabino ...	Av. Juarez # 128	Zacatecas, Zac.
Espinoza Olvera, Ydhelio ..	Nuevo León # 66 2/o. piso, Col. Hipódromo Condesa	México 11, D.F.
Faz Cole, Jose Roberto	Edif. Benavides Pino Suárez # 602 sur desp. 112	Monterrey, N.L.
Felguerez Mitra, Alejandro .	Bustamante # 112 desp. 112 ...	Oaxaca, Oax.
Fernandez Mc. Gregor, Jose Carlos	Antonio Caso # 28-3	México 14, D.F.
Figueroa Ortiz, Raymundo .	Cien fuegos # 665	México 14, D.F.
Flores Becerra, David	29 Southern Foreshore, Belico City	Centroamérica
Flores Castillo, Epigmenio .	Insurgentes Norte # 1333	México, D.F.
Flores Flores, Julio	Xola # 816	México 12, D.F.
Flores Hintz, Andres	Tehuantepec # 257 5/o. piso ...	México, D.F.
Flores Montalvo, Jose Maria.	Centro Médico de Altamira, Altamira 11 Pte. dpto. 303	Tampico, Tamps.
Foncerrada Benitez, Pedro .	PRivada 3 B # 3905, Col Pastor .	Puebla, Puebla
Fonte Barcenas, Anselmo ..	Av. Nuevo León # 66 2/o. piso ..	México 11, D.F.
Fonte Vazquez, Sanselmo ..	Av. Nuevo León # 66 2/o. piso ..	México 11, D.F.
Fromow Garcia, Jorge	Medellin # 43-206	México, D.F.
Gallegos Abrego, Arturo ...	Morelos # 604 Pte	Torreon, Coah.
Garcia Maravilla, Salvador ..	Justo Sierra # 2107	Guadalajara, Jal.
Garcia Mendez, Gonzalo ...	Dr. Galvez # 233-102, San Angel .	México 20, D.F.
Garcia Mendez, Oscar	6a SUR # 14	Tapachula, Chis.
Garcia Mondracon, Jose Pablo	División del Norte # 2748	México 21, D.F.
Garcia Roel, Alfonso	M. Arreola # 507 ote	Monterrey, N.L.

Garduño Ballesteros, Eduardo	Monterrey # 70 5/o. piso	México 7, D.F.
Garduño Espinoza, Leopoldo	Hegel # 228 6/o. piso	México 5, D.F.
Garibay Fernandez, Alfonso.	Allende # 305 ote	Torreon, Coah.
Garza Elizondo, Rogelio	Villagran # 424 ote	Monterrey, N.L.
Garza Treviño, Luis	Av. Pino Suárez # 440 sur	Monterrey, N.L.
Garza Zambrano, Felipe	Washington # 416 ote	Monterrey, N.L.
Garza Zambrano, Jorge	Washington # 416 ote	Monterrey, N.L.
Godinez Cejudo, Jorge	Arista # 19, Col. Guerrero	México 3, D.F.
Gomez Ballesteros, Rangel Efren	13 sur # 2510	Puebla, Puebla
Gomez Campaña, Humberto	Rosales # 318 pte	Culiacán, Sin.
Gomez Jimenez, Javier	Brillante # 26, Col. Estrella	México 14, D.F.
Gomez Leal, Alfredo	Reynosa # 22, Col. Hipódromo Condesa	México 11, D.F.
Gomez Verdin, Rodolfo	Ojinaga # 417 desp. 14	Chihuahua, Chih.
Gonzalez Campa, Alberto	Residencia Hospital 20 de Noviembre, Cuarto # 909	México 12, D.F.
Gonzalez De Vizcarra, Petra Maria	Av. col. del Valle # 419	México 12, D.F.
Gonzalez Garcia, Fernando	Aramberri # 506 ote	Monterrey, N.L.
Gonzalez Garza, Federico H.	5 de Mayo ote. # 438 'A'	Monterrey, N.L.
Gonzalez Lugo Tirso, Rene	Calle 57 # 471	Mérida, Yuc.
Gonzales Reynosa, Jorge A.	Centro Médico de especialidades # 201	Cd. Juárez, Chih.
Gonzalez Rubio, Estela	Matamoros # 413 ote	Monterrey, N.L.
Gonzalez y Gutierrez, Luis	Insurgentes sur # 662-204	México 12, D.F.
Graue Diaz, Gonzalez Enrique	Oaxaca # 46-103	México, D.F.
Guerra Cruz, Jose C.	Veracruz sur # 310	Cd. Obregón, Son.
Guerra De Fromow, Ana Maria	Medellin # 43-206	México, D.F.
Guerra Strop, Ricardo	Amsterdam # 271-103	México 11, D.F.
Guerrero Butron, Salvador	Sinaloa # 10	México 7, D.F.
Guerrero Murillo, Alberto	Obregon # 421	Aguascalientes, Ags.
Guevara Bautista, Evaristo	Insurgentes sur # 1194-403	México 12, D.F.
Gutierrez Gerrera, Jesus Vidal	Zacatecas # 44-5/10. piso	México, D.F.
Gutierrez Osuna, L. Alberto.	Av. Cuauhtemoc # 1424-5	México 13, D.F.
Gutierrez Perez, David	Hegel # 228 6/o. piso	México, D.F.
Gutierrez Zambrano, Miguel Angel	Av. Ridalgo # 25-36 pte., Col. Obispado	Monterrey, N.L.
Heatley Green, Jean	Durango # 33-32	México 7, D.F.
Hernandez Barrenechea, Gaspar	Jalapa # 13	México, D.F.
Hernandez Benavente, J. Manuel	Israel # 404, Col. León Moderna	Léon, Gto.
Hernandez Ceballos, Miguel.	Hegel # 228	México, D.F.
Hernandez Ibarra, Jorge	Guanajuato # 100-101, Coi. Roma	México, D.F.
Hernandez Ramirez, Carlos	Insurgentes sur # 1772	México, D.F.
Hernandez Reynante, Gaston	Av. Avila Cammacho # 125	Jalapa, Ver.

Hernandez Sanchez, Everardo .... Quevedo # 129-202, Col. Noroeste   México, D.F.

Hernandez Vazquez, Eustolio .... Van Dyk 40 # 120 'B' ....   México, 19, D.F.

Herreman Cornu, Rogelio .. Insurgentes sur # 1020-103 ....   México 12, D.F.

Herrera Urrutia, Manuel ... Galeana # 215 ....   Toluca, Edo. de México

Huesca Perez, Juan .... Morelos # 665 ote ....   Cd. Reynosa, Tamps.

Ibarra Lopez, Humberto ... Noé # 9-114, Col. Guadalupe
Tepeyac ....   México, 14, D.F.

Igartua Araiza, Jaime ..... Insurgentes sur # 753 7o. piso ..   México, D.F.

Iglesias Ortiz, Carlos ...... Alcalde # 383 ....   Guadalajara, Jal.

Isais Cortes, Hector .... Bucken # 16 2o. piso ....   México, D.F.

Kai Aguilar, Antonio ..... Av. Juarez # 78-5 ....   Jalapa. Ver.

Kulas Tejeda, Tasaki ...... López Velardo # 500 ....   Zacatecas, Zac.

Laustaunau Morles, Arturo . Plaza 5 de mayo y Av. Alvaro
Obregón, Edif. Isabel Dpto.
'A' ....   Navojoa, Sonora

Lara Mondragonm, Juan ... Hamburgo # 288-10, Col. Juárez   México 6, D.F.

Lara Sainz, Hector Antonio   Bolivar # 12-306 ....   Chihuahua, Chih.

Leal Bravo, Ricardo, Gabriel Estrella # 111 ....   México 3, D.F.

Lelo De Larrea, Rodriguez
Arturo .... Insurgentes sur # 753 7o. piso ..   México 18, D.F.

Leon Gonzalez, Andres
Francisco .... Central Médica Quirurgica .....   Los Mochis, Sinaloa.

Leon Rodriguez, Jorge .... 1a, av. sur # 254, Central Médica .   Tuxtla, Gutiérrez, Chis.

Limon de Brow, Ema ..... Oaxaca # 86 7o. piso, Col. Roma   México 7, D.F.

Lemelin Aragon, Jose Manuel .... T. Medina # 140 ....   México 8, D.F.

Lopez Alonso, Carlos ...... Calle 55 # 533 ....   Mérida, Yucatán

Lopez Bustillos, Jorge ..... Mario Molina # 469 ....   Veracruz, Ver.

Lozano Elizondo, David ... Patriotismo # 880 ....   México 19, D.F.

Loya Saldaña, Roberto .... Insurgentes # 303-201, Col. Hipó-
dromo Condesa ....   México, D.F.

Maya Fletcher, Maria Isabel . Guerrero # 512 ote. B ....   Cd. Mante, Tamps.

Mc. Gregor de La Fuente,
Juan Roberto .... Concepción Beistegui # 18, Col.
del Valle ....   México, D.F.

Mc. Gregor Fernandez, Luis . Tehuantepec # 204 ier. piso ....   México, D.F.

Macip Herrara, Moises ..... Rio Tuxpan # 5320, Col. San
Manuel ....   Puebla, Puebla

Madero Garza, German .... Centro Médico 2o. piso, Allende
351 ote ....   Torreón, Coah

Magro Garcia, Julio .... Aguscalientes # 201-704 ....   México 11, D.F.

Malacara Hernandez, Jose de
Jesus .... Coahuila # 5 int. 4, Col Roma ...   México 7, D.F.

Marin Jose, Maria .... Emilio Carranza # 103-102 .....   México 9, D.F.

Marquez Zavala, Genaro ... Havre # 7-702 ....   México 6, D.F.

Martin Lopez, Isela Frida .. Unidad Cuitlahuac Edif. # 13
desp 301 entrada 'A', Col
Naval ....   México 16, D.F.

Martinez Ballesteros, Luis .. Rio Neva # 28 ....   México 5, D.F.

Martinez Bracamontes, Julio Av. Hidalgo # 106 ....   Navojoa, Sonora

Martinez Castro, Guillermo
Francisco .... Concepción Méndez # 97 ......   México 12, D.F.

Martinez Olmos, Ricardo .. 20 de Noviembre # 28-125 .....   México, D.F.

Martinez Romo, Joaquin .. Insurgentes sur # 53-3 ....   México, D.F.

Martinez Treviño, Ramiro ..	Pino Suárez # 602-102	Monterrey, N.L.
Mascott Castro, Manuel ...	Campeche # 102 'A'	México, D.F.
Mata Flores, Felipe	Cien Fuegos # 678 desp. 1	México, D.F.
Marrufo Pavia, Eyder	Calle 21 # 281	México, Yucatán
Mejia Galderon, Sonia	Durango # 33-4, Col. Roma	México, 7 D.F.
Mejia Segundo, Julio	Alvaro Obregón # 64	Morelia, Michoacán
Menendez Esquivel, Rosalia .	Sixto Osuna # 23 pte	Mazatlán, Sinaloa
Mendez Fernandez, Ruperto	Monterrey # 172-1	México, 7 D.F.
Mendez Gutierrez, Antonio .	Av. Reforma # 1277	Mexicali, B.C.
Mendoza Tapia, Eduardo ..	Hacienda de San José Vistahermosa # 45	Bosuqes de Echegaray, Edo. de Méx.
Mesa Zamora, Ermando ...	Milwoauques # 62, Col. Nápoles .	México, D.F.
Meyran Garcia, Jorge	2a. de Juárez # 42, Col. San Alvaro	México 17, D.F.
Mijares Salinas, Ignacio	Padre Mier # 327 pte. 102	Monterrey, N.L.
Miranda Martinez, Aurora ..	Dakota # 308-3	México 18, D.F.
Miranda Rueda, Jorge	Centro Médico de especialidades .	Cd. Juárez, Chih.
Monares Garcia, Enrique ...	Cuauhtemoc # 545-1	México, 12, D.F.
Montellano Carrera, Francisco	Sonora # 49-201	México, D.F.
Montufar Borja, Apolinar ..	Av. California # 209-204	México 13, D.F.
Morales Jaramillo, Sergio Ernesto	Coronado # 10 desp. 6	Parral, Chih.
Morales Ledezma, Virgilio .	Leibnitz # 14-701	México 5, D.F.
Moreno Alvarez, Salvador ..	Independencia # 4 'A' A	Uruapan, Mich.
Moreno Armengual, Abelardo	Juárez # 62	Jalapa, Ver.
Montemayor Quintanilla, Jesuus Mario	Pino Suárez sur # 550-305	Monterrey, N.L.
Montemayor Salazar, Jesus .	Hidalgo # 2557 pte. desp. 604 ..	Monterrey, N.L.
Muñoz Flores Rosales, Sergio	Rivero y Gutiérrez # 301	Aguascalientes, Ags.
Murillo Fajardo, Renan	Nueva York # 32-303, Col. Nápoles	México 18, D.F.
Murillo Murillo, Leopoldo .	Nueva York # 32-303, Col Nápoles	México 18, D.F.
Malpica Aguilar, Eziquiel ...	Cuauhtemoc # 22-410	Acapulco, Gro.
Namba, Carlos	Arista # 19, Col. Guerrero	México 3, D.F.
Narvaez Angulo, Alberto ..	5 De Mayo # 114-104	Oaxaca, Oax.
Narvaez Angulo, Jose	Insurgentes sur # 300-510, Col. Roma	México, D.F.
Navarro Zimbron, Graciela .	Insurgentes sur # 605-502	México 18, D.F.
Navarro Zimbron, Mario ...	Insurgentes sur # 605-502	México 18, D.F.
Niño Ramos, Angel	Independencia # 433 Pte. 4	Los Mochis, Sinaloa
Nieto Pro, Maximiliano	Obregón # 113 ote.	Tampico, Tamps.
Noble Gtiérrez, Carlos	Tepic # 139 6o. puso, Col. Anzures	México 7, D.F.
Newton Sanchez, Jorge	Combate de las Juntas # 13 'A', Col. Residencial Militar	México, D.F.
Obregon Gonzalez, Oscar Emilio	6a. Av. calle # 72 'H'	Matamoros, Tamps.
O'Kelard Gonzalez, Pedro Pablo Rene	Séneca # 123	México 5, D.F.
Olivares del Castillo, Salvador	Av. Independencia # 318	Tehuacán, Pueb.

602   MEXICO

Oliver Aguirre, Porfirio	F.T.S. de Mier # 1028, Jardín Balbuena	México, D.F.
Olivera Lopez, Ramon	Toledo # 134	México 13, D.F.
Ortega Lojero, Jose Luis ...	Yang-Tse # 29-1	México, D.F.
Padilla de Alba, Francisco ..	Insurgentes sur # 363-303	México, D.F.
Paez Stille, Cecilio	Bartolome de las Casas # 636, Centro Médico	Morelia, Mich.
Palomino Dena, Feliciano ..	Londres # 44	México 6, D.F.
Paredes Salazar, Raul	Boulevard Benito Juárez # 300 ..	Cuernavaca, Morelos
Pasapera Ausenacc, Agustin	Marina Nacional # 123-104	México, D.F.
Paz Gutierrez, Miguel Angel .	Av. Universidad # 584-401	México, D.F.
Perez Fuentes, Isacc Julio ..	B. Garcia López G. calle 9	Guaymas, Sonora
Perez Valenzuela, Josue ...	Niño Perdido # 854	México 13, D.F.
Pintos Carvallo, Manuel ...	11 Pte. # 1302	Puebla, Puebla
Preza Martinez, Juan Antonio	Andador Juan Mancilla Ríos # 306-7, Cotoacan Col. Romero de Terreros	México, D.F.
Pizaña Guerra, Enrique	Morelos # 81	Matamoros. Tamps.
Poblano Ordoñez, Juvencio .	Irrigacion # 36, Col. Irrigación ..	México 10, D.F.
Ponce Arambula, Jose Arturo	Aquiles Serdán # 665 2o. piso ..	Morelia, Mich.
Prado Romaña, Rafael	Arista # 19, Col. Guerrero	México, D.F.
Prado Romaña, Vyeira Felipe	Arista # 19, Col. Guerrero	México, D.F.
Prieto Lopez, Hernandez ..	Monterrey # 172, Col. Roma ...	México 7, D.F.
Puig Solanes, Magin	Medellín # 94-6, Col. Roma	México 7, D.F.
Quiroz Barranco, Roberto	Insurgentes Centro # 23 'B'	México 4, D.F.
Quiroz y Carrasco, Jose Antonio	Colima # 220 desp. 301	México 21, D.F.
Quiroz Salgado, Carlos	Bajío # 203-204	México 7, D.F.
Rabinovitz Kroheim, Enrique	Chilpancingo # 51-501	México 11, D.F.
Ramirez Barreto, Antonio .	José María Velasco # 110-102, San Juan INN	México 19, D.F.
Ramirez Gilbon, Julio	Zacatecas # 230	México, D.F.
Ramirez Gonzalez, Armando	Monterry # 70 5o. piso	México, D.F.
Ramos Argote, Ricardo ...	16 de Septiembre de 1926	Cd. Juárez, Chih.
Ramos Renteria, Jose de Jesusu	Edif. 11 entrada 2 desp. 504, Tlatelolco	México, D.F.
Ramirez Lopez, Lucila	Calle 'A' # 70, Col Ampliacion Iganacio Zaragoza	México 9, D.F.
Rangel Galvez, Isidro	Constitución # 104 altos	Toluca, Mexico
Romolina Lopez, Emilio ...	Monterrey # 381 dpto. 101	México, D.F.
Renteria Perez, Jose Luis ..	Calle E. Manzana 2, Col. Educación	México, D.F.
Rico Rodriguez, J. Antonio .	Torcuato Taso # 335	México, D.F.
Rivero Borrell, V. Hector ..	Veracruz # 93	México 11, D.F.
Rocha Pellon, Jose	Sonora # 70 Pte	Hermosillo, Sonora
Rodriguez Cerda, Antonio .	Venustiano Carranza # 16	Zacapu, Mich.
Rodriguez Gomez, Juan de Dios	Zaragoza # 304-101	Coatzoacalcos, Ver.
Rodriguez Lara, Enrique ...	Boulevard Avila Camcho # 3219, Col Florida	Naucalpan, Edo. de México
Rodriguez Loaiza, Hector ..	Aldama # 523-202	Villahermosa, Tabasco

Rodriquez, Maria Luisa (Vendre)	Tabasco # 66, Col Roma	México, D.F.
Rodriguez Ramos, Rigoberto	Obregón # 240	Nogales, Sonora
Rodriguez Vazquez, Rodolfo	Chiapas # 91-401, Col. Roma ...	México 11, D.F.
Rojas Dorsal, Adrian Jose ..	Retorno # 811-15, Col. Centinela	México 21, D.F.
Rojas Moreno, Miguel	Privada # 7 sur 'A' No. 4504 ...	Puebla, Puebla.
Romero Apis, David	Descartes # 7	México 5, D.F.
Romero Venegas, Maria Teresa	Mezquitan # 1955	Gualdalajara, Jal.
Romero Villanueva, Ramon.	Hidalgo privada S/N	Zamora, Mich.
Romo Mora, Salvador	Gante # 15-125	México 1, D.F.
Romo Santos, Efrain	Ponciano Arriaga # 23 dpto. 200.	México 1, D.F.
Ross, Antonio	Torcuato Tasso # 321-101, Col. Polanco	México 5, D.F.
Romero Garcia, Rafael Maximiliano	Campo Matillas # 22, Ampliación San Antonio Azcapotzalco ..	México 16, D.F.
Rosales Tirado, Gilberto ...	Retorno # 45-51, Col. Jardin Balbuena	México, D.F.
Rosas Garcia, Roberto	Pedro Romero # 552 S.H.	Gudalajara, Jal.
Rosas Marin, Fernando E. ..	56 B # 498, Prolongación Montejo	Mérida. Yucatán
Rosas Santos, Gustavo	3a. sur # 103-101	Puebla, Puebla
Saenz Canales, Jose	Av. Obregón # 213 ote	Tampico, Tamps.
Sainz De La Fuente Casasa, Ricardo	Madero # 209	Cosamaloapan, Ver.
Saenz De Viteri, Manuel ...	Filadelfia # 119 4o. piso, Col. Nápoles	México 18, D.F.
Sahagun Barragan, Hector Javier	Hidalgo sur # 127	Zamora, Mich.
Salazar Lopez, Edmundo ..	Jalisco # 10 pte	Hermosillo, Son.
Salazar Salazar, Juan	Berlin # 31 6o. piso, Col. Juárez .	México 6, D.F.
Salazar Candell, Hugo	Av. Universidad # 375-3 'B'	México, D.F.
Salinas Rios, Carlos Rodolfo	Malecón M. Alemán # 23	Campeche, Camp.
Sanabria Madrid, Armando Hector	Matías Romero # 1353-1, Col. Vertiz Narvarte	México 13, D.F.
Sanchez Alarcon, Ignacio ..	Campana # 10	Mazatlán, Sinaloa
Sanchez Bulnes, Luis	Mérida # 119, Col. Roma	México 7, D.F.
Sanchez Davalos, Carlos ...	Hidalgo # 62 altos	Minatitlán, Ver.
Sanchez Fontan, Rafael ...	Mérida # 119, Col. Roma	Mexico 7, D.F.
Sanchez Gonzalez, Martha .	Av. Mutualismo # 706	Tijuana, B.C.
Sanchez Nuñez, Hector	Sinaloa # 9-409	México 7, D.F.
Santos Mazal, Ruel	Aristóteles # 98, Col. Polanco ..	México 5, D.F.
Sauter Treger, G. Alexander.	Reforma # 510-502	México 6, D.F.
Sayavedra Madrigal, Humberto	Alcalde # 3162	Guadalajara, Jal.
Serrano Anaya, Armando ..	Bravo # 611	La Paz, B.C.
Serrano Sanchez, Augustin .	Nte. # 56 'A' # 5403	México, D.F.
Silva Zeron, Sabino	Insurgentes sur # 1429-44	México 11, D.F.
Suarez Velazquez, Victor Manuel	Cuauhtemoc # 308 Nte	Cd. Mante, Tamps.
Takane Watanabe, Alvaro Shizo	Revolución # 156 'C', Col. Tacubaya	México 18, D.F.

Teran Garcia, Maria De Los Angeles	Av. Guanabana # 254, Col. Nueva Santa María	México, D.F.
Tirado Cruz, Jaime	Casa 5, Hospital Central Militar, Lomas de Sotelo	México 10, D.F.
Torres Estrada, Antonio ...	Soerre Paracaima # 1335, Col. Lomas de Chapultepec	México 10, D.F.
Tovilla Pomar, Jose Luis ...	Nueva York # 310, Col. Nápoles .	México 18, D.F.
Treviño Campuzano, Adolfo	Tepic # 139-604	México 7, D.F.
Treviño Guerreroa, Alonso Mario	Tapia # 150 ote	Monterrey, N.L.
Tuiran Vergara, Jose	Puerta de México Unidad 'B' dpto. 25	Piedra Negras, Coah.
Valdez Hernandez, Alberto L.	Clínica México, Terán y morales .	Piedras Negras, Coah.
Vazquez Nuñez, Gregorio ..	Oriente # 67 No. 2808	México 8, D.F.
Velez, O. Daniel	Aldama # 29, Col. Nápoles	México 18, D.F.
Torres Baquedano, Clementina	Crater # 441	México 20, D.F.
Ventosa Ortega, Federico ..	Residencia Médica # 404, Hospital 20 de noviembre	México 12, D.F.
Vyeira Martinez, Fernando .	Mirrano Sanchez # 20	Tlaxcala, Tlax.
Villanueva, Diaz, Gil	Cozumel 75	México 7, D.F.
Villarreal Ruiz, Roberto ...	Morelos # 818 pte.	Torreón, Coah.
Villaseñor Schwarz, Juan Horacio	Querétaro # 238-401	México, D.F.
Villegas Leon, Lucina	Rio Amoy # 13, Col. Cuauhtemoc	México 5, D.F.
Vivanco Avalos, Adrian Agustin	Av. Morelos # 3-20	Tlalnepantla, edo. de México
Valverde Gonzalez, Roman .	Morelos # 68, Inxtapalapa	México, D.F.
Wallentin Springer, Roberto.	Eucken # 16-202	México 5, D.F.
Warman Griyj, Alberto	Gelati # 29-111, Hospital Mocel .	México 10, D.F.
Washington Garza, Guillermo	Rosales # 15 Ote.	Culiacan, Sinaloa
Waxman Sherwin, Benjamin	Galápagos # 311, Col. Vistahermosa	Monterrey, N.L.
Zaldivar Bernal, Carlos	Plaza de la República # 51 2/o. piso	México 1, D.F.
Zamora Camacho, J. Francisco	Av. Cuauhtemoc # 95	Acupulco, Gro.
Zavala Bustillos, Raul	Aldama # 610	Villahermosa, Tab.
Zepeda Squer, Jaime	Luárez y 2a. Oeste	Cananea, Sonora
Zertuche Rodriguez, Abelardo	Durango # 296	México 7, D.F.

NOSCOMIA QUIBUS OCULIS AEGRI CURANTUR

Hospital de Nuestra Senora de la Luz, Ezequiel Montes # 135, Mexico 4, D.F.
Hospital Centro Médico Nacional des I.M.S.S. Sala de Oftalmología, Av. Cuauhtémoc 330-C, Mexico 7, D.F.

INSTITUTA SCHOLAEQUE CAECIS DESTINATAE

Escuela Nacional de Ciegos. Mixcalco No. 6. México 1, D.F.
Comité Internacional pro-ciegos Mariano Azuela No. 219, México 4, D.F.
Instituto Nacional Para la rehabilitación de los Ciegos. Viena No. 87, Coyoacán, México 21, D.F.

NORTVEGIA

SOCIETATES OPHTHALMOLOGICAE

Norsk Oftalmologisk Forening
President: Dr. Hans J. Holst
Secretary: Dr. Kaare Sandvig, Ringeriksveien 23, 1300 Sandvika
Number of members: 120

NOMINA ET DOMICILIA MEDICORUM AB OCULIS

Aalde, Ole	Øyeavdelingen, Bodø Sykehus ..	8000 Bodø
Aanesen, Nils T.	Øyeavdelingen, Tromsø Sykehus .	9000 Tromsø
Aanonsen, Alf B.	Epabygget	3900 Porsgrunn
Aasved, Henry	Øyeavdelingen, Haukeland Syke-hus	5000 Bergen
Abel, Hassa	Dronningensgt. 5	4000 Stavanger
Anseth, Arvid	Øyeavdelingen, Tromsø Sykehus .	9000 Tromsø
Arnesen, Prof. Kristen	Pat. Anat. Institutt, Ullevål Syke-hus	Oslo
Askelund, Per	Klostergt. 75	7000 Trondheim
Aulie, Kari	....	3600 Kongsberg
Berg, Tormod Holst	Arnebråtvn. 17 b, Smestad	Oslo 3
Bergaust, Bjørn	....	Lillehammer
Berger, Bjørn	Nordengveien 88	Oslo
Bertelsen, Prof. Torstein ...	Universitetets øyeavd., Haukeland Sykehus	5000 Bergen
Bjerke, Otto	....	2400 Elverum
Blomskøld, Gustav A.	....	8500 Narvik
Bore, John	Flatmyrgt. 173	5500 Haugesund
Borthne, Anders	Øyeavd., Bodø Sykehus	8000 Bodø
Braathen, Harald	Oyeavdelingen, Ålesund Sykehus .	6000 Ålesund
Braathen, Leif	Oyeavd., Namdal Sykehus	7800 Namsos
Braathen, Sverre	Kannikbakken 2	4000 Stavanger
Bulie, Tore	Øyeavd., Rikshospitalet	Oslo
Bull, Nicolai	Pilestredet 15	Oslo
Christensen, Gunnar	Sparebankgården	1600 Fredrikstad
Davanger, Martin	Rikshospitalet, øyeavd.	Oslo
Dybdahl, Tore	Teatergt 11	Oslo
Egeberg, Knut	....	4800 Arendal
Egge, Kjell	Fylkeshuset, Fylkeslegekontoret	3100 Tønsberg
Eitrem, Egil	....	3100 Tønsberg
Elstad, Kristian	....	2800 Gjøvik
Elvemo, Hans	....	8600 Mo i Rana
Flage, Thor	Øyeavdelingen, Rikshospitalet ..	Oslo
Forbord, Magnar	....	7600 Levanger
Foss, Bjørn	Bogstadveien 20	Oslo
Gjeruldsen, Sven	Øyeavdelingen, Rikshospitalet ..	Oslo
Granaas, Alf H.	Ødegaard i Randesund	4600 Kristiansand S.
Grøndahl, Jan	Gml. Drammensveien 33	1320 Stabekk
Gaarder, Ole	Storgt. 14	Oslo
Halseide, Reidar	Øyeavdelingen, Rikshospitalet ..	Oslo

Hansen, Egill	Øyeavdelingen, Rikshospitalet ..	Oslo
Hasne, Armand		3900 Porsgrunn
Hesselberg, Charles		1500 Moss
Hetland-Eriksen, Jens	Øyeavd., Ullevål Sykehus	Oslo
Hexeberg, Trygve N.	Slottsgt. 23	Oslo 1
Holst, Hans J.	Pilestredet 15	Oslo
Holst, Johan Collett	Pilestredet 15	Oslo
Horn, Einar	Karl Johansgt. 20	Oslo
Horne, Per	Nedre Storgt. 3	3000 Drammen
Hveding, Arnljot	Nedre Slottsgt. 23	Oslo
Hørven, Prof. Eivind	Teatergt. 3	Oslo 1
Hørven, Ivar	Øyeavd., Rishosp.	Oslo
Haarr, Marius	Øyeavd., Ålesund Sykehus	Ålesund
Ihler, Jon	Øyeavd., Telemark Fylkessykehus	3700 Skien
Jensen, Per	Romsøgården	4000 Stavanger
Johansen, Otto	Karl Johansgt.	Oslo
Kjensmo, Edel	Solhaugveien 94, Jongskollen ...	1300 Sandvika
Klouman, Otto	Strandgt. 27	4600 Kristiansand S.
Kolstad, Albert	Øyeavd., Ullevål Sykehus	Oslo
Kristiansen, Odd		2200 Kongsvinger
Lager, Reidar	Øyeavd., Haukeland Sykehus ...	5000 Bergen
Larsen, Jon	Øyeavd, Rikshospitalet	Oslo
Leira, Håkon	Kongensgt. 49	7000 Trondheim
Løche, Ragnar	Storgt. 12	3100 Tønsberg
Malling, Prof. Dirger	Teatergt. 11	Oslo
Mathiesen, Per Schjelderup	Karl Johansgt. 2	Oslo
Midtbø, Arne	Schwenckesgt. 5	3000 Drammen
Mohn, Arne	Grensen 3	Oslo
Moi, Ivar		3200 Sandefjord
Maartmann-Moe, Erik	Storgt. 17	3500 Hønefoss
Nicolaissen, Bjørn	Kirkeveien 64	Oslo
Nordhagen, Endre		3000 Drammen
Nyquist, Bengt	Valckendorffsgt. 1	5000 Bergen
Odd, Olaf		4800 Arendal
Odland, Magnus	Øyeavd., Haukeland Sykehus ...	5000 Bergen
Omvik, Per	Rosenbergsgt. 39	5000 Bergen
Opsahl, Roald	Øyeavd., Tromsø Sykehus	9000 Tromsø
Petersen, Finn		1700 Sarpsborg
Petersen, Hans Peter	Akersgt. 45	Oslo 1
Restan, Ludmilla	Arildsvei 28, Kjelsås	Oslo 4
Riise, Per	Kyhnsgt. 6	2300 Hamar
Riise, Dag	Øyeavd., St. Torfinns Klinikk ...	2300 Hamar
Rogge, Albert	Kaigt. 8	5000 Bergen
Ross, Reiulv	postboks 274	3001 Drammen
Røe, Oluf	Øyeavd., Namdal Sykehus	7800 Namsos
Sandberg, Hans Otto	Øyeavd., Ullevål Sykehus	Oslo
Sandvig, Kaare	Ringeriksveien 23	1300 Sandvika
Sato, Olav	Øyeavd., Rikshospitalet	Oslo
Saugstad, Arne	Akersgt. 41	Oslo
Schøne, Reier	Hegdehaugsveien 36	Oslo
Sellevold, Ole Jakob		4800 Arendal
Smith, Edvard	Waldemar Thranesgt. 14	Oslo
Standal, Brynjulv	Øyeavd., Molde Sykehus	Molde
Steinsvåg, Magnus		5500 Haugesund
Stuve, Arnold	Pilstredet 15	Oslo
Sunde, Olav Aga	Karl Johansgt. 20	Oslo

Syrdalen, Per	Øyeavdelingen, Rikshospitalet ..	Oslo
Syversen, Kjell	Øyeavdelingen, Haukeland Syke-hus	5000 Bergen
Saebø, Johan	....	3700 Skien
Saeteren, Torstein	Teatergt. 2	Oslo
Thomassen, Thore Lie, prof.	Øyeavd. Rikshospitalet	Oslo
Tjåland, Johan	Labben 9	Oslo
Torlei, Knut	Rådstueplass 2	5000 Bergen
Trumpy, Einar	Karl Johansgt. 13	Oslo
Tveiten, Berge	Markvn. 2a	Bergen
Tønjum, Asbjørn	Øyeavd., Rikshospitalet	Oslo
Tønjum, Knut	....	3100 Tønsberg
Uchermann, J. Albert	Svaneapoteket	5000 Bergen
Udjus, Ludvig G.	Wilses vei 10	Jar
Udnaes, Ingar	Øyeavdelingen, Molde Sykehus ..	6400 Molde
Valebjørg, Halvard	Korsvoll Terasse 12	Oslo 8
Vallersnes, Odd	....	5500 Haugesund
Weidemann, Johan	Idungården	7000 Trondheim
Westby, Reidar	Øyeavd., Fredrikstad Sykehus ..	1600 Fredrikstad
Wirsching, Johan	Nedre Vargvei 3	3100 Tønsberg
Wirsching, Ludvig sen.	Wergelandsveien 7	4600 Kristiansand S.
Wirsching. Ludvig jr.	Fruens Alle	4600 Kristiansand S.
Wium, Erling	....	1750 Halden
Waalen, Thorbjørn	....	2800 Gjøvik
Waaler, Paul	Kirkegt. 70	2600 Lillehammer
Yitteborg, Prof. Jan	Øyeavdelingen, Ullevål Sykehus .	Oslo

NOSOCOMIA QUIBUS OCULIS AEGRI CURANTUR

	No. of Beds
Universitetets Øyeklinikk, Rikshospitalet, Oslo, Prof. dr. med. Th. L. Thomassen	98
Ullevål Sykehus, Øyeklinikk, Oslo, Prof. dr. med. J. Ytteborg	38
Universitetets Øyeklinikk, Haukeland Sykehus, Bergen, Prof. dr. med. T. Bertelsen	50
Sentralsykehuset i Tromsø, Øyeklinikk, Tromsø, Prof. dr. med. Arvid Anseth	24
Bodø Sykehus, Øyeavdeling, Bodø, Overlege Ole Aalde	30
Namdal Sykehus, Øyeavdeling, Namsos, Overlege dr. med. Oluf Røe	25
Sentralsykehuset i Trondheim, Øyeavd., Trondheim, Overlege dr. med. Håkon Leira	28
Molde Sykehus, Øyeavdeling, Molde, Overlege Brynjulv Standal	28
Alesund Sykehus, Øyeavdeling, Ålesund, Overlege dr. med. Marius Haarr	33
Hamar Fylkessykehus, Øyeavdeling, Hamar, Overlege Dag Riise	35
Telemark Fylkessykehus, Øyeavdeling, Skien, Overlege Jon Øistein Ihler	25
Sentralsykehuset for Østfold, Øyeavdeling, Fredrikstad, Overlege Reidar Westbye	21

INSTITUTA SCHOLAEQUE CAECIS DESTINATAE

	inmates
Dalen offentlige skole for blinde, Trondheim	75
Huseby offentlige skole for blinde, Røa, Oslo	112
Hovseter forskole for svaksynte barn, Oslo	12
Emma Hiorths Hjem, Sandvika	36

NOVA ZEALANDIA

SOCIETATES OPHTHALMOLOGICAE

The Ophthalmological Society of New Zealand

President: A. C. Sandston
President-Elect: B. J. Bowden
Vice-President: R. J. Croke
Past President: A. N. Talbot
Secretary Treasurer: G. G. Powell, 274 A Remuera Road, Remuera, Auckland 5
Assistent-Secretary: J. C. D. Macdiarmid
Ed. of Transactions: J. C. Parr
Business Ed. of Transactions: R. M. P. Reynolds
Executives: R. F. Elliott, W. R. Holmes, L. W. Poole
Number of members: 70

NOMINA ET DOMICILIA MEDICORUM AB OCULIS

Ashbridge, M. R.	P.O. Box 664	Rotorua
Averill, T	110 Armagh Street	Christchurch 1
Bell, L. G.	Mayfair Chambers, 48 The Terrace	Wellington
Bowden, B. J.	107 Hatea Drive	Whangarei
Burns, W. L. B.	249 Papanui Road	Christchurch 1
Campbell, G. B.	363 Hardy Street	Nelson
Cox, S. D.	Thompson's Buildings, Ward St.	Hamilton
Croke, R. J.	251 Broadway Ave.	Palmerston North
Coop, H. V.	Cintra House, Whitaker Place	Auckland 1
Davidson, G.	Kelvin Chambers, 16 The Terrace.	Wellington
Doctor, J. A.	48 Winara Ave.	Waikanae
Elliott, R. F.	Wellington Club, Plaza, The Terrace	Wellington
Fenton, C. R.	Mayfair Chambers, 48 The Terrace	Wellington
Fenwick, G. de L.	17 Mount Street	Auckland 1
Ferguson, R. H. L.	Cinta House, Whitaker Place	Auckland 1
Hay, J. R.	80 Glandovey Road	Christchurch
Henderson, J. M.	39 Princes Street	Palmerston North
Hutton, W. G.	116 Cameron Road	Tauranga
Holmes, W. R.	Victoria Mansions, Victoria Street	Christchurch
Jameson, I. W.	3 Catherine Street	Invercargill
Johnston, D. G.	Thompson's Buildings, Ward St.	Hamilton
Kriechbaum, J. B.	45 Benson Road	Auckland 5
Le Grice, H.	122 Remuera Road	Auckland 5
Levien, G. H.	93a Victoria Avenue	Wanganui
Loughlin, J. M.	P.O. Box 294	Napier
Macdiarmid, D. C.	South British Insurance Buildings.	Hamilton
Macdiarmid, J. C. D.	South British Insurance Buildings.	Hamilton
Mac Donald, R. G.	500 George St.	Dunedin
Manson, N.	65 Nile Street	Nelson

Marchant, E. L.	15 Myrtle St.	Lower Hutt
Moore, G. J.	50 Perry Street	Masterton
Murdoch, D.	71 Browns Bay Rd., Browns Bay	Auckland 1
Nielsen, A. M. K.	27a Pukaki Street	Rotorua
Parr, J. C.	Dept. Ophthalmology, University of Otago	Dunedin
Pittar, C. A.	Wentworth Chambers, 74 Symonds St.	Auckland
Poole, L. W.	74 Symonds Street	Auckland 1
Potter, D. F.	Ryefield, Upper Place	Masterton
Powell, G. G.	274A Remuera Road	Auckland 5
Reynolds, R. M. P.	421 Malvern Street	Dunedin
Ring, C. C.	Suite 4, Ely Clinic, 102 Remuera Road	Auckland 5
Sabiston, D. W.	79a Emerson Street	Napier
Sandston, A. C.	Harley Buildings, 137 Cambridge Terrace	Christchurch
Stenhouse, C. M.	Dyers Pass Road	Christchurch
Sturman, D.	72 Messines Road, Karori	Wellington
Suckling, R. D.	137 Cambridge Terrace	Christchurch
Sutherland, A. L.	130 Hereford Street	Christchurch
Swanston, C.	Lister Buildings, Victoria Street East	Auckland 1
Talbot, A. N.	24 Robe Street	New Plymouth
Talbot, G. G.	69 Symonds Street	Auckland 1
Talbot, K. J.	80 Church Street	Timaru
Taylor, W.	Eye Dept., Public Hospital	Auckland
Tingey, R. E.	116 Cameron Road	Tauranga
Velvin, E. J.	Queen Street	Hastings
Wales, H. J.	173 Cambridge Terrace	Christchurch
Warden, N. J.	Brunette Buildings, Queen Street .	Lower Hutt
Warnock, D. C.	187 Broadway Ave.	Palmerston North
Weerekoon, L. M.	Public Hospital	Nelson
Wilson, R. P.	618 Highgate, Maori Hill	Dunedin

Associate members

Bowden, Katherine	107 Hatea Drive	Whangarei
Elliott, I. D.	Eye Department, Auckland Hospital	Auckland
Ellingham, T. R.	Dunedin Hospital	Dunedin
Greer, D. V.	69 Spottiswoods St.	Dunedin
Murdoch, Rosemary	71 Browns Bay Road, Browns Bay	Auckland 10
Tompkins, Sheena	28b Liverpool St.	Auckland
Wilson, D. G.	Lister Court, Francis Street	Blenheim

NOSOCOMIA QUIBUS OCULIS AEGRI CURANTUR

There are no special eye hospitals, all the larger hospitals have eye departments.

INSTITUTA SCHOLAEQUE CAECIS DESTINATAE

Royal New Zealand Foundation for the Blind, Parnell Road, Auckland 1.
This Foudation is a school in Auckland with approximately 120 pupils for primary and secondary
    education.
Administrative branches and welfare in the major cities.
Advisory Committees keep the Foundation in contact with the blind people in their areas.

PAKISTAN

SOCIETATES OPHTHALMOLOGICAE

Ophthalmological Society of Pakistan (Southern Region, Karachi)
President: Dr. A. D. Minhas
President-Elect: Dr. M. A. Farooqui
Hon. Gen. Secretary: Dr. Jamshed H. Wania, Anklesaria Nursing Home, Randal Road, Karachi
Hon. Joint Secretary: Dr. Haider Ali Mithani, Spencer Eye Hospital, Lea Market, Karachi
Hon. Treasurer: Dr. Taj Mohammed Soomro
Number of members: 28

Ophthalmological society of Pakistan (North Zone, Lahore)
President: Professor M. H. Alvi
Hon. General Secretary: Professor Raja Mumtaz, 22-C, Bahawalpur House, Lahore
Hon. Joint Secretary: Dr. Dil Muhammad Mirza
Hon. Treasurer: Prof. Dr. M. Latif Choudhary
Number of members: 60

NOMINA ET DOMICILIA MEDICORUM AB OCULIS

Southern Region:

Ahmed, M. M.	Cafe Persian Bldg., Preedy Street, Saddar	Karachi
Anklesaria, B. M.	Anklesaria Nursing Home, Randal Road	Karachi
Anklesaria, H. S.	53, Katrak Parsi Colony, M. A. Jinnah Road	Karachi
Anklesaria, S. D.	53, Katrak Parsi Colony, M. A. Jinnah Road	Karachi
Aqil Bin Qadir	Eye Hospital	Hyderabad
Farooqui, M. A.	Hasan Mazil, Arambagh	Karachi
Haider Ali Mithani	Spencer Eye Hospital, Lea Market	Karachi
Inam Ahsan	Hasan Manzil, Arambagh	Karachi
Javed Alam	Mahboob Chambers, Abdullah Haroon Road	Karachi
Khalid Naeem Baig	P. N. Shifa	Karachi
Khalil Rana M		Shikarpur (Sind)
Kirmani, T. H.	2, Rex Annexe, Abdullah Haroon Road	Karachi

Lodhi, A. R.	53, Katrak Parsi Colony, M. A. Jinnah Road	Karachi
Luther, H. N.	Mission Hospital	Quetta
Minhas, A. D.	Anklesaria Nursing Home, Randal Road	Karachi
Manazir Hassan, M.	Rex Annexe, 2nd floor, Abdullah Haroon Road	Karachi
Mohammed Akhtar		Shikarpur (Sind).
Mohammad Qamar Khan	Spencer Eye Hospital, Lea Market	Karachi
Nisar Pathan		Shikarpur (Sind).
Rizvi, M. H.	Spencer Eye Hospital, Lea Market	Karachi
Saleh Memon	Bambino Chambers, Garden Road	Karachi
Samad, A.	Opposite Lea Market	Karachi
Shah, M. A.	Victoria Mansion, Abdullah Haroon Road	Karachi
Taj Mohammad Soomro	Rahman Courts, Opp. Parsi Mama Girls School	Karachi
Wania, J. H.	Anklesaria Nursing Home, Randal Road	Karachi
Yahya, S. M.	Queens Road	Sukkur (Sind).
Yousuf Docrat	Edulji Dinshaw Chambers, Opp. Cafe George, Abdullah Haroon Road	Karachi
Zafar	Jinnah Post-Graduate Medical Centre	Karachi

North Zone, Lahore

Abdul Ghani	Shuja Abad	Multan
Abdul Majid	Aslam Eye Hospital, 89 Main Samanabad	Lahore
Abdul Rashid	Medical Superintendent, Civil Hospital	Gujranwala
Abrar Hussain, Prof.	Nishtar Medical College/Hospital .	Multan
Jabbar, Maj. A.	C. M. H. Lahore Cantt.	Lahore
Qazi, Prof. A. J.	7-A, University Town	Peshawar
Alim-Ud-Din, S. K.	Military Medical College, Hospital	Rawalpindi
Asghar Ali Syed	Ali Hospital, 21-Temple Road	Lahore
Asghar, Hamid Qureshi	M.O. I/C., Civil Hospital	Chakwal
Ashfaq, Ahmed	Civil Hospital	Okara
Bashir, Prof. Ahmed	27-Davis Road	Lahore
Bashir, Ahmed	P. W. R. Cairns Hospital	Lahore
Bashir, Ahmed Chohan	Central Government Polyclinic	Islamabad
Nizami, G. N. A.	Nizami Hospital, Kotwali Road	Lyallpur
Habib, Ahmed	Mayo Hospital	Lahore
Hafiz, Abdul Latif	M.O.I/C Civil Hospital	Daska (Sialkot)
Iwbal, Ahmed Choudhry	Aslam Eye Hospital, Main Samanabad	Lahore
Jalil-Ud-Daula, Prof.	King Edward Medical College	Lahore
Lal, Mrs.	Mission Hospital	Taxila
Maqsood Ahmad Cheema	Cheema Eye Hospital	Daska (Sialkot)
Malik, Aslam M.	Civil Hospital	Pindhi Gheb.
Masood, Ahmed Cheema	Cheema Eye Hospital	Daska (Sialkot)
Ullah, Col. M. Atta	18-G, Gulberg-III	Lahore
Mehboob Ahmed Cheema	Cheema Eye Hospital	Daska (Sialkot)
Alvi, Prof. M. H.	145 Shadman Colony, Jail Road .	Lahore

Iftikhar, Capt. M.	C.M.H.	Kharian
Mira Khan	Ordinance Factory	Wah Cantt.
Javed, M.		Lyallpur
Khurshid Kazmi, M.	Sargodha Eye Clinic, 146/A, Satellite Town	Sargodha
Latif Choudhary, Prof. M.	F. J. Medical College	Lahore
Ahmed, Col. M. M.	C.M.H.	Peshawar
Farooqi, M. M.	D.H.Q. Hospital	Lyallpur
Riaz Ahmed, M.	Eye Dept. Sir Ganga Ram Hospital	Lahore
Sadiq, M.		Daska (Sialkot)
Mohammad Afzal Sheikh	Eye Dept. Mayo Hospital	Lahore
Mohammad Ahsan Jamil	Sir Ganga Ram Hospital	Lahore
Mohammad Aslam Rai	Aslam Eye Hospital, Main Samanabad	Lahore
Mohammad Israr Khan	Amanat Eye Hospital, College Road	Rawalpindi
Mohammad Munir-Ul-Haq, Prof.	King Edward Medical College	Lahore
Mohammad Nawaz, Prof.	Khyber Medical College	Peshawar
Muhammad Asghar	D.H.Q. Hospital	Sargodha
Muhammad Yaqin	Data Darbar Hospital	Lahore
Munawar Ahmed Choudry	Civil Hospital	Bhalwal
Muzaffar Iqbal	Khyber Medical College	Peshawar
Nawazish Ali Bhutta	Medical Officer, Eye Dept., Mayo Hospital	Lahore
Christy, N. E.	Christian Hospital	Taxila
Parveen Munawar	Medical Officer, Eye Dept., Sir Ganga Ram Hospital	Lahore
Raja Mumtaz, Prof.	King Edward Medical College	Lahore
Ramzan Ali Syed, Prof.	Ali Hospital, 21-Temple Road	Lahore
Rashida Sultan, Prof.	F.J. Medical College	Lahore
Rehmatullah Choudhary		Lahore
Riaz Ali Shah	21-Nicholson Road	Lahore
Rehmat Ullah	Eye & General Hospital	Gojra (Lyallpur)
Sajjad Ahmed	27 Davis Road	Lahore
Qader, Maj. S. A.	New Market, Kashmir Road	Rawalpindi
Pirzada, Col. S. A. R.	C.M.H.	Lahore Cantt.
Imtiaz Hussain Bokhari, S.	Services Hospital	Lahore
Sardar Ali Sheikh, Prof.	Nishtar Medical College/Hospital	Lahore
Sultan Ahmad Cheema	Cheema Eye Hospital	Daska (Sialkot)
Burq, Z. A.	Quaid-i-Azam Medical College/Hospital	Bahawalpur

NOSOCOMIA QUIBUS OCULIS AEGRI CURANTUR

	No. of Beds
Civil Hospital, Karachi, Head of Ophth. Dept.: Dr. M. M. Hussain	45
Jinnah Post-Graduate Medical Centre, Karachi, Head of Ophth. Dept.: Dr. T. H. Kirmani	60
Masoomeen Hospital Trust, Karachi, Head of Ophth. Dept.: Dr. Jamshed H. Wania	10
Spencer Eye Hospital, Karachi, Head of Ophth. Dept.: Dr. M. H. Rizvi	200
Eye Hospital, Hyderabad, Head of Ophth. Dept.: Dr. Agil Bin Qadar	100
Mirpurkhas General Hospital, Ophthalmology Dept., Mirpurkhas	20

Sir Henry Holland Eye Hospital, Shikarpur, (This is a seasonal hospital), Head of Ophth.
Dept.: Dr. Ronnie Holland 200
Mission Hospital, Quetta. Head of Ophth. Dept.: Dr. H. N. Luther x
Nistar Medical College, Multan. Head of Ophth. Dept.: Dr. Abrar Hussain 40
King Edward Medical College Lahore. Head of Ophth. Dept.: Dr. Raja Mumtaz 50

INSTITUTA SCHOLAEQUE CAECIS DESTINATAE

Adult Blind Centre, Karachi.
Ida Ruy School for the Blind, Karachi.

PERU

SOCIETATES OPHTHALMOLOGICAE

Sociedad Peruana de Oftalmología
Secretary: Dr. Pedro Saenz, Camillo Carrillo 225, Lima

No data received.

PHILIPPINAE

SOCIETATES OPHTHALMOLOGICAE

Philippine Ophthalmological Society

President: Romeo B. Espiritu
Vice-President: Romeo V. Fajardo
Secretary: Alejandro S. de Leon, Philippine Eye Research Institute, PHG Compound, Taft Avenue, Manila
Treasurer: Corazon dela Cruz-Estrella
Councillors: Dr. Fortunato Y. Eusebio, Dr. Luciano U. Luczon, Dr. Cosme I. N. Naval, Dr. Vicente de la Paz Jr., Dr. Salvador R. Salceda, Dr. Emmanuel M. Almeda

Philippine Academy of ophthalmology and otolaryngology

President: Jose M. Marin
Vice-President: Vicente L. Santos
Secretary: Gloria Lim, 1336 Paz, Paco, Manila
Treasurer: Aurora A. Diaz
Past President: Conrado P. Banzon
Councillors: Mayorico H. Sandico, Eusebio E. Llamas, Alfredo R. Diaz, Sergio E. Mendoza, Romeo B. Espiritu, Manuel G. Lim
Bureau: P.O. Box 1510, Manila
Number of members: 89

NOMINA ET DOMICILIA MEDICORUM AB OCULIS

Abdon, Alfredo	Bautista Hospital	Cavite City
Abela, Augusto	Davao Doctors Hospital, Elpidio Quirino Avenue	Davao City
Alday, Adalberto	1860 F. Agoncillo	Malata, Manila
Alejo, Francisco	726-A delos Santos Ave	Cubao, Quezon City
Alianza, Likia C.	St. Elizabeth Center, Valeria St.	Ilio City, Ilio.
Almeda, Emmanuel M.	2178 Taft Avenue	Manila
Almeda, Ernesto M.	1808 Rizal Avenue	Sta. Cruz, Manila
Aquino, Mario V.	Liboro Clinic, 119 Rizal Avenue	Manila
Arribas, Nieva	133 Roman Street	San Juan, Rizal
Austria, Cresencio	171 Scout Fuentebella Kamuning	Quezon City
Ayuyao, Josefina	1999 Leon Guinto Sr.	Malate, Manila
Azurin, Jose Ma.	Sta. Ana Avenue	Davao City
Bailon, Andres	3 Sta. Maria St. Bo. Capitolyo	Pasig, Rizal
Baltazar, Eduardo	2242 Rizal Avenue, East Bajac-Bajac	Olongapo City
Banzon, Conrado	14 Baler St. San Francisco del Monte	Quezon City
Batungbacal, Ramon	34 Pili St., Forbes Park	Makati, Rizal
Bautista, Ariston	Makati Medical Center, 2 Amorsolo Street	Makati, Rizal

Bernardino, Vitaliano Jr. ..	15 Bayanihan St.	Quezon City
Bernardo, Romulo	Medalle Bldg., Osmeña Blvd.	Cebu City
Caparas, Edgardo	1814 M.H. del Pilar	Malate, Manila
Capulla, Fernando	152 Roosevelt Ave., San Francisco del Monte	Quezon City
Carbajal, Ulysses	789 Vito Cruz	Malate, Manila
Casilan, Alipio	104 Real Street	Tacloban City
Cezar, Lilia	330-A Ledesma St.	Iloilo City
Chan, Jose	1644 Rizal Avenue	Manila
Chanco, Leticia	450 Arguiza Street	Ermita, Manila
Cid, Corazon	A. Veles Street	Cagayan de Oro City
Cinco, Narciso	14 Acacia Street	Cebu City
Dabu, Floro	312 E. Angeles St.	Naga City
Degollacion, Salvador	New Manahan Bldg., Session Road	Baguio City
Diaz, Alfredo	1705 G. Tuazon	Sampaloc, Manila
Diaz, Aurora A.	Rm. 212 Don Santiago Bldg., Taft Avenue	Manila
Dizon, Concepcion	....	Porac, Pampanga
Espiritu, Romeo B.	Manila Doctors Hospital, United Nations Avenue	Manila
Estrella, Corazon C.	2301 Juan Luna	Tondo, Manila
Estrellado, Benjamin	....	Davao City
Eusebio, Fortunato	Bacolod Doctors Hosp.	Bacolod City
Eusebio, Jesus	41 P. Florentino, Sta. Mesa Heights	Quezon City
Evidente, Augusto	Bugallon Avenue	Dagupan City
Evidente, Virginia	Bugallon Avenue	Dagupan City
Fabie, Esteban	....	Tarlac, Tarlac
Fajardo, Romeo	Manila Doctors Hosp., Unit Nations Avenue	Manila
Feria, Quirico	C.I.W.	Mandaluyong, Rizal
Fernando, Antonio Jr.	1755 Taft Avenue	Manila
Fernando, Asuncion	1755 Taft Avenue	Manila
Fernando, Felisa	1755 Taft Avenue	Manila
Fuente, Jose dela	1550 Laong-Laan St.	Sampaloc, Manila
Gaerlan, Gavino	J. Reyes Memorial Hosp. Rizal Avenue	Sta. Cruz, Manila
Galang, Romeo	Pampanga EENT Infirmary Tagulod, Del Pilar	San Fernando, Pampanga
Garcia, Julian	Garcia Clinic, Guardia Nacional St.	Zamboanga City
Garcia, Rufo	Baguio General Hosp.	Baguio City
Gener, Terencio	32 Sta. Rosa Cor. Biak-na-Bato ..	Quezon City
Guanio, Ma. Luisa V.	6 Dr. Antonio Avenue	Pasig, Rizal
Hechanova, Manuel Jr.	Makati Medical Center, 2 Amorsolo Street	Makati, Rizal
Hembrador, Olympio	V. Luna Gen. Hospital	Quezon City
Hernandez, Bayani	1372 Rizal Ave. Ext.	Caloocan City
Hortaleza, Pedro	290 Naval Street	Navotas, Rizal
Ibañez, Ricardo	73 Detroit, Cubao	Quezon City
Icasiano – Santos, Caridad R.	Rm. 412 Sikatuna Bldg., Ayola Avenue	Makati, Rizal
Insilay, Marcelito	UERMM, Aurora Blvd.	Quezon City
Jalbuena, Alberto	Manila Contact Lens Clinic, 2030 A. Mabini	Malate, Manila

Javier, Vicente	1 Spencer St., Cubao	Quezon City
Jesus, Policarpio de	Baguio General Hosp.	Baguio City
Jimenez, Tim	Makati Medical Center, 2 Amorsolo Street	Makati, Rizal
Jose, Corazon	M.C.U. Hospital, Samson Road ..	Caloocan City
Lao, Han Liong	617 Condesa St.	Binondo, Manila
Lapitan, Romulo	1213 Lepanto St.	Sampaloc, Manila
Legasto, Mario	2060 Rizal Avenue Cor. Tayabas .	Manila
Legasto, Noe	2060 Rizal Avenue Cor. Tayabas .	Manila
Leon, Alejandro de	Phil. Eye Research Institute, PGH Cpd. Taft Avenue	Manila
Lcon, Jaime. de	276 Vicente Cruz	Sampaloc, Manila
Lim, Gloria	1336 Paz	Paco, Manila
Llamas, Eusebio	390 Columbia St. Cor. Lafayette Greenhills Subd.	Mandaluyong, Rizal
Luczon, Luciano	41 V. Luna Road	Quezon City
Macatangay, Galicano	881 Herran	Paco, Manila
Malvar, Basilio	23 Orange St.	Malabon, Rizal
Mangahas, Cayetano	Chinese Gen. Hospital, 286 Blumentritt	Sta. Cruz, Manila
Mangubat, Liborio	Medical Center Manila 1222 Gen. Luna St.	Manila
Marin, Jose	28 Badjao St., La Vista	Quezon City
Medalle, Ptolomeo	Medalle Bldg., Osmeña Blvd.	Cebu City
Mendoza, Dominador	Quirino Labor Hosp.	Quezon City
Mendoza, Jovito	Tabuco	Naga City
Mendoza, Perfecto	Laperal Bldg. Rizal Avenue	Manila
Mendoza, Sergio	24 Bright Hill, New Manila	Quezon City
Monfero, Leonida	940-C Lerma St.	Sampaloc, Manila
Nañagas, Pablo	2 Quezon Avenue	Lucena City
Naval, Cosme	1564 Dapitan St.	Sampaloc, Manila
Navarro, Jose	Mercedes Bldg.	Quiapo, Manila
Ocampo, Geminiano de ...	De Ocampo Eye Hosp., United Nations Ave	Manila
Ongsiako, Ramon Jr.	Makati Medical Center, 2 Amorsolo Street	Makati, Rizal
Paez, Tranquilino	Cuizon Memorial & Diagnostic Center	Cabanatuan City
Panganiban, Freddie	New Manubay Bldg., Peñafrancia Avenue	Naga City
Paz, Perfecto dela	97 N. Domingo	San Juan, Rizal
Paz, Vicente dela Jr.	998 N. dela Fuente	Sampaloc, Manila
Peñalosa, Eduardo	41 T. Azucena	San Pablo City
Perez, Abelardo	Batangas Doctors Hosp.	Batangas City
Perez, Antonio	Makati Medical Center, 2 Amorsolo Street	Makati, Rizal
Quilala, Francisco	Cebu Medical Center	Cebu City
Ramos, Emmanuel	San Fernando	Pampanga
Reyes, Andres	Nichols Airbase Hosp.	Pasay City
Reyes, Edmundo	Singian Clinic, 998 Gen. Solano .	San Miguel, Manila
Reyes, Godofredo	62 K-8 Kamias Kamuning	Quezon City
Reyes, Reynaldo	Zamboango Doctors Hosp., Veterans Avenue	Zamboanga City
Reyrao, Avelino	3567 Batas St., St. Mesa	Manila
Roasa, Ruperto	175 P. Guevara St.	Sta. Cruz, Laguna
Romero, Solon	Cagayan Prov'l. Hosp.	Tuguegarao, Cagayan

Roxas, Antonio L.	Tarlac Eye and Ear Clinic	Tarlac, Tarlac.
Rufino, Romeo	Taft Street, Daet	Camarines Norte
Salceda, Salvador	Phil. Eye Research Institute, PGH Cpd. Taft Avenue	Manila
Sandico, Mayorico	1808 Rizal Avenue	Sta. Cruz, Manila
Santayana, Robin	....	Iligan City
Santos, Caridad I.	Rm. 412 Sikatuna Bldg., Ayala Avenue	Makati, Rizal
Santos, Luis	Santos Clinic	Malolos, Bulacan
Santos, Rodrigo Jr.	Medical Center Manila Annex, United Nations Ave	Manila
Santos, Sabino	Santos Clinic	Malolos, Bulacan
Santos, Vicente	998 Gen. Solano, San Miguel ...	Manila
Sarabia, Antonio	North Drive	Bacolod City
Sayoc, Burgos	51 Scout Torillo Cor. Scout Madrinian	Quezon City
Sevilla, Carlos	Makati Medical Center, 2 Amorsolo Street	Makati, Rizal
Sison, Gregorio Jr.	Veterans Memorial Hosp. Hilaga Ave., Diliman	Quezon City
Songco, Vicente	....	Dagupan City
Soriano, Antonio	Baguio Medical Center	Baguio City
Tablante, Ronald	Makati Medical Center, 2 Amorsolo Street	Makati, Rizal
Tamesis, Jesus	Clinica Tamesis, Quezon Blvd. Ext.	Quezon City
Tan, Jesus	587 Rosario Street	Binondo, Manila
Tan. Macario	Oledan Bldg.	Makati, Rizal
Tan, Robert	587 Rosario Street	Binondo, Manila
Tan-Tiec, Vicente	587 Rosario Street	Binondo, Manila
Tionloc, Rafael	American Hosp. Bldg., Aduana St., Intramuros	Manila
Torralba, Benicio	213 B. Padilla St.	San Juan, Rizal
Torrejos, Jesus	1227 M. dela Fuente	Sampaloc, Manila
Triguero, Conrado	....	Legaspi City
Tuaño, Bernardo	647 Calderon	Mandaluyong, Rizal
Udasco, Rolando	519 P. Burgos Street	Cavite City
Uy, Vicente	House Int'l., Suite 208, 777 Ongpin St., Sta. Cruz	Manila
Valdez, Emilio Jr.	1556 Laong-Laan	Sampaloc, Manila
Valenzuela, Jose	46 San Luis	Pasay City
Velarde, Herminio Jr.	Makati Commercial Bldg.	Makati, Rizal
Velez, Jose	180 Jacinto Asiñas St.	San Juan, Rizal
Vera-Cruz, Ponciano	Clinica Tamesis, Quezon Blvd. Ext.	Quezon City
Victorio-Guano, Ma. Luisa B.	6 Dr. S. Antonio Avenue	Pasig, Rizal
Villafuerte, Cesar	1689 Maria y orosa	Ermita, Manila
Villar, Joaquin	Phil. Constabulary Station Hospital, Camp Crame	Quezon City
Vizcarra, Luis	Philippine Navy, Roxas Blvd. ...	Malate, Manila
Yambao, Carlos	1356 L. Guinto Sr.	Ermita, Manila
Yatco, Ismael	1302 V. Concepcion	Sampaloc, Manila
Zagala, Manuel	Southern Island Hosp.	Cebu City

NOSOCOMIA QUIBUS OCULIS AEGRI CURANTUR

De Ocampo Eye Hospital, United Nations Ave., Manila. Director: Dr. Geminiano de Ocampo. No. of Beds – 23

Philippine Eye & Ear Infirmary, 5890 S. de Guzman, Parañaque, Rizal, Director: Dr. Emmanuel M. Almeda. No. of Beds – 20

INSTITUTA SCHOLAEQUE CAECIS DESTINATAE

School for the Blind, 2620 F.B. Harrison, Pasay City. Supervisor: Mr. Geraldo Consolacion. No. of Pupils – 67

POLONIA

SOCIETATES OPHTHALMOLOGICAE

Nationalis

Polish Ophthalmological Society
Polskie Towarzystwo Okulistyczne
Address: ul. Lindleya 4, Warszawa
President: Prof. dr. Tadeusz Krwawicz
Secretary-Gen: Dr. Janina Krauss, ul Waryńskiego 28, Warszawa 00.650

Regionales

Ophthalmological Society Branches in:

No. of members

Białystok, ul. C. Sklodowskiej 24a, *Secretary:* Dr. K. Smoliźska 38
Gdańsk-Wrzeszcz, ul. Debinki 7a, *Secretary:* Dr. D. Fabiszewska 88
Katowice, ul. Francuska 20, *Secretary:* Dr. A. Karaszewska 177
Kraków, ul. Kopernika 38, *Secretary:* Doc. Dr. K. Krzystkowa 116
Lublin, ul. Chmielna 1, *Secretary:* Dr. Perekładowska-Jakubik 52
Lódz. ul. Narutowicza 118, *Secretary:* Dr. H. Rybus-Zelawska 49
Olsztyn, ul. Partyzantów 74, *Secretary:* Dr. A. Prusiewicz 32
Poznań, ul. Długa 1–2, *Secretary:* Dr. J. Kaluzny 88
Szczecin, ul. Powstańców 72, *Secretary:* Dr. W. Andrzejcwska 48
Warszawa, ul. Lindleya 4, *Secretary:* Dr. L. Mazurowska 121
Wrocław, ul. Chalubińskiego 2a, *Secretary:* Dr. H. Nizankowska 102

NOMINA ET DOMICILIA MEDICORUM AB OCULIS

Abłamowicz, Ryszarda	ul. Roswelta 4I	Bytom
Abramowicz, Ignacy	ul. Debinki 7a	Gdańsk-Wrzeszcz
Adamczewska, Irena	ul. Tatrzańska 2	Kamienny Potok
Adamczyk, Tadeusz	ul. Szpital Woj. Oddz. Ocz.	Stargard
Adamczyk, Adam	ul. Boczna 34	Katowice
Adamiec, Janina	ul. Kaszubska 3I	Szczecin
Adamowska Furtak, Krystyna	ul. Ogieńskiego 10	Szczecin
Adamska, Janina	ul. Słoneczna 26	Rabki Zdr
Adamski, Jan	ul. Kopernika 8	Kraków
Adler, Maria	ul. Styczyńska 16	Gliwice
Alberti, Teresa	ul. Narutowicza 2	Rzeszów
Alichniewicz, Halina	ul. Narutowicza 71/73	Łódz
Ambroszkiewicz, Irena	ul. Starobojarska 13	Białystok
Andrzejewska, Helena Wanda	ul. Grzegorza z Sanoka 60	Szczecin
Anbrzykowska, Helena	ul. Kołobrzeska 69	Gdańsk-Oliwa
Anisimowicz, Eugeniusz ...	ul. Debinki 7a	Gdańsk-Wrzeszcz
Antkowiak, Maria	ul. Brzezińska 12	Czarnków

Antoniszewska, Korona Maria	ul. Batorego 81 k	Nowy Sacz
Antonowicz, Kazimierz ...	ul. Kołobrzeska 13a	Olsztyn
Antowska, Romana	ul. Szpital Miejski Oddz. O.	Toruń
Arkin, Wiktor	Jerozolimskie 29	Warszawa A 1.
Atłasik, Bernadetta	ul. Sabinowska 129	Czestochowa
Attaman Wilczek, Barbara .	ul. Tyszki 13a	Katowice
Baborski, Ottoman	ul. Pułaskiego 5	Bytom
Bakkarewicz, Alicja	ul. Obozowa 85	Warszawa
Bałut Nowakowska, Alina ..	ul. Krasińskiego 29	Tarnów
Baran, Alina	ul. Chałubińskiego 2a K1.O.	Wrocław
Baran, Lech	ul. Kościuszki 32	Wrocław
Baranowska, George Teresa	ul. C. Skłodowskiej 72 K1.O. ...	Szczecin
Barański, Bronisław	ul. Wieczorka 49	Piekary Sl
Bartkowska, Klara	ul. Małeckiego 26	Poznań
Bartkowska-Orłowska, Maria	ul. Grochowska 9Ic	Poznań
Bartnik, Krystyna	Kościuszki 1	Dzbno pow. Czestochowa
Bartoszewicz, Inczewa	ul. Byszewskiego 50	Poznań
Barycki, Zbysław	ul. Dzierzyńskiego 12/3	Zamość
Basewicz, Elzbieta	ul. 1 Maja 4	Białystok
Baszczyńska Zielińska, Barbara	ul. Dubois 18	Zgierz
Bednorz Rduch, Eugenia ..	ul. Sienkiewicza 77	Radlin I
Bedyńska, Irena	ul. Kollataja 14	Opole
Bekier Wall, Elzbieta	ul. Powstańców Slaskick 177 ...	Wrocław
Berezowska, Ewa	ul. Boczna 3/26	Kraków
Bernardczykowa, Anna	ul. Grochowska 28	Poznań
Białas, Ewa	ul. Cicha 25/20	Tychy
Białecka, Alina	ul. Przychodnia Okulist.	Ketrzyn
Białkiewicz, Irena	ul. Dzierzyńskiego 70	Katowice
Białogłowska, Aleksandra ..	ul. Bol. Chrobrego 20/15	Rzeszów
Biedrońska, Maria	ul. Chałubińskiego 2a Kl. O.	Wrocław
Blegamowski, Lech	ul. Kraszewskiego 42	Toruń
Bieniewa, Henryka	Zjednoczenia 2/4	Chorzow A 1.
Biernacka, Mirosława	ul. Red. Ordona 58/3	Szczecin
Bieszczanin, Irena	ul. Waszyngtona 57/8	Czestochowa
Biniszkiewicz, Danuta	ul. Jagiellońska 30	Bytom
Binkiewicz, Elżbieta	ul. Fałata 16	Bytom
Biskup, Antoni	ul. Konarskiego 7/9	Kielce
Błasucka, Wanda	ul. Hrubieszowska 8L	Chełm
Błaszyński, Wojciech	ul. Roswelta 70	Gniezno
Błoniarz, Barbara	ul. Bociania 19	Oleśnica
Bobrowska, Karolina	ul. Rogójskiego 26c	Tarnów
Bochenek, Alina	ul. Pilarecka 2b	Kraków
Bocheńska, Nadzieja	ul. Puławska 28	Warszawa
Bogorodzki, Bazyli	ul. Narutowicza 46	Lódz
Boguslawska, Maria	ul. Prezydencka 4	Warszawa
Boguslawska, Zefiryna	ul. Inżynierska 10	Poznań
Boniecka Gawlik, Irena	ul. Grotgera 42	Gdynia
Borawska, Aleksandra	ZOR 80/3	Grajewo
Borkowska, Halina	ul. Karmelicka 2I	Warszawa
Borowicz, Zofia	ul. Czermiakowska 35	Poznań
Borowiecki, Jan	ul. Sienkiewicza 49/5	Kielce
Borowik Pyzińska, Helena .	ul. Chrzanowskiego 6	Gdańsk-Wrzeszcz
Borowski, Janusz	ul. Rogozińskiego 26	Łódź

Borzecka Teresa	ul. Mickiewicza 1/3	Gdańsk-Wrzeszcz
Borysiewicz, Barbara	ul. Marchlewskiego 5	Iława
Bosowska, Bogusława	ul. Chmielna 28/1	Włocławek
Branicka, Marianna	ul. Wojska Polskiego 2/5	Wroctaw
Brodziak, Kazimierz	ul. Chałubińskiego 2a Kl. O.	Słupsk
Browarska, Renata	ul. Zytnia 11/4	Wrocław
Brycz, Fryderyk	ul. Chodkiewicza 11	Bydgoszcz
Bryk, Edward	ul. Zaleskiego 11	Kraków
Brzykowa, Wanda	ul. Em. Plater 13	Bdygoszcz
Buchta, Barbara	ul. Dabrówki 13/15	Katowice
Bubień, Eleonora	ul. 1 Maja 2	Wrocław
Bujnowska, Teresa	ul. Konopnicka 2	Białystok
Bukowska, Renata	ul. Schillera 4	Warszawa
Bulanda, Maria	ul. Plac Mariacki 1/12	Kraków
Bularska, Barbara	Przych. przy Hucie	Skawina
Bulińska, Maria	ul. Rynek 6	Chrzanów
Bułhak, Irena	ul. Zajecza 25	Białystok
Burau, Jadwiga	ul. Kaprowa 8	Gdańsk-Oliwa
Burian, Barbara	ul. Nowomiejska 6	Elblag
Cabała Moszyńska, Danuta	ul. Grażyny 14	Warszawa
Cetkowska, Helena	ul. Gilów 18	Katowice
Cichocka, Anna	Os. Rydla bl. 9a	Kraków
Ciechanowska, Janina	ul. Dzierżyńskiego 8	Kraków
Cis-Bankiewicz, Hanna	ul. Szklanych Domów 11	Warszawa
Cwikliński, Jerzy	ul. Narutowicza 80/18	Lublin
Cybulska, Elźbieta	ul. Bracka 28	Łódz
Cylke, Leszek	ul. Kościuszki 5	Ozorków
Czabańska, Elźbieta	Szpital Woj. Oddz. O.	Koszalin
Czachar, Barbara	ul. Gwardii Ludowej 4Ia	Poznań
Czaplicki, Jaremi	ul. Brynowka 53	Katowice-Brynów
Czaplicki, Stefania	ul. Brynowska 53	Katowice-Brynów
Czarnomska, Zofia	ul. Bolecha 43	Warszawa
Czech, Jerzy	ul. Wyrzysko 9	Piła
Czech, Maria	ul. Nowowiejska 29	Kraków
Czechowicz, Janicka Krystyna	ul. Dobra 18/20	Warszawa
Czerniawska, Julia	ul. Czarnieckiego 11	Oświecim 4
Czerwińska, Włodzimiera	ul. Stołeczna 14	Warszawa
Czekańska, Danuta	ul. Powstańców 10	Mikołów
Czop, Elźbieta	ul. Skierki 1	Lublin
Czuruk, Stefania	Narutowicza 4I	Łódz
Chacińska, Grażyna	ul. Manny 20	Gliwice
Chetko, Edward	ul. Reymonta 22/23	Skierniewice
Chomiczewska, Eulalia	ul. Piotrkowska 56	Lódz
Chrapek Fajfer, Alicja	ul. Czarneckiego 23/4	Tychy
Chreszczyńska, Jadwiga	ul. Wojska Polsk. 1	Złotoryje
Chrzaliszewska, Stanisława	ul. Zeromskiego 17	Nowa Ruda
Chraznowski, Jan	ul. Karmelicka 33/3	Kraków
Chwirot, Roman	ul. Szpitalna 35a	Białystok
Chylimoniuk, Maria	ul. 15 Grudnia 2	Kraków
Dabrowska, Danuta	ul. Nowotki 26	Warszawa
Dabrowska, Krystyna	ul. Por. Okulist.	Oleśnica
Debicka, Alicja	Iłzecka 63	Ostrówiec Swietokrzyski
Delebińska, Barbara	ul. Konarskiego 8	Gliwice
Detko Kisielewska, Honorata	ul. Modzelewska 35	Czestochowa
Dobródzka, Anna	ul. Anki Krzywoń 1	Rzeszów

Domagalska, Helena	ul. Zdrowa 10	Wrocław
Domaszewicz, Wanda	ul. G. Curie 19 m. 7	Warszawa
Dominiak, Rybarczyk	ul. Marii Magdaleny 6/5	Poznań
Domżał, Barbara	ul. Miedzynarodowa 37a	Warszawa
Drabina, Creslaw	ul. Cieszyńska 2	Skoczów
Drozdowska, Stanisława	ul. Kościuszki 2I	Wrocław
Dróbecka Brydak, Ewa	ul. Gorlicka 10	Warszawa
Dugieło, Barbara	ul. Pasieczna 3/1	Opole
Dukat, Stefan	ul. Sienkiewicza 5/6	Wrocław
Dukat, Wanda	ul. Marksa 19	Zabrze 8
Dulewicz, Maria	ul. Sportowa 8	Bydgoszcz
Duszowa, Janina	ul. Górnicza 2I	Mysłowice
Dutkiewicz, Franciszek	ul. Rynek 16	Miksztat
Dziedzic, Elżanowska	ul. Młynarska 18	Kalisz
Dziegielewski, Konrad	ul. Kasprzaka 7a	Poznań
Dziewiecki, Grzegorz	ul. Osóbki Morawskiego	Strzelno
Dzikowski, Jan	ul. Zamenhoffa 24	Swidnica
Dziuba, Jadwiga	ul. Konopnickiej 6	Białystok
Dziunikowski, Krzysztof	ul. Mickiewicza 30	Katowice
Dziurkowska, Barbara	ul. Bat-Chłop. 42	Kwidzyń
Dybicka, Anna	ul. Fahrenheit 4	Gdańsk
Dybowa, Barbara	Os. Pokoju 5a	Kraków
Dymowski, Lechosław	ul. C. Skłodowskiej 38	Lublin
Elektorowicz, Andrzej	Przychodnia Okulist.	Giżycko
Fabian, Alojzy	ul. Łukaszewicza 8	Wrocław
Fabiszewska-Górny, Danuta	ul. Sportowa 15	Sopot
Falkowska, Zofia	ul. Widok 19 m 166	Warszawa
Federowicz, Amelia	Por. Okulist	Strzelce Opolskie
Federowicz, Teresa	ul. Solskiego 5	Szczecin
Ferenc, Alina	Szpital woj. Oddz. O.	Olsztyn
Filipiakowa, Zofia	ul. Prusa 16	Poznań
Filipowicz Banach, Alina	ul. Tagore 1	Warszawa
Filipowicz, Malgorzata	ul. Marszałkowska 111a	Warszawa
Filipowicz, Zofia	ul. Bagno 3	Warszawa
Foltyńska, Anna	ul. Niekłańska 42	Warszawa
Forfa, Grażyna	ul. Kopernika 10	Olsztyn
Formińska, Maria	ul. Piastów 18/4	Katowice
Frysz, Zygmunt	ul. Kościuzki 10	Brwinów
Fryczkowska, Alicja	ul. Wolności 35	Zabrze
Fryczkowski, Andrzej	ul. Narutowicza 107	Łódz
Frydrych, Urszula	ul. Bema 10	Raciborz
Furtak, Krystyna	ul. Ogińskiego 18	Szczecin
Gabrylewska, Anna	ul. C. Skłodowskiej 8	Białystok
Gagała, Danuta	ul. Bruna 14	Warszawa
Galewska, Zofia	ul. Nowowiejska 6	Warszawa
Gałecka, Krystyna	Osiedle Kopernika 4	Nowa Sól
Gardzilewicz Swica, Anna	ul. Pomorska 82a	Gdynia Oliwa
Garszewska, Barbara	ul. Pruszkowska 12	Warszawa
Gasińska, Ewa	ul. Sporna 83	Łódz
Gawrońska, Małgorzata	Szpital Oddz. O.	Koszalin
Gburek, Alina	Swidnicka 32	Katowice-Ligota
Gerkowich, Helena	ul. Wielopole 13/19	Kraków
Gerkowicz, Kazimierz	ul. Górna 3	Lublin
Gierczyńska, Alicja	ul. Grójecka 14a	Warszawa
Gierek, Ariadna	ul. Drozdów 3	Katowice
Giergielewicz, Nowicka	Górnoslaska 14	Kalisz

Glebisz, Zofia	ul. Chrobrego 25	Wałbrzych
Gluza Kłoszewska, Jadwiga	Plac Wojska Polsk. 16	Bielsko Biała
Głodzik, Tadeusz	Por. Okulist	Lubin
Głoszewska, Danuta	ul. Malczewskiego 17a	Szczecin
Głowacka, Irena	ul. Krasińskiego 12	Lublin
Głowacka, Jadwiga	ul. Szlak 39/7	Kraków
Glowacki, Zdżisław	ul. Malczewskiego 19b	Szczecin
Gontarska, Anna	ul. Rubinowa 32	Łódz
Gorczyca, Urszula	ul. Junoszy 16	Lublin
Gotz, Regina	ul. Mickiewicza 9	Poznań
Grabowski, Jan	ul. Snarskiego 12	Lublin
Grabska, Krystyna	ul. Zawadzkiego 6/80	Tarnów
Grałek, Mirosława	ul. Kilińskiego 26	Łódz
Greczko, Irena	Poradnia Okulist.	Sokółka
Grochowska Turek, Ewa	ul. Rejmonta 11a	Zabrze
Grochulska, Janina	ul. Obr. Stalingradu 21	Stalowa Wola
Gruszczyńska, Mieczysława	ul. Marksa 38	Zabrze Rokitnica
Grzesiuk, Jerzy	ul. Kruczkowskiego 9	Wałbrzych
Grzeszczuk, Helena	ul. Narutowicza 67	Łódz
Grzybowska, Danuta	ul. Marolewska 23	Inowrocław
Grzybowska, Lucyna	ul. Francuska 49	Warszawa
Gryglicka, Helena	1. Roswelta 39/4	Zabrze
Grys, Irena	ul. Wsterplatte 13	Leszno
Gumińska Faľdorowicz, Maria	ul. Nowotki 76	Zywiec
Górska, Zinajda	ul. Zwyciestwa 69	Gliwice
Guz, Jerzy	ul. Kościuszki 12	Gliwice
Gwis, Krystyna	ul. Sienkiewicza 22	Łódz
Gwizd, Aniela	ul. Kasprowicza	Czechowicze-Dziedzice
Gwóźdż, Eugeniusz	ul. Brazylijska 13a	Warszawa
Hafman Miszta, Maria	ul. Siemiradzkiego 28/37	Bielsko
Hałatak, Rajmond	ul. Czysta 3	Bielsko
Hamerski, Włodzimierz	ul. Grażyny 17	Lublin
Hańczyc, Piotr	ul. Chałubińskiego 2a	Wrocław
Harasiuk, Bronisława	Plac XX-lecia 2	Łapy
Harażna Charkowska, Amelia	ul. Zeromskiego 4d	Warszawa
Hause, Ewa	Poradnia Okulist.	Opole
Hauser, Hanna	ul. Piekarska 2	Legnica
Hauslinger, Gabriela	ul. Wojska Polsk. 9/16	Ciechocinek
Heczko, Paweł	ul. Grunwaldzka 6	Rzeszów
Helmanowa, Bożena	ul. Gen. Zajaczka 27	Warszawa
Hercel, Barbara	ul. Zurawia 43	Katowice
Herlich, Maria	ul. Słoneczna 12	Kalisz
Herniczek, Ewa	ul. Al. Pokoju 24/12	Kraków
Hierowska Przybył, Aleksandra	ul. Grunwaldzka 135	Poznań
Hofman, Maria	ul. Siemiradzkiego 28	Bielsko Biała
Hornung, Elżbieta	ul. Majowa 14	Gliwice
Horodeński, Jarosław	Szpital Ogólny Nr. 2	Toruń
Horodyński, Krzysztof	ul. Garbarska 5a	Białystok
Hryniewiecka, Danuta	ul. Fornalskiej 1/3	Białystok
Hryniewska, Halina	ul. Spiska 4	Warszawa
Huczyńska, Barbara	ul. Sw. Filipa 5/5	Kraków
Huszcza, Alfred	ul. Partyzantów 45	Wrocław
Hychar, Maria	Poradnia Okulist.	Gliwice

Hyla, Barbara	ul. Lella 24/5	Starachowice
Iglińska Szymańska, Irena	ul. Nowe Osiedle 29b	Inowrocław
Iwańczyk Czarnecka, Bogu-sława	ul. Hankego 19	Warszawa
Iwaszkiewicz Bilikiewicz, Barb.	ul. Siemiradzkiego 12	Gdynia Oliwa
Iwaszkiewicz, Ewa	ul. Broniewskiego 15	Warszawa
Iwaszkiewicz, Krystyna	Piastów 7-Osiedle 10	Wrocław
Jablkowska, Wanda	ul. Kościuszki 11	Piaski k Sosnowca
Jablońska, Barbara	ul. Miejska Por. Okulist.	Olsztyn
Jablońska, Eulalia	ul. Pocztowa 23	Szczecin
Jablońska, Walentyna	ul. Dzierzyńskiego 50	Gdynia
Jabloński, Alojzy	ul. Chudoby 11	Poznań
Jabloński, Janusz	ul. Ujejskiego 11	Gdynia
Jabloński, Piotr	ul. Bieruta 5I	Pila
Jabloński, Zbigniew	ul. Michalowskiego 43	Gdynia Oliwa
Jackowska, Dorota	ul. Slonimskiego 3I	Bialystok
Jackowska, Janina	ul. Starowiejska 10	Gdynia
Jaczynowska, Zofia	ul. Woronicza 46	Warszawa
Jagoda, Maria	ul. Górska 17	Warszawa
Jaguczańska, Halina	ul. Prusa 63	Wroclaw
Jaklewicz, Alfred	ul. Zjednoczenia 9	Gryfice
Jakubiec, Genowefa	ul. Wita Stwosza 1	Rybnik
Jakubowski, Feliks	nad Kania 20	Gostyń
Janc, Maria	ul. Czysta 12	Sosnowiec
Jańczak, Zdzislawa	Poradnia Okulist.	Lomza
Janczewska, Szczesna	ul. Dzierzyńskiego 40	Sopot
Janecka, Barbara	ul. Czysta 12	Sosnowiec
Janiak, Elzbieta	ul. Plac Wolności 26	Czeladz
Janiec, Jan	ul. Chalubińskiego 2a	Wroclaw
Janik, Jadwiga	ul. Dubois 8	Warszawa
Janiszewska, Grazyna	Al. Jerozolimskie 145	Warszawa
Janiszewski, Stanislaw	ul. Bialobrzeska 8	Warszawa
Janotka, Henryk	ul. Friedleina 25b	Kraków
Janukowicz, Halina	Zakopiańska 3	Gdynia Siedlce
Janusik, Henryka	ul. Spacerowa 6	Zgierz
Januszko, Iwona	Poradnia Okulist.	Ketrzyn
Jaroszyński, Grzegorz	ul. Marchlewskiego 15	Lublin
Jarzemska, Lidia	ul. Konarskiego 50	Poznań
Jastrzebska, Jadwiga	ul. Wieczysta 12	Nowa Huta Kraków
Jaworowska, Hanna	ul. Hoza 38	Warszawa
Jaworska Kozakowa, Krystyna	ul. 3-go Maja 22	Lublin
Jaworska, Zofia	ul. Mickiewicza 25	Warszawa
Jaworski, Wladyslaw	ul. Grzegórzecka 49	Kraków
Jedraszym, Maria	ul. Matejki 2	Poznań
Jedruszek, Krystyna	ul. Grunwaldzka 12b.	Bydgoszcz
Jelén, Dobrowolska	ul. Bukowa 3	Poznań
Jerzowiecka, Lidia	ul Chalubińskiego 2a K1.O.	Wroclaw
Jurkiewicz, Weronika	ul. Chrobrego 57	Zielona Góra
Juszczyk, Janina	ul. Szpitalna 8	Poznań
Juszko, Krystyna	Slowackiego 1	Piotrków Tryb
Juzwa, Józefa	ul. Swietokrzyska 6	Kraków
Kacala, Halina	ul. Krywki 4	Starachowice
Kaczarowska, Barbara	ul. Chalubińskiego 2a	Wroclaw
Kadlof, Wanda	ul. Rynek 6/2	Kozle

Kadlubowska, Krystyna ...	ul. Marcelińska 57	Poznań
Kadyj, Stanislaw	ul. Marchlewskiego 11	Jaslo
Kahlowa, Joanna	ul. Komandosów 12	Kraków
Kaluzna, Irena	ul. Modra 23	Poznań
Kaluzny, Józef	ul. Lidzka 8	Poznań
Kalymonowa, Eugenia	ul. Wroclawska 33	Jelenia Góra
Kamińska, Anna	ul. Dabrowskiego 5	Pskowice
Kamińska Olechowicz, Bozena	ul. Rew. Pazdziernikowej 182 ...	Tychy
Kamińska, Stefania	Poradnia Okulist.	Jelenia Góra
Kana, Emanuel	ul. Bieruta 16/8	Lublin
Kanas, Boguslaw	ul. 22 Lipca 29	Tarnowskieg
Kania Beldzińska, Maria ...	ul. Bema 19	Gdynia
Kapica, Jadwiga	ul. Zeglarska 17	Wroclaw
Kapuściński, Cezary	ul. Mickiewicza 10	Wroclaw
Kapuściński, Witold	ul. Mickiewicza 10	Wroclaw
Karaśkiewicz, Maria	ul. Kolorowa 19	Kraków
Karczewicz, Danuta	ul. Cegielskiego 2	Szczecin
Karczmarska, Danuta	ul. Grazyny 4	Szczecin
Karpowicz, Sergiusz	ul. Szenwalda 6	Opole
Karpowicz, Wanda	ul. Szenwalda 6	Opole
Kasprowicz, Tadeusz	ul. Pienieznego 13	Olsztyn
Kazanowska, Anna	ul. Dabrowska 87	Tychy
Kazigrotowska, Teodozja ..	ul. Wojska Polsk. 5	Gdańs-Wrzeszcz
Kecik, Tadeusz	ul. Prosta 4/18	Warszawa
Kicińska, Jadwiga	Lipowa 1	Lódzul
Kiewro, Jadwiga	ul. Pijarów 2b	Kraków
Kikiela, Marian	ul. Staffa 11	Zielona Góra
Kisiecki, Wlodzimierz	Poradnia Okulist.	Bielsko Biala
Kisiclewska, Anna	ul. Rymwida 8	Lublin
Klim, Leontyna	ul. Marchlewskiego 1	Olsztyn
Klimkiewicz, Krzysztof ...	Plac Leńskiego 10	Warszawa
Klinowski, Czeslaw	ul. Szpitalna 34	Kraków
Klomowska, Anna	ul. Hempla 4	Lublin
Klos Kosakowska, Alina ...	ul. Grunwaldzka 92	Gdańsk-Wrzeszcz
Klyko, Andrzej	ul. 50-cie Rw, Pazdziernik. 5 ...	Sochaczew
Koch, Kowalikowa	ul. Narciszewska 28	Nowy Sacz
Kodejszko, Jaroslaw	ul. Niemcewicza 9	Warszawa
Kokocińska Pokora, Janina .	ul. Rycerska 4	Choszczno
Kolodziej, Irena	ul. Nasyp 4	Gliwice
Kolodziej, Maria	ul. Moniuszki 8	Szczecin
Kolodziejczyk, Józef	ul. A. Pokoju 15	Czestochowa
Kolodyńska, Czeslawa	ul. Krasińskiego 4a	Kutno
Konopka, Barbara	ul. Armii Czerwonej 64/63	Zawiercie
Konopka Krogulska, Helena.	ul. Buczka 4	Chorzów
Kopeć Oleszyńska, Slawomira	ul. PKWN 5	Lublin
Koperski, Jerzy	ul. Miczurina 7	Czestochowa
Korkonowicz, Jadwiga	Swierczewskiego 26	Sopot
Kornacki, Boleslaw	ul. Grójecka 19	Warszawa
Koronczewska, Danuta	ul. Grazyny 4	Szczecin
Kościelniak, Helena	ul. Szklarska 7/3	Olkusz
Kościuk, Zenon	ul. Sportowa 9	Mlawa
Kossak, Ewa	ul. Batorego 39/38	Gdańsk
Kossakowski, Jerzy	ul. Zwierzyniecka 17/2	Bialystok
Kossowicz, Halina	Niepodleglości 157	Warszawa Al.

Kostro, Franciszek	ul. Hipoteczna 3	Lublin
Kostrubiec, Jadwiga	ul. Szamotulska 18	Lódz
Koszutska, Lidia	ul. Sobieskiego 26	Ursus
Kotania, Wladyslaw	ul. Szolca 6	Bedzin
Kotarska, Barbara	ul. Szeroka 1/2	Bydgoszcz
Kowalczyk, Julita	ul. Zawadzkiego 47	Wodzislaw
Kowalewski, Jan	ul. Zeromskiego 105	Radom
Kowanetr, Zofia	ul. Matejki 32a	Nowy Sacz
Kozacka, Halina	Poradnia Okulist.	Ostróda
Kozaczuk, Maria	ul. Kamienna 1	Legnica
Kozlowski, Andrzej	ul. Nowotki 1	Szrem
Kozlowski, Bogumil	ul. Wojska Polskiego 185	Lódz
Kozmińska, Wanda	ul. Partyzantów 16	Bedzin
Kozuchowska, Izabella	ul. Hibnera 9	Warszawa
Krassowska, Maria	ul. Powstańców Wkp. 11/7	Bydgoszcz
Krauss, Janina	ul. Waryńskiego 28	Warszawa
Krauze, Hanna	ul. Wyspiańskiego 4	Slupsk
Krawczuk, Olga	ul. Nowogrodzka 38	Bialystok
Krawczuk, Laryssa	ul. Lakowa 14	Bialystok
Krawczyk, Zofia	ul. Wojsk. Akademia Medyczna Okulis	Lódz
Krawczyńska, Irena	ul. Zakosy 38	Gdańsk-Sielce
Kroplińska, Anna	ul. Chalubińskiego 2a	Wroclaw
Krudysz, Jan	ul. Chalubińskiego 2a Kl. O.	Wroclaw
Krukowska, Krystyna	ul. Marszalkowska 27/35	Warszawa
Król, Wieslawa	ul. Naściszewska 84	Nowy Sacz
Królik, Halina	ul. Worcella 7	Czestochowa
Królowa, Anna	ul. 18 Stycznia 68/2	Kraków
Krulpolc, Bronislaw	ul. Poradnia Okulist.	Dzierzoniów
Kruszczyński, Tadeusz	ul. Kościuszki 33a	Sopot
Krwawicz, Tadeusz	ul. Krak. Przedmieście 49	Lublin
Krzystkowa, Krystyna	ul. Kościuszki 32	Kraków
Krzysztolik, Zofia	ul. Staromlyńska 3	Szczecin
Krzyzanowska, Zofia	ul. Plac Wolności 14/4	Rzeszów
Krzyzanowska, Zofia	ul. Spóldzielcza 8	Nowa Huta Kraków
Krygier, Zygmunt	ul. Chrobrego 8	Rybnik
Kubala Morcinek, Cecylia	ul. Marksa 7	Tarnowskie Góry
Kubatko, Eugeniusz	na Skarpie 59	Nowa Huta Osiedle
Kuczyk, Miroslawa	ul. Wojska Polskiego 27	Stargard
Kuczyńska, Barbara	ul. Sibelina 4I	Warszawa
Kuczyńska, Zofia	ul. Chalubińskiego 2a Kl. O.	Wroclaw
Kucharska, Irena	ul. Anczyca 11	Kraków
Kukawczyńska, Helena	ul. Swierczewskiego 30	Kedzierzyn
Kulesza, Janina	ul. Rajska 13	Lódz
Kulig, Maria	ul. Majowa 8	Gliwice
Kurianowicz, Wanda	ul. Spóldzielcza 2	Biala Podl
Kutkowska, Zofia	ul. Sikorskiego 3	Trzcianka
Kurowska, Teresa	ul. Swierczewskiego 27	Szczecin
Kwapiszewska Lachowicz, Barbara	ul. Sienna 66	Warszawa
Kwaskowski, Adam	ul. 23 Lutego 29/33	Poznań
Kwiatkowska Kawecka, Zofia	Osiedle Przyjaźń 32	Warszawa
Lange, Teresa	ul. Chalubińskiego 2a Kl. O.	Wroclaw
Langwińska, Maria	ul. Grotgera 1	Lublin
Larys-Blazejewska, Halina	ul. Baśniowa 5	Pruszków

Laśkiewicz, Maria	ul. Czapińskiego 2I	Dabrowa Górnicza
Laszczyk, Wieslawa	ul. Chocimska 29	Warszawa
Ledzińska, Krystyna	ul. Mickiewicza 32/23	Bialystok
Lenkiewicz, Edward	ul. Partyzantów 74	Olsztyn
Lenkiewicz, Zdzislaw	ul. Dabrowszczaków 14	Kraśnik
Leszczyńska, Barbara	ul. Kościuszki 12	Radomsko
Leszczyński, Mieczyslaw	ul. Prusa 1	Hrubieszów
Lewalski, Walenty	ul. Poradnia Okulist	Szczytno
Licowa, Halina	ul. Dobrzyńska 22	Wroclaw
Lipińska Chwiej, Eugenia	ul. Idzikowskiego 4	Warszawa
Loba, Barbara	ul. Wybickiego 11	Kościeszyna
Lowek, Janina	ul. Szpitalna 8	Limanowa
Lakota, Joanna	ul. Chalubińskiego 2a Kl. O.	Wroclaw
Lapiński, Marek	ul. Slawińskiego 13/15	Lublin
Laska Welfeld, Maria	ul. Królewska 2	Warszawa
Lodzińska, Izabella	ul. Jasnogórska 66	Czestochowa
Losowska, Wanda	ul. Zielna 3	Krosno. nad Wisloka
Luczyńska Anna	ul. Slowackiego 7	Bytom
Lukaszewicz, Benon	ul. Szpital Oddz. O.	Swidnica
Machowa, Helena	ul. Rynek Kleparski 6/2	Kraków
Maciazek, Halina	ul. 1 Maja 2I	Poréba
Maciejsz, Adam	ul. 18 Stycznia 12	Kraków
Maciejewska, Jolanta	ul. Chelmska 3/2	Bialystok
Maciejewski, Zbigniew	ul. Bitwy pod Lenino 5	Kraków
Maciszuk Mendecka, Zofia	ul. Dworcowa 26	Gliwice
Madroszkiewicz, Andrzej	ul. Lobzowska 4	Kraków
Madroszkiewicz, Marian	ul. Lobzowska 4	Kraków
Madziar, Danuta	ul. Niecala 6	Warszawa
Magnowska, Maria		Legnica Ośrodek Zdrowia
Majchrzak Karczyńska, Halina	ul. Folwarczna 7	Gdynia Orlowo
Majewska Cembrzyńska, Anna	ul. Czarnieckiego 70	Katowice
Majewska, Kalina	ul. Paryska 27	Warszawa
Majewska, Helena	ul. Sadowa 14a	Poznań
Maka, Alina	ul. Sukiennicza 1	Kalisz
Makiela, Teresa	ul. Plebiscytowa 17/10	Katowice
Makowska, Jadwiga	ul. Popiela 11	Kraków
Makszewska, Zdzislawa	ul. Zdrojowa 65	Warszawa
Maksymczuk, Halina	ul. Armii Czerwonej 61	Elk
Makuć, Renata	Szpital	Jelenia Góra
Makulec, Krystyna	Poradnia Okulist.	Olsztyn
Malanek, Maria	ul. Litewska 28	Kraków
Malec Luczywowa, Anna	Plac Wolności 17	Jelenia Góra
Maliczuk, Zofia	ul. Dworcowa 26	Gliwice
Malik, Alojzy	ul. Swierczewskiego 16	Katowice
Malinowska, Danuta	ul. Zlota 79	Warszawa
Malinowska, Elzbieta	ul. Kraszewskiego 1	Gdańsk-Wrzeszcz
Malinowska, Halina	ul. Marcinkowskiego 1c	Gorzów
Malinowska, Krystyna	ul. Swierczewskiego 1	Bartoszyce
Malus Stram, Maria	ul. Glowackiego 13	Lódz
Malecka, Alicja	Wyspiańskiego 37	Bielsko Biala
Malecka, Jolanta	ul. Marchlewskiego 68	Warszawa
Manna, Feliks	ul. Grunwaldzka 24	Gdańsk-Wrzeszcz
Marcinkowska, Teresa	ul. Zaleskiego 1	Szczecin
Marczak Klonowska, Jadwiga	ul. Henryka 4	Lublin

Markiewicz, Boleslaw	ul. Piotra Skargi 36	Szczecin
Markiewicz, Bozena	ul. Poradnia Okulist.	Biskupiec
Maślak, Maria	ul. Plac Wolności 4	Grodków
Matuszczyk, Irena	ul. Piastowska 2	Sosnowiec
Matuszewska, Bronislawa ..	ul. Zwirki i Wigury 13	Katowice
Matyja, Teresa	ul. 3 Maja 3	Dabrowa Górnicza
Matyjaszewska, Maria	ul. Stawowa 3	Katowice
Mazur Kolaczyńska, Maria .	ul. Pana Tadeusza 2	Lublin
Mazurek, Malgorzata	ul. Jaracza 3	Toruń
Mazurowska, Lidia	ul. Ludna 10	Warszawa
Melanowski, Wladyslaw ...	ul. Twarda 1	Warszawa
Miechowa, Stefania	ul. Grochowska 133	Poznań
Mieczkowska, Barbara	ul. Kościuszki 31	Olsztyn
Mielczarek, Bogda	ul. Lompy 18/10	Oledzko
Mierzyńska, Regona	ul. Kanoniczna 4	Czestochowa
Mietus Polak, Barbara	ul. Garlińska 12	Kraków
Mhalak, Janina Michalak ...	ul. Boczna 8	Barlinek
Michalek, Wieslawa	ul. Wieczorka 28	Bytom
Mikolajewski, Andrzej	ul. Szczecińska 7b	Pyrzyce
Mikucka, Zdzislawa	Szpital	Chelm
Milkowski, Stefan	ul. Raclawicka 32	Czestochowa
Misiewicz, Ryszarda	ul. Prusa 6	Toruń
Miszczuk, Halina	ul. Tysiaclecia 4/14	Elblag
Miszke Szantroch, Anna ...	ul. Pilarecka 24	Kraków
Moll, Danuta	ul. Skryta 10	Poznań
Mondelski, Stanislaw	ul. Jugoslowiańska 59	Poznań
Monies, Anna	ul. Leśna 12	Pulawy
Morawiecki, Jerzy	ul. Wasowskiego 8	Gdańsk-Wrzeszcz
Morawska, Helena	ul. Elblaska 49	Gdańsk
Moskal, Herman	ul. Slupska 2	Katowice
Mosoczy, Krystyna	ul. Kolobrzeska 58	Gdynia Oliwa
Moszczyńska, Alicja	ul. Marszalkowska 83	Warszawa
Mozolewska, Grazyna	ul. Niedzialkowskiego 20	Szczecin
Mozdzyńska, Eugenia	ul. 1 Maja 19	Bialystok
Mroczkowska, Halina	NBol. Chrobrego 28	Rzeszów
Mrozek, Alicja	C. Sklodowskiej 72	Szczecin
Mściszewska, Krystyna	ul. Tyszki 7a	Katowice
Muller, Elzbieta	ul. Zorzy 3	Warszawa
Murczkiewicz, Alina	ul. Polubska 1	Klodzko
Muszyńska, Maria	ul. Buczka 29	Kielce
Mrzyglód, Stanislaw	ul. Czerska 4	Wroclaw
Myga, Barbara	ul. Sloneczna 57	Tarnowskie Góry
Myga, Wieslawa	ul. Dzielna 17a	Warszawa
Myjakowa, Hanna	ul. Krasickiego 6	Gdynia
Myszkowska, Krystyna ...	ul. Spóldzielcza 13	Chelm
Naróg Wójcik, Alina	ul. Pulawska 1	Warszawa
Nasalska Musial, Janina ...	ul. Klodzka 58	Wroclaw
Nawrocki, Kazimierz	ul. Lipowa 5	Pruszków
Netzer, Irena	ul. Konopnickiej 13	Sopot
Niebrój, Tadeusz	ul. Warmińska 18	Katowice
Niechaj, Zofia	ul. Wallenroda 20	Lublin
Niemcewicz, Leszek	ul. Cyganerii 21	Tychy
Niepokojczycki, Piotr	Plac Grunwaldzki 4c	Katowice
Nieznański, Leszek	ul. Pustola 20	Warszawa
Nikiel, Antoni	ul. Cieszkowskiego 11a	Lódz
Nikosiewicz, Michal	ul. Filtrowa 59	Warszawa

Niklas, Zofia	ul. Wieczorka 158	Piekary Slaskie
Nizankowska, Hanna	ul. Plac PKWN 6	Wroclaw
Nowacki, Stanislaw	ul. Struga 14	Sosnowiec
Nowak, Antonina	ul. Zlota 69	Warszawa
Nowak Sobkowiak, Zuzanna	ul. Górnicza 15	Jaworzno
Nowak, Teodor	ul. Jerzyka 4	Wagrowiec
Nowakowska, Emilia	ul. Buczka 1	Szczecin
Nowakowski, Witold	ul. Mickiewicza 57	Sopot
Nowicka, Aldona	ul. Kilińskiego 1	Szczecin
Nowicka, Henryka	ul. Nowa 5	Parczew
Nowicka, Laryssa	ul. Hankego 23	Warszawa
Nowicka, Natalia	ul. Moniuszki 9	Gliwice
Nowicka, Stanislawa	ul. Konarskiego 7	Wroclaw
Nowiński, Andrzej	ul. Szopena 37	Lublin
Noyszewska Wylezyńska, Kazim.	ul. Sekocińska 3	Warszawa
Obermeyer, Wojciech	ul. Zacisze 7	Plońska
Obrebska, Klara	ul. Hoza 34	Warszawa
Ogielska, Eugenia	ul. Kasprowicza 17	Wroclaw
Ogrodowicz, Urszula	ul. Solna 4/6	Lublin
Olbromska, Wanda	ul. Szpitalna 35	Bialystok
Olchowa, Piotr	ul. Podwale 24	Jawotzno
Olekszyk, Maria	ul. Teczowa 8	Wroclaw
Olichnier, Barbara	ul. Chalubińskiego 2a Kl. O.	Wroclaw
Omeliarowicz, Halina	ul. Zeromskiego 14	Sopot
Omulecka, Danuta	ul. Przechodnia 2	Warszawa
Ordon, Alina	ul. Jerzykowa 3	Zielona Góra
Ordon Strawa, Alina	ul. Jagiellońska 41	Poznań
Ordon, Zofia	ul. Wojska Polskiego 50	Warszawa
Orlikowska, Aleksandra	ul. Piastowska 90	Gdynia Oliwa
Orlowska, Nadzieja	ul. Kredytowa 8	Warszawa
Orlowski, Witold	ul. Grochowska 9I c	Poznań
Ornatowska, Anna	ul. Jerzykowa 3	Zielona Góra
Orszewska, Otylia	ul. Kasprowicza 14a	Olsztyn
Orszulik, Anna	ul. Gliwicka 14a	Katowice
Orzel, Henryk	ul. Szamotulska 19	Lódz
Osetek, Tadeusz	ul. Slowackiego 30	Kielce
Osiecka, Halina	ul. Slowackiego 38	Warszawa
Osiecka, Krystyna	ul. Anielewicza 3I	Warszawa
Osikowska Smyk, Zofia	Ośrodek Zdrowia	Zamość
Osmański, Stanislaw	ul. Szeroka 36	Toruń
Ossowska, Anna	ul. Trybunalska 19	Lublin
Ostachowicz, Mieczyslaw	Oliwa. ul. Polanki 17	Gdynia
Ostrowska, Barbara	ul. Aleja 18/9	Czestochowa
Otrebski, Zbigniew	pow. Opoczno	Drzewica Stawowa
Ozdzyński, Henryk	ul. Swiatopelka 9	Chojnice
Pacewicz, Jadwiga	ul. Waszyngtona 18	Czestochowa
Pagieta, Malgorzata	ul. Swierczewskiego 29	Oleszyn
Pajak, Stefania	ul. Czysta 10/17	Kraków
Pakula, Danuta	ul. Oświecimska 6	Myslowice
Pakula, Krystyna	Rw. Pazdziernikowej 26	Lódz
Palacz, Olgierd	ul. Rynkowa 3I	Szczecin
Paluchiewicz, Jadwiga	ul. Zawadzkiego 46	Katowice
Palusiewicz, Wanda	ul. Armii Czerwonej 7	Dabrowa Górnicza
Palysewicz, Tadeusz	ul. Szopena 3	Lublin
Pancerz, Stanislawa	ul. Trynikarska 18	Kraków

Pankowska, Bozena	ul. Chodkiewicza 5	Gdańsk-Wrzeszcz
Parzuchowski, Andrzej	ul. Broniewskiego 87	Warszawa
Paryzek, Jósef	ul. Ostrowskiego 6	Rybnik
Pasierbiński, Stefan	Smoleńsk 3	Kraków
Pasternak, Danuta	ul. Jagiellońska 30	Bytom
Paszkiewicz, Alina	ul. Obr. Stalingradu 15	Stalowa Wola
Paszkowska, Maria	ul. Narutowicza 135	Lódz
Paszyc, Danuta	ul. Kościuszki 17	Rybnik
Pawlikowska Ichilczyk, Anna	ul. Zwyciesców 19a	Gdynia Orlowo
Pawlikowska, Bozena	ul. Wolborska 1	Lódz
Pecold, Krystyna	ul. Raszyńska 40a	Poznań
Pedzik Rajca, Barbara	ul. Piastowska 8	Radomsko
Peller, Krystyna	ul. Drukarska 34	Wroclaw
Penderecki, Janusz	ul. Kowalska 18	Zabrze
Pentak, Krystyna	ul. Nadrzecze 2	Zarkil Letnisko
Perekladowska, Maria	ul. Wallemroda 2	Lublin
Perz, Dominik	Kollataja 4	Szamotuly
Perz, Marian	ul. Dzialowa 16	Poznań
Petlak, Barbara	ul. Straganiarska 43	Gdańsk
Petrys, Alicja	ul. Marchlewskiego 48a	Kraków
Piasecka, Elzbieta	ul. Ciasna 19	Sosnowiec
Piasceka Kacperska, Krystyna	ul. Gospody 130	Gdynia Oliwa
Piatek, Henryka	ul. Tyszki 40	Katowice
Piatkiewicz, Zofia	ul. Osiedle Bloki 12	Nowa Huta
Piatkowska, Anna	ul. Nowowiejska 1	Lublin
Piech, Harry	ul. Zgrzebnicka 3	Chorzów
Piechowiak, Florentyna ...	ul. Winogrady 33	Poznań
Pieczka, Urszula	ul. Wita Stwosza 5	Gdynia Oliwa
Piestrzeniewicz, Wiesaw ...	ul. Parkowa 2	Mragowo
Pietrzyk, Elzbieta	ul. C. Sklodowskiej 14	Swinoujście
Pilecka Czekaj, Irena	ul. Piastowska 94	Gdynia Oliwa
Pilas Krol, Teresa	ul. Kościuszki 10	Bielsko Biala
Pilat, Maria	ul. Niedzialkowskiego 6a	Olsztyn
Pioruńska, Maria	ul. Rakowicka 12	Kraków
Piotrowski, Aleksander	ul. Kijowska 11	Warszawa
Piwońska, Stefania	ul. Grenadierów 12	Warszawa
Planda, Anna	ul. Wallenroda 2c	Lublin
Platakis, Krystyna	ul. Piastowska 3b	Bialystok
Plewińska, Halina	ul. Leśny Sad 1	Milanówek
Plonka, Maria	ul. Wiśniowa 33	Wroclaw
Poborc Godlewska, Janina .	ul. Hutowa 10	Lódz
Podziewska, Grazyna	ul. Niemcewicza 48	Suwalki
Pojda, Konrad	ul. Mieleckiego 4	Katowice
Pojda, Stefan	ul. Mieleckiego 4	Katowice
Pol, Wlalyslaw	ul. Barska 11	Warszawa
Polak, Salomea	ul. Okrzei 7	Katowice
Poludniewska, Maria	Szpital	Stargard
Pomykalska, Domicela	ul. Dubois 10a	Lublin
Poniszewska Kuczewska, Irena	ul. Swidnicka 11	Katowice-Ligota
Popek, Emilia Eva	ul. Karmelicka 52	Kraków
Popek, Irena	ul. Olszewskiego 77	Wroclaw
Popkowski, Jan	ul. Kościuszki 2I	Wloclawek
Portacha, Lidia	ul. Stoleczna 17	Warszawa

Prościewicz, Krystyna	ul. Grunwaldzka 7	Lebork
Protasiewicz, Stanisława	ul. Buczka 43	Szczecin
Protasowicka, Paulina	ul. Buczka 43	Szczecin
Pruchnicka, Maria	ul. Swierczewskiego 7	Cieszyn
Prusiewicz, Anna	ul. Wierzbowa 5	Olsztyn
Prustowska, Ewa	ul. Chalubińskiego 2a Kl. O	Wroclaw
Przadka, Leszek	ul. Bukietowa 17	Warszawa
Przepiórkowski, Ryszard	ul. Brodowicza 5a	Kraków
Przeworska, Ranata	ul. Zjednoczenia 18	Toruń
Przybyl, Ereńska K	ul. Hibnera 18	Poznań
Przybtlowicz, Anna	ul. Graniczna 30	Skarzysko Kamienna
Przyborowska, Helena	Swietojańska 36	Gdynia
Przybyslawska, Krystyna	ul. Narutowicza 24	Radom
Przyluska, Aleksandra	ul. Sarego 22	Kraków
Przysucha, Jerzy	ul. PKWN 15	Lublin
Przytulsko, Jan	Szpital Oddz. O.	Wieluń
Ptasińska, Maria	ul. Pulawska 111	Warszawa
Pukacz, Marianna	ul. 22 Lipca 4	Kedzierzyn
Pyzowski, Józef	ul. 1000-cia 43	Nowy Targ
Raczyńska, Krystyna	ul. Wyczólkowskiego 68	Gdańsk
Rajewska, Irena	ul. Bema 2	Kielce
Rawska, Barbara	ul. Przebendowskiego 9	Gdynia Orlowo
Reichelt, Anna	ul. Przybyszewskiego 9	Gdynia Orlowo
Reichert, Teresa	ul. Dekerta 2	Rzeszów
Rejnowicz, Ligia	ul. Lewartowskiego 18	Warszawa
Riedlowa, Sabina	ul. Olszańska 14	Kraków
Rogozińska, Danuta	ul. Murawska 5	Legnica
Rogowska, Danuta	Wojska Polskiego 128	Lódz
Roik, Aniela	ul. PPR 3I	Cieszyn
Romańczuk, Regina	Ligota. ul. Emerytalna 16	Katowice
Rościszewska, Bronislawa	Zawrat 25	Warszawaul
Rozanowicz, Izabella	ul. Warszawska 5	Katowice
Roznowski, Jan		Olsztyn PKP
Rudnicki, Jacek	ul. Belojanisa 18	Zabrze
Rudobielski, Romuald	ul. Nowy Swiat 10	Bialystok
Rudzińska, Anna	ul. Mickiewicza 32	Bialystok
Runge, Irena	ul. Chorzowska 22	Wroclaw
Rusek, Janusz	ul. Stelmacha 25	Raciborz
Rusin, Andrzej	ul. Sulkowskiego 19/1	Bydgoszcz
Rusin, Elzbieta	ul. Sulkowskiego 19/1	Bydgoszcz
Rutkowska, Alicja	ul. Bukietowa 15	Warszawa
Rutkowska, Leonia	Zrodlowa 4I	Lódzul
Rzepkowska, Lubomira	ul. 2 Mieczy 8	Rembertów
Rzeska, Henryka	ul. Kosińskiego 29	Poznań
Rypniewska, Helena	1 Maja 5/4	Zakopane
Sapka, Maria	ul. Zamenhoffa 1	Olsztyn
Sarama, Krystyna	ul. Mianowskiego 25	Wroclaw
Sawicka, Krystyna	ul. Borsucza 3	Bialystok
Sawińska Garstkowa, Bozena	ul. Brzeznicka 2	Poznań
Sciborowska, Krystyna	Poradnia Okulist.	Nowe Miasto
Semenicki, Krzysztof	ul. Broniewskiego 2	Warszawa
Semdyka, Maria	ul. Mazowiecka 125	Kraków
Sepiolo, Maria	ul. Kolberga 2a	Gdańsk-Wrzeszc
Serkowska, Halina	pow. Garwolin	Laskarzew
Sidorowicz Skrzypek, Leontyna	ul. Grójecka 122	Warszawa

Siemaszko Kobus, Jadwiga .	ul. Swierczewskiego 27	Slawécin
Sieradzka, Barbara	ul. Komandosów 5	Kraków
Sieroslawska, Feodozja	ul. Kościuszki 22	Wroclaw
Sikora, Urszula	ul. Ciencialy 1	Cieszyn
Sitkiewicz, Anna	ul. Legionów 4	Szczecin
Skalska Rakowska, Jadwiga .	Zywnego 16	Warszawa
Skapska Labedzka, Anna ..	ul. Boh. Stalingradu 39	Kraków
Skibińska, Rudolfowa Kazimiera	ul. Nowowiejska 1	Warszawa
Skorupska, Danuta	ul. Rudziszyńska 30b	Szczein
Skorus, Maria	ul. Rew. Pazdziernikowej 13	Tychy
Skowroński, Jerzy	ul. Ogrodowa 9	Lublin
Skrzynowska, Zofia	ul. Rodziewiczowej 2/3	Szczecin
Skrzyńska, Halina	ul. Lollka 2I	Gliwice
Sladkowska, Elzbieta	ul. Chalubińskiego 2a Kl. O.	Wroclaw
Sliwa, Stanislaw	ul. Manifestu Lipcowego 8/16 ..	Debica
Sliwińska, Halina	Poradnia Okulist.	Legnica
Sliwińska Osterczy, Hanna .	ul. Smoleńsk 48	Kraków
Slawińska, Wanda	ul. Kielecka 9	Kraków
Sluzewska, Teresa	ul. Zwirki i Wigury 3I	Katowice
Smajkiewicz, Zofia	ul. Szopena 2I	Szczecin
Smarzyńska, Helena	Os XX-cia PRL 14/15	Nowa Huta
Smielecki, Jan	Moniuszki 45	Gorzów
Smigiel, Grazyna	ul. Krasickiego 14	Gdynia
Smogulecka, Ewa	ul. Ostroroga 28	Poznań
Smoktunowicz, Irena	ul. Zelazna 58	Warszawa
Smolarska, Krystyna	ul. Sokolska 25	Bialystok
Smolarz, Janina	ul. Piotrkowska 107	Lódz
Smoleńska, Danuta	ul. Chrobrego 6	Bialystok
Smolińska, Krystyna	ul. Sokolska 25	Bialystok
Smulikowska, Krystyna ...	ul. Chalubińskiego 2a Kl.	Wroclaw
Sniezka, Krystyna	Poradnia Okulist.	Bartoszyce
Sobański, Janusz	ul. Narutowicza 119	Lódz
Sobańska, Maria	ul. Hipoteczna 18a	Lódz
Sobczyk, Jan	ul. Sowińskiego 24	Czestochowa
Sobczyński, Gerwazy	ul. Grunwaldzka 27	Jaroslaw
Sobieska, Clar Helena	ul. Bema 28	Elblag
Soboczyńska, Zofia	ul. Lodowa 20	Poznań
Sobusiak, Jan	ul. Lokietka 1	Chorzów
Sochańska Drewnowska, Alina	Sopocka 4	Szczecinul
Sokola, Henryka	ul. 15 Grudnia 157	Bobrowniki
Sokolowska, Barbara	ul. Zwyciestwa 10	Pulawy
Sokolowska, Jadwiga	ul. Kosmonautów 1d	Kedzierzyn
Sokolowska, Janina	ul. Smoleńsk 46	Kraków
Sokolowski, Tadeusz	ul. Zwyciestwa 4	Sosnowiec
Solarski, Zbigniew	Falata 16a	Bytom
Soroka, Daniela	ul. Swinoujska 12	Wroclaw
Sorokowska Traczuk, Natalia	ul. Polna 54	Warszawa
Sowina, Maria	ul. Kochanowskiego 2	Sopot
Srzednicka, Krystyna	ul. Westerplatte 7	Kraków
Staniak, Irena	ul. Rzeszowska 3	Nisko
Stankiewicz, Andrzej	Wrześniewska 46a	Lódzul
Starega, Bogdan	ul. Marchlewskiego 4	Gniezno
Starkiewicz, Witold	ul. C. Sklodowskiej 12	Szczecin

Starzycka, Maria	ul. Sw. Krzyza 3	Kraków
Stasińska Misiurewicz, Janina	ul. Kraszewskiego 12	Poznań
Staszewska, Zofia	ul. Stocka 9	Lódz
Stawicka, Anna	ul. Stawowa 15a	Bydgoszcz
Stawiński, Tadeusz	ul. Krasińskiego 29	Bielsko Biala
Stepak, Stanislaw	ul. Swobody 23	Poznań
Stepień, Tadeusz	ul. Zamenhoffa 11	Swidnica
Steplewska, Wilhelmina	ul. Brodzińskiego 5	Zabrze
Stepniewska, Barbara	ul. Bracka 25	Lódz
Stolarska, Helena	ul. Wawrzyniaka 2	Szczecin
Stolarzewicz, Cecylia	ul. Garibaldiego 6/5	Bielkos Biala
Straburzyński, Józef	ul. Niepodleglości 7	Walbrzych
Strzyzewski, Kazimierz	ul. Raclawicka 47	Wroclaw
Suchanek, Wieslawa	ul. Podchorazych 2	Bydgoszcz
Suliborska, Alicja	ul. Biegańskiego 8a	Lódz
Swatek, Miroslaw	ul. Wojska Polsk. 2a	Wadowice
Swiech, Wladyslaw	ul. Kollataja 21	Tarnów
Swierc Pawlik, Maria	ul. Poniatowskiego 30	Katowice
Swierzbińska, Danuta	ul. Armii Czerw. 25/34	Elk
Swietliczko, Irena	ul. Narutowicza 79	Lódz
Swietlik, Karol	ul. Kościuszki 3	Sanok
Swietlikowska, Anna	ul. Ketrzyńskiego 3	Olsztyn
Swistuń, Jerzy	ul. Buczka 15	Bydgoszcz
Switek, Teresa	1 Maja 14/5	Bielsko Biala
Szaflik, Jerzy	ul. Harcerska 13	Zabrze 4
Szafran, Leslaw	ul. Kasprowy 8a	Kraków
Szafranko, Romuald	ul. Kościuszki 2	Elk
Szafrańska, Anna	Szpital	Pisz
Szamborska, Wiktoria	ul. Buczka 4	Skierniewice
Szawlowska, Alina	ul. Wrzeciono 57	Warszawa
Szejca Dzuda, Teresa	ul. B. Czecha 7	Bielsko Biala
Szewera, Helena	ul. Krowodarska 3/6	Kraków
Szczepańczyk, Lidia	ul. Grunwaldzka 22a	Bielsko Biala
Szczupakm, Teresa	ul. Oświecimska 15	Brzeziny
Szczypiński, Józef	ul. Plomienna 5b	Poznań
Szmura, Zbigniew	ul. 22 lipca 1c	Kedzierzyn
Szpakiewicz, Irena	ul. Szopena 1	Kraśnik
Szpakowicz, Elzbieta	ul. Chalubińskiego 2 a Kl. O.	Wroclaw
Szpilewski, Stefan	ul. Sciegiennego 1	Kolobrzeg
Szostakiewicz, Helena	Walowa 26	Gdańsk
Szreterowa, Miroslawa	ul. Fabryczna 2	Warszawa
Szretter, Kazimierz	ul. Matwicka 8	Warszawa
Szubińska, Halina	ul. Staffa 7	Warszawa
Szumilas, Kazimiera	ul Brodzińskiego 2	Zabrze
Szumowska Trzmiel, Teresa	Ośrodek Zgr.	Zabkowice
Szusterowska, Martin Elzbieta	ul. Wojska Polsk. 11a	Lódz
Szwarc, Barbara	ul. Krucza 2/14	Lublin
Szyluk, Wombard	ul. Gwiazdista 10	Gorzów
Szymankiewicz, Stefania	ul. Marksa 28	Mikolow
Szymański, Andrzej	ul. Krótka 19	Knurów
Szymański, Józef	ul. Dabrowskiego 16	Slupsk
Szymańska, Krystyna	ul. Saklodowskiej 72	Szczecin
Sycha Warnecka, Helena	ul. Plebiscytowa 21	Rybnik
Tajchert, Jerzy	ul. Ujazdowskie 8	Warszawa

Taracha, Alina	ul. Skrzetuskiego 9	Warszawa
Tarantowicz, Wanda	ul. Grybowska 9	Warszawa
Tarnawska, Jadwiga	ul. Ordona 20	Katowice
Tarnowska, Krystyna	ul. Majowa 27/8	Gliwice
Tarnowska, Wieslawa	ul. Raclawicka 9/7	Gdańsk
Teppe, Stamarska	ul. Chalubińskiego 2a	Wroclaw
Tereferenko, Stefan	Szpital	Walcz
Teternak, Jadwiga	ul. Al. Niepodleglości 138	Warszawa
Toczolowski, Jerzy	ul. Rymwida 8	Lublin
Tokarz, Alicja	ul. 1 Maja 31	Bytom
Tomaszewska, Alicja	ul. Batorego 34	Gdańsk
Tomaszewska, Anna	ul. Marchlewskiego 72	Warszawa
Tomaszewska, Karolina	ul. Pradnicka 43	Kraków
Tomaszewska, Stefania	ul. Swierczewskiego Por.	Gdańsk
Toroń Charwat, Grazyna	Os. Strusia 3	Nowa Huta
Trapkiewicz, Lucja	ul. Szopena 5	Olsztyn
Trojanowska Klajnert, Ewa	ul. Pilicka 56	Warszawa
Trusiewicz, Lucja Danuta	ul. Pereca 13	Warszawa
Trzcińska Dabrowska, Zofia	ul. Dantyszka 2	Warszawa
Turowska, Wieslawa	ul. Kościuszki 3	Dabrowa Górnicza
Tuszewska, Renata	ul. Chalubińskiego 2a	Wroclaw
Twardzik Switlik, Danuta	ul. Sienkiewicza 28	Nowy Sacz
Tworek Budny, Danuta	ul. Nowotki 7/6	Zawiercie
Tymieniecka, Krystyna	ul. Grudziacka 33/6	Toruń
Uchta, Elzbieta	ul. Królowej Jadwigi 146	Dabrowa Górnicza
Ujazdowska, Anna	ul. Walecznych 77	Gdańsk
Urbaniak, Gustawa	ul. Przybyszewskiego 46	Poznań
Wachowiak, Kazimierz	ul. Zwyciestwa 80	Koszalin
Walewska, Ewa	ul. Cedlera 11	Sosnowiec
Warchalowska Pykala, Urszula	ul. Obornicka 41	Poznań
Warno, Gabriela	ul. Kasprzaka 39	Lódz
Was, Maria	ul. Swierczewskiego 9	Sosnowiec
Wasilec, Jadwiga	Chalubińskiego 2a	Wroclaw
Wasilewski, Mieczyslaw	ul. Swickiej 6	Gdańsk Wrzeszcz
Waśkowska, Maria	ul. Grazyna 8	Lublin
Wasowska, Malgorzata	Slowackiego 5	Warszawa
Waszkiewicz, Izabella	06r. Zdr.	Cieplice
Wawer, Pola	Swierczewskiego 82	Warszawa
Wazyński, Dariusz	ul. Sniadeckich 21	Poznań
Wdowska, Ewa	Leszka Czarnego 7	Lublin
Weglarz, Janina	N.D.M. 12	Kedzierzyn
Weglarz Wdowiak, Maria	ul. Wadowity 9	Wadowice
Weigensperg, Stefania	ul. Szopena 2	Rzeszów
Welke, Oskar	ul. Krakowska 15	Tarnów
Welsyng, Rózańska Katarzyna	Tetmajera 5	Gdynia Oliwa
Widomska, Ewa	ul. Leszka Czarnego 7	Lublin
Widinka, Józef	ul. Wyzwolenia 7	Skryszew
Wieckiewicz, Grazyna	ul. Brzozowa 9a	Gdańsk Wrzeszcz
Wieczorek, Bozena	ul. Powstańców 29a	Lubliniec
Wieczorek Baran, Irena	ul. Jagielońska 2	Dabrowa Tarnowska
Wieczorek, Renata	ul. Francuska 16	Katowice
Wieliczko, Jadwiga	ul. Zamenhofa 4	Zielona Góra
Wierzbowska, Anna	ul. Krótka 8	Lomza
Wieszczyczyńska, Maria	ul. Zabikowska 62	Luboń

Wilczak, Kazimierz	ul. Rydla 6	Kraków
Wilhelm, Elzbieta	ul. 22 Lipca 2	Swidnik
Winiarska, Alina	ul. Bystrzycka 4	Kraków
Winiarska, Krystyna	ul. Glebińska 9	Warszawa
Winogradzka, Wieslawa	ul. Parkowa 4a	Bialystok
Wiszniewski, Janusz	ul. 3 Maja 33/4	Zabrze
Witkiewicz, Jacek	1000-cia 37	Przemyśl
Witusik, Wladyslaw	ul. Kościuszki 20	Jaslo
Wlodarczyk, Ewa	ul. Bratnia 7	Pszczyna
Wnetrzak, Krystyna	ul. Wiwecka 24	Sosnowiec
Wojciechowska, Renata	ul. Debowa 8	Katowice
Wojciechowska, Zofia	ul. Ośr. Zdr.	Opole
Wojczak, Janina	ul. Rycerska 8	Poznań
Wojno, Barbara	Poradnia Okulist.	Orneta
Wojnowska, Ewa	ul. Marchlewskiego 74	Warszawa
Wojtas, Andrzej	ul. Musiala 2I	Czeladz
Wojtyczko, Danuta	ul. Hibnera 1	Siemianowice
Wolska, Barbara	ul. Dworcowa 9	Szczecin
Wolter Czerwińska, Halina	ul. Kopernika 8/18	Warszawa
Wolchowicz, Krystyna	ul. Chalubińskiego 2a Kl. O.	Wroclaw
Wolkow, Teresa	ul. Mydlana 63	Chrzanów
Woloszyn, Bogumila	ul. Pulaskiego 39	Rzeszów
Wolyniuk, Miroslaw	ul. Parkowa 8	Bialystok
Womaczkowa, Krystyna	ul. Padewskiego 13a	Warszawa
Wozniak, Irena	ul. Chalubińskiego 2a Kl. O.	Wroclaw
Wozny, Jerzy	ul. Rynek ... k/ Wroclawia	Domanice
Wroniecka, Maria	ul. Jeczmienna 1	Lódz
Wróbel, Maria	Por. Okulist.	Nidzica
Wrubel, Stanislaw	Por. Okulist.	Legnica
Wróblewska, Ewa	ul. PKWN 1	Pultusk
Wróblewski, Jerzy	Szpital	Gdynia Sielce
Wójcik Cieślak, Stefania	ul. Przyszkole 13	Lódz
Wójcik, Waclaw	ul. Brzezna 18	Lódz
Wójtowicz, Maria	Przychodnia	Tarnobrzeg
Wójtowicz, Stanislaw	ul. Bobrowskiego 3	Warszawa
Wrzask, Janina	ul. Chalubińskiego 2a Kl. O.	Wroclaw
Wyrwa, Urszula	ul. Dabrowskiego 35	Poznań
Wysocka, Danuta	ul. Warszawska 1	Sosnowiec
Wyrzysko, Krystyna	Slowackiego 3	Ostrów Mazowiecki
Zachert Dubel, Mieczyslawa.	ul. Wojzera 3	Zabrze
Zachwatowicz, Bozena	ul. Jagiellońska 10	Malbork
Zadrozna, Ewa	ul. Kollataja 14	Opole
Zagórski, Zbigniew	ul. Lubomelska 6	Lublin
Zajaczkowska, Anna	ul. Czwartaków 6	Lublin
Zajaczkowski, Tadeusz	ul. Czwartaków 6	Lublin
Zaleska Kopeć, Ewelina	ul. Koszykowa 3	Warszawa
Zalewska, Krystyna	ul. Zawadzkiego 14	Katowice
Zankiewicz, Alla	ul. Majowa 1	Bialystok
Zarebińska, Lidia	ul. Polna 18	Olsztyn
Zarosińska, Krystyna	ul. Kasztanowa 15	Augustów
Zaroski, Jerzy	ul. Piastowska 57	Poznań
Zawadzka, Alicja	ul. Ligonia 10	Katowice
Zawadzka, Janina	ul. 23 Lutego 19	Poznań
Zarzycka, Maria	ul. Nowotki 26	Warszawa
Zasucha, Zofia	ul. Nowotki 8	Mikolów
Zdeblarz Jerzy	ul. Kosmonautów 1	Skarzysko Kamienna

Zeydler-Grzedzielewska, Lucyna	ul. Franciszkańska 70	Lódz
Zen, Anna	Kilińskiego 18	Zduńska Wola
Zgoda, Leonia	Przychodnia	Strzelce Opolskie
Zientarska, Teresa		Biala Ośrodek Zdrowia
Ziobrowski, Szczesny	ul. Zamojskiego 12	Zakopane
Ziólkiewicz, Irena	ul. Saperska 18	Poznań
Zubczewska, Wanda	ul. Jaracza 8	Warszawa
Zwierzchowski, Andrzej	ul. Lodowa 16	Poznań
Zych, Irena	ul. Boh. Stalingradu 2I	Kraków
Zychowicz, Franciszka	ul. Dluga 33	Kraków
Zaczek, Maria	ul. Grunwaldzka 3	Kraków
Zelawska Rybus, Helena	ul. Lorentza 4	Lódz
Zeromuska Zbirska, Izabella	ul. Litewska 9	Poznań
Zmijewska, Miroslawa	ul. Debowa 15	Milanówek
Zukowski, Ludwik	ul. Grzybowska 6	Warszawa
Zulawiński, Czeslaw	Gostawicza 106	Prudnik
Zurek, Jadwiga	Poradnia	Gizycko
Zybaczyńska, Maria	Swierczeskiego 13	Nowe Debie
Zylka Mill, Lucja	ul. Pionierów 7	Kedzierzyn
Zychski, Jan	ul. Stroma 4	Tczew
Zywolewski, Boguslaw	ul. Zwyciestwa 42	Bialystok

NOSOCOMIA QUIBUS OCULIS AEGRI CURANTUR

Bialystok

No. of beds

Klinika Chorób Oczu Akademii Medycznej w Bialymstoku, ul. C. Sklodowskiej nr. 24a. Doc. R. Chwirot — 45
Oddzial Okul. Woj. Szpitala C. Sklodowskiej 14. Ord. Dr. R. Rudobielski — 36
Oddzial Okul. w Elku. Ord. Dr. H. Maksymczuk — 16

Gdańsk-Wrzeszcz

Klinika Chorób Oczu Akademii Medycznej w Gdańsku-Wrzeszczu, ul. Dębinki 7a Prof. dr. J. Morawiecki — 44
Oddzial Okul. Szpitala w Bydgoszczy. Ord. Doc. E. Rusinowa — —
Szpital Marynarki Woj. Gdańsk-Oliwa. Doc. Ostachowicz — —
Szpital Miejski w Gdyni. Dr. W. Jablońska — 25
Szpital Miejski w Elblagu. Ord. Dr. H. Clar-Sobieska — 25
Szpital Pow. w Chojnicach. Ord. Dr. H. Ozdzyński — 15
Szpital Miejski w Toruniu. Ord. Dr. J. Horodeński — 10
Szpital Miejski w Grudziądzu. Ord. Dr. A. Byczyński — —
Szpital Miejski w Kwidzyniu. Ord. Dr. A. Dziurkowska — —

Katowice

Klinika Chorób Oczu Akademii Medycznej w Katowicach, ul Francuska 20. Prof. dr M. Madroszkiewicz — —
Szpital w Bielsku. Ord. Dr M. Malecka — 10
Szpital Miejski w Bytomiu. Ord. Dr O. Baborski — 30
Szpital Miejski w Chorzowie. Ord. dr. H. Piech — 40
Szpital Miejski w Cieszynie. Ord. Dr M. Pruchnicka — 25

Szpital Miejski w Czeladzi. Ord. Dr I. Bialkiewicz 20
Szpital im. Biegańskiego w Czestochowie. Ord. dr S. Milkowski .... —
Szpital Tysiaclecia w Czestochowie ord. dr. A. Burghart 15
Szpital Miejski w Dabrowie Górniczej. Ord. dr H. Piatek 30
Szpital Miejski w Gliwicach. Ord. dr. M. Hychar 24
Szpital Miejski w Katowicach. Ord. dr. S. Polak .... —
Szpital Miejski w Myslowicach. Ord. dr D. Pakula 22
Szpital Miejski w Rudzie Slaskiej. Ord. dr A. Gburek .... —
Szpital Miejski w Rybniku. Ord. dr A. Kempińska 30
Szpital Miejski w Sosnowcu. Ord. dr T. Sokolowski 32
Szpital Woj. w Tychach. Ord. dr L. Niemcewicz .... —
Szpital Miejski w Zabrzu. Ord. dr K. Szumilas .... —
Szpital Miejski w Zawierciu. Ord. Dr T. Nowak 16
Centralny Szpital Górniczy w Bytomiu. Ord. Dr Z. Solarski 68
Szpital PKP Katowice-Ligota. Ord. dr I. Rózanowicz .... —

Kraków

Klinika Chorób Oczu Akademii Medycznej, Kopernika 38. Prof. H. Machowa .... —
Szpital Miejski w Krakowie. Ord. Prof. dr. M. Madroszkiewicz 26
Szpital Nowa Huta na Skarpie. Ord. dr E. Kubatko 55
Szpital Kolejowy. Ord. dr A. Maciejasz 15
Szpital Woj. Dla dzieci Kraków-Witkowice. Ord. Dr H. Janotka 251
Szpital w Tarnowie. Ord. dr Swiech 21

Lublin

Klinika Chorób Oczu Akademii Medycznej w Lublinie, ul. Chmielna 1 Prof. dr T. Krwawicz   1
Szpital Woj. w Lublinie. Ord. Dr F. Kostro 15
Szpital Miejski w Zamościu. Ord. Dr Z. Barycki 20
Szpital w Bialej Podlaskiej. Ord. Dr I. Domoradzka 30

Lódz

Klinika Chorób Oczu Akademii Medycznej ul Narutowicza 118. Prof. dr. J. Sobański 63
Klinika Chorób Oczu Akad. Med. Wojskowei. Doc. Z. Krawczyk 41
Szpital Miejski. Ord. Dr B. Kozlowski 90
Szpital w Wieluniu. Ord. Dr J. Przytulski 10
Szpital w Tomaszowie Maz 10
Szpital w Piotrkowie Tryb 10

Olsztyn

Oddzial Okul. Szpitala Miejskiego. Ord. Dr H. Kostrzweska 23
Oddzial Okul. Szpitala Woj.. Ord. Dr E. Lenkiewicz 40

Poznań

Klinika Chorób Oczu Akademii Medycznej, ul Dluga 1–2. Doc. dr Orlowski .... —
Szpital Dziec. Woj. Ord. Dr M. Perz 14
Szpital Miejski w Poznaniu przy ul. Szkolnej 46
Szpital Pow. w Koninie 25
Szpital Pow. w Kaliszu 25
Szpital Pow. w Ostrowiu Wkp 25
Szpital Miejski w Pile 21
Szpital Miejski w Poznaniu 36

Szczecin

Warszawa

Wroclaw

INSTITUTA SCHOLAEQUE CAECIS DESTINATAE

Szkola dla Niewidomych i Specj. Poradnia dla rodziców w Bydgoszczy ul. Krasińskiego 10
Państw. Zaklad Wychowawczy dla Niewidomych w Krakowie
Ośrodek Szkolenia Zaw. w Krakowie. ul. 18 Stycznia 86
Zaklad Specj. dla Ociemnialych Kobiet Zalów pow, Krasnystaw 62 kierownik:
    S. Rajmundo .... miejsc 62
Szkola dla dzieci niedowidzacych w Lodzi. ul. Tkacka 36
Zaklad Wychowawczy dla dzieci niewidomych, Lublin, Hirszfelda 6.
Kierownik: T. Piotrowski
Ośrodek szkolno-wychowawczy dla dzieci niewidomych w Owińskach k Poznania
Ośrodek rehabilitacji i wypoczynku wi Kiekrzu pow. Poznań

Szkola Podstawowa i Zaklad dla dzieci niedowıdzacych w Warszawie ul. Kozmińska 7
kierownik: mgr. A. Andyski .... miejsc 290
Zaklad dla dzieci niewidomych Laski warszawskie pow. Pruszków kierownik: mgr. dr pedag.
E. Bandych 350
Szkola dla dzieci niewidomych, Wroclaw, ul. Kasztanowa 3a ....
Zaklad Rehabilitacji Niewidomych w Chorzowie, Kier: mgr. S. Kotowski 60

Organ prasowy, miesiecznik; Klinika Oczna wydawca PZWL, redaktor naczelny: Doc. dr
W. Orlowski, ul. Dluga 1−2 Poznań

PORTUGALLIA

SOCIETATES OPHTALMOLOGICAE

Nationales

Sociedade Portuguesa de Oftalmologia

Presidente: Dr. Carlos da Maia
Secretário-Geral: Dr. João E. Lisboa, Av. da Liberdade, 12-1°D, Lisboa

Sociedade Portuguesa de Oftalmologia Social
(Secção da Sociedade das Ciências Medicas)
Av. da Republica 34, 1°, Lisboa 1

Presidente: Dr. H. Moutinho
Secretário: Dr. Jorge Monjardino

Liga Portuguesa de Profilaxia da Cegueira

Presidente: Dr. H. Moutinho
Secretário-Geral: Dr. Artur Anselmo, Av. Dr. Mário Moutinho, Restelo, Lisboa 3

NOMINA ET DOMICILIA MEDICORUM AB OCULIS

Afonso dos Santos, José Carvalho	Rua João A. Mourão	Castelo Branco
Afonso dos Santos, Maria Leonor	Rua do Arco do Cego, 75-5° Dt°.	Lisboa
Aguiar, Manuel de Sousa ...	Instituto Dr. Gama Pinto	Lisboa
Aires de Matos, José Coimbra	Hospital de S. João	Porto
Albarran, Eduardo		Setúbal
Albarran, Eduardo Bastos ..		Setúbal
Albergaria Pinheiro, Fernando	Rua Ferreira Borges, 42-2°	Coimbra
Albuquerque, Leovegildo dos Santos	Rua Ferreira Borges, 117-1°	Coimbra
Aleixo Pais, José Manuel ...	Ava. Sacadura Cabral, 25-2° Fr. .	Lisboa
Alexandre Katz, Walter	Rua da Victória, 38-1°	Lisboa
Almada e Melo, Artur José .	Ava da República, 22-1° Fr.	Lisboa
Almeida Ribeiro, Paulo Alexandre Soriano	Rua de Santa Catarina, 286-3° Dt°.	Porto
Azinheira Alves, Jaime Augusto	Ava. Duque d'Avila, 76-3° Dt°. .	Lisboa
Alves da Silva, Maria Cândida Santa Isabel de Farinha de Lourenço ...	Alameda das Linhas de Torres, 189-1° Dt°.	Lisboa

Alves, Fernando	Ava. da Liberdade, 224-R/C Esq..	Lisboa
Alves Pinto, Alcino Oliveira .	Praca Carlos Alberto, 110-1° ...	Porto
Alvo, Rogério dos Reis	Rua do Comércio	Portimão
Andrade, Dorvalina Tomé ..	Casa de Saúde de Alvaiazere	Alvaiazere
Andrade, Luiz	Ava. Defensores de Chaves, 23-1°	
	Dt°.	Lisboa
Andrade, Manuel Bizarro ..	Ava. Gomes Pereira, 50-4° Dt°..	Lisboa
Angelo, Miguel	Rua de Ceuta, 70-1°	Porto
Araújo, Fausto	Rua de S. Gonçalo, 885	Guimarães
Arede, Adelino Dias	....	Vizeu
Azevedo, Francisco de Jesus	Rua dos Lusiadas, 106-3° Esq. ..	Lisboa
Azevedo, Manuel Augusto da		
Costa	Ava. Marechal Gomes da Costa,	
Azevedo, Silvia dos Anjos	454-1°	Braga
Soares	Ava. da Liberdade, 73-1° Dt°. ...	Lisboa
Bento Xambre, José Pinto .	Ava. da Liberdade, 224- R/C Esq.	Lisboa
Branco da Cunha, José		
Manuel	Praceta Casal Brandão, 31-3° Dt°.	Reboleira-Amadora
Bravo de Oliveira, Joaquim		
José	Rua de Santa Catarina, 693-2° ..	Porto
Breda, Joaquim Ribeiro ...	Rua Dr. Alberto Souto, 20	Aveiro
Brinca, Manuel Esteves	Rua Ferreira Borges, 151-2°	Coimbra
Brites Moita, José Raimundo		
Martins	Hospital de Celas	Coimbra
Cachola, Manuel Pereira ...	Ava. Duque d'Àvila, 67-R/Dt° ..	Lisboa
Calçada, António Durão		
Viegas	Rua de Santa Marta, 33-1°	Lisboa
Campos, Milton de Oliveira .	Praça Carlos Alberto, 110-1° ...	Porto
Campos Costa, Eduardo ...	Rua da Junqueira, 16	Póvoa do Varzim
Candal, Manuel Dias da		
Costa	Ava. Dr. Lourenço Peixinho, 64 .	Aveiro
Carvalho, Joaquim Gomes .	....	Salvaterra de Magos
Carvalho, José Gouveia	Ava. da Liberdade, 236-1° Dt°. .	Lisboa
Castro Correira, José Fernan-		
do Barros	Ava. da Boavista, 975-6° Dt°. ...	Porto
Castro Silva, Pedro	Rua Miguel Bombarda, 31	Porto
Catarino, Manuel Francisco		
Cordeiro	Hospital de S. João	Porto
Cavaleiro de Ferreira, Aveli-		
no	Praça Marquês do Pombal, 4- R/C	
	Esq.	Lisboa
Cerveira, António	Rua Visconde da Luz, 27-2°	Coimbra
Cerveira, António José		
Melich	Rua Andrade Corvo, 31-1° B ...	Lisboa
Cordeiro, Carlos Alberto		
Nunes	Rua D. Maria Graça Lucia da Sil-	
	va, 2-2° Esq.	Leiria
Coroa, Emilio dos Campos .	Rua Filipe Alistão	Faro
Correia, Adelino Guerra ...	Rua Hilidoro Salgado, 15- R/C ..	Lisboa
Correia Anacleto, António		
Bento	Ava. da Liberdade, 73-2° Dt°. ..	Lisboa
Correia da Camara, Frede-		
rico	Rua Francisco Sanches, 43- R/C	
	Dt°.	Lisboa
Correia de Sousa, Luis	....	Lamego

Corte-Real, Maria Helena ..	Ava. D. Pedro, 8-1° Esq.-Bairro Falcão	Pontinha
Costa, Graça Louro Fernandes Pimenta Monteiro ..	Rua de Entre-Campos, 5-1° Dt°. .	Lisboa
Coutinho, Maria de Fátima Salvador	Hospital de S. João	Porto
Crato Monteiro, Telmo	Largo Luis de Camões, 36-1° ...	Lisboa
Cravo, Elias Tavares	Rua Sá da Bandeira, 61-1°	Coimbra
Crespo, Àlvaro Rui Machado Santos	Praça da Igreja, 11-3° Dt°.	Amadora
Cunha Vaz, António Manso .	Rua da Sofia, 23-1°	Coimbra
Cunha Vaz, José Guilherme Fernandes	Rua da Sofia, 23-1°	Coimbra
Diniz, António Joaquim Rodrigues Castanheira ..	Praça Rainha D. Filipa, 2-6° Dt°..	Lisboa
Fagulho, José Gonçalves ...	....	Beja
Falcão, Eduardo Albino ...	Rua Ferreira Borges, 62-2°	Coimbra
Faria, Ilidio Fernandes	Hospital de Celas	Coimbra
Faria de Abreu, José Rui ..	Hospital de Celas	Coimbra
Faria E Silva, Diogo	Ava. Frederico Ulrich, 9- R/C ...	Cascais
Fernandes, Hedwigo Lourdes	Rua das Amoreiras, 171-1°	Lisboa
Fernandes, Mário Rix Jesus .	Hospital de S. João	Porto
Ferrão, António Alves	Praça dos Restauradores, 48-1° ..	Lisboa
Ferrari de Almeida, João Carlos	....	Vizeu
Ferraz, Carlos Duarte	Rua Ferreira Borges, 155-2°	Coimbra
Ferraz de Oliveira, Luis Manso Coelho	Ava. Fontes Pereira de Melo, 11-1° A	Lisboa
Fialho de Moura, Fausto Teixeira	Hospital Militar Principal	Lisboa
Figueira Santos, Manuel Mascarenhas	Hospital de Celas	Coimbra
Figueiredo, Oscar Dionizio Gonçalves	Rua Gustavo de Matos Sequeira, 42-1° Esq.	Lisboa
Flor D'Oliveira, Ruth	Rua Pascoal de Melo, 150-1° Esq.	Lisboa
Fonseca, Dulcinia Coelho ..	Ava. Miguel Bombarda, 59-1° ...	Lisboa
Gil Duarte, Hermínio	Rua Rodrigo da Fonseca, 18-1° Esq.	Lisboa
Godinho Ferreira, Jorge Manuel	Rua Rodrigo da Fonseca, 24-1° Esq.	Lisboa
Gomes, Abel Cordeiro	Rua de Brito Capelo, 304-1°	Matosinhos
Gomes, António	Rua Dr. Magalhães Lemos, 111-1°	Porto
Gomes, Jorge Alberto	Rua Manuel Ferreira de Andrade, 6-1° Dt°.	Lisboa
Gonçalves, José António Baptista	Rua S. Domingos de Benfica, 5-1° Dt°.	Lisboa
Gravato, Maria Augusta Garcia Carrancho	Ava. Dias da Silva, 159-1°	Coimbra
Gonçalves, José Joaquim Calado Duarte	Hospital de Celas	Coimbra
Horta, Urgel	Rua Alexandre Braga, 24-1°	Porto

Izabelinha, Joaquim Duarte
Gonçalves .... Praça Marquês de Sá da Bandeira . Santarém
Jacinto Pinto, António .... Évora
Jales, Alfredo Gonçalves ... . Caldas da Rainha
Landeiro, Jorge .... Ava. da Liberdade, 202-1° Esq. . Lisboa
Leal Seruca, José Manuel .. Rua Sá da Bandeira, 784-2° .... Porto
Lebre, José Jacinto .... Beja
Leitão, Amândio Martins .. .. Covilhã
Leite, Alberto Marinho .... Hospital de Santo António ..... Porto
Leite, Mária Victória .... Santarém
Leite da Silva, Fernando ... Rua de Ilhavo, 12-1° B .... Aveiro
Lemos, Manuel .... Rua Cândido dos Reis, 100-1° .. Porto
Lima, Manuel Vieira da Cos-
ta .... Barcelos
Lisboa, João Eurico ...... Av. da Liberdade, 12-1° Dt.° ... Lisboa
Louceiro, Manuel Ferreira . Hospital de Celas .... Coimbra
Lopes de Andrade, Augusto
José .... Ava. da Liberdade, 164-R/C Dt°.. Lisboa
Lopes Godinho, Joaquim .. .. Évora
Luciano Torres, Joaquim .. Rua Sá da Bandeira, 706-2° .... Porto
Maia, Carlos da .... Rua Rodrigo da Fonseca, 18-1°
Esq. .... Lisboa
Maia Lima, Artur Rui ..... Rua de Santa Catarina, 519 .... Porto
Mancio dos Santos, André . Instituto Dr. Gama Pinto ...... Lisboa
Manso, Lúcio Contrand ... Ava. Defensores de Chaves, 23-1°
Dt°. .... Lisboa
Marques, Maria Celeste Bar-
bosa .... Rua do Almada, 262-1° ...... Porto
Marques dos Santos, João
Vasco .... Rua Alexandre Herculano, 11-1° . Lisboa
Martins, José Augusto ..... Palácio Atlântico, 1° .... Porto
Martins, José Augusto da
Costa .... Hospital de S. João .... Porto
Martins, José Ferreira .... Praça de Velasquez, 219-1° ..... Porto
Matos de Sousa, António .. Ava. Fontes Pereira de Melo, 5-2°
Esq. .... Lisboa
May Viana, Artur .... Faro
Mayer Garção, Pedro ..... Policlinica da Estefânia .... Lisboa
Melo de Menezes, João
Homem .... Rua Nossa Senhora do Egipto, 32-
1° .... Oeiras
Melo Tavares, António .... Rua Sá da Bandeira, 658-4° .... Porto
Mesquita, Albano .... Espinho
Miranda, Anacleto .... Misericórdia de Lisboa .... Lisboa
Monjardino; Jorge .... Misericórdia de Lisboa .... Lisboa
Montalvão Machado, Júlio . ... Guiné
Monteiro, Raul .... Praça Carlos Alberto, 123-2°, Sala
28 .... Porto
Monteiro Grilo, Eduardo .. Ava. da República, 45-4° Esq. .. Lisboa
Moreira Monteiro, José .... Praça Carlos Alberto, 123-2° Sala
28 .... Porto
Moreira, António Manuel
Martins .... Rua Passos Manuel, 71-2° ...... Porto
Moreira Pires, António .... Rua Eng°. José Bessa, 13 ...... Bragança
Moreno, Pompeu Nabais Bar-
reiros .... Ava. Infante Santo, 76-1° ...... Lisboa

Morgado, Elísio Carmona ..	....	Setúbal
Mouga Rodrigues, António José de Deus	Largo do Chiado, 15-1°	Lisboa
Moura Pinheiro, Artur Fernando Monteiro	Ava. da Liberdade. 224- R/C Esq.	Lisboa
Moutinho, Henrique	Ava. da Liberdade, 212- S/L	Lisboa
Murta, Amândio	....	Tomar
Neves, Elísio	....	Vila Real
Neves, Laura Amaral	....	Vila Real
Nobre da Silva, Orlando Elísio	Estrada do Calhariz de Benfica, 1-5° Esq.	Lisboa
Nolasco, Fernando	Ava. Duque d'Loulé, 94-R/C Esq.	Lisboa
Noronha, Alfredo Fernando Huclides	....	Guiné
Nóvoa, Waldemar	Rua Sá da Bandeira, 636-3°	Porto
Oliveira Correia, Gumercindo	Rua de St°. António, 22-1°	Abrantes
Paiva, José Monteiro	....	Guarda
Palma Nunes, Antero Diniz .	Hospital de Santa Maria	Lisboa
Peixoto, António Teixeira .	Praça Marquês do Pombal, 66-3° .	Porto
Perdigão, António José Dias.	Ava. dos Combatentes, 15-2° ...	Algés
Pereira, Altino Baptista	Rua Dr. Alberto Pinheiro Torres, 13-2°	Porto
Pereira, António Farinha ..	....	Abrantes
Pereira, Carlos Augusto	Rua 19, 364-1° Esq.	Espinho
Pereira, Joaquim Coloho ...	....	Leiria
Pereira, Ventura Azevedo ..	Hospital de S. João	Porto
Pereira Magalhães, António Pedro Roque de Lima ..	Hospital de S. João	Porto
Pina, Artur	Ava. Ant°. Augusto d'Aguiar, 15-1°	Lisboa
Pina, Maria Luisa de Sousa .	Hospital de Santo António	Porto
Pinho da Costa, Francisco ..	Hospital de S. João	Porto
Pinto Chambel, Maria Irene dos Santos	Hospital de Santa Maria	Lisboa
Pinto da Cunha, Abeldizindo	....	Viana do Castelo
Pinto da Rocha, Américo ..	Rua Alves Correia, 34-4°	Lisboa
Pinto de Figueiredo, Luis Eallermant	Rua Ivens, 49-2° Dt°.	Lisboa
Pita, António Rocha	....	Figueira da Foz
Prates, Jorge Maximo	Travessa do Pinheiro, 21-5° Esq. .	Lisboa
Proença, Mário Barreiros ...	....	Covilhã
Puga, José Coelho	Rua Braancamp, 88-R/C Esq. ...	Lisboa
Puga, Ruy	....	Santarém
Queiróz Marinho, António .	Rua de Santa Catarina, 132-1° ..	Porto
Quintela, José	Instituto Dr. Gama Pinto	
Ramos, Fernando Moura ..	Rua Sá da Bandeira, 405-1°	Porto
Rasteiro de Campos, Alfredo Jorge Martins	Rua Ferreira Borges, 15-2°	Coimbra
Rasteiro de Campos, António Júlio	Hospital de Celas	Coimbra
Rebelo Simões, José Manuel.	....	Leiria
Rebordão, José Maria Moreira	....	Cartaxo
Reich D'Almeida, Francisco .	Hospital de Santa Maria	Lisboa

Reis, António . . . . Ava. da Liberdade, 247-2° Esq. . Lisboa

Resende Rodrigues, Armando Luis . . . . Rua das Flores, 71-1° . . . . Lisboa

Ribeiro, Paulo . . . . Hospital Militar Principal . . . . . . Lisboa

Ribeiro da Silva, João Manuel . . . . Ava. da Liberdade, 100-2° . . . . . Lisboa

Robalo, Amândio Azevedo . Hospital de Celas . . . . Coimbra

Robles de Oliveira, Rui Alberto . . . . Instituto Dr. Gama Pinto . . . . . .

Rocha, Manuel Pinho . . . . . Rua Caldas Xavier, 38-1° C. . . . . Porto

Rocha Oliveira, Júlio Cesar . Rua Franaça Junior, 120-1° . . . . Matosinhos

Salvador, Maria José . . . . . . Rua Morais Soares, 114-1° . . . . . Lisboa

Sampaio e Melo, José de Almeida . . . . Praça Marquês de Pombal, 66-3° . Porto

Santana, João Vasco Fernandes . . . . Rua Rodrigo da Fonseca, 24-1° Esq. . . . . Lisboa

Santana Leite, João . . . . . . Ava. da Liberdade, 136- R/C . . . Lisboa

Santana Marques, Leonel . . Largo Hintze Ribeiro, 2-1° Dt°. . Lisboa

Santos, Anibal . . . . Hospital de Matosinhos . . . . Matosinhos

Santos, Olga . . . . Hospital de Matosinhos . . . . Matosinhos

Saraiva, João . . . . Ava. da Liberdade, 11-1° . . . . . . Lisboa

Seabra, Claudio . . . . Ava. Defensores de Chaves, 23-1°. Lisboa

Seabra, Octaviano Augusto Ferreira . . . . Hospital de Celas . . . . Coimbra

Silva Teixeira, António . . . . Tomar

Silva, Joaquim da . . . . Leiria

Silva e Sousa, António Júlio Coelho . . . . Ava. Guilherme Gomes Fernandes, 38-2° . . . . Porto

Silva Pinto, Joaquim Jorge . Hospital de Celas . . . . Coimbra

Silva Pinto, Manuel . . . . Hospital de S. João . . . . Porto

Simões, Maria do Rosário . . Ava. Elias Garcia, 194-1° andar . Lisboa

Simões de Sá, Amilcar . . . . Praça do Giraldo, 75 . . . . Évora

Soares Teles, Orlindo . . . . . Rua do Comércio, 10 . . . . Guarda

Sousa e Faro, Bernardo . . . . Ava. Ant°. Augusto d'Aguiar, 21-1° . . . . Lisboa

Sousa e Faro, Luisa . . . . Rua D. Maria Marques Pereira, 9-1° Esq. . . . . Lisboa

Sousa Fernandes, António Cândido . . . . Rua de Ceuta, 53-1° . . . . Porto

Sousa Fernandes, José Eduardo . . . . Praça Carlos Alberto, 110-1° . . . Porto

Sousa Ramalho, Paulo Eugénio . . . . Ava. Almirante Reis, 154- R/C Dt°. . . . . Lisboa

Sousa Nunes, Honorato . . . Hospital de S. João . . . . Porto

Soares, António Ferreira . . . Rua do Almada, 262-1° . . . . Porto

Soares de Matos, José Maria Hospital de S. João . . . . Porto

Sotto Morais, Carlos . . . . . . Praça Gonçalo Velho, 1 . . . . Viana do Castelo

Souto de Moura, José Alberto . . . . Rua de Ceuta, 60-3° . . . . Porto

Taborda, Mário Simão . . . . Leiria

Tarouca da Silva, Fernando . Praça da Figueira, 11-2° Esq. . . . Lisboa

Tavares, Assunção . . . . Beja

Tavares, Fernando Jorge Chiote .... Estrada da Ameixoeira, 33-2° Esq. .... Lisboa

Taveira, Gastão José Borges . Rua da Constituição, 871-4° Esq.. Porto

Tomé, Ernesto dos Reis ... Ava. Casal Ribeiro, 61-2° Esq. .. Lisboa

Toscano Rico, Fernando José Bastos .... Instituto Dr. Gama Pinto ...... Lisboa

Toste, José Nunes Ferreira . Rua Pedro del Negro, 1-2° Dt°. . Reboleira-Amadora

Trincão, Carlos Manuel Correia .... Rua D. Diniz, 64-1° Esq. ...... Cova da Piedade

Trindade Soares, Celestino . Rua de S. Marcos, 30-34-1° .... Braga

Vasconcelos, Maria Helena de Basto do Vale ...... Hospital de Santo António ..... Porto

Vaz Trindade, José Duarte Silva .... Hospital de Celas .... Coimbra

Vazão Trindade, José de Campos .... Rua Dr. José Alberto dos Reis, 3-1° Dt°. .... Portimão

Vendrell, Elmano .... Ava. da Liberdade, 224- R/C Esq. Lisboa

Viegas, José dos Santos .... Pombal

Vieira, José Gabriel Cardoso Rua da Constuição, 871-4° Esq. . Porto

Vieira, Ismael Mendonça ... Ava. 28 de Maio, 53-6° Esq. .... Lisboa

Villas-Boas e Alvim, António José .... Ava. Marechal Gomes da Costa, 819 .... Braga

Villas-Boas, Manuel Cabral . Rua Júlio Diniz, 867-3° Dt°. ... Porto

Açores

Arruda, Carlos Pacheco .... Rua Marquês da Praia e Monforte, 22 .... Ponta Delgada

Botelho de Melo, João Luis B. .... Rua Hintze Ribeiro, 26 .... Ponta Delgada

Brasil, Hélio Nunes Flores .. .. Angra do Heroismo-Terceira

Brasil, Manuel Nunes Flores Rua Rainha D. Amélia 38 2° ... Angra do Heroismo

Estrela Rego, José .... Rua de S. João, 20 .... Ponta Delgada

Freitas, José Pereira ..... Rua Conselheiro de Medeiros, 27 . Horta Faial

Machado, Octávio José Botelho .... Rua de S. João, 55 .... Ponta Delgada

Medeiros e Camara, Hermano Silveira de ...... Rua Marquês da Praia e Monforte. Ponta Delgada

Ormonde Aguiar, Jorge Manuel .... Angra do Heroismo-Terceira

Pimentel, Maria Francisca Pais Dias .... Rua Comendador Ernesto Rebelo, 16 .... Horta Faial

Vieira, João Alberto Pacheco Rua António José d'Almeida, 44 . Ponta Delgada

Angola

Menezes, José Luis Cardoso ....

Pereira Machado, Manuel Cordeiro ....

Rodrigues, Auibal da Silva . Avenida Sá da Bandeira, 53 .... Luanda

Sousa Dias, Mário .... Nova Lisboa

Texeira e Costa, Antonio Candido .... Benguela

Madeira

Araújo Alipio	Rua Ivens, 28-2° Dt°	Funchal
Falcão, Francisco de Sousa .	....	Funchal
Couveia, João	Rua Pimenta Aquiar, 2	Funchal
Jardim, Antonio Alberto Faria de França	Rua do Carmo, 6	Funchal
Natividade, António Jorge . Fernandez	Rua das Hortas, 10-1°	Funchal

Moçambique

Alves Martins, Antonio Manuel	Hosp. Rainha d. Amélia, C.P. 1517	Beira
Gustavo, Manuel Graça	....	
Sequeira, Victor Herbert ...	....	

Timor

Cayette, Fernando de Pratt .   ...

NOSOCOMIA QUIBUS OCULIS AEGRI CURANTUR

Lisboa

Clínica Oftalmologica Universitária, Hospital de Sta Maria.
Director: Prof. Dr. Ribeiro da Silva

Instituto de Oftalmologia Dr. Gama Pinto.
Director: Prof. Dr. Ribeiro da Silva

Servico de Oftalmologia do Hospital dos Capuchos.
Director: Dr. Sousa e Faro

Servico de Oftalmologia do Instituto Português de Oncologia.
Director: Dr. Artur Pina

Servico de Oftalmologia do Hospital da Misericórdia de Lisboa.
Director: Dr. J. Monjardino

Servico de Oftalmologia do Hospital de S. José.
Director: Dr. Carlos da Maia

Servico de Oftalmologia do Hospital do Ultramar.
Director: Prof. Dr. Ferraz de Oliveira

Servico de Oftalmologia do Hospital da Marinha.

Service de Oftalmologia do Hospital Militar da Estrêla.

Servico de Oftalmologia do Centro Sanatorial D. Carlos I (I.A.N.T.).
Director: Dr. Claudio de Seabra

Porto

Clinica Oftalmologica Universitária, Hospital S. João.
Director: Prof. Dr. Silva Pinto
Servico de Oftalmologia do Hospital de S. to Antonio.
Director: Dr. Queiroz Marinho

Servico de Oftalmolgia do Hospital Militar Regional.

Coimbra

Clinica dos Hospitais Universitários
  Director: Prof. Dr. J. Cunha Vaz

INSTITUTA SCHOLAEQUE CAECIS DESTINATAE

Lisboa

Centro Infantil 'Helen Keller'.
Centro de Aprendizagem pelo Tacto 'Anne Sulivan': Av. Dr. Mário Moutinho,ao Restelo, Lisboa 3.
Instituto Antonio Feliciano de Castilho, Rua Correia Teles, 45,Lisboa.
Instituto Branco Rodrigues, Parede.
Centro de Reabilitação de Nossa Senhora dos Anjos.
Centro de Reabilitação de Raquel e Martin Sain, Rua João Saraiva 11, Lisboa 5.
Lar da Boa-Hora.
Asilo Nossa Senhora da Saude, Rua Silva Carvalho, 36.
Asilo Nossa Senhora Auxiliadora, Rua Duarte Coelho, 1.

Porto

Instituto S. Manuel, Rua da Paz, 116.
Instituto S. José
Instituto de Campo Lindo.
Centro de Reabilitação Profissional da Granja.
Centro de Reabilitação Profissional da Areosa.
Centro Dr. Albuquerque e Castro (Imprensa Braille), Rua da Paz, 116.

Coimbra

Centro Dr. Oliveira Salazar.

Açores

Instituto S. Catarina, Ponta Delgada, S. Miguel.

Madeira

Instituto S. Antonio, Funchal.

Moçambique

Instituto Assis Milton, Beira.

ROMANIA

SOCIETATES OPHTHALMOLOGICAE

Nationalis

Societatea de Oftalmologie (de l'Union des Sociétés de Sciences Médicales)
President: Prof. Dr. I. Păcurariu
Secretary: Prof. Dr. M. N. David, Str. Progresului nr. 10, Bucureşti
Number of members: 480
Le Comité National:
   Prof. Dr. Ion Păcurariu, Facultatea de Medicină Cluj
   Prof. Dr. Mihai David, Facultatea de Medicină Bucureşti
   Prof. Dr. Vasile Săbădeau, Facultatea de Medicină Tg. Mureş
   Prof. Dr. Nicolae Zolog, Facultatea de Medicină Timişoara
   Prof. Agr. P. Petre Vancea, Facultatea de Medicină Taşi

Regionales

Secţia de Oftalmologie Bucureşti
President: Prof. Dr. M. N. David
Address: Str. Vulturi nr. 27, Bucureşti
Number of members: 170

Secţia de Oftalmologie Iaşi
President: Prof. Agr. Dr. P. P. Vancea
Address: Str. Decebal nr. 22, Iaşi
Number of members: 80

Secţia de Oftalmologie Cluj
President: Prof. Dr. I. Păcurariu
Address: Str. Racovitä nr. 16, Cluj
Number of members: 85

Secţia de Oftalmologie Timişoara
President: Prof. Dr. N. Zolog
Address: Str. Arsăneşti nr. 1, Timişoara
Number of members: 70

Secţia de Oftalmologie Tg. Mureş
President: Prof. Dr. V. Săbădeanu
Address: Str. Papiu Ilarion nr. 10, Tg. Mureş
Number of members: 60

NOMINA ET DOMICILIA MEDICORUM AB OCULIS

Anastasiu, Iordan	Str. I. L. Carageale nr. 56	Ploeşti
Anastasescu, Florian	Str. Păltiniş nr. 12	Timişoara
Andreescu, Emilia	Str. Compozjtorilor nr. 30	Bucureşti
Baciu, Otilia	Str. Vasile Lupu nr. 85	Iaşi
Begu, Dan	Str. Năvodari nr. 7	Craiova
Benia, Mircea	Str. Virgiliu nr. 13, sect. 7	Bucureşti
Boeraş, Fane	Str. Desişului nr. 12 Bl. 27 Sc. C et. I, ap. 45	Bucureşti
Bogdan, Ion	Spitalul de Adulţi Lugoj	Lugoj
Bolfa, Traian	Policlinica nr. 1 Braşov str. Brîncoveanu nr. 4	Braşov
Băgăluţ, Elvira	Spitalul Adulţi Baia Mare	Baia-Mare
Brucăr, Isac	Bd. A. I. Cuza nr. 10	Bucureşti
Bucur, Coriolan	Spitalul de Urgenţă	Bucureşti
Buiuc, Sergiu	Str. Victor Babeş nr. 10	Iaşi
Buiuc, Constanţa	Str. Victor Babeş nr. 10	Iaşi
Burloiu, Silvia	Policlinica Gara de Nord	Bucureşti
Buşneag, Tatiana	Str. Someş nr. 40	Craiova
Călin, Ada	Str. Cuza Vodă nr. 8	Iaşi
Carapancea, Mihai	Str. Prof. Bogdan nr. 21	Bucureşti
Carabiber, Constantin	Policlinica de Adulţi	Constanţa
Cathi, Gheorghe	Str. Morii nr. 51	Braşov
Cernea, Paul	Spitalul CFR	Iaşi
Cerchez, Vasile	Bloc S.3. Sc. B, ap. 7	Tulcea
Colev, Gheorghe	Spitalul nr. 1	Iaşi
Cînciu, Georgeta	Str. Academiei nr. 35–37	Bucureşti
Ciortoloman, Georgeta	Str. Popa Savu nr. 60 sect. 4	Bucureşti
Cuvin, Elena	Calea Victoriei nr. 139 et. I.	Bucureşti
David, Mihai	Str. Vulturi nr. 27	Bucureşti
Dumitrescu, Ana Maria	Bd. N. Bălcesu nr. 24, sct. I	Bucureşti
Eşanu, Iosif	Str. 9 Mai Bl. II Sc. 5 ap. 9	Petroşani
Fodor, Francisc	Str. Papiu Ilarion nr. 20	Tg. Mureş
Fugulyan, Gheorghe	Str. Gh. Marinescu 7 B.	Tg. Mureş
Gacichievici, Vasile	Bd. Gării nr. 5	Călăraşi
Gavriluţ, Mircea	Bd. Victoriei 4, bl. 41 sc. A. ap. 2	Braşov
Gîdescu, Petre	Str. Corbeni nr. 23 A	Bucureşti
Glăvan, I.Ion	Str. Brezoianu nr. 29 B. et. III, ap. 29	Bucureşti
Gyulai, Margareta	Clinica Oftalmologică	Timişoara
Harnagea, Emil	Str. Fluturilor nr. 8	Bîrlad
Haiduc, Maria	Str. Ardealului nr. 2 Bl. 4 ap. 4	Alba-Iulia
Hagiopol, Hoancă Victoria	Bd. Dacia nr. 16	Bucureşti
Horge, Ion	Spitalul Militar Central	Bucureşti
Ianopol, Jean	Spitalul Unificat	Suceava
Iofciulescu, Petre	Str. Pitar Moş nr. 29 et. VI ap. 63	Bucureşti
Iordănescu, Carmen	Bd. Carpaţi nr. 19 et. II. ap. 5	Constanţa
Karacaşian, Eduard	Str. Tomis nr. 1 Bl. 3 Sc. B. ap. 23	Constanţa
Kovacs, Magdalena	Str. Floreasca D. 4 ap. 10	Tg. Mureş
Leibovici, Mircea	Str. Zlatna Bl. S.2. Sc. B. et. 4	Timişoara
Lucian, Iosif	Str. Dobrogea nr. 32	Braşov
Lupuţiu, Ion	Str. Olga Bancic nr. 16	Ploeşti
Marinov, Ileana	Bd. Muncii nr. 28 Bl. 31 et. II ap. 9	Bucureşti

Macarie, Ion	Bd. N. Balcescu nr. 24, Sct. I	București
Manolescu, Dumitru	Bd. Hristo Botev nr. 6	București
Margescu, Felicia	Str. Republicii nr. 18	Cluj
Marinescu, Irena	Bd. Bălcescu nr. 36 sct. I	București
Michail, Sandu	Str. Izvor nr. 90	București
Micşa, Marius	Spitalul Unificat Piatra-Neamţ	Piatra-Neamţ
Mihu, Dumitru	Spital Intreprindere Copşa-Mică	Sibiu
Mîrza, Iulia	Str. Făurei nr. 1 et. III. ap. 101	București
Moisescu, Ion	Str. Negru Vodă nr. 53	Pitești
Moraru, Mircea	Spitalul Militar Central	București
Munteanu, Mircea	Bd. Tomis nr. 97, Sc. B, et. I. ap. 14	Constanţa
Niculiu, Ileana	Str. Postelnicului nr. 5 sct. I	București
Niculescu, Maria	Str. Plantelor nr. 50	București
Nuţă, Marcela	Str. Judeţului nr. 15 Sc. A. ap. 22	București
Oancea, Ion	Clinica Oftalmologică Cluj Str. Clinicilor 3	Cluj
Olteanu, Mircea	Str. Vasile Conta nr. 3–5 Sc. C et. VI, ap. 82	București
Orăşteanu, Dumitru	Spitalul Adulţi Victoria- Oraş	Victoria
Pangrati, Dinu	Str. Jianu nr. 2	Ploești
Payer, Francisc	Spitalul Adulţi Bistriţa Str. Viişoarei nr. 30	Bistriţa
Pîntea, Maria	Str. Pictor Stefan Luchian nr. 12	București
Păcurariu, Ion	Str. Racoviţa nr. 16	Cluj
Păcurariu, Lavinia	Str. Racoviţă nr. 16	Cluj
Pop, D. Popa Doina	Str. Lupeni nr. 4	Tg. Mureș
Popescu, Mircea	Str. Calea Griviţei nr. 232 Bl. 2 Sc. E, ap. 128	București
Popescu, Nicolae	Str. Poştei nr. 4	Ploești
Popovici, Mihai	Str. Belvedere nr. 6	Brăila
Radian, Alexandru	Cornişa II, Bl. 55 Sc. C. ap. 6	Bacău
Ratiu, Eugen	Str. Globului Bl. P. ap. 21	București
Răpiţeanu, Mircea	Pol. 1 Galaţi Str. Primăverii	Galaţi
Săbădeanu, Vasile	Str. Papiu Ilarion nr. 10	Tg. Mureș
Sandovici, Eva	Clinica Oftalmologică Str. Clinicilor nr. 3	Cluj
Săracăceanu, Lucia	Str. Eroilor nr. 25	Tg. Jiu
Schmidt, Gerhardt	Spitalul nr. 1	Baia-Mare
Schwartzenberg, Tikva	Str. Ion Creangă nr. 73 Bloc J.3 et. I. Sc. B	Iași
Segal, Notbert	Spitalul Adulţi Oradea	Oradea
Sîntion, Silvia	Spitalul Unificat Judeţean	Sibiu
Smatoc, Varvara	Bd. Hoşimin nr. 11 Dr. Taberii	București
Stănescu, Petre	Str. Stefan cel Mare nr. 1 Sc. 6 et IV, ap. 241	București
Stoica, Anastasia	Str. Impărat Traian nr. 8	Brăila
Sveţ, Nicolae	Str. Desrobirii Bl. F. I. Sc. 2	Craiova
Szeremy, Margareta	Spitalul Unificat Satu Mare	Satu-Mare
Taiachin, Vladimir	Spitalul de Adulţi	Alexandria
Tacorian, Doina	General A. Demostene nr. 5 sct. 6	București
Themo, Naim	Str. Marc Aureliu nr. 15	Constanţa
Tihani, Ladislau	Str. Zorilor nr. 2	Sf. Gheorghe
Vancea, Petre	Bd. Schitu Măgureanu nr. 3	Bucureţi
Vancea, P. Petre	Str. Decebal nr. 22	Iași
Vasinca, Mircea	Str. 30 Decembrie nr. 10	Cluj

Vicea, Ton	Spitalul Adulți Tr. Severin	Tr. Severin
Vlad, Petre	Bd. Nic. Bălcescu Bl. 11 ap. 29	București
Zolog, Nicolae	Str. Arsănești nr. 1	Timișoara

NOSOCOMIA QUIBUS OCULIS AEGRI CURANTUR

Serviciul de Oftalmologie Spitalul Adulți Pitești. Adress: Pitești Județul ARGES. Medic Primar: Dr. I. Moisescu.

Serviciul de Oftalmologie Spitalul Adulți Bacău. Adress: Bacău Județul BACAU. Medic primar: Dr. Al. Radian.

Serviciul de Oftalmologie Spitalul de Adulți Piatra-Neamț. Adress: Piatra Neamț Județul BACAU. Medic primar: Dr. V. Micșa.

Clinica de Oftalmologie Timișoara. Adress: Timișoara Județul TIMISOARA Director: Prof. Dr. N. Zolog.

Servicial de Oftalmologie Spitalul de Adulți Arad. Adress: Arad Județul ARAD. Medic primar: Dr. H. Lung.

Serviciul de Oftalmologie Spitalul de Adulți Lugoj. Adress: Spitalul de Adulți LUGOJ. Medic primar: Dr. S. Bogdan.

Serviciul de Oftalmologie Spitalul de Adulți Reșița. Adress: Reșița Județul CARAS-SERVERIN. Medic Primar: Dr. M. A. Friedenwald.

Serviciul de Oftalmologie Spitalul de Adulți Brașov. Adress: Spitalul de Adulți Brașov, Județul BRASOV. Medic primar: Dr. Gh. Cathi.

Serviciul de Oftalmologie Spitalul de Adulți Sibiu. Adress: Spitalul de Adulți Sibiu Județal SIBIU. Medic Primar: Dr. Sîntion Iulia.

Serviciul de Oftalmologie Spitalul de Adulți Sighișoara. Medic șef: Dr. Ciuzilă Emil.

Serviciul de Oftalmologie Spitalul de Adulți Sf. Gheorghe. Adress: Sf. Gheorghe Județul COVASNA. Medic Primar: Dr. L. Tihani.

Serviciul de Oftalmologie Spitalul de Adulți Bistrița. Adress: Spitalul de Adulți Bistrița Județul BISTRITA. Medic primar: Dr. F. Payer.

Clinica de Oftalmologie Cluj. Adress: Cluj. Director: Prof. dr. I. Păcurariu.

Serviciul de Oftalmologie Spitalul de Adulția Oradea. Adress: Spitalul de Adulți Oradea Județul BIHOR. Medic primar: Dr. N. Segal.

Serviciul de Oftalmologie Spitalul de Adulți Galați. Adress: Spitalul de Adulți Galați, Județul GALATI. Medic primar: Dr. V. Mărculescu.

Serviciul de Oftalmologie Spitalul de Adulți Brăila. Adress: Spitalul de Adulți Brăila, Județul BRAILA. Medic primar: Dr. M. Popovicin.

Serviciul de Oftalmologie Spital Adulți Deva. Adress: Deva, Județul HUNEDOARA. Medic Sef: Dr. Silviu Costea.

Serviciul de Oftalmologie Spitalul de Adulți Hunedoara. Adress: Spitalul Adulți Județul HUNE-DOARA. Medic primar: Dr. D. Jujescu.

Serviciul de Oftalmologie Spitalul de Adulți Petroșani. Medic primar: Dr. I. Eșanu.

Clinica de Oftalmologie Iași. Adress: Spitalul Sf. Spiridon Iași, Județul IASI. Director: Conf. dr. P. P. Vancea.

Serviciul de Oftalmologie Spitalul Neuropsihiatrie Iași. Adress: Spitalul de Neuropsihiatrie Iași, Județul IASI. Medic primar: Dr. S. Buiuc.

Serviciul de Oftalmologie Spitalul de Adulți Bîrlad. Adress: Spitalul de Adulți Bîrlad, Județul VASLUI. Medic primar: Dr. V. Harnagea.

Serviciul de Oftalmologie Spitalul de Adulți Satu Mare. Adress: Spitalul de Adulți Satu Mare, Județul SATUMARE, Medic primar: Dr. Margareta Szeremy.

Clinica de Oftalmologie Tg. Mureș. Adress: Tg. Mureș Județul MURES. Director: Prof. Dr. V. Săbădeanu.

Serviciul de Oftalmologie Spitalul de Adulți Craiova. Adress: Spitalul de Adulți Craiova, Județul DOIJ, Medic primar: Dr. V. Beta.

Serviciul de Oftalmologie Spitalul de Adulți Ploiești. Adress: Spitalul de Adulți Ploiești, Județul PRAHOVA. Medic primar: Dr. I. Anastasiu.
Serviciul de Oftalmologie Spitalul de Adulți Suceava. Adress: Spitalul de Adulți Suceava, Județul SUCEAVA. Medic Specialist: Dr. Ianopol Jean.
Clinica de Oftalmologie București. Adress: Spitalul Colțea, Bd. 1848 nr. 3 București. Director: Prof. dr. M. David.
Spitalul de Oftalmologie. Adress: Str. D. Bolintineanu nr. 9 BUCURESTI. Director: Dr. Ileana Marinov.
Serviciul de Oftalmologie Spitalul de Adulți Constanța. Adress: Spitalul de Adulți Constanța Județul CONSTANTA. Medic primar: Dr. Naim Themo.
Numărul total de paturi: 2.100

INSTITUTA SCHOLAEQUE CAECIS DESTINATAE

Scoala generală de 9 ani pentru copiii ambliopi. Str. Austrului nr. 33 București: clase 1 − 9 = 270 elevi.
Scoala profesională specială pentru orbi Nr. 1 (băeți+fete) Str. Vatra Luminoasă nr. 108 București: clase 1−9 = 533 elevi.
Scoala profesională specială de ambliopi. Str. Pantelimon nr. 299: clase 1−9 = 300 elevi.
Scoala profesională pentru orbi Arad. Str. Gheorghe Barițiu nr. 16 Arad: clase 1−9 = 252 elevi.
Scoala pentru orbi Cluj. Str. Buday Nagy Antal nr. 31 Cluj: clase 1−9 + grădiniță 205 elevi + 12 copii în grădiniță.
Scoala de nevăzători Timișoara. Str. Independenței nr. 25 Timișoara: clase 1−9 = 180 elvi.
Scoala de orbi fete Buzău. Str. Banghereanu nr. 1 Buzău: clase 1−9 = 164 elevi.
Căminul spital pentru orbi Dumbrăveni (Mediaș) 95 bărbați; 81 femei.
Scoala de orbi mixtă. Tg. Frumos Str. Cuza Vodă nr. 54 Tg. Frumos.

SVECIA

SOCIETATES OPHTHALMOLOGICAE

The Swedish Ophthalmological Society, Swenska Ögonlakareföreningen
President: Prof. S. E. Nilsson
Secretary: Dr. B. Svedbergh, Eye clinic, Akademiska sjukhuset, 750 14 Uppsala
Number of members: 307

NOMINA ET DOMICILIA MEDICORUM AB OCULIS

Ahrnberg, B.	Överåsgatan 5	412 66 Göteborg
Alani, Safwat	Dr. Linds Gata 1	413 25 Göteborg
Algvere, Peep	Ögonkl. Karol. sjukh. Fack	104 01 Stockholm
Andersson, Einar	Vilshärad	305 90 Halmstad
Andersson, Gerald	Götgatan 11 A	216 11 Malmö
Andersson, Ingrid	Viktoriagatan 2	302 46 Halmstad
Andersson, Lars	Ögonkl. Akad. sjukh. Fack	750 14 Uppsala
Andrén, Signe	Samariterhemmet	755 90 Uppsala
Anjou, Ingvar	Ögonklin. Lasarettet	551 85 Jöngköping
Arén, Åke	Ögonklin. Lasarettet, Fack	791 01 Falun
Aurell, Elisabeth	Lasarettet, Box 22	431 22 Mölndal
Aurell, Gert	Äppelviksvägen 9	161 36 Bromma
Amér, Birgitta	Visby Lasarett, Fack	621 01 Visby
Axelsson, Uno	Sabb. sjukh. Ögonkl. Box 6401	113 82 Stockholm
Bahr, Prof.-Gunnar von	Svartbäcksgatan 1 B	753 20 Uppsala
Barany, Prof. E.	Dag Hammarskjölds Väg 19	752 37 Uppsala
Barkamn, Yngve	Ögonklin. Lasarettet	972 00 Gällivare
Bartley, Margareta	Kyrkvägen 11	430 80 Hovås
Beijer, Frans	Askrikegatan 3, IItr.	115 29 Stockholm
Bengtsson, Bo	Frödingsvägen 19	245 00 Staffanstorp
Bengtsson, Jan	Ögonkl. Sabb. sjukh. Box 6401	113 82 Stockholm
Berg, Prof. F.	Kyrkogårdsgatan 27	752 35 Uppsala
Berggren, L.	Ogonklin. Lasarettet	901 85 Umeå
Berghagen, Hans	Handens sjukh. Dalaröväg. 12	136 44 Handen
Berglund, Anna-Berta	Lasarettet, Box 55	575 00 Eksjö
Bergman, Birgitta	Ögonkliniken, Lasarettet	451 01 Uddevalla
Bergmark, Bo	Luleåvägen 35	972 00 Gällivare
Bergquist, Birgitta	Ögonklin. Lasarettet, Fack	451 01 Uddevalla
Bergström, Bo	Ögonkl. Sabb. sjukh. Box 6401	113 82 Stockholm
Berns, W.	Hospitalstorget 1	582 27 Linköping
Beskow, Dag	Erik Dahlbergsgatan 14	411 26 Göteborg
Bill, Inga	Norby Källväg 7	752 45 Uppsala
Björk, Åke	Trädgårdsgatan 23, VItr	172 38 Sundbyberg
Björnberg, Kaj	Ögonklin. Lasarettet	521 00 Falköping
Björkman, Ingvar	Danderyds sjukhus, Fack	182 03 Danderyd
Blix, Magnus	Lasarettet, Fack	462 01 Vänersborg
Blomdahl, Sven	Östermalmsgatan 68 A	114 50 Stockholm
Blyme, Lars	Framnäsbacken 10	171 42 Solna
Boström-Smith, Inga-Lisa	Nygatan 24	803 55 Gävle

Brege, Claes-Göran	Ögonklin. Akad. sjukh. Fack ...	750 14 Uppsala
Brismar, Gudrun	Öppenv. c. ög. avd. Helgeandsg. 16	223 54 Lund
Brodén, Gunnar	Lasarettet, Box 101	542 01 Mariestad
Broman-Lindgren, Sonja ...	Botulfsgatan 2	223 50 Lund
Broström, Ingrid	Ögonkl. Sabb. sjukh. Box 6401 .	113 82 Stockholm
Brändstedt, G.	Kristineberg	451 00 Uddevalla
Bynke, Hans	Väpplingvägen 17 C	222 38 Lund
Calissendorff, Berit	Ögonkl. Karol. sjukh. Fack	104 01 Stockholm
Carlberg, O.	Strömsborgsvägen 7	902 23 Gävle
Carle, T.	Östergatan 24	230 10 Skanör
Cristiansson, John	Ögonklin. Lasarettet	291 00 Kristianstad
Cronqvist, Stig	Södergatan 13	211 34 Malmö
Cavallin-Sjöberg, Ulla	Barytongränd 14	223 68 Lund
Dahlberg-Parrow, Ragna ...	Åsgränd 4 B	752 35 Uppsala
Dahlqvist, Essie	Karlaplan 3 A	114 60 Stockholm
Dahlstedt, Erik	Ögonmottagn. sjukh. Fack	781 01 Borlänge
Dalén, Bengt	Drottninggatan 63 A	602 32 Norrköping
Daniels, B.	Drottninggatan 15	252 21 Helsingborg
Daunius, Carl	Ögonklin. Lasarettet, Fack	462 01 Vänersborg
Diderholm, Eva	Ögonklin. Akad. sjukh. Fack ...	750 14 Uppsala
Dohlman, C. H.	....	
Dymling, O.	Kungsportsavenyn 37	411 36 Göteborg
Dyster-Aas, Kjell	P. H. Lings Väg 2	223 65 Lund
Edler, Karin	Ilstorp 18	275 00 Sjöbo
Ehinger, Berndt	Ögonklin. Lasarettet, Fack	220 05 Lund
Ekvall, Karin	Skårängsvägen 10	803 60 Gävle
Elg, G.	Ögonklin. Lasarettet, Fack	381 02 Kalmar
Elzén, S.	Lasarettet, Box 143-144	771 01 Ludvika
Emilsson, T.	Ögonklin. Lasarettet	252 21 Helsingborg
Enoksson, Paul	Trollvägen 32	133 00 Saltsjöbaden
Ericson, L. A.	Lasarettet, Fack	451 01 Uddevalla
Ericson, Runo	Sotargatan 17	724 63 Västerås
Eriksen, Arne	Lasarettet, Fack	331 01 Värnamo
Eriksson, Anna-Stina	Lasarettet, Fack	961 19 Boden
Ervaeus, Sigrid	Ögonklin. Lasarettet, Fack	791 01 Falun
Esklund, Alf	Sommarvägen 1	171 40 Solna
Espegård-Wall, Gunnel	Mossvägen 7	182 74 Stocksund
Essen-Möller, L.	Drottninggatan 3	252 21 Helsingborg
Fabian, G.	Smedjegatan 8	722 13 Västerås
Finnström, Kerstin	Ögonklin. Lasarettet	901 85 Umeå
Forsmaru, E.	Styrmansgatan 9	114 54 Stockholm
Forsström, A.	Centralplan 1	691 00 Karlskoga
Frisén, Lars	Ögonklin. Sahlgrenska sjukh. ...	413 45 Göteborg
Gausland, T.	Tennisgatan 3	702 27 Örebro
Georgievska, Tatjana	....	
Germanis, Mirdza	Ögonklin. Danderyds sjukh. Fack.	182 03 Danderyd
Gjötterberg, Magnus	Gråhundsvägen 132	123 62 Farsta
Granath, Ulla	Storgatan 39, IIItr	871 00 Härnösand
Granit, Prof. Raguar	Eriksbergsgatan 14	114 30 Stockholm
Granstrom, Per Arne	Ögonkl. Sabb. sjukh. Box 6401 .	113 82 Stockholm
Grönwall, H.	Näsbychaussén 8	291 35 Kristianstad
Grönwall, Emy	Ögonklin. Lasarettet	291 85 Kristianstad
Gyllberg, Olof	Ögonklin. Lasarettet	371 00 Karlskrona
Hagbyhn-Gericke, A.	Ögonklin. Sabb. sjukh. Box 6401.	113 82 Stockholm
Halldén, Ulf	Östanväg 50	216 18 Malmö

Hallén, Barbro	Ögonkl. Södersjukhuset, Fack ..	100 64 Stockholm
Hannesson, O. B.	Domus Medica, Egilsgate 3	Reykjavik (Island)
Hanström, E.	Lasarettet, Fack	593 01 Västervik 1
Haptén, K. B.	Stora Nygatan 31	211 37 Malmö
Haagensen-Haptén, A. E. ..	Stora Nygatan 31	211 37 Malmö
Haelquist, Inger	Lasarettet, Fack	462 01 Vänersborg
Hasselgren, Jan	Medborgargatan 26	852 52 Sundsvall
Hauffman, Mårten	Heleneborgsgatan 5 A	117 31 Stockholm
Hedbeck, Krister	Bondegatan 13	593 00 Västervik
Hedbys, Bengt	Ögonklin. Sahlgrenska sjukh. ...	413 45 Göteborg
Hedensiö, Bertil	Drottninggatan 34 A	582 27 Linköping
Hedvall, Inger	Scheelegatan 10	112 28 Stockholm
Heldtander, Kristian	Ögonklin.-Lasarettet	721 89 Västerås
Hellberg, Anne-Marie	Knutstorpsgatan 12	216 22 Malmö
Hellum, Halvard	Ögonklin. Lasarettet, Fack	961 19 Boden
Henriksson, Marianne	Ögonklin. Allmänna sjukhuset ..	214 01 Malmö
Hiielo, Ants	Läkarhuset	162 90 Vällingby
Hjortzberg-Nordlund, U. ...	Vasa Kyrkogata 1	411 27 Göteborg
Holgén, Anna-Brita	Ögonavd. Lasarettet, Fack	891 02 Örnsköldsvik
Holm, K. K.	Lasarettet, Fack	521 01 Falköping
Holm, Olof	Äpplehagen 14	223 55 Lund
Holm, Stig	Vasagatan 14	411 24 Göteborg
Holmberg, Åke	Wirséns Väg 6	182 63 Djursholm
Huggert, Prof. A.	Småtuvegatan 7	431 39 Mölndal
Hörnsten, Gunnar	Neurolog. klin. Södersjukh. Fack .	100 64 Stockholm
Ivarsson, Gunilla	Tallvägen 25	183 62 Täby
Jahnberg, Peder	Grevgatan 37	114 53 Stockholm
Jansson, Folke	Falhemsvägen 2	791 00 Falun
Jansson, S.	Södra Torngatan 4	531 00 Lidköping
Jerndahl, Tord	Ögonklin. Sahlgrenska sjukh. ...	413 45 Göteborg
Johansson, Stig	Ögonklin. Falu Lasarettet, Fack .	791 01 Falun
Kallai, Karl	Ögonklin. Lasarettet	631 88 Eskilstuna
Kallai, Peter	Ögonklin. Lasarettet	601 82 Norrköping
Karlberg, Bo	Ogonpol. Sociala Huset	411 17 Göteborg
Karpe, Prof. G.	Ögonklin. Karolinska sjukh. Fack.	104 01 Stockholm
Kassman, Ture	Lasarettet, Fack	671 01 Arvika
Kjellner, G.	Drottningholmsvägen 39	112 42 Stockholm
Klang, Gunnar	Telestadsgatan 6	352 35 Växjö
Kling, Gunnar	Lasarettet, Fack	831 01 Östersund
Klingberg, S.	Tingsryds sjukstuga	360 20 Tingsryd
Knave, Bengt	Fysiolog Instit. II, K.I.	104 01 Stockholm
Kock, Erik	Ekbackevägen 11	181 46 Lidingö
Kristensen, Helge	Torvegate 59	Esbjerg (Danm.)
Kriisa, Viiu	Ögonklin. Sahlgrenska sjukh. ...	413 45 Göteborg
Kornerup, Tore	Solna Kyrkväg 7	171 64 Solna
Kronning, E.	Lasarettet, Box 52	931 01 Skellefteå
Kugelberg, Prof. I.	Nybrogatan 28	114 39 Stockholm
Kuljus, Ado	Jakobsbergs sjukh. Dackev. 1 ...	175 34 Järfälla
Källmark, Bo	Ögonklin. Regionsjukhuset	581 85 Linköping
Lagerlöf, Olof	Karlavägen 101	115 22 Stockholm
Lange, Göran	V. Långgatan 8	292 00 Karlshamn
Larsson, Lennart	Östra Hylievägen 2	216 21 Malmö
Larsson, Prof. S.	Dauderydsgatan 13	114 26 Stockholm
Latkovic, Stefan	Ogonklin. Regionsjukhuset	581 85 Linköping
Laurent, Ulla	Hävelvägen 9	752 47 Uppsala
Lehman, Birgitta	Fridkullagatan 27 D	412 62 Göteborg

660

SVECIA

Lennartz, Carsten	Ögonklin. Allmänna sjukhuset ..	214 01 Malmö
Lenti, Gösta	Ögonklin. Lasarettet	601 82 Norrköping
Lignell-Lundberg, Margareta.	Närlunda Gårdsväg 13	170 10 Ekerö
Lindberg, B.	Kungsvägen 13	633 49 Eskilstuna
Lindberg, Birgitta	Ögonklin, Lasarettet, Fack	220 05 Lund
Linde, Claes-Jahan	Lövnäsvägen 7	182 75 Stocksund
Linder, Bertil	Lasarettet, Fack	351 01 Växjö
Lindgren-Teague, Marg. ...	Wittstocksgatan 30	115 27 Stockholm
Lindorff, Helge	Ögonkliniken, Lasarettet	901 85 Umeå
Lindstedt-Jonson, Eva	Bergsvägen 10	133 00 Saltsjöbaden
Linnér, Prof. E.	Lövstigen 12	902 32 Umeå
Lithman, Rutger	Sturegatan 19 D	752 23 Uppsala
Ljungström, Stig	Danska Backarna 16	133 00 Saltsjöbaden
Lund, Rolf	Storgatan 11	114 44 Stockholm
Lundvall, Rune	Kullbergska sjukhuset, Box 110 .	641 00 Katrineholm
Lunt, Tönis	Ögonklin. Regionsjukhuset	581 85 Linköping
Låftman, B.	Lasarettet, Box 158	611 01 Nyköping
Löwegren, A.	Södra Förstadsgatan 1	211 43 Malmö
Magnusson, Loftur	Ögonklin. Regionsjukhuset	701 85 Örebro
Malmquist, Folke	Ö. Hamngatan 52	411 09 Göteborg
Mannerfelt, Thomasine	Karlavägen 7	802 23 Gälve
Marqvard, H.	Bollnäs sjukhus, Fack	821 01 Bollnäs
Mattson, R.	Backtjärnsgatan 5 H	416 78 Göteborg
Mertens, Ove	Ögonklin. Lasarettet	291 00 Kristianstad
Nilsson, Lilian	Smedjegatan 9	262 00 Ängelholm
Nilsson, Prof. Sven-Erik ...	Ögonklin. Regionsjukhuset	581 85 Linköping
Nordenfeldt, Lillebil	Ögonklin. Lasarettet, Fack	220 05 Lund
Norrby, Åke	Bergsgatan 14	881 00 Sollefteå
Norrlin, C. L.	Floragatan 10	114 31 Stockholm
Norrsell, Kerstin	Ögonklin. Sahlgrenska sjukh. ...	413 45 Göteborg
Nylander, Ulf	Ögonklin. Lasarettet, Fack	800 07 Gävle
Nyman, K. G.	Dalvägen 28	183 40 Täby
Nässén, Anna-Britt	Ögonklin. Lasarettet, Box 850 ..	501 15 Borås
Nässén, Bengt	Dr. Linds Gata 4	413 25 Göteborg
Odqvist, Bertil		
Ollers, J.	S:t Eriksgatan 65	113 32 Stockholm
Olsson, Gunnar	4; de Villagatan 37	502 44 Borås
Olsson, Gunvor	Ögonklin. Lasarettet, Fack	261 20 Landskrona
Olsson, Kim	Ögonklin. Sabb. sjukh. Box 6401.	113 82 Stockholm
Olson, Olof	Scheffersgatan 9	112 58 Stockholm
Olsson, Sven R.	Ögonklin. Lasarettet, Fack	941 01 Piteå
Ottow, Nelly	Slånvägen 5	133 00 Saltsjöbaden
Owe-Larsson, Alf	Sandbäcksgatan 25	653 40 Karlstad
Palikó, Béla	Ögonklin. Regionsjukhuset	701 85 Örebro
Pallin, Olof	Kungsladugårdsgatan 14	633 44 Eskilstuna
Pallin, Per	Slättvägen 6	161 36 Bromma
Palm, Prof. E.	Hills Väg 5	223 65 Lund
Palme, Leif	Ögonklin. Allmänna sjukh.	214 01 Malmö
Pandolfi, Maurizio	Koag. lab. Allmänna sjukhuset ..	214 01 Malmö
Patek, Eva	Ögonklin. Lasarettet	651 85 Karlstad
Peil, Mats	Ögonavd. Lasarettet	371 00 Karskrona
Permalm, Hugo	Läkarhuset, Drottninggatan 19 ..	652 25 Karlstad
Peterson, Hans	Gungbrinken 13	163 54 Spånga
Petrelius, Anders	Ögonklin. Sabb. sjukh. Box 6401.	113 82 Stockholm
Philipson, Bo	Långängsvägen 43	182 75 Stocksund
Piechocienski, Zbigniew ...	Ögonklin. Lasarettet	551 85 Jönköping

Prame, Göran	Ögonklin. Lasarettet	721 89 Västerås
Pücky, Gustav	Ögonklin. Lasarettet, Fack	351 01 Växjö
Pähn, Ilja	Ögonklin. Lasarettet	575 00 Eksjö
Ramgard, Barbro	Granitvägen 12	183 63 Vallentuna
Rehn, Nils	Stenhällsvägen 9	151 41 Södertälje
Reineck, Åke	Box 3309	733 00 Sala
Rendahl, Ilmari	Skogsfrugränd 39	161 38 Bromma
Rexed, Ursula	Attundavägen 16	183 36 Täby
Ribbing-Theoren, K.	Söderleden 37	582 64 Linköping
Rister-Lindberg, Marlene ..	Ögonklin. Lasarettet	851 86 Sundsvall
Rosengren, Prof. Bengt	Fridkullagatan 25 A	412 62 Göteborg
Rundqvist, Nils	Ögonklin. Lasarettet	651 85 Karlstad
Runesson, Sigvard	Ögonklin. Lasarettet	551 85 Jönköping
Rybeck, Karin	Skinnarviksringen 12	117 26 Stockholm
Ryberg, Jonas	Hornsgatan 62	117 21 Stockholm
Rydberg, Mats	Mogatan 22	702 13 Örebro
Rylander, Margareta	Skandiavägen 13	182 63 Djursholm
Rönström, Hjalmar	Högbergsgatan 25	891 00 Örnsköldsvik
Sahlström, Ingvar	Ljusstöparbacken 1	117 45 Stockholm
Sandström, Inger	Ögonklin. Sabb. sjukh. Box 6401.	113 82 Stockholm
Schele, Bengt	Ögonklin. Lasarettet	291 00 Kristianstad
Scherling, B.	Platensgatan 17	582 20 Linköping
Schwan, Helge	Läkarhuset	123 47 Farsta
Schüberg, Elof	Djurgårdsgatan 13	582 29 Linköping
Sellman, Anders	Drottninggatan 126	252 33 Helsingborg
Sendel, O.	Linnegatan 11	752 32 Uppsala
Sjöberg, Ulla	Öppenv.c. ög. Helgeandsg. 16 ...	223 54 Lund
Sjögren, Maria	Thulehem 6	223 66 Lund
Sjögren, Prof. H.	Thulehem 6	223 66 Lund
Skoog, Klas-Olav	Ögonklin. Regionsjukhuset	581 85 Linköping
Snöbohm, Jan	Ögenklin. Lasarettet	551 85 Jönköping
Sonnsjö, Bo	Läkarmottagningen	686 00 Sunne
Stankovic, Ljiljana		
Stenbeck, Anna	Nybrogatan 12, 5 tr	114 35 Stockholm
Stendahl, Lena	Ögonklin. Regionsjukhuset	581 85 Linköping
Stenkula, Göran	Ögonavd. Lasarettet, Fack	381 02 Kalmar
Stenkula, Staffan	Ögonklin. Regionsjukhuset	701 85 Örebro
Stenström, Bo	Ögonklin. Lasarettet	631 88 Eskilstuna
Stenström, S.	Vasa Kyrkogata 1	411 24 Göteborg
Stigmar, Göran	Barytongränd 18	223 68 Lund
Strecha, Radim	Ögonklin. Lasarettet, Fack	824 01 Hudiksvall
Strömberg, H. E.	Settervallsvägen 17	131 00 Nacka
Strömland, Kerstin	Ögonklin. Sahlgrenska sjukh. ...	413 45 Göteborg
Sundmark, Erik	Ögonklin. Lasarettet, Fack	301 01 Halmstad
Svedbergh, Björn	Ögonklin. Akad. sjukh. Fack ...	750 14 Uppsala
Swegmark, Gunnar	Rådjursgatan 21	510 54 Brämhult
Svensson, E.	Observatoriegatan 10, 5 tr.	113 29 Stockholm
Svensson, Torbjörn	Ögonklin. Akad. sjukh. Fack ...	750 14 Uppsala
Tengroth, Björn	Ellösgatan 4	416 74 Göteborg
Tengroth, S.	Geijersgatan 7 B	412 56 Göteborg
Thorburn, William	Ögonklin. Lasarettet	901 85 Umeå
Thyberg, Eva	Ögonklin. Sabb. sjukh. Box 6401.	113 82 Stockholm
Thylefors, Björn	Ögonklin. Lasarettet, Fack	301 01 Halmstad
Torgersruud, T.	Planetgatan 7	621 00 Visby
Törnquist, Ragnar	Ögonklin. Regionsjukhuset	701 85 Örebro
Törnqvist, Göran	Ögonklin. Lasarettet	901 85 Umeå

Ursing, Jan	Norrbäcksgatan 39	216 21 Lund
Wachtmeister, Lellemor ...	Ögonklin. Karol. sjukh. Fack ...	104 01 Stockholm
Wadensten, Lars	Ogonklin. Lasarettet, Fack	824 01 Hudiksvall
Wahlberg, Ivar	Floragatan 20	961 00 Boden
Vallhov, B.	Strandvägen 5 A, 6 tr.	114 51 Stockholm
Wanger, Peter		
Wargelius, Kristina	Ögonklin. Lasarettet, Fack	381 02 Kalmar
Wetrell, Karin	Bygglovsgränd 7	222 47 Lund
Widakowich, Johannes	Kvarnstugvägen 29	161 51 Bromma
Wiebert, Ove	Myntvägen 14	352 47 Växjö
Wikholm, Lauri	Ögonklin. Lasarettet	631 88 Eskilstuna
Wilke, Kenneth	Ritaregränden 8	222 47 Lund
Wold, Eivind	Ögonklin. Regionsjukh. Fack ...	701 85 Örebro
Wranne, Ingrid	Dalavägen 20	702 17 Örebro
Wulfing, Björn	Sjövägen 14	185 52 Täby
Wålinder, Per	Baldersvägen 14 B	852 33 Sundsvall
Zeidler, Inga	Floragatan 5, 4 tr.	114 31 Stockholm
Zetterlund, Olof	Ögonklin. Lasarettet, Fack	891 02 Örnsköldsvik
Zetterquist, Birgitta	Vesslevägen 4	183 40 Täby
Zetterström, Birgitta	Ögonklin. Karol. sjukh. Fack ...	104 01 Stockholm
Åberg-Ahrnberg, Brita	Överåsgatan 5	412 66 Göteborg
Åberg, Lennart	Ögonklin. C-lasarettet, Fack	381 02 Kalmar
Åborg, C. G.	Johan Skyttes Väg 11 C	552 59 Jönköping
Åkerblom, Torsten	Ögonklin. Lasarettet, Fack	301 01 Halmstad
Åkerskog, Gunnar	Dr. Linds Gata 4	413 25 Göteborg
Öberg, L.	Kungsportsavenyn 15	411 36 Göteborg
Öhman, Lena	Ögonklin. Akad. sjukh. Fack ...	750 14 Uppsala
Öhrström, Arne	Ögonklin. Allmänna sjukhuset ..	214 01 Malmö
Örtegren, Kerstin	Skogsbrynet 22	902 32 Umeå
Österlin, Sven	Allmänna sjukhuset	214 01 Malmö
Österlind, Prof. Göte	Gustaf Adolfs Torg 49	211 39 Malmö
Österman, Ann	Ogonklin. Sabb. sjukh. Box 6401.	113 82 Stockholm

NOSOCOMIA QUIBUS OCULIS AEGRI CURANTUR

There are no specific Eye Hospitals, but all major hospitals have eye departments.

	No. of beds
Karolinska sjukhuset, 104 01 Stockholm, Head: Professor G. Karpe	57
Sabbatsbergs sjukhus, 113 82 Stockholm, Head: Å. Holmberg	27
Södersjukhuset, 100 64 Stockholm, Head: P. Enoksson	19
Huddinge sjukhus, 141 86 Huddinge, Head: vacant	44
Akademiska sjukhuset, 750 14 Uppsala, Head: Professor G. von Bahr	46
Lasarettet i Eskilstuna, 631 88 Eskilstuna, Head: O. Pallin	22
Lasarettet i Nyköping, 611 01 Nyköping, Head: B. Låftman	12
Regionsjukhuset i Linköping, 581 85 Linköping, Head: Professor S-E. Nilsson	24
Lasarettet i Norrköping, 601 82 Norrköping, Head: G. Lenti	15
Lasarettet i Jönköping, 551 85 Jöngköping, Head: I. Anjou	34
Lasarettet i Växjö, 351 85 Växjö, Head: B. Linder	14
Västerviks sjukhus, 593 01 Västervik, Head: vacant	13

Lasarettet i Kalmar, 381 02 Kalmar, Head: G. Elg 20
Lasarettet i Visby, 621 01 Visby, Head: vacant 9
Lasarettet i Karlskrona, 371 00 Karlskrona, Head: M. Peil 19
Lasarettet i Kristianstad, 291 85 Kristianstad, Head: J. Cristiansson 32
Malmö Allmänna sjukhus, 214 01 Malmö, Head: Professor G. Österlind 28
Lasarettet i Lund, 221 85 Lund, Head: Professor E. Palm 49
Lasarettet i Helsingborg, 251 87 Helsingborg, Head: T. Emilsson 12
Lasarettet i Halmstad, 301 85 Halmstad, Head: E. Sundmark 21
Sahlgrenska sjukhuset, 413 45 Göteborg, Head: B. Tengroth 50
Lasarettet i Uddevalla, 451 01 Uddevalla, Head: L. Ericsson 30
Lasarettet i Vänersborg, 461 01 Vänersborg, Head: M. Blix 16
Lasarettet i Borås, 501 15 Borås, Head: G. Swegmark 25
Lasarettet i Falköping, 521 01 Falköping, Head: K. K. Holm 24
Karlstads sjukhus, 651 85 Karlstad, Head: N. Rundqvist 26
Regionsjukhuset i Örebro, 701 85 Örebro, Head: R. Törnquist 48
Lasarettet i Västerås, 721 89 Västerås, Head: G. Prame 30
Lasarettet i Falun, 791 01 Falun, Head: F. Jansson 51
Gävle sjukhus, 800 07 Gävle, Head: U. Nylander 24
Hudiksvalls sjukhus, 824 01 Hudiksvall, Head: L. Wadensten 23
Sundsvalls sjukhus, 851 86 Sundsvall, Head: P-E. Wålinder 26
Örnsköldsviks sjukhus, 891 01 Örnsköldsvik, Head: O. Zetterlund 14
Östersunds sjukhus, 831 01 Östersund, Head: G. Kling 20
Lasarettet i Umeå, 901 85 Umeå, Head: Professor E. Linnér 30
Lasarettet i Skellefteå, 931 00 Skellefteå, Head: E. Kronning 6
Lasarettet i Boden, 961 19 Boden, Head: A-S. Eriksson 29
Lasarettet i Gällivare, 972 00 Gällivare, Head: Y. Barkman 14

INSTITUTA SCHOLAEQUE CAECIS DESTINATAE

The Tomteboda Institute at Solna: special primary school for children (7-17 years old) suffering
from a visual defect. *110 pupils* + A consultant's section embracing 4 consultants for pre-school
age children.
Eskeskolan at Örebro: for children (5-21 years old), who, in addition to a visual defect, are
suffering from some other handicap, *100 pupils.*
The Annetorp Home at Lund: a special home for the care of mentally retarded blind over 16 years
of age (Activation, rehabilitation, ADC-training), *125 pupils.*
Special classes, so called 'sighted classes' exist in our three largest cities for teaching children with
defective sight, *62 pupils.*

(The rest of the children with defective sight (about 800) are being taught in an ordinary school
class with technical and pedagogical aids.)

Schools for adaptation training:
at
Kristinehamn   about 30 pupils
Växjö   about 30 pupils
Furulund   about 30 pupils
Norrköping   about 30 pupils
Uppsala   about 30 pupils
Skellefteå   about 30 pupils

(Short adaptation courses for elderly visually handicapped 4 weeks (12 pupils) are held at some
'people's university' or other suitable institute.)

About 80 visually handicapped students are studying at universities and university colleges helped by special services.

Preparatory courses for partially sighted students paving the way for secondary studies.

Gerdahemmet at Åby, Norrköping, special home for pre-school aged children with defective sight, 8 children for shorter periods.

SYRIA

SOCIETATES OPHTHALMOLOGICAE

Syrian Ophthalmological Society

President: Prof. Dr. Akram Anbari
Vice-President: Dr. Robert Jebejian
Secretary: Dr. Walid Joumra
2nd Secretary: Dr. Joudat Mandil
Accountant: Dr. Mouna El-Bezem
Treasurer: Dr. Adnan Attar
Member: Dr. Omar Shishakli
Address: Mouassat Hospital, Ophthalmic Dept., Damascus
Number of members: 43

NOMINA ET DOMICILIA MEDICORUM AB OCULIS

Abella, Alexander	Saint Louis Hospital	Aleppe
Anbari, Prof. Akram	Salhia St.	Damascus
Abrash, Hatem	Mahatta St.	Homs
Adib, Salah	Sheik Daher St.	Lattakia
Alsabeh, Fayez	Salhia St.	Damascus
Asmar, Leon	P.O. Box 795	Aleppe
Abou-oubeid, Mohamad	Hijaz St.	Damascus
Attar, Adnan	Raouda St.	Damascus
Bourak, Nizar	Youseef Azme place	Damascus
Chammeut, Nizar	29 Ayar St.	Damascus
El-Bezem, Mouna	29 Avar St.	Damascus
Faham, Zeki	Derwichye St.	Damascus
Farah, Eli	Bagdad St.	Damascus
Fatteuh, Joseph	Salhia St.	Damascus
Hajar, Mamoun	29 Ayar St.	Damascus
Hamarneh, Nashaat	Post 2650 Jiser Victoria St.	Damascus
Himmat, Hassan	Bagdad St.	Damascus
Hindaoni, Abdul-Majid	Mouassat Hospital	Damascus
Jebejian, Robert	Sabil	Aleppe
Joumra, Walid	Jiser Abiad St.	Damascus
Kanawati, Yassir	Chalan St.	Damascus
Kasuha, Fares	Military Hospital	Homs
Kawa, Salah	Youssef Azme place	Damascus
Kilsyeh, Abdul-Meuneim	Binaand Omran society	Aleppe
Kouzal, Fouad Sar	Tilal St.	Aleppe
Majbour, Malek	Military Hospital	Damascus
Mandil, Jaqudat	Military Hospital	Deir-ez-zer
Mateuk, Riad	Zahara building, Salhie	Damascus
Moheithawi, Shahine	Military Hospital	Damascus
Mora, Najib	29 Ayar St.	Damascus
Mott, Faez	Arabi Hospital, Bagdad St.	Damascus
Meusatat, Said	Baron St.	Aleppe
Mutlak, Schaker	Bab-Houd St.	Homs
Sabbagh, Prof. Mamdouh	29 Ayar St.	Damascus
Said, Prof. Adnan	Jiser Victoria St.	Damascus

Sahlul, Sami	Jouret el-Shayah St.	Homs
Sawaf, Adib	Bab el-Nasr. St.	Aleppe
Sehishakli Omar	Tawfiq Shishakli St.	Hama
Seffe, Abdul-Hadi	Bina and Omran Society	Aleppe
Serjieh, Fadel	Kistaki Homsi Azizie St.	Aleppe
Sibay, Houssni	Jouret el-Shayah	Homs
Sudan, Abdul-Rahman	Moujtaled St.	Damascus
Tabbash, Sharif	Bina and Omran Society	Aleppe

NOSOCOMIA QUIBUS OCULIS AEGRI CURANTUR

No. of beds
Mouassat Hospital, Dept. of Ophthalmology, Dir.: Prof. Dr. Akram Anbari, Damascus 63
Damascus Hospital, Dept. of Ophthalmology, Dir: Dr. Nizar Chammeut, Damascus 40
Military Hospital, Dept. of Ophthalmology, Dir: Dr. Nizar Bourak, Damascus ....

INSTITUTA SCHOLAEQUE CAECIS DESTINATAE

There is a school for the blind in Damascus with 105 pupils.

TAIWAN (Formosa)

SOCIETATES OPHTHALMOLOGICAE

Ophthalmological Society of the Republic of China
Address of Secretary: c/o Department of Ophthalmology, National Taiwan University Hospital, 1, Chang-Te Street, Taipei
President: Prof. Yen-Fei Yang
Vice-President: Prof. Jung-Mao Chang
Members: Yung-Hsin Chen, Yi Na, Nai-Huei Lin, Liang-Shi Ko, Chen-Kung Shi, Wu-Fu Chen
Secretary: Prof. Jung-Mao Chang, University Hospital, 1, Chang Teh St., Taipei
Number of Members: 97

Section of Ophthalmology, Formosan Medical Association
Secretary: K. H. Lin, 1, Jen Ai Rd., Taipei
Number of members: 90

NOMINA ET DOMICILIA MEDICORUM AB OCULIS

John Chang	148, Prince Edward Rd., 3rd Floor	Kow Loon, Hong Kong
Jung-Mao Chang	University Hospital, 1, Chang Teh St.	Taipei
Yi Hsiung Chang	Provincial Taichung Hospital, 48, Chi Juan St.	Taichung
Tse-Yu Chao	Provincial Chung Hsing Hosp., Chung Hsin Shin Chuang	Nan Tou Hsien
Chen-Wu Chen	Kao Hsiung Medical College	Kao Hsiung City
Eng-Ssu Chen	343 Chong Chung Rd.	Hwa Lien
Shin Lien Chen	38–4, Min Tzen Rd.	Pin Tong
Sow-Tseng Chen	84, Chung Cheng Road, Yeng Hsue Town	Tainan Hsian
Shiuh Ru Chen	17–1 Wen Chan St.	Sa Lo, Tai Chung Hsien
Tsau Chen	3, Alley 15, Lane 73, Peiton Rd.	Taichung
Wu-Fu Chen	108, Tong Ming Li Lo-Tong	I-Ran Hsien
Young-Hsin Chen	1–2, Small North St. Shiling	Taipei
Yuen-Chi Chen	313–1, Chang-Chun Rd.	Taipei
Kung-Hsing Cheng	154, Min Tzen Rd.	Taichung
Ping-Yang Cheng	69, Kuang Lin Li Nan Shan Rd., Lin Pien Shang	Pin Tong Hsien
Teh Shun Cheng	169–1, Sec. 2 Sin I Rd.	Taipei
Chi Li Chiang	84, Chong Chung Rd., Tao Yuan City	Tau Yuan Hsien
Chung- Lo Chie	5, Lane 16, Jung An St., Yen Ho Town	Taipei, Hsien
Fong-Siung Chiu	8, Yi 1st Road	Keelung City
Shen Pin Chou	237, Chung Chan Rd.	Yuan Lin
Tsai-Tsun Chou	214, Min Shen N. Rd.	Chiayi

Yu-Chin Chou	54-2, Pau-an St.	Taipei
Chao-Chang Chuang	100, Ping Ho Road, Kang Shan Town	Kao Siung Hsien
Dar-Min Chuang	27–1, Chung Tseng IVth Rd. ...	Kao Hsiung City
Chang-Sung Fan	4–2, Lane 157, Shin Shen S. Rd.	Taipei
Yun-Ching Han	6–5, Lane 210, Roosevelt Rd., Sec. 3	Taipei
Chih-Ying Ho	1, Lane 72, Section 1, Roosevelt Road	Taipei
Pin Kan Hou	Dept. Ophthalmology, University Hospital, 1, Chan Teh St. ...	Taipei
Yun Fan Hsieh	22, Lane 195, Sec. 2, Ho Ping E. Rd.	Taipei
Te-Yu Hu	53, Hsin 1st. Road	Kee Lung City
Chin-Chong Huang	68, Hsin Ming St., Tao Yuan City	Tau Yuan Hsien
Jung-Hue Huang	647, Pa Teh Rd., Sect. 4	Taipei
May Nwang Huang	Dept. Ophth. Provincial Taichung Hosp.	Taicnung
Por Tying Hung	Univ. Hosp., 1 Chan Teh St.	Taipei
Tsu-En Hung	19, Ningsia Road	Taipei
Kuang-Ching Kao	40, Hsi Men Road	Tainan
Liang Shi Ko	5, Lane 135, Sec. 1, Chung Shan North Road	Taipei
Fu-Chuan Ku	27, Kang Lien St., Tsu Tong Town	Hsin Tsu Hsien
Gen-Tung Ku	183, Si Zong St.	Chiayi
Fan-Mao Kuo	16, Sec. 1, Kai Hong St.	Taipei
Wun-Fang Lai	53, Pin Tung St.	Taichung
Sha-Suei Lai	188, Jen Ai Rd.	Chiayi
Chen-To Lee	5, Pass 8, Lane 123, Sec. 5 Nanking East Road	Taipei
Yiau-Cheng Lee	14, Yen Peng Li, Ching Ying Town	Tainan Hsien
Suei-Yen Lian	4–4, Fushin 1st. Rd.	Kao Hsiung
Kuei-Chen Liao	50, Ten Suei Road	Taipei
Shu-Jin Liao	87, Sect. 1, Yen Ho Road, Section 1, Yen Ho Town	Taipei Hsien
Chin Chi Lin	Dept. Ophth. Kao-Hsiung, Medical College	Kao-Hsiung
Ju-Yu Lin	70, Nan Chang Road, Sec. 1	Taipei
Keng Shen Lin	83, Erhlin Road, Erhlin Town ..	Changhwa Hsien
I-Hsin Lin	169, Yun Fu Rd.	Tainan
Nai-Huei Lin	45, Sec. 1, Chung San North Rd.	Taipei
Teng-En Lin	60, Min Tsan Road	Pin Tong
Tsi-Jung Lin	Chong Cheng Road, Fon Shan Town	Kao-Hsiung Hsien
Yi-Kuang Lin	115–5 Kui Lin Rd.	Taipei
Yi-Ming Lin	74, Ai 2nd Roaa	Keelung City
Chuan-Lai Liu	361, Chung Cheng Road	Chiayi
Ching Hung Liu	4–2, Lane 13, Li Sui St.	Taipei
Jung-Hsien Liu	79–5, Sec. 1, Chong Hua Road .	Taipei
Lin Schan Liu	55, Wu ru 4th Road, Dept. Ophth. G.E.C.C.	Kao-Hsiung
Seh Choung Liu	32, Lane 409, An Tong St., Jen Ai Road	Taipei
Sow-Ting Liu	91, Lu Tsuan St.	Taichung

Yu-Chiau Liu	55, Ming Tsu Road	Taichung
Hsue-Wang Lu	265, Chung San Road	Hwa Lien
We-Yen Lu	42, Chang Shoei Road	Chihu, Changhwa
Yi Na	16, Lane 8, Kuang Chou Rd.	Taipei
Lien-Fu Pan	47, Ta Gin Road	Kao Siung
Chi-Wen Shen	208, Ming Sun W. Road	Taipei
Yeong-Tai Shen	92, Sec. 2, Chung-Shan N. Rd.	Taipei
Chen-Kung Shih	288, Min-Chuan W. Road	Taipei
En Hsi Sun	P.O. Box 7835, Ton Shi	Taichung
Shen-Fa Tsai	82, Yeng Ping Road, Tong Kong Town	Ping Tong Hsien
Shyh Tzong Tsai	322, Chung-Tseng Road	Yan-Lin Town, Changhwa
Wu Fu Tsai	11, Lane 124, Chin Chiang St.	Taipei
Jung Hsiang Tseng	223, Fu Hsing Rd.	Ping Tong
San-Shung Tsan	152, Tso Ying Ta Road	Kao Hsiung City
Yi-Shung Wang	72, Kuang Hua Road	Chiayi
Wang-Pan Weie	52, Chung Cheng Road	Tainan
Ten-Hsien Wei	75, Min Tzo Rd.	Nan Tou
Wing-Tze Wong	2, B. King Tak St.	Kow Loon, Hong Kong
Chi-Fu Wu	169, Chong Chen 4th Road	Kao Hsiung City
Hsing-Chun Wu	73, Shu Fu Road	Taichung
Jiunn Shyong Wu	73, Shu Fu Rd.	Taichung
Tseng-Su Wu	70, Sec. 2, Yon Ho Rd., Yon Ho Town	Taipei Hsien
Tung-Yan Wu	36, Yen Ping Road	Sin Ying Town, Tainan
Lin Lian Wung	83–1, Wen Chan St.	Hsin Tsu City
Lin-Ying Wung	97, Chong Pin Road, Chong Li Town	Tau Yen Hsien
Hsien-Yung Wung	10–2, Kim men St.	Taipei
Jih-Huan Yang	31, Chang-An West Road	Taipei
Yen-Fei Yang	University Hosp., 1, Chang Teh St.	Taipei
Yu Yang	39, Kimber Ley Rd. 1st 71	Kow Loon, Hong Kong
Yu-Shian Yang	10, Chong Lin Tsung, Lin Pen Siang	Ping Tong Hsien
Long-Zuei Yeh	115, Wu Fu 4th Road	Hao-Shsiung City
Shaw Hsiung Young	125, Fu Tzen Rd.	Tainan
Tien Shieng Yu	3, Alley 41, Lane 407, Pei An Rd.	Ta-Tau, Taipei

NOSOCOMIA QUIBUS OCULIS AEGRI CURANTUR

National Taiwan University Hospital, Department of Ophthalmology. No. of beds: 50
Director: Jung-Mao Chang

INSTITUTA SCHOLAEQUE CAECIS DESTINATAE

Taiwan Provincial Taipei School for the Blind and Deaf, Chung Ching N.Rd., Taipei City
Taiwan Provincial Taichung Chi Ming School, 72 San Feng Rd., Holi, Taichung County Taiwan 421

The Home of Teaching and Training for the Blind Association for the welfare of the Blind of
    Taiwan, Pei-To, Taipei
Committee for the Blind of Taiwan, P.O. Box 10, Hsin Tsuan, Taipei Hsien
Hildesheim Blinden Mission, Ta-Ya, Taichung Hsien
Home for the Blind girls, Pin Tong, Taiwan
Home for the Blind girls, Hwa Lien, Taiwan
Mu-Kwang Blind Center, 11, Pei Chong St., Lo-Tung, Taiwan 265

THAILAND

SOCIETATES OPHTHALMOLOGICAE

Ophthalmo-Otorhinolaryngological Association

Secretary: Maj. General Luang, Mongkolbhaedyakom, 281 # 31
Swasdi. Sujumvit Rd., Bangkok

No data received.

TSECHO-SLOVAKIA

SOCIETATES OPHTHALMOLOGICAE

Czecho-Slovakian Ophthalmological Society
President: Prof. Dr. Rudolf Knobloch
Secretary: Dr. Hanus Kraus, U nemocnice 2, 128 08 Praha 2

This society is composed of the two national societies:

Czech Ophthalmological Society
President: Prof. Dr. Rudolf Knobloch
Vice-Presidents: Prof. Dr. Svatopluk Řehák. Dr. Otto Kühnel
Secretary: Dr. Hanuš Kraus, U nemocnice 2, 128 08 Praha 2

Slovak Opthalmological Society
President: Prof. Dr. Jozef Šuster
Vice-Presidents: Ass. Prof. Dr. Lúdovít Veselý, Dr. Anton Wachsmann
Secretary: Dr. Tomáš Mazalán, Mickiewiczova ul. 800 00, Bratislava

NOMINA ET DOMICILIA MEDICORUM AB OCULIS

No data received.

NOSOCOMIA QUIBUS OCULIS AEGRI CURANTUR

Ist Eye Department, Faculty of Medicine, Caroline University, Prague. *Director:* Prof. Dr. Emil Dienstbier, DrSc.
IInd. Eye Dept., Fac of Med., Caroline Univ., Prague. *Director:* Ass. Prof. Dr. Jaroslava Votočková, DtSc.
Eye Dept., Hyg. Epid. Fac. Caroline Univ., Prague. *Director:* Prof. Dr. František Vrabec, DrSc.
Eye Dept., Inst. for Postgrad. Med. Education, Prague *Director:* Ass. Prof. Dr. F. V. Michal, DrSc.
Eye Dept., Fac. of Med., Caroline Univ., Plzeň *Director:* Prof. Dr. Rudolf Knobloch, DrSc
Eye Dept. Fac. of Med. Caroline Univ., Hradec Králové. *Director:* Prof. Dr. Svatopluk Řehák, DrSc.
Eye Dept., Med. Fac. Komenský Univ., Martin. *Director:* Ass. Prof. Dr. Jozef Sevčik, CSc.
Eye Dept., Med. Fac. P. J. Šafarík Univ. and Inst. for Postgrad. Med. Educ. Košice. *Director:* Ass. Prof. Dr. Lúdovít Veselý
Eye Dept., Fac. of Med., Palacký Univ., Olomoue. *Director:* Ass. Prof. Dr. Václay Svec, CSc.
Eye Dept., Med. Fac., Univ. Jan Ev. Purkyně, Brno. *Director:* Ass. Prof. Dr. Otto Riebel, DrSc.
Eye Dept., Med. Fac., Komenský Univ., Bratislava. *Director:* Prof. Dr. Jozef Šuster

There are eye departments in all districts.

INSTITUTA SCHOLAEQUE CAECIS DESTINATAE

Schools for blind, partially sighted children and for children with defect vision are in *Prague, Bratislava, Levoča* and other places.

There are nursery schools, primary schools, secondary schools, high schools and schools for musical education.

TUNESIA

SOCIETATES OPHTHALMOLOGICAE

Société Tunisienne d'Ophthalmologie

Président: Dr. Mohamed Charfi
Secrétaire-Général: Dr. Taofik Daghfous, Institut d'Ophtalmologie, Bab Saâdoun, Tunis
Number of members: 20

NOMINA ET DOMICILIA MEDICORUM AB OCULIS

Azous, Mohamed Salah	Institut d'Ophtalmologie Bab Saâdoun	Tunis
Ben Amor Salem	Institut d'Ophtalmologie Bab Saâdoun	Tunis
Besaiess, Abdelmagid	Hôpital Régional de Bizerte	Bizerte
Bouttour, Abdelaziz	Hôpital Régional de Sfax	Sfax
Charfi, Mohamed	Hôpital Abib Thameur	Tunis
Daghfous, Mohamed Taoufik	Institut d'Ophtalmologie Bab Saâdoun	Tunis
Fakhfakh, Tabar	Hôpital Regional de Sfax	Sfax
Jaziri, Ammar	Institut d'Ophtalmologie Bab Saâdoun	Tunis
Mabrouk, Ridha	Institut d'Ophtalmologie Bab Saâdoun	Tunis
Messadi, Mohamed	Institut d'Ophtalmologie Bab Saâdoun	Tunis
M'rad, Ridha	Hôpital Charles Nicolles	Tunis
Nabli, Bechir	Institut d'Ophtalmologie Bab Saâdoun	Tunis
Petrov, Eftim	Hôpital Régional de Gabes	Gabes
Rais, Cherif	Institut d'Ophtalmologie Bab Saâdoun	Tunis
Romdhane, Khelil	Institut d'Ophtalmologie Bab Saâdoun	Tunis
Skandrani, Ali	Hôpital Régional de Sousse	Sousse
Slimane, Ben	42 Bd Bab Menara	Tunis
Trabelsi	Institut d'Ophtalmologie Bab Saâdoun	Tunis
Zaghedane, Mohamed	Hôpital Régional de Sousse	Sousse
Zeghal, Mohamed	Institut d'Ophtalmologie Bab Saâdoun	Tunis

NOSOCOMIA QUIBUS OCULIS AEGRI CURANTUR

Institut d'Ophtalmologie Bab Saâdoun
Directeur: Dr. Daghfous Taoufik .... 150 lits

Dispensaires Ophtalmologiques dans les Hôpitals Régionaux

INSTITUTA SCHOLAEQUE CAECIS DESTINATAE

Institut des Aveugles de Bir El Kassâa, Tunis.
Institut des Aveulges de Bir El Kassâa, Sousse.

TURCIA

SOCIETATES OPHTHALMOLOGICAE

Nationales

Türk Oftalmologi Cemiyeti (Societé d'Ophtalmologie Turque)
Président: Prof. Dr. Demir Başar
Sécrétaire-Général: Dr. Arif Atli
Trésorier Général: Dr. Fevzi Akkan
Bureau: Clinique Ophtalmologique, 28 Yeni Çarçi, Galatasazay, Istanbul
Membres: 136

Türk Ergoftalmologi Cemiyeti (Societé d'Ergophtalmologie Turque)
Président: Dr. Bülent Artuner
Vice-Président: Prof. Dr. Demir Başar
Sécrétaire-Général: Dr. Arif Atli, Yeminahalle Havlucular S.I/2, Istanbul
Trésorier Général: Dr. Rana Ergun

Türk Göz Sagligi Dernegi (Societé d'Hygienique Ophtalmologique Turque)
Président: Prof. Dr. Demir Başar
Vice-Président: Prof. Dr. Muhsin K. Idil
Sécrétaire Général: Prof. Dr. Ünal Bengisu
Membre: Dr. Turhan Sezer

Regionales

Ankara Oftalmologi Cemiyeti
Président: Prof. Dr. Ümit Emüler
Instanbul Oftalmologi Cemiyeti
Président: Dr. Fevzi Akkan
Izmir Oftalmologi Cemiyeti
Président: Prof. Dr. Selahattin Erbakan
Erzurum Oftalmologi Cemiyeti
Président: Prof. Dr. Gülham Slem

NOMINA ET DOMICILIA MEDICORUM AB OCULIS

Abadan, Prof. Sabahat	Kavaklidere Kibris sok. Efes Ap. .	Ankara
Acargil, Özşen	Yeşilyurt İstasyon cad. 20-3/9 ..	İstanbul
Ahi, Kemal	Hakki Cankat sok. Öğretmen evleri	Gaziantep

Akaraz, Zaven	Cumhuriyet cad. 87/3 Elmadağ .	İstanbul
Akkan, Fevzi	Osmanbey Tavukçu fethi sok. 26 .	İstanbul
Akkan, Ulviye	Cihangir Tavuk uçmaz 14/6	İstanbul
Aksoy, Ahmet	Meşrutiyet mah. Yeniyol sok. 12 .	Zonguldak
Aksoy, Şükrü	Kardeşler apartimani	Edremit
Aksu, Erdoğan	Gazi cad. Özboyaci ap. No: 3 ...	Burdur
Akyol, Cihad	Kadiköy. Bahariye cad No: 48/3	İstanbul
Aleksiyadis, Sokrat	Taksim Neşelik sok. 36/10	İstanbul
Algun, Prof. Talàt	Beşevler. 2. sok 4/8 Bahçelievler .	İstanbul
Alpaslan, Hayrettin	İstiklal cad No: 68/I İzmit	Kocaeli
Altay, Lale	Cerrahpaşa Tip Fak. Göz Klin. ..	İstanbul
Andaç, Kutay	Üniversite loj. C/3 Bornava	İzmir
Ara, Abidin	Yenişehir Meşrutiyet cad. 32/5 ..	Ankara
Aralp, Hikmet	Bahariye cad. 98/5 Kadiköy	İstanbul
Arslan, Okan	S.S.K. Beyoğlu Hast. Şişli. Okmeydani	İstanbul
Artuner, Bülent	Yeniçarşi 28 Artuner göz Kliniği .	İstanbul
Ataç, Azmi	Etem efendi Nur sok. 10/5 Erenköy	İstanbul
Ataç, Kemal	Çekrige Çukurköşkü yani 58	Bursa
Ataç, Muhsin	Altiyol. Kadiköy. Mürver çiçeği sok	İstanbul
Atik, Dündar	Trahom hast. Baştabıbi	Kilis
Atilla, İ Hakki	Askeri Hast. Baştabibi	Manisa
Atli, Arif	Yenimahalle Haclucular S.I/2 ...	İstanbul
Atukalp, Ahmet	S.S.K. Hastanesi Baştabibi	Konya
Ayberk, Prof. Nejat	Taksim Cumhuriyet cad. 27/i ...	İstanbul
Ayberk, Nuri F.	Taksim Cumhuriyet cad. 27/I ...	İstanbul
Aygün, Selahattin	Şair Nedim cad. 54-3/5 Beşiktaş .	İstanbul
Aytek, Prof. Muaffak	Bilir sok 17/10	Ankara
Bamyaci, Rahmi	Hastane Cad. No: 44/A	Denizli
Basa, Mazhar	Göz mütehassisi	Rize
Başar, Prof. Demir	Harbiye valikonaği cad 19/21 ...	İstanbul
Bayar, Şeref	S.S.K. Beyoğlu disp. Tepebaşi ...	İstanbul
Bayramoğlu, Cafer	Kanatli cad. 21	Antakya
Bayramoğlu, Namik	Yenilevent 10. cad No: 9	İstanbul
Bengisu, Prof. Naci	Taksim. MeşelikAbdullah sok 2/5.	İstanbul
Bengisu, Prof. Ünal	Taksim, MeşelikAbdullah sok 2/2.	İstanbul
Bilger, İzzet	Cumhuriyet cad. 249/8 Harbiye .	İstanbul
Canbakan, Nizami	Bedesten sok. Şen Ap.	Konya
Çitkaya, Fahri	İstasyon cad. 19/5 Göztepe	İstanbul
Çoruk, Cavidan	Bahariye cad. 44 Kadiköy	İstanbul
Danişman, Hulusi	Karşiyaka 1746 sok. 12/9	İzmir
Ege, Fahriye	Bağdat cad. 156/4 Feneryolu ...	İstanbul
Eke, Arif	Bahariye cad. 86/I Kadiköy	İstanbul
Elbeyli, Şefik	Öğretmen evleri 27	Gaziantep
Emüler, Prof. Ümit	Yenişehir sağlik sok. 46/II	Ankara
Engin, Günay	S.S.K. Hastanesi	Ordu
Erbakan, Prof. Selahattin	Alsancak Atatürk cad. 220/3 ...	İzmir
Ercan, Macit	Devlet Hast. Göz Müt	Samsun
Ercan, Müfit	Göktürkler cad A-2/3 Karabük ..	Zonguldak
Erçikan, Prof. Celal	Babiali cad. 16/3	İstanbul
Erdinç, Sami	S.S.K. Hastanesi	İzmir
Erdoğan, Mehmet	Karşiyaka 1690 sok 75/3	İzmir
Ergun, Rana	Ayazpaşa kutlu sok. 39/4	İstanbul
Erhan, İsmail	S.S.K. Göztepe Hastanesi	İstanbul

Erker, Haluk	Göztepe şair arşi sok 4/1	İstanbul
Firat, Prof. Tanju	Osmanpaşa Halici sok. 10/3	Ankara
Fridman, Albert	Taksim Gümüşsuyu cad (5/5)	İstanbul
Germen, Prof. Melek	S.S.K. Eyüp Hästanesi	İstanbul
Görk, Haydar	Ortabahçe Çelik iş hani beşiktaş	İstanbul
Göze, İbrahim	Yeni sülün tekirler sok 2 levent	İstanbul
Gözonar, Prof. Semih	Etiler Nispetiye cad. Kervan Ap. 7	İstanbul
Güleç, Süleyman	Istasyon cad Güleç ap. 53/3	Eskişehir
Gümüş, İsmet	Semerciler mah. Küçük sok No: 10	Adapazari
Günalp, Zeren	Vali Doktor Reşit cad. 9/9 Kavaklidere	Ankara
Haznedaroğlu, Günay	Cumhuriyet bulvari Gündoğdu Ap 198/6	İzmir
Hepgüler, Tahsin	İstasyon cad Akman Ap. 43	Eskişehir
Isik, Mahmut	S.S. Yardim Bakanliği Trahom Savaş Gen. Md.	Ankara
İdil, Prof. Muhsin Kaya	İst. Üniversitesi Çapa göz kliniği	İstanbul
İkizoğlu, Oğuz	S.S.K. hast. Göz Müt.	Antalya
İlday, Nazif	Zafer meydani Küçükköylü Ap. 9	Konya
İlhan, Nurettin	Birinci Harput cad. 53	Elaziğ
İspir, Nevzat	Fabrika sok No: 27	Elaziğ
İzgür, Mustafa	Altiparmak cad. Başari Ap 4	Bursa
Kafescioğlu, Süreyya	Birincibeyler sok No: 35	İzmir
Karabiyik, Meral	Güzelyali Mithatpaşa cad. 995	İzmir
Karamete, Cemalettin	Sirer cad No: 27/i	Sivas
Kaptonoğlu, İzzet	Cumhuriyet Bulvari 1448 sok 6/3	İzmir
Kayali, Mihraver	Küçük bebek cad. 55/9	İstanbul
Kendiroğlu, Gürhan	İç Levent Yenikaranfil Haci İdil sok 75/2	İstanbul
Kiliçli, Mükrimin	Cengiztopel cad. 90/5 D:12	Samsun
Konturopis, Sotiri	HalaskarGazi cadHuzur Ap. 209 /211	İstanbul
Kösebay, Baha	Taksim. Talimhane. Şehitmuhtar 43/6	İstanbul
Kurşunluoğlu, Raşit	Recai güreli cad. 7/2	Muğla
Kutucuoğlu, Kemal	Tabaklar mah. İstanbul cad No: 4	Bolu
Manavoğlu, Asim	Abidin Paşa cad. 61/4	Adana
Manzakoğlu, Adil	Fatih Fevizipaşa cad. 16/5	İstanbul
Mayoğlu, Yakovas	Beyoğlu Mis sok. 6/4	İstanbul
Menderes, Gönül	Çankaya Güvenlik sok. 76/B	Ankara
Mengüç, Fikri	Atatürk şafak sok. No: 1	Balikesir
Meriç, Faruk	Utku. M. Gençlik sok No: 122	Manisa
Mirzataş, Çolpan	Cerrahpaşa tip fak. Göz Kliniği	İstanbul
Mutlu, Prof. Fikret	Gülhane Tip Akademisi Göz Kl. Dir.	Ankara
Nayman, Selçuk	Atatürk cad No: 10	Bursa
Oktar Torumtay	S.S.K. İstanbul Hast. Göz Kliniği	İstanbul
Oykut, Ziya	Devlet Hastanesi Göz Kliniği	Giresun
Öner, Rifat	Fabrika cad No: 13	İsparta
Öner, Prof. Cemal	Nispetiye c. Peker sok. Tuğ Ap. Levent	İstanbul
Özden, Ratip	İstiklal cad. 54	İstanbul
Omay, Ruşen	Cerrahpaşa Tip fak göz klin.	İstanbul
Öğretmengil, Mahmut	Atatürk cad. Vali yolu karşisi	Adana
Örgen, Prof. Cahit	Tip Fak. Göz Klin. Direktörü	Ankara

Özerengin, Tarik	Osmanbey Ebekizi sok Aydin Ap 7	İstanbul
Özkeskin, Mehmet	S.S.K. İstanbul Hast. Cerrahpaşa .	İstanbul
Papadopulos, Aleksandir ...	İstiklal c. 65/1 Beyoğlu	İstanbul
Saltoğlu, Zekai	Kilicaslan Ap. D:5	Malatya
Sayrun, Adnan	Cihangir Güneşli sok. 12/5	İstanbul
Sezen, Fazil	Çapa göz kliniği	İstanbul
Sevimli, Zeki	Cumhuriyet cad. 161	Erzurum
Slem, Prof. Gülhan	Tip Fak. Göz Kli. Direktörü	Adana
Sökmen, Ayhan	Hatay cad. 344/7	İzmir
Sözen, Kamil	Kenedi cad. 40/7 Küçükesat	Ankara
Sürer, Prof. Zeki	Ahmetvefik paşa c. 70/A Şehremini	İstanbul
Şerifoğlu, Arif	Kizilirmak c. 27/14 Yenişehir ...	Ankara
Saysel, Ülkü	S.S.K. İstanbul Hast. Cerrahpaşa .	İstanbul
Şima, Halim	Birinci Beyler s, 22 Konak	İzmir
Tahinci, Emil	Istiklal c. 475 Tünel	İstanbul
Tansi, Muammar	Babiali cad 21/3 Çağaloğlu	İstanbul
Tolun, Nahit	İlkyardim Hastanesi Beyoğlu ...	İstanbul
Tarhan, Ertuğrul	Akkaranfil sok. No: 5 Levent ...	İstanbul
Teksur, Neriman	Kadieminefendi sok No: 11	İstanbul
Tugay, Rafet	Bahçelievler	Antalya
Tüzmen, Prof. Behiç	Selanik cad. 46/19 Yenişehir ...	Ankara
Urgancioğlu, Meri	Bozkurt c. 28/4 feriköy	İstanbul
Uygur, Aydin	Çark caddesi No: 21	Adapazari
Ünal, Aysun	Cerrahpaşa göz kliniği Aksaray ..	İstanbul
Ünlüçerçi, Cahit	İstiklal cad. Taksim palas	İstanbul
Ürgenç Sefa	Mermerli mah. 36 sok. 21	Adana
Yemeniciler, Necip	İstasyon cad. No: 49	Manisa
Yilmaz, Eyüp	Mecidiyeköy Sakizağaci 30/8 ...	İstanbul
Yiğitsubay, Prof. Vedat ...	Göztepe cavitpaşa s. 17/7	İstanbul
Zeytinoğlu, Hasan	İstasyon cad 63/8	Eskişehir
Zografos, Mina	Mete cad. 24/2 taksim	İstanbul

NOSOCOMIA QUIBUS OCULIS AEGRI CURANTUR

Ankara:
Ankara Üniversitesi Göz Kliniği, Direktör: Prof. Dr. Cahit Örgen.
Hacettepe Üniversitesi Göz Kliniği, Direktor: Prof. Dr. Behiç Tüzmen.
Gülhane Tip Akademisi Göz Kliniği, Direktör: Prof. Dr. Fikret Mutlu.
Ankara Hastanesi Göz Kliniği, Direktör: Dr. Abidin Ara.
Ankara Numune Hastanesi Göz Kliniği, Direktör: Dr. Arif Şerifoğlu.

İstanbul:
İstanbul Üniversitesi Çapa Göz Kliniği, Direktor: Prof. Dr. Naci Bengisu.
İstanbul Üniversitesi Cerrahpaşa Göz Kliniği, Direktör: Prof. Dr. Nejat Ayberk.
Numune Hastanesi Göz Kliniği, Direktör: Dr. Rana Ergun.
Şişli çocuk Hastanesi Göz Kliniği, Direktör: Dr. Ertuğrul Tarhan.
Haseki Belediye Hastanesi Göz Kliniği, Direktör: Dr. Baha Kösebay.
Beyoğlu Belediye Hastanesi Göz Kliniği, Direktör: Dr. Fevzi Akkan.
Guraba vakif Hastanesi Göz Kliniğği, Direktör: Dr. Tarik Özerengin.
S.S.K. Istanbul Hastanesi Göz Kliniği, Direktor: Dr. Bülent Artuner.
S.S.K. Beyoğlu Hastanesi Göz Kliniği, Direktör: Dr. Natik Esin.
S.S.K. Eyüp Hastanesi Göz Kliniği, Direktör: Doç. Dr. Melek Germen.

Clinique Privèe, Artuner Göz Kliniği, Direktör: Dr. Bülent Artuner.
Ege Üniversitesi Göz Kliniği, Direktör: Prof. Dr. Selahattin Erbakan.

Erzarum:
Atatürk Üniversitesi Göz Kliniği, Direktör: Prof. Dr. Gülhan Slem.

Diyarbakir:
Diyarbakir Üniversitesi Göz Kliniği, Direktör: Prof. Dr. Fikret Mutlu.

Au dehors des Cliniques il y ont:
40 Services Ophtalmologiques de la Ministère de la Sante
17 Services Ophtalmologiques de l'Assurance Sociale (S.S.K.)
11 Services Ophtalmologiques des Hôpitaux Utilitaires
5 Services Ophtalmologiques des Grands Fondations Officielles (D.D.Y. – P.T.T. – E.K.I.)
4 Services des Hôpitaux Privees.

INSTITUTA SCHOLAEQUE CAECIS DESTINATAE

Sociétés pour bien des aveugles:
I.   Alti Nokta Körler Vakfi (Fondation six points)
      A.   Ankara Şubesi: Dr. Mathat Enç – Gazi Terbiye Enstütüsü.
      B.   İstanbul Şubesi: Yeni çarşi No: 28, Galatasaray.
      Centre de rehabilitation: Emirgan Reşitpaşa, Istanbul.
II.   Körler Okulu: Gaziantep.
III. Körler Okulu: Ankara.

VENEZUELA

SOCIETATES OPHTHALMOLOGICAE

Sociedad Venezolana de Oftalmología

Secretary: Dr. G. Ascamio Escobar, Apart. del Este no. 50.150, Caracas

No data received.

ACTA PERIODICA AD OPHTHALMOLOGIAM
PERTINENTIA

ACTA PERIODICA AD OPHTHALMOLOGIAM PERTINENTIA

AEGYPTUS

BULLETIN OF THE OPHTHALMOLOGICAL SOCIETY OF EGYPT
Dar El Hekmah, 42 Kasr El Ainy Street, Cairo

AFRICA MERIDIONALIS

SOUTH AFRICAN ARCHIVES OF OPHTHALMOLOGY
Main Editor: Prof. M. H. Luntz, Department of Ophthalmology, Medical School, Hospital Street, Johannesburg

AMERICA SEPT. (U.S.A.)

No data received.

AUSTRALIA

THE AUSTRALIAN JOURNAL OF OPHTHALMOLOGY
Editor Dr. R. Hertzberg, 27 Commonwealth Street, Sydney, N.S.W. 2101

AUSTRIA

Die Sitzungsberichte der ÖSTERREICHISCHEN OPHTHALMOLOGISCHEN GESELLSCHAFT erscheinen als eigener Band. Verlag Gebrüder Hollinek, Steingasse 25, 1030 Wien

Die Sitzungsberichte der OPHTHALMOLOGISCHEN GESELLSCHAFT IN WIEN erscheinen in:
WIENER KLINISCHE WOCHENSCHRIFT, Springer-Verlag, Mölkerbastei, Wien
WIENER MEDIZINISCHE WOCHENSCHRIFT, Verlag Gebrüder Hollinek, Steing. 25, 1030 Wien
KLINISCHE MONATSBLÄTTER FÜR AUGENHEILKUNDE, Verlag Ferdinand Enke, Stuttgart
KLINISCHE MEDIZIN, Verlag Urban & Schwarzenberg Ges.m.b.H., Wien-Innsbruck

BELGICA

BULLETIN DE LA SOCIÉTÉ BELGE D'OPHTALMOLOGIE
Editeur: Prof. P. Danis, 15 Ave de la Folle Chanson, Bruxelles B-1050
Le Bulletin parait 3 foix par an

BRASILIA

REVISTA BRASILEIRA DE OFTALMOLOGIA
Rua Mexico, 111 salas 1406/07/08, Centro Rio de Janeiro, Guanabara
Editor Chefe: Dr. Cláudio Humberto Savastano Ramalho

ARQUIVOS BRASILEIROS DE OFTALMOLOGIA
Caixa Postal 4086, São Paulo, Est. De Sâo Paulo
Editor Chefe: Prof. Rubens Belfort Mattos

BOLETIN DO CENTRO DE ESTUDOS IVO CORRÉA MEYER
Enfermaria n° 25 da Santa Casa de Misericordia, Porto Alegre, Rio Grande do Sul
Editor Chefe: Prof. Luis A. Osório

ARQUIVOS DO INSTITUTO PENIDO BURNIER
Caixa postal 284, Campinas, Est. De Sâo Paulo
Editor Chefe: Prof. Francisco Arthur Mais

BOLETIN DO CENTRO BRASILEIRO DE ESTRABISMO
Rua Cincinato Braga, 59, São Paulo, Est. De Sâo Paulo
Editor Chefe: Dr. Carlos Souza Dias

BRITANNIA

ANNALS OF OPHTHALMOLOGY
7-8 Henrietta Street, London, W.C.2.

BRITISH JOURNAL OF OPHTHALMOLOGY
British Medical Association, Tavistock Square, London, WC1H 9JR

OPHTHALMIC LITERATURE
British Medical Association, Tavistock Square, London, WC1H 9JR

OPHTHALMIC RESEARCH
John Wiley and Sons Limited, Baffins Lane, Chichester, Sussex

OPHTHALMOLOGICA
John Wiley and Sons Limited, Baffins Lane, Chichester, Sussex

OPTHALMOLOGY
Excerpta Medica, Chandos House, 2 Queen Anne Street, London, W.1.

SURVEY OF OPHTHALMOLOGY
7-8 Henrietta Street, London, W.C.2.

TRANSACTIONS OF THE OPHTHALMOLOGICAL SOCIETIES OF THE UNITED KINGDOM
104 Gloucester Place, London, W. 1.

CANADA

THE CANADIAN JOURNAL OF OPHTHALMOLOGY
Editor: Dr. H. N. Reed, 425 St. Mary Avenue, Winnipeg, Manitoba, R3C ON2

DANIA

ACTA OPHTHALMOLOGICA
Main editor: Professor P. Braendstrup
Address: Kommunehospitalets øjenafdeling, Ø. Farimagsgade 3, 1399 København K.

HIBERNIA (Eire)

YEARBOOK OF THE IRISH FACULTY OF OPHTHALMOLOGY
Editor: G. P. Crookes, 18 Fitzwilliamplace, Dublin 2

GALLIA (la France)

ANNALES D'OCULISTIQUE
Rédacteur en Chef: Dr. P. V. Morax, 14, Avenue Pierre-Ier-de Serbie, 75008 Paris

ARCHIVES D'OPHTALMOLOGIE
Rédacteur en Chef: Pr. G. Offret, Hôtel-Dieu, Service d'Ophtalmologie, 1, Place du Parvis-Notre-Dame, 75004 Paris

BULLETIN DES SOCIÉTÉS D'OPHTALMOLOGIE DE FRANCE
Directeur de Rédaction: Dr. J. P. Bailliart, 47, rue de Belle-chasse, 75007 Paris

BULLETINS ET MÉMOIRES DE LA SOCIÉTÉ FRANÇAISE D'OPHTALMOLOGIE
Directeur de Rédaction: Mr. le Secrétaire Général de la Société Française d'Ophtalmologie, 9, rue Mathurin-Régnier, 75015 Paris

L'OPHTALMOLOGIE FRANÇAISE
Rédacteur en Chef: Dr. J. Mergier, 12, Avenue P. V. Couturier, 92150 Suresnes

REVUE INTERNATIONALE DU TRACHOME
Rédacteur scientifique: Dr. R. Pages, Résidence 'Le Richelieu', 50, Avenue Albert-Camus, 86100 Chatellerault

GERMANIA (D.B.R.)

ALBRECHT V. GRAEFES ARCHIV FÜR KLINISCHE UND EXPERIMENTELLE OPHTHAL-MOLOGIE
Schriftleitung: Professor E. Schreck, 852 Erlangen, Prof. W. Straub, Marburg/Lahn
Verlag: Springer-Verlag, 69 Heidelberg

KLINISCHE MONATSBLÄTTER FÜR AUGENHEILKUNDE
Schriftleitung: Prof. Dr. F. Hollwick, Münster
Verlag: F. Enke-Verlag, 7 Stuttgart

ZENTRALBLATT FÜR DIE GESAMTE OPHTHALMOLOGIE
Schriftleitung: Prof. Dr. W. Kreibig, Homburg, Dr. O. Käfer, Heidelberg
Verlag: Springer-Verlag, 69 Heidelberg

BERICHTE DER DEUTSCHEN OPHTHALMOLOGISCHEN GESELLSCHAFT
Redaktion: Prof. Dr. W. Jaeger, Heidelberg
Verlag: J. F. Bergmann, München

GRAECIA

BULLETIN OF THE HELLENIC OPHTHALMOLOGICAL SOCIETY
Published by the Council of the Society, Athens

BULLETIN OF THE OPHTHALMOLOGICAL SOCIETY OF NORTHERN GREECE
Published by the Council of the Society, P.O. Box 497, Thessaloniki

ANNALS OF OPHTHALMOLOGY (Ofthalmologika Hronika)
Quarterly publication
Editor-in-Chief: G. Chilaris, 14 Navarinou St., Athens 144

HELVETIA

OPHTHALMOLOGICA
Journal International d'Ophtalmologie
Redactores: J. Francois, Gand (Belgique), M. M. J. Schweitzer, Groningen (Nederland), E. B.
Streiff, Lausanne (Suisse)
Siège: Karger Verlag, Basel (Suisse)

HISPANIA

ARCHIVOS DE LA SOCIEDAD ESPAÑOLA DE OFTALMOLOGIA
Main Editor: Dr. J. M. Aguilar, C. Alcalá Galiano 8, Madrid, 4

ANALES DEL INSTITUTO BARRAQUER
Main Editor: Prof. J. Barraquer, Muntaner 314, Barcelona

REVISTA ESPAÑOLA DE OTO-NEURO-OFTALMOLOGIA
Main Editor: Prof. J. J. Barcia Goyanes, C. Cirilo Amorós, 86, Valencia

HOLLANDIA

TRANSACTIONS OF THE NETHERLANDS OPHTHALMOLOGICAL SOCIETY
are published in Ophthalmologica (Karger Verlag, Basel, Suisse)

DOCUMENTA OPHTHALMOLOGICA
Edited by Harold E. Henkes
Publ.: Dr. W. Junk b.v. Publishers, 13 van Stolkweg, the Hague

INDIA

INDIAN JOURNAL OF OPHTHALMOLOGY
Editor: Dr. S. N. Cooper, Land Mansion, 21 Queens Road, Bombay 400.004

INDIAN ARCHIVES OF OPHTHALMOLOGY
Editor: Dr. L. P. Agarwal, Centre for Ophthalmic Sciences, A.I.I.M.S., New Delhi 16

ITALIA

ANNALI DI OFTALMOLOGIA E DI CLINICA OCULISTICA
Editor: Maccari Editore, Parma

JAPONICA

ACTA SOCIETATIS OPHTHALMOLOGICAE JAPONICAE: (Nippon Gankagakukai Zasshi)
c/o Nippon Ishikaikan, No. 5, 2-Chome, Kanda-Surugadai, Chiyoda-ku, Tokyo
Editor: Otsuka, Jin

JAPANESE JOURNAL OF CLINICAL OPHTHALMOLOGY: (Rinsho Ganka)
c/o Igaku Shoin, No. 29–11, 5-Chome, Hongo, Bunkyo-ku, Tokyo
Editor: Nakaizumi, Yukimasa

JAPANISCHE MONATSCHRIFT FÜR PRAKTISCHE AUGENHEILKUNDE: (Ganka Rinsho Iho)
No. 12–27, 3-Chome, Kugayama, Suginami-ku, Tokyo
Editor: Kato, Kaku

FOLIA OPHTHALMOLOGICA JAPONICA: (Nihon Ganka Kiyo)
c/o Ophthalmological Department, Osaka University Medical School, Fukushima-ku, Osaka
Editor: Mizukawa, Takashi

JAPANESE JOURNAL OF OPHTHALMOLOGY
c/o Ophthalmological Department, Tokyo University Medical School, Hongo, Tokyo
Editors: Mishima, Saiichi; Shikano, Shin-ichi

OPHTHALMOLOGY: (Ganka)
c/o Kanehara Shuppan, No. 31–14, 2-Chome, Yushima, Bunkyo-ku, Tokyo
Editors: Ohashi, Kohei; Otsuka, Jin; Kato, Ken; Kunitomo, Noboru; Matsuo, Harutake

OPHTHALMIC PRACTICE: (Nihon no Ganka)
c/o Nippon Gankaikai, 1-Chome, Suga-cho, Shinjuku-ku, Tokyo
Editors: Mita, Hiroshi; Ueno, Eiichi

KOREA

THE JOURNAL OF THE KOREAN OPHTHALMOLOGICAL SOCIETY
Chief editor: Koo, Bon Sool, Department of Ophthalmology, Sacred Heart Hospital, Chung Ang
University Medical School, Pil-Doug 2-Ka, Seoul

MAROCCO

REVUE 'VOIR', ORGANE OFFICIEL DE LA BANQUE DES YEUX DU MAROC
6 Rue Mohamed Diouri, Casablanca
Editeurs: Mr. Gabriel Gauthey, 8 Rue Voltaire, Casablanca

NOVA ZEALANDIA

TRANSACTIONS OF THE OPHTHALMOLOGICAL SOCIETY OF NEW ZEALAND
Editor: Prof. J. Parr, Department of Ophthalmology, Public Hospital, Dunedin

PHILIPPINAE

PHILIPPINE JOURNAL OF OPHTHALMOLOGY
Editor in Chief: Dr. Romeo V. Fajardo, Manila Doctors Hospital, United Nations Ave., Manila
Managing Editor: Dr. Liborio L. Mangubat, Department of Ophthalmology, Phil. General
Hospital, Taft Ave., Manila
Associate Editor: Dr. Salvador R. Salceda, Phil. Eye Research Institute, PGH Compound, Taft
Avenue, Manila

PORTUGALLIA

ARQUIVOS PORTUGUESES DE OFTALMOLOGIA
Instituto Oftalmologico Dr. Gama Pinto
Director: Prof. Dr. Ribeiro da Silva

REVISTA PORTUGUESA DE OFTALMOLOGIA SOCIAL
Director: Dr. H. Moutinho, Av. da Liberdade, 212-S/L Dto, Lisboa

SCANDINAVIA
(DANIA, FINLANDIA, NORTVEGIA, SVECIA)

ACTA OPHTHALMOLOGICA
Vide sub Dania

TAIWAN (Formosa)

TRANSACTIONS OF THE OPHTHALMOLOGICAL SOCIETY OF THE REPUBLIC OF CHINA
Main Editor: Jung-Mao Chang
Address: Department of Ophthalmology, National Taiwan University Hospital, 1, Chang-Te
Street, Taipei

TSECHO-SLOVAKIA

ČESKOSLOVENSKÁ OFTALMOLOGIE (bimonthly)
Main Editor: Ass. Prof. Dr. J. Votočková, U. nemocnice 2, 128 08 Praha 2
Publishing House: Avicenum, Tomášská ul., 110 00 Praha 1

ADVERTISEMENTS, ANNONCES, ANUNCIOS

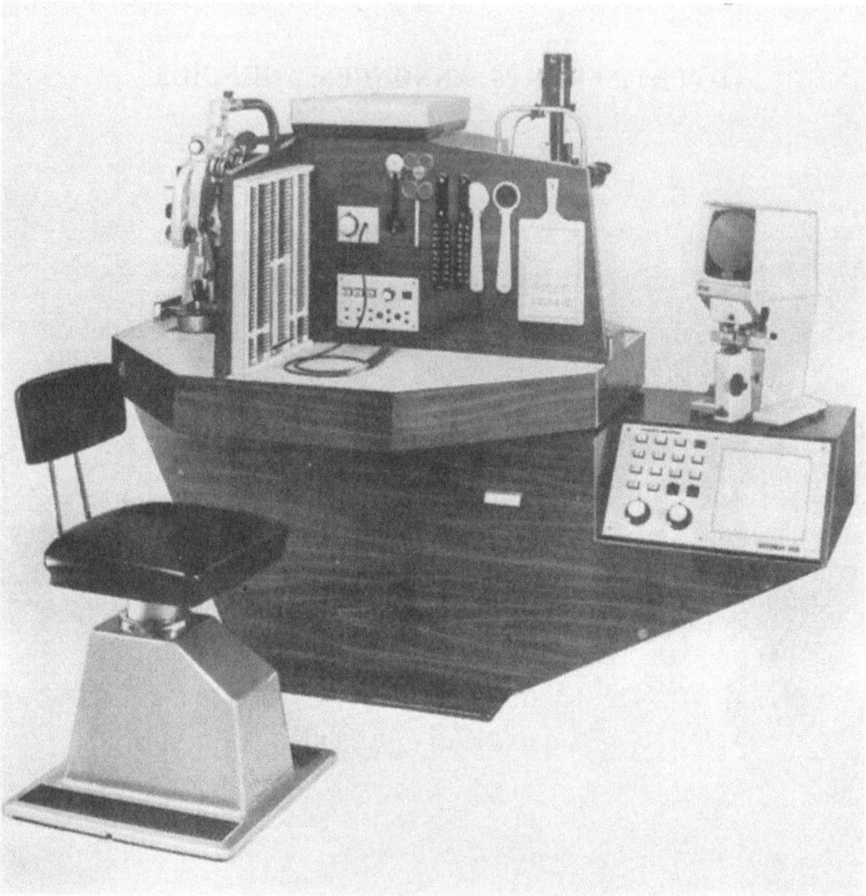

OCTOMAT 300

CONSULTATION UNIT
left and right hand models

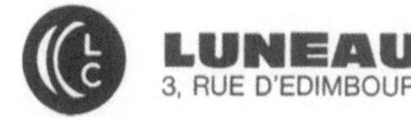

LUNEAU & COFFIGNON
3, RUE D'EDIMBOURG - 75008 PARIS - TEL. (1) 292 20 35

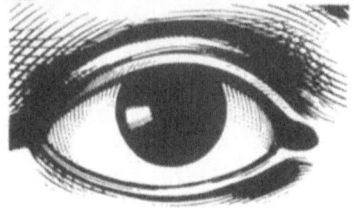

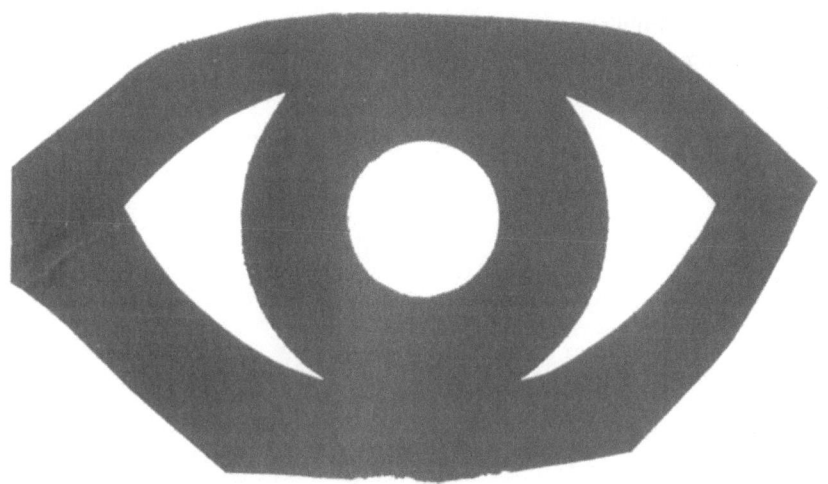

Documenta Ophthalmologica Proceedings Series

Edited by Harold E. Henkes

Publishes: Proceedings of international meetings. Authorative reviews on special subjects. Volumes dedicated to particular events.

Volume 1.
"Symposium on light-coagulation", Ghent 1972. 1973, X, 95 pp., 53 Figs.
ISBN 90 6193 141 X. Dutch Guilders 35.—

Volume 2.
Xth Symposium of the International Society for Clinical Electroretino-graphy, Los Angeles 1972. 1973, VI, 290 pp., 158 Figs.
ISBN 90 6193 142 8. Dutch Guilders 75.—

Volume 3.
"Photography, Electro-ophthalmology and Echo-ophthalmology in ophthalmic practice".
3rd post-graduate course of the Netherlands Ophthalmological Society, Rotterdam 1973. 1973, VI, 318 pp., 285 Figs.
ISBN 90 6193 143 6. Dutch Guilders 80.—

Volume 4.
XIth Symposium of the International Society for Clinical Electroretino-graphy, Bad Nauheim 1973. 1974 in press.

Dr. W. Junk b.v. Publishers — The Hague — The Netherlands.

Dr W. Junk, b.v. - Publishers
13 van Stolkweg, The Hague, The Netherlands

Since its start, over 35 years ago, our publications on ophthalmology have gained an ever increasing importance amongst our scientific publications.
About our series "Documenta Ophthalmologica",
Sir Stewart Duke-Elder wrote in the British Medical Journal of April 18th, 1959:
The Opthalmological — and physiological — world has learned to look forward to each successive volume of „Documenta Ophthalmologica"
The series succeeds in fulfilling an aim difficult of realization, the publication of some length of articles of considerable scientific or clinical importance which would with difficulty be accommodated in the current clinical journals.
Fifteen years have past since, in which "Documenta Ophthalmologica" has convincingly flourished and succeeded in its purpose. From 1970 it is published as a journal in two volumes of two issues per year under the editorship of Prof. Dr. H. E. Henkes.
To facilitate the publication of proceedings of international meetings, authorative reviews on special subjects and articles dedicated to particular events, we started a new book series in 1973:
Documenta Ophthalmologica Proceedings Series, also under the editorship of Prof. Dr. H. E. Henkes. (See our advertisement elsewhere in this issue).
If you want to get fully informed about more of our publications on ophthalmology, please let us know.
Dr. W. Junk, b.v. - Publishers, hope to extend their list of ophthalmic titles and to start new project in this field in the near future. Authors are invited to send their manuscripts; all contributions are considered for publication.

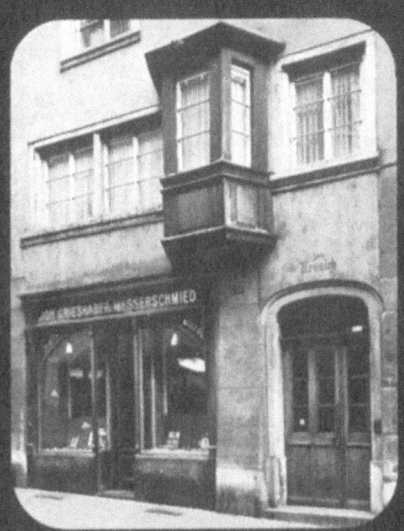
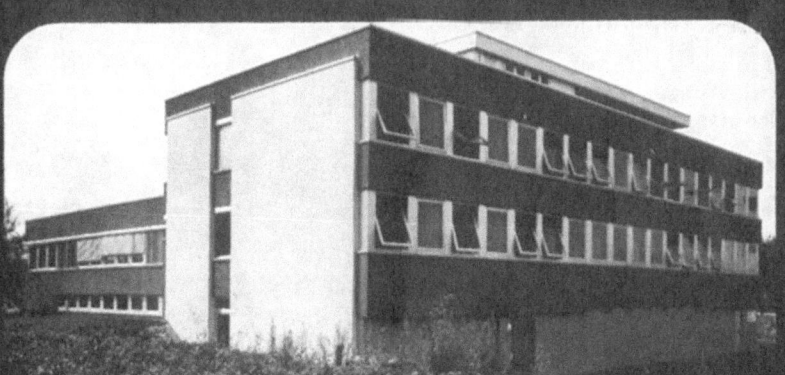
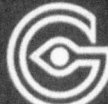

A new adjustable biomicroscopy contact glass with erect imagery

The new contact glass features one fixed and one adjustable mirror.

Developed by Lars Frisén, MD
Department of Ophthalmology
University of Gothenburg Sweden

Mirror adjustments are made by turning an easily accessible knurled ring enveloping the lens housing. The main advantages are non-reversed fundus and anterior chamber imagery, and a meridional direction of scan. A built-in scale permits approximate indications of positions. The design minimizes microscope manipulations.

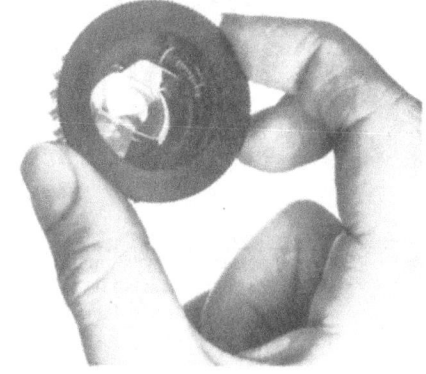

Lens housing is held between thumb and forefinger, middle finger engages ring to adjust mirror inclination. Scale adjacent to spring guide is seen at right of adjustable mirror.

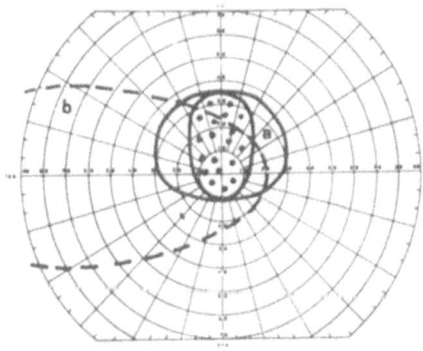

Approximate limits for field of view

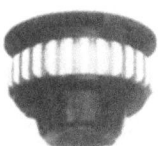

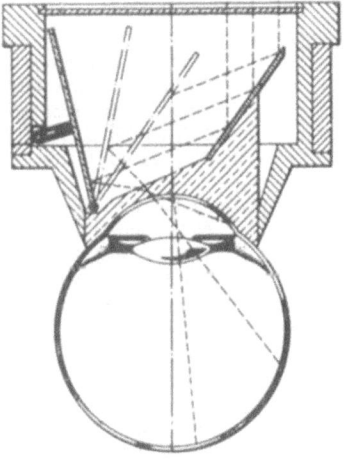

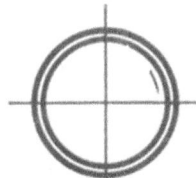

The Contact Glass will be equipped with a device for depressing the sclera

Delivery of the new biomicroscopy contact glass—Frisén will start September 1974

Patent Pending Made in Sweden

JUNGNER INSTRUMENT AB

Svetsarvägen 15
Fack
S-171 20 Solna 1
Stockholm—Sweden
Telephone: 08-28 90 10
Telegram: Jungnerinstrum Stockholm
Telex: 1592 Jungner S

Welcome to our stand TI-1 in Ternes Hall at the XXIInd International Ophthalmological Congress in Paris May 26—31 1974

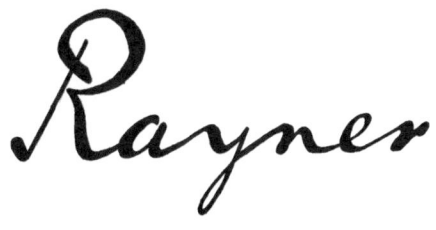

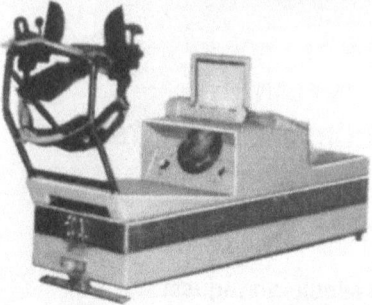

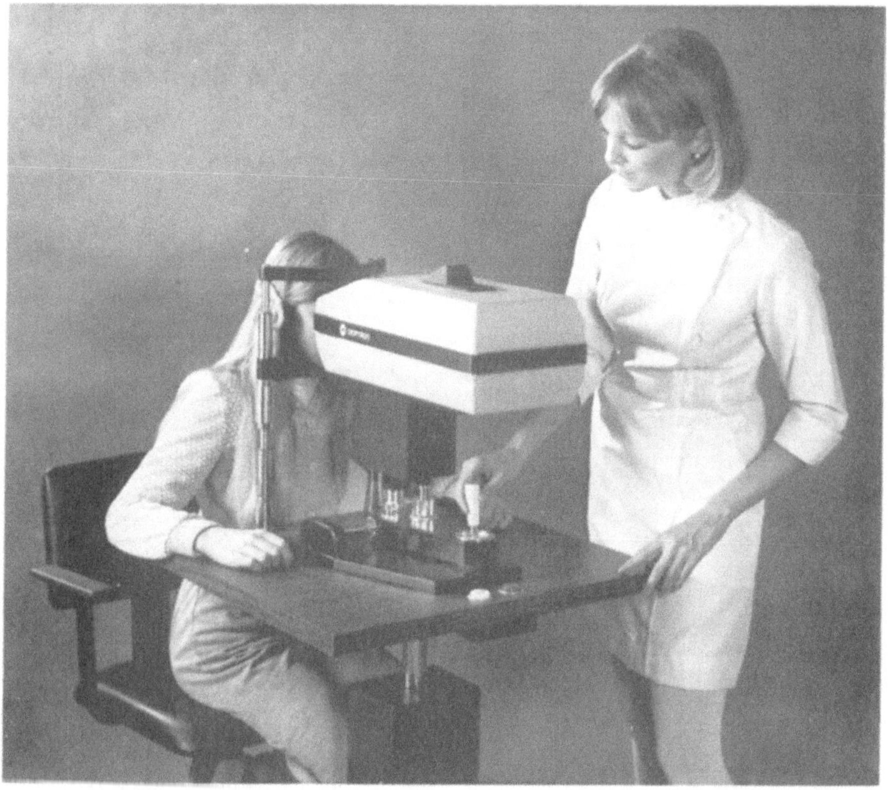

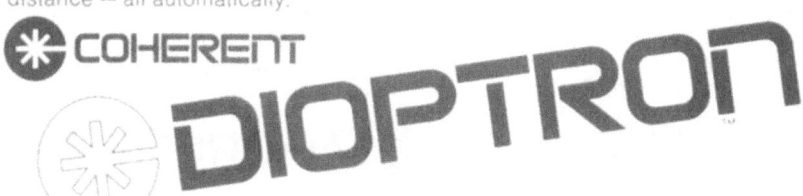

Why buy an automatic refractor?
An auto-refractor adds valuable time to your day by transferring routine measurements to an assistant.

Why buy a Dioptron™ auto-refractor? This newest auto-refractor is a second generation instrument designed to *fully* automate the objective refraction. It fogs the patient — automatically. It ignores blinks — automatically. It detects which eye is being measured — automatically. It even prints the results corrected for vertex distance — all automatically.

The operator presses two buttons. One to view while aligning with the simple slit-lamp style controls and a second to initiate the measurement.

Why Dioptron™? Because making the operator's job simpler benefits you. It eliminates clerical errors, minimizes training time and requires a less skilled operator.

Write or call us. 3210 Porter Drive, Palo Alto, CA 94304 (415) 493-2111, Dept. A. **Dioptron™ . . . look into it.**

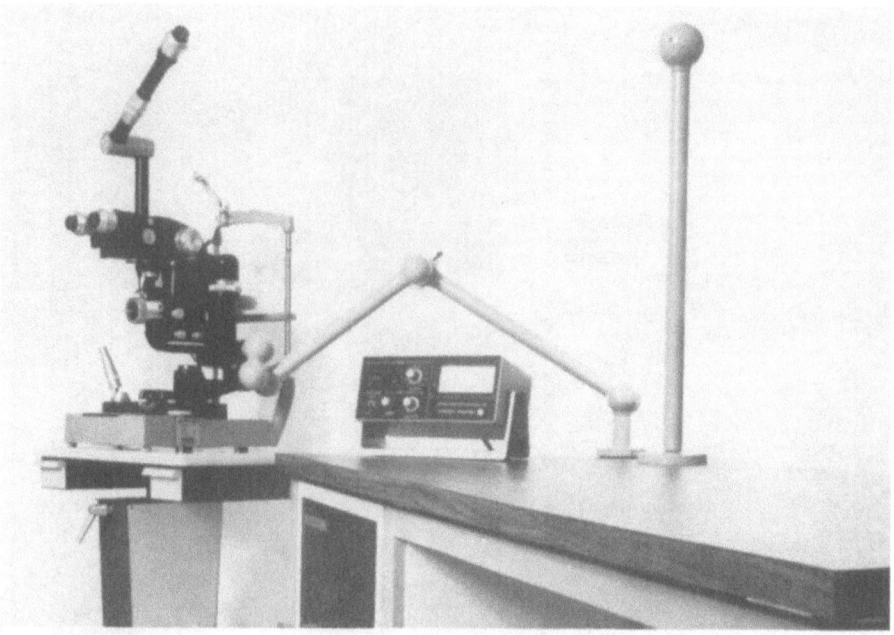

The Coherent Argon Laser Photocoagulator — First and Still Finest.

Several years ago, Coherent laser engineers teamed with top retinal surgeons and biophysicists to design the first argon laser photocoagulator. Now, the Model 800 is working in hundreds of clinics throughout the world. The equipment has earned an unrivaled reputation for design excellence and day-to-day reliability

Excellence doesn't just happen. It results from having command over all inter-related technologies in a sophisticated system Coherent is the only argon supplier that produces lasers, optics, thin-film coatings, electronics, and optical power measurement equipment. In the Model 800, each of these critical technologies is integrated and fine-tuned with the others to optimize the total system design. Every detail from the special laser optics needed to form the retinal spot to the sophisticated attenuators used to create the coaxial aiming beam has been ana-

lyzed carefully and verified clinically.

The Coherent 800 is offered with either a slit lamp or direct ophthalmoscope delivery system Power delivered to the cornea is continuously variable from 0 to 1-watt. Pulses from 10 milliseconds to 5 seconds can be preselected electronically. And, of course, the Model 800 is protected by interlock systems and back-up systems to insure the safety of both practitioner and patient.

Coherent also offers a complete line of versatile laser accessories. Expanded scale power meters, observation tubes, camera attachments, and AR coated fundus lenses. All designed with a total technology concept, all tested clinically, and all backed with a world wide sales and service network.

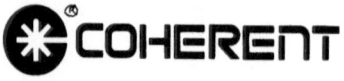

Coherent Radiation 3210 Porter Drive, Palo Alto, California 94304, (415) 493-2111
Coherent Radiation LTD P O Box 12 Royston, Herts SG8, 9 EQ, United Kingdom, Royston 43565
Coherent Radiation GmbH D-6056 Heusenstamm, Industriestrasse 48, West Germany, 06104-2092

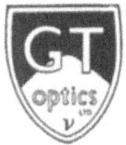

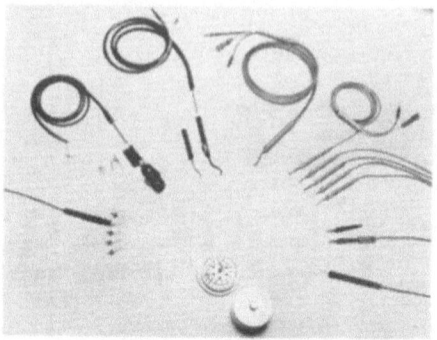

Syncron Optikon

Eye surgery unit with the following possibilities:

Cryo section

* with probes for cataract, vitreous, retinal detachment and special self-illuminated probe

Diathermy section

* with completely solid state generator, especially designed for eye surgery
* more than 20 different electrodes
* bipolar forceps for coagulation

Light section

* cryo and diathermy probe for retinal detachment
* for ophthalmoscopy
* for ocular angioscopy
* for gonioscopy etc.
* for the illumination of STRAMPELLI's cryo probes

Thermocautery section

* with the possibility of epilation

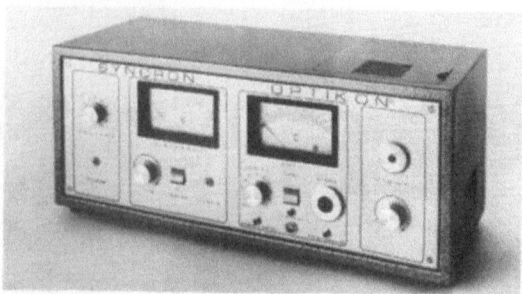